NOVAK'S
Textbook of Gynecology

NOVAK'S
Textbook of

Ninth Edition

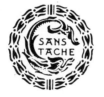

THE WILLIAMS
& WILKINS COMPANY

Gynecology

EDMUND R. NOVAK, M.D.

Associate Professor, Gynecology and Obstetrics,
Johns Hopkins Medical School; Gynecologist, Johns Hopkins Hospital,
Union Memorial Hospital and Greater Baltimore Medical Center.

GEORGEANNA SEEGAR JONES, M.D.

Professor, Gynecology and Obstetrics,
Johns Hopkins Medical School, Baltimore.

HOWARD W. JONES, JR., M.D.

Professor, Gynecology and Obstetrics, Johns Hopkins
Medical School, Baltimore.

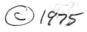 © 1975

Made in the United States of America

First Edition, 1941

Second Edition, 1944

Third Edition, 1948
Reprinted February, 1950
Reprinted March, 1951

Fourth Edition, 1952
Reprinted June, 1953
Reprinted February, 1954
Reprinted July, 1955

Fifth Edition, 1956
Reprinted September, 1957

Sixth Edition, 1961
Reprinted May, 1962

Seventh Edition, 1965

Eighth Edition, 1970

Ninth Edition 1975
Reprinted 1976

Novak, Edmund R
    Novak's Textbook of gynecology.

    1. Gynecology. I. Jones, Georgeanna Seegar, 1912–   joint author. II.
Jones, Howard Wilbur, 1910–   joint author. III. Title. IV. Title: Textbook
of gynecology. [DNLM: 1. Gynecologic diseases. WP100 N935t]
RG101.N69 1974   618.1   74-19377
ISBN 0-683-06187-9

Composed and Printed at the
Waverly Press, Inc.
Mount Royal and Guilford Avenues
Baltimore, Md.   21202   U.S.A.

TO OUR FAMILIES

Preface to the Ninth Edition

Since the appearance of the eighth edition, and even before, medical education has been undergoing evolutionary changes. Particularly noteworthy is the widespread adoption of the core program, one where the medical student receives very scant exposure to any aspect of medicine except the one which is planned as a specialty. Many medical schools offer only a four- to six-week block in obstetrics and gynecology accompanied by perhaps a short series of lectures. This seems rather short-sighted, for unless one should elect to go into male urology, approximately 50 percent of his practice will consist of women. Four to six weeks is hardly sufficient to learn about female diseases. Right or wrong, the core program is here.

In the core programs, the students usually opt to purchase concise textbooks for study of those subjects where the four- to six-week blocks are presented. The comprehensive textbook is sought only in the elective specialty chosen. For this reason, we published with our eighth edition a student paperback edition which selectively was a reduction in size and which proved to be popular. This pattern will be repeated, for a new student edition will be published simultaneously with the ninth edition of the comprehensive book. The individual chapters of the student edition conform to the chapter layout of this ninth edition; in effect, the student can draw upon this ninth edition for additional information and references.

For those students who wish to learn gynecology in depth or who elect to specialize in gynecology, those residents who have made the choice, and those practitioners who encounter diseases peculiar to women, be they generalist or specialist, this ninth edition will serve to update the subject. Major revisions will be noted in the sections on endocrinology, cytogenetics, oncology, and population control. Modernization, however, is part and parcel of all chapters and their references.

We shall continue to avoid the so-called TNM classification for many gynecological lesions; while cognizant of its purpose, nevertheless we feel that TNM is often cumbersome and impractical. We shall likewise take two other liberties. On occasion, we may abbreviate references, being careful not to change the context. Further, where papers are published by multiple authors, we shall list the lead author. Perhaps these innovations will not be misleading nor offensive.

Where graphics are an integral part of the learning process, a supporting textbook should strive to present the best available. We are constantly trying to improve these via our own photographic department, ably staffed by competent professionals such as Mr. Chester Reather, and Mr. Raymond Lund. On occasion, we choose to use illustrations sent to us by cooperative friends. In some instances these may depict only a subtotal hysterectomy, a rare procedure in our own clinic. However, we give the reader a knowledge which otherwise may not be communicated, albeit not of the quality of reproduction consistent with our own.

We authors are sincerely grateful to Dr. John K. Frost for his truly remarkable chapters on cytopathology, which have received highly laudatory remarks in reviews of previous editions. Dr. J. Donald Woodruff has been responsible for the chapters on the vulva and vagina, and in addition has been generally invaluable by means of various suggestions and criticisms. To this truly fine clinician and pathologist, who is an even better friend, go our sincere thanks. We specifically thank Dr. Hyman Strauss (Brooklyn) for his excellent color plates of the vulva. Cooperation and helpfulness by The Williams and Wilkins Company in the preparation of this and every edition has been superb; we express our appreciation to them and to the W. B. Saunders Company, both of whom have kindly permitted generous interchange of various prints, plates, and tables without always specific notation. Lastly, sincere thanks go to Miss Helen Clayton and Mrs. Katheryn Frederick in our offices, and to Dr. Theodore Baramki for his tireless proofreading; without their frequent and unselfish efforts, preparation of this edition would have been impossible.

E.R.N.
G.S.J.
H.W.J., Jr.

Preface to the First Edition

SINCE THE PLAN and scope of this book represent something of a departure from those followed in other textbooks of gynecology, the author feels impelled to state the ideas which furnished the incentive for the preparation of this work, and which dictated its character and scope.

First of all, no especial apology seems necessary for the combined title. While gynecology was formerly often spoken of as a branch of surgery, this is certainly not its present status. Only a small proportion of gynecological patients require surgical treatment. On the other hand, the biological aspects of gynecology have assumed vast importance, chiefly because of the amazing developments in the field of reproductive physiology and endocrinology. Many of these advances find daily application in the interpretation and management of functional disorders in women. In other words, female endocrinology is now an integral and important part of gynecology, and it is so considered in this book.

Secondly, it has always seemed to me that the great majority of readers of textbooks on gynecology must be not at all interested in the details of operative technique, to the consideration of which most authors have devoted many pages. Certainly this applies to the general practitioner, while medical educators are now generally agreed that the medical student should not be burdened with such details in his undergraduate years. Since this book is designed for these two groups primarily, the indication seemed clear to omit the consideration of operative details. The plan followed is to carry the patient up to the point of operation, and to discuss the indications, scope and purpose of the latter, without going into descriptions of the technique itself.

Diagnosis and treatment have been accented throughout the book, as I believe most readers would wish. The traditional chapters on anatomy, history-taking and methods of examination have been boiled down to the essentials. On the other hand, functional disorders, including especially the large group of gynecological endocrinopathies, have been treated rather elaborately, in keeping with the avowed plan of covering the combined fields of gynecology and female endocrinology. The list of references appended to each chapter makes no pretense of exhaustiveness, and preference has been given to publications most worth while, those most recent, and those written in English. The pathological aspects of gynecological disease, so fundamental to a proper understanding of the whole subject, have received adequate but not disproportionate consideration.

In the consideration of various endocrine disorders a disturbing problem presented itself. In the discussion of endocrine preparations which might be indicated in treatment, there is no doubt that the mention of various products by their commercial names would have had some advantages. On the other hand, these have appeared to be definitely outweighed by the disadvantages of such a plan, apart from its questionable delicacy. These proprietary preparations are constantly multiplying, and their commercial names are being changed from day to day. For example, there are now well over forty estrogenic preparations on the market. It would be almost impossible, in any enumeration of such therapeutic products, to avoid omission of some of them, and this might be very unfair to products perhaps just as effective as those which might be included. A complete list published today is quite likely to be very incomplete within a few months.

The sensible plan seemed to be to rely on the intelligence and initiative of the reader, who should have no difficulty in ascertaining good commercial preparations of estrogen, progesterone, chorionic hormone or any other hormone principle to which reference is made in the treatment of various disorders.

It will be noted that the work is devoted to "straight" gynecology and female endocrinology, and that it does not include a consideration of disorders in allied fields which concededly obtrude themselves frequently into the practice of the gynecologist. For example, many gynecologists include female urology in their practices, while anorectal and abdominal surgical problems are often encountered, as may be problems in almost any field of medicine. For textbook purposes, however, the line must be drawn fairly sharply, and the reader will naturally expect to go to the proper sources for information in any of these allied fields.

In short, the purpose of this book is to present to the reader as much information as is possible in as practical a fashion as possible on the subjects of gynecology and female endocrinology. Whether right or wrong, the ideas behind the book represent the crystallization of many years of teaching and practice in gynecology. The author's goal has been to produce a book which would not only be suited to the needs of the medical student, but which could be carried with him into the practice of his profession.

It is a pleasant obligation to express my indebtedness to those who have been helpful to me in the preparation of this book. To a number of my friends, especially Dr. R. B. Greenblatt, of Augusta, Georgia, I am grateful for the loan of illustrations; to Dr. E. L. Krieg for the excellent colored illustrations as well as for other photographic work; to Mr. Chester Reather, for most of the photomicrographs; to Miss Eva Hildebrandt, technician in the Laboratory of Gynecological Pathology at The Johns Hopkins Hospital and to Sister Mary Lucy, technician at Bon Secours Hospital, for help in the preparation of sections for microscopic illustration; to my artist, Miss Frances Shultz, for many of the illustrations; and to my faithful secretary, Miss Helen L. Clayton, for much help throughout the project. For permission to use illustrations which have appeared in previously published articles of my own I am indebted to the publishers of the Journal of the American Medical Association; the American Journal of Obstetrics and Gynecology; Surgery, Gynecology and Obstetrics; and the Bulletin of The Johns Hopkins Hospital.

Certain illustrations which appeared in one of my previous books, Gynecological and Obstetrical Pathology, do not have a credit line in the caption. For permission to use these I wish to thank W. B. Saunders Company, the publishers.

Finally, it is a genuine pleasure to acknowledge the efficient and wholehearted cooperation of the publishers, Little, Brown and Co., throughout the preparation of this work.

Baltimore   EMIL NOVAK

Contents

chapter 1

Anatomy

The female reproductive organs are divisible into two groups, the external and internal. The former comprise the vulva and vagina; the latter the uterus, tubes, and ovaries.

THE VULVA

The vulva, representing the part of the genital apparatus visible externally, is a composite structure, its constituent parts being the following: (1) the labia majora, (2) mons pubis or mons veneris, (3) labia minora, (4) clitoris, (5) vestibule, (6) urethral meatus, (7) vaginal orifice, (8) hymen (in virgins), and (9) vulvovaginal or Bartholin's glands.

Labia Majora

The labia majora are two longitudinal raised folds of adipose tissue covered by skin which, especially in brunettes, is rather heavily pigmented. They are markedly developed at puberty, as one of the secondary sex characters. Before puberty the vulva is rather flat, and the labia minora are much more conspicuous than the labia majora. In the postpubertal female, the latter extend posteriorly toward the perineum. On separating them pos- teriorly, a slightly raised connecting ridge, the *fourchette,* is seen. Just anterior to this, between it and the vaginal orifice, is a shallow, boat-shaped fossa, the *fossa navicularis.* The external surface of the labia shows a heavy growth of hair, usually curly, but the hair on the inner surface is much more sparse.

The substance of the labia majora is adipose tissue, although it contains also a light fascial layer which is the analogue of the dartos in the male. The labia themselves are to be looked upon as corresponding to the scrotum of the male. Mistakes in the diagnosis of the sex of pseudohermaphrodites have not infrequently been made because of the resemblance of the split scrotum to the labia majora of the vulva.

Mons Pubis

The mons pubis is a mound of fat covered by hair, situated just above the level of the symphysis pubis, at the lowest portion of the anterior abdominal wall.

Labia Minora

The labia minora are two firm pigmented folds which extend from the clit-

1

oris posteriorly to about two-thirds of the distance toward the perineum. Anteriorly they subdivide, one fold covering the clitoris to form its prepuce (preputium clitoris), the other passing beneath the glans to form, with its fellow of the opposite side, the frenulum clitoridis.

The skin covering the labia minora is devoid of hair follicles, but is very rich in sebaceous glands. Sudoriferous glands are exceedingly sparse, and, according to some, completely absent. The substance of the labia minora is described as being of the erectile type, though the degree of erectility is not comparable to that of the clitoris. It contains many venous spaces with much involuntary muscle tissue.

Clitoris

The clitoris is a small, cylindrical, erectile organ corresponding to the male

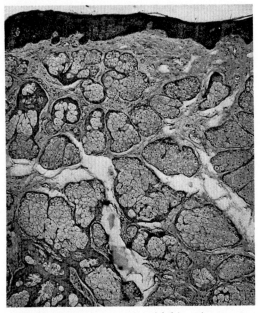

1.2. Histological structure of labia minora, near clitoris, showing large number of sebaceous glands.

penis. Like the latter it consists of a glans, a corpus or body, and the crura. Only the *glans clitoridis,* about 6 to 8 mm. in diameter, is visible externally between the two folds into which the labia minora bifurcates anteriorly, the upper fold

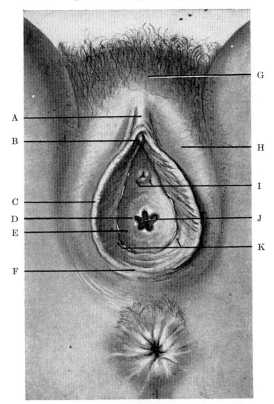

1.1. The vulva. *A,* prepuce; *B,* clitoris; *C,* labia minora; *D,* hymen; *E,* vestibule; *F,* posterior commissure; *G,* mons pubis; *H,* labia majora; *I,* opening of Skene's ducts; *J,* vagina; and *K,* vulvovaginal (Bartholin's) glands.

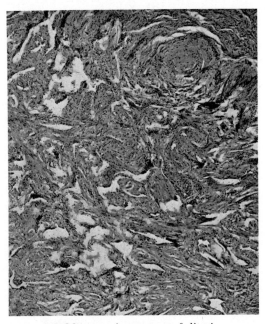

1.3. Microscopic structure of clitoris

forming the *prepuce* and the lower the *frenulum* of the clitoris. The *body* extends upward toward the pubis beneath the skin dividing into two *crura* which are attached to the pubic bones. The clitoris is made up of erectile tissue, with many large and small venous channels surrounded by large amounts of involuntary muscle tissue. The erectile tissue is arranged in two corpora cavernosa, and there is no corpus spongiosum as in the case of the male organ.

Vestibule

The vestibule is the boat-shaped fossa which becomes visible on separation of the labia. In it are seen the vaginal orifice and, anterior to this, the meatus urinarius. In the virgin the former is partly occluded by the *hymen,* a rather rigid membrane of firm connective tissue covered on both sides by stratified squamous epithelium. It is most frequently of annular crescentic shape, but it may be cribiform or sievelike. Under abnormal conditions it may be imperforate, occluding the vaginal orifice completely and leading to retention of the menstrual discharge.

Urethra

The urethral meatus is the small slitlike or triangular external orifice of the urethra. It is visible in the vestibule, at about two-thirds of the distance from the glans clitoridis to the vaginal orifice. At each side of the meatus one usually sees a small pitlike depression in which there are a number of mucous glands, called the lesser glands of the vestibule, to distinguish them from the greater glands, which are the glands of Bartholin.

Just below the outer part of the meatus are the orifices of the *paraurethral or Skene's ducts,* which run in a tortuous fashion below and parallel to the urethra for a distance of about 1.5 cm. Except near the orifice, where one finds stratified epithelium, the paraurethral ducts are lined by a transitional type of epithelium.

The *female urethra,* opening externally at the meatus, is lined proximally by a stratified transitional type of epithelium, whereas its distal portion is covered with stratified squamous epithelium which extends into the canal for a variable but considerable distance. The studies of Huffman have shown that the canal is surrounded by a labyrinth of *paraurethral glands* which he considers to be the homologues of the male prostate. Some of these paraurethral canals enter into the urethra and some into Skene's ducts which open just below the urethral meatus. Their chief clinical importance lies in the fact that they frequently harbor the Gonococcus, the infection often being intractable to any treatment except excision or destruction of the ducts. In addition, *suburethral diverticula* may occur as a sequel to infection and cystic enlargement of these glands.

Vulvovaginal or Bartholin's Glands

The vulvovaginal or Bartholin's glands are lobulated racemose glands situated one on each side of the vaginal orifice, at about its middle, and placed deeply in the perineal structures. They are frequently the seat of gonorrheal or other infections.

The main duct of the gland is lined by a stratified transitional type of epithelium, except for a very short distance within the orifice. As the ducts become smaller and smaller, the epithelium is flatter and flatter, so that in the finest branches it consists of a single layer of flat cells. The acini are lined by a layer of cuboidal cells with basal nuclei. The function of the gland is the secretion of mucus for lubrication of the vaginal orifice and canal, especially during coitus.

THE VAGINA

The vagina is a musculomembranous canal which connects the vulva with the uterus. It is about 9 or 10 cm. in length, and, in the erect position of the woman, its direction is in general upward and backward from its vulvar to its uterine end. Its upper end expands into the cup-shaped *fornix,* into which the cervix uteri is fitted. The portions of the fornix in front of, behind, and at the sides of the cervix are designated as the anterior, pos-

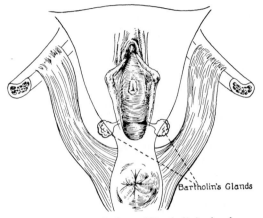

1.4. The deep relations of Bartholin's glands.

terior, and lateral fornices. The posterior fornix is of special surgical interest because it gives ready access to the peritoneal cavity, as the upper fourth or so of the posterior wall of the vagina is covered by peritoneum.

In the virgin, the *mucous membrane* of the anterior vaginal wall is horizontally corrugated, with a central vertical ridge, thus producing the arbor vitae appearance. These ridges are absent in the widened canal of the woman who has borne children.

The mucous membrane of the vagina is reddish pink, and is lined by a stratified squamous epithelium into which project many tiny subepithelial papillae of the subjacent fibrous tissue. In the young child the epithelium shows only perhaps six or eight layers of cells, but in the postpuberal phase many more layers are present.

Beneath the mucous membrane is the muscular coat, made up of an inner circular and an outer layer. The outermost layer is the fibrous, derived from the pelvic connective tissue.

The not infrequent finding of certain glands, probably paramesonephric, in the vagina, producing the so-called "adenosis," will be noted in subsequent chapters. The recent review by Forsberg adequately discusses the derivation of the cervico-vaginal epithelium.

Cervix

The cervix is separated from the corpus externally by a slight constriction cor-

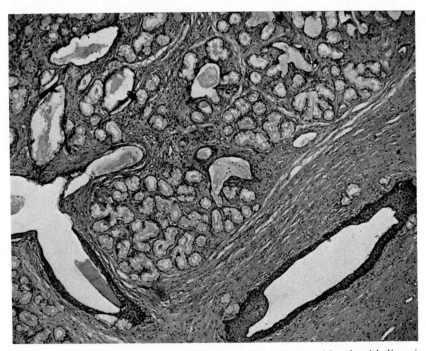

1.5. Microscopic appearance of normal Bartholin's gland. Note the transitional epithelium in the large ducts, the flattened epithelium in the small ducts, and the cuboidal secretory epithelium in the gland acini.

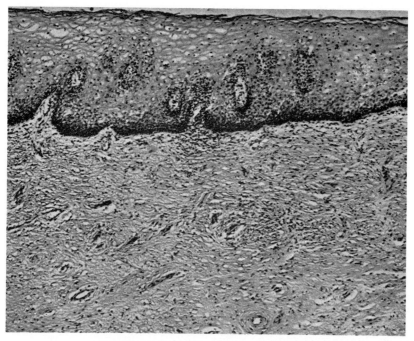

1.6. Histological structure of normal vagina

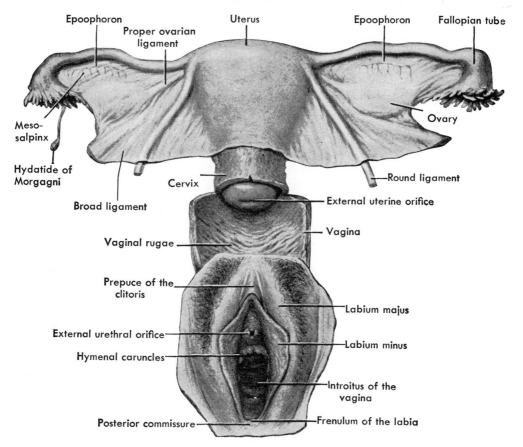

1.7. The female reproductive organs. (From Rubin, I. C., and Novak, J.: *Integrated Gynecology, Principles and Practice,* Vol. 1. Blakiston Division, McGraw-Hill Book Company, Inc., New York, 1956.)

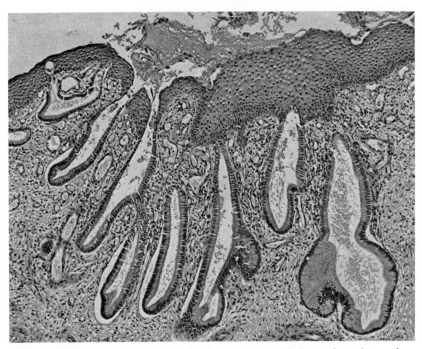

1.8. Showing cervical glands opening on stratified squamous epithelium of cervix, as they often do in chronic inflammatory conditions (see Chapter 11).

responding to the region of the internal os. The portion of the cervix above the level of the vagina is the supravaginal portion, that protruding into the vagina is the *pars* or *portio vaginalis.* The *cervical canal* is somewhat spindle-shaped, terminating below at the *external os,* a small round or transversely slitlike opening averaging in the nulliparous woman about 5 mm. in diameter. At its upper end the cervical canal communicates with the uterine cavity through a constricted orifice called the *internal os.*

The *mucous membrane* covering the external or vaginal surface is of the stratified squamous variety, a continuation of that covering the adjacent vagina. From it arises the squamous cell or epidermoid carcinoma of the cervix, the most common of all gynecological forms of cancer. The cervical canal, on the other hand, is lined by an entirely different type of mucous membrane, the endocervix, which is distinguished by the following features.

(1) A tall, "picket" variety of columnar epithelium, with deeply stained nuclei placed close to the basement membrane, and a cytoplasm which is rich in mucin.

There is a rather abrupt transition between this epithelium and the stratified squamous epithelium of the pars vaginalis at or near the external os, and it is at this transition area that cancer is most apt to develop.

(2) Glands of the racemose variety, lined by epithelium like that found on the surface. Studies by Fluhmann indicate that there is in reality a complex system of tunnels and clefts that appear like glands.

(3) Stroma of fibrous tissue type, rich in spindle cell elements.

The muscular coat of the cervix is well developed in the region of the internal os, but becomes increasingly sparse at a lower level, so that only a thin outer layer is present in the lower portion of the cervix, with a corresponding increase in the proportion of connective tissue. Glandlike vestiges of the mesonephric duct are occasionally observed deep in the cervical musculature.

THE UTERUS

The uterus is a hollow, thick-walled muscular organ which is situated in the pelvis, between the bladder anteriorly and

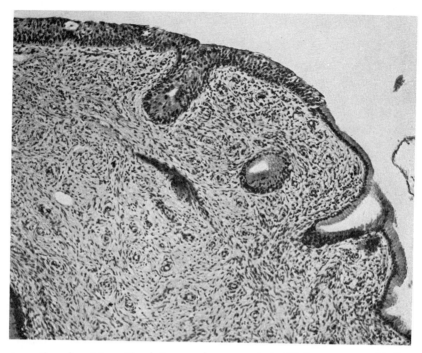

1.9. Showing rather abrupt transition between columnar and stratified squamous epithelium of cervix in vicinity of external os.

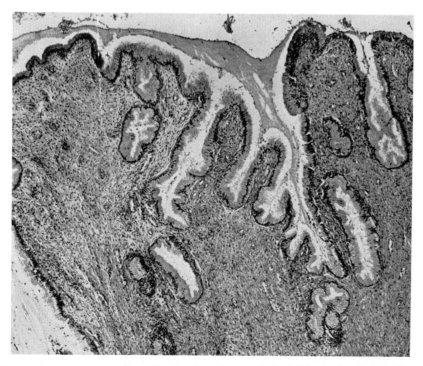

1.10. Microscopic appearance of cervix, showing characteristic "picket" gland epithelium, racemose glands, and spindle-celled fibrous stroma.

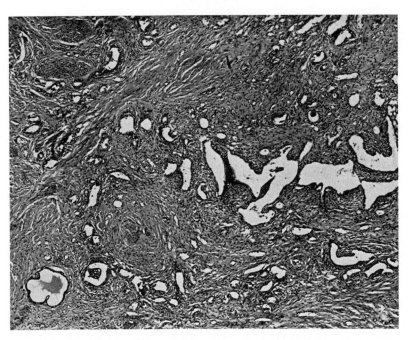

1.11. Mesonephric tubules deep in the cervical substance

the rectum posteriorly. It is placed almost at right angles to the vagina, with the bladder below and in front of it. It is somewhat pear-shaped, and measures in

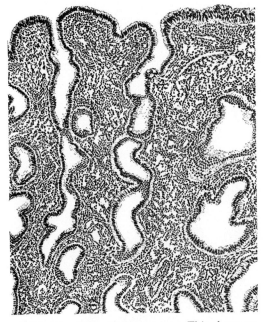

1.12. Histology of endometrium. This, however, undergoes striking cyclical changes, which are described and illustrated in Chapter 4.

the nulliparous woman about 8 to 9 cm. in length, 6 cm. in its widest portion, and about 4 cm. in thickness. It is divisible into a *corpus* or body and a *cervix* or neck. In the prepubertal and post menopausal female the corpus is extremely small, but in the menstrual era, it is usually considerably increased in size and much larger than the cervix as a result of ovarian hormonal stimulation. The upper domelike portion of the corpus is called the *fundus,* whereas the angle marking the attachment of the tube at each side is the *cornu.* The *uterine cavity* is rather conical, with the base above at the fundus and the apex, corresponding to the narrow internal os, leading into the cervical canal. Externally the corpus is covered with peritoneum.

The mucous membrane of the uterine body is the *endometrium.* This varies in thickness not only in individual women, but even more at different phases of the menstrual cycle. In general it is thinnest just after the periods, gradually increasing in thickness until just before the beginning of the next menstrual period, as will be described subsequently.

The *stroma* is a characteristic immature type of connective tissue, made up of a homogeneous mass of small cells with round or slightly oval nuclei and, in the early stages of the cycle, almost no cytoplasm. They are supported by an almost invisible light fibrillary supporting structure. The vascular supply of the endometrium is through two sets of vessels, the spiral or coiled arterioles and the basal arterioles. The latter are the chief nutritional vessels, supplying especially the basal layers. The spiral arterioles, on the other hand, play an important part in the mechanism of the menstrual cycle and especially in menstrual bleeding.

The *muscular* coat of the uterus is made up of involuntary muscle fibers arranged in an interlacing fashion which, at least in the nonpregnant woman, is not disposed in any definite layer pattern. The serous coat consists of the peritoneum, which covers the entire corpus uteri.

The Ligaments of the Uterus

These are three in number on each side, as follows.

Broad Ligaments. Each of these consists of a broad double sheet of peritoneum which extends from the lateral surface of the uterus outward to the pelvic wall. At its upper border the broad ligament encircles the fallopian tube, and beyond the tube continues on the pelvic wall as the *infundibulopelvic ligament,* through which the ovarian vessels make their way toward the tube and ovary. From the lower edge of the tube the broad ligament extends downward to surround the round ligament, this portion constituting a sort of tubal mesentery, or *mesosalpinx.* In this portion is found the parovarium (epoophoron or organ of Rosenmüller), which represents the lateral portions of the vestigial remains of the mesonephric tubules. To its medial side lies the paroophoron, likewise made up of vestigial mesonephric tubules, which, like those of the epoophoron, empty into the main mesonephric, or Wolffian, duct. It is the latter which in the male develops into the vas deferens. At its lower border the broad

ligament is thickened, with a condensation of connective tissue and some muscle fibers, forming the thonglike *cardinal ligament or ligamentum colli of Mackenrodt.* This structure has always been considered to be of prime importance in the support of the uterus, and its elongation as the chief cause of uterine prolapse. The earlier study by Range and Woodburne would suggest that this structure termed the transverse cervical ligament is much less important in maintaining uterine position than the retroperitoneal connective tissue.

Between the two layers of peritoneum which make up the broad ligament there is to be found, in addition to the structures already mentioned, a considerable amount of connective tissue, a small amount of involuntary muscle tissue, blood vessels, and nerves. Weed has summarized the important role of the uterine ligaments (especially the cardinal) in the prevention of procidentia or in the operative management of this problem.

The Round Ligaments. These are two round, muscular bands which arise from the lateral aspect of the fundus on each side, a short distance below and anterior to the insertion of the tube. They course outward between the broad ligament layers in a curved fashion to the internal inguinal ring, passing then through the inguinal canal, and spreading out in a fanlike fashion to fuse with the connective tissue of the groin. The thickness of these ligaments is very variable, but averages about 5 to 6 mm. They are made up of involuntary muscle continuous with that of the uterus itself, and their function seems to prevent retrodisplacement. They are probably more important during pregnancy, when they undergo marked hypertrophy.

Uterosacral Ligaments. The uterosacral ligaments are peritoneal folds containing, in addition to connective tissue, a considerable amount of involuntary muscle. They arise on each side from the posterior wall of the uterus at about the level of the internal os, and pass backward toward the rectum, around which they extend to their insertion on the sacral wall at about the junction of the second and third sacral vertebrae. In their course backward they describe an arclike curve, the concavity being directed toward the midline. They play an important part in the support of the uterus and cervix, so that when they are elongated the cervix sags abnormally downward and forward. In addition, they probably contain sensory nerve fibers which play a part in the production of dysmenorrhea.

Blood Supply

The blood supply of the uterus is derived from the ovarian and uterine arteries. The former, which correspond to the spermatic arteries of the male, arises from the abdominal aorta, passing down behind the peritoneum to the infundibulopelvic ligament, through which it enters the mesosalpinx to supply the tube and ovary, finally anastomosing with the uterine artery to complete the utero-ovarian vascular arch.

The uterine artery arises from the anterior branch of the hypogastric artery, passing toward the uterus through the parametrium. It turns upward about 1.5 or 2 cm. lateral to the cervix, coursing upward in an extremely tortuous fashion to anastomose with the ovarian and giving off many branches to the uterine wall as it courses upward. As it turns upward at the level of the cervicovaginal juncture it is in close relation to the ureter, which passes *downward and inward,* behind the artery, on its course to the bladder. This is an exceedingly important relationship for the surgeon to bear in mind, as injury to the ureter is the chief bugbear in the operation of total hysterectomy.

The veins correspond in a general way with the arteries. The ovarian veins, on their way from the hilum of the ovary toward the vena cava, form, between the

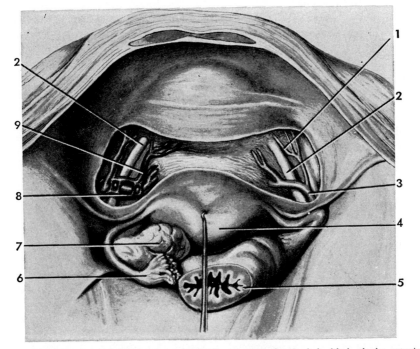

1.13. The topic relationship between ureter and uterine vessels. *On the left side* both the arteries and veins are drawn; *on the right side,* only the arteries. *1,* Cervical branch of uterine artery; *2,* ureter; *3,* uterine artery; *4,* uterus; *5,* rectum; *6,* fallopian tube; *7,* ovary; *8,* uterine veins; and *9,* vesical vein. (From Rubin, I. C., and Novak, J.: *Integrated Gynecology, Principles and Practice,* Vol. 1. Blakiston Division, McGraw-Hill Book Company, Inc., New York, 1956; as redrawn from Tandler, J.: In *Handbuch der Gynäkologie,* Ed. 3, edited by W. Stoeckel, Vol. 1. J. F. Bergmann, Munich, 1930.)

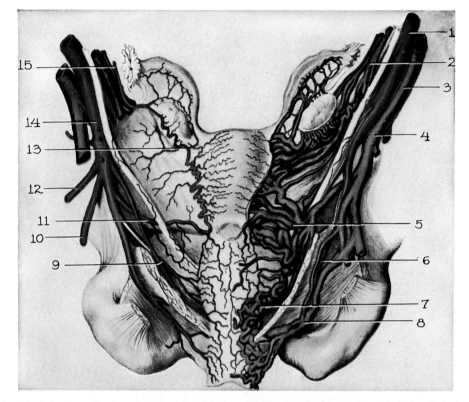

Plate 1.1. Arteries and veins of the female genital organs as seen from the dorsal side. *1,* Common iliac artery; *2,* ovarian plexus; *3,* common iliac vein; *4,* internal or hypogastric iliac vein; *5,* uterine venous plexus; *6,* internal pudendal artery; *7,* vaginal venous plexus; *8,* internal pudendal vein; *9,* vaginal arteries; *10,* caudal or inferior gluteal artery; *11,* uterine artery; *12,* cranial or superior gluteal artery; *13,* anastomosis between uterine and ovarian arteries; *14,* internal iliac or hypogastric artery; and *15,* ovarian artery. (From Rubin, I. C., and Novak, J.: *Integrated Gynecology, Principles and Practice,* Vol. 1. Blakiston Division, McGraw-Hill Book Company, Inc., New York, 1956.)

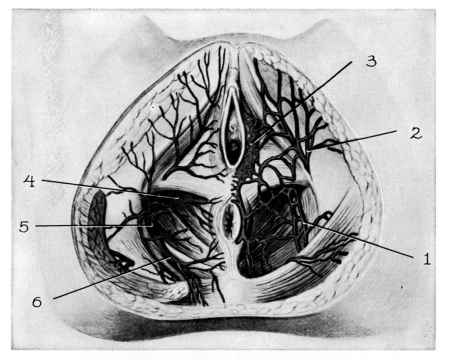

Plate 1.2. The blood vessels of the pelvic floor. The *left half of the plate* demonstrates the ramification of the internal pudendal artery; *the right side* shows the tributaries of the internal pudendal vein. *1,* Internal pudendal vein; *2,* anastomoses between pudendal and cutaneous veins; *3,* bulbus vestibuli; *4,* transverse perineal artery; *5,* internal pudendal artery; and *6,* inferior hemorrhoidal artery. (From Rubin, I. C., and Novak, J.: *Integrated Gynecology, Principles and Practice,* Vol. 1. Blakiston Division, McGraw-Hill Book Company, Inc., New York, 1956; as redrawn from Tandler, J.: In *Handbuch der Gynäkologie,* Ed. 3, edited by W. Stoeckel, Vol. 1. J. F. Bergmann, Munich, 1930.)

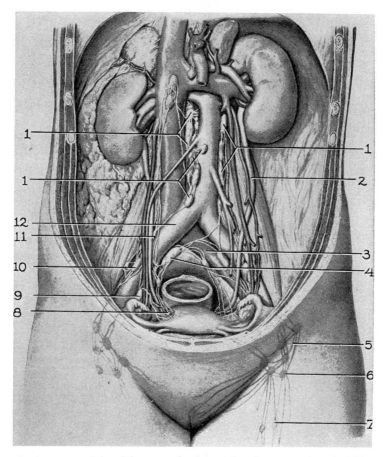

1.14. The lymphatic system of the abdomen and pelvis. *1,* Lumbar or aortic nodes; *2,* ureter; *3,* common iliac vein; *4,* sacral lymph nodes; *5,* inguinal lymph nodes; *6,* subinguinal or inguinofemoral lymph nodes; *7,* femoral lymph nodes; *8,* parametric gland of Championière; *9,* hypogastric lymph node; *10,* external iliac lymph nodes; *11,* common iliac lymph nodes; and *12,* common iliac artery. (From Rubin, I. C., and Novak, J.: *Integrated Gynecology, Principles and Practice,* Vol. 1, Blakiston Division, McGraw-Hill Book Company, Inc., New York, 1956.)

layers of the broad ligament, a rich network called the *pampiniform plexus.* On the right side the ovarian vein empties into the inferior cava itself, on the left into the left renal vein. The uterine veins follow the arteries and empty into the internal iliac veins.

Nerve Supply of the Female Genitalia

The genital tract is supplied by branches of both the autonomic and spinal nerve pathways. In the human certain higher centers as well as the *tuber cinereum* are of importance in regulating various sexual and menstrual functions, and one must always be cognizant of the highly important hypothalamic-hypophysial domination of ovarian function.

Various sympathetic and parasympathetic fibers of the *autonomic* system below the bifurcation of the aorta form the superior hypogastric plexus or presacral nerve, which is the chief supply of the uterus. As they pass caudal, they form the ganglion of Frankenhäuser or uterovaginal plexus located near the base of the uterosacral ligaments.

The clinician should be aware that the presacral nerve as it crosses the sacral promontory has fibers immediately adherent under the posterior peritoneum

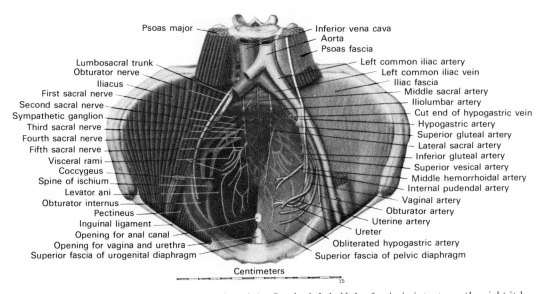

Psoas major — Inferior vena cava
Aorta
Psoas fascia
Lumbosacral trunk — Left common iliac artery
Obturator nerve — Left common iliac vein
Iliacus — Iliac fascia
First sacral nerve — Middle sacral artery
Second sacral nerve — Iliolumbar artery
Sympathetic ganglion — Cut end of hypogastric vein
Third sacral nerve — Hypogastric artery
Fourth sacral nerve — Superior gluteal artery
Fifth sacral nerve — Lateral sacral artery
Visceral rami — Inferior gluteal artery
Coccygeus — Superior vesical artery
Spine of ischium — Middle hemorrhoidal artery
Levator ani — Internal pudendal artery
Obturator internus — Vaginal artery
Pectineus — Obturator artery
Inguinal ligament — Uterine artery
Opening for anal canal — Ureter
Opening for vagina and urethra — Obliterated hypogastric artery
Superior fascia of urogenital diaphragm — Superior fascia of pelvic diaphragm

Centimeters

1.15. The vessels and nerves of the female pelvis. *On the left half* the fascia is intact, *on the right* it has been removed.

as well as others which directly overlie the bony protuberance. Both of these must be divided in the surgical procedure of presacral neurectomy, which is utilized in treating difficult cases of dysmenorrhea. The ovary is supplied not by the sacral fibers, but rather by branches of the renal and aortic plexuses which are located in the suspensory ligaments of the ovary.

The pudendal nerve of the *spinal* nervous system is the primary source of motor and sensory activation of the lower genital tract. This is derived from roots of the second, third, and the fourth sacral nerves. It passes out of the pelvis via the greater and lesser *sciatic foramina,* and enters the pudendal canal of the *obturator fascia.* Various branches supply vulva, vagina, and perineum. Other nerves such as the ilioinguinal, genitofemoral, and cutaneous femoral nerve also contribute to the lower genital tract and perineum, but for details one is urged to consult appropriate neuroanatomical texts.

THE FALLOPIAN TUBES

The tubes are two musculomembranous canals which transport the ova from the ovaries to the uterus. They are about 11 or 12 cm. in length, and are divisible, for purposes of description, into four parts.

(1) The *interstitial portion* is the narrow portion contained in the muscular wall of the uterus, which the tube penetrates to reach the uterine cavity. The uterine os of the tube is extremely minute, being about the diameter of a hairbrush bristle. (2) The *isthmus* is the narrow portion of the tube close to its insertion into the uterine cornu. (3) The *ampulla* is the wider, baggier middle portion of the tube. (4) The distal third or so is the *fimbriated extremity,* which is rather funnel-shaped, the small orifice being surrounded by a number of peaked fringes or fimbriae.

Histologically, the tube consists of three coats, as follows: (1) the *serous coat,* which is formed by the encircling peritoneum of the upper margin of the broad ligament; (2) the *muscular coat,* arranged for the most part in an inner circular and an outer longitudinal layer; and (3) the *mucosa,* or endosalpinx, which is disposed in longitudinal folds or rugae, usually only three or four in number at the isthmus, but branching and subbranching longitudinally toward the fimbriated extremity, so that a cross section of the latter presents a very arborescent appearance as compared with the few folds at the isthmus. The lining *epithelium* is composed of a single layer of cells,

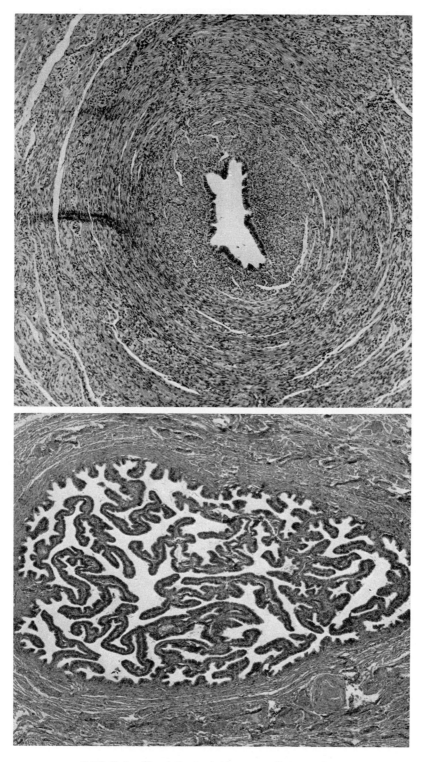

1.16. Tube. *Top,* isthmic; *bottom,* ampullary portion

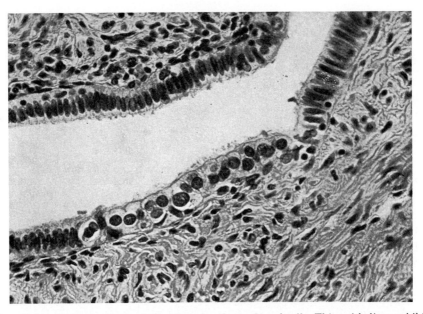

1.17. The tubal epithelium, showing both ciliated and nonciliated cells. This epithelium exhibits definite cyclical changes in height and other characteristics.

superimposed on a rather cellular tunica propria. Like the uterine epithelium, the epithelium of the tube undergoes definite cyclical changes, although these are much less conspicuous than in the uterus.

THE OVARIES

The ovaries are two ovoid bodies which constitute the genital glands of the female. They are placed, one in each side of the pelvis, just below the tubes, the outer ends of which are curved over them in an arclike fashion. They measure about 3.5 by 2 by 1.5 cm., although there is considerable variation. Anteriorly, the ovaries are set in the posterior surface of the broad ligament much as a diamond is set in a ring. At the line of attachment is the *hilum*, through which blood vessels and nerves enter and leave the ovary. In a very small number of cases (five in the report by Pearl and Plotz) supernumerary ovaries have been documented.

The *external surface* of the ovary is of dull, whitish, opaque appearance. In the young child it is smooth, in the adult woman pitted from previous ovulations, and in the old woman it may be shrunken and corrugated, like the surface of a peach stone. The ovary is attached to the uterus by a well developed *ovarian ligament,* while the upper outer pole is suspended to the side of the pelvis by that portion of the broad ligament beyond the tube (infundibulopelvic ligament or suspensory ligament of the ovary).

On section, the ovary is seen to be divisible into an outer cortex and a central portion or medulla. Covering the *cortex* is the so-called *germinal epithelium,* made up of a single layer of cuboidal epithelium. It is usually absent in the adult ovary, but often appears in the presence of chronic inflammation. Under such conditions the epithelium may show metaplastic changes. Beneath the epithelium is the cortical stroma, which, just beneath the epithelium, shows a slightly condensed layer called the *tunica albuginea.* The stroma itself is made up of compactly placed spindle cell connective tissue cells, in which are to be seen the follicular elements and their derivatives.

In the ovary of the young child the follicles are exceedingly numerous, being estimated at about 100,000 in number in the ovary of the newborn child, but becoming progressively less numerous after puberty. The histological structure of the mature

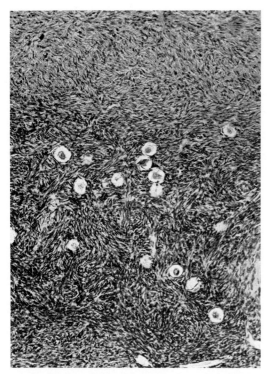

1.18. Section of ovary showing primordial follicles and typical spindle-celled stroma.

follicle, as well as of the *corpus luteum* in its various stages is described in Chapter 3 under "Cyclical Changes in the Ovary." Only a small proportion of primordial follicles reach full maturity, the majority being blighted at various phases of development by the process known as *astresia folliculi*. This is characterized by death of the ovum, followed by degeneration and disappearance of the granulosa, so that in this *cystic stage* the atretic follicle appears as a tiny cyst, with or without a lining epithelium. With increasing age, the follicle count drops progressively as indicated by Winter.

Hilus Cells

In the hilus of the ovary one not infrequently finds small nests and occasionally rather large fields of ovoid or polyhedral cells, usually arranged in rather mosaic fashion. They were originally spoken of by Berger as sympathicotrophic cells, but these hilus cells, as they are more commonly designated, are now looked upon as the homologues of the

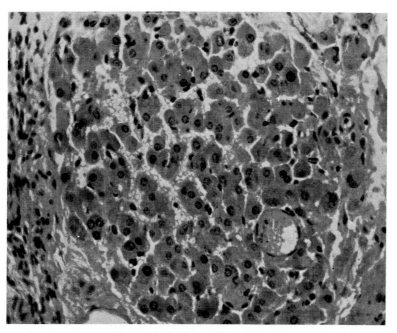

1.19. Cluster of hilus cells in the ovary

interstitial or Leydig cells of the testis, which they indeed resemble histologically. The peculiar rectangular crystalloids of Reincke may be found in both, although by no means invariably. The remarkable similarity, if not identity, between hilus and theca cells has been discussed by Loubet and Loubet.

The Pelvic Floor and Perineum

This is described in the section on relaxations and fistulas (Chapter 13).

REFERENCES

Berger, L.: La glande sympathicotrope du hile de l'ovaire; ses homologies avec la glande interstitielle due testicule; les rapports nerveuses des deux glandes. Arch. Anat. (Strasb.), *2:* 255, 1923.

Fluhmann, C. F.: The developmental anatomy of the cervix uteri. Obstet. Gynec., *15:*62, 1960.

Forsberg, J. G.: Cervico-vaginal epithelium; its origin and development. Amer. J. Obstet. Gynec., *115:* 1025, 1973.

Huffman, J. W.: Detailed anatomy of paraurethral ducts in adult female. Amer. J. Obstet. Gynec., *55:* 86, 1948.

Huffman, J. W.: Mesonephric remains in cervix. Amer. J. Obstet. Gynec., *56:* 23, 1948.

Huffman, J. W.: Mesonephric remains in human female. Quart. Bull. Northwest Univ. Med. Sch., *25:* 1, 1951.

Loubet, R., and Loubet, A.: Le systeme des cellules hilaires de l'ovaire: hyperplasies et tumeurs. Soc. Franc. Gynec., *33:* 589, 1963.

Pearl, M., and Plotz, E. J.: Supernumerary ovary. Obstet. Gynec., *21:* 253, 1963.

Range, R. L., and Woodburne, R. T.: The gross and microscopic anatomy of the transverse cervical ligament. Amer. J. Obstet. Gynec., *90:* 460, 1964.

Rubin, I. C., and Novak, J.: *Integrated Gynecology, Principles and Practice,* Vol. 1. Blakiston Company, Division of McGraw-Hill Book Company, Inc., New York, 1956.

Weed, J. C.: Pelvic anatomy from the point of view of a gynecologic surgeon. Clin. Obstet. Gynec., *15:* 1035, 1972.

Winter, G. F.: Follicle counts in the ovaries of healthy nonpregnant women. Zbl. Gynaek., *84:* 1824, 1962.

Zacharin, R. F.: The anatomic supports of the female urethra. Obstet. Gynaec., *32 754, 1968.*

Physiology of Menstruation and Pregnancy

HISTORICAL

The advances which have been made in our knowledge concerning the mechanism and significance of menstruation can best be appreciated by placing our present concepts against the background of an earlier day.

Before the turn of the century, Pflüger suggested that menstruation was due to a pelvic hyperemia evoked reflexly through the nervous system by the ripening of Graafian follicles in the ovary. This was considered a great advance over the previous so-called lunar theory which related the cause of menstruation to the cycle of the moon.

Precisely in 1900 Knauer demonstrated the endocrine nature of the ovary by surgical extirpation and transplantation experiments. In 1903, Fraenkel clarified the function of the corpus luteum as an endocrine organ by showing that removal in the first few days of pregnancy invariably caused resorption of rabbit embryos. The life history of the follicle and the corpus luteum soon became the subject of intensive study and, when Hitschmann and Adler in 1908 described the histological cycle in the endometrium, it was almost immediately possible to correlate the ovarian and endometrial cycle chronologically.

In 1912 Adler was able to report the first successful experiments with an ovarian extract which would repair the atrophic changes in the uterus of a castrate guinea pig. The event, however, which more than any other furthered the study of the reproductive cycle was the discovery by Stockard and Papanicolaou, in 1917, that the vagina, as well as the uterus of animals, undergoes definite cyclic changes. It was this laboratory technique which really allowed for the isolation and final identification of the ovarian hormones.

Estrogens

In a brief communication in 1915, shortly after Adler's report with crude whole ovarian extracts, Frank and Rosenbloom called attention to the estrus-producing effects of an extract of follicular fluid. However, Allen and Doisy really deserve the credit for making a thorough investigation of the hormone which has come to be known as estrogen, the generic name applied to derivatives of the female sex hormone.

In 1927 Zondek and Aschheim found pregnancy urine to be rich in estrogenic substances and thus furnished the chemists with not only a ready source of material but one far easier to work with than the ovarian or placental tissue previously used. Three years later, four laboratories almost simultaneously announced the crystallization from human pregnancy urine of an estrogenic substance which was later designated as estrone. In 1930 Browne isolated from the placenta a much less potent estrogenic steroid which has since been called estriol, and in 1936 MacCorquodale, Thayer, and Doisy, in Doisy's laboratory, crystallized the active ovarian hormone known as estradiol. A number of derivatives all more or less estrogenic have since been demonstrated as urinary metabolites.

Progesterone

In 1929 Corner and Allen established the presence of a hormone principle in the corpus luteum which they named progestin to indicate its specific concern with gestation. Butenandt identified the hormone as a sterol and suggested the chemical nature be indicated by the suffix sterone, thus the term progesterone. Although two other progestational steroids were isolated from the corpus luteum by Zander and his associates in 1958, their progestational activity is substantially less than that of progesterone and there is little evidence that there is any other naturally occurring progestational substance of physiological significance.

Marrian in 1929 and Butenandt in 1930 identified a sterol which was excreted in large amounts in the urine of pregnant women. For this reason the name pregnanediol was assigned to it. However, it remained for Venning and Browne in 1937 to establish that pregnanediol, excreted as sodium pregnanediol glucuronide, was a metabolite of progesterone and furnishes a reasonably accurate measure of progesterone secretion. Although other lesser metabolites have since been described, pregnanediol remains the major excretion product of progesterone.

Pituitary Gonadotropins

It is interesting that almost simultaneously with the unraveling of the relationship between the ovarian cycle and the endometrial cycle another relationship was unfolding, this time in an area far removed from the pelvic organs.

It has been known, certainly since the report of Fröhlich in 1901 of a 14-year-old boy with infantilism associated with a destructive lesion of the pituitary, that this gland was in some way concerned with the development of the reproductive organs. However, it was not until 1910, when Crowe, Cushing, and Homans performed the first experimental hypophysectomy on dogs, that active laboratory investigation of the control of the reproductive function by the pituitary was really begun. This experimental operation began an era of investigation of the effects of ablation which in turn led to the experimental work of Smith and Engle with hypophysial implants and extracts. In 1927 these authors postulated two gonadotrophic hormones for the control of ovarian function in an effort to explain the follicular growth and luteinization which invariably occurred following implantation or injection of pituitary extracts.

To Evans *et al.* goes the credit for the major contributions towards the separation and purification of the pituitary hormones, a work ably continued by Evans' successor Li. In 1936 the first publication appeared from this laboratory describing the separation, from hypophysial extracts, of two gonadotrophic principles identified as luteinizing hormone (LH) and follicle-stimulating hormone (FSH). Purification of LH from swine pituitaries was accomplished in 1940 by Shedlovsky *et al.*, working at the Squibb Institute.

Hypothalamus

The dominance of the ovary by the pituitary is not, however, altogether one-sided, the functional relationship being a reciprocal one. In 1932 both Severinghaus and Wolfe independently reported that the gonadotrophic potency of the pituitary was enhanced by castration.

The closely integrated pituitary-ovarian relationship, the "feedback" control, is largely regulated by the central nervous system through the region of the hypothalamus, although in many instances the exact role of hypothalamus and pituitary in the modulation mechanism is still disputed.

The possibility of pituitary-hypo-thalamic control was established by the demonstration of Adams *et al.* of a pituitary-portal system by which hypothalamic hormones could reach the anterior pituitary. Transplantation experiments of Harris showed that the pituitary cells from an immature animal, if placed in the fossa of an adult animal, are capable of producing gonadotrophic hormones and maintaining normal ovarian function. This suggested that the initiation of puberty is caused by maturation of the nervous system, not the pituitary. Observations of Elwers and Critchlow on the production of precocious puberty in rats after damage to the amygdala or the stria terminalis (the tract of communication with the hypothalamus) further substantiate this fact. As the higher centers mature, the hypothalamic centers are released from inhibitory influences and puberty is initiated by the subsequent pituitary stimulation. The function of the hypothalamus is apparently made possible by excitory and inhibitory stimuli from the central nervous system which influence cells in the hypothalamus through neurotransmitters such as serotonin, norepinephrine or dopamine (Fig. 2.1).

An important consideration in the understanding of hypothalamic neurophysiology comes from the work of Nagle *et al.* in 1972, who showed that a neurotransmitter, serotonin, is synthesized in the retina. Nerve tracts have been traced directly from the retina to the posterior hypothalamus by O'Stein and Baughan. Along these tracts, serotonin is transmitted from its synthetic source to the hypothalamic cells. The content of serotonin in the hypothalamus increases with maturity. If one assumes that serotonin is necessary for positive secretion of hypothalamic gonadotrophic hormones and that some other inhibitory neurotransmitter is dominant in the im-

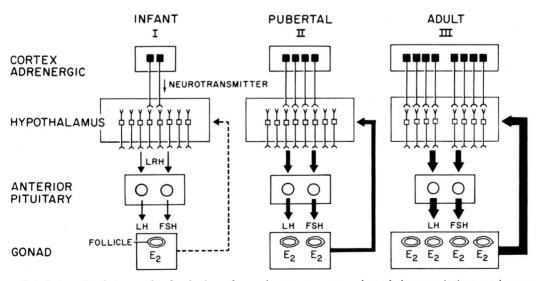

2.1. Interaction between the developing adrenergic nervous system, hypothalamus, pituitary and ovary from infancy to adulthood. (Derived from the theory of K. B. Ruf, Z. Neurol., *204:* 95, 1973).

mature organism and that this inhibitory transmitter enters the hypothalamus through a tract from the amygdaloid nucleus by way of the stria terminalis, the basic mechanism for a positive and negative control system is established as a rationale for the onset of puberty.

A series of unrelated investigations has demonstrated that three major types of stimuli exert an influence on ovulation and mating behavior. These are (1) sensory stimuli from all of the four senses (*sight, smell, touch,* and *hearing*); (2) emotional (*adrenergic* and *cholinergic agents* which are released during emotional stress); and (3) chemical (ovarian *steroids,* and *related compounds* or *drugs*). *Visual* control of the reproductive cycle is highly developed in birds and a review of the subject by Farner indicates that in certain species the hypothalamus relies almost entirely on day length as the source of environmental information in its control of the gonadotrophic function of the anterior pituitary gland. Fiske and Greep present evidence that the effect of light on ovulation is mediated through the supraoptic nuclei. Work by Bruce demonstrates the role of *olfactory* stimulation; mice placed in cages which had previously housed strange males showed pregnancy blocking. The characteristic of the rabbit to ovulate only on coital stimulus is an example of *tactile sensibility* as a control of the reproductive system. An ingenious experiment of Zondek with high frequency sound waves has indicated that *auditory stimuli* also exert an influence on ovulation and mating in the rat. Markee has shown that *cholinergic* and *adrenergic agents* will cause release of pituitary LH and that this reaction can be blocked by a sympathetic or para-sympathetic nervous system antagonist. This type of reaction could explain a possible mechanism for the influence of *emotional factors* on ovulation. The effect of *steroid hormones* on the anterior pituitary gland has also been shown to be mediated at least in part by the hypothalamus. Thus, Flerko demonstrated that estrogen-producing ovarian grafts had no effect when placed directly in contact with the pituitary cells, but if placed in specific hypothalamic areas, inhibition of FSH production was obtained.

McCann and his colleagues are responsible for much of the early physiologic work with the hypothalamic hormones. Purification of luteinizing release hormone (LRH) was accomplished almost simultaneously by Schalley *et al.* and Guillimaine. This hormone is sometimes referred to as GnRH, gonadotrophin release hormone, as it stimulates both LH and FSH release. Although Johansson *et al.* reported the identification of a specific FSH-RH, their work has not been confirmed. LRH has since been synthesized and is a decapeptide (Fig. 2.19).

Igarashi and his colleagues used a partially purified extract of beef hypothalamus LH-RH for the first time in humans for the induction of ovulation. They obtained ovulation in 3 of 14 women and pregnancy in 1. They indicated that the hypothalamic hormones are not species specific.

In the rat three centers have been demonstrated which are specifically concerned with control of the ovarian cycle. These are the tonic FSH and LH release centers in the posterior hypothalamus in the region of the arcuate nucleus, and the cyclic-LH release center in the anterior hypothalamus in the suprachiasmatic area. The cyclic-LH center which controls the sudden release of LH at mid-cycle resulting in ovulation has been shown to be blocked in the male. This is apparently by the action of androgen from the fetal testis. Although irreversible in the rat, this block is apparently reversible in the primate.

The negative feedback mechanism, the long-loop, by the gonadal steroids on the hypothalamus and pituitary seems to be the major regulatory control for the rhymicity of the ovarian cycle. Shalley *et al.* have shown that women who have suppression of baseline gonadotrophin secretion by steroids, nevertheless have a brisk LH release following LRH administration. They interpret this as indicative that the major steroid modulation is at the hypothalamic level. Experimental work with LRH by Taymor *et al.* indicates that estrogen affects the release of LH at the pituitary level as well.

Although all three gonadotrophic centers can apparently be suppressed by estrogen, the FSH-release center is the most sensitive in the human. Testosterone is a potent LH inhibitor, but a poor FSH inhibitor. Although synthetic progestational drugs, which are used as oral contraceptives, are efficient cyclic-LH inhibitors, this activity may depend upon the inherent or added estrogen in these drugs as well as the androgenicity of most. If progesterone *per se* is effective, either as a stimulator for LH release or a tonic LH inhibitor, it apparently requires a preliminary estrogen priming action. For further documentation, see the discussion under 17α-hydroxylase deficiency (Chapter 30).

A number of investigators have shown that estrogen at a specific dosage stimulates rather than suppresses LH release. This is the so-called "positive" estrogen feedback and is evoked to explain the cyclic LH surge. The intracellular mechanisms by which estrogen can elicit a suppression at one dosage and a stimulation at another has not been explained. A helpful working hypothesis is the assumption that the anterior hypothalamic cyclic-LH center is secreting an LH-inhibitory hormone (LH-IH). This obviates the necessity for postulating a positive estrogen feedback (Fig. 2.2).

It has also been thought that the pituitary LH surge is stimulated by a concomitant LRH surge. A bioassay for LRH has been devised by Reichert and an im-

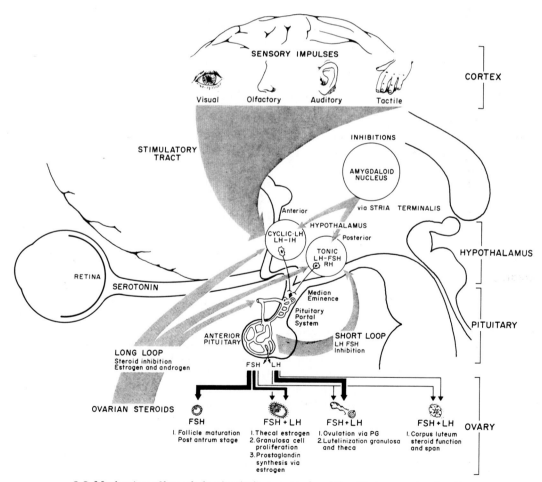

2.2. Mechanism of hypothalamic-pituitary control and the effect on ovarian function

munoassay by Shalley, but there are conflicting reports regarding the serum content of LRH during the normal menstrual cycle. These investigators both report increased LRH secretion at midcycle, while others report no discernible variation.

The Pineal. The relation of the pineal gland to reproductive function has been recognized since 1896 when Gutzeit first described the association of precocious puberty and a pinealoma in a small boy. Impetus for further study of this relationship came in 1950, when Lerner reported the isolation of an indole compound, melatonin, from the cow pineal gland. Wurtman has summarized the current concepts which indicate that the pineal acts as a transducer, receiving nervous stimuli, and secreting a neural hormone, melatonin.

In the rat, constant light depletes the pineal of its indole stores, while darkness causes increased pineal melatonin. There is some reason to believe that day-oriented animals may show a reverse pattern from the rat, a nocturnal animal. The nervous pathway for the pineal stimulus is through fibers which originate in the retina and are carried in the inferior accessory optic tracts into the spinal cord. These nerves reach the pineal not through the stalk but by way of the sympathetic nervous system from the superior cervical ganglia. Thus the pineal may act as a regulator between the environment and the physiological factors which control the rythmicity of the reproductive function.

Ovarian Factors

During the past decade a great deal of experimental work has helped to clarify ovarian development and the factors which determine the ability of the ovary to respond to the various gonadotrophic stimulations. Jones, Ferguson-Smith and Heller, from a study of a number of individuals with abnormal sex-chromosome complements, including the 45,X, suggested that two normal sex chromosomes were necessary for the maturation of germ cells and that streak gonads, *e.g.*, gonads without follicles, resulted whenever there was an absence of germ cells. Singh and Carr, in a study of eight human embryos between the ages of five weeks and four months with the XO karyotype, described the effect of a missing X chromosome on the development of the gonads. Embryos with a 45,X karyotype had gonads similar to normal 46,XX embryos up to the third month of intrauterine age. However, these fetuses after the third month of intrauterine life failed to show the expected normal sequence of primary follicle formation. This finding suggests that although mitotic division in the abnormal germ cell is normal, meiotic division, which begins at about two months of embryonic life (Baker) and proceeds at an increasing rate until all germ cell have been converted, is impossible. The observations of Singh and Carr suggest that the germ cells with an abnormal complement of sex chromosomes begin to disappear more rapidly than usual as they enter into the meiotic division stage. It seems likely that crossing over, which is a normal process during prophase of meiosis I, cannot occur unless there are two normal chromosomes between which the exchange of genetic material can take place.

The oocytes must be competent to organize a layer of granulosa cells by which they are surrounded as they reach the end of meiosis I. These cells comprise the primordial follicles which, in turn, organize the stroma into the theca. If, for any reason, these reactions cannot be induced, the ovary is intrinsically incapable of responding normally to an ovulatory stimulation.

To recapitulate, a normal 46,XX karyotype is necessary for normal numbers of oocytes. If ovarian stromal cells are normal, the oocyte induces granulosa cell formation which, in turn, stimulates a theca reaction, the whole comprising a normal antrum stage follicle. If these cells contain normal gonadotrophin receptor proteins, gonadotrophic hormones, FSH plus the addition of small amounts of LH, are then able to induce follicle growth past the antrum stage and estrogen secretion. After an adequate FSH growth stimulus, an adequate LH stimulus will induce ovulation and corpus luteum formation.

The usual 14-day life span of the corpus luteum is dependent upon minimal tonic LH stimulation. As human prolactin, LTH, has become available for testing, no luteotrophic activity has been demonstrated for this hormone. Factors influencing follicular atresia and corpus luteum lysis are as yet still undetermined. Ross *et al.* have shown in the rat that follicular atresia is dependent upon the local concentrations of FSH and estrogen. With estrogen present, FSH causes follicular growth and decreases atresia. With estrogen concentration, low FSH causes increased atresia. Lysis of the corpus luteum may be caused by prostaglandin which in turn may be synthesized in the luteal cells under estrogen stimulation.

Prolactin (Mammotrophin, Luteotrophin, Lactotrophin)

The possibility of a pituitary lactogenic hormone was first suggested in 1928 by Stricker and Grueter who found that lactation could be induced in the pseudopregnant rat by injection of an anterior pituitary extract. In 1931 Riddle and Braucher described the production of milk in the pigeon crop sac following the injection of pituitary extracts. This observation laid the foundation for the bioassay and nomenclature of the hormone which persists today. In 1941 Astwood, and Evans and his co-workers simultaneously described a pituitary hormone, luteotrophin (LTH), capable of initiating progesterone secretion in the functionless corpus luteum of the hypophysectomized rat. Shortly thereafter it was agreed, however, that luteotrophin was identical with prolactin.

Although luteotrophic action in the rat suggested an additional role which prolactin might play in the mammal, no luteotrophic activity has been demonstrated for the human.

The antigonadotrophin effect of prolactin was first noted by Riddle and Bates in 1933 in experiments on adult pigeons. The testicular weights were reduced by 90% following 10 days of prolactin injection. This activity has since been confirmed in mice and rats by Dresel and Greep and Jones.

The established functions of prolactin then can be named as (1) stimulation of lactation, and (2) antigonadotrophic activity. Both of these physiological actions are seen in pure culture, clinically, in patients having a prolactin-secreting pituitary adenoma associated with the Ahumada-del Castillo syndrome (see Chapter 22).

In 1937 Lyons isolated prolactin in a fairly pure form and chemically characterized it. It has since been extensively investigated by Li, Simpson, and Evans and unlike the two gonadotrophins, FSH and LH, it is alcohol-soluble, and not a glycoprotein. It is closely related to growth hormone and adrenocorticotrophic hormone (ACTH). There is some evidence from the immunological cross reaction that human growth hormone and prolactin have the same basic molecular structure with probably only one or two dissimilar groups.

The major control of prolactin production is apparently through a hypothalamic inhibitory hormone, the prolactin inhibiting factor, PIF. Thyrotropic release hormone, TRH, exerts a positive stimulation on prolactin production. This hypothalamic hormone, a tripeptide, seems to be as efficient for prolactin stimulation as for pituitary thyrotropic hormone stimulation (Fig. 2.3). Estrogen causes hypertrophy of the pituitary lactotrops and thereby increases prolactin. Dopamine is the neurotransmitter which stimulates the release of PIF, therefore decreases pituitary prolactin.

In the human the PIF hypothalamic center can be poisoned by phenothiazine derivatives which are commonly used as tranquilizers. This blocks the effect of dopamine preventing the release of prolactin inhibiting factor and increases the production of prolactin. Under these circumstances, one sees the clinical syndrome of amenorrhea, uterine hypoplasia, and breast secretion. Pituitary stalk section in the human is also associated

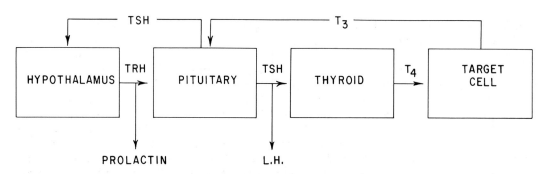

2.3. Interrelation between thyroid and gonadotrophic function. TRH stimulates prolactin which usually inhibits LH. However, if TSH is unusually elevated, an LH-like effect will be induced because of the chemical similarity between TSH and LH (see Fig. 2.13).

with excessive prolactin release, further indicating that the neural control in the human is similar to the one described for experimental animals.

The reason for the inverse relation of pituitary gonadotrophin hormones, LH and FSH, to prolactin is not clear. Although no change occurs in prolactin when depressed LH levels are elevated by LRH administration, when elevated prolactin levels are lowered by ergocornine administration, there is a prompt rise in gonadotrophins (see Chapter 30).

CURRENT STATUS OF THE PHYSIOLOGY OF MENSTRUATION

Sexual maturation is apparently a gradual, not a cataclysmic, process which is dependent upon maturation of the central nervous system. Specifically, this seems to involve the concentration of neural hormones, adrenergic and cholinergic transmitters in the hypothalamus. The process is accomplished by transmission of the hormones from the site of origin, along nerve tracts which have their endings in the hypothalamus. An example of this mechanism, which has been nicely documented by neurophysiology, is illustrated (Fig. 2.2). Serotonin is synthesized in the retina, presumably under light stimulation and transmitted through nerve tracts to the posterior hypothalamus in the region of the arcuate nucleus, the area closely associated with the cells which produce tonic FSH and

LH releasing hormone (LH-RH). The concentration of these neurotransmitters in the hypothalamus, as in the cerebral cortex, can be shown to increase with the age of the individual, presumably related to the quality or quantity of sensory stimuli exposure. As the amount of stimulatory transmitters reaches the level compatible with physiologic activity, the effects of the gonadotrophic stimulation of the pituitary by the hypothalamus are evidenced in the response of the end organs, and pubertal development begins.

In the experimental animal an inhibitory control seems to be operational in the immature individual. Thus, if lesions are made in the amygdaloid region or the stria terminalis, the tract leading from this complex to the hypothalamus, precocious development is initiated. The occurrence of precocious puberty in children with central nervous system scars would seem to be compatible with the same type of early inhibitory control in the human. The actual presence of such inhibitory neural hormones in the hypothalamus of infancy and preadolescence has not been demonstrated.

The hypothalamus can be shown to have two anatomically distinct nervous systems (1) the tubero-infundibular tract, which originates within the basal hypothalamus, secretes dopaminergic transmitters, which stimulate, and indolamines, which inhibit, LRH synthesis, and (2) the noradrenergic (catecholaminergic) neurons, which have cell bodies outside the hypothalamus and axons only within the hypothalamus. These neurons also stimulate LRH synthesis. Estrogen has been shown to inhibit catecholamine stimulation of LRH release.

The noradrenergic neurons (catecholaminergic system) have the ability to grow postnatally and actively regenerate by sprouting after injury or when given access to areas previously innervated by other fibers. They can be stimulated in a dose-dependent relation by neural growth factor. These characteristics of ontogenicity and plasticity of the central monoaminergic neurons has led Ruf to hypothecate that when the adrenergic neurons reach the limit of their growth potential, puberty is initiated by the adult level of terminal arborization (and possibly definitive numbers of cells) of adrenergic neurons synapsing with neurons of hypothalamic cells synthesizing GnRH. This results in increased GnRH, increased FSH and LH, increased follicle growth and estrogen production (Fig. 2.1).

The appearance of precocious puberty following brain injury or lesions in amygdala or stria terminalis therefore can be due not so much to interruption of inhibition as to the capacity of the aminergic fiber system to show increased sprouting and regeneration after injury and to its ability to avidly innervate areas previously innervated by injured neural fibers.

Gonadal control by the hypothalamus is dependent upon cells in the posterior hypothalamus in the region of the arcuate nucleus which synthesize tonic FSH and LH release hormone designated as LRH, LH-RH and FSH-RH. Sometimes these hypothalamic hormones are referred to as GnRH, gonadotrophic release hormone because, at the present time, it has not been determined if there is one or two different hypothalamic hormones which cause the synthesis and release of pituitary LH and FSH. LRH has been isolated and synthesized and can be shown to cause LH stimulation in a reproducible manner. It also causes stimulation of FSH but usually to a lesser

degree and in a more unpredictable fashion. Johannson *et al.* have attempted to isolate an FSH-RH and, although initial investigations looked promising, no confirmation has been forthcoming. This work indicated that the FSH-RH might also contain the potential for stimulating both FSH and LH, but in reverse ratios to that seen by LRH. The hypothalamic hormones, two of which have been synthesized, are small polypeptides, LRH being a decapeptide and are, therefore, not species specific and are active by all routes of administration.

In the anterior hypothalamus in the region of the supraoptic nucleus, a group of cells, the mechanism of action of which is not well understood, control the cyclic release of LH responsible for ovulation. It is this center which is especially responsive to steroid modulation. Cells of the anterior hypothalamus, in addition to containing estrogen receptor protein, have the capability of aromatizing C-19 steroids to estrogens. This center is blocked in the male during embryonic life apparently by androgen. In the rat, but not the primate, the block is permanent.

Modulation of hypothalamic function occurs by way of (1) steroid feedback, the long loop, (2) pituitary feedback, the short loop, and (3) the ultra short loop, the intra-hypothalamic feedback. All of these mechanisms can be demonstrated under special conditions, but the importance of the specific control mechanism varies with the specific hypothalamic and pituitary hormone complex in question.

The functional hypothalamic unit requires a cell or cells which are programmed to synthesize hypothalamic hormones, neurotransmitters to initiate the release of these hormones and perhaps to regulate the synthesis by both stimulation and inhibition. The cells must also contain steroid receptor proteins to allow for modulation by the long loop steroid feedback and a membrane receptor for the pituitary hormones to permit the short loop feedback.

Both tonic FSH and LH are suppressed by estrogen, FSH being most responsive and LH secondarily so. LH is suppressed by testosterone and certain of the progestational drugs. However, progesterone *per se* is not effective in inhibiting pituitary gonadotrophins in humans. Kraftin *et al.* have postulated that the major site of steroid suppression of pituitary gonadotrophins occurs at the hypothalamus or higher, because pretreatment with oral contraceptives, estrogen and progestational drugs (Lyndiol) did not prevent the release of LH and FSH after the administration of LRH. However, as modulation of pituitary gonadotrophin production also occurs at the pituitary level, it has been extremely difficult to pinpoint the exact site of action. FSH is also suppressed by some non-steroidal substance or substances secreted by the testicular tubules and the Graafian follicles in the ovary.

LH and, to a lesser extent, FSH are secreted by the pituitary in an episodic fashion. Reichert and Ward have presented evidence using a bioassay for LRH that the LRH hypothalamic secretion is likewise episodic and the periodicity is in an inverse relation suggesting that the short loop feedback is operational.

The so-called positive estrogen feedback is the initiating of the LH surge by the anterior hypothalamic cells apparently under the influence of a specific amount of estrogen. In addition to the effect on the anterior hypothalamus, estrogen also apparently exerts an effect on the ability of pituitary cells to release LH. Arimura *et al.,* using a sensitive immunoreactive LH-RH assay in plasma, have demonstrated an apparent increase in this hypothalamic hormone at midcycle, substantiating these authors' belief that an increased LRH is responsible for the LH surge. Other authors, Nett *et al.,* Keye *et al.,* have been unable to demonstrate this relationship. Whatever the etiology, however, the important facts are that given a specific amount of estrogen at the mid-cycle, some mechanism is initiated in the anterior hypothalamus which triggers a flood of LH from the pituitary.

The ensuing corpus luteum function after ovulation results in production of sufficient estrogen and, perhaps, progesterone to inhibit the posterior hypothalamic centers decreasing pituitary FSH and LH. As the corpus luteum regresses, approximately 2 to 4 days prior to menstruation, steroid levels reach a sufficiently low concentration to allow the pituitary to increase FSH secretion. This initiates the growth of follicles for the next cycle. FSH continues to rise during the first 7 to 10 days of the follicular phase associated with a slightly delayed LH rise. This rising LH in the first part of the follicular phase is responsible for the production of estrogen by the theca surrounding the developing follicles. However, during this phase of the cycle, the estrogen remains relatively low. In the preovulatory swelling phase, approximately 4 days prior to ovulation, there is a rapid increase of estrogen apparently from the ovulatory follicle in the "active ovary," and it is this estrogen surge which then triggers the LH surge.

The LH surge which is associated with ovulation initiates luteinization of the granulosa cells and corpus luteum formation. Ovulation *per se* is dependent upon a vascular phenomenon, the stigmata that can be shown in experimental animals to depend upon prostaglandin which, in turn, may be stimulated by estrogen.

The ability of the ovary to respond to the pituitary gonadotrophins depends primarily upon the normalcy of the chromosomal content. In the absence of two normal X chromosomes, it has been shown that meiosis does not occur and, as oocytes begin to go into meiotic division during the second or third month of embryonic life, the germ cells disappear from the genital ridge leaving only stroma and forming a "streak ovary" (Chapter 8). Given two normal X chromosomes and a normal complement of oocytes, these eggs organize around them granulosa cells, which in turn organize the theca. The normally programmed granulosa cell contains FSH gonadotrophic receptor sites, as the follicle will not proceed beyond the antrum stage in the absence of pituitary stimulation. Channing has presented some evidence which indicates that the FSH stimulation is also responsible for the induction of LH receptor sites in the granulosa and theca cells. The theca cells, under the stimulation of LH, are responsible for estrogen production and use as their preferential substrate in the follicular phase of the cycle dehydroepiandrosterone, a Δ^5 steroid. In the luteal phase, the preferential substrate has been shown to be progesterone, a Δ^4 steroid. Immediately after the estrogen surge which triggers the LH surge and ovulation, there is a fall in the estrogen concentration followed by a secondary rise which parallels the serum progesterone elevation. The etiology of this interruption of estrogen secretion at midcycle is as yet undetermined, but because of temporal relationships with the assay of serum 17α-hydroxyprogesterone, an intermediate metabolite between the synthesis of progesterone and estrogen, it can be postulated that this hiatus is due to the lag which occurs in the change over from the Δ^5 to the Δ^4 substrate.

The normalcy of corpus luteum function depends upon the initial programming of the granulosa cells to contain proper gonadotrophin receptor sites and the necessary enzymes for progesterone production, secondly upon a proper FSH stimulation beginning in the prior cycle to initiate normal numbers and composition of granulosa cells, and finally adequate residual tonic LH stimulation during the luteal phase to insure an adequate 14-day span. It is as yet unresolved whether the corpus luteum fixed life span depends upon its failing response to minimal LH, or upon some active luteolytic factor. Prostaglandin $F_{2\alpha}$ has been suggested as such an agent. Under the aegis of estrogen production, the corpus luteum cells also apparently produce prostaglandin $F_2\alpha$ and both of

these substances can be shown to be luteolytic in the experimental animals.

CHEMISTRY OF STEROID HOMONES

Nomenclature

The ovarian, testicular, and adrenal hormones are steroids derived from the same basic molecular structure as cholesterol. The steroid nuclei from which these hormones derive their names, *estrane, androstane,* and *pregnane,* with the designation of the rings and the numbering of the carbon atoms, are shown in Figure 2.4. The major structural differences are the *absence of the side chain* (C_{20} and C_{21}) *in the androstane nucleus,* from which the androgens are derived, and the *absence of both the side chain and a methyl group at C_{19}, in the estrane nucleus,* from which the estrogens are derived. Progesterone and the adrenal corticoids belong to the pregnane series.

Stereoisomerism can occur at any of the asymmetric carbon atoms, 5, 8, 9, 10, 13, and 14, and is important as it affects the biological activity of the compound. The Greek letters, α and β, are used to designate the stereometric position of the hydrogen atom or substituents in relation to the angle of the methyl groups at carbon atom 18 or 19 or both, β being in the same plane and α in the opposite. When drawn on a formula, solid lines are used for the β position and dotted lines

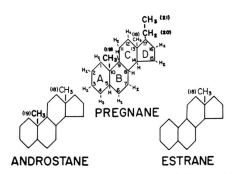

2.4. The steroid hormone parent nuclei from which the nomenclature is derived. The ring designations and the carbon atom numbers are shown in the pregnane nucleus. Hydrogens are not shown on the androstane or estrane nuclei.

are used for the α position. The β position, which is present in biologically active steroids, is also referred to as *cis* while the α position may be called *trans*. The terms *allo* and *epi* are sometimes used to denote the α and β positions. However, *allo* is used only in relation to the hydrogen atom at C_5, while *epi* can be used in relation to any other carbon atom.

The presence of a double bond is noted in the nomenclature by changing the suffix "ane" to "ene." Two double bonds are denoted by the suffix "diene" and three by "triene." The number of the lowest sequential carbon designates the position of the bond and this number should be placed between the name of the parent nucleus and the prefix. The Greek letter, Δ, placed before the parent nucleus

name, with the superior carbon number, *e.g.,* (Δ^5), has also been used for this purpose.

The presence of a hydroxyl group is denoted by the prefix "hydroxy" or the suffix "ol" and a ketone group by the prefix "oxo" or the suffix "one." The absence of a substituent group or a carbon is designated by the prefixes des or nor.

Biosynthesis

As might be expected from the chemical similarity of their formulae, the biosynthetic pathways for the production of estrogens, progesterone, androgens, and adrenal corticoids seem to be equally interrelated. The ovary, adrenal, and testis apparently all possess, in some

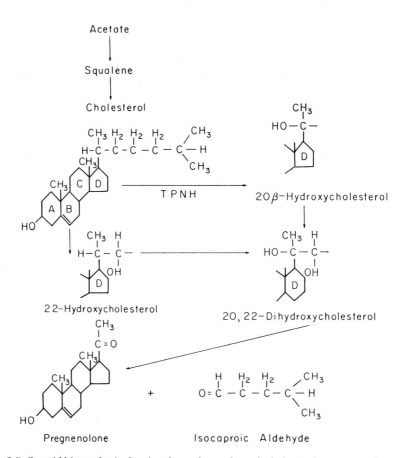

BIOSYNTHESIS OF STEROIDS

2.5. Steroid biosynthesis showing the pathway through cholesterol to pregnenolone degree, capabilities for biosynthesis of all steroids.

In general, two major pathways seem to exist. The first utilizes cholesterol as the substrate (Fig. 2.5). After hydroxylation at C_{20} and C_{22}, the sidechain is split off with the formation of pregnenolone and isocaproic acid. Reduced nicotinamide adenine dinucleotide phosphate (TPNH) is an essential cofactor. By and large,

TPNH is necessary wherever an hydroxylation occurs. Nicotinamide adenine dinucleotide (DPN) seems to be essential for certain of the dehydrogenase reactions, *e.g.,* removal of hydrogen.

Progesterone is formed from pregnenolone by removal of the hydrogen at the three position and shifting of the double bond from the B ring to the A ring (Fig. 2.6). The first reaction utilizes a 3β-

STEROID BIOSYNTHESIS OF ANDROGEN

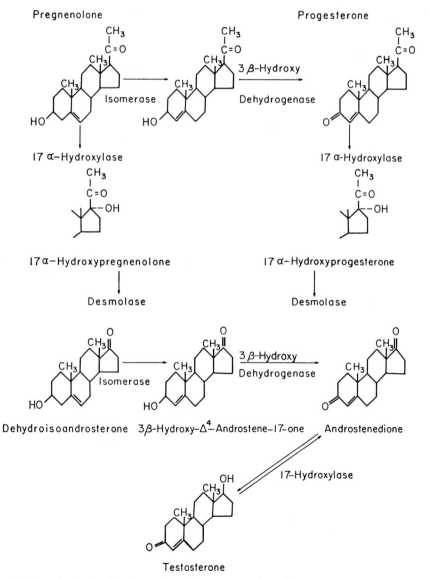

2.6. Steroid biosynthesis showing the pathway from pregnenolone through progesterone to androstenedione or testosterone.

hydroxydehydrogenase which is catalyzed by DPN. The isomerization reaction which shifts the double bond from the Δ^5 to the Δ^4 position can be accomplished either enzymatically or chemically.

Progesterone has been said to be the precursor of all sex steroids, as it is possible to proceed from progesterone to corticoids, testosterone, or estrogens through 17α-hydroxyprogesterone. This has been called the Δ^4 pathway. Following the formation of 17α-hydroxyprogesterone the side chain can be removed, forming Δ^4-androstene-3, 17-dione which can be converted readily to either testosterone (Fig. 2.6) or estrogens (Fig. 2.7). Evidence for the occurrence of this pathway in the human corpus luteum and luteinized follicle was furnished by Zander who identified both of these steroids, and Baggett *et al.* who demonstrated the in vitro conversion of testosterone to estradiol by human ovarian slices. While studying this reaction, Longchampt *et al.* identified a steroid with an hydroxyl group at C_{19}, Δ^4, *19-hydroxyandrostene-3, 17-dione,* and it now appears proved that before the A ring can be aromatized, *i.e.,* unsaturated, it is necessary to change the methyl group at C_{19} to an hydroxyl radical (Fig. 2.7). The aromatization mechanism has not been elucidated although Morato *et al.,* in 1962, suggested several theoretical pathways.

The second pathway, the Δ^5 pathway, demonstrated by in vitro experiments with human Graafian follicles is through dehydroisoandrosterone, DHA, rather than through pregnenolone and progesterone. This pathway has become more interesting since it has become apparent that the dehydroisoandrosterone pool in the blood represents a constant source of steroid substrate.

Currently it seems that the Δ^5 pathway, directly through DHA, is probably most active in estrogen production by the theca and interstitial cells of the ovary during the proliferative stage of the cycle, while the Δ^4 pathway, through pregnenolone and progesterone, is probably the one of choice following luteinization and corpus luteum formation.

With a better understanding of the chemical reactions involved in the production of the various steroids, it is easy to understand the amount of interconversion which can and does occur. The final synthetic potential of the adrenal, ovary, or testis depends upon the amount of enzymes and cofactors present which, in turn, is probably under the control of pituitary hormones. These factors determine to what extent estrogens, androgens, progesterone, or corticoids are to be produced by the gonads and adrenal.

In addition to these sources, however, it has been shown by MacDonald and Siiteri and others that for estrogens and androgens peripheral conversion of steroid substrates occurs in the skin and appendages. The presence of subcutaneous fat has a positive influence on the efficiency of these mechanisms.

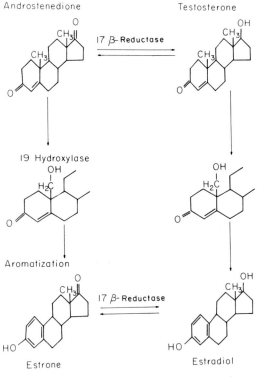

2.7. Steroid biosynthesis showing the pathway from androstenedione to estrone and estradiol. Androstenedione may be derived from either progesterone through 17α-hydroxyprogesterone or from dehydroepiandrosterone.

HORMONE CONTENT OF TISSUE AND BODY FLUIDS, METABOLISM FUNCTION AND MECHANISMS OF ACTION

Estrogens

Tissue Content and Metabolism

Estrogens have been recovered from follicular fluid, human placenta as well as urine, blood, feces, and bile of pregnant and menstruating women. Free circulating estrogens are bound to a specific protein for transport and are conjugated in the liver for excretion into the urine or feces as glucuronides or sulfates. Estradiol and estrone are the major components of Graafian follicle fluid; estriol represents the largest urinary estrogen component. Although all three major estrogens have been identified in placental extracts, estriol seems to be the predominant placental estrogen.

Definitions. Secretion rates equal the estimated contribution of a gland to the total blood hormonal concentrations. Production rates equal the total blood hormone concentration from whatever source. The metabolic clearance rate equals the volume of blood which is cleared of hormone per unit of time.

Ovary. *Follicular Fluid.* Since 1935, when MacCorquodale working in Doisy's laboratory first crystallized estradiol from follicular fluid of sow ovaries, this estrogen has been considered to be the naturally occurring ovarian hormone. Zander and his associates isolated and chemically identified estradiol and estrone from human ovaries in 1959. Estrone is found in lesser amounts and since the conversion reaction between the two hormones is apparently completely reversible, an equilibrium is probably established.

Nakayama *et al.* concluded, from experiments with perfused human ovaries, that estradiol might be the sole estrogen synthesized. Baird and Fraser have published estrone and estradiol values for peripheral blood and ovarian vein blood with simultaneous studies on follicular fluid (Table 2.1) throughout the normal menstrual cycle. From these they have calculated blood production and ovarian secretion rates (Fig. 2.8).

Table 2.1

Concentration (ng/100 ml) of estrone (E1) and estradiol (E2) in follicular fluid

Patient No.	Right Ovary		Left Ovary	
	E1	E2	E1	E2
1	—	—	2.86*	11.44*
2	2.40*	44.1*	1.04	10.19
	6.39*	130.7*	—	—
	8.95*	166.0*	—	—
	5.90	88.63	—	—
	5.37	83.12	—	—
3	—	—	4.94*	127.5*
4	—	—	1.55	7.35
5	0.33	2.23	0	0.80
6	0	1.46	0	0
7	0.42*	12.78*	—	—
8	24.4*	380.5*	—	—
9	16.5*	375.0*	—	—

*All follicles of diameter 1 cm or greater.

(Baird and Fraser: J. Clin. Endo. Metab., *38:* 1009, 1974.)

Blood. Knowledge of estrogen transportation in the blood has been handicapped, prior to immunoassay, by the extremely low amounts of physiologically active circulating estrogen. As early as 1925, Loewe and Frank independently reported estrogen activity in human blood, and Frank and Goldberger in 1926, with bioassay techniques, were able to describe the double peak found during the normal menstrual cycle.

Using a sensitive radioimmunoassay, Thorneycroft *et al.* measured estrone and estradiol in the normal menstrual cycle in relation to other steroids, as well as to pituitary FSH and LH (Fig. 2.9). The range for estradiol is between 20 and 500 pg/ml and for estrone between 50 and 400 pg/ml. Menopausal values for estradiol are below 10 pg/ml and below 30 for estrone. Male values are in the range of 15

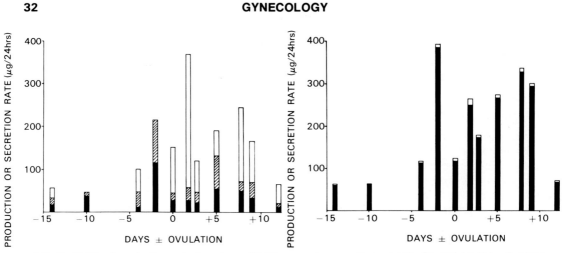

2.8. (*Left*) Blood production rate for estrone ($P_B{}^{E_1}$) or ovarian secretion rate ($S_{ov}{}^{E_1}$). (*Right*) Estradiol (E_2) throughout the normal menstrual cycle. Values have been plotted by the estimated day of ovulation (O) for each subject. Total blood production rate for each subject is indicated by the height of the bar. The amount of estrone or estradiol from each steroid is indicated by the corresponding codes:

Estrone

■ = ovarian E_1
▨ = E_1 derived from E_2
☐ = E_1 derived from other sources

Estradiol

■ = ovarian E_2
☐ = E_2 derived from E_1

(From Baird and Fraser, J. Clin. Endocrinol. Metab., *38:* 1009, 1974.)

through 25 pg/ml for estradiol and 40 through 75 for estrone.

The metabolic clearance rate of estradiol is reported by Longcope *et al.* to be 1,360 L/day for females and 1,600 L/day for males, while the clearance rate of estrone is the same for males and females, approximately 2,000 L/day.

Urine. A number of urinary metabolites of estradiol have been recovered. These are apparently conjugated as glucuronides or sulfates or double conjugates: glucuronide sulfates. Only the three classic estrogens, estradiol, estrone, and estriol, have been measured throughout the menstrual cycle. However, some idea about the relative importance of each metabolite can be obtained by the work of Gallagher and his co-workers who have measured the various fractions after administering radioactive carbon-labeled estradiol. The percentage recovery in the individual fractions is shown in Figure 2.10. The urinary estrogen curve parallels the serum levels. There is a gradual rise after menstruation, reaching a peak prior to ovulation after which a drop in the hormone levels occurs. This is followed by a

secondary rise, corresponding to maximum corpus luteum function with a fall just before menstruation. The amounts of estriol, estrone, and estradiol recoverable from the urine during the various phases of the menstrual cycle can be seen in Table 2.2.

Bile and Feces. The recovery of substantial amounts of estrogen from the

Table 2.2

Estrogen Levels Found at Various Times during Menstrual Cycle

Time in Cycle	Estrogens Excreted (μg. per 24 hr.)					
	Average			Range		
	Estriol	Estrone	Estradiol	Estriol	Estrone	Estradiol
Onset of menstruation....	6	5	2	0–15	4–7	0–3
Ovulation peak........	27	20	9	13–54	11–31	4–14
Luteal maximum........	22	14	7	8–72	10–23	4–10

From Brown, J. B.: Lancet, *1:* 320, 1955.

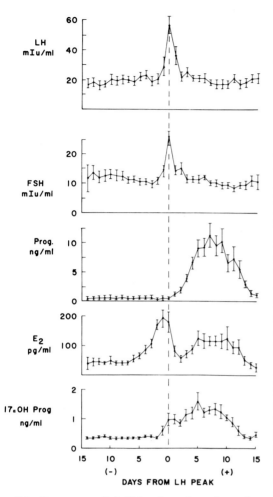

2.9. Serum estradiol (E_2) values throughout the normal menstrual cycle, related to gonadotrophin FSH and LH and progesterone values. (From Thorneycroft et al., Amer. J. Obstet. Gynec., 111: 947, 1971.)

feces has been reported following estrogen administration. Siebke and Schuschania reported equal amounts of estrogen in the feces and the urine of normally menstruating women. Dohrn and Faure report high estrogen titers in the feces of pregnant women. Autopsy findings indicate that the liver of pregnant women is high in estrogen content and Cantarow et al. report that the bile content is 3 times that of the blood in human term pregnancy. These combined experimental observations suggest an enterohepatic estrogen circulation. A consideration of the enterohepatic circulation is of importance in determining the biologic effect of administered estrogenic drugs. Either the mode of administration or the chemical configuration of the drug can change its circulation time and the access of liver cells to the steroid.

Contribution of Androgenic Steroids to Estrogen Milieu. Testosterone is secreted presumably by the hilus cells of the ovary. Abraham has confirmed a midcycle peak and slightly higher values in the luteal phase as compared to the follicular phase (Fig. 2.11). The range for normal menstruating females is between 20 and 50 μg/ml. The ovarian contribution to the peripheral testosterone value is estimated at 33% during the follicular and luteal phases and 60% at the mid-cycle. The remainder is due to adrenal function. Testosterone contributes relatively little to the E_2 blood production rate.

Androstenedione, ADD, is the steroid preferentially secreted by the ovarian stromal cells, according to Rice et al. Ovarian vein studies of Lloyd et al. indicate it is the major androgen secreted by the ovary, and Abraham has confirmed this. The range for normal menstruating females is between 100 and 220 μg/ml. An appreciable amount of ADD is also secreted by the adrenal but, under normal conditions, the contribution of the ovary makes up as much as 70% of peripheral ADD at mid-cycle (Table 2.3). ADD is an important steroid, as it is a precursor for estrone. In the menopause little or no estrogen is secreted by the ovary. All of the serum estrone is derived by peripheral conversion of ADD which at this time of life is thought to come mainly from the adrenal.

ADD can also be aromatized to estrogen by cells of the anterior, but not posterior, hypothalamus furnishing the ovary with a differential feedback control mechanism of the cyclic and tonic centers.

Summary. In summary, the theca cells of the ovary apparently produce estradiol which is immediately in equilibrium with estrone. It is transported in the

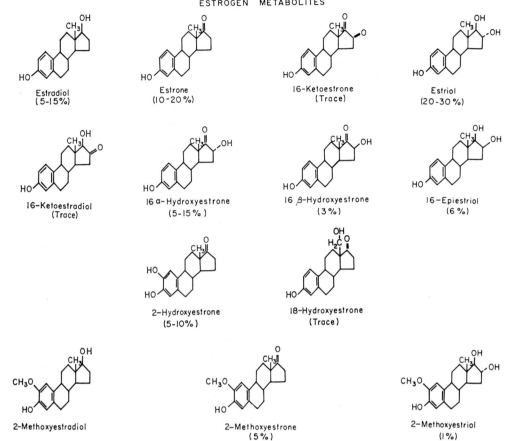

ESTROGEN METABOLITES

2.10. Human urinary metabolites of estrogen with the estimated total urinary radioactivity found on recovery experiments. (Compiled with the assistance of F. Gallagher.)

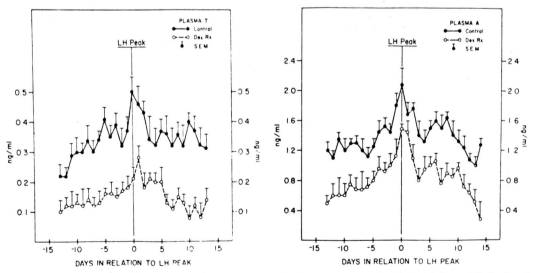

2.11. Patterns and levels (mean + SEM) of serum testosterone (*T*) and androstenedione (*A*) during 2 consecutive menstrual cycles in 6 premenopausal women. The first cycle served as control and the adrenal cortex was suppressed with dexamethasone (*Dex Rx*) during the second cycle.

Table 2.3

Ovarian and adrenal contribution to peripheral androgens (ng/ml)

Steroid	Ovarian contribution			Adrenal contribution
	F	M	L	
T	0.1 (33%)	0.3 (60%)	0.1 (33%)	0.2 (40-66%)
DHT*		0.1 (50%)		0.1 (50%)
A	0.5 (45%)	1.5 (70%)	0.8 (60%)	0.6 (30-55%)
DHEA*		0.8 (20%)		3.2 (80%)
DHEA-S	80 (4%)	200 (10%)	80 (4%)	2000 (90-96%)

( ) = percent contribution calculated by comparing control cycles with a cycle in which the adrenal cortex was suppressed by dexamethasone.

* = ovarian contribution not influenced by phase of menstrual cycle.

F = early follicular; M=midcycle; and L=late luteal phase.

T = testosterone, A=androstenedione,

DHT = dihydrostestosterone, DHEA=dehydroepiandrosterone, DHEAS=dehydroepiandrosterone sulfate.

blood by a specific estrogen binding protein. The liver is the site of conjugation and conversion of estradiol and estrone to estriol glucuronide through 16-ketoestrone. This conjugated steroid is the major metabolite excreted in the urine. Substantial amounts of estrone are excreted in the bile and feces as estrone sulfate, or estrone glucuronide sulfate.

Androstenedione, which is the major steroid secreted by ovarian interstitial cells, is the steroid precursor for estrone by peripherial conversion. Estrone constitutes the major estrogen in menopausal women.

Functions

Estrogen is commonly regarded as the "female sex hormone" and perhaps rightly so as it is indeed responsible for many of the typical female characteristics: fat deposition, breast growth and development, and the external female genitalia. It also has a selective growth ef-

fect upon all tissues derived from the Müllerian ducts. It does, however, have a rather widespread effect on general physiology, controlling blood proteins and lipids, and exerting some influence on the supportive tissues, the vascular and skeletal systems specifically. Different tissues show different sensitivity to similar "estrogen" doses. Therefore, it is important to define a dose response in terms of a specific tissue.

Uterus. Under estrogen stimulation the cervix becomes patulous, the os open, and the mucus abundant, acellular, fluid, with ferns of crystallization and capable of supporting sperm motility. There is a marked increase in the size of the uterus which comprises both the endometrium and the uterine musculature. This growth effect is associated with an increase in the blood supply of the affected tissues. The rhythmic muscular contractility of the uterine musculature reaches its peak under estrogen dominance.

Fallopian Tubes. The motility of the fallopian tubes is also under the control of estrogen, the greatest activity being in the estrogen dominant phase.

Vagina. The cornification of the vagina described many years ago by Stockard and Papanicolaou is so characteristic of estrogenic activity that it has been used to define an estrogen. These changes are described in Chapter 36, "Clinical Cytology."

Breasts. The growth of the duct system of the breast is stimulated by estrogen. The nipple erectility and pigmentation of the areolae are also estrogen dependent.

Ovary. There is evidence that estrogen *per se* is necessary for the normal development of the ovaries. The development of primordial follicles with progress through the antrum stage is facilitated by estrogen, and Greep and Jones have demonstrated that estrogen aids in the deposition of cholesterol in the interstitial cells and theca interna of the rat ovary.

Pituitary. The ability of estrogen to suppress the secretion of pituitary gonadotrophins, FSH and LH, has long been recognized. However, the locus of action at the pituitary level *per se* has been clouded by the finding that estrogen also decreases the secretion of hypothalamic gonadotrophic hormones. The presence of specific estrogen receptor proteins in the cytosol of pituitary cells as well as the suppression of the LH response to LRH, when estrogen is given, indicate that there is probably an action of estrogen at the pituitary level *per se* and perhaps on the pituitary cell membranes (Fig. 2.12). Both pituitary and plasma LH were decreased in the rat by acute experiments with high dosage estrogen (Kulkarni *et al.*).

The most striking effect of estrogen on

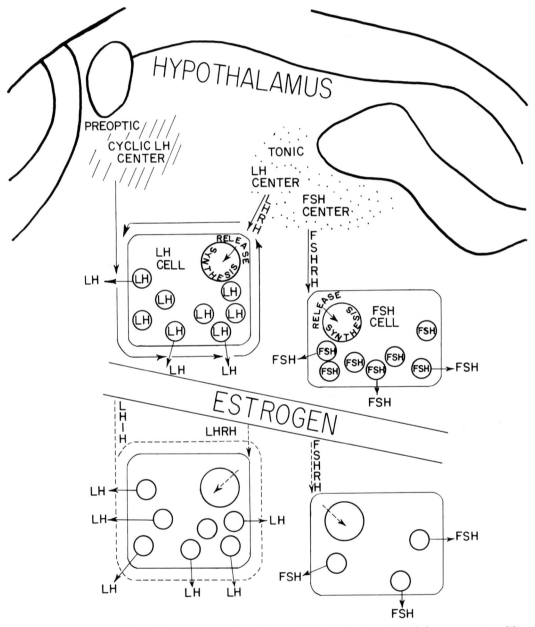

2.12. Effect of hypothalamic hormones on the pituitary LH cell. Explanation of the apparent positive estrogen feedback on the anterior cyclic-LH center by assuming that these cells are producing an inhibitory LH-releasing hormone (LH-IH). Estrogen can then be assumed to have an inhibitory effect in both anterior and posterior hypothalamic centers. (From S. Aksel and G. E. S. Jones, Obstet. Gynec., *44:* 1, 1974.)

the pituitary, however, is seen in the lactotropic cells. Although Greep and Jones found no significant change in prolactin production after estrogen administration, it has recently been shown that prolactin production is enhanced by estrogen. This accounts for the increased size of the pituitary gland during pregnancy and also during the administration of oral contraceptive drugs containing estrogenic activity. Assay of somatotropin, pituitary growth hormone (Merimee *et al.*) indicates that estrogen stimulation enhances the pituitary response of this hormone to any inciting stimulation; again, however, the effect may be mediated through the hypothalamus.

Hypothalamus. The estrogen effect on pituitary gonadotrophin secretion, although initially thought to be a direct one, was later ascribed by neurophysiologists to the hypothalamus. The characteristic effect is a suppression of both FSH and LH presumably due to suppression of GnRH in the posterior tonic release center. FSH is most sensitive to estrogen suppression in the human, if not the rat. LH suppression requires a longer estrogen administration. This is the long-loop negative feedback. If estrogen is given acutely in high dosage or chronically at intermediate levels, a "so-called" positive feedback or stimulation of LH occurs. This effect is thought to be mediated by the anterior hypothalamic cyclic-LH center, as it is abolished by destruction of these cells or interruption of axons between the suprachiasmatic area and the median eminence. It is probably via the hypothalamus rather than pituitary, because no acute stimulation effect of estrogen on LH release occurs after an LRH infusion. As discussed elsewhere the "positive" feedback could be the result of a negative feedback of an inhibition, *e.g.*, an inhibition of an inhibition.

Thyroid. The clinical observation that women are more prone to hyperthyroidism and myxedema than men and that these conditions often have their onset at puberty, in pregnancy, or at the menopause has fostered the belief among gynecologists and obstetricians that there is a close relationship between thyroid and ovarian function. The recently discovered fact that thyrotropic stimulating hormone (TSH) has a limited cross-reactivity, both immunologically and biologically, with LH may help to explain some of these apparent relationships (Fig. 2.13). The LH-like action of TSH is seen only when excessively high values of TSH are present. This cross-reactivity may explain the hyperestrogenism which is occasionally associated with thyroid pathology. If in addition to an elevated pituitary TSH, there is also an elevated TRH, prolactin production with lactation may occur due to the prolactin stimulating effect of TRH (see Chapter 30). Estrogens also cause an increase in the serum thyroxin binding protein, thus increasing the amount of bound thyroxin circulating. The bound hormone, however, is inactive and, therefore, this mechanism has little significance in abnormal physiologic states.

Adrenal. Estrogen increases the cortisol binding protein, transcortin, and, therefore, causes an increased circulation of bound cortisol. Experimental work indicates that estrogen can block cortisol synthesis in the adrenal.

Pancreas. Houssay, a number of years ago, reported a marked improvement in experimental diabetes in the rat after estrogen administration. Funk *et al.* found that estrogen enhanced the production of insulin probably through a pituitary pathway. However, Barnes and his associates demonstrated that estrogen will check glycosuria in a pancreatectomized dog or monkey indicating that the effect may be through the liver rather than an increased insulin output.

Thymus. Atrophy of the thymus following estrogen administration has been described by Selye.

General Systemic Effects. *Skeletal Growth.* Estrogen has a marked effect on skeletal growth, estrogen stimulation being associated with epiphysial closure at puberty and estrogen deprivation with osteoporosis. In an article on the pathogenesis of osteoporosis, Nordin concludes that the sensitivity of the bone to parathyroid hormone seems to be

ALIGNMENT OF THE CHAINS OF THE TSH AND LH TO SHOW MAXIMUM HOMOLOGY

a (TSH and LH) NH_2-Phe-Pro-Asp-Gly-Glu-Phe-Thr-Met-[8]

TSH-β NH_2-Phe-Cys-Ile-Pro-Thr-Glu-Tyr-Met-Met-His-Val-Glu-Arg-[13]

LH-β   Acyl-Ser-Arg-Gly-Pro-Leu-Arg-Pro-Leu-Cys-Gln-Pro-Ile-Asn-Ala-Thr-Leu-Ala-Ala-Glu-Lys-[20]   (CHO)

a   Gln-Gly-Cys-Pro-Glx-Cys-Lys-Leu-Lys-Glu-Asn-Lys-Tyr-Phe-Ser-Lys-Pro-Asx-Ala-Pro-[28]

TSH-β   Lys-Glu-Cys-Ala-Tyr-Cys-   Leu-Thr-Ile-Asn-[23] (CHO)

LH-β   Glu-Ala-Cys-Pro-Val-Cys-   Ile-Thr-Phe-Thr-[30]

a   Ile-Tyr-Gln-Cys-Met-Gly-Cys-Cys-Phe-Ser-Arg-Ala-Tyr-Pro-Thr-Pro-Ala-Arg-Ser-Lys-[48]

TSH-β   Thr-Thr-Val-Cys-Ala-Gly-Tyr-Cys-Met-Thr-Arg-Asx-Val-Asx-Gly-Lys-Leu-Phe-Leu-Pro-[43]

LH-β   Thr-Ser-Ile-Cys-Ala-Gly-Tyr-Cys-Pro-Ser-Met-Lys-Arg-Val-Leu-Pro-Val-Ile-Leu-Pro-[50]

a   Lys-Thr-Met-Leu-   (CHO sα) Val-Pro-Lys-Asn-Ile-Thr-Ser-Glx-Ala-Thr-Cys-Cys-Val-Ala-Lys-[67]

TSH-β   Lys-Tyr-Ala-Leu-Ser-Gln-Asp-Val-Cys-Thr-Tyr-Arg-Asp-Phe-Met-Tyr-Lys-Thr-Ala-Glu-[63]

LH-β   Pro-   Met-Pro-   Gln-Arg-Val-Cys-Thr-Tyr-His-Glu-Leu-Arg-Phe-Ala-Ser-Val-Arg-[68]

a   Ala-The-Thr-   Lys-Ala-Thr-Val-Met-Gly-Asn-Val-Arg-Val-Glx-Asn-His-Thr-Glx-Cys-[86] (CHO sβ)

TSH-β   Ile-Pro-Gly-Cys-Pro-Arg-His-Val-Thr-Pro-Tyr-Phe-Ser-Tyr-Pro-Val-Ala-Ile-Ser-Cys-[83]

LH-β   Leu-Pro-Gly-Cys-Pro-Pro-Gly-Val-Asp-Pro-Met-Val-Ser-Phe-Pro-Val-Ala-Leu-Ser-Cys-[88]

a   His-Cys-Ser-Thr-Cys-Tyr-Tyr-His-Lys-Ser-COOH[96]

TSH-β   Lys-Cys-Gly-Lys-Cys-Asx-Thr-Asx-Tyr-Ser-Asx-Cys-Ile-His-Glu-Ala-Ile-Lys-Thr-Asn-[103]

LH-β   His-Cys-Gly-Pro-Cys-Arg-Leu-Ser-Ser-Thr-Asp-Cys-Gly-Pro-Gly-Arg-Thr-Glx-Pro-Leu-[108]

TSH-β   Tyr-Cys-Thr-Lys-Pro-Gln-Lys-Ser-Tyr-Met-COOH[113]

LH-β   Ala-Cys-Asx-His-Pro-Pro-Leu-Pro-Asp-Ile-Leu-COOH[119]

2.13. Pituitary LH and TSH contain many similar configurations. This chemical similarity is indicated by underlines. (From R. H. Williams (editor), *Textbook of Endocrinology,* p. 41, W. B. Saunders Co., Philadelphia, 1974, from data supplied by J. G. Pierce and D. N. Ward.)

increased in the absence of estrogen. This results in increased bone resorption and hypercalcemia. Thus the effect of estrogen to increase bone density may be mediated through an inhibiting effect of parathormone (Herrmann *et al.*).

Proteins. Estrogen augments the amount of many specific blood proteins; the thyroxin-binding globulin, transcortin, angiotensin, aldosterone-binding protein, coagulation Factor IX and plasma fibrinogen among those studied.

Vascular. The effect on lipid metabolism and the circulatory system has been of interest in relation to the possible role estrogens may play in protecting against arteriosclerotic cardiovascular disease. In man as well as in some experimental animals, estrogens lower the cholesterol to phospholipid ratio. In the rat they have been shown to enhance the respiration of the aorta and to decrease experimentally produced atherosclerosis in the cardiac but not thoracic arteries. Davis *et al.* have experimental evidence that estrogen decreases the incidence of coronary atherosclerosis and hypertension in the menopausal woman.

Hematology. Although there is a great deal in the literature concerning the effect of estrogens on the hematopoietic system, very little of a positive nature has been found in the human. Witten and Bradbury in 1951 reported a definite increase in blood volume but no change in actual red blood cell count after estrogen administration. This experimental hemodilution effect seemed to mimic that found in pregnancy. The authors speculate that the extravascular fluid as well as the intravascular fluid might be increased under estrogen domination. Such a finding might account for preovulatory and premenstrual edema.

Skin Appendages. Estrogens oppose the effect of androgens on sebaceous glands and hair follicles in the sexual regions.

Mechanisms of Action

The current theory for the intracellular mechanism of estrogenic action is that of gene activation. Estrogen target cells contain specific loci, receptor proteins, which bind estrogens. These proteins have a sedimentation rate of approximately 8S. As the hormone is bound, the protein splits to form a hormone complex and a 4S (S = Svedberg unit) protein. The hormone receptor complex must then be activated in order for it to move into the nucleus where it combines with an acceptor protein. This nuclear receptor protein is not hormone specific. It will accept other molecules such as insulin, glucagon and aminopeptides. Once in the nucleus, the hormone acceptor complex can act as a gene derepressor by combining with a repressor protein on the surface of the gene; it removes the repression and allows gene activation. This results in replication of RNA polymerase, which in turn increases ribosomal RNA and transfer RNA, thus setting into motion all of the necessary reactions for the synthesis of proteins (enzymes) which are characteristic of the target cell response to estrogen (Fig. 2.14).

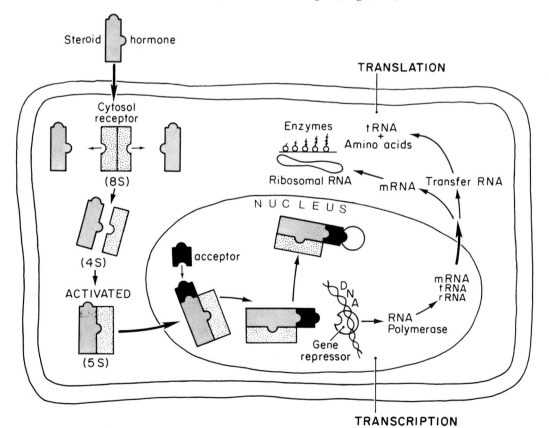

2.14. Intracellular mechanisms of action of estrogen by gene activation

Progesterone

Tissue Content and Metabolism

Progesterone has been isolated from ovarian tissue, placental tissue, adrenal, and testis.

Ovary: Corpus Luteum. In 1948, Hoffmann and Van Lam assayed human corpora lutea of different ages and found a measurable amount of progesterone on the first ovulatory day. This increased to a maximum by the 16th cycle day and remained elevated until the 24th cycle day. Appreciable amounts of progesterone were, however, still present at the onset of menstruation and traces were detectable in the corpora of the previous cycle. Zander, studying the corpus luteum of pregnancy, identified two additional pregestational steroids (Table 2.4). However, there is some question as to the physiological activity of these compounds in the human. The 20 β-ol steroid is said to be inactive and the activity of the α compound may depend upon the ability of the body to convert it to progesterone. Thus, although there are many naturally occurring steroids which are estrogenic to some degree, there seems to be only one naturally occurring steroid which has appreciable progestational activity.

Blood. Progesterone is transported in the blood as are other steroids by a specific binding protein. Radioimmunoassay or a competitive protein binding method, adapted from the Murphy technique, indicates a low baseline serum progesterone level in the follicular phase of the menstrual cycle

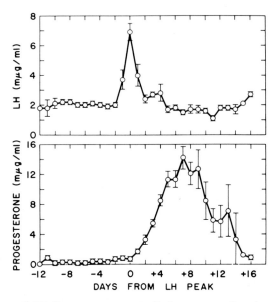

2.15. Serum progesterone during menstrual cycle. (From Neill, *et al.*: *J. Clin. Endocr., 27:* 1167, 1967.)

compatible with adrenal function. Just prior to ovulation, a slight increase can be detected, apparently due to luteinization of the granulosa cells of the preovulatory follicle. Following ovulation, there is a gradual rise to a plateau between days 19 and 21 and a rather sharper decline to baseline values again at the time of menstruation (Fig. 2.15). The value of approximately 0.5 ng/ml in males and menopausal women is the same as that in the follicular phase of the cycle and represents the adrenal component.

The metabolic clearance rate of progesterone in males and ovariectomized females, according to Little *et al.*, is 2,100 L/day. The rapid removal of progesterone from the blood and its equally rapid conversion to a biologically inactive steroid must be obviated for effective administration of this hormone. This has been accomplished by frequent intramuscular administration, vaginal absorption or chemical changes in the molecule which protect it from metabolism.

Urine. In 1937, Venning and Browne presented evidence that sodium pregnanediol glucuronide was the metabolic product of progesterone and published their result on the urinary ex-

Table 2.4

Progestational Compounds Isolated from Human Corpora Lutea

Progesterone = Δ^4-3-ketopregnene-20α-one[a]

$\frac{1}{2}$–$\frac{1}{3}$ activity of Progesterone
= Δ^4-3-ketopregnene-20α-ol[b]

$\frac{1}{5}$–$\frac{1}{10}$ activity of Progesterone
= Δ^4-3-ketopregnene-20β-ol[b]

[a] Isolated by Corner and Allen, 1929, and identified by Butenandt and Schmidt, 1934.

[b] Isolated by Zander, Forbes, Von Munstermann, and Neher, 1958.

cretion throughout the menstrual cycle. Before ovulation, between 0.2 and 1 mg of pregnanediol per 24 hours can be excreted. This amount presumably represents the contribution from the adrenal gland. After ovulation, the excretion rapidly rises to between 3 and 6 mg per 24 hours at the peak of the luteal phase and falls again before menstruation. When measured as free pregnanediol, this metabolite represents approximately 20% of injected progesterone. Although other metabolic products of progesterone have been isolated from human urine (Fig. 2.16), only one, pregnanolone, is of any importance.

Bile and Feces. Sodium pregnanediol glucuronide has been identified in the blood and has also been isolated from bile. However, in the feces pregnanediol is found in the free form, indicating that hydrolysis occurs in the gut.

Summary. In summary, progesterone is probably the only naturally occurring progestational agent of any significance. Small amounts may be synthesized by the cells of the follicle in the preovulatory swelling phase; however, the major production is by the corpus luteum cells of the ovary during the luteal phase of the cycle. It is constantly produced in small amounts by the adrenal gland and by the testis in the male. In the adrenal and the testis, it probably serves as the precursor for corticoids and androgens. It is transported in the blood by a specific binding protein and metabolized and conjugated in the liver into sodium pregnanediol glucuronide which also circulates in the blood. Approximately 20% is excreted in the urine as sodium pregnanediol glucuronide; pregnanolone represents a minor metabolic product. The pregnanediol which is excreted in the bile is enzymically hydrolyzed by the gut so that the pregnanediol recovered in the feces is in the free form.

Functions

The major functions of progesterone are the preparation of the endometrium for implantation and the maintenance of pregnancy. Its effects, therefore, are almost entirely confined to the uterus, unlike estrogen which has such widespread physiological actions. A peculiarity of progesterone activity is that usually an initial estrogenic stimulation is required before the progestational stimulation if an effect is to be attained. This estrogen dependence may be due to the necessity for estrogen in order to induce the specific progesterone receptor protein.

Uterus. The cervical os is contracted, the mucus is scanty and thick. The endometrium shows the progestational changes classically described by Hitschmann and Adler and elaborated upon by Noyes *et al.* The normal menstrual flow occurs from such a progestational endometrium. The amount of progesterone necessary to produce these typical endometrial changes is influenced by the previous estrogenic stimulation as well as by the duration and the continuity of the progesterone dosage.

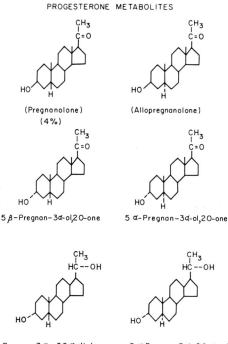

PROGESTERONE METABOLITES

(Pregnanolone) (4%)

(Allopregnanolone)

5 β-Pregnan-3α-ol,20-one

5 α-Pregnan-3α-ol,20-one

5 β-Pregnan-3α, 20α-diol (Pregnanediol) (15-20%)

5 α-Pregnan-3α,20α-diol Allopregnanediol (0.6%)

2.16. The metabolic products of progesterone isolated from human urine.

In addition to deposition of glycogen in the endometrium under the influence of progesterone, the carbonic anhydrase is increased. Böving believes that it is this enzyme which, in conjunction with the carbonate from the blastocyst, disrupts the epithelial cement substance allowing the trophoblast to implant. A protein, blastokinin, specifically induced by progesterone without previous estrogen stimulation, has been described in the rabbit uterus and tentatively identified in the human. This protein seems to be one of the first manifestations of progesterone stimulation. It is apparently necessary for normal implantation of the rabbit blastocyst. If induction of this same type of protein can be substantiated in the human, this may well be the most important action of progesterone. The uterine musculature under the influence of progesterone becomes quiescent, thus allowing for the continued growth and development of the implanted trophoblast.

Fallopian Tubes. Like the uterine musculature the fallopian tubes show a decreased motility under progesterone dominance.

Breasts. The development of acinar buds from the breast milk ducts is stimulated by progesterone administration.

Vagina. The vaginal epithelium following progesterone stimulation shows an increased number of precornified cells, mucus shreds and aggregates of cells (see Chapter 36).

Pituitary and Hypothalamus. As previously stated, the effects of steroids on the pituitary function are at least partially mediated through the hypothalamus. Many of the synthetic progestational compounds used in oral contraception apparently have a marked suppressive effect upon the cyclic pituitary secretion of LH, the LH surge. Progesterone *per se,* however, has very little gonadotrophic suppression activity. McCann concluded that progesterone exerts only a feeble inhibitory effect on the secretion of LH, unless it is preceded by estrogen stimulation. Wallach *et al.* have also shown by LRH stimulation studies that estrogen is essential for the suppressive action of at least some progestational drugs. Stimulation of LH by progesterone is apparently not physiologic in the human.

General Systemic Effect. *Thermogenetic Effect.* The ability of progesterone to induce a rise in the basal body temperature is conveniently used as an index of ovulation in the human. This effect is apparently mediated through the central nervous system.

Anesthetic Action. Selye noted that progesterone, given in massive doses, caused an anesthetic-like reaction in rats. Rothchild and Rapport confirmed this effect in the human using intravenous progesterone in a therapeutic trial for patients with hopeless endometrial carcinoma.

Mechanisms of Action

Progesterone has been shown in experiments by O'Malley and Means to exert its action in exactly the same way that estrogen does. One specific progesterone induced protein is blastokinin. This can be synthesized by endometrial cells in response to progesterone stimulation, even in an absence of prior estrogen exposure. Another interesting intracellular metabolic effect has been shown by Wade and Jones. The resynthesis of high energy phosphate in the electron transport chain is blocked by progesterone. In the process the hormone is metabolized. The experiments indicated that one locus of the steroid inhibition, and perhaps metabolism, is between reduced diphosphopyridine nucleotide (DPNH) and cytochrome *c* in the electron transport chain. This effect would lead to energy storage rather than energy utilization and account for many of the known properties of progesterone such as the accumulation of glycogen in the endometrial cells, the inhibition of muscle contractility, and the anesthetic action which occurs when massive dosage of progesterone is given.

Gonadotrophic Hormones

Chemistry

The three pituitary hormones which are glycoproteins, follicle-stimulating hormone (FSH), luteinizing hormone (LH) and thyrotrophic hormone (TSH), as well as the placental hormone, human chorionic gonadotrophin (HCG), are water-soluble, heat-labile and orally inactive. They are composed of three basic units, an α and β peptide chain which are non-covalently bonded, both of which have a carbohydrate moiety with sialic acid. Biologic activity is dependent upon the presence of the two protein chains. However, the specificity of biologic activity is determined by the β subunit. The α subunit is interchangeable among the four hormones. There is some evidence to indicate that the units are synthesized by the pituitary independently and secondarily combined. This might explain the extremely infrequent occurrence of gonadotrophinor thyrotropin-secreting pituitary tumors and the hormonally inert chromophobe adenoma. The sialic acid moiety protects the molecule from metabolic destruction by the liver, thus increasing the circulation time and enhancing biologic activity.

Some pituitary hormones, somatotrophin and prolactin, are species specific. However, the gonadotrophins are not. Although certain animal preparations are physiologically active in the human, their antigenicity makes them unsuitable for therapeutic agents.

Tissue Content and Metabolism

The pituitary gonadotrophins, follicle-stimulating hormone, and luteinizing hormone have been isolated from human pituitaries, serum and urine. Prolactin, perhaps to be regarded in the human as an antigonadotrophin, has also been isolated from these sources.

Pituitary. FSH and LH are produced by a small basophilic type of cell (β type) in the anterior pituitary. Hellbaum *et al.*, using special stains described by Remels, have correlated a purple staining cell with FSH production and storage, and a red staining cell with LH. Both types of cells are located in the angles adjacent to the pars intermedia as well as in clumps in the central zone. Midgley has identified the LH-producing cells by immunofluorescence, and believes that there is

good evidence for the conclusion that LH and FSH are distinct hormones stored and synthesized in different cells. These must be differentiated from a rather similar type of β cell which apparently produces thyrotrophic hormone. Recent investigations have indicated that the α and β subunits of these glycoprotein pituitary hormones are made in separate cells and combined at different sites.

Emmart *et al.* demonstrated the localization of prolactin in the pituitary cells of rats and cats by using a fluorescent antibody technique. The findings are confirmatory of earlier works by Pearse and Severinghaus which indicate it is formed in the acidophilic or α cell.

Currie and Dekanski assayed human pituitaries for gonadotrophic and prolactin activity and found increasing amounts of both LH and FSH with age, confirming the earlier work of Severinghaus. The pituitary of menstruating women contains approximately 700 I.U. of LH and 200 I.U. of FSH. After the menopause, the LH is 1,700 I.U. and the FSH approximately 450 I.U. As the LH production rate in menopausal women has been calculated as between 3 and 4,000 I.U./day, the turnover rate of stored gonadotrophins is between 12 and 24 hours. No detectable gonadotrophin is found in the pituitary during pregnancy. The prolactin content, however, is increased, perhaps accounting for the increased pituitary size in pregnancy.

Blood. Serum gonadotrophin levels are elevated in infancy. FSH values in female infants tend to be higher than LH values falling to the lowest level at about 2 years. A gradual secondary rise then begins at about the age of 5 years and continues until adult levels are reached. The rise in LH values occurs approximately 2 years prior to puberty, at about 8 years but the change is not really significant until the menarche at approximately the age of 12 years. Rhythmic, cyclic FSH patterns and an elevation during sleep are characteristic of the pubertal gonadotrophic function. Just prior to the menarche, an LH pulse is seen during sleep. Following the menarche, no further sleep elevations are seen, and the cyclic changes associated with ovulation are manifest, the cyclic LH surge being the most dramatic.

In cyclic women, the FSH shows a rise in the first part of the follicular phase which begins prior to menses at approximately day 25 or 26 of a 28-day cycle and declines after day 7, reaching a nadir just prior to the ovulatory LH surge at day 13. With this surge, there is an associated but lesser FSH surge, the importance of which is not well documented (Fig. 2.17). It is possibly related to the response of FSH, as well as LH, to the hypothalamic LRH stimulation and may have no physiologic significance.

In the perimenopause, as the numbers of oocytes and follicles in the ovary decrease, the FSH begins to rise. When the follicular estrogen values fall associated with failing ovulatory function, LH rises, and both gonadotrophin levels remain elevated during the rest of the individual's life span. Thus, it is the change in FSH pattern which first signals a change in ovarian function at both extremes of menstrual life, the menarche and the menopause.

As LH is secreted or released in a pulsatile manner, frequent sampling is necessary to assure a proper baseline value. The cause of this periodicity has not been explained. The half-life of both FSH and LH is estimated to be between 30 and 60 min. The metabolic clearance rate of LH is calculated to be about 25 ml/min.

Urine. Fractionation of the gonadotrophin into LH and FSH activity during a normal menstrual cycle indicates that the urinary pattern closely approximates that in serum. There is a single sharp peak for LH just before ovulation with low values throughout the remainder of the cycle whereas FSH values tend to be higher immediately prior, during, and after menstruation. Total gonadotrophins are elevated postmenopausally or in the castrate woman and tend to remain so for the duration of life. Christiansen's work indicates that although FSH rises slightly with age in the male, there is no significant rise in the LH.

The renal clearance of LH is estimated at 7 ml/min. Although approximately 35% of administered FSH can be recovered in the urine, only 5% of LH is detectable.

Function

The purification of the pituitary hormones allowed the group at the Squibb Institute, Chow *et al.,* to define the biological activities in rats quite precisely.

Follicle-stimulating Hormone. Follicle-stimulating hormone (FSH) in the female rat will cause growth of the Graafian follicles past the antrum stage but no estrogen secretion. In the male rat it causes testicular tubular development and maturation of spermatozoa but no androgen secretion. In women the initial FSH stimulation of the developing

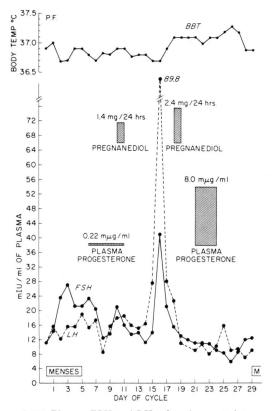

2.17. Plasma FSH and LH values in an ovulatory cycle of a normal fertile woman in relation to clinical parameters of the basal body temperature (BBT), urinary pregnanediol excretion and plasma progesterone. (From Cargille, C. M., Ross, G. T., and Yoshimi, T.: J. Clin. Endoc., *29:* 13, 1969.)

Graafian follicle must be adequate to insure normal luteal span and function. It has been suggested by Channing that FSH may be responsible for the induction of LH receptor protein.

Luteinizing Hormone (LH) or Interstitial Cell-stimulating Hormone (ICSH). In the female rat, LH causes stimulation of ovarian interstitial cells and, in conjunction with FSH, estrogen secretion. It appears that, at least in the rat, neither pituitary hormone alone is able to initiate estrogen secretion. In the male, however, LH causes testicular interstitial cell stimulation and androgen secretion. Everett has indicated by histochemical studies that LH is also responsible for the accumulation in the corpus luteum of a progesterone precursor substance, presumably cholesterol. It is apparently the LH surge, following an adequate FSH stimulation, which is the trigger mechanism for luteinization of the granulosa at ovulation. The normalcy of corpus luteum function is also conditioned by the adequacy of the cyclic-LH stimulation and luteal function is maintained by a minimum LH stimulation.

Mechanism of Action

The pituitary gonadotrophins, FSH and LH, are protein hormones and exert their biologic effect by interacting with cyclic AMP, the so-called second messenger. These hormones have their receptor proteins on the outer cell membrane and never enter the cytoplasm. The hormone protein complex on the outer membrane reacts with adenylcyclase, an enzyme on the inner cell membrane which in turn catalyzes the conversion of adenosine triphosphate, ATP, to cyclic adenosine monophosphate, cAMP. cAMP, by activation of protein kinase, is then able to phosphorylate all enzymes necessary to induce the reponses characteristic of the hormones. The release of calcium ions in the first step of conversion of ATP to cAMP is possibly a key reaction, as the free calcium ions increase cell membrane permeability and therefore allow access to the cell of extracellular elements necessary to generate the energy for protein synthesis. Calcium ions may also provide a mechanism for intracellular feedback which blocks the synthesis of cAMP. An additional intracellular control mechanism is the enzyme diphosphodiesterase which likewise inhibits the synthesis of cAMP (Fig. 2.18).

Hypothalamic Hormones

Chemistry of Luteinizing Release Hormone (LRH, LH-RH or GnRH)

Two hypothalamic hormones have been purified and synthesized. LRH, the luteinizing-release hormone, sometimes referred to as GnRH, gonadotrophic releasing hormone, because both LH and FSH release are stimulated, is a decapeptide with the formula as illustrated (Fig. 2.19). TRH, thyrotropic release hormone, which has also been purified and synthesized, is a tripeptide. Both are species non-specific and physiologically active by any mode of administration.

Tissue Content

Both biological and immunological assays have been developed for LRH. Nevertheless, the sensitivity is such that the exact measurements in human serum are still in doubt. Reichert and Ward believe that LRH is secreted in an episodic pattern inversely related to LH episodic secretion. Schalley *et al.* think their assay shows an elevated LRH at mid-cycle in the normal menstrual cycle, accounting for the mid-cycle LH surge. Ramirez and Sawyer have reported an increase in LRH content of the medial basal hypothalamus during proestrus in the rat.

Function

LRH is associated with a stimulation of both LH and FSH, albeit FSH is stimulated less consistently and to a lesser degree. The best evidence is that LRH stimulates both synthesis and release of pituitary gonadotrophins. Johansson *et al.* have reported the isolation of an FSH-RH which also stimulates both FSH and LH, but in a reverse ratio to LRH. This finding has not been confirmed.

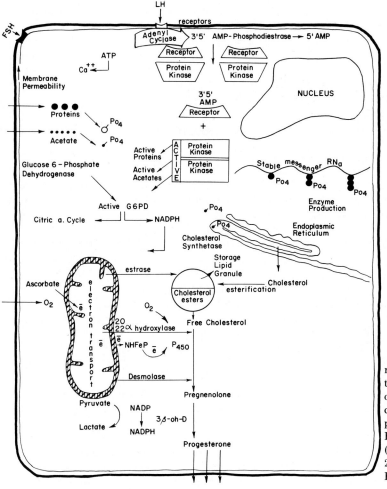

2.18. Intracellular mechanism of action of protein hormones by activation of "the second messenger" cyclic adenosine monophosphate, cAMP. (From S. J. Behrman and R. W. Kistner (eds.), *Progress in Infertility,* 2nd Ed., Little Brown & Co., Boston, 1975.)

Mechanisms of Action

The mode of action of the hypothalamic hormones which are polypeptides is probably quite similar to that of the pituitary gonadotrophins. The intranuclear action of these protein and polypeptide hormones, however, is unclear but, as both categories of hormones can cause cellular hyperplasia as well as intracellular synthesis, an intranuclear action must exist.

Vascular Phenomena of Menstruation

Menstruation is in the last analysis a vascular phenomenon; it has been shown that two groups of blood vessels supply the endometrium: (1) the straight arteries and (2) the coiled arteries. The straight

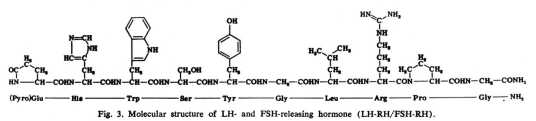

Fig. 3. Molecular structure of LH- and FSH-releasing hormone (LH-RH/FSH-RH).

2.19. Hypothalamic luteotrophic releasing hormone is a decapeptide. (From A. V. Schally *et al.*, Science, *179:* 341, 1973.)

vessels undergo no fundamental change during menstruation, supplying the basal third or so of the endometrium (See Fig. 3.14).

Much more important are the coiled arterioles, which alone supply blood to the superficial third and most of the middle third of the endometrium. As endometrial growth advances, the arteries become more and more coiled because their length increases more rapidly than the endometrium thickens. This increased coiling is accentuated by a regression in endometrial growth beginning some days before the onset of menstrual bleeding, and leading to a stasis, with or without vasodilatation. For these observations we are indebted to Markee, who observed that following this phase of slowed circulation, there occurs an intense vasoconstriction, beginning 4 to 24 hours before the onset of any bleeding. As a matter of fact, throughout the earlier part of the cycle the endometrium exhibits a rhythmic alternating vasoconstriction and vasodilatation, each phase of which lasts from 60 to 90 seconds.

The actual bleeding of menstruation occurs from one of the branches of a coiled artery which has been constricted for a number of hours. It has been suggested that prostaglandin, synthesized in the endometrium under progesterone stimulation, is released at this time and produces further vasoconstriction. The dissolution of the endometrium releases acid hydrolases which have been hitherto confined in the cell lysosomes. These liberated enzymes are then able to further disrupt the endometrial cell membranes and thus complete the process of menstruation.

Markee's method of study was the direct observation of endometrial tissue implanted in the anterior chamber of the eyes of monkeys. He was thus able to observe the actual mechanism of the bleeding. "Five types of hemorrhage were observed in the transplants: (1) blood escaping through a break in the wall of an arteriole or capillary may form a hematoma which ruptures, or (2) it may break through the uterine epithelium and escape without forming a hematoma, (3) diapedesis may occur through the wall of a capillary and the escaping blood may or may not form a hematoma, (4) there may be either a direct flow or a reflux of blood from the veins in fields of previous hemorrhage and destruction of tissue, and (5) secondary bleeding may occur from an arteriole following experimentally induced fright or violent movement" (Markee). The first mechanism appears to be the most frequent. The vasoconstriction which precedes and accompanies menstrual bleeding is believed by Markee to prevent loss of an excessive amount of blood.

Endocrine Mechanism of Menstruation

Having considered the various hormones which are concerned in the menstrual cycle, we may proceed to a consideration of the rather intricate menstrual mechanism which they motivate.

Preovulation: Follicular Phase

A convenient starting point in our discussion is the phase immediately prior to onset of a menstrual period. At this time the corpus luteum is regressing and the decreased steroid production releases pituitary FSH inhibition. The stimulus of the increased FSH causes a burst of follicular activity in the ovary. This increased FSH activity continues during the first 7 days of the follicular phase causing continual follicle maturation. As LH rises after a slight lag period, it stimulates the theca cells to produce increased amounts of estrogen. However, only in the 4 days preovulatory is there a marked increase in estrogen secretion. This change is synchronous with the preovulatory swelling stage of the follicle. As a rule, only one follicle in each cycle reaches complete maturity and comes to ovulation, the remainder of the partially mature follicles undergo the process known as follicular atresia.

Ovulation

Ovulation takes place at approximately the 14th day of the cycle. The migration of a follicle to the cortex of the ovary is apparently dependent upon pituitary hormone stimulation and determined by the vascular and stromal composition of the ovary. The loose syncytial stromal arrangement in the medulla and the spiral arteries allows growth of the young antrum follicle. However, as the follicular size increases, it impinges on the cortex stretching the straight arterioles and branching arcades (Fig. 2.20) which are unable to compensate. The ensuing impairment in the blood supply, perhaps in conjunction with vasoconstriction of prostaglandin, induces the stigma, an avascular area on the surface of the follicle through which ovulation occurs. In the rabbit, it has been possible to induce a corpus luteum with a trapped ovum by inhibiting the action of prostaglandin. This clearly supports the theory that the pituitary LH action is responsible for luteinization of the granulosa cells, while prostaglandin is responsible for stigma formation and ovulation.

The extruded ovum is directed toward and into the fimbriated end of the tube by two forces, *viz.*, (1) the ciliary current in the peritoneal fluid produced by the cilia of the epithelium of the fimbria ovarica and (2) the motility of the tube.

Postovulation: Luteal Phase

With the rupture of the follicle, there occurs a temporary drop in the production of estrogen. The reason for this decrease in estrogen is unexplained, but it may be dependent upon the lag period associated with the change in preferential substrate from the Δ^5 steroid, DHA, to the Δ^4 steroid, progesterone. The collapsed follicle soon launches on its second or corpus luteum phase of development. The stratum granulosa cells, hitherto functioning as nurse cells for the ova, have begun to show luteinization and lipid droplets signifying progesterone production some 24 hours before ovulation and shortly after the LH flood begins. Under previous LH stimulation, the progesterone precursor, cholesterol, has been laid down and the cells are now rapidly luteinized, blood vessels infiltrate, organization of the central blood clot occurs, and increased amounts of progesterone are secreted. Estrogen also is produced, perhaps by the same corpus luteum cells, but more probably by the stimulated theca interna cells. The fixed life span of the corpus luteum (in the absence of pregnancy) which usually averages between 14 to 16 days, may be determined by the inability of the cells to augment precursor substances laid down in the preovulatory phase, or by the inability of the minimal amount of LH available in the luteal phase of the cycle to stimulate steroid synthesis for a longer period of time. However, a luteolytic action, perhaps related to estrogen and/or its effect on the luteal synthesis of prostaglandin may be responsible for the demise of the cyclic corpus luteum.

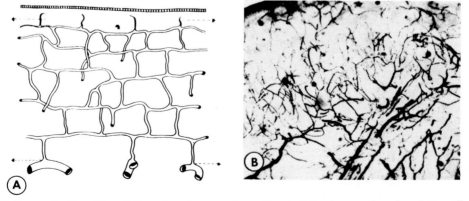

2.20. Demonstration of the relation of ovarian vascular pattern to follicular growth and ovulation. (From G. Reeves, Obstet. Gynec., *37:* 832, 1971.)

Paralleling the corpus luteum phase in the ovary, the endometrium in the postovulatory phase shows increasing evidence of the characteristic progesterone effects, such as increasing thickness and edema, increased tortuosity of the glands, steadily increasing secretory activity of the glandular epithelium, and decidua-like hypertrophy of the stromal cells. These histological changes are described in the chapter on cyclical changes in the endometrium (Chapter 3).

Menstruation: Menstrual Phase

The height of the progestational phase is reached, not at the beginning of the next menstrual bleeding, but probably 4 to 6 days before this, when regression of the corpus luteum begins. In general it may be said that so long as the endometrium is receiving a steady, supporting supply of the ovarian hormones, it shows no tendency to bleed. When this endocrine support is rather abruptly withdrawn, however, retrogression occurs in the previously built-up endometrium. It has been long known that estrogen deprivation of this sort can produce bleeding, and this is perhaps the hormone mechanism concerned in the production of dysfunctional bleeding of the anovulatory type. On the other hand, the evidence indicates that in the usual ovulatory type of cycle the deprivation of progesterone plays a more important role than does estrogen withdrawal. With the decline of corpus luteum function approximately 2 to 4 days before menstruation, the estrogen and progesterone inhibition of the pituitary gonadotrophic hormones is released and another crop of follicles begins to mature as the next cycle begins.

The endometrium, under the influence of progesterone, synthesizes prostaglandin and, as the endometrium breaks down with the withdrawal of ovarian estrogen and progesterone steroid support, prostaglandin is released causing further vasoconstriction and endometrial disruption. Lysosomes, intracellular packets which contain acid hydrolase enzymes, are also increased under progesterone influence and, as the cell membranes are disrupted, these enzymes are released and cause further cellular dissolution.

Significance of Menstruation

Whereas to the lay mind the monthly bleeding is the conspicuous feature of the cycle, this really is only an expression of the frustration of the purpose of the cycle, which is to prepare the endometrium for the reception and nidation of the egg in the event that the latter is fertilized.

Much more frequently, however, the ovum is not fertilized, in which case the elaborate progestational endometrial preparation goes for naught. The endometrium is dismantled, with bleeding which we call menstruation, and another cycle is hopefully begun. With every cycle, therefore, the endometrium prepares for a possible pregnancy, and its progestational phase represents, as it were, a flying start toward the changes characteristic of the pregnant uterine mucosa.

Endocrines in Pregnancy

If, however, the egg is fertilized, the corpus luteum continues to produce increasing amounts of progesterone and the endometrium is not only not cast off but continues to develop further, becoming the decidua of early pregnancy. The corpus luteum of pregnancy probably continues to function for several months. According to Hoffmann and Van Lam, progesterone is detected in appreciable amounts in the corpus luteum of pregnancy until the 19th day, after which the secretion decreases. Regressive changes in the corpus luteum of pregnancy noted histologically a number of years ago by Marcotty substantiate the biochemical findings. Progesterone secretion may be taken over by the placenta at this relatively early date. Ask-Upmark, a number of years ago, noted that abortion occurred in only 17 of 51 women in whom the corpus luteum was removed before the second missed period. Thus one may conclude that although corpus luteum activity probably continues through at least the first trimester, substantial placental take-over of progesterone production may occur prior to the second missed period.

The prolonged luteal function in pregnancy is caused by a third gonadotrophin, chorionic gonadotrophin (HCG). This hormone was first isolated from pregnancy urine in 1927 by Zondek and Aschheim, who initially considered it to be a pituitary hormone. Tissue culture experiments by Jones *et al.* demonstrated it was produced by trophoblastic cells. HCG is closely related both biologically and chemically to the pituitary hormone LH. The α chain is interchangeable with that of pituitary FSH and LH. The β chain is immunologically distinguishable from both FSH and LH, allowing for a specific radioimmunoassay. Plasma clearance of HCG is relatively slow, a half-life in human serum is estimated at 38 hours by radioimmunoassay. The renal clearance rate reported by Wide *et al.,* is approximately 1 ml/min, considerably slower than the estimated 7 ml/min for LH. The function of HCG to prolong the corpus luteum life span in the early part of pregnancy is well documented. To this end, the amount of hormone produced increases rapidly from just prior to the first missed period to a peak at the 60th day (Fig. 2.21). Thereafter it falls somewhat less precipitously until about 90 days, at which point it maintains a fairly stable level until delivery. Chorionic gonadotrophin is the basis for most of the biological and immunological pregnancy tests. The values in the serum are slightly higher than those in the urine as shown by Foote and Jones and, as the hormone is heat labile, when accurate quantitative values are necessary for diagnostic purposes, serum is preferable to

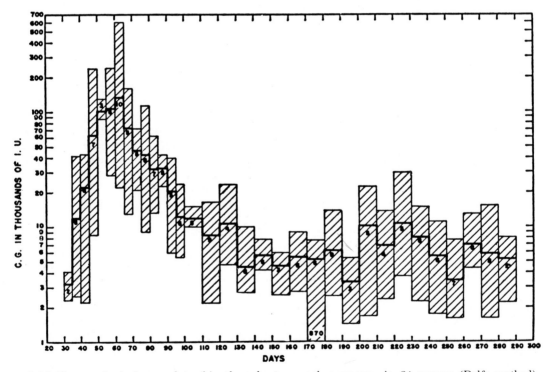

2.21. Serum chorionic gonadotrophin throughout normal pregnancy in 24 women (Delfs method). Gonadotrophin in international units (I.U.) is plotted against duration of pregnancy in days, counting from Day 1 of the last menstrual period. *Heavy black line* shows average gonadotrophin level. *Cross-hatched area* indicates extreme variation for the period with the number of determinations in each. Plotted on semilogarithmic graph scale. (From Jones, G. E. S., Delfs, E., and Stran, H. M.: Chorionic gonadotrophin and pregnanediol values in normal pregnancy. Bull. Johns Hopkins Hosp., *75:* 359, 1944.)

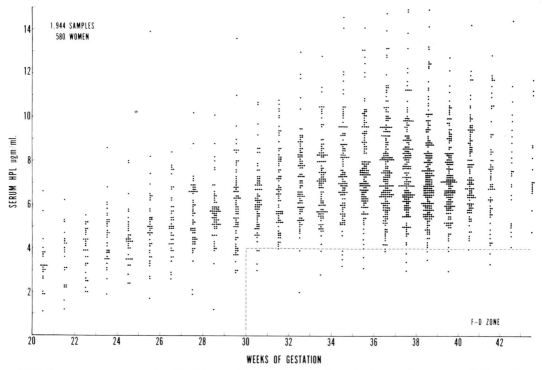

2.22. Serum somatomammotrophin (placental lactogen) values throughout normal pregnancy. F-D zone indicates the area of concern for fetal danger. (From W. N. Spellacy and J. E. Cohn, Obstet. Gynec., *42:* 330, 1973.)

urine. The quantitative serum chorionic gonadotrophin levels are helpful in the evaluation of the normalcy of fetal growth and development in the first trimester of pregnancy (Chapter 29). Assays are also important in the diagnosis and follow-up examinations of patients who have had trophoblastic disease, hydatidiform moles or chorionepithelioma.

Because of the thyroid stimulating activity sometimes seen in conjunction with the presence of trophoblastic tissue, it has been postulated that the placenta produces a chorionic thyroid-stimulating hormone. Nisula and Ketelslegers have presented evidence that the "large thyroblastic thyrotropin" found in association with trophoblastic tumors, when HCG titers are high, is in fact HCG. They suggest that it is the chorionic hormone *per se* which is responsible for the clinical hyperthyroidism sometimes seen in association with these conditions.

Another specific placental hormone is placental lactogen or placental somatomammotrophin. The values during pregnancy are shown (Fig. 2.22). The functions of this hormone are as yet undetermined. It can be used as a measure of placental competence after the first trimester.

The placenta is also responsible for steroid production and, as previously indicated, as early as 36 days may have assumed sufficient progesterone production to allow a pregnancy to progress following ablation of the corpus luteum. Pearlman and Thomas have estimated that the placenta in the last trimester of pregnancy is able to secrete 250 mg of progesterone per 24 hours. Kumar *et al.* found 2.5 to 3.9 μg of progesterone per gram of placenta. Blood levels of progesterone in pregnancy roughly approximate the rise in progesterone production previously indicated by studies of the urinary pregnanediol excretion (Fig. 2.23). It is assumed that the

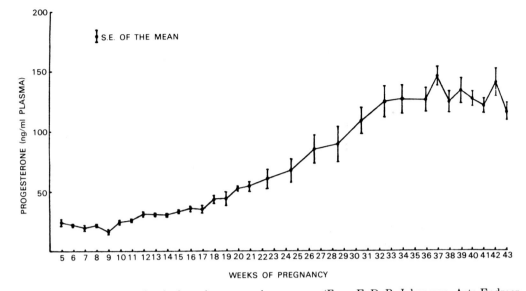

2.23. Plasma progesterone levels throughout normal pregnancy. (From E. D. B. Johansson, Acta Endrocr., *61:* 692, 1969.)

function of progesterone in pregnancy is to maintain the quiescence of the uterus. The pregnanediol excretion after the third month can serve as an index of placental competence.

Placental cells are also capable of synthesizing estrogens and the rising urinary estrogen values for estrone, estradiol, and estriol (Fig. 2.24) reflect this function. The tremendous amounts of estriol which are found in pregnancy urine have, however, been shown to be an index of fetal well being. Zondek and Goldberg first suggested that fetal distress or death can be predicted by the urinary estriol values. Cassmer showed that although the urinary excretion of gonadotrophin and pregnanediol was independent of the fetus, estriol excretion depended upon an intact fetal circulation. Frandsen and Stakemann found that women who carried anencephalic fetuses, having small adrenal glands, also showed very low urinary estriol values. These authors therefore postulated that the estriol excretion in pregnancy was somehow related to the elaboration of steroids from the fetal adrenal cortex. Ryan has added the last step in our knowledge by isolating a 16-hydroxydehydroepiandrosterone from fetal cord blood which is converted by the placenta to estriol. Therefore, it seems clear that urinary estriol, at least during late pregnancy, is for the most part derived from fetal adrenal substrates and is a sensitive measure of fetal health after the first trimester.

Measurement of these steroids in amniotic fluid has been accomplished and the findings are more closely related to the actual status of the fetus as no consideration need by given to the maternal liver and kidney function. If 16α-hydroxydehydroepiandrosterone is measured the factor of aromatization by the placenta is also eliminated, giving an even closer approximation of the actual fetal physiology (Schindler and Ratanasopa).

As previously stated, the determination of blood estrogens is to date still fraught with such technical difficulties that the clinical value is limited. The importance of evaluation of both urinary and blood estriol levels under specific circumstances is however apparent.

The subject has recently been reviewed by Smith and Arai. Diczfalusy found 122 μg of estriol and 17 μg of presumed "estrone" per kilogram of blood immediately postpartum; Preedy and Aitken report values of 2 to 10 μg of

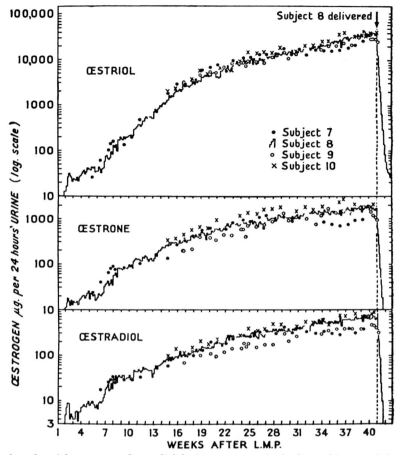

2.24. Excretion of estriol, estrone, and estradiol during pregnancy in the four subjects, and during the puerperium in Subject 8. (From Brown, J. B.: Urinary excretion of estrogens during pregnancy, lactation, and reestablishment of menstruation. *Lancet, 1:* 704, 1956.)

estrone and 4 to 18 μg of estriol per 100 ml of late pregnancy plasma. Dawood and Ratnam have reported serum estradiol values throughout normal pregnancy (Fig. 2.25).

Pregnancy Tests

The chorionic hormone in pregnancy urine or serum is the basis for the validity and accuracy of the biological and immunological pregnancy tests. The tests may be expected to be positive when the trophoblast is living and functioning, and when the hormone has access to the maternal circulation. Even if trophoblast is present, the test will be negative if the trophoblastic cells have degenerated and ceased to function or if the physiological level is too low to detect by the assay

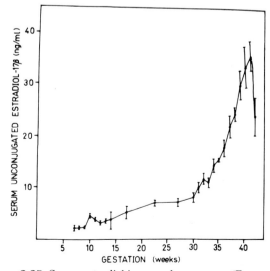

2.25. Serum estradiol in normal pregnancy. (From M. Y. Dawood and S. S. Ratnam, Obstet. Gynec., *44:* 194, 1974.)

method used. Although the chorionic hormone is present throughout pregnancy, it reaches its greatest concentration between 50 and 90 days, following which there is a decline to a low level which is maintained throughout pregnancy.

The biological urine pregnancy tests have been replaced by the immunological assay. Barr reports a 97.4% accuracy rate, the disadvantage being that there were 2.3% false-positive reactions.

When the diagnosis is uncertain and true complications of pregnancy are suspected, such as a missed abortion or an hydatidiform mole, or when one wishes to evaluate the normalcy of the developing trophoblast, an accurate quantitative serum test is indicated. Vaitukaitis has described a specific immunoassay, based on an HCG β subunit which eliminates reactivity with LH and thereby allows greatly improved sensitivity.

When trophoblastic disease, hydatid mole or chorionepithelioma is present, it is also desirable to have a bioassay, such as the Delfs assay, for comparison with the immunoassay. If an abnormal molecule is present, it may not react with the specific radioimmunoassay system, whereas a serum bioassay may detect such structurally abnormal hormones.

REFERENCES

Abraham, G. E.: Ovarian and adrenal contributions to peripheral androgens during the menstrual cycle. J. Clin. Endocr., *39:* 340, 1974.

Adams, J. H., Daniel, P. M., and Prichard, M.: Distribution of hypophysial portal blood in the anterior lobe of the pituitary gland. Endocrinology, *75:* 120, 1964.

Adler, L.: Zur Physiologie und Pathologie der Ovarial Funktion. Arch. Gynaek., *95:* 349, 1912.

Allen, I., and Doisy, E. A.: An ovarian hormone; preliminary report on its localization, abstraction, and partial purification, and action in test animals. J.A.M.A., *81:* 819, 1923.

Antaki, A., Somma, M., Wyman, H., and Campenhout, V. J.: Hypothalamic-pituitary function in the olfactogenital syndrome. J. Clin. Endocr., *38:* 1083, 1974.

Arthur, A. T., and Chang, M. C.: Induction of blastokinin by oral contraceptive steroids; implications for fertililty control. Fertil. Steril., *25:* 217, 1974.

Ask-Upmark, M. E.: Le corps jaune est-il necessaire pour l'accomplishment physiologique de la gravidite humaine? Acta Obstet. Gynec. Scand., *5:* 211, 1926.

Astwood, E. B.: The regulation of corpus luteum function by hypophysial luteotrophin. Endocrinology, *28:* 309, 1941.

Baggett, B., Engel, L. L., Balderas, L., Lanman, G., Savard, K., and Dorfman, R. I.: Conversion of C^{14}-testosterone to C^{14}-estrogenic steroids by endocrine tissues. Endocrinology, *64:* 600, 1959.

Baird, D. T., and Fraser, I. S.: Blood production and ovarian secretion rates of estradiol-17β and estrone in women throughout the menstrual cycle. J. Clin. Endocr., *38:* 1009, 1974.

Bartelmez, G. W., Corner, G. W., and Hartman, C. G.: Phases of menstrual cycle in macaque monkey. Anat. Rec., *94:* 512, 1946.

Benjamin, F.: Basal body temperature recordings in gynecology and obstetrics. J. Obstet. Gynaec. Brit. Comm., *67:* 177, 1960.

Bjorkman, N.: A study of the ultrastructure of the granulosa cells of the rat ovary. Acta Anat. (Basel), *51:* 125, 1962.

Böving, B. G.: Implantation. Ann. N. Y. Acad. Sci., *75:* 700, 1958.

Bower, A., Hadley, M. E., and Hruby, J.: Biogenic amines and control of melanophore stimulating hormone release. Science, *184:* 70, 1974.

Bowers, C. Y., Friesen, H. H., Hwang, P., et al.: Prolactin and thyrotropin release in man by synthetic pyroglutamyl-histidyl-prolinamide. Biochem. Biophys. Res. Commun., *45:* 1033, 1971.

Brown, J. B.: Urinary excretion of estrogens during pregnancy, lactation, and the reestablishment of menstruation. Lancet, *1:* 704, 1956.

Bruce, H. M.: A comparison of olfactory stimulation and nutritional stress as pregnancy-blocking agents in mice J. Reprod. Fertil., *6:* 221, 1963.

Burr, I. M., Sizonenko, P. C., Kaplan, S. L., and Grumbach, M. M.: Observations on the binding of human TSH by antisera to human chorionic gonadotropin. J. Clin. Endocr., *29:* 691, 1969.

Burnstein, S., and Dorfman, R. I.: Biosynthesis of C_{19} steroids from 4-^{14}C-cholesterol and 7-^{3}H-pregnenolone in vivo: consideration of new pathways. Acta Endocr. (Kobenhavn), *40:* 188, 1962.

Butenandt, A., and Westphal, U.: Zur isolierung und Charakterisierung des Corpusluteum-Hormons. Ber. chem. Ges., *67:* 1440, 1934.

Cantarow, A., Rakoff, A. E., Paschikis, K. E., Hansen, L. P., and Walkling, A. A.: Excretion of exogenous and endogenous estrogen in bile of dogs and humans. Proc. Soc. Exp. Biol. Med., *52:* 256, 1943.

Cassmer, O.: Hormone production of the isolated human placenta. Acta Endocr. (Kobenhavn). (Suppl.), *45:* 7, 1959.

Catt, K. J., Dufau, M. L., and Tsuruhara, T.: Studies on a radioligand-receptor assay system for luteinizing hormone and chorionic gonadotropin. J. Clin. Endocr., *32:* 860, 1971.

Chow, B. F., van Dyke, H. B., Greep, R. O., Rothen, A., and Shedlovsky, T.: Gonadotropins of the swine pituitary. Endocrinology, *30:* 650, 1942.

Christiansen, P.: Urinary follicle stimulating hormone and luteinizing hormone in normal adult men. Acta Endocr., *71:* 1, 1972.

Corner, G. W., and Allen, W. M.: Physiology of the corpus luteum. 11. Production of a special uterine reaction (progestational proliferation) by extracts of the corpus luteum. Amer. J. Physiol., *88:* 326, 1929.

Crowe, S. J., Cushing, H., and Homans, J.: Experimental hypophysectomy. Bull Hopkins Hosp., *21:* 127, 1910.

Currie, A. R., and Dekanski, J. B.: Gonadotrophins and prolactin in human pituitary glands. Acta Endocr. (Kobenhavn), *36:* 185, 1961.

Davidson, J. M., and Sawyer, C. H.: Effects of localized intracerebral implantation of oestrogen on reproductive function in the female rabbit. Acta Endocr. (Kobenhavn), *37:* 3, 1961.

Davis, M. E., Jones, R. J., and Jarolim, C.: Long-term estrogen substitution and atherosclerosis. Amer. J. Obstet. Gynec., *82:* 1003, 1961.

DeFeo, V. J., and Reynolds, S. R. M.: Modification of the menstrual cycle in rhesus monkeys by reserpine. Science, *124:* 726, 1956.

Delfs, E.: An assay method for human chorionic gonadotrophin. Endocrinology, 28: 196, 1941.

Diczfalusy, E.: Chorionic gonadotropin and estrogens in the human placenta. Acta Endocr. (Kobenhavn) (Suppl.), 12: 1, 1953.

Doe, R. P., Mellinger, G. T., Swain, W. R., and Seal, U. S.: Estrogen dosage effects on serum proteins: a longitudinal study. J. Clin. Endocr., 27: 1081, 1967.

Dohrn, M., and Faure, W.: Uber die Ausschiedung des weiblichen Sexualhormons. Klin. Wschr., 7: 943, 1928.

Donini, P., Puzzuoli, D., D'Alessio, I., Bergesi, G., and Donini, S.: Purification and properties of human urinary follicle-stimulating and luteinizing hormones. In Gonadotropins, edited by Rosenberg, Geron-X, Inc., Los Altos, Calif., 1968.

Downie, J., Poyser, N. L., and Wunderlich, M.: Levels of prostaglandins in human endometrium during the normal menstrual cycle. J. Physiol., 236: 465, 1974.

Dresel, I.: The effect of prolactin on the estrus cycle of nonparous mice. Science, 82: 173, 1935.

Dugger, G. S., Van Wyk, J. J., and Newsom, J. S.: The effect of pituitary stalk section on thyroid function and gonadotrophic hormone excretion in women with mammary carcinoma. J. Neurosurg., 19: 589, 1962.

Eleftherian, B. E., and Zolovick, A. J.: Effect of amygdaloid lesions on plasma and pituitary levels of LH. J. Reprod. Fertil., 14: 33, 1967.

Elwers, M., and Critchlow, V.: Precocious ovarian stimulation following interruption of stria terminals. Amer. J. Physiol., 201: 281, 1961.

Emmart, E. W., Spicer, S. S., and Bates, R. W.: Localization of prolactin within the pituitary by specific fluorescent antiprolactin globulin. J. Histochem. Cytochem., 11: 365, 1963.

Evans, H. M., Korpi, K., Simpson, M. E., Pencharz, R. I., and Wonder, D. H.: On the separation of the interstitial cell-stimulating luteinizing, and follicle-stimulating fraction in the anterior pituitary gonadotropic complex. Univ. Calif. Publ. Anat., 1: 255, 1936.

Everett, J. W.: Hormonal factors responsible for the deposition of cholesterol in the corpus luteum of the rat. Endocrinology, 41: 364, 1947.

Faiman, C., and Ryan, R. J.: Gonadotropins in human pregnancy and puerperium. Clin. Res., 15: 413, 1967.

Farner, D. F.: Photo periodic control of reproductive cycles in birds. Amer. Sci., 52: 137, 1964.

Fiske, V. M., and Greep, R. O.: Neurosecretory activity in rats under conditions of continuous light or darkness. Endocrinology, 64: 175, 1959.

Flerko, B.: Hypothalamic control of the hypophyseal gonadotrophin function in the rat. Acta Physiol. Pharmacol. Neerl., 8: 545, 1959.

Flerko, B., and Szentagolhai, I.: Oestrogen sensitive nervous structures in the hypothalamus. Acta Endocr. (Kobenhavn), 26: 121, 1957.

Foote, E. C., and Jones, G. E. S.: An evaluation of the Hogben pregnancy test. Amer. J. Obstet. Gynec., 51: 672, 1946.

Fraenkel, L.: Die Funktion des Corpus Luteum. Arch. Gynaek., 68: 438, 1903.

Frandsen, V. A., and Stakemann, G.: The site of production of estrogenic hormones in human pregnancy. Acta Endocr. (Kobenhavn), 38: 383, 1961.

Frank, R. T., and Goldberger, M. A.: The female sex hormone. Its occurrence in the circulating and menstrual blood of the human female. J.A.M.A., 86: 1686, 1926.

Frank, R. T., and Rosenbloom, J.: Physiologically active substances contained in the placenta and corpus luteum. Surg. Gynec. Obstet., 21: 646, 1915.

Frank, R. T., and Salmon, U. J.: Effect of administration of estrogenic factor upon hypophysial hyperactivity in the menopause. Proc. Soc. Exp. Biol. Med., 33: 311, 1935.

Fraschini, F., Mess, B., Piva, F., and Martini, L.: Brain receptors sensitive to indole compounds: function in control of luteinizing hormone secretion. Science, 159: 1104, 1968.

Fröhlich, A.: Wien. Klin. Rundschau, 15: 883, 906, 1901.

Funk, C., Chamelin, I. M., Wagreich, H., and Harrow, B.: Study of hormonal factors which influence production of insulin. Science, 94: 260, 1941.

Goldenberg, R. L., Vaitukaitis, J. L., and Ross, G. T.: Estrogen and follicle stimulating hormone interactions on follicle growth in rats. Endocrinology, 90: 1492, 1972.

Greep, R. O., and Jones, I. C.: A Symposium on Steroid Hormones, p. 330. University of Wisconsin Press, Madison, 1950.

Gutzeit, J. P.: Dissertation, Konigsberg, Gilatis, 1896. Cited by Tharndrup, Precocious Sexual Development. Charles C Thomas, Springfield, Ill., 1961.

Halász, B., and Réthelyi, M.: Data on the Site of Production of Hypothalamic Release and Inhibiting Factors of the Hypothalamus. In Polypetide Hormones, edited by E. Góth and J. Fövenigi. Publishing House of the Hungarian Academy of Science, Budapest, 1971.

Harman, S., and Ross, T.: New light on follicular atresia; interaction of estrogen and gonadotrophins (abstract). J. Clin. Endocr., 94: A166, 19.

Harris, G. W.: The Neural Control of the Pituitary Gland. Edward Arnold & Company, London, 1955.

Hembree, W. C., Bardin, C. W., and Lipsett, M. B.: A study of metabolic clearance rates and transfer factors. J. Clin. Invest., 48: 1809, 1969.

Hitschmann, F., and Adler, L.: Der Bau der Uterusschleimhaut des Geschlechtesreifen Weibes mit besonderer Berücktigung der Menstruation. Mschr. Geburtsh. Gynaek., 27: 1, 1908.

Hoffmann, F., and van Lam, L.: Uber die Progesteronbildung im Zyklus und in der Schwangerschaft. Zbl. Gynaek., 70: 1177, 1948.

Hyppa, M., Motta, M., and Martini, L.: "Ultra short" feedback control of follicle-stimulating hormone-releasing factor secretion. Neuroendocrinology, 7: 227, 1971.

Igarashi, M., Yokota, N., Ebara, Y., Mayuzumi, R., Hirano, T., Matsumoto, S., and Yamasaki, M.: Clinical effects with partially purified beef hypothalamic FSH-releasing factor. Amer. J. Obstet. Gynec., 100: 867, 1968.

Ito, Y., and Higashi, K.: Studies on the prolactin-like substance in human placenta. II. Endocr. Japn., 8: 279, 1961.

Job, J. C., Garnier, P. E., Chaussain, J. L., Scholler, R., Toublanc, J. E., and Canlorbe, P.: Effect of synthetic luteinizing hormone-releasing hormone (LH-RH) on the release of gonadotropins in hypophyso-gonadal disorders of children and adolescents. V. Agonadism. J. Clin. Endocr., 38: 1109, 1974.

Johansson, K., Currie, B. L., and Folkers, K., and Bowers, C. Y.: Biosynthesis and evidence for the existence of the follicle stimulating hormone releasing hormone. Biochem. Biophys. Res. Commun., 50: 8, 1973.

Johnson, S. G.: A clinical routine method for the quantitative determination of gonadotrophins in 24-hour urine samples. II. Normal values for men and women and all age groups from puberty to senescence. Acta Endocr. (Kobenhavn), 31: 209, 1959.

Jones, G. E. S., Delfs, E., and Stran, H. M.: Chorionic gonadotrophin and pregnanediol values in normal pregnancy. Bull. Johns Hopkins Hosp., 75: 359, 1944.

Jones, G. E. S., Gey, G. O., and Gey, M. K.: Hormone production by placental cells maintained in continuous culture. Bull. Hopkins Hosp., 72: 26, 1946.

Jones, H. W., Ferguson-Smith, M., and Heller, R.: Pathology and cytogenetics of gonadal aplasia. Amer. J. Obstet. Gynec., 87: 578, 1963.

Josimovich, J. B., and Atwood, B. L.: Human placental lactogen (HPL), a trophoblastic hormone synergizing with chorionic gonadotropin and potentiating the anabolic effects of pituitary growth hormone. Amer. J. Obstet. Gynec., *88:* 7, 1964.

Kaiser, I. H.: Histologic appearance of coiled arterioles in the endometrium of rhesus monkey, baboon, chimpanzee, and gibbon. Amer. J. Obstet. Gynec., *55:* 699, 1948.

Kanematsu, S., Hilliard, J., and Sawyer, C. H.: The effect of reserpine on pituitary prolactin content and its hypothalamic site of action in the rabbit. Acta Endocr. (Kobenhavn), *44:* 467, 1963.

Kingsley, T. R., and Bogdanove, E. M.: Direct feedback of androgens; localized effects of intrapituitary implants of androgens on gonadotrophic cells and hormone stores. Endocrinology, *93:* 1398, 1973.

Klooper, A., Strong, J. A., and Cook, L. R.: The excretion of pregnanediol and adrenocortical activity. J. Endocr., *15:* 180, 1957.

Knauer, E.: Die Ovarientransplantation. Experimentelle Studie. Arch. Gynaek., *60:* 322, 1900.

Kobayashi, T., Kigawa, T., Mizuno, M., and Amenomani, Y.: Influence of rat hypothalamic extracts and rat pituitary cells in tissue culture. Endocr. Jap., *10:* 1, 1963.

Kumar, D., Azoury, R. S., and Barnes, A. C.: Studies on human premature births. I. Placental progesterone concentrations. Amer. J. Obstet. Gynec., *87:* 126, 1963.

Lazo-Wasem, E. A., Neher, G. M., Shoger, R. L., and Zarrow, M. V.: Gelbkörperhormon in Blute männlicher Wirbeltiere. Endokrinologie, *31:* 166, 1954.

Levan, A. B., and Szanto, P. B.: Frequency of anovulatory menstruation as determined by endometrial biopsy. Amer. J. Obstet. Gynec., *48:* 75, 1944.

Little, B., Tait, J. F., Tait, S. A., and Erlenmeyer, F.: Metabolic clearance rate of progesterone in males and ovariectomized females. J. Clin. Invest., *45:* 901, 1966.

Loewe, S., and Lange, F.: Der Gehalt des Frauenharnes an brunsterzeugenden Stoffen in Abhängigkeit vom ovariellen Zyklus. Klin. Wschr., *5:* 1038, 1926.

Longchampt, J. E., Gual, C., Ehrenstein, M., and Dorfman, R. I.: 19-Hydroxy-Δ^4-androstene-3, 17-dione an intermediate in estrogen biosynthesis. Endocrinology, *66:* 3, 1960.

Longcope, C., Layne, D. S., and Tait, J. F.: Metabolic clearance rates and interconversions of estrone and 17β-estradiol in normal males and females. J. Clin. Invest., *47:* 93, 1968.

MacCorquodale, D. W., Thayer, S. A., and Doisy, E. A.: The isolation of the principal estrogenic substance of liquor folliculi. J. Biol. Chem., *115:* 435, 1936.

Macht, D. I.: Further historical and experimental studies on menstrual toxin. Amer. J. Med. Sci., *206:* 281, 1943.

Magendantz, H. G., and Ryan, K. J.: Isolation of an estriol precursor, 16β-hydroxydehydroepiandrosterone from human umbilical sera. J. Clin. Endocr., *24:* 1155, 1964.

Malacara, J. M., Seyler, L. E., Jr., and Reichlin, S.: Luteinizing hormone releasing factor activity in peripheral blood from women during the midcycle luteinizing hormone ovulatory surge. J. Clin. Endocr., *34:* 271, 1972.

Marcotty, A.: Uber das Corpus Luteum menstruationis und das Corpus Luteum graviditatis. Arch. Gynaek., *103:* 63, 1914.

Markee, J. E.: Menstruation in intraocular endometrial transplants in the rhesus monkey. Contrib. Embryol., *28:* 219, 1940.

Markee, J. E.: Morphological basis for menstrual bleeding. Anat. Rec., *94:* 481, 1946.

Markee, J. E., Sayer, C. H., and Hollinsdead, W. H.: Adrenergic control of release of luteinizing hormone from hypophysis of rabbit. Recent. Progr. Hormone Res., *2:* 117, 1948.

Marrian, G. F.: The chemistry of oestrin. I. Preparation from urine and the separation from an unidentified solid alcohol. Biochem. J., *23:* 1090, 1929.

Mason, N. R., and Savard, K.: Conversion of cholesterol to progesterone by corpus luteum slices. Endocrinology, *75:* 215, 1964.

McCann, S. M.: A hypothalamic luteinizing-hormone-releasing factor. Amer. J. Physiol., *202:* 395, 1962.

McCann, S. M.: Effect of progesterone on plasma luteinizing hormone activity. Amer. J. Physiol., *202:* 601, 1962.

McCann, S. M., Taleisnik, S., and Friedman, H. M.: LH-Releasing activity in hypothalamic extracts. Proc. Soc. Exp. Biol. Med., *104:* 432, 1960.

Meites, J., Kahn, R. H., and Nicoll, C. S.: Prolactin production by rat pituitary "in vitro." Proc. Soc. Exp. Biol. Med., *108:* 440, 1961.

Merimee, T. J., Burgess, J. A., and Rabinowitz, D.: Sex-determined variation in serum insulin and growth hormone response to amino acid stimulation. J. Clin. Endocr., *26:* 791, 1966.

Mess, B.: Releasing and Inhibiting Factors of the Hypothalamus. In *Polypetide Hormones,* edited by E. Goth and J. Fövenigi. Publishing House of the Hungarian Academy of Sciences, Budapest, 1971.

Midgley, A. R., Jr.: Human pituitary luteinizing hormone: An immunohistochemical study. J. Histochem. Cytochem., *14:* 159, 1966.

Milgrom, E., Atger, M., and Baulieu, E.-E.: Studies on estrogen entry into uterine cells and on estradiol-receptor complex attachment to the nucleus; is the entry of estrogen into uterine cells a protein-mediated process? Biochim. Biophys. Acta, *340:* 267, 1973.

Morato, T. K., Raab, H. J., Brodie, M., Hyano, M., and Dorfman, R. I.: The mechanisms of estrogen biosynthesis. J. Amer. Chem. Soc., *84:* 3764, 1962.

Myer, R.: Anovulatory cycle and menstruation. Amer. J. Obstet. Gynec., *51:* 39, 1946.

Nisula, B. C., and Ketelslegers, J.: Thyroid-stimulating activity and chorionic gonadotropin. J. Clin. Invest., *54:* 494, 1974.

Noall, M. W., Alexander, F., and Allen, W. M.: Dehydroisandrosterone synthesis by the human ovary. Biochem. Biophys. Acta, *59:* 520, 1962.

Novak, E.: Superstition and folklore of menstruation. Bull. Hopkins Hosp., *29:* 270, 1916.

Noyes, R. W., Hertig, A. T., and Rock, J.: Dating the endometrial biopsy. Fertil. Steril., *1:* 3, 1950.

O'Malley, B. W., and Means, A. R.: Female steroid hormones and target cell nuclei. Science, *183:* 610, 1974.

Parkes, A. S., and Bruce, H. M.: Pregnancy block in female mice placed in boxes soiled by males. J. Reprod. Fertil., *4:* 303, 1962.

Pearlman, W. H., and Thomas, M.: The progesterone content of human placental blood. Endocr., *52:* 590, 1953.

Pflüger, E.: *Über die Bedentung und Ursuche der menstruation.* Berlin, 1865.

Purves, H. D., and Griesbach, W. E.: The site of thyrotropin and gonadotrophin production in the rat pituitary studies by McManus-Hotchkiss staining for glycoprotein. Endocrinology, *49:* 244, 1951.

Reeves, G.: Specific stroma in the cortex and medulla of the ovary; cell types and vascular supply in relation to follicular apparatus and ovulation. Obstet. Gynec., *37:* 832, 1971.

Reichert, L. E., Jr., and Ward, D. N.: On the isolation and characterization of α and β subunits of human pituitary follicle-stimulating hormone. Endocrinology, *94:* 655, 1974.

Reiter, R. J.: Comparative effects of continual lighting and pinealectomy on the eyes; the harderian glands and reproduction in pigmented and albino rats. Comp. Biochem. Physiol., *44A:* 503, 1973.

Riddle, O., and Bates, R. W.: Concerning anterior pituitary hormones. Endocrinology, *17:* 689, 1933.

Riddle, O., and Braucher, P. F.: Control of the special secretion of the crop-gland in pigeons by an anterior pituitary hormone. Amer. J. Physiol., 97: 617, 1931.

Root, A. W.: Endocrinology of puberty. I. Normal sexual maturation. J. Pediat., 83: 1, 1973.

Rothchild, J., and Rapport, R. S.: The thermogenic effort of progesterone and its relation to thyroid function. Endocrinology, 50: 580, 1952.

Rowlands, I. W., and Parkes, A. S.: Inhibition of the gonadotropic activity of the human pituitary by anti-serum. Lancet, 1: 924, 1937.

Ruf, K. B.: How does the brain control the process of puberty? Z. Neurol. 204: 95, 1973.

Ryan, K. J.: The conversion of pregnenolone-7-³H and progesterone-4-¹⁴C to oestradiol by a corpus luteum of pregnancy. Acta Endocr. (Kobenhavn), 44: 1, 1963.

Schindler, A. E., and Ratanasopa, V.: Profile of steroids in amniotic fluid of normal and complicated pregnancies. Acta Endocr., 59: 239, 1968.

Schroder, R.: Der mensuelle Gentialzyklus des Weibes und seine Storungen. In Handbuch der Gynakologie, edited by W. Stoecket, Vol. 1, Part 2. J. F. Bergmann, Munich, 1930.

Segal, H. L.: Enzymatic interconversion of active and inactive forms of enzymes. Science, 180: 25, 1973.

Selye, H.: Textbook of Endocrinology. University of Montreal Press, Montreal, 1947.

Severinghaus, A. E.: The effect of castration in the guinea pig upon sex-maturing potency of the anterior pituitary, Amer. J. Physiol., 101: 309, 1932.

Shedlovsky, T., Rothen, A., Greep, R. O., van Dyke, H. B., Chow, B. F.: The isolation in pure form of the interstitial cell stimulating (luteinizing) hormone of the anterior lobe of the pituitary gland. Science, 92: 178, 1940.

Shiino, M., Arimura, A., Schally, A. V., and Rennels, E. G.: Ultrastructural observations of granule extrusion from rat anterior pituitary cells after injection of LH-releasing hormone. Z. Zellforsch., 128: 152, 1972.

Siebke, H., and Schuschania, P.: Ergebnisse von Mengen-bestimmungen des Sexualhormons; Sexualhormon in Harn und Kot bei regelmassigem mensuellem Zyklus Zyklusstorungen und bei Hormontherapie. Zbl. Gynaek., 54: 1734, 1930.

Singh, R. P., and Can, D. H.: The anatomy and histology of XO human embryos and fetuses. Anat. Rec., 155: 369, 1966.

Smith, P. E., and Engle, E. T.: Experimental evidence regarding role of anterior pituitary in development and regulation of the genital system. Amer. J. Anat., 40: 159, 1927.

Stein, S., Spelsberg, T. C., and Kleinsmith, J.: Nonhistone chromosomal proteins and gene regulation. Science, 183: 817, 1974.

Stockard, C. R., and Papanicolaou, G. N.: The existence of a typical oestrous cycle in the guinea-pig with a study of its histological and physiological changes. Amer. J. Anat., 22: 225, 1917.

Stricker, P., and Grueter, F.: Action du lobe anterieur de l'hypophyse sur la montee laiteuse. Compt. rend. Soc. Biol., 99: 1978, 1928.

Taleisnik, S., and McCann, S. M.: Effects of hypothalamic

lesions on the secretion and storage of hypophyseal luteinizing hormone. Endocrinology, 68: 263, 1961.

Talwalker, P. K., Ratner, A., and Meites, J.: In vitro inhibition of pituitary prolactin synthesis and release by hypothalamic extract. Amer. J. Physiol., 205: 213, 1963.

Tenny, B., Jr., and Parker, R., Jr.: Estrogenic content of cirrhotic livers. J. Clin. Endocr., 2: 293, 1942.

Thomas, K., and Ferin, J.: Suppression of the midcycle LH surge by a low-dose mestranol-lynestrenol oral combination. Contraception, 6: 17, 1972.

Thorneycroft, I. H., Mishell, D. R., Jr., Stone, S. C., Kharma, K. M., and Nakamura, R. M.: Serum gonadotrophin and steroid patterns in early human gestation. Amer. J. Obstet. Gynec., 111: 947, 1971.

Tixier-Vidal, A., Kerdelhue, B., and Jutisz, M.: Kinetics of release of luteinizing hormone (LH) and follicle stimulating hormone (FSH) by primary cultures of dispersed rat anterior pituitary cells; chronic effect of synthetic LH and FSH releasing hormone. Life Sci., 12: 499, 1973.

Toole, P.: Cyclic AMP phosphodiesterase in cloned astrocytoma cells; norepinephrine induces a specific enzyme form. Science, 180: 304, 1973.

Venning, E. H., and Browne, J. S. L.: Urinary excretion of sodium pregnandiol glucuronidate in the menstrual cycle (an excretion form of progesterone). Amer. J. Physiol., 119: 417, 1937.

Wade, R., and Jones, H. W.: Effect of progesterone on oxidative phosphorylation. J. Biol. Chem., 220: 553, 1956.

Wallach, E. E., de Cherney, A. H., Russ, D., Duckett, G., Garcia, C., and Root, A. W.: Episodic secretion of LH and FSH after ovariectomy. Obstet. Gynec., 41: 227, 1973.

Weicke, R. F., Dierschke, D. J., Karsch, F. J., Yamaji, T., and Knobil, E.: The refractory period following estrogen-induced LH surges in the Rhesus monkey. Endocrinology, 91: 1528, 1972.

Westman, A.: Investigations into transit of ova in man. J. Obstet. Gynaec. Brit. Comm., 44: 821, 1937.

Witten, C. L., and Bradbury, J. T.: Hemodilution as a result of estrogen therapy. Estrogenic effects in the human female. Proc. Soc. Exp. Biol. Med., 78: 626, 1951.

Wolfe, J. M.: The action of a synthetic estrogenic agent on the anterior pituitary of the castrated female rat. Amer. J. Physiol., 115: 665, 1936.

Wurtman, R.: Neuroendocrinology, Vol. 2, p. 641. Academic Press, New York, 1967.

Yen, S. S. C., Vanden Berg, G., and Siler, T. M.: Modulation of pituitary responsiveness to LRF by estrogen. J. Clin. Endocr., 39: 170, 1974.

Zacharias, L., and Wurtman, R.: Blindness: its relation to the age of menarche. Science, 144: 1154, 1964.

Zander, J., Forbes, T. R., von Munstermann, A. M., and Neher, R.: Δ⁴-3-Ketopregnane-20α-ol and Δ⁴-3-ketopregnane-20β-ol, two naturally occurring metabolites of progesterone. J. Clin. Endocr., 18: 337, 1958.

Zondek, B., and Aschheim, S.: Das Hormon des Hypophysenvorderlappens Testobjekt zum Nachweis des Hormones. Klin. Wshr., 6: 248, 1927.

Zondek, B., and Goldberg, S.: Placental function and foetal death. J. Obstet. Gynaec. Brit. Comm., 64: 1, 1957.

chapter *3*

Cyclical Histology of the Genital Tract

Thorough familiarity with the appearance of the endometrium at different stages of the cycle will permit the experienced pathologist to approximate the time of the menstrual cycle. It is our own feeling that there is so much variation among different women as to make it impossible to date the endometrium to the day, although certain pathologists make this statement (Noyes and co-workers).

Nevertheless we approximate the date within a 48 hour span (as day 18–19 or day 23–24) and feel that this is quite accurate provided the patient is not taking contraceptive pills. Our criteria are essentially those of Noyes *et al.* with slight modifications as noted in Table 3.1. Dating the endometrium prior to ovulation is of no practical importance.

To recapitulate what has been presented in Chapter 2, Figure 3.1 is appended with the hope that the reader, when studying the endometrium, will always be cognizant of the behavior of the ovary and pituitary. The important role of the hypothalamus and its release factors is just beginning to be recognized, as noted in other chapters.

The endometrium, under the immediate influence of the two ovarian hormones, estrogen and progesterone, exhibits certain characteristic cyclical changes, which may be most conveniently divided into four phases.

Postmenstrual Phase

The endometrium is thin, measuring ordinarily only 1 or 2 mm. in thickness. The surface epithelium, as well as that lining the glands, is of cuboidal type (Fig. 3.2). The glands are straight, narrow, and collapsed, whereas the stroma is dense and compact. This phase may arbitrarily be put as including the four or five days immediately following cessation of a period. There is some evidence to indicate that a period of *rest* may at times occur just after menstruation, but this applies chiefly to women with abnormally long cycles, with marked prolongation of the preovulatory phase.

Proliferative Phase

By a gradual transition the postmenstrual phase is followed by the interval stage, during which the continued

Table 3.1

A. Endometrial Dating

Day	Criteria
16	Subnuclear vacuoles. Pseudostratification. Mitoses, glands and stroma.
17	More or less orderly row of nuclei. Cytoplasm above nuclei and subnuclear vacuoles below. Gland and stromal mitoses. Very minimal secretion.
18	Vacuoles above and below nuclei. Improved linear arrangement of nuclei. Gland mitoses rare. Stromal mitoses rare. Bubbles of secretion seen at luminal border.
19	A few vacuoles remain in cell. Mainly active evacuation with intraluminal secretion. No gland or stromal mitoses. May look like day 16 but *NO* pseudostratification.
20	Peak secretion with "ragged" luminal border. Vacuoles are rare—all subnuclear vacuoles gone. Inspissation may be beginning.
21	Abrupt onset of stromal edema. Gland secretion prominent (inspissated). "Naked" stromal nuclei begin to appear.
22	Peak edema. Marked appearance of "naked" stromal nuclei. Stromal cells small and dense filamentous cytoplasm. Active secretion, but subsiding. Rare stromal mitoses.
23	Prominent spiral arterioles. Periarteriolar cuffing with enlargement (earliest predecidual change) of stromal cell nuclei and cytoplasm. Stromal mitoses. Glands with secretory "exhaustion"—low columnar cells, luminal edges ragged.
24	Definite predecidual cells around arterioles with early subepithelial changes. Greater stromal mitoses. Ragged cell borders; *i.e.*, secretorily exhausted.
25	Definite subcapsular predecidua. Inspissated secretion noted to begin. Early stromal infiltration with lymphocytes and occasional polymorphonuclear leukocytes.
26	Generalized decidual reaction—decidual islands in stroma. Polymorphonuclear leukocytic invasion (lymphocytes may accompany or precede).
27	Solid sheet of decidua. Marked leukocytic infiltrate. Polymorphonuclear leukocytes. Inspissated secretion with variable intracellular secretory activity.

Table 3.1—Continued

Table 3.1—Continued

Day	Criteria
28	Focal necrosis and hemorrhage. Peak leukocytic infiltration. Polymorphonuclear leukocytes prominent. Cells may show secretory exhaustion or may show active secretion. Beginning stromal clumping and fragmentation of glands. *Menstruating* Disruption of capsular layer. Stromal clumping. Glandular break-up and hemorrhage. Variable leukocytic infiltration. Edema. After 24 hours, metaplastic alterations on surface.

B. Dating the Corpus Luteum

Stage	Criteria
Proliferation (days 14–15)	Collapsed follicle. Unluteinized granulosa. Absence of blood vessels in granulosa. Vascularized theca with ovoid or polyhedral cells. No blood in lumen.
Vascularization (16–17 days)	Invasion of granulosa by thin blood channels. Blood in lumen next to granulosa. Large polyhedral granulosa cells.
Maturity (day 18)	Mitosis in granulosa ends in day 18. Broad lutein zone traversed by trabeculae of theca interna with numerous blood vessels. Presence of paralutein cells. Fibrous layer lining lutein zone.
Retrogression (begins about day 22–23)	Increase in lipids in and fibrosis of lutein zone. Presence of "mulberry" cells (vascularized lutein cells). Theca cells smaller in size, resemble ordinary connective tissue. Hyalinization occurring over several weeks, cicatrization and formation of corpus albicans over several months.

action of estrogen brings about increased thickness of the uterine mucosa. The surface epithelium becomes taller and columnar, as does that of the glands, while mitotic figures are quite numerous, more so than in the immediately postmenstrual phase. Ciliated cells are a normal finding according to Fleming *et al.* and Schueler. The *early interval* phase antedates ovulation, and during this period no evidence of secretory activity is to be seen in the gland epithelium (Fig. 3.3), as the secretion of progesterone has not yet begun. This non-secretory portion of the cycle is usually spoken of as "proliferative" and is characterized primarily by growth.

Secretory or Progestational Phase

After ovulation, in the *late interval* or *secretory* phase, the evidence of secretory activity in the gland epithelium becomes more and more marked (Fig. 3.4). If differential staining for glycogen is carried

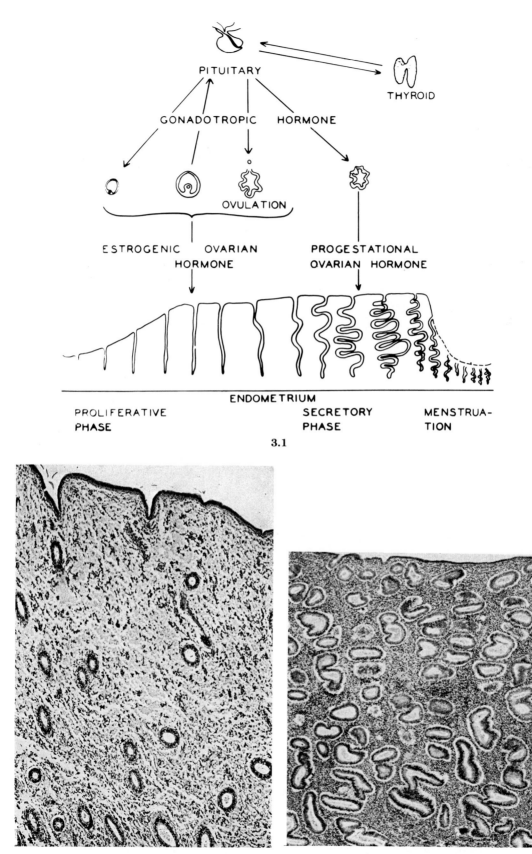

PITUITARY

THYROID

GONADOTROPIC   HORMONE

OVULATION

ESTROGENIC   OVARIAN
HORMONE

PROGESTATIONAL
OVARIAN HORMONE

ENDOMETRIUM

PROLIFERATIVE
PHASE

SECRETORY
PHASE

MENSTRUA-
TION

3.1

3.2. Postmenstrual endometrium

3.3. Early proliferative endometrium

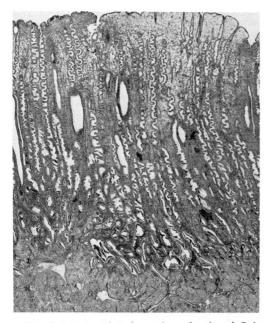

3.4. Late interval endometrium showing definite secretory activity.

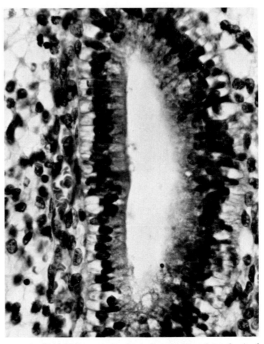

3.6. Subnuclear vacuoles, the earliest histological evidence of secretory activity (high power).

out, granules of glycogen are demonstrable, at first only few in number and within the cytoplasm of the cells, but later more abundant in the cells and in increasing amount in the gland lumina. Subnuclear vacuoles (Figs. 3.5, 6), which

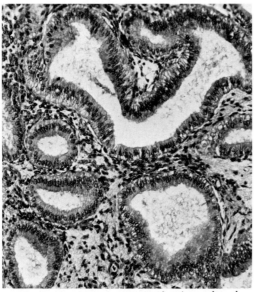

3.5. Early secretory pattern showing subnuclear vacuoles.

are believed to represent a prosecretion phase, begin to crowd the nuclei from the base of the cells toward the lumen. Despite some uncertainty, it is generally assumed that these prosecretion vacuoles represent the earliest stages of progesterone activity. The stroma is more abundant and more vascular than in the postmenstrual phase, particularly in the later stage of the interval, which extends to within a week of the next menstrual phase.

Premenstrual Phase (Figs. 3.7–9)

During this stage the secretory function of the now fully mature corpus luteum brings about a full-blown secretory response in the endometrium, which now is soft, velvety, and edematous, measuring from 4 or 5 mm. to as much as 6 or 7 mm. in thickness. Whereas the surface epithelium is still tall and cylindrical, that of the glands is now low, the nuclei having receded toward the base of the cells, and the cytoplasm appearing to melt into the lumen, so that the edge is apt to appear frayed.

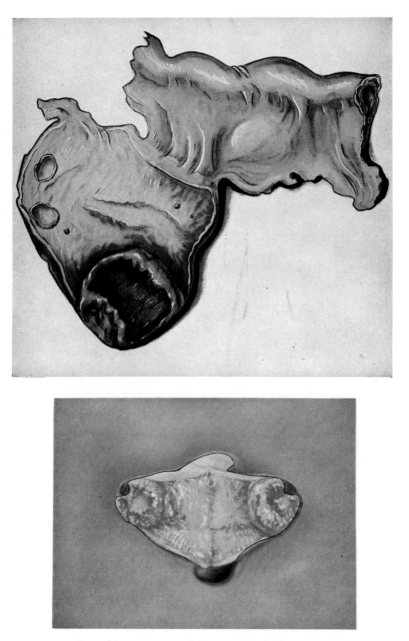

Plate 3.1. *A* (*top*), corpus luteum in stage approaching maturity; *B* (*bottom*), mature corpus luteum

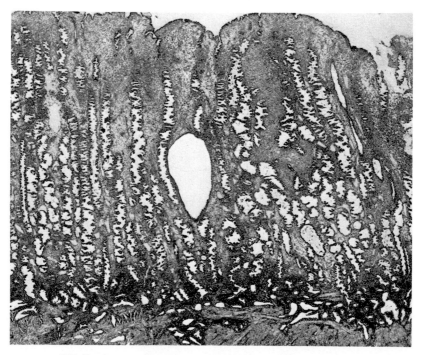

3.7. Premenstrual or progestational endometrium (25th day)

The glands are wide and assume a characteristic corkscrew pattern, the convolutions producing tuftlike accumulations of epithelium on either longitudinal or cross section. The necks of the glands often remain rather narrow and straight, the tortuosity involving chiefly the middle or spongy zone of the endometrium. The growing tips of the glands in the basalis, in immediate contact with the musculature, are lined by an immature type of epithelium which is apparently unresponsive to progesterone, so that a secretory reaction is lacking.

The stroma becomes edematous and loose textured, especially in its superficial layer, and the constituent cells undergo hypertrophy, with an increased amount of cytoplasm. This gives them an appearance suggesting decidual cells, and in many cases the resemblance is so striking that one might well suspect the existence of early gestation. Wienke *et al.* note that the stroma shows an increased ability to respond to hormonal stimuli as the cycle progresses.

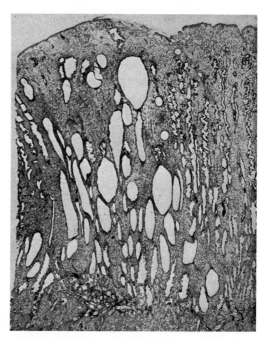

3.8. Large area of unripe endometrium in an otherwise progestational endometrium. Curettings from such a uterus reveal at least one variety of so-called mixed endometrium.

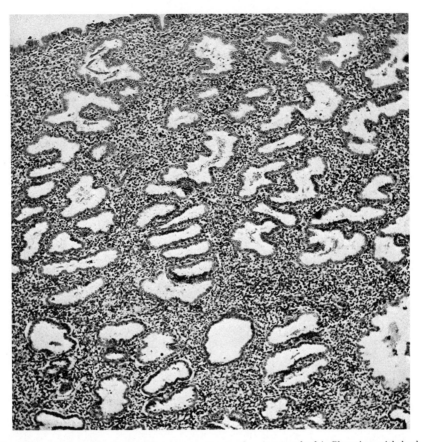

3.9. Endometrium from patient just about to menstruate showing marked infiltration with leukocytes and wandering cells.

In this phase one can distinguish the same three layers which one sees even more sharply delimited in the young decidua. The uppermost layer is compact in appearance, consisting of broad fields of hypertrophied stromal cells between the rather narrow necks of the glands. It is called the *stratum compactum*. The *stratum spongiosum* (middle zone) presents a lacy, labyrinthine appearance because of the preponderance of dilated and tortuous glands, with very little intervening stroma. Finally, the deepest layer (*basalis*) in contact with and often penetrating the muscularis for short distances is made up of the growing tips of the glands, with a dense, compact stroma surrounding them. Because it is composed of an immature refractory tissue it may exhibit only a proliferative pattern even in the premenstrual phase of the cycle, in as much as this undifferentiated endometrium has not acquired the ability to respond to progesterone despite a biphasic cycle.

The compacta and spongiosa together make up the portion of the endometrium chiefly participating in the cyclical phenomena of menstruation, so that together they comprise the so-called *functional* zone. The basalis, on the other hand, is the layer responsible for growth and regeneration of the endometrium.

It is not uncommon to find even large areas of unripe endometrium, often showing the Swiss cheese pattern of hyperplasia (see Chapter 14) in endometria which otherwise are typically secretory or progestational in character. It is apparent that curettings from such a uterus would show a mixture of secretory and unripe endometrium, constituting the so-called *mixed endometrium.* Such localized areas of unripe or hyperplastic endometrium seem to produce no such menstrual excess as is so often seen in association with diffuse Swiss cheese hyperplasia of the endometrium.

Differential staining in the progestational phase reveals increasing quantities of *glycogen,* the first appearance of which, in the form of small intracellular granules, is noted immediately after ovulation, but which in the progestational phase are much more richly distributed, not only within the cells but also in the gland lumina. Quantitative studies on this point have been made by a number of investigators who conclude that *mucin* is also present but appears to be independent of hormonal influence and is found, not in the cells, but only in the gland lumina or in the uterine cavity.

The blood vessels of the endometrium are most conspicuous in the premenstrual phase, and this applies especially to the coiled or spiral arterioles, which are best seen in the lower and middle zones of the endometrium. The relationship of prostaglandin to the blood vessels has been discussed in the preceding chapter.

Degenerative changes make their appearance in the endometrium well before the onset of menstrual bleeding. The immediately premenstrual phase is characterized especially by a rather massive infiltration by polymorphonuclear and mononuclear leukocytes, producing a *pseudoinflammatory* appearance. The staining reaction of the upper layer becomes impaired, suggesting their impending dissolution.

Menstrual or Bleeding Phase (Figs. 3. 10–14)

On the first day of the period the tissue loss is quite patchy and only slight and fragmentary. The factor responsible for both the death of tissue and the bleeding is the ischemia produced by the prolonged

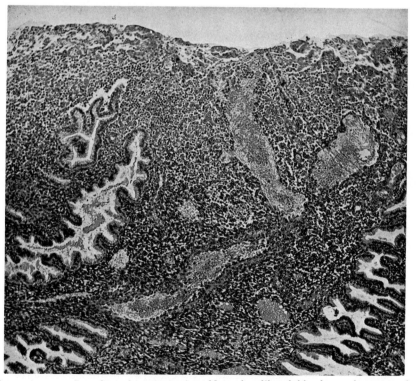

3.10. Endometrium on first day of menstruation. Note the dilated blood vessels, some of which are opening directly on the surface. There is marked infiltration of the upper layers, and small particles of the surface are being cast off. There are considerable differences in the degree of tissue loss on the first day.

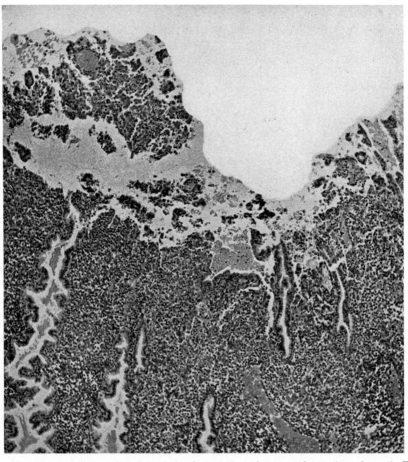

3.11. More extensive crumbling of surface at another portion of same endometrium shown in Figure 3.10.

and intense vasoconstriction of the coiled arterioles as described in Chapter 2. Page pointed out over a decade ago that fibrinolytic activity is increased in the premenstrual and menstrual phases of the cycle and may be related to endometrial desquamation and the fluidity of menstrual blood.

The area supplied by each of these vessels exhibits its own individual degenerative and bleeding changes, and the sum total of many such localized phenomena produces the composite changes characterizing menstruation. Because of the constrictive occlusion of the arterioles, the blood from the endometrial veins backs up into the venules and capillaries, and many of these venous channels rupture, so that small lakes of blood are produced which often cause the

appearance of subepithelial hematomas. Strips of tissue are cast off in scattered areas as the process advances, whereas bleeding increases not only as a result of actual rupture of blood vessels but also from increased permeability of the blood vessel walls.

By the second day of bleeding the tissue loss is extensive, practically the entire surface being denuded. There is much individual difference in the amount of endometrium thrown off, but as a rule the entire compacta and a considerable portion of the spongiosa are lost, although the deeper portions of the latter are left behind.

Even while desquamation is still proceeding, evidences of *regeneration* of the surface are usually apparent. This takes place from the epithelium of the

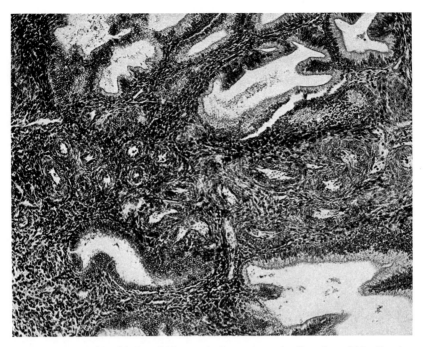

3.12. Photomicrograph of a buckled, coiled, or spiral artery on the first day of bleeding in an ovulatory cycle (monkey). (From Markee, J. E.: Contrib. Embryol., *28:* 219, 1940.)

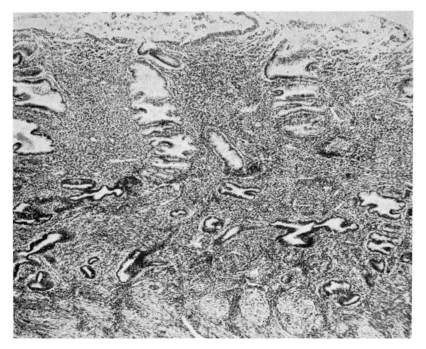

3.13. Endometrium at end of menstruation showing epithelialization of surface by outgrowth of epithelium from stumps of glands.

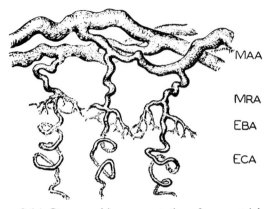

3.14. Stereographic representation of myometrial and endometrial groups of arteries in the Macaque monkey. Above are shown parts of myometrial arcuate arteries (*MAA*) from which proceed myometrial radial arteries (*MRA*) toward the endometrium, in which two types of arteries are found: the larger endometrial coiled arteries (*ECA*) and the smaller endometrial basal arteries (*EBA*). (From Okkels, H., and Engle, E. T.: Acta Path. Microbiol. Scand., *15:* 150, 1938.)

gland stumps in the basalis and the shrunken retracted portions of compacta which may remain. The surface is restored with amazing rapidity, apparently by a process of amitotic division of cells, as nuclear figures are not seen. Baggish *et al.* indicate that the superficial stromal cells may actually undergo metaplasia into epithelium. The regeneration of the endometrium is so rapid that if a uterus, removed immediately after the cessation of the flow, is examined, the surface is complete.

The Endometrium of Pregnancy (Decidua)

In the event of pregnancy the hypertrophic and secretory changes of the pregravid phase become even more marked, so that there is an insensible transition between the premenstrual picture in the nonpregnant and the very early decidua of the pregnant woman. In fact, it is not always easy to make the distinction in the laboratory unless embryonic elements, such as villi or trophoblast are present in the section. The *glands* of the decidua present marked sawtooth convolution and scalloping, and

the *epithelium* is low, pale staining, and actively secretory. At a little later stage the tortuosity of the glands is much less and the epithelium becomes very flat, so that there may be difficulty in distinguishing the glands from lymphatics or venules.

The *stromal* cells become large and polygonal, with a wide zone of cytoplasm surrounding the nucleus. They now constitute the characteristic *decidual cells,* and are arranged in mosaic or tile-like fashion, occurring in large fields in the superficial or compact layer of the endometrium, where the gland elements are sparsest. In the middle or spongy zone (Fig. 3.15), on the other hand, the hypertrophy and convolution of the glands are most pronounced, and the interglandular septa are thin and delicate, so that an intricate lacy pattern is produced.

In certain cases of pregnancy, both intrauterine and extrauterine, the endometrium exhibits an intensely adenomatous, hypersecretory response with the cells lining the glands mimicking malignant cells by marked mitotic activity, hy-

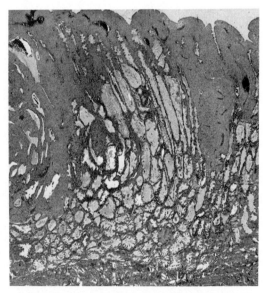

3.15. Decidua of early pregnancy showing the superficial compact zone in contrast with the spongy middle portion. The basalis is not well shown in this field.

perchromatic nuclei, and bizarre abnormal cell types. This *Arias-Stella* reaction is further described and depicted in Chapter 26. Finally, the basalis stands out in even sharper contrast with the upper layers of the endometrium than in the nonpregnant woman, the tips of the glands being lined by a cuboidal non-secretory type of epithelium quite different from that in the upper reaches of the gland.

Progesterone Therapy

In recent years there has ensued a widespread tendency to utilize various progestogens, combined or sequential, in treating bleeding problems, endometriosis, dysmenorrhea, etc., as well as providing contraception. That it is effective in many instances seems apparent; whether it should completely replace the infinitely cheaper stilbestrol is controversial, although it is admittedly more physiological if often no more effective. Nevertheless, it is important to become familiar with the appearance of the endometrium that has been subjected to prolonged progesterone therapy.

There is a striking conversion of the endometrial stroma into typical decidual cells (Fig. 3.16) with simultaneous suppression of the glandular components so that these undergo almost complete exhaustion. This "glandular atrophy" is much more striking with the combined than with sequential hormones. It is apparent that progesterone affects only the functional zone of the endometrium, with the basal layer of the endometrium exhibiting only an estrogen response.

Clomiphene Therapy

In past years there was no hormone or chemical agent that was really instrumental in inducing ovulation, but today there are at least two, clomiphene citrate (Clomid) and various combinations of gonadotrophins; as well as luteinizing hormone-release factor (LRF). A fuller discussion of all these agents will be found in subsequent chapters of this text. Clomiphene, however, is available to all physicians, and it may be fitting to simply

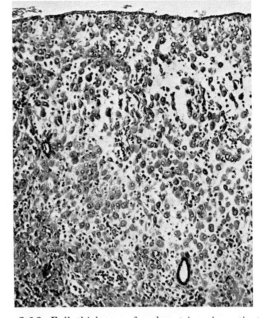

3.16. Full thickness of endometrium in patient treated by prolonged continuous progesterone. There is almost complete absence of glands along with marked edema of the decidualized stroma. Changes are less pronounced in the lower (basal) portion.

mention what its action may be on the endometrium, for this pathological information is of considerable importance to the clinician.

Ovulation may occur after an appropriate course of clomiphene, as manifested by temperature charts, and progestational changes may be found in the endometrium. In our experience, however, after seeing many biopsies of clomiphene-stimulated endometrium, there might be considerable difficulty in interpreting the approximate temporal status of the tissue. The stromal cells may show an advanced progesterone effect with a marked decidua-like pattern. On the other hand, the glands seem to "lag behind" with only such early evidence of ovulation as subnuclear vacuoles in mildly tortuous glands (Fig. 3.17). This sequential disparity between glands and stroma has been a relatively constant feature in these clomiphene-treated patients; we have seen insufficient en-

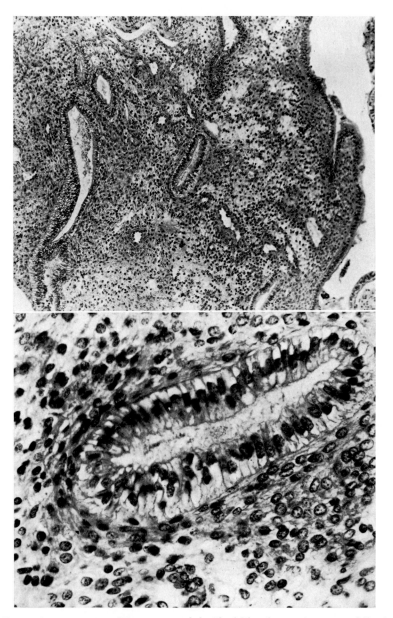

3.17. (*top*) Postovulatory pattern with pronounced decidual-like changes in stroma following clomiphene therapy. (*bottom*) High power of gland showing prominent vacuoles, but little tufting and budding. Clomiphene-induced changes seem less advanced in glands than in stroma. (From *Novak's Gynecologic and Obstetric Pathology*, 7th Ed., W. B. Saunders Co., Philadelphia, 1974.)

dometria in women treated by gonadotrophins to know if the same pattern is present.

Although the precise mechanism of clomiphene is unexplained, its action would seem to be at the hypothalamic-pituitary level as an anti-estrogenic agent. The usual dosage of 50–100 mg for 5–7 days may be increased with ovulation occurring 7–10 days after beginning therapy. Ovarian overstimulation with as many as 14 corpora lutea and massive ascites has been recorded by Scommegna and Lash. Multiple pregnancy is common.

The Senile Endometrium

After the menopause the endometrium may undergo shrinkage, becoming thin and atrophic. This is what one would expect from the withdrawal of the estrogenic hormone which supplies the normal growth stimulus to the genital mucosa. The surface epithelium becomes lower, whereas the glands are narrow and sparsely distributed in the stroma, which with increasing years assumes a more and more fibrotic appearance (Fig. 3.18). The thinned out atrophic mucosa is prone to superficial punctate ulceration and infection, resulting in the so-called *senile endometritis,* a not infrequent lesion which is of importance because it sometimes produces postmenopausal bleeding which calls for diagnostic differentiation from that produced by adenocarcinoma of the uterus. However, atrophic vaginitis rarely co-exists with adenocarcinoma which is characterized by a well supported mucosa and a shift to the right in the maturation index (MI).

Although the atrophic changes described above are common, it must be remembered that for a considerable time after the last menstruation, the endometrium may show little atrophy and it may actually present a hyperplastic appearance (Fig. 3.19). In other words, the disappearance of an estrogen influence is not always abrupt, and we know now that even after complete cessation of menstrual function, estrogen may still be produced by some ovarian or extragenital source, most likely the adrenal cortex.

It is not surprising, therefore, that even many years after the menopause one may at times find a typical hyperplasia of the endometrium, sometimes in a very active phase, sometimes retrogressive (Fig. 3.20). These variations are more fully described in the discussion of "Hyperplasia of the Endometrium" (Chapter 14).

Histochemical Studies of the Endometrium

It is becoming increasingly apparent to all gynecological pathologists that study of hematoxylin-eosin preparations is often

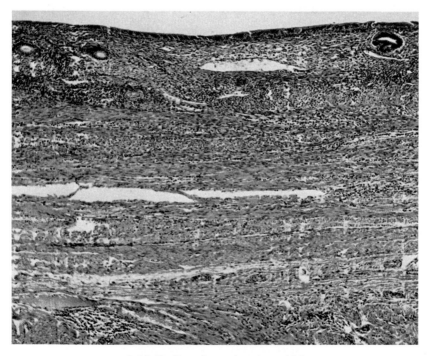

3.18. Senile endometrium (atrophic)

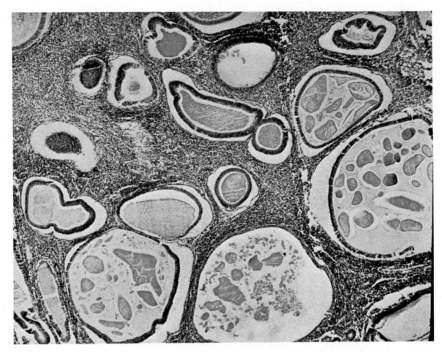

3.19. Hyperplasia of endometrium in patient 87 years old

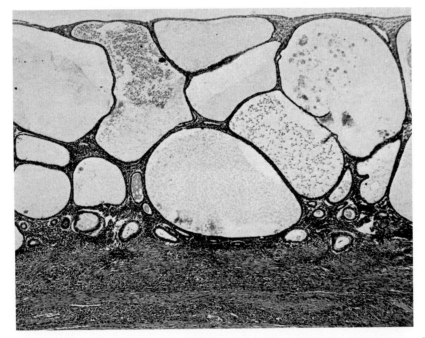

3.20. Cystic enlargement of glands in senile endometrium (patient aged 57), a persistence of the Swiss cheese pattern of hyperplasia, but of inactive or retrogressive type.

insufficient for adequate distinction and evaluation of tissues. Consideration of their various biochemical properties is often necessary along with differential stains capable of detecting certain histochemical characteristics.

Appropriate techniques have led to determination of a great many important metabolites at various stages of the menstrual cycle. Because these sequential changes involve glands, stroma, lining epithelium, and the blood vessels in differential fashion, it would seem unwise to attempt a complete discussion of the many phases of histochemistry. Instead the interested reader is referred to the studies of McKay (with various coworkers), Atkinson and Gusberg, and Boutbelis, DeNeet, Ullery, and George. The striking color plates of the last authors illustrate more vividly than words the precise results of their studies.

It would appear that the *proliferative* (estrogen-influenced) stage of the cycle is characterized by increased activity in alkaline phosphatase, β-glucoronidase, ribonucleic acid (RNA), and reduced triphosphopyridine nucleotide (TPNH). In the *secretory* phase (progesterone plus estrogen) there is an increased formation of acid phosphatase, glycogen, glycoproteins, lipids, reduced diphosphopyridine nucleotide (DPNH) and certain dehydrogenases, lactic (LDH) and succinic (SDH) acids. All of these enzymes have specific roles in the metabolism and reaction to the ovarian steroids.

Study of abnormal endometria by McKay suggests that postmenopausal atrophy showed a general decrease in the histochemical activity of the epithelial cells. Cystic hyperplasia surprisingly showed similar inactive properties, although there was extreme variability. On the other hand, adenocarcinoma, even of the incipient variety, showed histochemical similarities to a progestational endometrium, which may be somewhat surprising to those who believe in a frequent although not inevitable association with estrogen stimulation. Atkinson and Gusberg have also carried out determination of alkaline phosphatase in abnormal endometria, and their studies indicate variations compatible with an estrogen effect. Levine feels that undifferentiated tumors show a decreased alkaline phosphate and suggest an increasing inability to produce alkaline phosphatase as the malignancy progresses.

On the other hand, Atkinson and Hall state that glycogen study in endometrial adenocarcinoma show results similar to a normal secretory endometrium. Since β-glucoronidase activity is high with estrogen stimulation, but decreases after ovulation, determination of this in the woman with corpus cancer might help to pinpoint any specific endocrine influence.

It is impossible to become involved in all of the ramifications of histochemical and biochemical study of cell metabolism in this text. It is one of the most dynamic but constantly changing facets of our specialty, and we have attempted to mention only a few of the many articles pertaining to it. Unfortunately, there has been relatively little new that has truly advanced our knowledge of the endometrial behavior, although the studies by Roddick *et al.* and Gross deserve some mention.

Cervical Mucosa

Like the endometrium, the endocervix is of Müllerian origin, and it would seem quite certain that it must show some sort of cyclical response to the ovarian hormones. One of the most complete studies thus far made is that of Sjövall, who concluded that the cervical epithelium, under the influence of the ovarian estrogenic hormone, increases in height until after ovulation, becoming lower and increasingly secretory thereafter under the influence of the progesterone then operative. The glands become increasingly large and tortuous, but no evidence of menstrual desquamation is found. Topkins has not been impressed by cervical cyclic changes although cytopathological smears indicate that some type of cycle undoubtedly exists in the lower genital tract. Study of the cervical mucus is of importance in the study of infertility.

Crystallization of Cervical Mucus. Papanicolaou in 1946 first pointed out that cervical mucus, if spread on a slide and allowed to dry, forms *fernlike crystals,* which he associated with estrogen activity and the changes thus produced in the viscosity of the mucus. The phenomenon has excited a good deal of interest. In one of the early papers on the subject Rydberg expressed the opinion that the crystals are due to the presence of sodium chloride, this form being influenced by the mucin components of the secretion. Campos da Paz found that progesterone inhibits this crystallization process, so that it is not

surprising that this "palm leaf" (PL) reaction has been suggested as a test for various functional disorders, and even the early diagnosis of pregnancy. There are, however, a good many authors who are skeptical as to its value. In their evaluation of the test, Zondek and Rozin expressed the belief that it can for some indications replace endometrial biopsy, as, for example, in the differentiation of ovulatory from anovulatory cycles. At the present writing it would seem to us that the PL test can scarcely be recommended over the more clearly established techniques, such as cytological study and endometrial biopsy. (Chapter 29)

Pregnancy Changes in Cervix. It is apparent that the *endocervical glands increase strikingly in size and tortuosity*

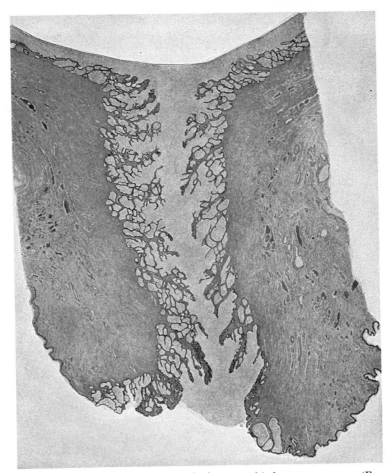

3.21. Section of cervix late in pregnancy showing the hypertrophied, spongy mucosa. (From Stander, H. J. (Editor): *Williams' Obstetrics.* D. Appleton-Century Company, New York, 1941.)

in pregnancy, producing a lacy adenomatous pattern of the thickened mucosa (Fig. 3.21). Similar but more striking changes mimicking adenocarcinoma, although reversible, may be produced by contraceptive pills (Graham *et al.*). Microcystic mucoid metaplasia is frequent.

There have been numerous reports of *decidual changes* in the cervix, so that the occurrence is not longer considered rare. Estimates as to the frequency vary greatly, but Epperson and his co-workers, on the basis of a large series of cervical biopsies in pregnant women, found an incidence of 10.4 per cent. Sometimes the decidual change occurs in the form of small patches, but often large fields of typical decidual cells are observed, as in Figure 3.22. The decidual change is limited to the stromal elements, so that it would be illogical to assume that the decidua is merely a pregnancy response of a preceding cervical endometriosis. For some reason the cervical stromal elements of such cervices show a sensitivity to the pregnancy hormones, as may connective tissue elements in the ovary and pelvic peritoneum in the fairly frequent instances of ectopic decidua, of which cervical deciduosis must be considered a form.

It is the changes in the *squamous epithelium of the pars vaginalis* which show atypicality approaching that seen with *in situ* carcinoma. Current opinion, however, as influenced by the studies of Greene and Peckham, would indicate that if the pattern of intraepithelial cancer unfolds during pregnancy, it is the real entity and not a mere artifact caused by the pregnancy.

It is vital that the extent of cervical atypia be clarified even though the patient may be pregnant. Nesbitt has emphasized that observations of the cervical epithelium should be more frequent in the gravid woman, and some 15 to 20 per cent of the everted infected endocervices often seen in pregnancy will show microscopic evidence of a hyperactive surface epithelium. This will generally regress following termination of the pregnancy, but may persist postpartum. A small percentage of women (less than 5 per cent) will manifest marked degrees of cervical dysplasia as evidenced by cytopathological determination and confirmed by biopsy.

It is important in certain equivocal cases to exclude the presence of intraepithelial cancer which may of course co-exist in conjunction with the more marked degrees of atypical epithelium (see Chapter 12). On occasion conization of the cervix during pregnancy may be necessary, and although certain authors speak very blithely of this "minor procedure," to us it is a potentially for-

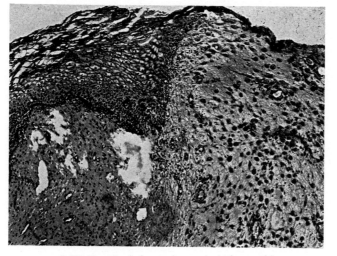

3.22. Decidual change in cervix (4th month)

midable operation. The later trimesters of pregnancy give rise to a large hyperemic cervix, and even though hemostatic sutures are applied, bleeding can be rather profuse. Although required on occasion, when invasive carcinoma is suspected, this procedure may frequently be replaced by *directed colposcopic biopsy.* It should be understood that most cases of mild cervical atypia are not extreme, are reversible, and need only repeat cytopathological study. Only a few are sufficiently abnormal to warrant biopsy, and only a proportion of these require conization; yet this should not be deferred if there is any possibility of invasive cervical malignancy.

CYCLICAL CHANGES IN THE OVARY

Following menstruation a number of follicles begin to mature in the ovary, but, with rare exceptions, only one of these undergoes full maturation, as evidenced by ovulation. The remainder of the follicles are blighted at various phases of development, through the process known as *atresia folliculi.* The process of maturation of the follicle from its early primordial phase (Fig. 3.23) to that of the full development which is attained just before ovulation is characterized by the following chief features.

(*a*) The originally flat follicular epithelium or *membrana granulosa* becomes cuboidal, with later stratification and multiplication of cells, so that at maturity it consists of several layers. The *granulosa* possesses no blood vessels of its own, receiving its nutrition from the *theca interna;* after ovulation the thecal blood vessels grow into the granulosa layer.

(*b*) The ovum becomes embedded in a well marked peninsula of granulosa cells, the *cumulus oophorus* (Fig. 3.24) or *discus proligerus.* Call-Exner bodies (small folliculoid areas resulting from cystic degeneration with a surrounding rosette of granulosa cells) are frequent, as they are in certain granulosa cell tumors (Chapter 24).

(*c*) The follicle develops a central cavity or *antrum* filled with a clear fluid or *liquor folliculi.*

(*d*) The *theca interna* (Fig. 3-25), at first poorly developed, becomes a conspicuous zone, the cells of which, as maturity is approached, become large and polyhedral, with abundant lipoid content, presumably going to the nutrition of the nonvascular granulosal layer.

The fully mature follicle, as shown in Figures 3.26 and 3.27, consists of the following layers, from without inward.

(*a*) The *theca externa,* a layer of

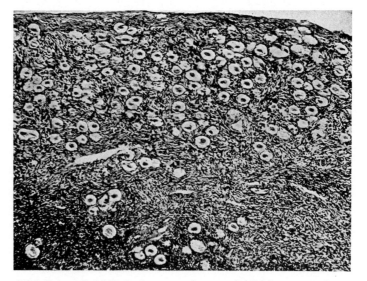

3.23. Primordial follicles in cortex of ovary of child four years of age

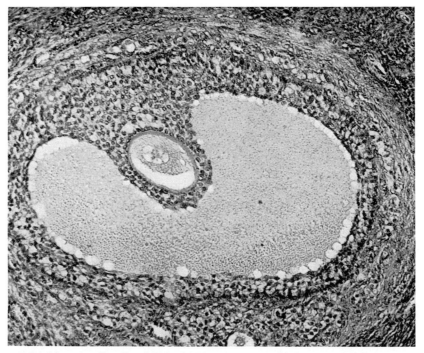

3.24. Maturing Graafian follicle showing ovum embedded in cumulus oophorus

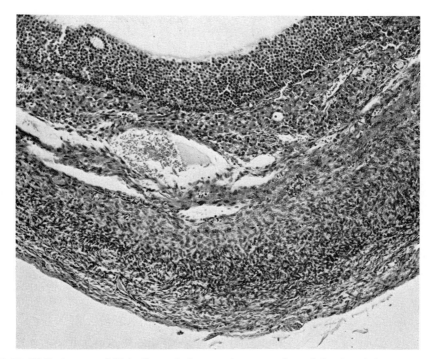

3.25. Wall of mature follicle. Beneath the granulosa, note the well developed theca interna.

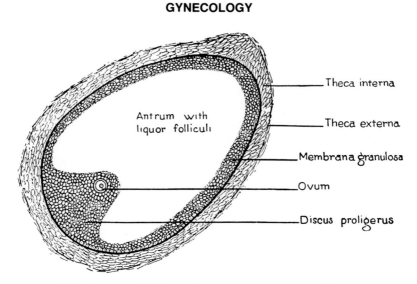

3.26. Diagram of chief constituent elements of mature follicle

condensed ovarian tissue merging imperceptibly with the stroma.

(*b*) The *theca interna,* as above
described. It has been established that
these are the cells which are responsible
for estrogen production, and the granulosa
are more concerned with progesterone
formation.

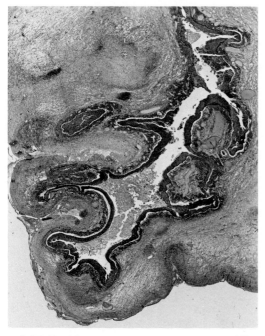

3.27. Freshly ruptured follicle showing crumbling
of wall.

(*c*) The *membrana granulosa.*

(*d*) The central cavity or *antrum,* filled
with the liquor folliculi.

(*e*) The *cumulus oophorus* or *discus
proligerus.*

(*f*) The *corona radiata,* the layer of cells
of the discus immediately surrounding the
egg, and arranged in radial fashion.

(*g*) The *zona pellucida,* a thin,
refractile, amorphous zone just within the
corona radiata.

The rupture of the follicle is attended
by extrusion of the egg and, with it, of the
zona pellucida, corona radiata, and a
considerable number of the cells of the
cumulus. No one but a pathologist will
understand the extreme difficulty in distinguishing between a mature follicle and
an early corpus luteum, because the
lutein changes in granulosa and theca
cells are not abrupt but very gradual in
their evolution. The collapse of the follicle
(Fig. 3.27) with the subsequent crumbled
festooned pattern is probably the most reliable index of ovulation.

Metabolic studies suggest that the
granulosa cells which convert to true lutein
cells lack 17α-hydroxylase, so that the
biosynthetic pathway cannot progress beyond progesterone. Theca cells, currently
presumed to be estrogenic, apparently
contain this enzyme, allowing further metabolism to estrogen production. The
absence of blood vessels in the preovula-

tory granulosa layer of the follicle suggests that progesterone manufactured by these, passes through the theca zone to be excreted as estrogen; when there is a direct (postovulation) vascular supply the luteinized granulosa cells secrete progesterone into the circulation unchanged.

Strassman has shown that the theca interna forms a wedgelike cone directed toward the surface of the ovary and thus playing an important mechanical role in ovulation. The cavity collapses with the escape of the follicular fluid, and the second or *corpus luteum phase* of development now begins, reaching its maximum several days before the onset of the next menstrual period. It should be stressed, however, that the corpus luteum is only a modified follicle, and an exact line of demarcation is histologically impossible. For purposes of description, its life cycle can be divided into the following stages, according to the plan originally suggested by Meyer.

(*a*) The stage of *proliferation* immediately following rupture of the follicle. As might be expected, therefore, the wall of the corpus luteum in its earliest stage is identical with that of the fully mature follicle. The granulosal layer, however, soon shows evidence of beginning transformation into the large, polyhedral, often vacuolated cells known as lutein cells (Figs. 3.28, 29). Between the granulosa and theca there is a zone of

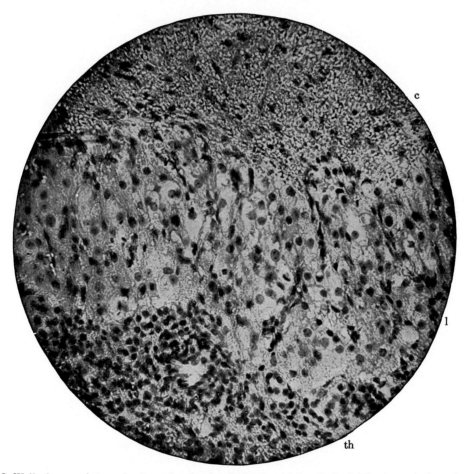

3.28. Wall of corpus luteum in stage of early vascularization (sixteenth day). Blood vessels from the theca are pushing into the granulosa layer (*l*) which now shows definite lutein characteristics. The theca cells (*th*) have undergone retrogression. The blood now in the cavity (*c*) is beginning to be invaded by endothelial cells. (From *Novak's Gynecologic and Obstetric Pathology*, 7th ed., W. B. Saunders Co., 1974.)

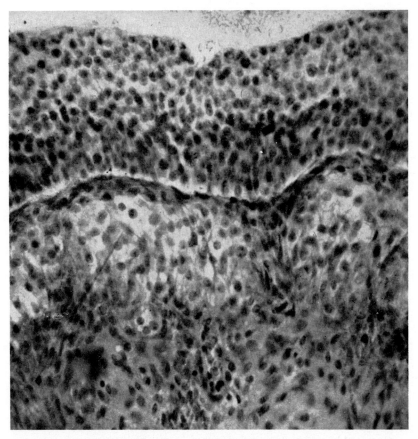

3.29. Higher power of wall of early corpus luteum

blood vessels known as the perigranulosal vascular wreath.

Grossly the corpus luteum in this early stage is a very inconspicuous structure, its thin wall being crenated and folded on itself because of shrinkage of the cavity. There is no such festooning of the wall as is seen in later stages, and its color is a grayish yellow instead of the bright carroty yellow of late stages.

(b) The stage of *vascularization* (Fig. 3.30). This phase is so designated because its chief characteristic is an invasion of the layer of now definite lutein cells by blood vessels from the theca. These channels extend to the very lumen, and hemorrhage into the latter is a normal feature of this phase. Characteristically it is of limited amount, the blood forming a zone along the lumen edge of the lutein zone. At times, however, the cavity may be distended with blood. The theca interna has

undergone retrogressive changes, its cells having shrunken through disappearance of the rich lipoid content of the earlier phase.

Grossly, the corpus luteum is now a rather large structure of hemorrhagic appearance. It may measure 10 or 12 mm. in diameter, and is usually recognizable on the surface of the ovary, where it often forms a slight mound. On section the bright yellow lutein zone is seen to be fairly wide and moderately festooned, its color contrasting sharply with the blood which is present in the lumen.

(c) The stage of *maturity,* which parallels the progestational phase in the endometrium. The broad yellow lutein zone is thrown into festoon-like bunting, the color being due to the presence of the pigment carotene. The theca pushes down into the lutein zone in wedgelike septa which divide the lutein into broad folds and alveoli. The cells of the theca themselves often show luteinization, constituting the theca lutein or paralutein cells (Fig. 3.31), although these are always much smaller than the granulosa lutein cell. Along the inner edge of the lutein zone a layer of fibroblastic tissue appears to shut off the lutein cells from the cavity. The latter contains a varying amount of fluid, including usually unresorbed blood elements from the preceding stage.

The gross appearance of a mature corpus luteum is not always the same, nor is its size, which varies from 10 to 20 mm. in diameter. Its yellowish color can often be seen shimmering through the surface of the ovary, above which it may project as a more or less conspicuous mound, at times actually polypoid. In other cases the corpus may seem to lie beneath the surface, being revealed only by cutting into the ovary. The cavity may be small, with only a scant amount of fluid, or it may be very large and distended with a yellowish liquid.

(d) The stage of retrogression (Fig. 3.32). The maximal development of the corpus luteum is attained, not a day or two before the onset of menstruation, as was formerly believed, but probably as early as the fourth to the sixth day before the appearance of menstrual bleeding. This has been well established by the study of Brewer on this subject. The retrogression of the corpus is marked by fatty degeneration, fibrosis, and later by hyalinization of the lutein zone, with increase of the cicatricial tissue within the cavity. The yellowish color may persist for a long time, even several months, but ultimately it disappears.

The end product is the corpus albicans (Fig. 3.33) appearing as a whitish, hyalinized, convoluted structure which slowly decreases in size. Its morphology has been discussed by Joel and Foraker. It is not difficult to "date" the corpus luteum of the present cycle; to ascertain whether it is 2 or 6 months old may be more of a problem.

Although as a rule only one follicle each month reaches full maturation, many others advance to various stages of incomplete maturation and then are blighted (atresia folliculi). The ovum dies, and this is followed by degeneration and later

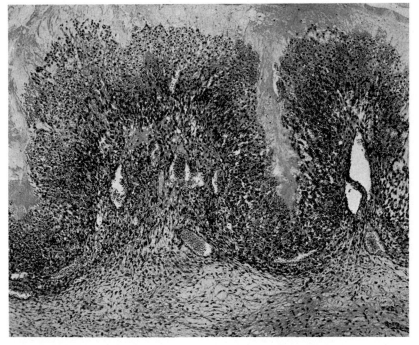

3.30. Corpus luteum in stage of vascularization

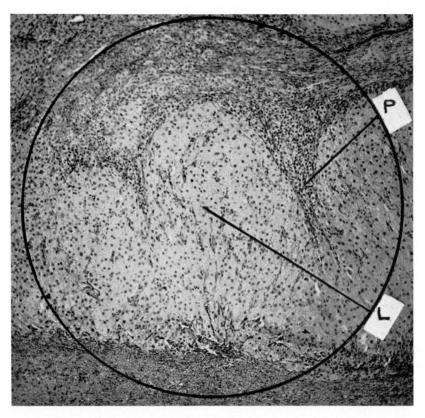

3.31. Wall of mature corpus luteum (27th day). Showing lutein (*L*) and theca-lutein or paralutein (*P*) cells. The latter are not always so well marked.

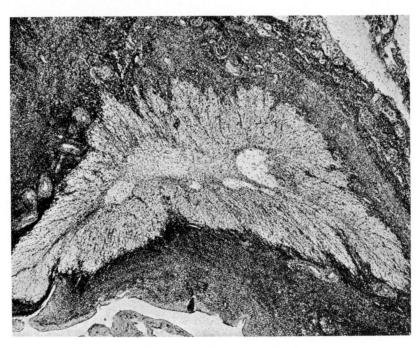

3.32. Retrogressive corpus luteum

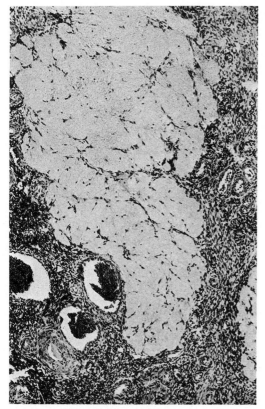

3.33. Corpus albicans

stages of the cycle, and their preliminary work has provided a firm background for much of the recent application of biosynthetic properties. Their contributions were concerned primarily with the close association of alkaline phosphatase and steroid activity, at the same time indicating certain histochemical similarities and differences between various steroid-producing cells. The observations seemed to indicate certain enzyme deficiencies as a probable cause of abnormal steroid function.

Their visionary work has been enlarged on by many biochemists who have pointed out certain biosynthetic pathways to the formation of the various ovarian hormones. Unquestionably, the generally accepted scheme is that proposed by Smith and Ryan (see Fig. 3.34). From cholesterol (derived from acetate) there are two alternate pathways (via pregnenolone or progesterone) by which testosterone may be produced. There is very possibly an equilibrium between this and the estrogenic hormones which may vary in certain physiological and neoplastic disorders. Kase and Conrad have suggested that in most cases of estrogen and androgen formation, the "progesterone route" is bypassed with production of the end products occuring via pregnenolone.

Hence, knowing the probable pathways to steroid formation it is possible to incubate fresh frozen tissue with different substrates, and by utilizing an indicator dye, to detect certain enzymes deemed essential in steroidogenesis. As indicated in Figure 3.34, steroid 3β-ol-dehydrogenase is an enzyme whose action is necessary for many important steps in steroid formation. By utilizing a number of substrates, this and other similar enzyme systems can be demonstrated, and hormone-producing cells can thus be demonstrated, although complete specificity is uncertain.

A comparison of normal ovaries and testes, and abnormal gonads permits a semi-quantitative estimate of the enzymatic reaction of certain component cells, and we have utilized these to study potential hormone action in various normal and abnormal conditions. Many

disappearance of the granulosa, with not infrequently distention of the cavity with fluid. Such small follicular cysts are found in all normal ovaries during reproductive life, but under some conditions, such as chronic pelvic inflammatory disease, they may be so numerous that they produce the so-called "cystic ovary." The process of atresia is also exaggerated during pregnancy.

The cystic stage is followed by cicatricial obliteration proceeding slowly from the periphery toward the center (obliterative phase). The end result is the *corpus fibrosum,* a convoluted zone of hyalinized tissue surrounding a small central cicatrix. Its much smaller size and the narrow and usually less hyalinized fibrous wall make it easy to distinguish the corpus fibrosum from the corpus albicans.

Histochemical Study of the Ovary

McKay *et al.* have performed extensive histochemical studies on the ovary at all

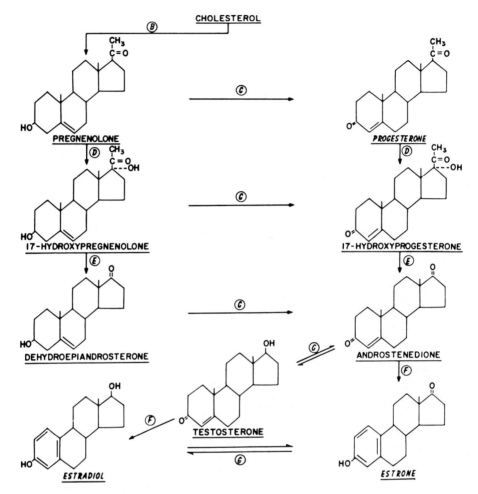

3.34. Pathway of steriod biosynthesis in the ovary. *Step C* is dependent on steroid 3β-ol-dehydrogenase plus isomerase. (From Smith, O. W., and Ryan, K. J.: Amer. J. Obstet. Gynec., *84:* 141, 1962.)

previous authors have employed these methods in studying ovarian tumors, and the usual techniques utilized have been reviewed recently by Goldberg *et al.* Similar observations have been made on various virilizing neoplasms such as Brenner tumor (Ullery *et al.*), Krukenberg tumor (Ober *et al.*), and others as reported by Scully and Cohen. The latter have published a recent comprehensive summation of the behavior of ovarian stromal cells which are enzymatically active and are referred to as "enzymatically active stromal cells." These are closely related if not identical to the luteinized thecal stromal cell. Deane, Lobel, and Romney have also provided excellent references to histochemical study of cellular biosynthesis; Dorfman points out the probability that many other unknown biosynthetic pathways to steroids probably exist.

By utilizing various substrates and determining the reaction exhibited by normal cells of the testis and ovary, it is then possible by a comparative study to determine enzyme activity related to steroidogenesis in certain equivocal cells in ovarian tumors or dysfunctions. For example, it has been shown possible to demonstrate considerable activity in many postmenopausal ovaries, and the cells in which steroidogenesis is strongly suggested by the enzymatic activity are the hilus cell and the so-called "luteinized thecal stromal" cell, although the latter seems to show certain striking differences from the theca cell of the normal follicle (Novak *et al.*).

It is currently impossible to conclude whether any demonstrated enzymatic activity is indicative of estrogen and androgens, but it is probably only a matter of time before specific distinction can be made between the C_{19} and C_{18} steroids. However, many histochemical studies would seem to suggest that the postmenopausal ovary produces an androgenic steroid which may be converted to an estrogen at another area such as the skin, striated muscle, or adrenal (Plotz). Mattingly and Huang believe that the postmenopausal ovary produces androgenic steroids but minimal estrogen presumably due to absence of follicles. Study from our own laboratory has correlated

histochemical activity with clinical data in pointing out that certain "nonendocrine" types of tumors are not infrequently associated with steroid activity, and such observations strongly suggest the possible importance of the stromal cells of the tumor matrix. Leventhal and Scommegna have likewise contributed an excellent publication on histochemical techniques in evaluating possible steroidal function in a variety of tumors and abnormal conditions.

Corpus Luteum of Pregnancy

In the event of fertilization of the egg, the corpus luteum does not undergo retrogression, but continues to develop, becoming considerably larger than the corpus luteum of menstruation, and comprising sometimes one-third or even one-half of the ovarian volume. The large size is often due to cystic distention, but

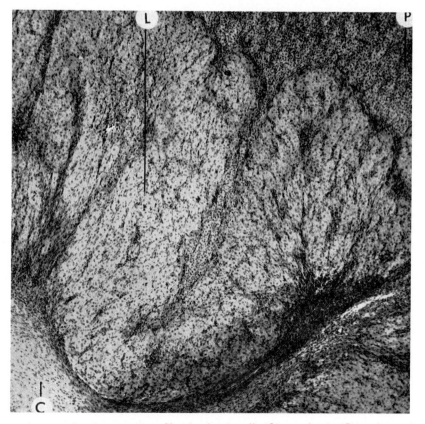

3.35. Corpus luteum of early pregnancy. Showing lutein cells (*L*), paralutein (*P*), and organization along inner wall to lutein layer (*C*).

there is considerable variation in this respect, some corpora lutea of pregnancy being of rather solid structure. The lutein cells are large and tilelike in appearance, and paralutein cells are often conspicuous (Fig. 3.35). The maximum of histological development is reached at about 10 to 12 weeks. *Chorionic gonadotrophin* (HCG) maintains the corpus luteum which produces sufficient estrogen and progesterone to inhibit further ovulation, and it is the gonadotrophin which is utilized for the different pregnancy tests. By 10–12 weeks, the placenta acquires the capability of progesterone and estrogen excretion, and there is regression of the corpus luteum as well as a decreased level of HCG (see Chapter 2).

Fraenkel's early work on the function of the rabbit corpus luteum in pregnancy led him to conclude that the removal of this structure in the early stages of pregnancy invariably results in abortion. The results of his studies were erroneously applied to humans, for it has now been abundantly shown that early removal of the corpus luteum does not usually lead to abortion in women. Collective study of cases of corpus luteum removed in early pregnancy showed an abortion rate of approximately 20%.

Since the procedure is apparently not wholly devoid of risk of terminating pregnancy, the majority of surgeons still prefer to defer the removal of apparently benign ovarian tumors, when discovered in the pregnant woman, until after the first trimester, unless some such complication as torsion of the pedicle makes the indication for operation seem more imperative. By the same token, most surgeons follow such operations in early pregnancy with progesterone substitutional therapy, but, with some skepticism as to its value; there is no doubt that this would not always be essential.

Other Pregnancy Changes in the Ovary

Aside from the presence of the *corpus luteum* of pregnancy, the following histological changes may be noted in the ovaries during pregnancy.

(1) An inhibition of follicle maturation, and the presence of an increased number of atretic follicles. Govan has reported that new follicles develop after 11 and up to 20 weeks, which is about the time when the gonadotrophic level begins to decline. The significance of this observation is not fully understood.

(2) Toward the end of pregnancy, the theca interna cells of atretic follicles often undergo extensive luteinization, sometimes forming large fields which invade the ovarian stroma. Such accumulations were formerly often spoken of as the interstitial gland of pregnancy, the constituent "interstitial" cells being believed by some to be the analogues of the interstitial cells of the testis.

(3) In a considerable portion of cases the ovarian surface shows the presence of ectopic decidual cells, appearing grossly as light pinkish gray deposits of fluffy tissue, as seen in many cases at cesarean section.

REFERENCES

Atkinson, W. B., Engle, E. T., Gusberg, S. B., and Buxton, C. L.: Histochemical studies on abnormal growth of human endometrium; cytoplasmic ribonucleic acids in normal and pathological glandular epithelium. Cancer, *2:* 132, 1949.

Atkinson, W. B., Gall, E., and Gusberg, S. B.: Histochemical studies on abnormal growth of human endometrium; deposition of glycogen in hyperplasia and adenocarcinoma. Cancer, *5:* 138, 1952.

Atkinson, W. B., and Gusberg, S. B.: Histochemical studies on abnormal growth of human endometrium; alkaline phosphatase in hyperplasia and adenocarcinoma. Cancer, *1:* 248, 1948.

Baggish, M. S., Pauerstein, C. J., and Woodruff, J. D.: Role of stroma in the regeneration of the endometrial epithelium. Amer. J. Obstet. Gynec., *98:* 459, 1967.

Bartelmez, G. W., Corner, G. W., and Hartman, C. G.: Phases of menstrual cycle in macaque monkey. Anat. Rec., *94:* 512, 1946.

Besch, P. K., Barry, R. D., Byron, R. C., Teteris, N. J., Hamwi, G. J., Vorys, N., and Ullery, J. C.: Testosterone synthesis by a Brenner tumor. Amer. J. Obstet. Gynec., *86:* 1021, 1963.

Blandau, R. J.: Ovulation in living Albino rat. Fertil. Steril., *6:* 391, 1955.

Boutselis, J. G., DeNeet, J. C., Ullery, J. C., and George, O. T.: Histochemical and cytologic observations in the normal human endometrium. Obstet. Gynec., *21:* 423, 1963.

Buchholz, R.: Researches on the influence of sex hormones on gonadotrophin excretion in humans. Geburtsh. Frauenheilk., *10:* 851, 1959.

Corner, G. W.: Events of primate ovarian cycle. Brit. Med. J., *2:* 403, 1952.

Craig, J. M., and Danzigen, S.: Histological distribution and nature of stainable lipoids of the human endometrium. Amer. J. Obstet. Gynec., *93:* 1018, 1965.

Deane, H. W., Lobel, B. L., and Romney, S. L.: Enzyme histochemistry of normal human ovaries of the menstrual cycle, pregnancy, and the early puerperium. Amer. J. Obstet. Gynec., *83:* 281, 1962.

Dorfman, R. I.: Steroid hormones in gynecology. Obstet. Gynec. Survey, *18:* 65, 1963.

Epperson, J. W. W., Hellman, L. M., Galvin, G. A., and Busby, T.: Morphologic changes in cervix during pregnancy, including intraepithelial carcinoma. Amer. J. Obstet. Gynec., *61:* 50, 1951.

Fischel, A.: Uber die Entwicklung der Keimdrüsen des Menschen. Z. Ges. Anat., *92:* 34, 1930.

Fleming, J., Tweedale, D. N., and Roddick, J. W.: Ciliated endometrial cells. Amer. J. Obstet. Gynec., *102:* 186, 1968.

Fluhmann, C. F.: Clinical and clinicopathologic study of lesions of cervix uteri during pregnancy. Amer. J. Obstet. Gynec., *55:* 133, 1948.

Fraenkel, L.: Die Funktion des Corpus luteum. Arch. Gynaek., *68:*438, 1903.

Goldberg, B., Jones, G. E. S., and Woodruff, J. D.: A histochemical study of 3-beta-ol dehydrogenase activity in some steroid-producing tumors. Amer. J. Obstet. Gynec., *86:* 1003, 1963.

Govan, A. D. T.: The human ovary in early pregnancy. J. Endocr., *40:* 421, 1968.

Graham, J., Graham, R., and Hirabyashi, K.: Reversible "cancer" and the contraceptive pill. Obstet. Gynec., *31:* 190, 1968.

Greene, R. R., and Nelson, W. W.: Decidual reaction in ovary. Quart. Bull. Northwest. Univ. Med. Sch., *26:* 197, 1952.

Greene, R. R., and Peckham, B. M.: Preinvasive cancer of the cervix and pregnancy. Amer. J. Obstet. Gynec., *75:* 551, 1958.

Gross, S. J.: Histochemistry of the normal and abnormal endometrium. Amer. J. Obstet. Gynec., *88:* 647, 1964.

Hall, J. Alkaline phosphatase in human endometrium. Amer. J. Obstet. Gynec., *60:* 212, 1950.

Henderson, S. R. and Schalch, D. S.: Estrogen receptors in the human uterus. Amer. J. Obstet. Gynec., *112:* 762, 1972.

Huffman, J. W.: Mesonephric remains in cervix. Amer. J. Obstet. Gynec., *56:* 23, 1948.

Joel, R. V., and Foraker, A. G.: Fate of the corpus albicans: a morphologic approach. Amer. J. Obstet. Gynec., *80:* 314, 1960.

Kase, N., and Conrad, S. H.: Steroid synthesis in abnormal ovaries. Amer. J. Obstet. Gynec., *90:* 1251, 1964.

Lapan, B.: Deciduosis of cervix and vagina simulating carcinoma. Amer. J. Obstet. Gynec., *58:* 743, 1949.

Leventhal, M. L., and Scommegna, A.: Multiglandular aspects of the Stein-Leventhal syndrome. Amer. J. Obstet. Gynec., *87:* 445, 1963.

Levine, B.: Sex steroids, alkaline phosphatase, and endometrial carcinoma. Obstet. Gynec., *22:* 563, 1963.

Markee, J. E.: Menstruation in intraocular endometrial transplants in the rhesus monkey. Contrib. Embryol., *28:* 219, 1940.

Markee, J. E.: Morphological basis for menstrual bleeding. Anat. Rec., *94:* 481, 1946.

McBride, J. H.: Normal postmenopausal endometrium. J. Obstet. Gynaec. Brit. Comm., *61:* 691, 1954.

Mattingly, R. F., and Huang, W. N.: Steroidogenesis of the menopausal and postmenopausal gonad. Amer. J. Obstet. Gynec., *103:* 679, 1969.

McKay, D. G., Hertig, A. T., Bardawil, W. A., and Velardo, J. T.: Histochemical observations on the endometrium. 1. Normal endometrium. Obstet. Gynec., *8:* 22, 1956.

McKay, D. G., Hertig, A. T., Bardawil, W. A., and Velardo, J. T.: Histochemical observations on the endometrium. 2. Abnormal endometrium. Obstet. Gynec., *8:* 140, 1956.

McKay, D. G., Pinkerton, J. H. M., Hertig, A. T., and Danzigen, S.: The adult human ovary: a histochemical study. Obstet. Gynec., *18:* 13, 1961.

McLennen, M. T., and McLennen, C. E.: Estrogenic action of menstruating and menopausal women assessed by cervico-vaginal smear. Obstet. Gynec., *37:* 325, 1971.

Meyer, R.: Über Corpous Luteumbildung beim Menschen. Zbl. Gynaek., *46:* 1206, 1911.

Nesbitt, R. E. L.: Benign cervical changes in pregnancy. Clin. Obstet. Gynec., *6:* 381, 1963.

Novak, E., and Richardson, E. H., Jr.: Proliferative changes in senile endometrium. Amer. J. Obstet. Gynec., *42:* 564, 1941.

Novak, E. R., Goldberg, B., Jones, G. E. S., and O'Toole, R. W.: Enzyme histochemistry of the postmenopausal ovary associated with normal and abnormal endometria. Amer. J. Obstet. Gynec., *93:* 669, 1965.

Noyes, R. W.: Underdeveloped secretory endometrium. Amer. J. Obstet. Gynec., *77:* 929, 1959.

Noyes, R. W., and Haman, J. O.: Accuracy of endometrial dating. Fertil. Steril., *4:* 504, 1953.

Noyes, R. W., Hertig, A. T., and Rock, J.: Dating the endometrial biopsy. Fertil. Steril., *1:* 3, 1950.

Papanicolaou, G. N., Traut, H. F., and Manchetti, A. A.: *Epithelia of Woman's Reproductive Organs: A Correlative Study of Cyclic Changes. Commonwealth Fund,* New York, 1948.

Plotz, E. J., Wiener, M., Stein, A. A., and Hahn, R. D.: Enzymatic activities related to steroidogenesis in postmenopausal ovaries of patients with and without endometrial carcinoma. Amer. J. Obstet. Gynec., *99:* 182, 1967.

Pommerenke, W. T., and Viergiver, E.: Cyclic variations in viscosity of cervical mucus and its correlation with amount of secretion and basal temperature. Amer. J. Obstet. Gynec., *51:* 192, 1946.

Riley, G. M.: Endocrinology of the climacteric. Clin. Obstet. Gynec., *7:* 432, 1964.

Roddick, J. W., Ing, G. K. C., and Midboe, D.: Isozymes of lactic dehydrogenase in normal endometrium. Amer. J. Obstet. Gynec., *95:* 439, 1966.

Ryan, K. J.: Synthesis of hormones in the ovaries. *The Ovary,* edited by H. G. Grady and D. E. Smith, p. 69. The Williams and Wilkins Company, Baltimore, 1963.

Rydberg, E.: Observations on crystallization of cervical mucus. Acta Obstet. Gynec. Scand., *28:* 172, 1948.

Schrüder, R.: Anatomische Studien zur normalen und pathologischen Physiologie des Menstruationzyklus. Arch. Gynaek., *104:* 27, 1915.

Schueler, E. F.: Ciliated epithelium of the human uterine mucosa. Obstet. Gynec., *31:* 215, 1968.

Schueler, E. F.: Human endometrial ciliated cells. Obstet. Gynec., *41:* 188, 1973.

Schwarz, O. H., Young, C. C., Jr., and Crouse, J. C.: Ovogenesis in adult human ovary. Amer. J. Obstet. Gynec., *58:* 54, 1949.

Scommegna, A., and Lash, S. R.: Ovarian overstimulation, massive ascites and singleton pregnancy after clomiphene. J.A.M.A., *207:* 753, 1969.

Scully, R. E., and Cohen, R. B.: Oxidative-enzyme activity in normal and pathological ovaries. Obstet. Gynec., *23:* 667, 1964.

Sjövall, A.: Untersuchungen uver die Schliemhaut der cervix uteri. Acta Obstet. Gynec. Scand. (Suppl. 4), *18:* 4, 1938.

Strassman, E. O.: Theca interna cone and its role in ovulation. Surg. Gynec. Obstet., *67:* 299, 1938.

Topkins, P.: Histologic appearance of endocervix during menstrual cycle. Amer. J. Obstet. Gynec., *58:* 654, 1949.

Wallach, E. E.: Physiology of menstruation. Clin. Obstet. Gynec., *13:* 366, 1970,

Wienke, E. C., Jr., Cavazos, F., Hall, D. G., and Lucas, F. V.: Ultrastructure of the human endometrial stroma cell during the menstrual cycle. Amer. J. Obstet. Gynec., *102:* 65, 1968.

Zondek, B., and Rozin, S.: Cervical mucus arborization. Obstet. Gynec., *3:* 463, 1954.

chapter *4*

Clinical Features of Menstruation

Menstruation may be defined as a periodic physiological hemorrhage, occurring at approximately four-week intervals, and having its source from the uterine mucous membrane. There are some who add to this definition the requirement that the bleeding be preceded by ovulation with progestational changes in the endometrium, but this stipulation seems unjustified.

Interval

Although the traditional menstrual interval is about 28 days, there are wide variations from this rule, not only in different women, but in the individual, although the most frequent interval lengths fall between 25 and 32 days. Under abnormal conditions, not necessarily of serious import, intervals of far longer or shorter duration are encountered, and it is by no means infrequent to observe spontaneous changes of the interval. Irregular intervals rarely have such potential pathological significance as intermenstrual or prolonged or heavy bleeding. The first day of bleeding should be counted as the first cycle day.

Duration and Amount

Here again wide variations are seen, the usual duration being 3 to 5 days, with normal extremes of 1 or 2 days, and 7 or 8 days. In any one woman, however, the duration of the flow is usually uniform. Hallberg *et al.* in a study of 476 randomly selected Swedish women, report a mean value of 33.2 ± 1.6 ml. for blood loss during the menstrual period. The younger age women, 15 years, showed less loss while the 30-year-old group had higher losses. Women with signs of iron deficiency anemia also had slightly higher losses than the mean loss of the series. Blood loss above 80 ml was regarded as pathological.

A rough estimate of blood loss can be made from the number of pads soiled or tampons used and from a hematocrit taken before and immediately after the flow. On rare occasions it is necessary to observe the patient during menstruation. Blood loss during the normal menstrual cycle is enough to lower the hemoglobin slightly among women on an adequate diet. If there is a deficient nutritional state, a chronic anemia may ensue.

Hervey, McIntire, and Watson found that 13 per cent of women blood donors were rejected due to anemia in contrast to only 1 per cent of men.

It should be emphasized that many women state that they "are hemorrhaging," although the blood count is normal. What may seem to be heavy bleeding to the patient may in reality be rather insignificant if hematological studies are performed.

Subjective Symptoms

The line of demarcation between the normal and the abnormal is often a shadowy one. Although actual pain is not normal, a moderate sense of heaviness and weight in the pelvic region would be within the bounds of normality. Slight nervous instability is also often seen, with occasional bladder irritability and a tendency to constipation. On the whole, however, the menstrual function should entail no appreciable discomfort and cause no interference with normal activities.

It has been shown during recent years that *the basal body temperature exhibits a characteristic course during the ovulatory cycle* with a slight but definite dip and subsequent rise of from 0.5° to 1° at about ovulation time, remaining thus elevated throughout the luteal phase. The significance and clinical application of this basal temperature variation is more fully discussed in the chapter on sterility, but it is fitting to note that temperature charts as assembled by an unintelligent woman may be difficult to interpret.

Character of Menstrual Discharge

The menstrual discharge is characteristically a dark reddish color like that of venous blood. The offensiveness of the discharge is due not only to decomposition of the blood elements but also to the admixture of the increased secretions of the vulvar sebaceous glands. When menstrual bleeding is profuse, the discharge is often of brighter red color. The flow contains not only blood elements, but also cervical mucus, degenerated particles of endometrium, vaginal mucosa, and numerous bacteria.

The characteristic of menstrual blood which has excited the greatest interest is its *noncoagulability*. This is not to say, however, that occasional small clots are not within normal limits. During the past few years a number of studies have been made which indicate that menstrual blood does actually clot, but then undergoes intrauterine liquefaction because of certain fibrinolytic enzymes. Huggins, Vail, and Davis showed that the menstrual discharge contains serum, but lacks prothrombin and fibrinogen, like the serum of clotted blood. They believe, therefore, that the blood in the menstrual discharge has already clotted, but that most of the clot has been dissolved in utero by fibrinolytic enzymes, which were demonstrable in some specimens. There seems to be no real evidence for a menstrual *toxin* as was once suggested.

PUBERTY AND MENARCHE

The term puberty refers to the transitional developmental phase between childhood and full maturity. One of the manifestations of this phase, but only one of many, is the appearance of the first menstrual period, to which the term menarche is applied. This distinction is stressed because the mistake is often made of referring to the occurrence of the first menstrual period as the age of puberty.

Phenomena of Puberty

Precisely what initiates puberty is uncertain. However, long before the onset of menstruation there is beginning secretion of a hypothalamic hormone, the so-called luteinizing hormone-release factor (LRF), which stimulates the pituitary to produce both follicle stimulating hormone (FSH) and luteinizing hormone (LH). Consequently estrogen production at an increasing level begins and on occasion follicle cysts may occur despite any clinical bleeding. At some time, however, sufficient estrogen is present to incur menstruation, although this initially is almost uniformly anovulatory in nature as noted recently by Altchek. Only at a later date, perhaps a year or two, is there sufficient LH production and LH surge to induce ovulation, and a complete reproductive potential. The causes for the onset of puberty are enormously complicated and incompletely understood at this writing. However, a fully functioning and responsive hypothalamus and reciprocal feedback mechanism seems essential.

Inauguration of the Menstrual Function (Menarche). The age at which the first period occurs varies between wide limits, but an average age for girls of the North American Continent is 12 1/2 years. It may, in individual cases, be as low as 10 or as high as 16 years. When the menarche occurs below or above these limits, it is to be considered as abnormally premature or delayed.

Statistical data indicate that the age of the menarche is a heritable characteristic which is influenced by general hygiene rather than racial or climatic factors. Just as women are having later menopauses today, it seems that the age of the menarche has steadily decreased in all parts of the world according to Thoma who quotes Semmelweis as estimating 100 years ago that the menarchal age of Viennese women was between 15 and 19 years.

Studies by Brown indicate that two types of changes have occurred to account for this difference. There has been a reduction in the numbers of girls who have a significantly delayed menarche. This might be accounted for by improved general hygiene, nutrition, and a decrease in chronic disease processes. However, there is another more general trend which indicates a decrease in several months for the age at menarche for all girls. This would best be explained on the basis of a change in some more universal biological mechanism. These should be factors which would influence the maturation of the nervous system, and thereby release the hypothalamic inhibitory influence described in Chapter 2.

Secondary Sex Characteristics. These embrace a large group of changes, some general and others local. The sequence of events reported by Young and his co-workers for 11 Florentine school girls has been divided into four stages: (1) *prepuberal:* downy pubic hair; little, if any growth spurt; elevation of nipples; (2) *first stage puberty:* pubic hair, coarse and curly, in small quantities; budding of breasts with areolar enlargement; marked growth spurt; enlargement of labia; (3) *second stage puberty:* pubic hair as described above in moderate quantity; filling out of breasts, a projection of areolae and papilla to form a secondary mound; axillary hair in small quantities; menarche usually begins in this phase; growth spurt already decreasing; further labial growth; and (4) *third stage puberty:* pubic hair further increased and approaching or reaching adult type and configuration with recession of areolae to level of breasts; labia approaching or reaching adult type; annual growth less than prepuberty; menstruation usually well established.

Timewise it appears that the first prepuberal changes may begin as early as two years prior to the menarche, closely correlated with the appearance of urinary gonadotrophins. The growth spurt ordinarily lasts about six months, reaching its peak approximately two months prior to the menarche at an average age of 12.3 years. The growth rate than steadily declines and ceases at approximately 2.5-years postmenarche, this average age being 14.8 years.

It should be noted that although the labial growth is marked, the growth of the fundus may not be as rapid and although the configuration of the uterus may change as demonstrated in Figure 4.1, the actual size of the fundus may not be appreciably increased for several years.

Psychological Changes. The nervous and psychological manifestations of puberty are not comparable to those seen at the menopause but are caused by the difficulty and concern of the individual in changing from the sheltered, secure state of childhood into the self-responsible, independent realm of adulthood. The most noticeable feature of this transition may be the development of self-consciousness;

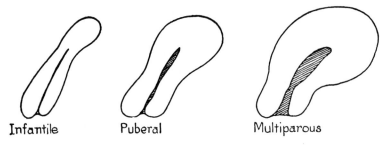

Infantile   Puberal   Multiparous

4.1. Changes in contour of uterus at different age periods. Note the increased size of the corpus at puberty.

as the young girl becomes conscious of sex differences she is apt to develop a shyness toward members of the opposite sex not noted in very early life. However, the most important psychological change is the shifting of the emphasis from a self-centered one to a consideration of others. It is the successful accomplishment of this transition which assures a normal, well adjusted adult both sexually and socially.

There are enormous pressures and tensions involved in today's teenage females, such as were not seen a generation ago. The change in sex mores, usage of drugs, etc., may make the young girl exceedingly unsure, and totally confused about what is expected of her. Close and sympathetic parental guidance is of utmost importance.

Management and Hygiene of Puberty

Every girl should be prepared for her first menstruation and, as it is preceded by the general development and changes noted above, there is sufficient advance warning for the parent or guardian to see that this is properly done. Such preparation entails a simple explanation of the anatomy and physiology of both male and female reproductive organs. It can be supplemented by books and charts, if necessary. Corner's books, *Attaining Manhood* and *Attaining Womanhood*, are still the best references which can be given. In the discussion it is important to emphasize that menstruation is a normal function and does not handicap or materially interfere with her life or activities. Although violent exercise is not advisable, if the flow is not too profuse, reasonable exercise is quite ac-

ceptable. One would not think that it is necessary today to advise patients or parents that bathing and hair washing are not contraindicated during menstruation.

Fortunately many of today's schools provide an adequate sex education program so that the young female usually has at least some knowledge of what to expect with the onset of menstruation, a distinct change from our former rather rigid and straight-laced attitudes.

In addition to preparing the individual intellectually and emotionally for menstruation, it is well to keep on hand a kit of items necessary for menstrual hygiene. These are commercially available in most attractive packages to maintain as esthetic an air as possible about the menstrual function which many young girls find very unesthetic. Although the young girl at puberty will certainly find the sanitary pad the most acceptable menstrual protection, there has been an increasing popularity of intravaginal menstrual tampons. These offer certain obvious advantages of convenience over the external pad, and there is no objection to their employment in most patients, although they are hardly practical where there is a tight virginal hymeneal ring. Certainly there are no adverse sequelae, such as endometriosis or infection. Another method which may be helpful, especially while traveling, is the use of the intravaginal cup. Douching is not necessary unless recommended by a physician for a specific reason.

The Anovulatory Cycle

Menstruation may occur without ovulation, and a large proportion of such anovulatory cycles are noted in young adolescents and in women approaching the menopause. During active reproductive life such cycles are relatively uncommon.

It is known that a certain degree of follicle maturation and estrogenic function begins a considerable time, often several years, before the appearance of the first menstrual period. When estrogenic function reaches a sufficiently high point, periodic bleeding without follicular rupture or corpus luteum formation may ensue.

Menstruation in such cases may be more or less irregular for many months, but not infrequently it is of approximately the four-week type, with a flow which, in amount and duration, is within normal limits.

While anovulation is compatible with rather regular bleeding, all types of abnormal bleeding, often heavy, and occasionally alarming, may be associated with failure to ovulate, and this will be discussed more fully in Chapters 14 and 31. It should be stressed, however, that abnormal bleeding in the teen-age girl should not be presumed to be functional in type, and warrants careful investigation by the appropriate techniques noted in subsequent chapters. This is especially true if there is a history of maternal stilbestrol ingestion during pregnancy, because of the not infrequent occurrence of adenosis along with vaginal and cervical mesonephroid adenocarcinoma. In addition Acosta, Kaplan and Kaufman, and Smith, Rutledge and Sutow have assembled separate excellent studies on other malignant pelvic tumors in children.

A study by Döring, using the basal temperature record as a guide to ovulation, shows a high rate of anovulatory cycles before the age of 21 years. The difficulty with this investigation is that it was made on institutionalized girls, not on a population living under normal conditions. In addition, one wonders how conscientious youngsters can be relied upon to take their temperatures over prolonged periods of time. The other side of the picture is depicted by Benjamin who had three children record their temperatures before, and through, their first menstrual cycles. All three charts showed an ovulatory rise prior to the initial menstrual period.

As the end of menstrual life approaches, divergence of menstruation and ovulation is again frequently noted, and on this point it is easily possible to secure definite evidence by the simple method of premenstrual or menstrual endometrial biopsy. Here again, it is impossible to speak of the statistical incidence of anovulatory cycles, although the numerous reports on this subject leave no doubt as to their comparative frequency. It is now fully justified to say that while probably the great majority of women ovulate until the end of menstrual life, and occasionally beyond, there are many in whom the cycle becomes anovulatory or aluteal for a variable time before its cessation.

Between the two extremes of menstrual life, and therefore during the greater portion of reproductive life, there can be no doubt that the overwhelming majority of cycles are of the characteristic ovulatory type, but even here one finds exceptions.

MENOPAUSE OR CLIMACTERIUM

The average duration of menstrual life is about 38 years. Frommer determined that the median age of the menopause of women in Great Britain was 50 years. This represents an increase of about four years since 1850. No very clear relationship has been established between the age of puberty and that of the menopause, although there are some who believe that women who begin to menstruate early are apt to retain the function rather longer. The statistical evidence for this is not convincing. The most important influencing factor is probably heredity, as unusually early to unusually late menopauses do seem to be characteristic of the women of certain families. It is difficult to state any specific age at which the woman should be expected to cease physiological bleeding. Continued bleeding after the age of 55 warrants a Papanicolaou smear at six-month intervals. Curettage should be performed if there is the slightest irregularity.

Just as the inauguration of menstrual function is only one manifestation of a general developmental process, so the cessation of menstruation is only a part of a general retrogressive change. For this reason the term *climacterium* is a better one for this transitional phase than the term menopause, which has reference only to the cessation of the menstrual function. The word climacterium, on the other hand, is derived from a Greek word meaning "rung of a ladder," and expresses better the idea of this transitional step which every woman, provided she lives long enough, must take in her progress from the cradle to the grave.

Phenomena of the Climacterium

The phenomena characteristic of the climacterium may conveniently be discussed under the following headings.

Cessation of Menstruation. As already stated, the average age at which menstruation ceases is somewhat less than 50 years, with wide individual variations. In some women the function ceases very abruptly, but more often its disappearance is gradual. A period or two is skipped, then menstruation recurs more or less normally from one to several times, with again a period of amenorrhea which may last several months, and so on, until complete cessation of the function. This "dodging period" of the menopause may last a year or two. The amount and duration of the periods may be normal until the very end, but frequently there is a gradual diminution in both.

There should normally be no excessive flow, contrary to the prevalent lay belief that flooding at the menopausal epoch has no significance, a belief which has been responsible for the death of many women. Nor is intermenstrual bleeding a characteristic of the menopause. Neither of these two is necessarily due to serious causes, but not infrequently the etiological factor is cancer, and hence the need for prompt investigation in every case. While a smear should be performed, cytopathology is of limited value in evaluating the endometrium. On the other hand, excessive menstruation may be due to comparatively simple functional causes, and milder forms not infrequently go on to spontaneous disappearance of the function. The fact remains, however, that marked menstrual excess and intermenstrual bleeding are not any more normal at the menopause than they are at other ages, and always call for proper investigation (see chapter on uterine bleeding).

Cessation of Ovulation. Ovulation as well as menstruation cease at the climacterium, but the disappearance of the two functions is not necessarily synchronous. Not infrequently the woman may cease to ovulate long before she stops menstruating. In other words, the terminal cycles may be of the anovulatory type.

The fact that the final cessation of menstrual life is often preceded by rather long periods of amenorrhea gives rise to many interesting diagnostic problems because of the fear of many such patients that they are pregnant. As a matter of fact, unexpected pregnancy may occur in the terminal years of menstruation chiefly because contraceptive vigilance is apt to be relaxed at this period due to a false sense of security regarding the possibility of impregnation. Although ovulation rarely occurs after from six months to a year following the last menstruation, we have found a typical progestational endometrium six years after the menopause in one case, and in another fully 10 years post-irradiation at the age of 46 because of dysfunctional bleeding. Such instances, however, are exceedingly rare. It is well to advise the menopausal woman to continue contraception for one year after her last menstrual period.

Vasomotor Symptoms. The most characteristic symptoms of the climacterium are the so-called *vasomotor group:* hot flushes, which involve chiefly the head, neck, and upper part of the thorax and the sweats, often profuse, which frequently immediately follow the flushes.

The frequency and severity of these vasomotor symptoms are exceedingly variable, being almost absent in some women, very moderate in most, and severe in a minority of patients. In the latter case, hormone treatment is often called for, and usually is successful in ameliorating the symptoms, as is discussed in the chapter on treatment of menopausal symptoms.

The *cause* of the vasomotor symptoms is the cessation of ovarian function with estrogen withdrawal and a resultant elevated FSH. The characteristic flush certainly involves a vasomotor mechanism, perhaps not unlike that concerned in the phenomenon of blushing. Just what pathways are involved in the production of the vasomotor phenomena is not known.

Other Symptoms. Aside from the vasomotor phenomena such a legion of other symptoms has been ascribed to the menopause, that the public is apt to attribute almost any symptom that happens to occur in the middle-aged woman to the "change of life." In this connection we wonder whether many of our colleagues are not at times to blame in suggesting to the woman, or in acquiescing in her own ready suggestion, that the menopause is responsible for all sorts of indefinite symptoms, especially when a more likely cause for the latter is not patently clear.

A distinction should be made between (1) those symptoms which are clearly menopausal in origin, in the sense that they are the physiological results of the cessation of ovarian activity, and (2) those frequently seen in women passing through the menopause, but which are only indirectly or secondarily of menopausal origin and therefore not characteristic. To illustrate what is meant, let us take the example of an average uninformed woman who approaches the menopause with a considerable degree of apprehensiveness. The occurrence of frequent hot flushes and sweats, often disturbing her rest at night and awakening her with a panicky feeling, increases her nervous instability and makes her irritable. Why should not such a woman have headaches, vertigo, depression, a tendency to insomnia, loss of appetite, other digestive symptoms, or any of many other subjective manifestations? These are certainly not the direct result of any endocrine disturbance, but a part of this particular woman's menopausal disturbance.

There is no question, however, that there is a tremendous psychogenic overlay in many of these women who are beginning to miss periods, and it is often difficult to be certain what problems are bona fide and what are fictitious. Most stress should be placed on the aforesaid vasomotor symptoms, especially if there is an elevated FSH and an atrophic smear.

Postmenopausal Ovarian Function

There is growing evidence that the postmenopausal ovary is not necessarily the atrophic, functionless organ it has been presumed to be. Randall and Harkins have indicated a persistence of estrogen effect in a considerable percentage of women who have had no vaginal bleeding for years. Although the adrenal can on occasion manufacture estrogen, it is difficult to deny that the ovary is also of some importance, perhaps by virtue of certain hyperplastic stromal cells (ovarian stromal hyperplasia). Poliak *et al.* were able to show substantial increases in urinary estrogen production of menopausal women following chorionic gonadotrophic stimulation as long as 20 years after the last menstrual period. The ovaries of these women had stromal cells which appeared active by both histological and histochemical examinations. A more complete discussion is found in Chapter 33.

As noted elsewhere, it seems likely that the steroid produced may be an androgen (androstenedione) which is converted to an estrogen at diverse areas. Our own studies suggest that both androgenic and estrogenic hormones may be present in the aging female for many years after cessation of the menses.

Treatment

See Chapter 33.

REFERENCES

Acosta, A., Kaplan, A. L., and Kaufman, R. H.: Gynecological cancer in children. Amer. J. Obstet. Gynec., *112:* 944, 1972.
Albright, F.: Studies on ovarian dysfunction; menopause. Endocrinology, *20:* 24, 1936.

Altchek, A.: Dysfunctional menstrual disorders in adolescence. Clin. Obstet. Gynec., *14:* 975, 1971.

Arey, L. B.: Degree of normal menstrual irregularity. Amer. J. Obstet. Gynec., *37:* 12, 1939.

Brown, P. E.: The age at menarche. Brit. J. Prev. Soc. Med., *20:* 9, 1966.

Corner, G. W.: *Attaining Manhood.* Harper & Brothers, New York, 1939.

Corner, G. W.: *Attaining Womanhood.* Harper & Brothers, New York, 1939.

Engle, E. T., and Shelesnyack, M. S.: First menstruation and subsequent menstrual cycles of pubertal girls. Hum. Biol., *6:* 431, 1934.

Frommer, D. J.: Changing age of the menopause. Brit. Med. J., *2:* 549, 1964.

Glueck, H. I., and Mirsky, I. A.: Clotting mechanism of menstrual blood. Amer. J. Obstet. Gynec., *42:* 267, 1941.

Hallberg, L., Högdahl A-M., Nilsson, L., and Rybo, G.: Menstrual blood loss: a population study. Variation at different ages, an attempt to define normality. Acta Obstet. Gynec. Scand., *45:* 320, 1966.

Hervey, G. W. McIntire, R. T., and Watson, V.: Low hemoglobin levels in women as revealed by blood donor records. J.A.M.A., *149:* 1127, 1952.

Huffman, J. W.: *Gynecology of Childhood and Adolescence.* W. B. Saunders Co., Philadelphia, 1968.

Huggins, C., Vail, V. C., and Davis, M. E.: Fluidity of menstrual blood; a proteolytic effect. Amer. J. Obstet. Gynec., *78:* 46, 1943.

Kennedy, W. P.: Menarche and menstrual type; notes on 10,000 case records. J. Obstet. Gynaec. Brit. Comm., *49:* 792, 1933.

Lozner, E. L., Taylor, J. E., and Taylor, F. H. L.: So-called coagulation defect in menstrual blood. New Eng. J. Med., *236:* 481, 1942.

Novak, E. R.: The menopause. J.A.M.A., *156:* 575, 1954.

Poliak, A., Jones, G. E. S., Goldberg, B., Soloman D., and Woodruff, J. D.: The effect of human chorionic gonadotrophin on postmenopausal women: ovarian histochemistry and urinary hormone excretion. Amer. J. Obstet. Gynec., *101:* 731, 1968.

Randall, C. L.: Ovarian function and women after the menopause. Amer. J. Obstet. Gynec., *73:* 1000, 1957.

Randall, C. L., and Harkins, J. L.: Ovarian function after the menopause. Amer. J. Obstet. Gynec., *74:* 719, 1957.

Simmons, K., and Graulich, W. W.: Menarchal age and height, weight and skeletal age of girls age 7 to 17 years. J. Pediat., *22:* 518, 1945.

Smith, J. P. Rutledge, F., and Sutow, W.: Malignant gynecological tumors in children. Amer. J. Obstet. Gynec., *116:* 261, 1973.

Thoma, A.: Age at menarche, acceleration and heritability. Acta Biol. Acad. Sci. Hung., *11:* 241, 1960.

chapter 5

Gynecological History, Examination, and Operations

GYNECOLOGICAL HISTORY

The aim of each history should be to obtain a complete picture of the patient and her illness at the time of her examination. Indeed, a strongly presumptive diagnosis can frequently be made from the history alone, before examination. The history, however, obviously should not supercede the more important pelvic examination. Various methods of taking histories are employed, but should always include the patient's full name along with her husband's, age, social condition (single, married, divorced, or separated), social security number, address, referring physician, and health or hospital insurance. Index files by name and history number are desirable. A complete and accurate history is of extreme value for defense of the physician involved in today's frequent medico-legal problems.

Patient's Complaint

The general nature of the patient's complaint should be ascertained at the beginning of the consultation, and should be stated as nearly as possible in the patient's own language. This may not always be very precise, or even literate, but it will at least be authentic, and will often point the way to later questioning.

Family History

Special attention should be directed to familial diabetes, tuberculosis, or cancer. It should be emphasized that cancer is not directly hereditary. However, the woman in whom there is a strong family background of this disease stands a better than average chance of contracting it.

History

A record of the patient's previous illnesses, and especially of any operations is of obvious importance. It is remarkable how little many women know as to the nature of previous surgery. This information is often of such significance in the diagnosis and treatment of later gynecological disease that it is often wise to

Sample Case History

No.: 21875
Name: Smith, Mary A. (John C.)
    36 N. Main Boulevard
    Johnston, S. C.

Date: March 18, 1973
Referred by: Dr. Paul A. Brown
    262 N. Centre St.
    Jonesville, S. C.

Age: 64

C.C.: "Bleeding after the change of life."

F. H.: Mother died of cancer of the cervix; otherwise negative.

P. H.: D. & C. 1970, "Bleeding," Johns Hopkins Hospital. Appendectomy approximately 1928. Possible rheumatic fever without cardiac involvement as child. Otherwise only c.c.d.

G. U.: History of apparent cystitis 30 years ago with only pregnancy. No present hematuria, dysuria, urgency, etc.

G. I.: Chronic constipation; otherwise negative.

M. H.: LMP 1972 after uneventful menstrual life. (1 D. & C. as noted above).

Ob. H.: Para 1-1-0.0.1. One uncomplicated pregnancy at age 32 after 8 years involuntary sterility; no other pregnancies; never contraception.

P. I.: LMP 16 years ago. No further bleeding until 1 month ago when noticed bright red spotting, at first intermittent, but now more or less constant, so requires pad. Never excessive flow and no pain of any kind. No known estrogen therapy although is taking indocin for arthritis.
Menses generally normal though D. & C. in premenopausal area for flooding. No sequelae and LMP about 1 year later. Para 1 after 8 years sterility and no other pregnancies. G. U.-G. I. essentially negative as above.

P. E.: Shows an obese rather flushed W. F. 64. (Wt. 220; B.P. 210/120). *Thyroid* not enlarged. *Breasts* pendulous without masses. *Abdomen*—marked panniculus. No masses or tenderness. C.V. angles nontender. *Pelvic*—external genitalia normal. Outlet parous with no relaxation anterior or posterior. Cervix small and smooth, almost flush with the vault. Fundus normal postmenopausal size, midposition, regular, and free. Adnexa not palpable. *Speculum*—no present bleeding. Cervix clean. Vaginal mucosa well supported. *Rectal*—small hemorrhoids at 3, 6, and 10 o'clock. Otherwise essentially negative and confirmatory.

Impression: (1) Postmenopausal bleeding.
    (2) Adenocarcinoma fundus (?).

Rx: Papanicolaou smear with maturation index and cervical biopsy taken.
    Urine (cath.) for microscopic and culture taken.
    Old D. & C. specimen to be reviewed.
    To be admitted 3/28/73 for glucose tolerance, cholesterol, and routine laboratory studies.
    Medical consultation (EKG, chest x-ray, etc.) 3/29/73. For D. & C. and possible subsequent hysterectomy.

secure more accurate information from the previous surgeon or hospital. Patients who have had malignancies seem predisposed to other primary lesions.

Menstrual History

Since menstrual symptoms are of more significance than any other in gynecological patients, a complete menstrual history should be obtained in every case. Countless women today are taking contraceptive pills which may modify the periods. The history should note any forms of contraception and include the following data.

Age at Onset. An unusually early menarche, especially when accompanied by general developmental changes, may be indicative of certain endocrinopathies, whereas others are characterized by the late appearance of puberty.

Interval. Although the traditional menstrual interval is 28 days, there are wide individual variations even in normal women. Departures from the woman's norm, however, are frequently produced by either functional or anatomical abnormalities.

Duration. The same general statement may be made concerning the duration of the flow. Most frequently this parallels the quantity, a prolonged flow being usually an excessive one, and a very short period being scanty, but a two- to seven-day flow represents normal variation.

Amount. Although variations in the

amount of blood lost at menstruation by different women are wide, a marked diminution is suggestive of an endocrine or constitutional abnormality of some sort, whereas menstrual excess is produced by either functional or structural lesions, often the latter. A rough idea as to the amount of menstrual flow may be obtained by inquiry as to the number of napkins or tampons required daily.

Character of Menstrual Discharge. The menstrual blood is characteristically of dark venous appearance, and normally is unclotted. When menstruation is excessive, however, the blood may be bright red with clots. It is not unusual to find some clotting even with normal menstruation but when clots are numerous and large, dysmenorrhea is usually a complaint.

Menstrual Pain. Pain with menstruation is one of the most common of gynecological symptoms, and many factors may be responsible. These need not necessarily be of anatomical or structural character, for often constitutional, psychogenic, and other general factors may be concerned. In questioning patients, it is wise to inquire as to the character of the pain, which is usually of either a bearing down or colicky character, and also as to the time of its onset and its duration. For example, in the common type or primary dysmenorrhea, it most characteristically begins a day or two before the onset of the period, and disappears after menstruation has been well established. In other cases, it may persist throughout the flow or even beyond. Any increased dysmenorrhea should require further elucidation.

Intermenstrual Bleeding. It is important to ascertain whether or not there is bleeding between the menstrual periods, and whether this is apt to occur after coitus or other contact. Bleeding of this type is the most characteristic symptom of early cervical cancer, although it is also common with such innocuous lesions as cervical polyp or erosion.

The Date of the Last Menstrual Period. When this is inquired for, the physician will often find the patient's memory very hazy, and this item in the history is sure to be inaccurate in many cases. Yet it is often of great importance, as in cases of possible early gestation, intra- or extra-uterine. When possible, it is desirable also to secure the menstrual data preceding the last period, as well as information as to the normalcy of the period, subsequent spotting, etc. One should be prepared for certain women harboring an undesired pregnancy who will fabricate a story of abnormally profuse bleeding with the hope of a curettage, although liberal abortions in many areas make this unnecessary.

Vaginal Discharge

Leukorrhea is such a common gynecological symptom that it merits a special heading. The duration of the leukorrhea, the character, color, possible odor, and possible irritativeness of the discharge are among the items of inquiry. The budding physician will soon learn that certain fastidious women will complain bitterly about a minor discharge. Others are seemingly oblivious to a copious leukorrhea.

Obstetrical History

Whether the patient is single or married, and, if the latter, how long, is of obvious significance. Even more so is the history of the pregnancies and labors, with especial reference to their number, character, and possible complications. Other important items concern miscarriages or abortions, either spontaneous or induced. On the other hand, a history of sterility, when there has been no contraception, may be of significance.

Urinary Symptoms

The great frequency of urinary symptoms among women, not only in association with urinary tract disease but also with various gynecological disorders, makes it important to inquire as to such items as increased frequency, pain, incontinence, nocturia, and hematuria. A history of previous urinary tract disease, such as cystitis or pyelitis, may likewise be of much value in the interpretation of existing urinary symptoms.

Gastrointestinal Symptoms

Anorexia, bloating, belching, and discomfort after eating, may be secondary to gynecological disease, or they may suggest functional or organic abnormalities of the abdominal viscera. The same statement may be made concerning nausea and vomiting. The latter symptoms, when associated with amenorrhea, would naturally make the physician think of the possibility of pregnancy, to give only one illustration of their possible significance. Constipation is especially common in gynecological patients but may be a rather direct result of certain pelvic lesions associated with pressure or rectal pain. Bleeding on defecation is often due to hemorrhoids, but procto-sigmoidoscopy may be necessary.

Present Illness

Last and perhaps most important comes the most comprehensive heading, that of the history of the present illness, which constitutes a summation of those previously mentioned. Chronological appearance of all gynecological symptoms is particularly desirable with brief mention only of the many irrelevant problems that many women include. Evaluation of the sexual habits are of particular importance in the infertility problems.

GYNECOLOGICAL EXAMINATION

Although the gynecologist's examination will naturally be directed chiefly toward the pelvic and abdominal organs, it must include a general survey of the entire physical make-up. The most important function of examination should be to exclude the presence of malignant or premalignant lesions, and Table 5.1 and Figures 5.1 and 5.2 have been included to present certain statistical features as to age, sex, site, mortality, and various other aspects of this frequent gynecological problem.

General

Among the general items to be included are the height, weight, and general build of the patient, and, in the case of obese patients, the regional distribution of the adipose tissue, as well as any abnormalities of hair distribution. The thyroid should be examined, and at least a superficial examination of the heart and lungs made. The blood pressure should be taken, and the urine examined for albumin and sugar, with, usually, a microscopic examination.

Examination of the Breast

Certain gynecological textbooks have attempted to include sections on the diag-

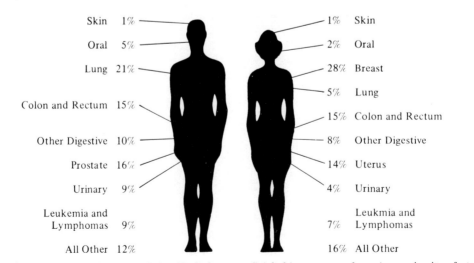

5.1a. Cancer incidence by sex and site. Excludes superficial skin cancer and carcinoma *in situ* of uterine cervix. (American Cancer Society.)

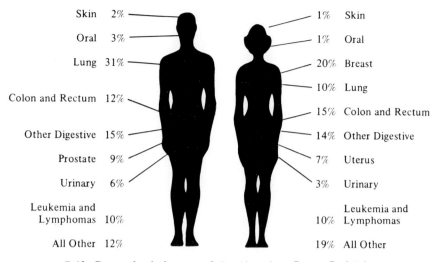

5.1b. Cancer deaths by sex and site. (American Cancer Society)

nosis and treatment of this common type (Fig. 5.1) of female malignancy. Breast disease is so complex and so highly specialized that it warrants not a chapter but a textbook of its own. In our own locale, breast surgery is the domain of the general surgeon; in many areas it falls within the realm of the gynecologist and, indeed, operative surgery on the breast is fully sanctioned by the American Board of Obstetrics and Gynecology. Whether he performs mammary surgery himself, or refers it to a fellow surgeon, palpation of the breast by the gynecologist is mandatory as part of a gynecological "checkup," for mammary cancer is more common than any other form of carcinoma which the female may acquire. We are very impressed by the value of mammograms, especially in the obese patient when palpation is difficult; thermography seems equally promising.

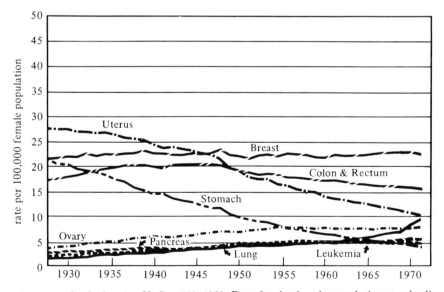

5.2 Female cancer deaths by site, U. S., 1930–1969. Rate for the female population standardized for age on the 1940 U. S. population. Sources of data: National Vital Statistics Division and Bureau of the Census, U. S.

Table 5.1

Mortality for the Five Leading Cancer Sites by Age, Sex and Site, U. S.—1969

Total		Under 15		15–34		35–54		55–74		75+	
Male	Female	Male	Female	Male	Female	Male	Female	Male	Female	Male	Female
Lung 50,481	Breast 28,830	Leukemia 986	Leukemia 759	Leukemia 691	Breast 443	Lung 9,129	Breast 8,613	Lung 32,838	Breast 13,966	Prostate 9,184	Colon and rectum 9,307
Colon and rectum 22,069	Colon and rectum 23,178	Brain, etc. 516	Brain, etc. 403	Hodgkin's disease 511	Leukemia 410	Colon and rectum 2,450	Uterus 3,335	Colon and rectum 11,915	Colon and rectum 11,057	Lung 8,342	Breast 5,805
Prostate 16,836	Uterus 12,475	Lymphosarcoma, etc. 151	Bone 99	Brain, etc. 408	Uterus 355	Pancreas 1,434	Lung 2,911	Prostate 7,336	Lung 6,175	Colon and rectum 7,520	Stomach 2,808
Stomach 10,000	Lung 11,362	Bone 79	Kidney 83	Testis 388	Hodgkin's disease 309	Brain etc. 1,339	Colon and rectum 2,663	Pancreas 5,777	Uterus 6,092	Stomach 3,379	Pancreas 2,802
Pancreas 9,932	Ovary 9,788	Kidney 72	Lymphosarcoma, etc. 55	Lymphosarcoma, etc. 238	Brain, etc. 291	Stomach 1,202	Ovary 2,643	Stomach 5,352	Ovary 5,146	Pancreas 2,678	Uterus 2,689

Source: Vital Statistics of the United States, 1969.

Although we feel that a gynecological textbook should not include a short and incomplete chapter on breast disease, we should like simply to list *verbatim* an old but important set of rules, advocated by Montgomery, Bowers, and Taylor, which exemplify our own feelings in regards to palpation of the breast. Incidently, evaluation of the breast, particularly in the obese woman, is one of the greatest problems with which the gynecologist comes in contact.

"1. There is some safety in numbers: to wit, bilateral diffuse induration of the breast is rarely cancerous and offers no site of selection for biopsy. Such cases should be observed periodically.

"2. Cancer may appear in an area of chronic mastitis by coincidence, or possibly as a result of cause and effect. Any local change of texture or development of a 'dominant' lesion should therefore be biopsied promptly.

"3. Unilateral persistent fibrocystic disease, such as appears frequently in the upper and outer quadrant of the breast, should be freely excised and studied in multiple section.

"4. Enlarged glands of the axilla adjacent to such areas of induration should also be excised for study, even though the breast area itself is benign.

"5. In the case of patients appearing with a well defined mass in the breast, arrangements should be made for prompt biopsy and mastectomy at the same sitting if the tissue is positive.

"6. In a slender undernourished woman, the whole fabric of the breast may be revealed to a degree suggesting fibrocystic disease or even small neoplasms.

"7. Lipoma-like masses in the breast of aged women often harbor scirrhous carcinoma. *Be strongly suspicious of any lesion of the breast after the menopause* (italics ours), especially if there is no hormone therapy.

"8. Questionable areas of nodulation in the breasts of pregnant women should be biopsied under local anesthesia, the biopsy examined in paraffin section, and the definitive therapy carefully planned.

"9. Small apparent lesions of the breast discovered at examination just before menstruation should be rechecked after the period is over; they may disappear.

"10. Minute and doubtful lesions which seem scarcely deserving of biopsy even though they persist after the period should be rechecked every 6 to 8 weeks until the problem is resolved.

"11. The patient with serous discharge from the nipple should be biopsied whenever the secretion can be traced or whenever induration is palpable at any point around the areola or adjacent breast tissue.

"12. A patient with fibrocystic disease may have to be biopsied several times in the course of years to satisfy the physician that cancer is not developing. In some such cases, simple mastectomy becomes the ultimate solution.

"13. The patient who complains most of pain is least likely to have carcinoma, unless she has an enormous lesion.

"14. The patient with extensive fibrocystic disease or adenosis of the breast, and a strong family history of cancer, had better have a simple mastectomy.

"15. Postmenopausal patients should be discouraged in the prolonged use of estrogens because of the untoward effect on the breasts."

With all of the dicta so specified, we are in full accord. Like Montgomery, Bowers, and Taylor, we are inclined to wonder how deleterious to the patient simple biopsy may be, and why immediate mastectomy must be carried out if frozen section, frequently of poor quality and not always representative, should suggest carcinoma. An equally important and related question is whether the young menstruating woman should be castrated. Although there is no certain answer, it would seem unwise to utilize any *exogenous hormones* as *estrogen* in the menopausal patient or "*birth control pills,*" either combined or sequential, because of the uncertainty as to whether a neoplasm might be stimulated rather than suppressed by steroids.

The Relation of the Ovary to

Breast Cancer. Like the uterus, the breast is an end organ insofar as stimulation by the ovarian hormone is concerned. It has been pointed out by Randall and Harkins that a significant number of women continue to show evidence of estrogen effect on the vaginal mucosa for many years after the cessation of the menses, and there is general agreement with this observation. It has been well documented that in certain animals, even of the male sex, breast cancer can be produced by protracted doses of estrogen. It has likewise been noted that women with breast cancer who are subjected to oophorectomy reveal a considerable degree of so-called "ovarian stromal hyperplasia," and thus such gonads seem to harbor cells morphologically akin to the theca cells which normally secrete estrogen. It would therefore seem highly rational, as noted by Rosenberg and Uhlmann, to advocate *routine castration in the menstruating woman* to avoid further stimulation of an already proved malignant end organ. Patterson and Russell suggest irradiation as an effective and simple method of ablating ovarian functions.

The study of Feinleib would suggest that early castration for gynecological problems in the woman *less than* forty markedly decrease the expected incidence of subsequent breast cancer. *After* forty years the difference is less striking, and it is suggested that removal of the cyclic stimulation of the functioning ovary may be of importance.

Unfortunately, the problem is not nearly so simple, for it is well established that the adrenal gland is quite capable of estrogen secretion. Review by Brown, Falconer, and Strong indicates that *castrated* patients treated with adrenocorticotrophin (ACTH) have a large measurable amount of urinary estrogen, almost certainly of adrenal origin. For this reason, certain gynecologists, surgeons, and endocrinologists have adopted a policy of oophorectomy for the young menstruating patient and adrenalectomy for the older patient, especially when there has been evidence of metastatic disease. That this approach is not entirely satisfactory is suggested by a series of recent articles by Bulbrook and Greenwood. In a limited number of patients with advanced breast cancer, who had been subject not only to oophorectomy and adrenalectomy but also to hypophysectomy, the level of urinary estrogen was nearly equivalent to that found at certain stages of the cycle in normally menstruating women. We can merely speculate as to what is the source of this estrogenic substance; but is it too far-fetched to wonder if it may be ingested by female and male alike as part of the daily diet, perhaps as cholesterol which can be synthesized to the steroidal hormones.

Castration with Breast Cancer. The National Surgical Adjuvant Breast Project (Ravdin *et al.*) has reached the following conclusions. "There seems no justification for prophylactic oophorectomy in the treatment of operable breast cancer. Its use therapeutically in advanced breast carcinoma is not contested." Fortunately this text need not become involved in the current problems concerning radical or simple mastectomy, with or without irradiation, as summarized by Haagensen.

The same study group could find no particular difference in the duration between observed recurrence and survival in patients treated by castration, chemotherapy, and placebos where there was operable breast disease. Thus it might seem that castration may be restricted to premenopausal women with recurrent or metastatic disease. In the postmenopausal woman, oophorectomy might be beneficial where there is a hormone-dependent lesion, as noted by Maas *et al.* The problems of estrogen receptivity will be discussed in Chapter 15.

Approximately 60,000 of all annual female cancers will originate in the breast, and although all women are susceptible, about 25,000 of these women will be in the *premenopausal age group.* Although a minority of these females will have a cancer that is hormone dependent, approximately 30 per cent of young women seemingly exhibit a beneficial response if immediate therapeutic surgical castration is carried out for advanced or metastatic disease. Results with irradiation are more variable, slower to appear, and less convincing than comparable patients treated surgically.

Lewison points out the current difficulties in ascertaining which lesion will respond to castration, and indicates that it cannot as yet be equated with estrogen assay or cytological maturation index. In any case, the possibility of exacerbation of the disease by castration may be discounted, but the relative frequency (25% noted by Kasilag and Rutledge) with which terminal metastatic breast cancer spreads to the ovary would likewise warrant consideration.

Currently *irradiation* to the breast is utilized primarily where there is extensive or metastatic disease, but not if the process is localized. An excellent report by Goldenberg would suggest a 20% remission rate in advanced or metastatic cancer with the use of androgens. The use of progesterone, effective in certain cases (33%) of endometrial recurrences, seems logical in the treatment of recurrent breast cancer, but this particular hormone has received only cursory trial.

As a consequence of the above opinions, we have formulated certain generalizations for women with breast cancer, which we hope will be verified by further clinical trials. (1) Conservation of ovaries in the young patient where there is no evidence of metastatic disease, but castration if there is proved evidence of major axillary involvement. (2) Castration, even in the premenopausal woman who has had recurrence or metastasis after radical mastectomy. (3) Castration in the postmenopausal woman with metastatic or recurrent cancer *only* if the vaginal smear shows evidence of sustained high estrogen effect. (4) Pregnancy is to be avoided, and if other than simple curettage is indicated for therapeutic abortion, probably hysterectomy with castration is preferable to hysterotomy. Indeed, if hysterectomy by any approach or for any reason is contemplated, probably it is well to practice simultaneous oophorectomy, except in the very youthful woman.

Although these tenets must not be regarded as absolute, and although there are unquestionably certain exceptions, they have at least provided a general working rule in regard to the management of a highly controversial subject. Obviously certain religious and individual indications on occasion influence our expressed intentions, and we would be the first to admit that our opinions are by no means based on firmly established facts.

Steroid therapy of advanced breast cancer is likewise highly unpredictable. Brilliant results have sometimes been obtained by usage of large dosage of testosterone proprionate (100 mg. three times a week) where there is local or soft tissue involvement. Similar large dosage of estrogenic substances for bony metastasis may be utilized in the older patient. Since breast cancer like endometrial adenocarcinoma is on occasion presumed to be estrogen-dependent, it would seem that mammary cancer might show the striking remission often exhibited by fundal disease to large dosage progesterone. Opinion, however, is far from uniform.

That there are occasional dramatic remissions of the disease following hormone therapy is undeniable. Certainly cure is infrequent, and in any case, the critical physician will recall that on occasion there may be dramatic spontaneous remission of malignancies. Where there is no overt evidence of continued estrogenic function, however, we are in full accord with a trial of large dosage steroid therapy where there is advanced or recurrent cancer if only to alter the hormone milieu. The role of corticiods, as well as such ablation procedures as *adrenalectomy* and *hypophysectomy,* can be beneficial but requires careful clinical judgment in the total treatment of advanced breast cancer.

Abdominal Examination

Simple inspection will reveal such abnormalities as undue prominence or asymmetrical contour, as well as variations in abdominal and pubic hair distribution. Any masses or tenderness should be carefully noted. Particular attention should be directed toward certain cardinal areas, especially the adnexal regions, McBurney's point, the gall bladder region, the epigastrium, and the kidney areas. Previous surgical scars should be noted.

If an abnormal mass of any kind is felt, its position and its relation to any abdominal or pelvic organ or region should be noted, together with its size, shape, contour, consistency, movability, and tenderness or lack of tenderness. Percussion is of special value in the case of certain large tumors, such as ovarian cysts, which must be distinguished from ascites. Sonar is often helpful.

Pelvic Examination

It is in the examination of the pelvic organs proper that the special training of the gynecologist comes into play. The more experienced, thorough, and methodical he is, the more he will learn from the examination.

Preparation and Position of the Patient. The clothing having been removed, the patient lies in the dorsal recumbent position, with flexed thighs and knees, the feet resting on the stirrups of the examining table, and the limbs and lower abdomen being draped with a sheet. The presence of a nurse, or of a female relative or friend, should be looked upon as essential for obvious reasons. It is of great importance that the patient's bladder be emptied just before the examination.

The examining hand is covered with a rubber or "throw-away" plastic glove, for the protection of the physician perhaps even more than of the patient, and the index finger is well lubricated. The traditional examining hand of the gynecologist is the left, and the expert gynecologist soon learns to feel both sides of the pelvis equally well with the left hand. A reason for use of the left hand is that the stronger and more useful right hand is left free to handle the instruments which are at times called for during the examination.

Careful inspection of the external genitalia is the first step of the pelvic examination. This will take cognizance of the presence of any anatomical or pathological abnormalities, the presence of any skin lesions or of any inflammation or irritation of the vulvovaginal mucosa and urethra, the presence or absence of the hymen, the size of the clitoris, etc.

Before proceeding with the vaginal examination, the presence of urethral or Bartholin's gland disease should be ex-

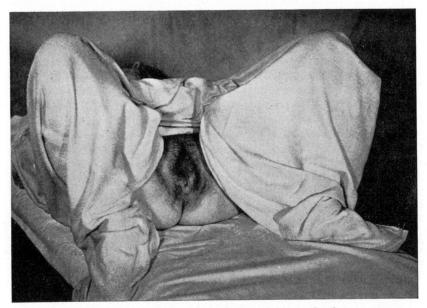

5.3. Position of patient for ordinary pelvic examination

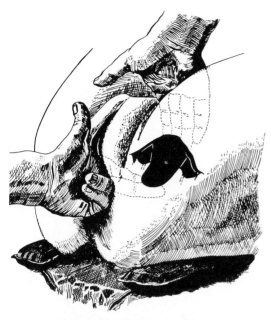

5.4 Bimanual palpation of pelvic viscera

cluded. Urethral caruncle or erosion will usually be evident on inspection, but the distal portion of the urethra should be gently stripped to ascertain whether a purulent exudate can be milked from either the urethra, the subjacent Skene's ducts, or a suburethral diverticulum infection.

Speculum examination of the cervix is performed before pelvic examination, since any type of lubricant will make evaluation of a cytopathological smear more difficult. Smear should be performed at least annually; in addition visualization of the cervix may provide certain information. The presence of polyps, erosion, eversion, or retention cysts must be looked for, and the character, amount, and probable source of any discharge noted. The vaginal mucosa should likewise be inspected. The Gonococcus may be sought for and cultured from the secretion from the cervical canal or urethra, whereas the Trichomonas can be found in the exudate obtained from the speculum in the posterior fornix. This technique for these various tests is described in the appropriate chapters.

Perhaps the most important field for very careful and painstaking speculum inspection of the cervix is in cases of suspected malignancy of the cervix. Although the later stages of cancer are ordinarily unmistakable, the early lesions are not characteristic and present no specific appearance. One must suspect any cervical lesion and settle the question definitely, as it can practically always be settled, by subsequent *biopsy*, although a *smear* suffices if there is no discrete lesion. These and other special diagnostic methods are discussed in Chapters 12 and 15.

One or more fingers well lubricated, are

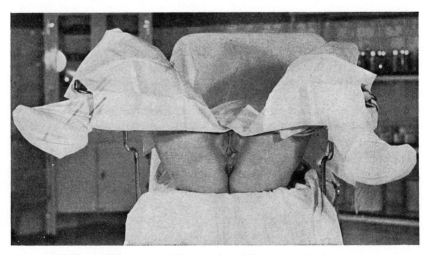

5.5. Dorsal lithotomy position employed for most vaginal operations

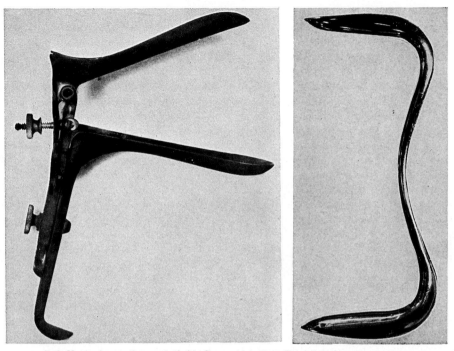

5.6. Vaginal speculums. *A (left)*, Graves' bivalve; *B (right)*, Sims' speculum

then introduced into the vagina, and as the fingers pass into the vagina one can note the degree of relaxation if any is present. Ordinarily the patient is asked to bear down for a moment, as this will indicate the degree of any cystocele, rectocele, or uterine descensus which may be present.

In the case of unmarried patients in whom an intact hymen would render digital examination of the vagina impossible or very painful, the examination of the pelvic organs should be made *per rectum*. Occasionally examination under anesthesia is desirable, especially in the case of young girls.

The examination of the internal genitalia begins with careful *palpation of the cervix*, making note of such data as its size and shape, the direction in which the cervix points, whether or not there is any laceration or hypertrophy, and whether such digital contact with the cervix causes bleeding, as it so commonly does with certain lesions (polyp, cancer).

The examining fingers now seek to determine the size, shape, and position of the uterus, and the external hand is called into play, and the real *bimanual procedure* begins. The purpose is to map out the organs between the internal fingers and the hand externally, and the cooperation of the patient is indispensable for good results. When the abdominal wall is very thick and obese, one can scarcely expect to be able to outline the organs as clearly and sharply as in the case of women with thin and flabby abdominal walls.

A common complaint of beginners is that the fingers are too short to permit satisfactory outlining of the internal genital organs. During the examination the fingers should hug the posterior rather than the anterior wall, for pressure against the urethra may cause much discomfort. On the other hand, the perineum can be pressed backward toward the rectum quite freely and painlessly. By passing the finger along the front of the cervix one comes to the anterior surface of the uterine body, which can be felt through the anterior vaginal fornix, especially if the external hand gently presses the uterus down toward the internal. Between the two the fundus can then be clearly felt, and one can determine its size, contour, and movability quite accurately. An irregular, knobby outline, combined with enlargement of the uterus, for example, makes it quite certain that the uterus contains myomatous tumors. The posterior wall can likewise be readily palpated in most cases.

When, on the other hand, the fundus cannot be felt anteriorly, the finger passed upward along the posterior surface of the uterus encounters the firm uterine body posteriorly, so that *retroversion* or *retroflexion* can be easily diagnosed.

The idea, in other words, is simply to play one hand against the other, groping gently about to outline the various normal or abnormal pelvic contents. In palpating behind the cervix one incidentally notes any tenderness or thickening in the uterosacral region, sometimes due to inflammatory thickening of the ligaments themselves but often due to the presence of prolapsed, inflamed, and adherent adnexa.

The sides of the pelvis are then carefully and gently explored by the external hand in an effort to feel the lateral organs between the two hands. In most cases the normal ovaries are readily palpable and are tender to palpation. Any enlargement is noted, as well as the movability of fixation of the organ. Although the normal tube cannot be felt, any noteworthy enlargement, as with pyosalpinx, leads to a definite, usually fixed and adherent mass of varying size, inseparable from the ovary.

Examination of the Rectum

Finally, examination of the rectum is of importance, especially in those cases in which rectal symptoms, especially bleeding or pain, have been complained of. External hemorrhoids, fissures, and fistulous openings are readily seen, but other abnormalities require digital or proctoscopic examination. We do not perform routine proctoscopy as advocated by the American Cancer Society, since most rectal carcinomas are low enough to be felt by the examining finger. Frequently, combined examination, with one finger in the vagina and one in the rectum, will be informative.

GYNECOLOGICAL OPERATIONS

A textbook on clinical gynecology cannot satisfactorily include adequate coverage of operative gynecology. Attempts to achieve this have invariably resulted in rather obvious shortcomings in discussion of the surgical methods or of such aspects as pathology or endocrinology—which are more important to the student or general practitioner than is operative technique. However, it seems advisable to describe only a few gynecological operations which, with certain variations, comprise probably 90% of most standard surgical procedures. This attempt should in no way be construed as a half-hearted portrayal of operative technique, but only as a realistic effort to illustrate and explain a few methods which are referred to repeatedly throughout this text.

Dilatation and Curettage

This is unquestionably the most common operation performed by the gynecologist, for it is standard procedure to investigate *any atypical* or *irregular bleeding* by simply "scraping out" the lining endometrium when no cause for bleeding has been found in preliminary office examination and biopsy. This procedure is sometimes omitted in the case of young girls whose bleeding is rarely of serious cause and frequently amenable to hormone therapy. It should be emphasized that cytopathological detection of endometrial lesions does not approach the accuracy found with cervical diseases and indeed, in many reports, does not achieve even an 80% incidence of accuracy. If a 50-year-old woman who has a normal pelvis is bleeding abnormally, it may be very well to assume that the bleeding is of functional origin and related to an incipient menopause. However, *curettage* should never be omitted, for one simply cannot be certain of the contents of an externally normal uterus without exploration of the interior. This same procedure will be of extreme aid in outlining the contour of the cavity for such entities as submucous myomas, generally precluding the use of a hysterogram or hysteroscopy in the usual case.

Although curettage (with previous or concomitant cervical biopsy) is the most important diagnostic procedure available to us, its value as a therapeutic agent is not fully appreciated. Despite uncertainty as to the mechanism, a significant number of patients with bleeding of either functional and, occasionally, organic cause seem improved or cured after curettage. The incidence of such cases, approximately 50%, is so striking that it has sporadically evoked speculation as to whether the endometrium might not harbor some hormonal or toxic agent, the removal of which, by curettage, might allow return of normal menstruation. Attempts to isolate such an agent have been unsuccessful despite the good clinical response to curettage.

Curettage may yield many ancillary benefits. It is our custom to perform routine preoperative *examination under anesthesia,* because a much more accurate assessment of the female organs is afforded in the completely relaxed patient. *Dilatation of the cervix* is a preliminary procedure to curettage, and this is not infrequently of certain value in the control of dysmenorrhea. *Rubin's test, cauterization of the cervix,* and *application of radium* for benign or malignant disease are frequently utilized in conjunction with curettage, according to specific indication.

In most instances it is logical to perform certain minor operative procedures as curettage on an outpatient basis. Good risk patients simply report in the morning with an empty stomach, have the minor surgery performed under sodium pentothal anesthesia, and are allowed to leave in the early afternoon after a few hours of observation in a recovery bed. Such complications as infections or bleeding are minimal, and if

perforation of the uterus is suspected hospital admission overnight is arranged. This innovation has resulted in a tremendous saving in expense to the patient and in hospital beds. It should be emphasized that this is not an office procedure and should be performed only in a hospital atmosphere on patients who have had adequate medical clearance although in some areas, even incomplete and therapeutic abortions are treated as office procedures; this seems risky.

The technique of curettage is simple. After preliminary examination under anesthesia a vaginal retractor is inserted and the cervix is grasped with a tenaculum clamp. The uterine cavity is then measured by a sound, after which the cervix is dilated by various methods. Thorough curettage is then accomplished, after which the cavity is probed by certain types of *"polyp forceps."* Pregnancy and acute infections are obvious contraindications to curettage. Care must be taken to avoid perforation of the uterus, especially when it is soft as with a bleeding incomplete abortion, or sharply retroflexed; actually, however, uterine perforation is rarely attended by any significant complication, with expectant therapy the rule, and laparotomy the exception (Radman and Korman). Where early therapeutic abortion is performed, curettage is preceded by suction.

Laparoscopy

Since the last edition of this text, use of the laparoscope for diagnostic and therapeutic measures has become increasingly popular, and there have been many publications with regard to the results of its use; because of the large number only a few will be included in the references, and naturally these will be those pertaining to the methods and results utilized in our own clinic. Of the various different techniques, either the two-incision techniques in which the laparoscope and biopsy tong are utilized through separate incisions, or the one-incision technique with the fibre-optic operating laparoscope with an electric coagulation forceps may be used. The latter is currently the technique of choice in our own institution.

The abdomen is insufflated with carbon dioxide, after which a trocar is introduced through the lower portion of the umbilicus. The laparoscope is then inserted, and the pelvic organs can be visualized. Previous surgery or obesity can make visualization difficult, but the well trained operator can generally overcome these. It is our clinic policy to handle these women as out-patients, allowing them to go home in the late afternoon. However, various medical complications may dictate overnight admission.

The pelvic organs in any case can be visualized more adequately than with culdoscopy and without the knee-chest position necessitated by the culdoscopic approach. Use of the laparoscope lends expediency to the diagnosis of such diseases as ectopic pregnancy, inflammatory disease, ovarian neoplasms, etc. It is extremely useful in the study of infertility patients, particularly where there is a contradictory Rubin's test and hysterosalpingogram; indigo carmine can be injected through the cervix via a cannula; and, if the tubes are patent, the dye can be visualized passing out the fimbriated end of the tube; if there is tubal blockage, stoppage of the dye will indicate at approximately what area of the tube the obstruction is located.

Perhaps the most widespread use of the laparoscope is as a method of providing sterilization of the patient by coagulation of the tubes. In our area this is done on an out-patient basis, and is colloquially referred to as "band aid" surgery, since the patient leaves the same afternoon with a simple dressing over the umbilicus.

It is of course imperative that the fallopian tube be thoroughly visualized and recognized as such. For the novice it is easy to confuse the tube with the round ligament or other structures, but the problem lessens with experience. The tube is grasped and coagulated, but at the same time a small portion of the tube is removed. Care should be taken that adequate coagulation is achieved (Fig. 5.7).

It is still too early to know precisely the

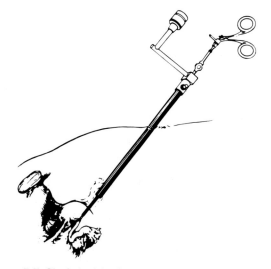

5.7. Single incision laparoscopic sterilization.

long-term pregnancy rate following laparoscopic tubal sterilization. In our own first 666 patients there were 5 who were apparently already pregnant at the time of laparoscopy, and were subsequently aborted. There were, however, two subsequent pregnancies, one of which was an ectopic gestation, and the other an intrauterine pregnancy which was thought to be due to cauterization of the round ligament rather than the tube.

Laparoscopy is not without complication, even when performed by a skilled operator. Bleeding may be a problem which is generally controlled by recoagulation, but on occasion laparotomy may be necessitated. Uterine perforation may occur if the intrauterine cannula, which is utilized to mobilize the uterus, is manipulated too briskly. Burn at the trocar site may occur, as may infection or cardiac arrhythmia. Far and away the most serious complication, however, is damage to the bowel, which is generally in the nature of a burn, leading to subsequent bowel perforation, and peritonitis. While the exact mechanism of this is uncertain, it has happened in at least a half a dozen cases in this community, and unfortunately this is the type of problem that leads to medicolegal intervention. For this reason various clinics are utilizing various types of clips to the tube, but the results seem uncertain at this writing. However, the complication rate is quite low, and laparoscopic sterilization has become an efficient and extremely safe adjunct to family planning.

Hysterectomy

The most common major gynecological operation is removal of the uterus by either the *abdominal* or *vaginal* route. Each approach has various indications and contra-indications, and we deplore a rigid insistence on either procedure, preferring individualization as dictated by various findings. *Hysterectomy* is an operation which, in some quarters, has acquired an onerous reputation, due perhaps to a small minority of overzealous surgeons (frequently not gynecologists) who have seemed inclined to believe that removal of the uterus would be the panacea for every pain or discomfort which might afflict the woman. A constructive but critical report by D'Esopo would indicate that most hysterectomies performed by specialists are justifiable, even though the uterus shows no evidence of a pathological condition (as in prolapse, recurrent bleeding, etc.).

Similarly, to many women, *hysterectomy* has always been construed as a worse fate than decapitation. Massive obesity, hirsutism, loss of mental faculties, and above all, cessation of any real or assumed sexual proficiency, have been considered to be a certain sequel to this operation, as is the dread "change of life." If the gynecologist will take the time to explain a few fundamental facts to the patient, it will be possible to make her understand that no dire consequences will occur. She will not, of course, become pregnant again, but this often welcome news. Nor will she have further menstruation, but adequate control of abnormal bleeding is frequently the main reason for surgery.

Aside from these two sequelae, no drastic results are found following removal of the uterus. Concomitant oophorectomy may of course produce genuine menopausal symptoms, and illogically these may occur as a mild, transient phenomenon of hysterectomy alone. If, however, some explanation of their nonpathological and evanescent character is afforded, most patients will be very willing to accept their minor difficulties, with only a few requiring hormone therapy.

Elective Hysterectomy

Within the last five years there has been increasing enthusiasm among many gynecologists for hysterectomy, especially vaginal, as an elective method of sterilization. The matter is not completely settled but seemingly revolves around two points.

1) Hysterectomy is admittedly a more tedious and complicated procedure than tubal ligation, with a higher morbidity and mortality, and a more prolonged and expensive hospitalization. Most statistics, however, with regard to vaginal hysterectomy, include patients of all age groups who have an associated repair; where hysterectomy alone is performed on young good-risk patients without repair, the mortality probably is very little more than with tubal ligation. Certain psychologists suggest that hysterectomy will lead to a loss of femininity and to sexual frigidity. This seems unlikely if the procedure is explained, and if the continued ovarian function is stressed to the woman. It seems well ascertained that even total hysterectomy does not lead to any appreciable shortening of the vagina with resultant dyspareunia.

2) Many gynecologists feel very strongly that vaginal hysterectomy is much preferred over tubal ligation, and can advance the following rather convincing arguments. Most statistics on tubal ligation indicate an approximate 2 per cent pregnancy rate following the procedure even though the technique may be adequate, for certain tubes can apparently become recanalized. Only a very few pregnancies have been observed after hysterectomy, as noted in Chapter 26. In addition, many reports on patients who have been treated by tubal ligation indicate that anywhere between 25 and 50 per cent of them will subsequently need some type of pelvic

surgery, generally hysterectomy, because of various bleeding problems, myomata, uterine cancer, prolapse, etc. If these secondary procedures are considered and added to the immediate mortality and morbidity from tubal ligation, this figure would unquestionably be considerably higher than simple hysterectomy for an essentially normal uterus. Menstruation is a nuisance to most women, and if this can be abolished without impairing ovarian function, it would probably be a blessing to not only the woman but to her husband. Finally, many women who undergo vaginal hysterectomy might have minor degrees of outlet relaxation and descensus which could be corrected, thus obviating the need for subsequent secondary surgery.

Thus one can make a rather convincing case for the value of elective hysterectomy, and there seems definitely a trend in this community, as well as in the country as a whole for this to be the procedure of choice. Obviously this should be qualified by the fact that surgery be done by a competent, well-trained gynecologist. We might hesitate at the utilization of vaginal hysterectomy on the pregnant uterus as a means of abortion and sterilization, as has been advocated by some, for on occasion this might be a rather formidable and sometimes bloody surgical procedure. Ballard, however, has reported a rather respectable morbidity on abortion-sterilization by vaginal hysterectomy in women less than 15 weeks pregnant.

Abdominal Hysterectomy (Fig. 5.8, *A, B,* and *C*). In past years there was considerable debate as to the relative desirability of total or subtotal hysterectomy (preservation of the cervix). Today no one will question preference for the total operation as a prophylaxis against

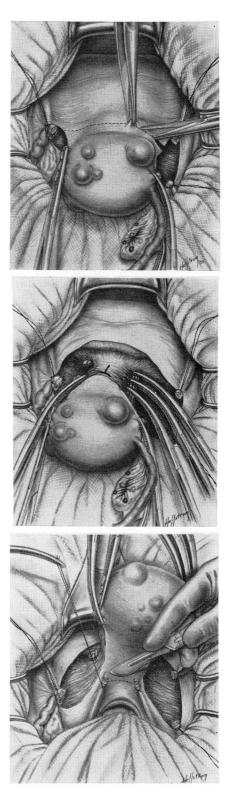

5.8A. Abdominal hysterectomy. *Top,* left tube, utero-ovarian and round ligaments divided and doubly ligated; bladder peritoneum mobilized. *Middle,* uterine vessels doubly ligated. *Bottom,* division of uterosacral ligaments and posterior peritoneum; an inverted T-incision has been utilized anteriorly to push the pubocervical fascia laterally along with the ureter (as per Richardson).

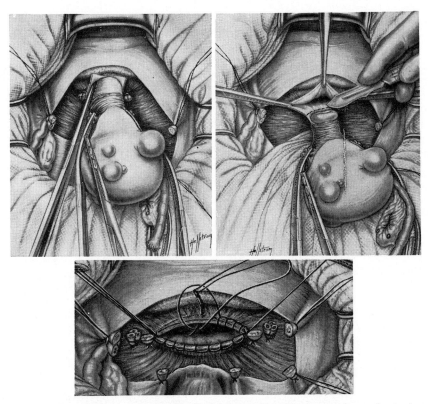

5.8B. Abdominal hysterectomy (*continued*). *Top left,* cardinal ligaments clamped, staying within the fascia reflected by the T-incision. *Top right,* cervix excised, clamp at both angles as well as anterior and posterior, according to individual technique. *Bottom,* lock, or some kind of hemastatic suture, of vaginal cuff.

cervical stump cancer as well as persistent leukorrhea. At our clinic over 95% of all hysterectomies are complete, but we prefer to praise rather than condemn our house staff for utilizing the lesser operation in poor risk or difficult cases in which morbidity and mortality would be increased by insistence on total hysterectomy. In many instances preliminary subtotal hysterectomy with removal of a bulky myomatous tumor or large adnexal masses will improve exposure and facilitate removal of the cervix (this will explain why certain figures in this text show only a uterine fundus). Howkins and Williams indicate that the mortality of total hysterectomy is 0.2%; in some areas the incidence is higher for the subtotal procedure which is reserved for more difficult cases.

The abdominal approach is favored for large myomatous tumors, ovarian lesions, and for certain conditions in which the uterus is apt to be fixed, as in endometriosis, inflammatory disease, certain types of previous surgery, etc. Desire to repair a ventral hernia, remove the appendix, or explore for pain are suggestions for laparotomy when hysterectomy seems indicated. Cancer of the endometrium is best treated by abdominal hysterectomy, and this is the usual approach for *stage I.C.O. cancer of the cervix* only if there is a suggestion of micro-invasion in preoperative biopsy or (cryostat) conization. We are not convinced that the so-called modified Wertheim hysterectomy, which is merely an extended total abdominal hysterectomy, is preferable to vaginal excision of the uterus, and we do not hesitate to individualize.

Oophorectomy with Benign Disease? Although it is generally accepted that complete removal of all pelvic organs is the preferred treatment in most cases of pelvic malignancies (with such

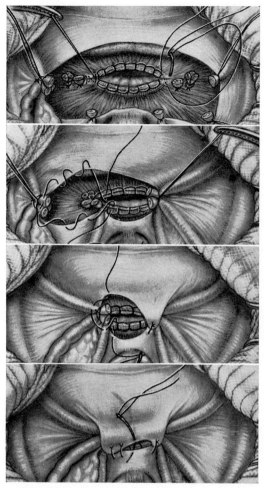

5.8C. Abdominal hysterectomy (*continued*). *Top,* attachment of uterosacral and cardinal ligaments to angles. *Second from top,* round ligaments, tubes, and utero-ovarian ligaments attached to angles. *Third from top,* also *bottom,* complete peritonealization. (From Gray, L. A.: Techniques of abdominal total hysterectomy. Amer. J. Obstet. Gynec., *75:* 33, 1958.)

exceptions as certain dysontogenetic ovarian tumors or intraepithelial cervical cancer in the youthful woman), there is the greatest difference of opinion as to removal of the gonads in the fifth decade woman who is having abdominal hysterectomy for a benign disease such as myomata, recurrent bleeding, etc.

One can find no set criteria for removal or preservation of the adnexa, and although Randall has presented all of the questions pertinent to the removal or con-

servation of the gonads, he has unfortunately not provided any certain formula for the harassed gynecologist to follow. This is of course understandable, because of our relative ignorance of gonadal function in the postmenopausal woman.

The problem revolves around several points. (1) Although it is generally accepted that ovarian cancer will afflict less than one of every 100 40-plus-year-old-woman, it is nevertheless an extremely insidious and usually fatal disease. (2) The importance of the aging gonad is not fully understood, especially its possible role in preventing certain cardiovascular changes. One may find the greatest difference of opinion, Parrish *et al.* emphasizing that castration 10 years before the usual menopausal age of 50 years is attended by a high incidence of atherosclerosis. On the other hand, Plotz and Novak and Williams are not impressed by such an association. Actually today it might appear that protracted exposure to estrogen is associated with increased cardiovascular problems. (3) A not infrequent occurrence is an enlarged cystic ovary, generally functional, but not always, which is extremely worrisome to the conscientious gynecologist who will be aware of the fact that 5 to 10 per cent of all ovarian cancers will develop in the posthysterectomy female. Grogan has always stressed the frequency of posthysterectomy functional cysts of the ovary, but we regard them as infrequent.

Although we will propose no inviolable routine, preferring to individualize according to the patient's psyche, familial history for cancer, etc., our inclination is toward the radical approach, namely removal of the gonads. Where vasomotor symptoms appear, these are generally controlled by various oral hormones with minimal complications if the uterus is out. Although *not* advocating replacement therapy for every aging female, we are certainly more inclined to utilize it *when necessary* if the uterus is absent.

Vaginal Hysterectomy (Fig. 5.9, *A* and *B*). This procedure has enjoyed a tremendous surge of popularity in the last 30 years, and has considerable to recommend it. Postoperative discomfort is

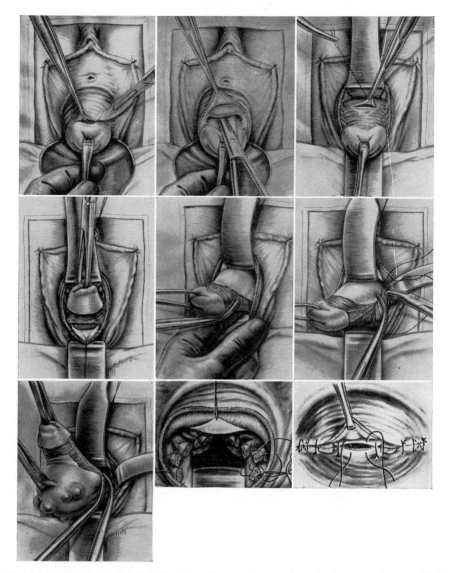

5.9A. Vaginal hysterectomy. *Top left,* incision above and around cervix, low enough to avoid damage to bladder. *Top middle,* separation of bladder from cervix up to peritoneal reflection; note bladder pillars with ureters in close proximity. *Top right,* peritoneal cavity entered anteriorly so that long Heaney retractor may be inserted beneath bladder. *Center left,* entry into posterior cul-de-sac (this is frequently preferable initially, because early division of the uterosacral ligaments will increase mobility of uterus). *Center middle,* division and suture of uterosacral ligaments. *Center right,* ligation of uterine vessels, preferably double. *Bottom left,* fundus delivered, either posteriorly or anteriorly, with suture of tubes, utero-ovarian and round ligaments. *Bottom middle,* suture of ligaments to provide support for vagina. Heaney method utilizes peritoneum, tube, utero-ovarian and round ligaments to respective anterior vaginal apex. Mayo-Simpson suspension interposes ligaments from both sides in midline under bladder. In either plication of uterosacral ligaments with posterior vagina is utilized to prevent enterocele (illustrated before approximation of ligaments). *Bottom right,* suture of mucosa, if no repair.

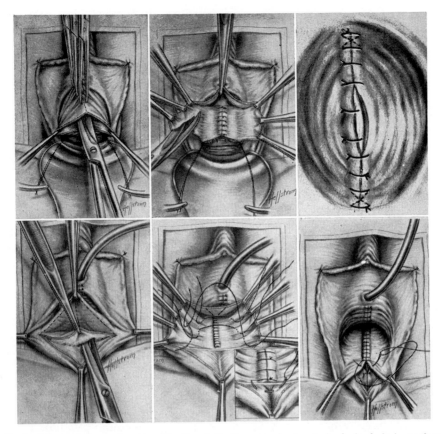

5.9B. Vaginal hysterectomy (*continued*). *Top left,* if cystocele repair is desired, it is performed after suspension of the vagina; note separation of mucosa from bladder and fascia. *Top middle,* excision of redundant mucosa after approximation of pubocervical fascia (plication of sphincter where necessary). *Top right,* closure of vault with excision of redundant vaginal mucosa. *Bottom left,* posterior repair begun by elevating mucosa. *Bottom middle,* approximation of levator ani (repair of perirectal fascia is often desirable). *Bottom right,* running lock suture of posterior vaginal wall. (From Gray, L. A.: *Vaginal Hysterectomy,* Charles C Thomas, Springfield, Ill., 1955.)

minimal and mortality is low, although morbidity is not uncommon, particularly when cystocele repair is also carried out. Pratt has recently compiled the complications, dividing them into vascular, urinary, and pyogenic varieties, as well as indicating that morbidity is increased in the woman less than 35 years old because of pelvic vascularity, and more than 60 years due to the problems associated with increasing age.

Specific indications for a vaginal approach are prolapse and outlet relaxation, with associated rectocele, enterocele, and urinary incontinence. Appropriate reparative procedures are then combined with hysterectomy. However, cases of recurrent functional bleeding, painful retropositions, and small myomas are also amenable to surgery by the vaginal route. Lack of descensus or even nulliparity is not a contra-indication, but large tumors (especially ovarian), endometriosis, or inflammatory disease should suggest laparotomy. A previous lower midline scar is not in itself a contraindication (as noted by Coulam and Pratt), but dictates sober discretion. Such procedures as ventrofixation and other types of suspension can make subsequent vaginal hysterectomy of considerable difficulty. One of the nicest features of the vaginal approach to hysterectomy is that it spares the surgeon the decision as to how to handle the ovaries. These are rarely removed during the course of the average vaginal operation, although this would often technically be easy. Vaginal hysterectomy (with or without adnexectomy) is occasionally expedient in treating endometrial adenocarcinoma as noted by Pratt, Symmonds, and Welch.

We cannot justify morcellation of large, myomatous uteri so that hysterectomy may be achieved vaginally, nor can we advocate ovarian or tubal surgery as a routine by the vaginal approach. There are certain individual patients with large fibroids whose problems may include the desirability of vaginal surgery. When there is any doubt as to whether all of the operation can be accomplished from below, we generally post the patient for a combined procedure.

Combined Procedure. This generally implies the necessary vaginal repair followed by laparotomy. If, however, hysterectomy is deemed desirable and can be accomplished easily from below, this is performed. If the uterus is too bulky or fixed for satisfactory removal from below, we complete the vaginal repair and then redrape the patient for laparotomy without undue delay.

POSTOPERATIVE COMPLICATIONS

Most posthysterectomy patients will be ambulatory the day following surgery and will be discharged in about a week. Nevertheless a certain proportion of these will develop complications, which will prolong their hospitalization, and on occasion tax the ingenuity of the surgeon in charge. Although all respective operative procedures are done in basically the same fashion, there is no denying the fact that a small but inevitable proportion will develop certain complications as noted below.

In a recent review Mattingly and Wilkinson described the high risk patient, wherein such features as advanced age, obesity, such intercurrent disease problems as diabetes, various pulmonary and cardiac disorders, and certain others increase the possibility of a postoperative complication. If these features are recognized and put into proper proportion, certain precautions may be taken preoperatively to minimize the possibility of serious postsurgical sequelae.

1. Hemorrhage

This may occur immediately postoperative as a result of inadequate hemostasis at the time of surgery. Bleeding may be very slight, and indeed self-limited, or may be massive at times, producing varying degrees of shock. Ideally this should be recognized while the patient is still in the operating suite or recovery room.

Vaginal surgery may be followed by either abdominal or vaginal bleeding; the latter of these, if minor, may be controlled by a pack or, on other occasions, by simple vaginal suture. However, if not adequate, laparotomy must be carried out with ligation of any observed bleeding point. *Abdominal* hysterectomy may likewise be associated with severe intraperitoneal bleeding, and massive degrees of hemoperitoneum. Laparotomy should not be deferred too long while the patient is gotten into adequate condition. Where bleeding points are easily visualized, ligation should be carried out, but on occasion this is not always as easy as it sounds, for clamping of any poorly visualized vessel might impair the integrity of the ureter. On occasion ligation of the hypogastric vessels may be carried out as a life-saving procedure.

Bleeding may occur as late as 10 to 14 days postoperatively, after either an abdominal or vaginal procedure, and probably is a result of absorption of the catgut sutures. This is often slight and transitory, being manifested by minor degrees of vaginal bleeding, which usually responds to simple packing—occasionally more profuse bleeding may occur so that secondary surgery is necessary.

2. Hematoma

A rather common but somewhat delayed postoperative complication, after either vaginal or abdominal surgery, is the hematoma. This is more common in the younger woman with an abundant blood supply, but is particularly frequent following radical surgery as for cervical cancer. On occasion there is relatively little in the way of symptomatology, but a rising temperature along with a drop in the postoperative hematocrit is suggestive. The hematoma may frequently be palpated in the lower pelvis; and if it should dissect down into the cul-de-sac, and be sufficiently soft, posterior colpotomy is often curative. In utilizing this approach, however, one must use extreme caution to avoid injuring bladder or bowel, with resultant fistula formation. An excellent resume of the role of hemorrhage in gynecologic surgery has been published by Twombly.

3. Urinary Complications

A. Urinary Retention. This is a rather common sequel to hysterectomy, particularly where this has been vaginal with associated anterior repair. Catheter drainage is generally instituted for about 5 days, after which the catheter is removed. Inability to void following removal is often of serious nuisance value, necessitating repeated catheterization, and reinsertion of an indwelling catheter with resultant infection. Today, however, many clinics utilize suprapublic drainage via a small polyethylene catheter or tube, introduced via a large bore needle or trocar, with no urethral drainage. Many of these patients will void spontaneously once the tube is clamped off (after about 3 days), so that it can be removed. This seemingly has minimized the incidence of infection. Tidal drainage is often helpful.

B. Infection. *Cystitis* or infection of the bladder is quite common following vaginal surgery with repair where catheterization has been utilized, but it usually subsides promptly following chemotherapy or antibiotics. Culture with sensitivity tests should of course be carried out, and response is usually rapid.

Pyelitis may occur and produce a high fever along with chills and flank pain. This too generally responds promptly to medication; failure to do so should indicate intravenous pyelograms to exclude the possibility of any type of operative damage to the urinary tract.

C. Fistula. Damage to the ureters or bladder is most common where radical hysterectomy has been performed for a malignant disease, particularly in the patient who has had previous irradiation. It may, however, occur even after the easiest type of vaginal or abdominal hysterectomy, and this is always distressing since the surgeon may have no idea as to why it happened. It is perhaps the most common cause of malpractice suits despite careful and medically appropriate surgical techniques. If recognized at the time of surgery, appropriate reparative measures should be carried out, and are generally successful. If not, leakage of urine immediately postoperative will indicate the probability of a fistula, although sometimes this leakage does not occur until several weeks later due to a compromised blood supply, rather than trauma directly to the urinary tract itself. Pre-operative ureteral catheterization is often helpful in identifying the ureter at surgery.

4. Lung Complications

Certain patients present with obstructive pulmonary diseases, such as chronic bronchitis, asthma, and emphysema. These represent a much higher hazard of respiratory difficulties postsurgery, but they also lead to a much higher incidence of wound disruption. It has been suggested that these patients should be admitted for several days preoperative for antibiotics and aerosol therapy.

In any case postoperative *atelectasis* or collapse of the lungs may occur immediately postoperative, and necessitate bronchoscopic removal of any mucus plugs. Despite prophylactic antibiotics, postoperative bronchitis and pneumonitis occur in a certain proportion of cases, as evidenced by x-ray. Prompt ambulation, particularly of the elderly patient, is highly desirable. Deep breathing should be encouraged, and occasional respiratory support may be necessary. Close surveillance of such patients in an intensive care therapy is mandatory.

5. Bowel Complications

A. Paralytic Ileus. This extremely troublesome problem generally occurs following a complicated abdominal hysterectomy, although it may ensue after vaginal surgery. Extreme distention and vomiting may occur, and on occasion it may be very difficult to distinguish this from a true mechanical obstruction. However, bowel sounds are usually absent, and there is not the colicky, crampy pain that ensues with obstruction. X-ray may show dilated small bowel, but there is generally gas present in the large bowel as well. Judicious use of a nasogastric tube along with periodic x-rays as well as bowel stimulants and enemas may be required for the proper diagnosis and treatment.

B. Mechanical Obstruction. This is much more common following abdominal hysterectomy, although it may occur following the vaginal approach if a loop of bowel is agglutinated to the vaginal wall. Nausea, vomiting, distention, and high pitched bowel sounds (in contrast to the lack of bowel sounds with a paralytic ileus) should lead to the diagnosis, and periodic x-rays with search for fluid levels are helpful. If a true mechanical obstruction is suspected, initial trial with nasogastric tubes is indicated; but if there is not prompt improvement, laparotomy seems indicated. This may on occasion be quite difficult, and the possibility of various intestinal fistulae must always be considered. With today's improved forms of anesthesia, gastric dilatation is not so common as in previous decades. However, profuse vomiting should warrant an x-ray, and, if a dilated stomach is found, gastric suction should be instituted. It should be emphasized that in the postoperative patient mechanical obstruction is rarely an acute emergency so that one may generally temporize with intestinal suction and the usage of intravenous fluids.

6. Thromboembolism

This represents an extremely disturbing problem as far as postoperative complications are concerned. Since thrombosis of the deep veins of the lower extremities is often silent in nature, diagnosis may be difficult. Any trauma to the pelvic veins or lower extremity, which occurs most commonly with radical surgery, may lead to thrombosis and infection. On occasion the thrombophlebitis is relatively asymptomatic, and the first sign is the development of a pulmonary embolus. Mattingly and Wilkinson have pointed out the type of patient who is most apt to develop thromboembolic phenomena (obese, diabetic, cachectic, etc.), in which case prophylactic therapy may be instituted. Anticoagulant therapy may be instituted preoperatively, but this must be observed quite carefully to prevent the possibility of subsequent hemorrhage.

Thrombophlebitis generally ensues about a week postoperatively, but may occur later. A low grade elevation of temperature, with discomfort in the thigh, and a positive Homan's sign as well as occasional swelling of the legs, all may be noted. In many instances, however, the possibility of venous problems is not noted until emboli occur, with chest pain, hemoptysis, and occasional shock with large emboli. It is not, however, always easy to make a distinction between this and various pulmonary infections. X-rays, lung scan, and pulmonary arteriography are recommended for diagnosis, although other adjuvant studies may be necessary. Prompt heparinization with subsequent dicumarol and dextran seem indicated. If emboli are major and recurrent, the possibility of vena cava or ovarian vein ligation should be considered. For details the reader is urged to study the review by Mattingly and Wilkinson.

7. Infection

Incisional infection may occur following abdominal hysterectomy, particularly in the obese or diabetic individual, and this may be obviated by placing a small drain in such a patient, particularly when there has been a previous laparotomy. Local heat, antibiotic therapy, and drainage of any abscess are generally utilized. Significant infection seems less common after vaginal procedures, although an infected cuff hematoma is a not infrequent sequel.

More serious infection such as peritonitis may occur following abdominal procedures, especially where there is such a process as an acute inflammatory disease or appendicitis. Adequate chemotherapy and drainage of any localized abscess is indicated. Pelvic abscesses may occur or be secondary to an infected hematoma.

Severe infection, especially postabortal gas gangrene, may lead to endotoxic shock. This term is applied to the characteristic clinical picture associated with a gram-negative infection, often in the absence of any observed blood loss. Patients so afflicted are extremely ill, and indeed on occasion the shock may be irreversible. The initial therapy should be supportive with adequate fluids and blood replacement, antibiotic therapy as indicated, vasomotor drugs, and judicious use of cortisone. Drainage of any abscess should strongly be considered and the clinician should be prepared to face the possibility of ensuing thrombophlebitis. Emergency "pelvic cleanout" may be required if there is no response to drug therapy.

Numerous studies including one from our own clinic by Wheeless seem to indicate that prophylactic antibiotic therapy in any type of major surgery may significantly decrease the incidence of postoperative infection. There seems little question that the morbidity following major surgery has been cut approximately in half, with judicious use of prophylactic antibiotic therapy, and there have been no adverse results. This has led to a significant saving in hospital time and expense. We would doubt that routine use of antibiotics would predispose patients to other types of infection, particularly since newer and more effective antibiotics are being evolved every day.

8. Electrolyte Imbalance

This generally occurs in complicated postoperative patients, particularly where there has been sustained nausea or vomiting, with the necessity for continuous intravenous fluids. It is extremely important in such patients that the blood chemistry be followed quite closely with administration of the necessary fluids and electrolytes. On the other hand, overenthusiastic use of intravenous fluids may put a border-line cardiac patient into heart failure. Close observation of sodium, potassium, chlorides, etc., is extremely important to avoid any problems of hypernatremia or hyponatremia, as indicated in the recent comprehensive study by Herbert.

9. Evisceration

Complete or partial disruption of the incision may occur following any type of abdominal procedure, but this is most common in extremely obese or very thin individuals, where there is an associated respiratory problem, such as bronchiectasis, or in the irradiated patient with malignant disease. A serosanguineous discharge from the incision in the patient with a low grade elevation of temperature should make the surgeon concerned about the possibility of ensuing evisceration. Prompt recognition and surgery with through and through closure of the abdomen with silver or stainless steel wire should be considered. The wires may be removed two to three weeks postoperatively, after the patient has left the hospital. Evisceration through the vagina or postoperative vaginal vault is a rare occurrence, but may occur particularly in an elderly individual as a result of coitus after prolonged celibacy.

In a recent discussion Pratt has outlined the importance of incisional hematomas, particularly those large ones deep to the fascia as an etiological factor in the development of dehiscence. These are extremely prone to become infected, and lead to disruption of the suture line. Evisceration is a serious complication with a mortality rate in the range of 20 per cent, although fortunately it is relatively rare, occurring in less than 0.5 per cent of all patients who have had gynecologic laparotomy. Careful hemostasis is obviously imperative at the time of initial surgery, and even though the surgeon may be fatigued after a long and difficult procedure, painstaking closure of the abdomen may prevent subsequent complications.

10. Foreign Bodies

Now and then even in the most efficient operating rooms some kind of foreign body may be left in the abdomen. In past years an intriguing variety of objects found in the abdomen have been recorded, such as eye glasses, false teeth, pencils, etc., but fortunately such instances are a rarity today. However, foreign bodies may likewise be noted after vaginal surgery, for once the peritoneal cavity is opened from below, this is likewise subject to involvement by instruments or sponges. Although sponge and instrument counts are the rule in most hospitals, the careful physician will be extremely mindful of any loose sponges. Fortunately many of these are radiopaque, and if there is any such postoperative complication as incisional break down or fistula formation, flat plate should always be obtained. Nevertheless the utmost care should be taken to avoid such problems, for the medical-legal implications are unlimited.

11. Nerve Injury

A rare patient may exhibit damage to the femoral nerve subsequent to surgery with numbness, paresthesia, and weakness of the thigh. The neuropathy may be caused not by the surgery itself but by prolonged pressure from the lateral blades of a self-retaining retractor. Similar trauma to the peroneal or sciatic nerve may occur at the time of vaginal surgery when the dorsal lithotomy position leads to pressure by the bar of the leg holder. This nerve damage is usually transient and the treatment is nonspecific.

12. Prolapse of the Tube (Fig. 5.10)

A rather rare postoperative problem is prolapse of the tube through the apex of the vaginal vault. Sapon and Solberg record 48 cases following hysterectomy, only 12 abdominal. This superficially re-

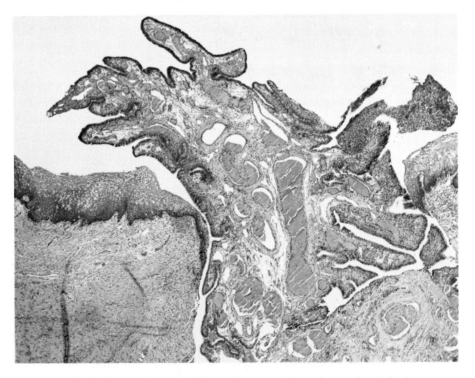

5.10. Prolapse of the tube with marked congestion and secondary infection.

sembles granulation tissue but is quite painful if biopsied. Varying degrees of discharge and discomfort may be noted (Ellsworth).

Many other postoperative complications will inevitably occur even for the most proficient surgeon; the only method of avoiding these is to avoid the practice of surgery. However, these unfortunate accidents can be minimized by adherence to strict surgical technique and good operative judgment.

REFERENCES

Allen, J. L., Rampone, J. F., and Wheeless, C. R.: Antibodies in gynecological operations. Obstet. Gynec., 39: 218, 1972.

Ballard, C. A.: Therapeutic abortion and sterilization by vaginal hysterectomy. Amer. J. Obstet. Gynec., 118: 891, 1974.

Birnbaum, S. J.: Prolapsed vagina. Amer. J. Obstet. Gynec., 115: 411, 1973.

Brown, J. B., Falconer, C. W. A., and Strong, J. A.: Urinary estrogens of adrenal origin in women with breast cancer. J. Endocr., 19: 52, 1959.

Bulbrook, R. D., and Greenwood, F. C.: Persistence of urinary estrogen excretion after oophorectomy and adrenalectomy. Brit. Med. J., 1: 662, 1957.

Cavanagh, D., and Rao, P. S.: Septic shock (endotoxic shock). Clin. Obst. Gynec., 16: 26, 1973.

Cohn, I., Slack, N. H., and Fisher, B.: Complications and toxic manifestations of surgical adjuvant chemotherapy for breast cancer. Surg., Gynec. Obstet., 127: 1201, 1968.

Coulam, C. B., and Pratt, J. H.: Vaginal hysterectomy—is previous operation contraindicated. Amer. J. Obst. Gynec., 15: 252, 1973.

D'Esopo, D. A.: Hysterectomy when uterus is grossly normal. Amer. J. Obstet. Gynec., 83: 113, 1962.

Ellsworth, H. S., et al.: Prolapse of the tube following vaginal hysterectomy. J.A.M.A., 224: 891, 1973.

Falk, H. C.: Abdominal and vaginal hysterectomy (edited by Falk, H. C.) Clin. Obstet. Gynec., 15: 695, 1972.

Feinleib, M.: Breast cancer and artificial menopause, J. Nat. Cancer Inst., 315: 1968.

Fisher, B., Ravdin, R. G., Ausman, R. K., Slack, N. H., Moone, G. E., and Noer, R. J.: Surgical adjuvant chemotherapy in cancer of the breast. Ann. Surg., 168: 337, 1968.

Goldenberg, I. S.: Testosterone proprionate therapy in breast cancer. J.A.M.A., 188: 117, 1964.

Gray, L. A.: Vaginal Hysterectomy. Charles C Thomas, Springfield, Ill., 1955.

Gray, L. A.: Techniques of abdominal total hysterectomy. Amer. J. Obstet. Gynec., 75: 334, 1958.

Gray, L. A.: The place of vaginal hysterectomy in gynecological surgery. Western J. Surg., 67: 153, 1959.

Greenwood, F. C., and Bulbrook, R. D.: Effect of hypophysectomy on urinary oestrogen in breast cancer. Brit. Med. J., 1: 666, 1957.

Grogan, R. H.: Reappraisal of residual ovaries. Amer. J. Obstet. Gynec., 97: 124, 1967.

Haagensen, C. D.: A great leap backward in the treatment of brease carcinoma. J.A.M.A., 224: 1181, 1973.

Haynes, A. M., and Wolfe, W. M.: Tubal sterilization in an indigent group. Amer. J. Obstet. Gynec., 106: 1044, 1970.

Hebert, L. A., and Lemann, H. Jr.: Operative risk: clinical evaluation and management of disorders of water and electrolyte balance. Clin. Obstet. Gynec., 16: 195, 1973.

Howkins, J., and Williams, D.: Total abdominal hysterectomy; 1000 consecutive operations. J. Obstet. Gynaec. Brit. Comm., 70: 20, 1963.

Jones, H. W.: Prophylactic castration for cancer of the breast. Obstet. Gynec. Survey, 14: 774, 1959.

Kasilag, F. B., Jr., and Rutledge, F. N.: Metastatic breast carcinoma in the ovary. Amer. J. Obstet. Gynec., 74: 989, 1957.

Laufe, L. E., and Kreutner, F. K.: Vaginal hysterectomy for abortion and sterilization. Amer. J. Obstet. Gynec., 110: 1096, 1971.

Maas, H., et al.: Estrogen receptors in human breast cancer. Amer. J. Obstet. Gynec., 113: 377, 1972.

Mattingly, R. F., and Wilkinson, E. J.: Thromboembolism in pelvic surgery. Clin. Obst. Gynec., 16: 162, 1973.

Montgomery, T. L., Bowers, P. A., and Taylor, H. W.: Breast lesions. Obstet. Gynec., 1: 394, 1953.

Novak, E. R., and Williams, T. J.: Autopsy comparison of cardiovascular changes in castrated and normal women. Amer. J. Obstet. Gynec., 80: 863, 1960.

Parrish, H. M., Carr, C. A., Hall, D. G., and King, T. M.: Time interval from castration to development of excessive coronary arteriosclerosis. Amer. J. Obstet. Gynec., 99: 155, 1967.

Parrot, M. H.: Elective hysterectomy. Amer. J. Obstet. Gynec., 113: 531, 1972.

Patterson, R., and Russell, M. H.: Clinical trials in malignant disease. II. Breast cancer; value of irradiation of the ovaries. J. Fac. Radiol., 10: 130, 1959.

Plotz, E. J., Wiener, M., Stein, A. A., and Hahn, B. D.: Enzymatic activities related to steroidogenesis in postmenopausal ovaries in patients with and without endometrial carcinoma. Amer. J. Obstet. Gynec., 99: 182, 1967.

Pratt, J. H.: Operative and postoperative difficulties of vaginal hysterectomy. Obstet. Gynec., 21: 220, 1963.

Pratt, J. H.: Wound healing—evisceration. Clin. Obstet. Gynec., 16: 126, 1973.

Pratt, J. H. and Galloway, J. R.: Vaginal hysterectomy in patients less than 30 or more than 60 years of age. Amer. J. Obstet. Gynec., 93: 812, 1965.

Pratt, J. H., Symmonds, R. E., and Welch, J. S.: Vaginal hysterectomy for carcinoma of the fundus. Amer. J. Obstet. Gynec., 88: 1063, 1964.

Radman, H. M., and Korman, W.: Uterine perforation during dilatation and curettage. Obstet. Gynec., 21: 210, 1963.

Randall, C. L.: Ovarian conservation. Obstet. Gynec., 20: 880, 1962.

Randall, C. L.: The risk of gynecological malignancies in older women. Clin. Obstet. Gynec., 7: 545, 1964.

Randall, C. L., and Harkins, J. L.: Ovarian function after the menopause. Amer. J. Obstet. Gynec., 74: 719, 1957.

Ravdin, R. G., et al.: Results of prophylactic oophorectomy for breast carcinoma. Surg. Gynec. Obstet., 131: 1055, 1970.

Rosenberg, N. F., and Uhlmann, E. M.: Prophylactic castration in carcinoma of the breast. Arch. Surg., 78: 376, 1959.

Sapon, I. P., and Solberg, N. S.: Prolapse of the uterine tube after hysterectomy. Obstet. Gynec., 42: 26, 1973.

Schlueter, D. P.: Pulmonary risks. Clin. Obstet. Gynec., 16: 91, 1973.

Silverberg, S. C., and Frable, W. J.: Prolapse of the fallopian tube into the vaginal vault after hysterectomy. Arch. Path., 97: 100, 1974.

Sinclair, E. H., and Pratt, J. H.: Femoral neuropathy after pelvic operation. Amer. J. Obstet. Gynec., 112: 404, 1972.

Smith, R. D., and Pratt, J. H.: Serious bleeding following vaginal or abdominal hysterectomy. Obstet. Gynec., *26:* 592, 1965.

Thompson, B. H., and Wheeless, C. R.: Complications of laparoscopic sterilization. Obstet. Gynec., *41:* 669, 1973.

Twombly, G. H.: Hemorrhage in gynecological surgery. Clin. Obstet. Gynec., *16:* 135, 1973.

Wheeless, C. R.: Postoperative pelvic infection. Clin. Obstet. Gynce., *16:* 111, 1973.

Wheeless, C. R.: Elimination of second incision at laparoscopic sterilization. Obstet. Gynec., *39:* 134, 1972.

Wheeless, C. R.: Outpatient and laparoscopic sterilization under local. Obstet. Gynec., *39:* 767, 1972.

Williams, E. A.: Vaginal hysterectomy, J. Obstet. Gynaec. Brit. Comm., *69:* 590, 1962.

chapter *6*

Embryology

GENETIC FACTORS OF SEX DETERMINATION

Sex is basically an inherited characteristic which is carried by the genes of the X and Y chromosomes. The combination of the sex chromosomes is fixed at fertilization and is normally transmitted unchanged to all subsequent cells of that individual. Although a specific sex is thus built into the cells, it may be said that many of the manifestations of sex, such as the presence or absence, in whole or in part, of the internal and external genitalia and other characteristics of sex, are dependent upon influences other than the mere presence of the proper chromosomes.

The Sex Chromatin

The understanding of the genetic background of sex at the clinical level was greatly stimulated and aided by the discovery of Barr and Bertram of a simple technique for the recognition of sexual dimorphism in interphase nuclei. This imprint of sex is found in the so-called X-chromatin which is distinctive for the human female as well as for many other mammals (Fig. 6.1). Equally helpful is the Y-chromatin, visible in interphase

cells by fluorescence microscopy and found in patients with a Y chromosome (Fig. 6.2).

The X-chromatin is one of the two X chromosomes which has become stainable and therefore visible during interphase. Because of certain X-linked characteristics, Lyon suggested that the visible X chromosome was of maternal origin in a fixed portion of cells and the remainder of paternal origin. Furthermore the Lyon proposal suggested that the X-chromatin was partially genetically inactive and that all descendents of a given cell whose maternal or paternal X chromosome was randomly inactivated will have inactivated the X chromosome of the same parent.

The Sex Chromosomes

For many years it was thought that the human diploid chromosome number was 48. However, in 1956 Tjio and Levan using a tissue culture technique found but 46. In addition to the establishment of the chromosome number, newer techniques allow further study of chromosome morphology. Using a variety of nuclear stains the identification of most chromosomes including both X and Y is reasonably clear (Fig. 6.3). With fluorescence or

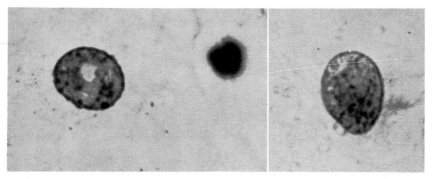

6.1. Photomicrograph of cells from buccal smear prepared for examination for sex chromatin. *Left,* presence of sex chromatin at about 5 o'clock just beneath the nuclear membrane. *Right,* the absence of specific sex chromatin makes this a negative examination.

banding techniques, the identification of each chromosome is possible (Fig. 6.4).

Sex Determination

All mature eggs are alike in their chromosomal constitution, and the human assortment consists of 22 autosomes and 1 X sex chromosome. Spermatozoa, on the other hand, are of two kinds: one half contains 22 autosomes and 1 X sex chromosome, and the other half contains 22 autosomes and 1 Y sex chromosome.

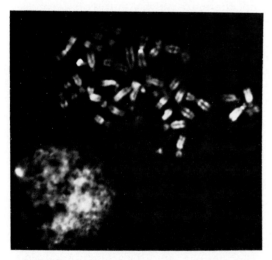

6.2. Photomicrograph by fluorescence microscopy of interphase cell (*lower*) and metaphase chromosomes (*upper*) from same patient. In interphase cell note the brilliant spot (10 o'clock) which is the Y-chromatin. Near the left side of the metaphase chromosome spread (inward from chromosome No. 1) may be seen the brilliant long arms of the Y chromosome.

Fertilization of any egg (22 + X) by one kind of sperm cell (22 + X) results in a female (44 + XX). Fertilization by the other kind of sperm cell (22 + Y) results in a male (44 + XY). As will be related, the role of the chromosomes seems to be limited to the determination of the sex of the gonad which in turn apparently controls the direction of development of the sex ducts and external genitalia.

DEVELOPMENT OF THE OVARY

The Indifferent Stage

The first gonadal structures are recognizable in human embryos when they measure about 5-mm. crown rump length (approximately four weeks). It is not possible to assign a specific sex to this first gonadal primordium and the so-called indifferent stage lasts until the embryo has reached about 15 mm. (between six and seven weeks) when, according to Gillman, testicular differentiation begins.

The germ cells have an extra-gonadal origin. McKay *et al.* were able to observe the migration of the germ cells from early stages by their high alkaline phosphatase activity. These cells can first be identified in the endodermic wall of the primitive gut from which they migrate to the gonadal site. Germ cells never persist outside of the genital ridge.

By an examination of a section through the gonadal structure of a 7.4-mm. embryo (approximately five weeks) (Fig.

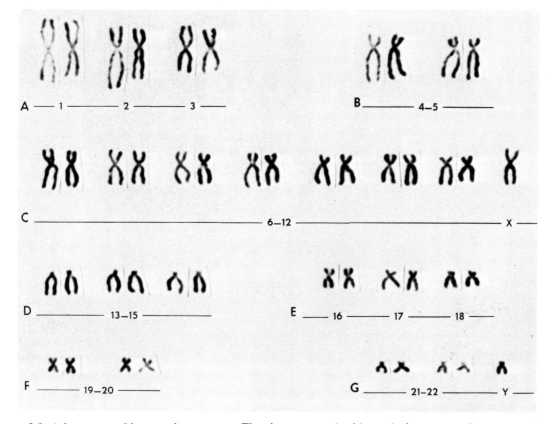

6.3. A karyotype of human chromosomes. The chromosomes in this particular case are from a normal male used to illustrate both the X and Y chromosomes.

6.5) several different components may be recognized: (1) germinal epithelium, a well established name but misleading in that it apparently does not have the capacity to produce germ cells; (2) underlying loose embryonic connective tissue; (3) cellular condensations lying at right angles to the celomic epithelium in the mesenchyme and referred to as medullary cords; and (4) germ cells which have wandered in from the outside as previously described and which seem to accumulate beneath the germinal epithelium.

The derivation and subsequent development of the structures referred to above have been the subject of considerable difficulty and controversy. For purposes of simplicity the views of Witschi will be followed. According to this authority the cellular cords referred to above constitute the *medulla* of the gonads. Further condensation of cells in the upper portions of the gonad establishes solid connection between these cords and mesonephric tubules, the primordial efferent ductules (Fig. 6.6).

According to Witschi, when the migrating germ cells enter the primitive gonad they selectively accumulate under the celomic epithelium but the cords, which may now be referred to as medullary cords, do not contain many germ cells in embryos of 8-mm. length (five weeks). Suddenly the behavior of the germ cells changes and at this time many of them pass from the cortex to the medulla along the medullary sex cords. During this transit they seem to carry with them some somatic cells from the cortex which, according to Witschi's view, later become Sertoli cells. The significance of this observation lies in the attempt to explain the estrogenic production

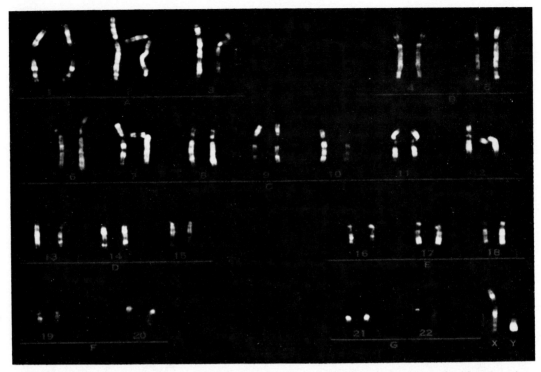

6.4. A karyotype by fluorescence microscopy after treatment of the metaphase spread with quinacrine. Note the distinctive pattern of each chromosome and the usefulness of the method for distinguishing between chromosomes which are morphologically similar, *e.g.*, between chromosomes 21 and 22.

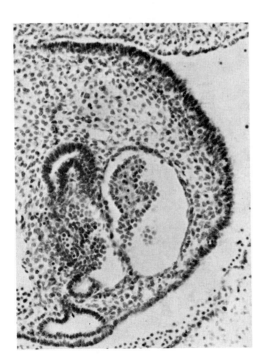

of the Sertoli cells in the adult testis, which is primarily the development of the medulla of the primitive gonad. This explanation assumes that estrogenic production must be of cortical origin. Finally, by the 14-mm. stage (slightly older than six weeks) the indifferent gonad is composed of an outer cortex containing many germ cells and an internal medulla

6.5. Human embryo 7.4 mm. Cross section through left urogenital fold at indifferent gonad stage. The cortex consists of the much thickened celomic epithelium and contains several germ cells. The medulla is composed of a nucleus of blastema cells, more or less distinctly organized as cords radiating from the mesonephros toward the cortex. A narrow albuginea with a few mesenchyme cells separates cortex and medulla. (Reprinted by permission from Jones, H. W., Jr., and Scott, W. W.: *Hermaphroditism, Genital Anomalies and Related Endocrine Disorders*, 2nd ed., The Williams & Wilkins Company, Baltimore, 1971.)

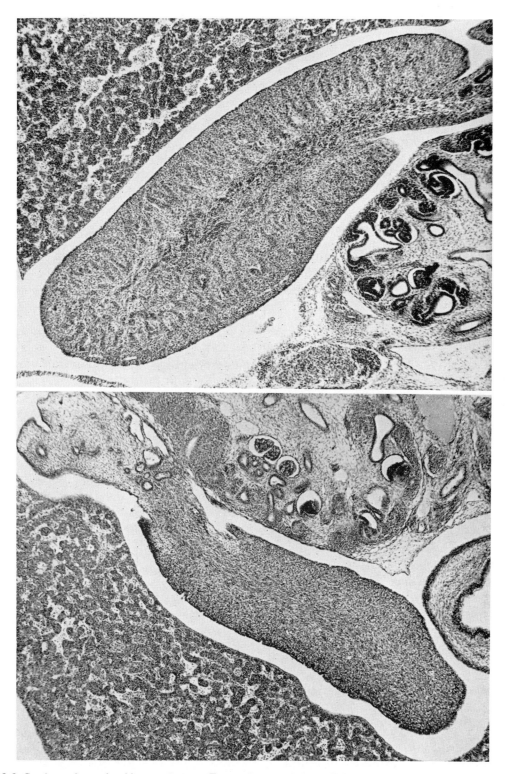

6.6. Sections of gonads of human fetuses. *Top,* male 27 mm. long. This section shows short, straight testicular tubules connected with the rete testis which are darker in the center. *Bottom,* female embryo 25 mm. long. Note the cellular cortex with the poorly developed rete and the inconspicuous medulla. (Reprinted by permission from Jones, H. W., Jr., and Scott, W. W.; *Hermaphroditism, Genital Anomalies and Related Endocrine Disorders,* 2nd ed., The Williams & Wilkins Company, Baltimore, 1971.)

comprising sex cords also provided with germ cells.

Differentiation of the Testis

According to Gillman the differentiation of the testis first becomes recognizable in an embryo with a crown rump length of 14 to 16 mm. (six to seven weeks). The medullary cords which become the seminiferous tubules of the testis acquire a prominence. During this same time the cortex degenerates, the germ cells disappear from the cortex, the cells of the outer epithelium flatten, and a connective tissue layer develops between the sex cords and the covering epithelium. In a male fetus the sex gland of a 27-mm. embryo (about eight weeks) is a typical testis (Fig. 6.6).

According to Gillman's studies the interstitial cells show their first signs of specialization in a fetus of about 31-mm. crown rump length (about 10 weeks). By the time the fetus reaches 50 mm. (about 11 weeks), they begin to increase enormously and the medullary tubules now properly called seminiferous tubules, are separated by large areas of hypertrophied cells with abundant cytoplasm. This increase continues until the fetus reaches a length of 160 or 190 mm. (five to six lunar months), when the interstitial cells suddenly shrink or degenerate. The possible functional significance of these with respect to the development of the sex ducts should be kept in mind.

Differentiation of the Ovary

After the embryo reaches 14 to 16 mm. (six to seven weeks), the conversion of the gonad into an ovary is not so prominent as its conversion into a testis. The young ovary seems to remain in the indifferent stage for a longer period of time. The main feature of ovarian development is the progressive importance and increase in size of the cortex at the expense of the medulla. The germinal epithelium becomes thicker and more prominent (Fig. 6.6). In places, massive clumps of sex cells are visible and cortical sex cords push into the gonad. The cortical cords seem to contain or produce certain somatic cells which later become the granulosa cells. The first follicles, constituted of ovocytes surrounded by recognizable layers of granulosa cells, appear initially in the central part of the ovary when the fetus measures about 150-mm. crown rump length (slightly younger than five lunar months). During cortical differentiation and development the medullary cords gradually become smaller and crowded to a central position. According to Forbes some medullary tubules located in the hilum of the ovary and even containing germ cells may be found in all ovaries until the fetus attains a length of 280 mm. (approximately eight lunar months). It is the persistence of this medullary material which has been implicated in the development of virilizing tumors in adult females.

As described above, the primitive germ cells have an extra-gonadal origin and migrate to the indifferent gonad. After arrival in the gonad of the female the germ cells may be called oogonia. They are noted as early as the fifth week although the gonad cannot be identified as an ovary at that time. According to Baker, whose account is followed, oogonia may be found through the seventh month of fetal life. They undergo mitotic division with great frequency and their maximal number is at the fifth month when their estimated number is about 2.6 million.

The oogonium is said to become an oocyte when it enters the first of its two meiotic divisions. The first oocyte may be recognized at about eight weeks and their maximum number is likewise at about five months when their number approximates 4.2 million. At birth no oogonia remain and the oocytes have been reduced to 2.0 million. By the seventh postnatal year there remain only about 300,000.

The primary oocyte remains in a kind of hibernation in the prophase of the first meiotic division for many years. Completion of the first meiotic division is simultaneous with preovulatory follicular maturation and ovulation. The second meiotic division usually occurs after ovulation and is completed only if there is sperm penetration.

Considerations of Ovarian Development

The descriptive account of the development of the ovary given above is purely in morphological terms and gives no understanding of the mechanisms involved or their causes. Understandably there are no data on experimental studies of human embryos, but there is an enormous amount of animal work which shows that the normal development of the gonad can be altered in important ways by suitable experiments. The application of these data to the human is, of course, only speculative, but from a theoretical point of view does shed some light on certain clinical situations.

It seems clear that the genetic sex factors are responsible for the prevalence of either the cortex or the medulla but the exact mechanism by which this is translated into an ovary or a testis, as the case may be, remains obscure. However, for reasons which will be given later, it is likely that this determination is the only specific duty of the sex determining genes.

Among the many experiments bearing upon this subject the data on amphibians reviewed by Jost may be cited as an example. In amphibian larvae, which are either united in heterosexual parabiosis or receive heterosexual gonadal grafts from other individuals, the medullary sex inductor of the genetic male usually predominates and inhibits the ovarian cortex of females. Depending upon the stage of development, the ovary may become quite reduced or even undergo a complete sex reversal if the medullary component is able to develop. It thus appears that such sex reversal may be attributed to damage to one part of the corticomedullary system.

On a more fundamental level it may be inquired as to the circumstances of the establishment of the indifferent gonad. Many efforts have been made to determine whether the gonadal anlage could be established in the absence of germ cells. Witschi is of the opinion that a true cortex cannot differentiate in the complete absence of germ cells. His opinion is based in part on the study of the sex glands of frogs and toads which came from overripe eggs.

Delayed fertilization constitutes another cause of gonadal abnormalities. Most of the germ cells degenerate under this condition and the gonads are quite abnormal and often develop only small sterile medullary sections resembling the rudimentary testes found in the Klinefelter syndrome.

In the lower animals the sex hormones also exert a profound influence on the developing gonad. For example, complete sex reversal of genetic males to functional females which were reared and mated with normal genetic males was obtained under the influence of estradiol in the newt *T. pleurodles Waltlii* by Gallien. For the most part such studies have been carried on in species below mammals. However, Burns has succeeded in reversing the differentiation of the testis of young opossums treated with small doses of estradiol dipropionate. In the treated males the cortex of the indifferent gonads persisted and proliferated ovarian cords with germ cells after the atrophy of the testicular tubules.

In placental mammals gonadal reversal studies have met with limited success. By transplanting fetal ovaries and testes of rats under the kidney capsule of a castrate host, MacIntyre, Baker, and Wykoff demonstrated that the testes could suppress ovarian development and vice versa depending upon the relative age of the transplants. Somewhat similar studies by Turner and Asakawa in mice showed that an ovotestis could be produced in this way. The germ cells in the ovarian portion exhibited the morphological characteristics of oocytes while the germ cells in the testicular portion exhibited the characteristics of spermatocytes. These experiments confirmed in the placental mammal the findings in lower animals that the germ cells assume the role of the germ cell of the organ in which they develop, while retaining their original genotype.

It is obvious that more information is needed to define clearly the mechanism of genic action in the determination of gonadal sex.

DEVELOPMENT OF INTERNAL AND EXTERNAL GENITALIA

The Morphological Differentiation of the Fallopian Tubes and Uterus

The genital tract appears later than the sex glands. At about the time when differentiation of the indifferent gonads begins (between 14 and 16 mm. at six to seven weeks), the various structures which ultimately contribute to the internal genitalia are recognizable. At this time the mesonephros is the functioning kidney. The mesonephric urinary duct, generally known as the Wolffian duct, opens at its posterior end into the urogenital sinus, a specialized part of the cloaca formed when the urorectal septum divides the cloaca into rectum and urogenital sinus.

About this same time a second pair of ducts, the Müllerian ducts, are developing anterior and external to the mesonephros. Cranially they appear as a funnel of the celomic epithelium and later this funnel will become the ostium of the fallopian tube. The blind end of this funnel proliferates posteriorly and pushes a cord of cells lateral to the Wolffian duct. The Müllerian ducts reach the urogenital sinus at about 32-mm. crown rump length (about 10 weeks). At this stage the fetus may be considered to be provided with both Müllerian and Wolffian structures and is sexually undifferentiated and bisexual with respect to the gonaducts. Near the cloaca the two urogenital ridges approach medially and fuse into the so-called genital cord. At this level the Müllerian ducts, originally lateral in position in the cephalic area as described, are medial to the mesonephric ducts and brought side to side in the midline where they fuse and end blindly at the Müllerian tubercle. This tubercle is a median protuberance into the dorsal wall of the urogenital sinus but at this time contains no lumen or opening into the sinus (Fig. 6.7).

In the female, when somatic sex differentiation begins somewhere around the 10th week, the Wolffian ducts retrogress, perhaps due to failure of androgen support. In the adult female these structures are sometimes represented as tiny tubules near the ovaries, called the epoophoron. On the contrary, the Müllerian ducts persist and differentiate into tubes and uterus. The fallopian tubes are derived from those portions of the Müllerian ducts which remain unfused and the uterus is derived from the fused caudal portion of the Müllerian ducts.

The Morphological Differentiation of the Vagina

It should be recalled that when the posterior ends of the Müllerian ducts reach the urogenital sinus they make contact with the epithelium of the sinus at the level where the Wolffian ducts open into the sinus. This point of contact with the dorsal wall of the sinus is known as the Müllerian tubercle. At the time and place of contact the two Müllerian ducts have fused into a genital canal and end blindly against the sinus as already noted. Progressively this united blind core of cells which now might be called the vaginal cord or the vaginal plate lengthens and becomes the vagina when a lumen appears in it (Figs. 6.8-6.10).

There has been considerable debate about the origin of the cells comprising the vaginal cord. The description here will largely follow that of Vilas which was confirmed by Meyer and which fits in well with what would be expected from the comparative study of the development of the vagina.

As has been said, the Wolffian ducts open into the sinus whereas the Müllerian ducts are only in contact with the urogenital sinus. As development proceeds the epithelium from the urogenital sinus progressively extends around the posterior part of the Wolffian ducts and between the Wolffian and the Müllerian ducts. Therefore, the ends of the degenerating Wolffian ducts are embedded in a mass of cells coming from the sinus. In earlier

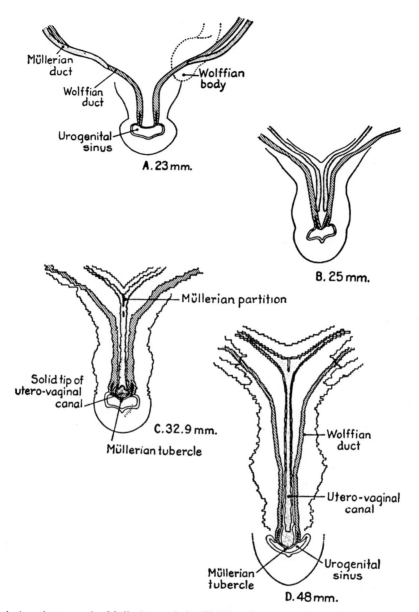

6.7. The relations between the Müllerian and the Wolffian ducts at various phases of early embryonic development. (From Koff, A. K.: Contrib. Embryol., No. 140, 1933.)

works this led to the misinterpretation that the Wolffian ducts contributed to the vaginal plate. Later studies have shown that they degenerate inside this outgrowth of sinus cells. As development progresses the Müllerian ducts which contain a lumen end against the solid cord of cells constituting the vaginal plate which in turn ends against the urogenital sinus which progressively becomes smaller as development continues. The vaginal plate acquires a lumen first at the end nearest the urogenital sinus at the stage of about 150 mm. (slightly less than five months). The fornices and a continuous lumen all through the canal appear at about the stage of 200 mm.

From this course of events it is clear

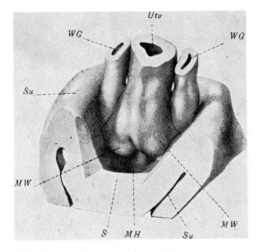

6.8. Human female embryo 42 mm. reconstruction. This shows from the dorsal side the contact between (1) the posterior wall of the urogenital sinus (*Su*) which is locally depressed into a cuplike concavity projecting into the urogenital sinus, (2) the Wolffian ducts (*WG*), and (3) the Müllerian swellings are in contact with the sinus wall only laterally (*dotted line*); in the middle, connective tissue separates them from the sinus which here appears hollow since the connective tissue was not reconstructed. (Reprinted by permission from Jones, H. W., Jr., and Scott, W. W.: *Hermaphroditism, Genital Anomalies and Related Endocrine Disorders,* 2nd ed., The Williams & Wilkins Company, Baltimore, 1971.)

endocervical and endometrial mucosa joined.

The Morphological Differentiation of the External Genitalia

Like the other portions of the genital tract, the external genitalia pass through a bisexual period before specialized differentiation appears at about 50 mm. (two months) (Fig. 6.11).

At early stages the external genitalia are constituted by (1) a genital tubercle or phallus, (2) the urethral groove which is limited laterally by the two urethral folds, and (3) the genital swellings (scrotolabial swellings) which appear on either side of the phallus.

The urogenital sinus opens into the urethral groove. The under surface of the phallus is composed of a urethral plate which is a proliferation of sinus epithelium.

Sex differences become recognizable when the fetus measures about 50 mm. (two months). In males the urethral folds fuse first in the pelvic region, progressively bringing the urogenital os-

that there has been a junction between the epithelium of the urogenital sinus and that of the Müllerian ducts. The exact site of this junction has been the subject of considerable discussion. Vilas and Meyer have held that the junction is marked in the adult by the squamocolumnar junction in the cervix. Both Vilas and Meyer felt that they had demonstrated that the sinus epithelium actually invaded the cervical canal, but that these squamous elements were forced out by the proliferating endocervical cells which descended from the uterine cavity. On the other hand Koff concluded from his studies that the junction was in the upper third of the vagina. Fluhmann, in a more recent study, reviewed the previous evidence and presented some of his own which he believed showed that the junction was in the internal os where the

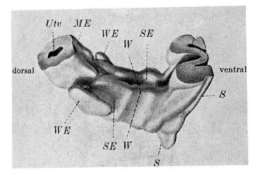

6.9. Human female embryo, 60 mm. Reconstruction of the vaginal anlage viewed from the right side. The "uterovaginal canal" (*Utv*) made of Mullerian epithelium (*ME*), is connected to the urogenital sinus (S) by a plate of sinusal epithelium (*SE*) the limits of which are shown by the *dotted contour*. The Wolffian ducts made of Wolffian epithelium (*WE*) are reducted; their posterior part is embedded in the sinusal epithelium and extends inside the vaginal plate approximately to the level indicated by the discontinued line (*W---W*). (Reprinted by permission from Jones, H. W., Jr., and Scott, W. W.: *Hermaphroditism, Genital Anomalies and Related Endocrine Disorders,* 2nd ed., The Williams & Wilkins Company, Baltimore, 1971.)

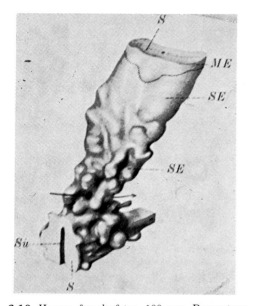

6.10. Human female fetus, 100 mm. Reconstruction of vaginal plate, viewed from the dorsal side. The sinusal vaginal plate (*SE*) has now an appreciable length (940 μ) in this specimen between the Mullerian epithelium, *ME,* and the sinus, Su). The *arrow* shows a hole in the vaginal plate, filled with connective tissue. (Reprinted by permission from Jones, H. W., Jr., and Scott, W. W.: *Hermaphroditism, Genital Anomalies and Related Endocrine Disorders,* 2nd ed., The Williams & Wilkins Company, Baltimore, 1971.)

the genetic determination of sex may be confined to its influence in controlling the sex of the gonad. For various reasons which will now be elaborated, sexual differentiation of the ducts and external genitalia are greatly influenced by and normally seem to depend upon the proper hormonal environment at a specific time in embryonic life. This hormonal theory of sexual differentiation has been firmly established by a large number of investigators working primarily on convenient laboratory animals. It is, of course, not at all sure that such data apply to the human, but clinical data are such that it seems very likely that sexual differentiation in the human is hormonally controlled.

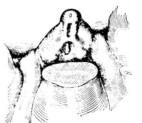

tium onto the phallus toward the glans penis. The fusion of the folds results in the formation of a perineal raphe which extends from the anus to the urogenital ostium. The genital swellings which may now be called scrotal swellings have migrated toward the anus and no longer flank the base of the phallus.

In female embryos the urethral groove remains open and becomes the vestibule. The urethral folds do not fuse but form the labia minora. The genital swellings which may now be called labial swellings become elongated and flank the base of the clitoris. The external genitalia are definitely female in character in a three-month fetus.

Experimental Considerations in the Development of the Internal and External Genitalia

As was mentioned in discussing the experimental data on gonadal development,

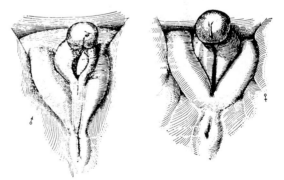

6.11. Development of the human external genitalia. *Upper,* undifferentiated external genitalia of an embryo 16.8 mm. long. *Lower,* external genitalia during the period of sexual differentiation. *Lower left,* male embryo (45 mm. long.); *lower right,* female embryo (49 mm. long). (Reprinted by permission Jones, H. W., Jr., and Scott, W. W.: *Hermaphroditism, Genital Anomalies and Related Endrocrine Disorders,* 2nd ed., The Williams & Wilkins Company, Baltimore, 1971.)

Effect of Castration on the Differentiation of the Genitalia. Alfred Jost in a series of brilliant experiments elucidated the role of the developing gonads in the differentiation of the sex ducts in the rabbit. It was found possible to open the uterus of the pregnant doe, surgically castrate fetuses at various stages of pregnancy, and to replace them in the uterus until near term when they were delivered by cesarean section. Castration did not interfere with feminine differentiation of female rabbit fetuses; ovariectomized females developed a complete feminine genital tract. Thus, feminine organogenesis does not depend upon the presence of the ovaries. In the earliest castrated females the Müllerian ducts were somewhat reduced in size, indicating that some growth-contributing influence might arise from the ovaries.

Castration of male fetuses, on the contrary, showed the primordial import of the testis as a body sex differentiator, and in fetuses castrated before initiation of somatic sexual differentiation (day 19), no male characteristic developed and the whole genital tract became feminine similar to that observed in castrated female fetuses. In other words, in the absence of the testis the Wolffian ducts disappeared, the Müllerian ducts were retained, and differentiated into fallopian tubes, uterine horns, and Müllerian vagina. The urogenital sinus and the external genitalia became feminine (Fig. 6.12).

From such experiments arose the following concept about somatic sexual differentiation of the mammalian fetus. The neutral or gonadless type which develops in the absence of any sex gland (or in the presence of ovaries) is feminine. The testis prevents male embryos from acquiring a female body by suppressing very early the Müllerian ducts and by stimulating masculine organogenesis of the other parts of the genital tract. The Wolffian ducts are taken into the sexual sphere and all masculine structures are stimulated to grow.

It might be conjectured whether feminine organogenesis of the genital tract

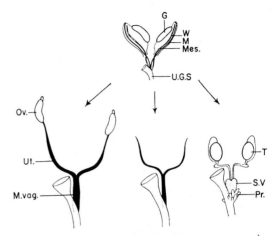

6.12. Schematic representation of sexual differentiation of the sex ducts in the rabbit embryo. From the undifferenitated condition shown in the *upper part* may rise either the female structure (*lower left*) or the male structure (*lower right*) or the gonadless structure (*lower center*) in castrated embryos of either sex. G, gonad; M, Müllerian duct; *MES*, mesonephros; *M vag*, Müllerian vagina; *Ov*, ovary; *Pr*, prostate; *S.V.*, seminal vesicle; *T*, testes; U.G.S., urogenital sinus; Ut, uterine horn; *W*, Wolffian duct. (Reprinted by permission from Jost, A.; *Memoir No. 7 of the Society for Endocrinology.* Cambridge University Press, 1960.)

in the absence of the testis is not imposed by maternal or extratesticular hormones. In vitro experiments (Jost, 1950) showing that isolated pieces of embryonic genital tract of rats also differentiate as in females seem to rule out such a surmise.

In the above mentioned experiments after early removal of the testis, the entire organogenesis of the genital tract took place in the absence of the testicular morphogenetic secretion. Under other experimental conditions, it is possible to allow the testis to influence the genital tract to a reduced extent, thus simulating a partial testicular deficiency. Three series of experiments may be considered: (1) removal of both testes at various stages during sexual differentiation; (2) unilateral castration at various stages; and (3) hypophysectomy.

Castration at Various Stages. Rabbit fetuses were castrated at one-day intervals between day 19 and 24, and it was observed that critical stages occur for each part of the genital tract during which the testes definitely mark them as masculine structures for the remainder of life. Castration before this critical stage prevented masculine organogenesis. Castration after this critical stage no longer interfered with masculine differentiation even though at the time of castration sexual specialization was not yet morphologically obvious.

The critical stage was observed to occur on day 20 for the two anterior prostatic buds, on day 23 for the other prostatic buds, the seminal vesicles, and the external genitalia, and on day 24 for the deferent ducts. Thus, fetuses castrated on day 21 or 22 bear variable sections of the Müllerian ducts, sometimes small remnants of the Wolffian ducts, a reduced prostate, and feminine or hypospadic external genitalia. Those embryos in which the testes were allowed to remain until day 23 exhibit a generally masculine organization but lack deferent ducts. Finally, when the testes are removed on day 24 or later, all masculine features develop

although they may display some reduction in size.

An important point which should be retained from these experiments is that the testicular impulse toward masculinity occurs during a very limited time of development and is a crucial phase. From what is known about morphological differentiation of the genital tract in the human fetus, the crucial period should extend approximately between the stages of 30 and 50 mm. (roughly 50 to 60 days of fertilization age). It is noteworthy that the interstitial cells almost completely disappear when the male organogenesis is established.

Unilateral Castration. The effect of unilateral castration in rabbit fetuses also depends upon the stage at which it is done. When one testis is removed at a relatively late stage, for example on day 23, the remaining single testis is able to complete, on the opposite side, the sexual specialization which had been started, and both deferent ducts may be retained.

In early castrated embryos the single

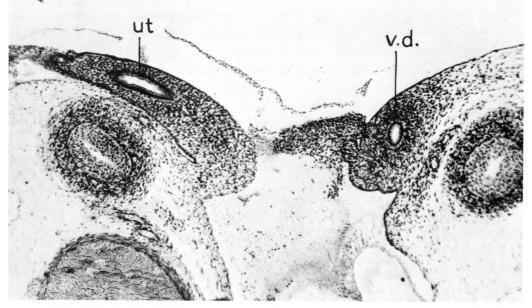

Fig. 6.13. Sections of the genital tract of a 28-year-old male rabbit fetus unilaterally castrated on day 19. Between the two ureters the genital ducts are seen. On the intact right side of the body the vas deferens is seen (v.d.); on the gonadless left side a uterine horn (*ut*) developed creating a lateral asymmetry. (Reprinted by permission from Jones H. W., Jr., and Scott, W. W.: *Hermaphroditism, Genital Anomalies and Related Endocrine Disorders*, 2nd ed., The Williams & Wilkins Company, Baltimore, 1971.)

remaining testis produces a completely masculine organogenesis at the level of the urogenital sinus with its dependents, as well as the external genitalia, but it often does not succeed in masculinizing the anterior part of the genital tract on the opposite side. The Wolffian duct may disappear and the Müllerian duct may differentiate into a uterine horn; thus, a lateral asymmetry of the genital tract is realized, one side being normally masculine and the other normally feminine. Of course, intermediary degrees may be found (Fig. 6.13).

This indicates that the activity of the fetal testis is restricted, a fact which is also clear in grafting experiments (Fig. 6.14), in which a testis is inserted on the feminine genital tract. Such cases of lateral asymmetry resemble the condition observed in certain types of patients with hermaphroditism.

The Effect of Hypophysectomy. Decapitation of the rabbit fetus is in effect a simplified technique for hypophysectomy and allows the observation of the result of decreased testicular activity. The sexual abnormalities displayed by the decapitates were not the same as those found in castrates. The epididymides and deferent ducts, the structures which developed in the closest vicinity of the testes, were seemingly normal and the Müllerian ducts retrogressed. The impaired seminal vesicles were present but somewhat poorly developed. True abnormalities were found at the level of the prostate which was rudimentarily developed in fetuses castrated on day 21 or day 22 and at the level of the external genitalia which were feminine in form as in the castrated fetuses. This male pseudohermaphroditism could be avoided if gonadotrophic hormones were given to the decapitates, thus strongly suggesting that the signs of feminization resulted from testicular impairment. In decapitates, the testis again displayed a spatially restricted activity influencing only the structures nearest to it. The far removed external genitalia were not prevented from becoming feminine.

Finally, it should be added that the external genitalia were only hypospadic in

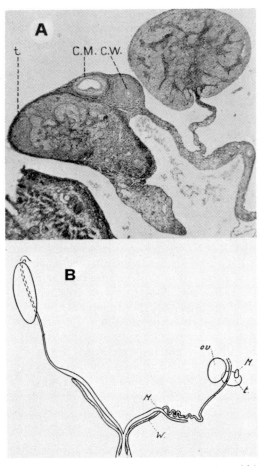

Fig. 6.14. Testicular graft on a female rabbit fetus and masculinization of the genital tract. A, histological section, showing the testicular graft (*t*) inserted on the mesosalpinx which contains the Wolffian duct (*CW*) and a Müllerian cyst (*C.M.*). B, reconstruction of the genital ducts showing the grafted testis (*t*); near to the ovary (*Ov*); the Müllerian duct (*M*) is locally unhibited. The Wolffian duct (*W* punctate) is unilaterally persistent. The fetal testis was grafted on the female fetus on day 20 and this fetus sacrificed on day 28. (Reprinted by permission from Jones, H. W., Jr., and Scott, W. W.: *Hermaphroditism, Genital Anomalies and Related Endocrine Disorders*, 2nd ed., The Williams & Wilkins Company, Baltimore, 1971.)

those fetuses which were decapitated during the course of sexual differentiation (day 22). Decapitation at a still later stage was without effect on the external genitalia.

Chemical Nature of Testicular Morphogenetic Secretion. From the preceding experiments it seems quite clear that the fetal testis produces a morphogenetic secretion responsible for two effects during sexual differentiation: (1) suppression of Müllerian ducts which, in the absence of the testes, would otherwise persist, and (2) stimulation of the development of male structures.

Interestingly enough in all experiments so far recorded no synthetic chemically pure androgen ever tried has been able to exert in the mammalian fetus all the effects produced by the fetal testis. Such synthetic androgenic substances are very potent in stimulating male organogenesis

of the Wolffian ducts and particularly the male organogenesis of the urogenital sinus and external genitalia, but they do not inhibit the feminine development of the Müllerian ducts (Fig. 6.15).

Effect of Androgen on the Differentiation of the Genitalia. The hormonal theory of sexual differentiation inspired a great number of researchers destined to explore the possibility of reversing sex in the mammalian fetus by sex hormones. It is important to remember that experiments were made on animals as different as the opossum, the

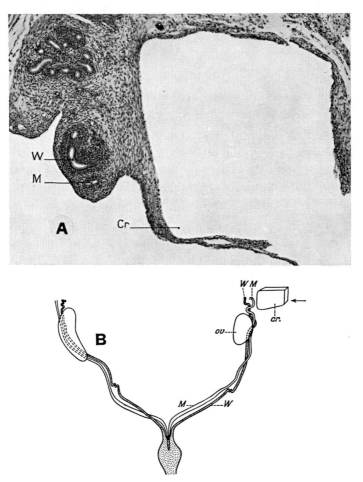

Fig. 6.15. Masculinization of the genital tract of the female rabbit fetus by a crystal (*Cr*) of testosterone propionate implanted on day 20 and sacrificed on day 28. A, histologic section showing the quadrate area which was occupied by the crystal of androgen; Müllerian (*M*) and Wolffian (*W*) derivatives are present. B, reconstruction of the genital tract showing the persistence of the complete Wolffian duct (*W* punctate); no inhibition of the Müllerian duct occurred. The *arrow* indicates the level of the section seen in A. (Reprinted by permission from Jones, H. W., Jr., and Scott, W. W.: *Hermaphroditism Genital Anomalies and Related Endocrine Disorders.*, 2nd ed., The Williams & Wilkins Company, Baltimore, 1971.)

guinea pig, the rat, the mouse, the field mouse, the golden hamster, the rabbit, the hedgehog, and the Rhesus monkey. To this list should now be added the human who has inadvertently been exposed to powerful androgens during fetal life (Wilkins and Jones).

As a rule, androgens were found not to alter the type of male embryos but to masculinize female embryos. When they reach the female embryo before the initiation of somatic sexual differentiation their maximal effect can be summarized in the following manner. The Wolffian ducts are fully developed from the epididymides to the seminal vesicles. The urogenital sinus furnishes male accessory glands (such as prostate) and is definitely masculine as are the genitalia. Besides the male structures stimulated by androgen, the masculinized females exhibit normal or almost normal ovaries and the Müllerian ducts are not inhibited. The vagina does not develop in a normal manner from the urogenital sinus and the Müllerian ducts connect with that position of the urogenital sinus which normally develops in the male urethra (Fig. 6.16).

If low doses of androgens are used, only those parts of the genital tract respond which have a low threshold of sensitivity.

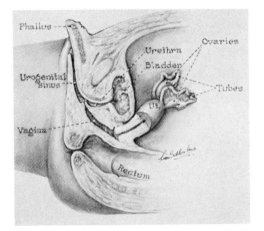

Fig. 6.16. Drawing showing the relation of the urogenital sinus to the vagina and the female urethra of an 18-month-old patient with female hermaphroditism. (Reprinted by permission from Jones, H. W., Jr., and Wilkins, L.: Fertil. Steril., *11:* 148, 1960.)

The most sensitive parts, in almost all animals tested, were the urogenital sinus and external genitalia which may to some extent explain why these parts respond almost selectively in cases of human hermaphroditism caused by exposure to androgens.

Effect of Estrogen on the Differentiation of the Genitalia. The effect of estrogen administered to the mother upon the sexual differentiation of male fetuses has also been studied in several different animal species such as the opossum, rat, mouse, field mouse, golden hamster, mole, and others. Changes are generally produced in the developing male genital tract. The derivatives of the Wolffian ducts are more or less diminished and the Müllerian ducts retained in part or in their entirety. Although there is variation from animal to animal, the prostate is completely inhibited in the opossum and less so in the rat and mouse. The external genitalia may be feminized.

Many of these effects could be interpreted by assuming that the fetal testis has been more or less impaired by the estrogen, allowing a certain "feminization" of the genital tract. Oddly enough, in the rat and in the mouse, estrogens produce some paradoxical effects such as the slight stimulation of the prostate or of the posterior part of the Wolffian ducts.

Although no alteration in the sexual development of male fetuses has been reported from the administration of rather large doses of diethylstilbestrol to mothers for various complications of pregnancy, Bongiovanni, Di George, and Grumbach have reported a few cases of paradoxical masculinization of the female fetus.

REFERENCES

Baker, T. G.: A quantitative and cytological study of germ cells in human ovaries. Proc. Royal Soc. (Biol.), *158:* 417, 1963.

Barr, M. L., and Bertram, E. G.: A morphological distinction between neurones of the male and female and the behavior of the nucleolar satellite during accelerated nucleoprotein synthesis. Nature, *163,* 676, 1949.

Bongiovanni, A. M., Di George, A. M., and Grumbach, M. M.: Masculinization of the female infant associated with estrogenic therapy alone during gestation: four cases. J. Clin. Endocr., *19:* 1004, 1959.

Burns, R. K., Jr.: Transformation due testicule embryonnaire de l'action de l'hormone femelle, le dipropionate d'oestradiol. Arch. Anat. Micr. Morph. Exp., *45:* 173, 1956.

Fluhmann, C. F.: The developmental anatomy of the cervix uteri. Obstet. Gynec., *15:* 62, 1960.

Forbes, T. R.: On the fate of medullary cords of the human ovary. Contrib. Embryol., *30:* 9, 1942.

Gallien, L.: Inversion experimentale du sexe sous l'action des hormones sexuelles chez le triton Pleurodeles Waltlii Michah. Analyse des consequences genetiques. Bull. Biol. France Belg., *88:* 1, 1954.

Gillman, J.: The development of the gonads in man, with a consideration of the role of fetal endocrines and the histogenesis of ovarian tumors. Contrib. Embryol., *32:* 81, 1948.

Jost, A.: Sur le role des gonades foetales dans la differenciation sexuelle somatique de l'embryon de Lapin. C. R. Assoc. Anat., *34:* 255, 1947.

Jost, A.: Recherches sur la differenciation sexuelle de l'embryon de Lapin. II. Action des androgenes de synthese sur l'histogenese genitale. Arch. Anat. Micr. Morph. Exp., *36:* 242, 1947.

Jost, A.: Le controle hormonal de la differentiation du sexe. Biol. Rev., *23:* 201, 1948.

Jost, A.: Sur le controle hormonal de la differenciation sexuelle du Lapin. Arch. Anat. Micr. Morph. Exp. *39:* 577, 1950.

Jost, A.: A new look at the mechanisms controlling sex differentiation in mammals. Johns Hopkins Med. J., *130:* 38, 1972.

Koff, A. K.: Development of the vagina in the human fetus. Contrib. Embryol., *24:* 59, 1953.

Lyon, M. F.: Sex chromatin and gene action in the mammalian X-chromosome. Amer. J. Hum. Genet., *14:* 135, 1962.

MacIntyre, M. N., Baker, L., Jr., Wykoff, T. W.: Effect of the ovary on testicular differentiation in heterosexual embryonic rat gonad transplants. Arch. Anat. Micr. Morph. Exp., *48:* 141, 1956.

McKay, D. G., Hertig, A. T., Adams, E. C., and Danziger, S.: Histochemical observations on the germ cells of human embryos. Anat. Rec., *117:* 201, 1953.

Meyer, R.: Zur Frage der Entwicklung der menschlichen Vagina, Teil IV. Arch. Gynaek., *165:* 504, 1938.

Tijo, J. A., and Levan, A.: The chromosome number of man. Hereditas (Lund), *42:* 1, 1956.

Turner, C. D., and Asakawa, H.: Experimental reversal of germ cells in ovaries of fetal mice. Science, *143:* 1344, 1964.

Vilas, E.: Uber die Entwicklung der Menschlichen Scheide. Z. Anat. Entwicklungsgesch., *98:* 263, 1932.

Wilkins, L., and Jones, H. W., Jr.: Masculinization of the female fetus. Obstet. Gynec., *11:* 355, 1958.

Witschi, E.: Embryogenesis of the adrenal and the reproductive glands. Recent Progr. Hormone Res. *6:* 1, 1951.

chapter *7*

Genetics (Including Cytogenetics)

Although the important principles of genetics, including cytogenetics, have been mastered long before the student enters medicine, the details of these principles have often become a little hazy to medical students or to those in their internship and residency years, not to mention to those who are even more senior. In addition, genetics rightfully has become of importance for the gynecologist in understanding certain disorders in his daily work, in counseling potential parents about genetic hazards of reproduction, in offering therapy to those who might be pregnant with a genetically handicapped child, and in supervising the pregnant patient in whose uterus one genetic message is being decoded and another one is being coded. For these reasons, it has been thought appropriate to include in this textbook suitable minimal material for reference and review for a working knowledge of this important speciality.

MENDELIAN PRINCIPLES

Although the familial occurrence of disease has been described since an-

tiquity, any discussion of contemporary genetics must begin with Gregor Mendel who realized several basic truths which have helped elucidate certain types of inheritance.

Dominance and Such

Mendel wrote "These characteristics which are transmitted entire or almost unchanged in the hybridization and, therefore, in themselves constitute the characteristics of the hybrid are termed the *dominant*, and those which become latent in the process, the *recessive*."

These definitions of dominant and recessive, as applied to traits, are as valid today as when written, although in human genetics by no means all alternate gene pairs express themselves according to the dominant-recessive concept, but they may have an *intermediate*, or even a *co-dominant* expression. If alternate forms of a gene at the same locus be designated A and A', the two forms are called *alleles*, or *allelic genes* for this particular locus and the *genotype* of an individual with respect to the alternate form of this gene may be AA, AA' or A'A'. The genotypes AA and A'A' are called *homozygotes* and AA' a heterozygote. It sometimes happens that the heterozygote AA′ is indistinguishable from the homozygote AA. It may then be said (and was said by Mendel in other words as quoted above) that allele A is dominant over A′ or that A′ is recessive to A. In this circumstance, the *phenotypes* of AA and AA′ are indistinguishable. By convention, the capital letter A (or other letter) is used to designate the dominant allele and the lower case a (or other letter) to designate the recessive allele. If each allele has a distinct recognizable effect, there may be three distinguishable *phenotypes*. Sickling of red cells is an example of such an *intermediate* expression. AA individuals are normal and A′A′ have sickle cell anemia, whereas AA′ individuals have the sickle cell trait. On the other hand, the A and B alleles of the ABO blood groups are examples of genes which have *co-dominant* expression, as each gene has an antigen and both can be recognized in AB individuals.

The original observations of Mendel also had important and still pertinent quantitative aspects. The crossing of heterozygotes (Aa) provide three genotypes, but, because of dominance, two phenotypes in the ratio of three (AA + 2 Aa) to one (aa).

Mendel's Law of Segregation

One of Mendel's most significant conclusions was that, during germ cell formation in the hybrid, the discrete and unmodified characteristics representing alternate forms of an hereditary trait segregated from each other. In other words, during gametogenesis, alleles segregate.

Mendel's Law of Independent Assortment

Mendel's second significant conclusion was that during germ cell formation in a hybrid, the discrete and unmodified characteristics of each of two or more alternate characteristics assorted independently of each other, *i.e.,* nonalleles assort. Thus, with two genotypes Aa and Bb, there are 11 possible recombinant genotypes but, because of dominance, only four phenotypes.

Altogether there are 11 different genotypes, but because of certain duplications, the four phenotypes fall out in the ratio 9:3:3:1 as may be seen from the 16 possible recombinations listed:

AB	AB	Ab	Ab	aB	aB	ab	ab
Ab	AB	ab	Ab	ab	aB		
aB	AB	Ab	ab	aB	ab		
ab	AB						
AB	Ab						
AB	Ab						
aB	aB						
Ab	aB						
AB	ab						

However, each phenotype expressed by the dominant A or B independently assorted with its recessive a or b in the ratio of 3:1.

Many exceptions to the two cardinal Mendelian principles, especially to that of independent assortment, seem to have been noted. Problems with the law of segregation are usually explainable by failure of survival due to genetic disadvantage of one of the genotypes. For the most part, exceptions to the principle of independent assortment may be explained by *linkage* by which is meant the occurrence of two gene loci sufficiently close together on one chromosome so that independent assortment cannot take place.

THE CHROMOSOMES

The hereditary message of man is carried by the desoxyribonucleic acid (DNA) of the 46 chromosomes. A haploid set of 23 chromosomes, consisting of 22 autosomes and one sex chromosome, is contributed by each parent. Each of the 22 autosomes has a homologous partner and each gene locus in the diploid set of autosomes is duplicated by an allelic gene for the given paired characteristic and located on the homologous chromosome.

The sex chromosomes represent a special situation in this regard. The basic facts of sex determination and the inactivation of the X chromosome in the female with the genetic consequences according to the hypothesis of Lyon have been discussed in the chapter on Embryology. At this point it is only necessary to mention that the result of this inactivation is the reduction in the amount of active genetic material in female cells to approximately the amount of active genetic material in male cells. This has been referred to as *dosage compensation*. There are genetic reasons, which will be discussed in the appropriate sections, to believe that the inactivation of the X chromosome in man is not complete. Furthermore, cytological studies of meiosis in the human male indicate end to end pairing of the X and Y chromosomes (Fig. 7.1). Therefore, it is currently believed that there are pairs of allelic genes on at least parts of the X and Y chromosome. Although recombination of genes may occur during meiosis from these parts of the sex chromosomes, it is obvious that no recombination can occur between the sex determining genes of the X and Y chromosomes or else sex determination would not be precise. Thus, the X and Y chromosomes in part have

genes which are unpaired and nonallelic and to which the term hemizygosity may be applied.

The chromosomes may be seen by the light microscope best during mitosis. When first visible in prophase but when better seen in metaphase, they consist of two identical chromatids attached only at the centromere. At anaphase the centromere will split to form two daughter chromosomes.

Three types of human chromosomes have been described according to the location of the centromere and the relative arm lengths: (1) the metacentric chromosome where the centromere is approximately near the center, (2) the submetacentric where the centromere is nearer one end than the other, and (3) the acrocentric where the centromere is very near the extremity so that one arm of each chromosome is very short.

Chromosomes may be conveniently cultured from the peripheral blood for most clinical observations but can be obtained

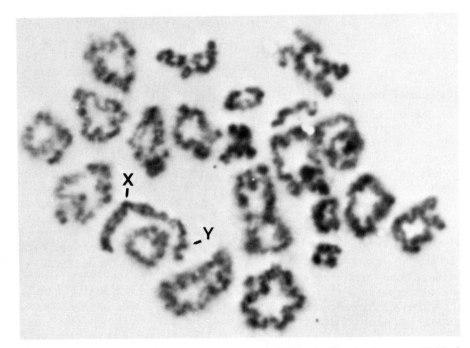

7.1. Photomicrograph of primary human spermatocyte at diakinesis. Clearly shown are 23 bivalents, the pairing in the autosomes being longitudinal and the pairing in the XY bivalent clearly shown to be end to end. The centromeres of the X and Y chromosomes are indicated by appropriate letters (courtesy of Dr. Malcolm Ferguson-Smith).

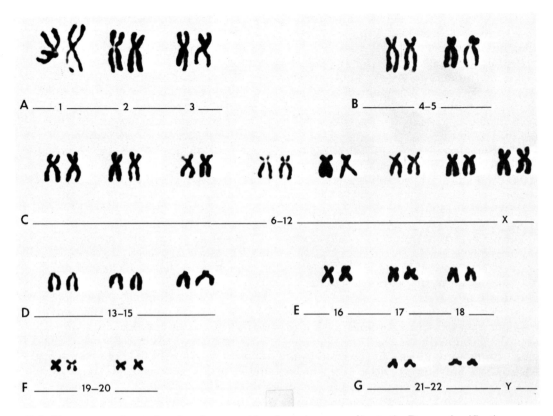

7.2. Chromosomes from a female cell arranged in a karyotype according to the Denver classification.

from other tissues. After fixation, staining, and photography, the chromosomes of an individual cell may be arranged in a karyotype in seven groups in order of descending length according to a standard arrangement (Fig. 7.2).

MITOSIS AND MEIOSIS

The division of the cell cycle into interphase and mitosis is well known. It may be recalled that, in interphase, DNA synthesis occurs during the S (synthesis) period which is preceded by a gap (G 1) and followed by a second gap (G 2). During the S period, the amount of DNA increases from the diploid to tetraploid amount in preparation for mitosis when two cells are formed, each with a diploid amount of DNA. The net result of mitosis is two cells which are genetically identical to their parent.

The final two nuclear divisions of the germ cells, the two meiotic divisions, differ from mitosis in two important respects: (1) the recombination of maternal and paternal genetic material to form genetically unique chromosomes, and (2) the reduction of the number of chromosomes from the diploid 46 to the haploid 23, so that the union of the female gamete with the male gamete will result in a zygote with a normal diploid chromosome number for the next generation.

In contrast to the situation in mitosis, no major DNA synthesis takes place during meiosis, but each cell enters meiosis with the tetraploid amount of DNA by virtue of the synthetic period immediately following the last mitotic division.

During the prophase of the first meiotic division referred to as meiosis I, the interchange of the genetic material derived from mother and father takes place. The events of prophase I provide the biological basis of Mendelian inheritance. Five stages of prophase I may be conveniently described.

Leptonema is characterized by polarization of the chromosomes. They are no longer distributed randomly throughout the nucleus but lie clumped to one side with a clear space at the opposite pole of the nucleus.

The homologous pairs of chromosomes come to lie parallel to each other during the second stage or *zygonema*. The pairing process, called synapsis, seems to begin at any of several places along the length of the chromosomes.

During the third stage, or *pachynema*, the chromosomes become thicker; at this time there seems to be considerable activity between the various strands of chromatin material.

During the succeeding phase or *diplonema*, paired chromosomes begin to split longitudinally so that the homologous chromosomes begin to separate from each other, but, nevertheless, seem to be held together at one or up to four points along their length. These points called chiasmata are thought to represent sites of exchange of maternal and paternal genetic material which result in a reshuffling of genes from mother and father.

The special situation of the sex chromosomes during meiosis was discussed in the preceding section on the chromosomes.

In many mammals the diplotene stage is said to be followed by a prolonged period of resting referred to as the *dictyate* stage. However, according to Baker, the dictyate stage is not observed in the human, and the maturation of the germ cells rests in diplonema, in which stage they are seen in the fixed sections of human ovary and may stay so for from 10 to 50 years. Further division in the female does not take place until sexual maturation of the individual.

Diakinesis is a relatively brief stage, during which the chromosomes are greatly contracted, the chiasmata terminalized, the nucleolus begins to disappear, and the nuclear membrane begins to break down. The metaphase of Meiosis I now begins;

this differs from mitotic metaphase in that in meiosis the chromosomes are lined up at the equatorial plate of the cell by homologous pairs instead of singly. Thus, homologous chromosomes apparently lie side by side on the fibers of the spindle.

In anaphase, the second important purpose of meiosis is achieved. During this phase a reduction in the number of centromeres, and therefore of chromosomes, takes place. One of each of the 23 chromosome pairs migrates to one of the two centrioles, so that there is an accumulation of 23 chromosomes at each of the poles of the cell.

Telophase of the first meiotic division results in the formation of two cells, each of which now has 23 chromosomes. It should be mentioned that, while the distribution of the chromatin material seems to be equal, meiosis I in the female is really an asymmetrical division. The main portion of the cytoplasm of the cell remains with one of the daughter ovocytes and a small polar body is extruded. The polar body is essentially a group of 23 chromosomes and little else.

The second meiotic division now takes place much as a normal mitotic division, except that there are now only 23 chromosomes along the equatorial axis of the cell. During the second meiotic division the centromeres divide and each new centromere takes with it one short arm and one long arm of the chromosome and migrates in opposite directions along the meiotic II spindle to the dispersed centrioles with the net result that there are now two cells, but with quite unequal division of the cytoplasm. The larger cell, which at the end of the process just described might be properly called an ovum, retains most of the cytoplasm, with the result that the second polar body contains little more than the chromatin material. It should be mentioned that the conversion of the ovocyte into a gamete cannot occur until after ovulation and is always incomplete unless the ovocyte is penetrated by a sperm. It is only after fertilization that the secondary ovocyte will complete its division, giving rise to an ovum and a second polar body. In the event that fertilization does not take place, the maturation of the secondary ovocyte seems to stop in metaphase II.

MENDELIAN INHERITANCE

From a clinical view, the identification of the type of Mendelian inheritance is made by an examination of the pedigree pattern. There are three principal types: autosomal dominant, autosomal recessive, and X-linked.

The Language of Pedigree Patterns

There is more or less general agreement on the method of representing the family of the individual who is affected with the particular disorder. The index person is often referred to as the propositus (female: proposita) (Fig. 7.3).

AUTOSOMAL DOMINANT INHERITANCE

Although the gynecologist, in his role as physician to the fetus, is interested in all genetically affected children, there are relatively few conditions which directly affect the female genitourinary tract and which are inherited by autosomal dominance.

However, one frequently seen condition which has been suspected of being transmitted by autosomal dominant inheritance is the Stein-Leventhal syndrome. Cooper *et al.* (1968) suggested an autosomal dominant mode of inheritance on the basis of high frequency of hirsutism in the fathers, high frequency of hirsutism and oligomenorrhea in female sibs, the culdoscopic identification of ovaries which appeared to be affected by the Stein-Leventhal Syndrome in 8 out of 12 sibs and elevated 17-ketosteroids in other related individuals. Although this may be so, as is often the situation in the human, it requires an assumption of considerable variation in the expressivity of the gene to account for the data. A representative pedigree pattern from Cooper indicates the type of information with which it is necessary to work in many areas of human genetics (Fig. 7.4).

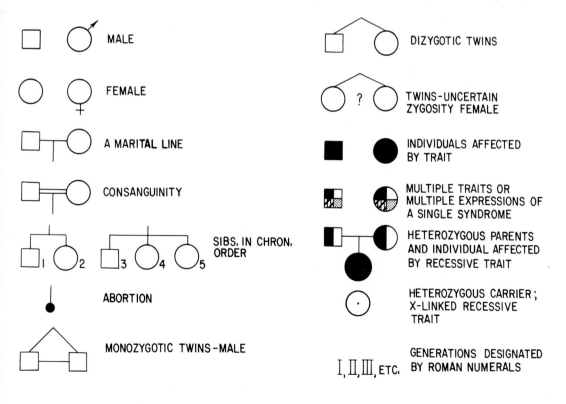

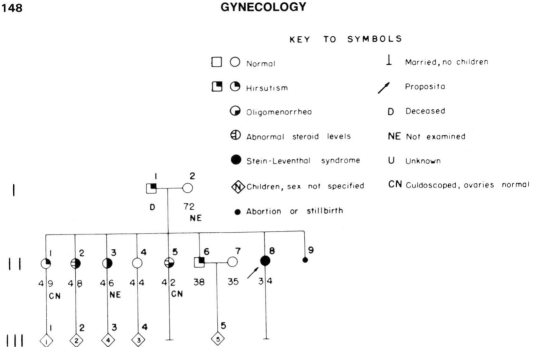

7.4. A pedigree pattern which indicates the mode of inheritance of patients with the Stein-Leventhal Syndrome (from Cooper, H. E., *et al.* Amer. J. Obstet. Gynec., *100:* 361).

A more clear cut dominantly inherited condition with important obstetrical implications is achondroplasia.

As a rule of thumb, autosomal dominant conditions are not sex related and have their source in but a single parent. If there is but one affected heterozygous parent, one-half the children will be affected heterozygotes and the other half will be normal. A thrice-married achondroplastic patient illustrates the mode of inheritance (Fig. 7.5).

AUTOSOMAL RECESSIVE INHERITANCE

Autosomal recessive traits occur without reference to sex and are inherited from both mother and father both of whom are of necessity heterozygous. Consanguinity predisposes to this type of inheritance.

Congenital, virilizing, adrenal hyperplasia is a classic example of an autosomally recessive trait which is of great familiarity to the gynecologist. It should be noted that the various forms of the disorder, *e.g.*, 21-hydroxylase deficiency or 11-hydroxylase deficiency, etc., seem to behave genetically as distinct entities.

An example of a very rare disorder, which seems to be trasmitted in a recessive manner, is that of transverse vaginal septum (Fig. 7.6).

According to Mendelian principles, one-fourth of all offspring of heterozygous parents are affected homozygotes and one-half will be carriers whereas one-fourth will be unaffected homozygotes. This information is exceedingly useful in counseling patients with virilizing adrenal hyperplasia or other such disorders and it is important to know that, if an affected homozygote marries a normal mate, none of their children will be affected, but all will be carriers. If an affected homozygote, who is treated, happens to marry an heterozygote, one-half of all their children will be affected and the other half will be carriers. The practicality of such information can be seen when it is realized that the gene for congenital virilizing adrenal hyperplasia seems to occur in the frequency of about 1 in 100 in Caucasians.

X-Linked Inheritance

The genes on the X chromosome may be expressed in either a dominant or a

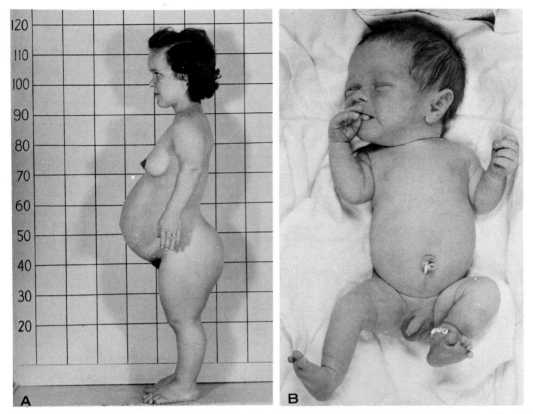

7.5. A. Photograph of pregnant patient with achondroplasia. (See **7.5C.**) **B.** Photograph of unaffected child of achondroplastic patient.

recessive manner. However, this is true only in the female. In the male, who is hemizygous for the major part of the X chromosome, all genes of the hemizygous portion are expressed irrespective of their action in the female.

No X-linked dominant condition with

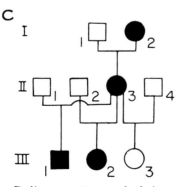

7.5.C. Pedigree pattern of thrice-married achondroplastic patient shown in **A**. The patient is II-3 (courtesy of Dr. V. A. McKusick).

disorders of the genitourinary tract of special interest to the gynecologist has been described.

Hemophilia is a very well known example of an X-linked recessive trait and, although it does not specifically affect those organs normally dealt with by the gynecologist, he is very much concerned in caring for patients affected by hemophilia and is particularly concerned with the possibility of the intrauterine diagnosis of this condition.

Another disorder of special interest to the gynecologist is the androgen insensitivity syndrome or testicular feminization. As in all X-linked conditions, the inheritance is always through the mother and there is no male to male transmission. In the androgen insensitivity syndrome, there is a second reason for no male to male transmission in that affected males are incapable of reproduction. The children in such a family may

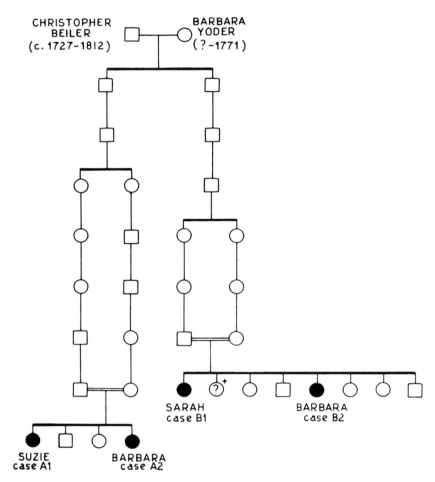

7.6. Pedigree pattern suggesting female limited autosomal recessive inheritance for patients with transverse vaginal septum. Drawing of the patient Barbara in the above pedigree pattern (from McKusick, V. A., J.A.M.A. *189:* 813, 1964) is shown in Fig. 8.5 (next chapter).

be affected male, normal male, carrier female, or normal female (Fig. 7.7).

It is noted that, although the androgen insensitivity syndrome has been included among the X-linked recessive disorders, the theoretical possibility exists, on the basis of the pedigree pattern, that the condition might be an autosomal dominant disorder limited to males. However, in view of the rarity of this mode of inheritance, the clear-cut X-linked transmission of a comparable condition in rodents, and the relative frequency of X-linked recessive disorders, it is most convenient to consider the androgen insensitivity syndrome as an example of the latter condition.

CHROMOSOMAL DISORDERS

Chromosomal disorders which, after all, concern the maldistribution of genetic material are certainly a proper part of genetics. However, chromosomal disorders, save for exceptional circumstances, are not inherited in a Mendelian sense. Their etiology is often obscure, although they are known to occur under certain specific circumstances as exemplified by the aging factor in the Down syndrome.

In rare circumstances, Medelian-type inheritance of chromosomal disorders is a possibility. For example, an unaffected carrier mother with a 14/21 translocation

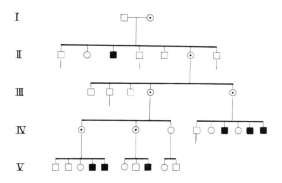

■ Testicular feminization

7.7. Pedigree pattern of family showing several members in several generations affected with testicular feminization. The patient illustrated in Figure 8.24 is the patient represented by IV-6 in the above pedigree.

where all or almost all of a number 21 chromosome is translocated to a number 14 chromosome has the theoretical possibility of transmitting this abnormal 14/21 chromosome to one-half her offspring. She has four types of oocytes with respect to

the 14 and 21 chromosomes: one 14/21, two 14,21 three 14/21, 21 and four 14. Fertilization of one would result in a 14/21 translocation carrier, of two in a normal child, of three in a mongol child and fertilization of four would result in a lethal zygote due to autosomal monosomy. Thus, theoretically there is a one in three chance of having an affected child and, according to Lejeune's data, this corresponds closely to practical experience.

Interestingly enough, if the father is the 14/21 carrier, although he too has the same theoretical chance of one in three of an affected child, Lejeune's data show that only about 2 per cent of children of such matings are affected. The discrepancy is apparently due to a disadvantage suffered by the spermatozoa burdened by the extra genetic material.

Repeated miscarriage has also been implicated, under rare circumstances, as a result of the Mendelian-type transmission of an abnormal chromosome usually a 13/14 translocation of the D group (Fig. 7.8).

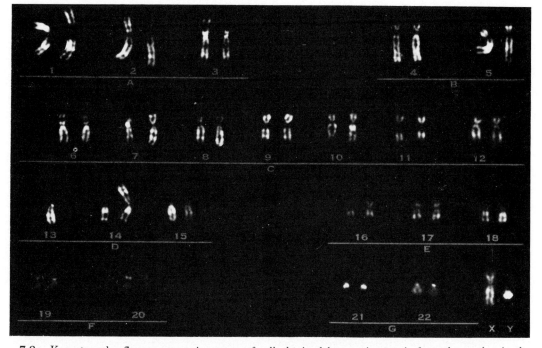

7.8a. Karyotype by fluorescence microscopy of cell obtained by amniocentesis from the mother in the pedigree pattern shown in **7.8b.** Note the translocation involving two D chromosomes which, by the fluorescence technique, can be identified as chromosomes No. 13 and No. 14: 45,XY,-13,-14,+t(13q14q).

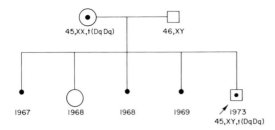

7.8b. Pedigree pattern of a patient who had three spontaneous miscarriages. During the last pregnancy, an amniocentesis revealed the karyotype shown in **7.8a.** A karyotype of the mother showed that she was a balanced carrier: 45,XX,-13,-14,+t(13q14q). The miscarriages were most likely due to an unbalanced chromosoal complement, probably a D trisomy.

Specific chromosomal disorders will not be further discussed at this point as they are considered in appropriate chapters where such disorders affect the genitourinary tract in women.

INTRAUTERINE DIAGNOSIS

As physician to the fetus, the gynecologist may find it appropriate to attempt to make a diagnosis of genetic disease in the unborn child in high risk pregnancies.

At the present time, the only therapy which can be offered to the pregnant patient with a genetically affected child is therapeutic abortion. As two or three weeks or longer may be required to make a suitable determination after obtaining material by amniocentesis and as a range of 20–26 weeks gestation has been established by law in most states for considering therapeutic abortion, it is important that diagnostic purposes of this type be carried out as soon as possible. It is difficult to obtain sufficient amniotic fluid before about 16 weeks.

About 30 ml. of amniotic fluid may usually be obtained from about the 16th week of pregnancy up to the 20th week without disturbing the course of the pregnancy. Using the supernatant fluid, it is possible that assays for enzyme defects or steroid disorders might be useful in diagnosing fetal disease. However, up to the moment, investigation of the supernatant fluid has produced very little of practical value except for alpha-feto protein.

The cells obtained by amniocentesis can be used for a variety of purposes. They may be used to determine the sex of the fetus by examination for the X- and Y- chromatin. This is of obvious importance in a variety of X-linked conditions. For example, a known hemophilia carrier may wish to be aborted if she carries a male child, half of whom could be expected to be affected.

The cells may also be cultured to determine the chromosome complement of the fetus. The principal usefulness here is when the Down syndrome is suspected, from a previously affected child, or as a screening procedure in women above the age of about 38.

Several other types of chromosomal disorders have been diagnosed by this technique.

In addition to the chromosomal disorders, a number of inborn errors of metabolism can be diagnosed by a determination of the specific activity of the enzyme, the deficiency of which is responsible for the syndrome in question. If the heterozygous carrier state is determinable, as in the Tay-Sachs syndrome, the mating of two carriers is a clear indication for a prenatal assay of the first pregnancy. In situations where heterozygosity is not determinable, the need for amniocentesis is not evident except after the birth of an affected child. At the time of writing, there are about 40 inborn errors of metabolism for which suitable assay techniques exist.

Curiously enough, there is no autosomal dominant condition for which there exists a suitable test which lends itself to prenatal diagnosis.

Table 7.1 lists the indications for the first 200 odd cases monitored by amniocentesis at Johns Hopkins.

GENETIC COUNSELING

Genetic counseling in all its ramifications requires information far beyond that outlined in this chapter. Nevertheless, a discussion of the principles involved and the citing of a few examples may be worthwhile.

First and foremost, to provide in-

Table 7.1

Indications for Amniocentesis (203 Cases)

Chromosomal Disorders	
Previous Down syndrome................	68
Maternal age...........................	83
Known translocation carrier..............	5
Previous E-18 trisomy...................	3
Previous D_1 trisomy.....................	2
Other................................	2
X-Linked Disorders	
Muscular dystrophy (Duchenne)...........	5
Hemophilia............................	2
Metabolic Disorders	
Tay-Sachs disease.......................	20
Generalized gangliosidosis................	4
Metachromatic leukodystrophy...........	3
Hunter disease.........................	2
Gaucher disease........................	1
Hurler disease.........................	1
Norrie disease.........................	1
Pelizaeus-Merzbacher disease..............	1

telligent counseling, a precise and accurate diagnosis of the alleged genetic condition is an absolute necessity. To this end, in the event there is a child, parent, prospective parent, or other relative with an alleged genetic defect, sophisticated cooperation from the appropriate pediatrician or internist or other consultant will most often be required. In the event the patient is pregnant, amniocentesis may be desirable to secure cytological or biochemical information about the unborn child.

The task of the counselor has been rendered infinitely more simple by *"Mendelian Inheritance in Man,"* a catalogue of autosomal dominant, autosomal recessive, and X-linked phenotypes compiled by McKusick and published by the Johns Hopkins Press and frequently revised. This is a thumbnail sketch of over 3000 conditions with their type of inheritance and pertinent references to the literature. With an accurate diagnosis and by the use of this magnificent compendium and a knowledge of the basic principles of Mendelian inheritance and an estimate of the frequency of the gene, it is often possible to formulate the probabilities of inheritance of a given trait.

A single example will suffice. The older sister of a patient who was treated for congenital adrenal hyperplasia is married and contemplates pregnancy. Recalling the difficulties of her sister as a child, she wishes to know what chance she has of producing an affected child. The counselor knows that this is an autosomal recessive disorder and that there are two chances out of three that unaffected sibs of such affected individuals are carriers. He also knows that one child out of four of two carrier parents is an affected homozygote. He also knows that in round figures, among Caucasians, the gene for congenital virilizing adrenal hyperplasia has a frequency of about one in 100. Therefore, the probabilities that the normal sister will produce an affected offspring are $\frac{2}{3} \times \frac{1}{4} \times \frac{1}{100}$ or 1 in 600.

Much more troublesome are problems involving congenital anomalies such as anencephaly, cleft palate, hare lip and the like, or mental retardation where genetic advice is very frequently sought. Such diseases are apparently multifactorial and are not inherited in a strict Mendelian fashion although it is recognized that familial occurrence is above mere chance. So-called empirical risk figures for the disease in question must be used to predict the probabilities of trouble.

It has already been stated that chromosomal disorders are not inherited in the Mendelian sense except in special circumstances. However, the Down syndrome has been much studied and certain risk factors are known. For example, Carter and McCarthy collected data giving the approximate risk of mongolism with age and have shown that, after the mother has reached 45, there is one chance in 40 that she will produce a mongoloid infant. However, in the translocation variety, Mendelian transmission does occur as referred to above for the D-G type. With a G/G translocation where the translocation is apparently 21/22 with either the father or the mother as the carrier, interestingly enough Lejeune's figures show that there is an exceedingly low probability of a mongoloid infant. On the other hand, where there is a 21/21 translocation, there is 100 per cent probability of a mongoloid.

Although the diagnosis of genetic defects may require the skill of a variety of physicians, and while there is constant improvement in the treatment of patients with congenital defects, as for example, control of the adrenal hyperplasia with cortisone or the use of a suitable diet for phenylketonuria, it is nevertheless true that the gynecologist is often the critical physician in handling genetic defects in that it is he who advises about the intelligent selection of methods of prevention of pregnancy and it is he who must make an intrauterine diagnosis and it is he who must carry out the therapeutic abortion, if this seems indicated.

For these and other reasons, the gynecologist must be well informed about genetics.

REFERENCES

Carter, C. and McCarthy, D.: Incidence of mongolism and its diagnosis in the newborn. Brit. J. Prev. Soc. Med., 5: 83, 1951.

Cooper, H. E., Spellacy, W. N., Prem, K. A., and Cohen, W. D.: Heredity factors in the Stein-Leventhal syndrome. Amer. J. Obstet. Gynec., 100: 371, 1968.

Lejeune, J.: The 21 trisomy-current stage of chromosomal research. Progr. Med. Genet., 3: 144, 1964.

McKusick, V.: Mendelian Inheritance in Man. Johns Hopkins Press, Baltimore, 1974.

Nowell, P. C., and Hungerford, D. A.: Chromosome studies in human leukemia. II. Chronic granulocytic leukemia. J. Nat. Cancer Inst., 27: 1013, 1961.

Rary, J. M., Park, I. J., Heller, R. H., Jones, H. W., Jr., and Baramki, T. A.: Prenatal cytogenetic analysis of women with high risk for genetic disorders. J. Hered., 65:209, 1974.

chapter 8

Congenital Anomalies and Hermaphroditism

It is scarcely necessary to emphasize that an intelligent interpretation of the many congenital anomalies which are encountered in the female generative organs is not possible without some understanding of the embryology of these organs. For a brief review of the latter subject the reader is referred to Chapter 6.

EXTERNAL GENITALIA

Agglutination of the Labia

Properly speaking, agglutination of the labia is not a congenital anomaly of the external genitalia, but it is so often confused with an anomaly that it is properly considered at this point. The labia minora and the labia majora may be held together in the midline by such dense adhesions that at first glance one seems to be viewing the median raphe of a male perineum. Occasionally this fusion is so complete as to prevent normal voiding. The labia are adherent because of a mild childhood inflammatory process which has been insufficient to attract attention. Treatment consists of separation of the labia and the use of petroleum jelly or an estrogenic ointment to prevent the recurrence of the adhesions. Anderson has pointed out that although labial adhesions are not uncommon in childhood, they are rarely, if ever, seen in adults. For this reason he considers it unnecessary to separate fused labia if they are asymptomatic, pointing out that the prevention of recurrence is troublesome and apt to draw undue attention to the genitalia.

Masculinization of the External Genitalia

This subject is covered later in this chapter and will not be further considered at this point.

Imperforate Hymen

The hymen is the area where the embryonic vagina buds from the urogenital sinus. It is not to be confused with the so-called transverse vaginal septum. The hymenal area is entirely of urogenital sinus origin. If a lumen fails to develop at the point where the budding vagina arises from the urogenital sinus, the result is an

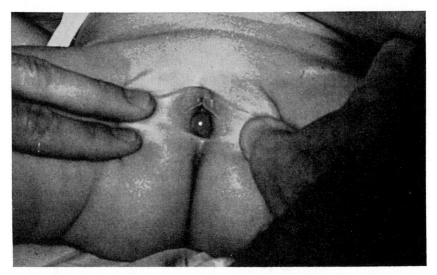

8.1. A 1½ -year-old child with cystic mass extending from the vagina. This proved to be an imperforate hymen, the excision of which released 8 ml. of clear, sterile mucus. (From Jones, H. W., Jr., and Scott, W. W.: *Hermaphroditism, Genital Anomalies and Related Endocrine Disorders,* 2nd ed. The Williams & Wilkins Company, Baltimore, 1971.)

imperforate hymen, a relatively rare condition.

It is unusual for an imperforate hymen to be discovered before the onset of puberty. If the condition is discovered before the onset of the menarche, the hymen should nevertheless be incised. At that time the vagina may be found to contain a clear, mucoid fluid which is apparently accumulated cervical secretion. On occasion the mucocolpos may reach considerable proportions (Fig. 8.1). If the condition is not discovered until after the onset of puberty, symptoms arise from the accumulation of menstrual blood. Although cyclic lower abdominal pain is the common symptom, it is sometimes remarkable that a large amount of blood can accumulate in the vagina, uterus, and tubes and cause relatively little discomfort (Plates 8.1 and 8.2). In rare instances, flank pain due to urinary retention is a presenting symptom.

The treatment of this condition consists of simple incision of the hymen with excision of a triangular flap. Because of the presence of old blood and the potentiality of bacterial infection, antibiotics can be routinely advised (Fig. 8.2). The admixture of blood, of course, changes the diagnosis to hematocolpos.

VAGINA

Congenital Absence of Vagina

Patients with congenital absence of the vagina usually also have absence of the

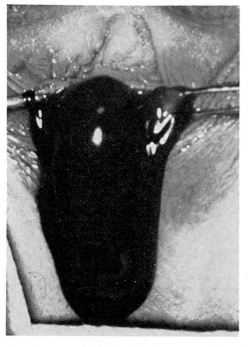

8.2. Escape of tarry retained menstrual blood after incision of imperforate hymen.

uterus. Therefore, a more accurate term might be aplasia or dysplasia of the Müllerian ducts, for it is the absence of the Müllerian portion of the vagina that we are here concerned with. However, by common usage the term "congenital absence of the vagina" is used to describe the condition. Such patients may have a normally developed lower vagina which is derived from the urogenital sinus. However, the usual lesion includes absence of the middle and upper vagina, the uterus, and sometimes the fallopian tubes. The ovaries are normal, anatomically and functionally. Such patients seek the physician after puberty because of the failure of the onset of menstruation. The external genitalia are normal except that the vaginal opening is absent or there may be a very shallow vagina. In a review of 100 cases at the Gynecological Clinic of The Johns Hopkins Hospital, 71 patients had no suggestion of a vagina. In the remaining 29 the vagina was very shallow, the longest being 5 cm. These findings are to be compared with those of McIndoe, who found 58 of 61 women with complete vaginal absence.

Four of the patients in the Hopkins series had exploratory operations for reasons unrelated to the anomaly. In each instance the findings were similar (Fig. 8.3). The ovaries appeared grossly normal as did the fallopian tubes. There seemed to be a failure of fusion and development of the Mullerian ducts, and at the proximal end of each tube there were muscular thickenings which were joined in the midline by palpable and visible strands suggesting a diminutive and undeveloped double uterus (Fig. 8.4). Most often nothing resembling a uterus can be felt on rectal examination, although the above case illustrates that recognizable undeveloped uteri may be present.

Absence of uterus and vagina is associated with anomalies of the urinary tract in a significant number of cases. Among 17 patients reported by Thompson, Wharton, and Te Linde from our clinic, eight were found to have major urological anomalies (two with absent single kidneys, two with pelvic kidneys, two with crossed ectopia, one with ipsilateral ectopia, and one with bilateral

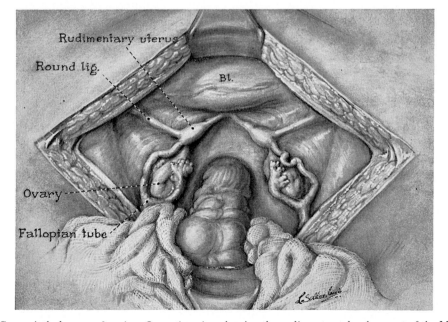

8.3. Congenital absence of vagina. Operative view showing the rudimentary development of the Mullerian ducts. This is the common finding in this condition and indicates that the disorder is more extensive than a simple anomaly of the vagina. (From Jones, H. W., Jr., and Scott, W. W.: *Hermaphroditism, Genital Anomalies and Related Endocrine Disorders,* 2nd ed. The Williams & Wilkins Company, Baltimore, 1971.)

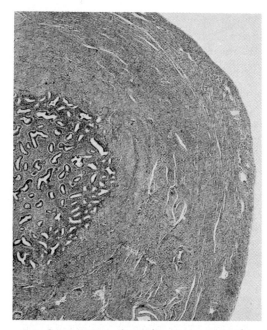

8.4. Cross section of a rudimentary uterus from the patient (Fig. 8.3) with congential absence of vagina. There is no real lumen, but there is a small amount of endometrium. (From Jones, H. W., Jr., and Scott, W. W.: *Hermaphroditism, Genital Anomalies and Related Endocrine Disorders,* 2nd ed., The Williams & Wilkins Company, Baltimore, 1971.)

ureteropelvic obstruction). Among 41 patients examined by Bryan, Nigro, and Counseller (1949), 21 had anomalies of various sorts. All patients with genital anomalies should have intravenous pyelograms.

Bony anomalies of the spine seem to be unduly common. Among 11 cases in the Hopkins series there was one case of lumbarization of the first sacral segment; and Bryan *et al.* reported six such instances in their series of 100 patients.

Azoury and Jones were unable to demonstrate any cytogenetic abnormality in such patients.

McIndoe has ingeniously used a split thickness skin graft over a mold in vaginal reconstruction. A space is developed between the bladder and rectum and the mold is left in place initially for about one week and then with decreasing frequency for a span of about six months. The skin graft usually takes

without difficulty. McIndoe reported in 1959 the results of 105 such operations and found that the results were satisfactory in 95%. Jones and Wheeless reported similar success.

A small but special group of patients is encountered with congenital absence of most of the vagina but with normal development of the uterus and most often with a very small part of the upper vagina. Such patients may be looked upon as having an extraordinarily long transverse vaginal septum (see below). After the menarche they accumulate retained menstrual blood. A special technique for handling this situation was described by Jones and Wheeless.

Transverse Vaginal Septum

A patient with a transverse vaginal septum can easily be mistaken for a patient with congenital absence of the vagina and uterus if the examiner misinterprets the septum as the vaginal apex. This is a rather rare condition and there are only a few pertinent reports in the literature. Bowman and Scott recorded four patients with this abnormality and briefly reviewed the literature.

The symptoms will depend entirely on whether the septum is imperforate or has a small opening. In the latter case, menstruation may be apparently normal and no difficulty is suspected until vaginal obstruction is encountered at marriage, or, as in a case reported by Bowman and Scott, until pregnancy occurs. If the septum is imperforate, external menstrual bleeding is, of course, impossible and symptoms will arise soon after the menarche because of retention of the blood. In rare circumstances a large mucocolpometra will collect behind an imperforate transverse septum, as in an unpublished case of Dr. Roger Scott (Fig. 8.5). Any child with amenorrhea and a lower abdominal mass should have cervical dilatation prior to laparotomy.

The transverse vaginal septum occurs most often at about the junction of the upper and middle third of the vagina, although it has been described at other points along the vaginal canal (Fig. 8.6).

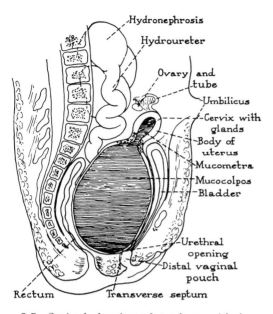

Labels on figure:
Hydronephrosis
Hydroureter
Ovary and tube
Umbilicus
Cervix with glands
Body of uterus
Mucometra
Mucocolpos
Bladder
Urethral opening
Distal vaginal pouch
Rectum
Transverse septum

8.5. Sagittal drawing of newborn with huge mucocolpos due to transverse vaginal septum. This is an unpublished observation of Dr. Roger Scott. The child had marked urinary obstruction due to the pressure of the mass. The patient did not present any bulging at the outlet as would be expected from the mucocolpos due to an imperforate hymen. The source of the mucus is apparently the cervical glands, but why some newborns with complete obstruction of the vagina collect great quantities of mucus and others do not is completely unknown (see Fig. 7.5). (From Jones, H. W., Jr., and Scott, W. W.: *Hermaphroditism, Genital Anomalies and Related Endocrine Disorders,* 2nd ed., The Williams & Wilkins Company, Baltimore, 1971.)

McKusick and his associates described two distant Amish cousins with this malformation. He was able to trace them to a common ancestor and felt that autosomal recessive inheritance was a very likely explanation for at least some of these abnormalities (Fig. 7.6).

Either manual dilatation or surgical excision of the septum is necessary and usually not difficult.

Double or Septate Vagina

A double vagina may occur with an entirely normal uterus and tubes. On the other hand, a complete double uterus and vagina are sometimes encountered. It is not uncommon to have a double vagina and double cervix and a single corpus. The septum, which is longitudinal and anterior-posterior, may be only partial or it may extend almost to the vaginal outlet. Both sides are usually patent but, in rare instances, the septum may be off center and fused with the lateral vaginal wall in such a way that one side of the vagina and uterus are obstructed and distended by retention of menstrual blood (Fig. 8.7).

The vaginal septum is generally asymptomatic and undiscovered until marriage when it may be found to be a cause of dyspareunia. In other instances it may not be discovered until labor. Most obstetricians can relate cases they have seen or heard about in which a breech has straddled a septate cervix or vagina. If one side of the vagina is obstructed, symptoms from the retention of the menstrual blood will obviously occur.

Excision of the vaginal septum is usually rather simple but sometimes bloody. If the septum causes obstruction, dyspareunia, or dystocia it should be removed.

UTERUS AND TUBES

Although a great variety of anomalies of the uterus has been described, they may be grouped under five heads: (1) absence of the uterus; (2) unicornuate uterus; (3) rudimentary uterine horn; (4) blind uterine horn; and (5) symmetrical double uterus.

Absence of the Uterus

In an otherwise normal female, absence of the uterus but with a vagina of normal length is almost unheard of. For the most part such individuals also have greater or lesser degrees of absence of the vagina and this condition is essentially that of congenital absence of the vagina which has been previously discussed.

Unicornuate Uterus

If the development of one Müllerian duct is completely arrested, the uterus and fallopian tube may be formed entirely from the other. This so-called uterus unicornus or unicorn uterus

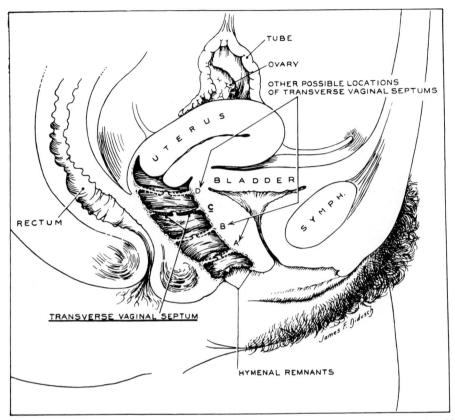

8.6. Drawing of congenital transverse vaginal septum with other possible locations in the vagina. Note that these locations are not related to the position of the hymenal remnants. (From Bowman, J. A., Jr., and Scott, R. B.: Obstet. Gynec., *3:* 441, 1954.)

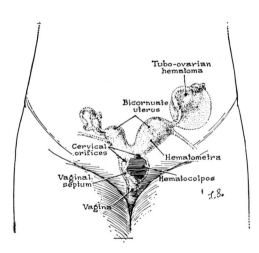

8.7. Sketch of situation in a patient with double uterus and double vagina with obstruction of the left half of vagina.

seldom causes any clinical abnormality (Fig. 8.8, *left*).

Rudimentary Uterine Horn

When the development of one Müllerian duct is normal and the other very imperfect, various degrees of rudimentary uterine horns are produced. Most rudimentary horns are non-communicating and are connected to the opposite unicornuate uterus by fibrous bands (Fig. 8.8 *right*). In some instances the endometrium is nonfunctional, so that no clinical symptoms are present. A clinical situation may arise from the retention of menstrual blood in a rudimentary horn which does not communicate and where the endometrium is functional. It is amazing how large these may become and how long they may go before compelling

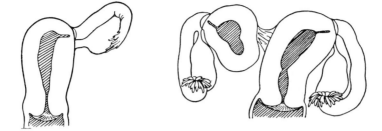

8.8. *Left,* sketch of uterus unicornus; *right,* sketch of a uterus with a rudimentary horn.

symptoms are present. In some instances the endometrial cavity of the rudimentary uterine horn may communicate through a narrow channel to a more normal opposite cavity. Under these circumstances pregnancy has been observed in such a rudimentary organ. If pregnancy does so occur, the patient may present the classic picture of an ectopic pregnancy, including rupture.

As with all examples of maldevelopment of the Müllerian ducts, anomalies of the urinary tract may be present. With rudimentary horns this is especially common. The anomaly of the urinary tract is, as a rule, on the same side as the most serious underdevelopment of the Müllerian duct. Although the kidney may be malrotated, low lying, or actually within the bony pelvis, complete agenesis is not uncommon.

Blind Uterine Horn

If the two Müllerian ducts develop about equally well but one fails to communicate, either with the other or exteriorly, the condition of a blind uterine horn results. The usual history is that of increasing dysmenorrhea with the development of a mass which presents in the lower abdomen and vagina lateral to the cervix. Pelvic endometriosis is a not uncommon accompaniment. Under this circumstance it is often possible to anastomose the blind horn with the opposite half of the uterus (Fig. 8.9). Anomalies of the urinary tract are also common in this disorder.

Symmetrical Double Uterus

When the two Müllerian ducts develop side by side without communicating with each other, there is produced a so-called double uterus. Each duct forms one cervix and one uterine body with one fallopian tube attached to each. The duplication may continue down into the vagina in that part of the vagina formed by the Müllerian ducts. Such complete duplication may be referred to as the *uterus didelphys* (Fig. 8.10 *left*). However, most reduplicated uteri are not so complete and the fusion may be only in the upper portion so that there will be a double uterus with a single cervix and a single vagina. If the two horns of such a partially fused uterus are recognizable, the uterus is designated as a *bicornuate uterus* (Figs. 8.10 *right* to 8.12, inclusive). Sometimes, however, the external configuration of the uterus is relatively normal and the malfusion is represented only by a septum within the uterus. In that case the uterus may be referred to as a *septate uterus* (Fig. 8.13). If the condition is minimal, an *arcuate uterus* occurs.

These various degrees of reduplication of the uterus may be associated with reproductive failure. However, it should be emphasized that an anomalous uterus may be compatible with a normal reproductive history. Only about one-fourth of all women with this anomaly have reproductive problems. If it can be demonstrated by suitable tests that the double uterus is, in fact, responsible for the reproductive problem, surgical reconstruction of the uterus to form a single uterine cavity is entirely feasible. Various other factors which might lead to abortion should first be investigated by suitable studies. It is interesting that a septate uterus is more apt to cause difficulty than a true bicornuate uterus although re-

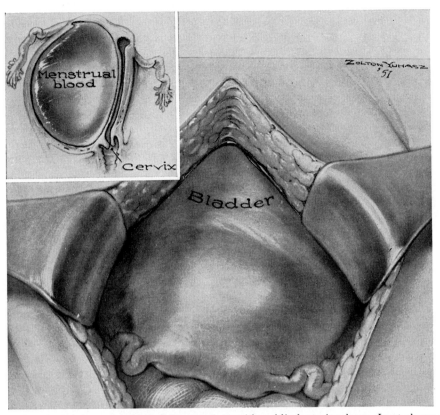

8.9. Appearance of uterus at operation in a patient with a blind uterine horn. *Inset* shows diagram representing a transverse section through the uterus. In this case it was possible to anastomose the blind horn to the patent horn. (From Jones, H. W., Jr., and Jones, G. E. S.: Amer. J. Obstet. Gynec., *65:* 325, 1953.)

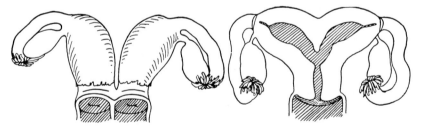

8.10. *Left,* sketch of uterus didelphys; *right,* sketch of a mild form of bicornuate uterus.

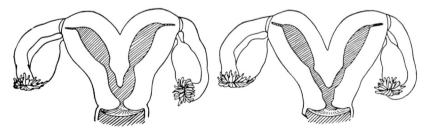

8.11. *Left,* sketch of a moderate form of bicornuate uterus; *right,* sketch of a more severe form of a bicornuate uterus.

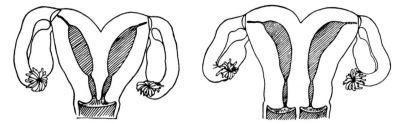

8.12. Sketch of a bicornuate uterus. *Left,* with a double cervix but a single vagina; *right,* with a double cervix and a double vagina.

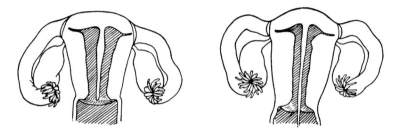

8.13. Sketch of a septate uterus. *Left,* with a double cervix; *right,* with a double cervix and a double vagina.

productive failure may be associated with either. Jones and Wheeless reported the problems encountered and the results of treatment in 173 patients with double uterus. In properly selected cases, the results of treatment for reproductive failure are quite good.

OVARIES

Ovarian Aplasia

The subject of congenital absence of the ovaries, or ovarian aplasia or gonadal aplasia, is essentially a problem in hermaphroditism and is considered later in this chapter.

Supernumerary and Accessory Ovaries

Ectopic ovarian tissue is an extremely rare condition. Wharton has thoroughly reviewed this subject. *Supernumerary ovaries* include those cases in which one or more normal extra ovaries are entirely separate from the normally placed ovaries (Fig. 8.14). They would seem to arise through an embryological process accessory to that which was responsible for the normally placed ovaries. According to Wharton there are only four such acceptable cases in the literature.

Accessory ovaries include those cases in which excess ovarian tissue is situated near the normally placed ovary, may be connected with it, and seems to have developed from it. Such accessory tissue is invariably located near the normally placed ovary. Generally speaking, these

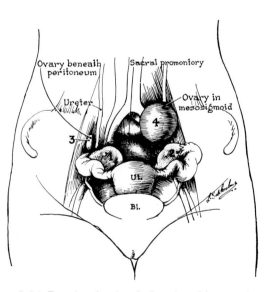

8.14. Drawing showing the location of four ovaries removed from a single patient. (From Wharton, L. R.: Amer. J. Obstet. Gynec., *78:* 1101, 1959.)

accessory ovaries are small and almost always less than 1 cm. in diameter. Most frequently they have been found attached to the broad ligament near the normal ovary. They have been described near the cornu of the uterus and between the leaves of the broad ligament. These small bits of tissue have usually been grossly mistaken for lymph nodes and their true nature has been revealed only by microscopic examination. For the most part they have been solitary, but a few cases of two and even of three such accessory ovaries have been reported. They have universally been an incidental finding, although we have recently seen a granulosal thecal tumor arising from aberrant gonadal tissue well removed from the normal ovary.

In addition to supernumerary and accessory ovaries, there are other examples of heterotopic ovarian tissue. Very rarely, an ovary will be located at a position higher than normal, *e.g.,* at the lower pole of the kidney.

Absence of One Tube and a Corresponding Ovary

In addition to cases in which the heterotopic ovarian tissue seems to be the result of an embryonic aberration, ectopic ovaries might be the result of mechanical causes. An ovary is occasionally encountered which is parasitic to the omentum or other intraabdominal structure and is completely separate from its normal attachments. This condition is caused by torsion of the ovarian pedicle. At times, the parasitic ovary is represented only by a small calcified nodule in the omentum. At first glance in such a condition, there seems to be congenital absence of the tube and ovary. However, a small stump of tube and a tiny omental nodule indicates the true condition.

HERMAPHRODITISM

Sex identification may be described in terms of at least seven characteristics. The first five of these are organic and the last two psychological: (1) chromosomal arrangement and chromatin pattern; (2) gonadal structure; (3) morphology of the external genitalia; (4) morphology of the internal genitalia; (5) hormonal status; (6) sex of rearing; and (7) gender role. The meaning and implications of these criteria are well known except, perhaps, for chromosomal arrangement, chromatin pattern, and gender role.

Chromosomal arrangement and *chromatin pattern* have been discussed from the biological viewpoint in Chapter 6 "Embryology" and in Chapter 7 "Genetics and Cytogenetics" to which the reader is referred for this and other matters which give essential background for understanding the anomalies of sex differentiation.

As a screening test, a determination of the X- and Y-chromatin gives valuable information about the sex chromosome composition of the patient, and tests should be made on all patients with a problem of sex differentiation.

In the normal female, the percentage of cells showing the chromatin varies with the technique of preparations and the tissue used. In clinical work, cells from the buccal mucosa are readily obtained and 20 to 50 per cent of them show a single X-chromatin body. From a study of pathological states, it has been found that the number of X-chromatin bodies per cell is one less than the number of X chromosomes in each cell. Thus, a cell with three X chromosomes has two sex chromatin bodies during interphase (Fig. 8.15). Chromosomal mosaicism is said to exist when cell lines with variance in the quantity or quality of the chromosomes are found in the same individual. An example of a type of mosaicism may be represented 45,X/46,XX. When there is dilution of the normal cell line by a strain of cells which does not have a positive X-chromatin, the quantitative count will be reduced. Therefore, in patients with a low quantitative X-chromatin count, chromosomal mosaicism of the sex chromosomes must be suspected.

Not only have abnormal numbers of chromosomes been found, but structural abnormalities of individual chromosomes have been encountered. This may take

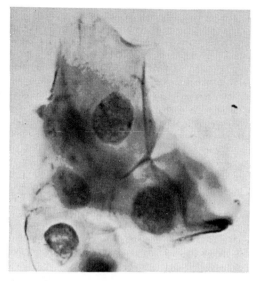

8.15. Buccal smear showing two sex chromatin bodies in a single cell. This patient was found to have three X chromosomes in a total of 47 (aceto-orcein, ×1500).

the form of deletion of a portion of the chromosome, translocation of one part of a chromosome to another chromosome, or the formation of an isochromosome by an error in mitosis, *e.g.,* an abnormal X chromosome may be composed of four long arms or four short arms instead of the normal configuration of two long and two short arms. In these abnormal forms, the size of the sex chromatin body is affected; an isochromosome of the long arms of an X chromosome gives a large chromatin body and an isochromosome of the short arms gives a small sex chromatin body.

"Drumsticks" of polymorphonuclear leukocytes are also an expression of the X-chromatin but are not as convenient or reliable as a study of the chromatin bodies of a smear made from the buccal mucosa.

Of equal importance, in problems of sexual differentiation, is a determination of the Y-chromatin. This is readily determinable in interphase cells, but does require fluorescence microscopy. It is, however, a very simple way to determine the presence or absence of a Y chromosome or, more specifically, of the distal long arms of a Y chromosome. The

presence or absence of the Y is a critical point in the differential diagnosis and treatment of patients with problems of sexual development.

Gender role may be defined as all those things a person says or does to disclose himself or herself as having the status of boy or man, girl or woman, respectively.

In a normal person all five organic and the two psychological criteria correspond to one sex. The hermaphroditic state may be said to exist when there is a contradiction of one or more of the four morphological criteria: chromosomal arrangement or chromatin pattern, gonad structure, morphology of external genitalia, and morphology of internal genitalia. A sex contradiction of hormonal dominance may exist without hermaphroditism, as for example with a virilizing tumor in a female. However, as a matter of experience the hormonal sex is often contradictory in hermaphroditism. Although the two psychological criteria of sex are of extreme importance, especially in regard to therapy, a contradiction of these criteria does not imply a diagnosis of the hermaphroditic state. In fact, their contradiction in the face of agreement of all the organic characteristics of sex is entirely a psychiatric problem of transvestism and transsexualism quite beyond the scope of hermaphroditism *per se.* Table 8.1 lists the various groups of hermaphrodites and their abnormalities with respect to the criteria of sex identification.

Although any of the several criteria of sex might be the basis of a classification of ambisexual individuals, the well established nomenclature of Klebs is based upon the microscopic character of the gonad. According to this view the state of hermaphroditismus verus (true hermaphroditism) can be considered to exist only if both testicular and ovarian elements can be identified in a given patient. Klebs further specified that ambisexual individuals with entirely male gonads should be identified as male pseudohermaphrodites and ambisexual individuals with entirely female gonads should be identified as female pseudohermaphrodites. Although long usage justifies the

Table 8.1

Hermaphroditic Abnormalities and Criteria of Sex Identification

Etiology	Group	Chromosomal Arrangement	X-Chromatin	Gonadal Structure	Criteria of Sex			Sex of Rearing		Gender Role
					Morphology of External Genitalia	Morphology of Internal Genitalia	Hormonal Dominance	Actual	Preferred	
Chromosomal aberration in most cases	Ovarian agenesis and dysgenesis	45,X 45,X/46,XX etc.	Negative or positive	None	Female	Female	None	As women	As women	As women
Unknown	Hermaphroditismus verus	46,XX etc.	Positive or negative	Testis and ovary	Mixed	Mixed	Mixed	Either	Either	Either
Chromosomal aberration	Klinefelter's syndrome	47,XXY etc.	Positive	Testis	Male	Male	Mixed	As men	As men	As men
Chromosomal aberration	Multi X females	47,XXX 48,XXXX etc.	Multiple positive	Ovary	Female	Female	Female	As women	As women	As women
Genetic or chromosomal	Male hermaphroditism with virilization	46,XY 45,X/46,XY etc.	Negative	Testis	Mixed	Mixed	Male	Either, but mostly as women	Either, but mostly as women	Either, but mostly as women
Genetic	Male hermaphroditism with feminization	46,XY	Negative	Testis	Female	None	Female	As women	As women	As women
Congenital adrenal hyperplasia (genetic)	Female hermaphroditism with virilization	46,XX	Positive	Ovary	Mixed	Female	Male	Either, but mostly as women	As women	Either, but mostly as women
Maternal androgen in some cases	Female hermaphroditism with feminization	46,XX	Positive	Ovary	Mixed	Female	Female	Either, but mostly as women	As women	Either, but mostly as women

continuation of the Klebs emphasis on the importance of the gonadal structures as a basis for classification, the multitudinous Latin subdivisions of this scheme are best omitted as being both unnecessary and inaccurate. Furthermore, the use of male hermaphrodite or female hermaphrodite is permissible in place of the obsolete pseudohermaphrodite. This point of nomenclature stems from the thought that *pseudo* is redundant in describing an individual with an entirely male or entirely female gonad if *true* be retained to describe the patient with the mixed gonads of *hermaphroditismus verus.*

CLINICAL GROUPS OF HERMAPHRODITES

Ovarian Agenesis and Dysgenesis

One of the most striking developments in the field of intersexuality in recent years has been the discovery that a majority of patients with ovarian agenesis exhibit a negative chromatin pattern. Furthermore, it has been shown that most

of these chromatin-negative individuals are lacking in one of the pair of sex chromosomes and have only a single X chromosome (Fig. 8.16). Patients exhibiting the syndrome of ovarian agenesis have feminine external genitalia, although a few have been described with a slightly enlarged clitoris (Fig. 8.17). Without exception they are thought to be girls at birth and have uniformly been reared as girls and women. The Müllerian ducts develop entirely along female lines and the uterus and tubes are present although in a prepubertal condition throughout life. Menstruation and secondary female sex characteristics never appear. The gonads do not develop and are represented only by collections of connective tissue (Figs. 8.18 and 8.19). Considerable experimental work has given an excellent understanding of the factors responsible for such development. This is discussed in Chapter 6, "Embryology."

The failure of ovarian development is often associated with a variety of somatic

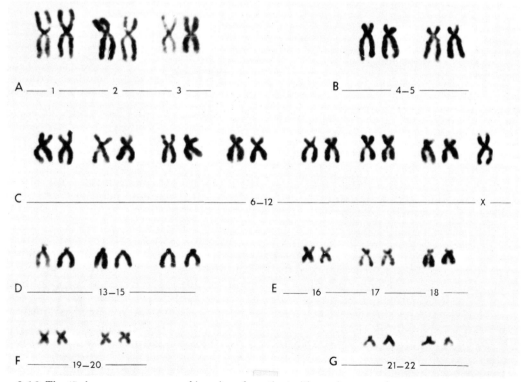

8.16. The 45 chromosomes, arranged in pairs, of a patient with ovarian agenesis.

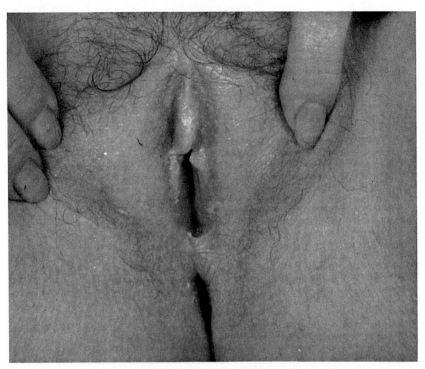

8.17. External genitalia of patient with gonadal aplasia. The buccal smear of this patient was negative. (From Jones, H. W., Jr., and Scott, W. W.: *Hermaphroditism, Genital Anomalies and Related Endocrine Disorders,* 2nd ed. The Williams & Wilkins Company, Baltimore, 1971.)

anomalies. Turner in 1938 described seven female patients with sexual infantilism, (later shown to be due to ovarian agenesis), retardation of growth, webbed neck, and cubitus valgus. Patients who exhibit such findings are said to have Turner's syndrome (Fig. 8.20). Since Turner's description many other somatic anomalies have been encountered in patients with ovarian agenesis. Haddad and Wilkins described shield chest, overweight, high palate, micrognathia, epicanthal folds, low set ears, hypoplasia of nails, osteoporosis, pigmented moles, hypertension, lymphedema, cutis laxa, keloid formation, coarctation of the aorta, mental retardation, intestinal telangiectasis, deafness, and others. Urinary tract anomalies have also been frequently encountered. Abnormalities of the bone are common; in general these have to do with loss of density and deviation of the angles and joints. Shortness of the fourth metacarpal

bone is often seen and quite characteristic.

Because a variety of somatic abnormalities have been associated with streak gonads, terminology has become confused. Jones, Ferguson-Smith, and Turner attempted to redefine *Turner's syndrome* and suggested that this eponym be confined to those patients with the key findings of streak gonads and short stature. Such patients with Turner's syndrome often have one or more of the somatic abnormalities listed above.

There are others with streak gonads who are normally tall. Such patients sometimes have no noticeable somatic difficulties and are referred to as examples of *pure gonadal dysgenesis.* However, careful examination often reveals some somatic problem so that most "pure" patients are not so "pure."

There are other syndromes under the large umbrella of streak gonads. Milet *et al.* (1967) found that those with a chromosome constitution of 46, X, i(Xq) (isochromosome for the long arm of the X) are a specific group characterized by short stature, streak gonads, absence of major somatic anormalities, but with an increase in the total digital ridge count and a high incidence of thyroid abnormalities. Another variant of this disorder is characterized by a few menstrual periods usually measured in weeks or, at the most, a few months. A final variant is characterized by some enlargement of the phallus and is referred to as *gonadal dysgenesis with phallic enlargement.*

A large number of sex chromosomal aberrations have been found associated with streak gonads. The collective review of Malcolm Ferguson-Smith has furnished us important data, not only on the types of sex chromosomal anomalies, but on the correlation between these anomalies and the phenotype. Approximately 82 per cent of patients with streak gonads have short stature and, therefore, can properly be considered to have Turner's syndrome as defined herein. Some 44 per cent have 45,X karyotype and the second most common pattern (14%) is a mosaic 46,XX/45,X. Some 40% of patients are mosaic and structural abnormalities of the sex chromosomes are involved in 22% of patients. In the karyotype-phenotype correlation, it seems clear that shortness of stature, the key manifestation of Turner's syndrome, is associated with deficiency (technically monosomy) of the short arm of one X chromosome. Thus, nonmosaic 45,X, 46,

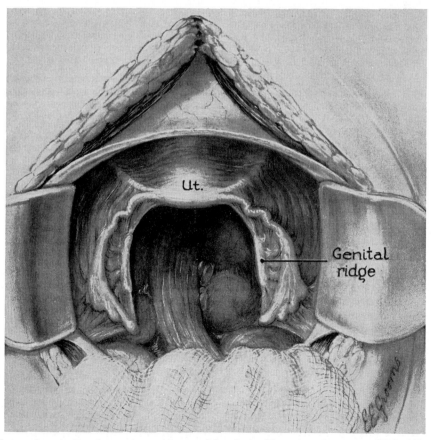

8.18. Internal genitalia of a patient with gonadal aplasia. Note that the uterus (*Ut.*), fallopian tubes and round ligaments are normally formed but relatively undeveloped. The gonads are represented by thickenings or streaks. This patient had a negative chromatin pattern.

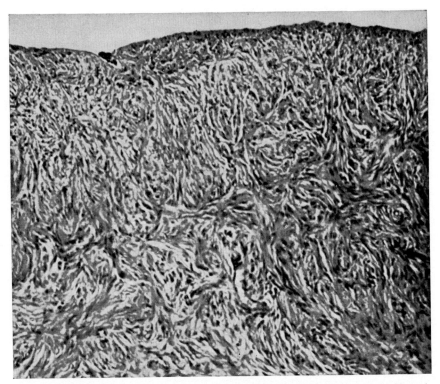

8.19. Microscopic section through the genital ridge of a patient with ovarian agenesis. Note that there is abundant stroma resembling ovarian stroma but no evidence of structures which would allow identification of either an ovary or a testicle. This patient's X-chromatin was also negative.

X,i(Xq) or 46,XXp− cases have Turner's syndrome, whereas 46,X,i(Xp) and 46, XXq− cases do not. In the structural X aberration group, the phenotype clearly depends on the extent and location of the deletion, because the complete Turner's syndrome occurs only when the short arm of the X is deficient.

The presence of streak gonads does not depend on a specific sex chromosomal arrangement, but rather seems to depend on the fact that there is an absence of two normal sex chromosomes.

Thus, the syndrome under discussion may be considered to be the result of two independent variables. One of these, *i.e.,* monosomy for the short arm of the X chromosome or its corresponding loci on the Y results in somatic abnormalities, and the second variable, *i.e.,* absence of two normal sex chromosomes, results in failure of normal gonadal development. Patients may be found with all varieties of these two independent variables.

Treatment consists of estrogenic replacement therapy.

Hermaphroditismus Verus

In rare instances there is both male and female gonadal tissue combined as an ovotestis on one or both sides, or an ovary on one side and a testis on the other. Several hundred such cases have been described in the literature during the current century. The external genitalia are mixed. In some cases the development of the genital ducts may follow the sex of the adjacent gonad. In general, however, there are innumerable variations in the degree of female and male development of both the external and internal genitalia. At puberty, hormonal dominance may be either male or female, depending upon the preponderance of functioning tissue.

The majority of patients with true hermaphroditism have a normally positive sex chromatin pattern and an XX sex chromosome complement. However, a

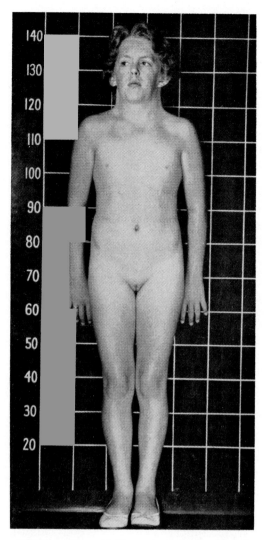

8.20. A patient with Turner's syndrome. Note the short stature, the webbed neck, and the sexual infantilism in spite of the fact that the patient was 17 years of age. The buccal smear in this patient also was negative. (From Jones, H. W., Jr., and Scott, W. W.: *Hermaphroditism, Genital Anomalies and Related Endocrine Disorders,* 2nd ed., The Williams & Wilkins Company, Baltimore, 1971.)

number of other patterns have been encountered including an intriguing group of chimeras with the finding of 46, XX/46,XY. Van Niekerk has a very complete review of this interesting problem.

Multi-X

A few females have been observed with two sex chromatin bodies apparently in all cells. An examination of the chromosomes in these patients has revealed three X chromosomes with a total of 47 in all. For the most part, these patients have normal periods and some have delivered normal children. Amenorrhea has been noted in a few individuals. Several of them have been mentally deficient.

Other patients with similar symptoms have been found to have up to five X chromosomes. All patients with more than three X chromosomes have had severe mental deficiency.

Male Hermaphroditism (with Virilization or Feminization)

Male hermaphroditism taken as a whole is one of the two most common types of intersexuality and occurs with a frequency equal to that of female hermaphroditism due to adrenal hyperplasia. The X-chromatin is uniformly negative and the gonadal structure is male although the gonads may be markedly deformed. The testicular tubules are quite atrophic but in some instances may consist of well developed Sertoli cells. Leydig cells seem to be relatively hyperplastic in most cases. For practical purposes, these patients fall into two groups: those who masculinize and those who feminize.

Male Hermaphrodites with Virilization. Individuals in this group have varied degrees of development of the phallus and fusion of the scrotolabial folds. In rare instances there may seem to be completely normal male genitalia and the hermaphroditic state arises only with the unexpected discovery of well developed Müllerian structures. For the most part, however, the genitalia are so ambiguous that considerable doubt exists as to the sex of the patient. Some patients may be difficult to distinguish from simple cryptorchid boys with hypospadic urethras, and indeed such anomalies have sometimes been considered the simplest forms of hermaphroditism. In some instances, the phallus is only moderately developed and the scrotolabial folds are partly fused.

Anatomically, the external genitalia of

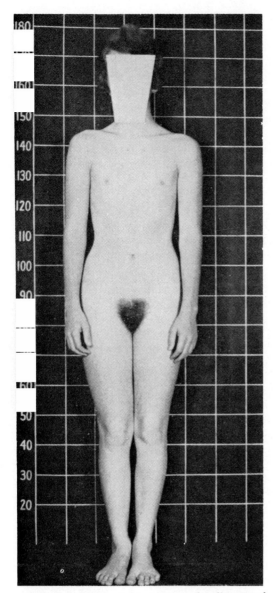

8.21. Photograph of a male hermaphrodite reared quite successfully as a girl. (From Jones, H. W., Jr., and Scott, W. W.: *Hermaphroditism, Genital Anomalies and Related Endocrine Disorders,* 2nd ed., The Williams & Wilkins Company, Baltimore, 1971.)

these subjects may be identical with female hermaphrodites due to congenital adrenal hyperplasia. Most male hermaphrodites of this category are considered and reared as girls, although some with marked masculine genitalia are rightfully considered to be boys (Figs. 8.21–8.23).

These patients virilize to a greater or less degree at puberty and may develop hair which is quite troublesome if they are being reared as women. Menstruation never occurs even though the Müllerian ducts may sometimes be well developed. The endometrium, when present, is quite capable of responding, as may be demonstrated by the uterine bleeding following the exogenous exhibition of estrogen.

From an etiologic and pathogenetic point of view, male hermaphrodites with virilization represent a heterogeneous group. Some of these patients suffer from a mutation resulting in a specific enzymatic defect which in turn causes a blockage of testosterone synthesis. Park and Jones reviewed several examples of this such as 17α-hydroxylase deficiency, 17β-ketosteroid reductase deficiency, etc. Other patients are examples of chromosomal defects which result in gross failure of gonadal development and, therefore, in deficiencies of testosterone synthesis and Müllerian inhibiting factor, which in turn cause failure of development of Wolffian duct structures, normal male external genitalia and persistence of the Müllerian ducts.

Male Hermaphrodites with Feminization. This is a most striking group of patients who are often mistaken for normal females. At puberty well developed feminine secondary sex characteristics appear. The general body habitus and body contours are markedly feminine. The breasts develop along female lines and the vaginal mucosa is thoroughly estrogenized (Fig. 8.24). Menstruation does not occur, as the development of the Müllerian ducts is arrested and well developed uterus and tubes do not occur in this group of patients. The patients may marry as women and have satisfactory sexual intercourse. The external genitalia are entirely feminine (Fig. 8.25). The testes may be in the inguinal canals or labial folds but most often are situated intraabdominally at the position of normal ovaries (Fig. 8.26). These testes generally have well developed Sertoli cells. Large clumps of

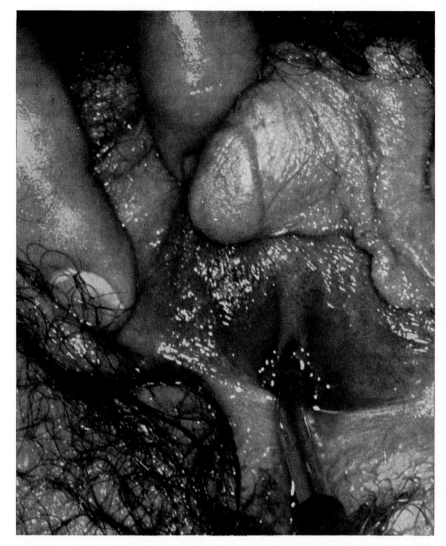

8.22. External genitalia of same patient shown in Fig. 8.21. (From Jones, H. W., Jr., and Scott, W. W.: *Hermaphroditism, Genital Anomalies and Related Endocrine Disorders,* 2nd ed. The Williams & Wilkins Company, Baltimore, 1971.)

interstitial cells may also be present (Fig. 8.27).

Removal of the testes results in a fall of the estrogen values as well as a fall in the 17-ketosteroid excretion which may be elevated to as much as 30 mg. per 24 hours even in well feminized individuals. The fact that the urinary gonadotrophins rise to menopause levels after castration is additional evidence that both the major androgens and estrogens in these cases are of testicular origin. One of the characteris-tics of some patients with this syndrome is the relative absence of pubic and axillary hair.

This disorder is inherited as an X-linked recessive or a male-limited auto-somal dominant. It is not due to a defi-ciency of testicular secretions but rather to an inability of the end organs to respond to testosterone. The end organ deficiency is due to the relative absence of the androgen binding protein in the target cells. It has been suggested that it be

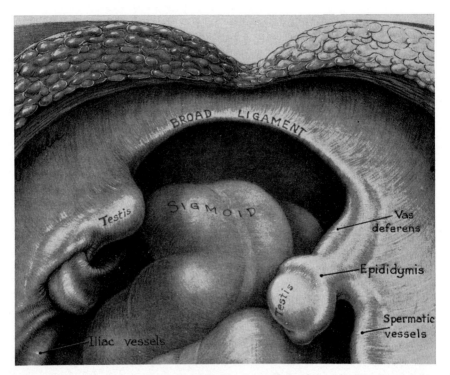

8.23. Internal genitalia of same patient shown in Fig. 8.21. (From Jones, H. W., Jr., and Scott, W. W.: *Hermaphroditism, Genital Anomalies and Related Endocrine Disorders,* 2nd ed. The Williams & Wilkins Company, Baltimore, 1971.)

called the *androgen insensitivity syndrome,* although it is frequently referred to as *testicular feminization.*

The sex chromosomes in this variety of abnormality have been found to be uniformly XY.

Female Hermaphroditism with Virilization

The virilization of this group of patients is caused by an enzymatic defect probably in the fascicular zone of the adrenal cortex. The defective adrenals are incapable of producing a normal amount of cortisol when stimulated by a normal amount of adrenocorticotrophic (ACTH) hormone. This deficiency stimulates an excessive secretion of ACTH by the pituitary, which stimulates the normal reticular zone of the adrenal to marked hyperplasia. This latter zone is apparently responsible for the production of a preponderance of virilizing adrenal steroids which cause the virilization of the

patient. The excess sex steroids in turn suppress the pituitary gonadotrophins.

This chain of events begins in early intrauterine life and is of varying levels of severity. The result is that the external genitalia of female fetuses exhibit varying degrees of masculine development of the phallus and fusion of the scrotolabial folds. Most often there is a hypospadic meatus, but in an occasional instance there is a completely phallic urethra (Fig. 8.28). The vagina enters the urogenital sinus and in severe degrees of the anomaly is not visible externally. The Müllerian ducts differentiate into well formed uterus and tubes. The ovaries are present in their usual position and are microscopically normal, but are unstimulated because of the absence of pituitary gonadotrophins. The excessive adrenal androgens, which may be identified by an elevated urinary 17-ketosteroid excretion, result in precocious growth; therefore these children are larger than normal for their age until

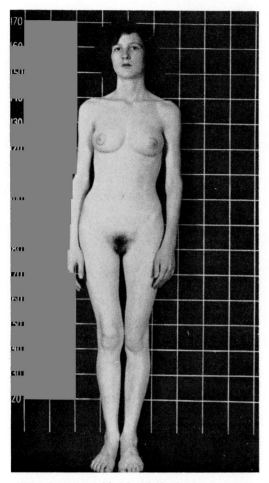

8.24. A 17-year-old girl with the feminizing variety of male hermaphroditism. (From Jones, H. W., Jr., and Scott, W. W.: *Hermaphroditism, Genital Anomalies and Related Endocrine Disorders,* 2nd ed., The Williams & Wilkins Company, Baltimore, 1971.)

about 10 or 11 years, when the epiphysial closure gives them an adult height which is less than normal (Fig. 8.29).

These patients are chromatin positive and have a normal XX sex chromosome complement. The disorder is inherited as an autosomal recessive. In round numbers the gene for this disorder occurs with a frequency of about one in 100.

A portion of cases is associated with the loss of electrolytes and death may result from this cause in severe instances. In the untreated case, feminization does not take place, menstruation never occurs, and

there is excessive growth of the hair on the face, body, and extremities. Several of these patients have lived and married as men, although the majority are recognized as virilized women. Since the advent of cortisone this unhappy chain of events can be completely prevented, and by early treatment these patients will feminize at the time of puberty and develop and grow as relatively normal girls and women (Fig. 8.30).

Female Hermaphroditism with Feminization

A small group of patients has been described with normal female internal genitalia and normal ovaries without any of the virilizing influences of adrenal hyperplasia but with external genitalia which have developed toward the male configuration. A penile urethra has been observed, although, for the most part, the deformity is limited to what seems to be a simple hypospadias and fusion of the scrotolabial folds (Fig. 8.31). Contrary to the situation with female hermaphrodites who virilize, this group of patients shows no manifestation of androgenic secretion and they menstruate and develop secondary female sexual characteristics at the usual age of puberty. The mothers of most of these patients have received an androgenic steroid during pregnancy. Some mothers received androgens for nonobstetrical causes but the majority received synthetic steroids given for their progestational effect. A few patients in this category have had no obvious exposure to androgenic substances. The mothers of some of these patients have had androgenic tumors.

TREATMENT OF HERMAPHRODITISM

Study has shown that the sex of rearing is a primary consideration in the formation of the gender role of the individual. It has been demonstrated that this is as important as such obvious signs as the morphology of the external genitalia, the hormone dominance, and gonadal structure. Furthermore, it has been shown that there are serious psychiatric conse-

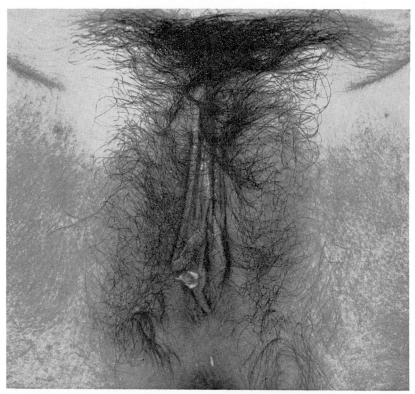

8.25. The external genitalia of the same patient shown in Fig. 8.24. (From Jones, H. W., Jr., and Scott, W. W.: *Hermaphroditism, Genital Anomalies and Related Endocrine Disorders,* 2nd ed. The Williams & Wilkins Company, Baltimore, 1971.)

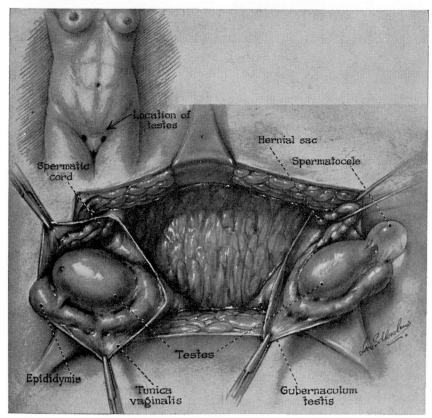

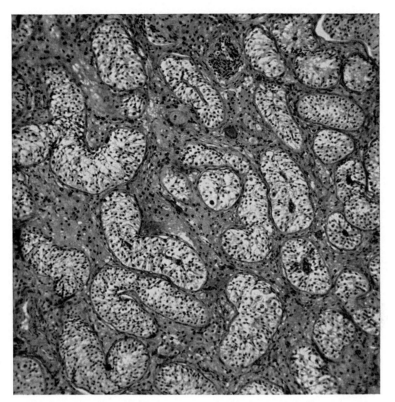

8.27. Microscopic appearance of the testes from the same patient shown in Fig. 8.24. (From Jones, H. W., Jr., and Scott, W. W.: *Hermaphroditism, Genital Anomalies and Related Endocrine Disorders,* 2nd ed. The Williams & Wilkins Company, Baltimore, 1971.)

quences from changing the sex of rearing after the age of infancy. Except in rare instances, it is no longer proper to advise a change of sex after infancy to conform with the gonadal structure, external genitalia, and the like; instead the physician should exert his efforts to complete the adjustment of the individual to the sex in which the child finds itself. For the surgeon this means reconstruction of the external genitalia to more nearly conform with the sex of rearing. It also means the removal of any contradictory sex structures which may be functioning in an antagonistic manner. In our opinion, the testes should always be removed from male hermaphrodites reared as women, regardless of hormone production. This thought is prompted not only by their contradictory hormone production in some instances but by the incidence of seminoma and other tumors in these deformed retained testes.

Manuel, Katayama and Jones have reviewed the age at which gonadectomy is desirable. In patients with a Y chromosome with ovarian agenesis, asymmetrical gonadal differentiation, or masculinizing male hermaphroditism, the frequency of tumors rises abruptly at about the age of puberty. It is, therefore, desirable that in these circumstances the gonads be removed prior to that time. On the other hand, the expectancy of tumor is somewhat delayed in patients with the testicular feminization syndrome, so that if a risk of about 4 per cent is acceptable, gonadectomy can be delayed until the

8.26. The operative findings in the patient shown in Fig. 8.24. (From Jones, H. W., Jr., and Scott, W. W.: *Hermaphroditism, Genital Anomalies and Related Disorders,* 2nd ed. The Williams & Wilkins Company, Baltimore, 1971.)

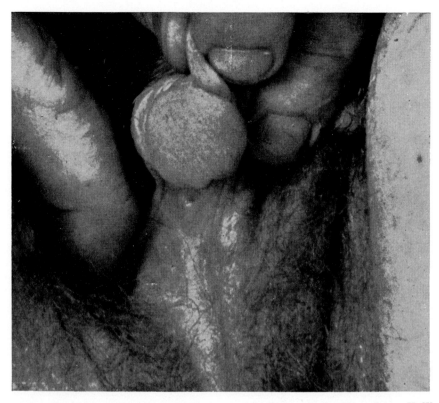

8.28. Characteristic genitalia of patient with congenital adrenal hyperplasia. (From Jones, H. W., Jr., and Scott, W. W.: *Hermaphroditism, Genital Anomalies and Related Endocrine Disorders,* 2nd ed. The Williams & Wilkins Company, Baltimore, 1971.)

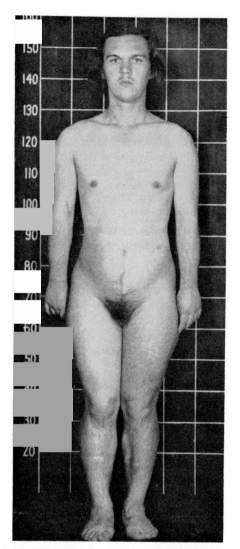

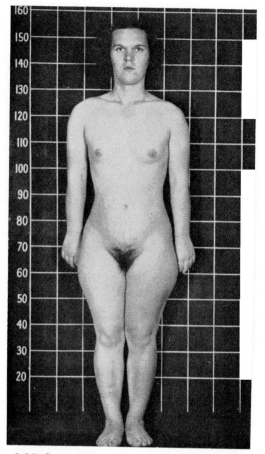

8.30. Same patient shown in Fig. 8.29 after three months of cortisone therapy. Note the alteration in the body habitus to the feminine configuration and the diminution in the hirsutism. (From Jones, H. W., Jr., and Scott, W. W.: *Hermaphroditism, Genital Anomalies and Related Endocrine Disorders,* 2nd ed. The Williams & Wilkins Company, Baltimore, 1971.)

8.29. Photograph of patient with congenital adrenal hyperplasia. Note the rather characteristic stature of short arms and short legs. Also note the absence of breast development and the growth of hair on the face and body. This patient was 16 years old when the photograph was taken. She had been untreated and had not menstruated. (From Jones, W. H., Jr., and Scott, W. W.: *Hermaphroditism, Genital Anomalies and Related Endocrine Disorders,* 2nd ed. The Williams & Wilkins Company, Baltimore, 1971.)

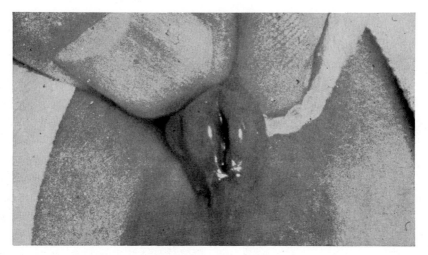

8.31. External genitalia of female patient whose mother received an androgenic steroid during pregnancy. The fusion of the scrotolabial folds is ordinarily not so complete.

20's in this condition. This is not undesirable in this situation, in order to allow secondary female sexual characteristics to develop spontaneously.

In the case of *virilized female hermaphrodites due to adrenal hyperplasia,* the suppression of adrenal androgen production by the administration of cortisone from an early age will result in completely female development, including the onset of puberty at the expected time and normal menstruation. It is no longer necessary to explore surgically the internal genitalia in this well delineated syndrome, and the surgical effort is confined entirely to reconstruction of the external genitalia along female lines. It cannot be overemphasized that the exhibition of cortisone must be carefully and properly supervised. The urinary 17-ketosteroids must be followed serially, with suppression to a level consistent with the onset of puberty at the expected time.

Patients with *ovarian agenesis* who are invariably reared as girls and women require the exhibition of exogenous estrogen at the expected time of puberty. Other hermaphrodites reared as women who will not feminize also require the use of estrogen to promote the development of a female habitus and breasts. In patients with a well developed Müllerian system,

cyclic uterine bleeding may be produced although reproduction is, of course, out of the question.

Hermaphrodites reared as boys and men may require exogenous androgen as well as plastic reconstruction of ambiguous external genitalia. It is much easier to excise a phallus and lengthen a vagina than to build up adequate organs in the child reared as a male.

REFERENCES

Anderson, W. O.: Treatment of labial adhesions in children. J. A. M. A., *162:* 951, 1956.
Azoury, R. S., and Jones, H. W., Jr.: Cytogenic findings in patients with congenital absence of the vagina. Amer. J. Obstet. Gynec., *94:* 178, 1966.
Bowman, J. A., Jr., and Scott, R. B.: Transverse vaginal septum. Obstet. Gynec., *3:* 441, 1954.
Bryan, A. L., Nigro, J. A., and Counseller, V. S.: One hundred cases of congenital absence of the vagina. Surg. Gynec. Obstet., *88:* 79, 1949.
Ferguson-Smith, M. A.: Karyotype-phenotype correlations in gonadal dysgenesis and their bearing on the pathogenesis of malformations, J. Med. Genet., *2:* 142, 1965.
Haddad, H. M., and Wilkins, L.: Congenital anomalies associated with gonadal aplasia. Pediatrics, *23:* 885, 1959.
Jones, H. W., Jr., Delfs, E., and Jones, G. E.: Reproductive difficulties in double uterus. Amer. J. Obstet. Gynec., *72:* 865, 1956.
Jones, H. W., Jr., Ferguson-Smith, M. A., and Heller, R. H.: Pathology and cytogenetics of gonadal agenesis. Amer. J. Obstet. Gynec., *87:* 578, 1963.
Jones, H. W., Jr., and Jones, G. E. S.: Double uterus as an etiological factor in repeated abortion; indications for surgical repair. Amer. J. Obstet. Gynec., *65:* 325, 1953.

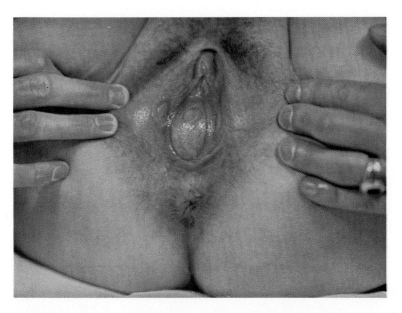

Plate 8.1. Imperforate hymen in a patient 27 years of age, showing the marked bulging due to retained menstrual accumulation of many years (Courtesy of Dr. James E. Brown, Baltimore).

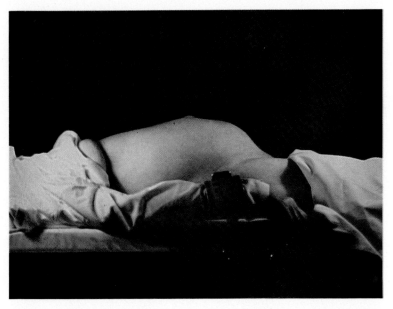

Plate 8.2. Abdominal enlargement due to enormous uterine distention is same patient as shown in Plate 8.1.

Jones, H. W., Jr., and Jones, G. E. S.: The gynecological aspects of adrenal hyperplasia and allied disorders. Amer. J. Obstet. Gynec., *68:* 1330, 1954.

Jones, H. W., Jr., and Scott, W. W.: *Hermaphroditism, Genital Anomalies and Related Endocrine Disorders,* 2nd ed. The Williams & Wilkins Company, Baltimore, 1971.

Jones, H. W., Jr., Turner, H. H., and Ferguson-Smith, M. A.: Turner's syndrome and phenotype. Lancet, *1:* 1155, 1966.

Jones, H. W., Jr., and Wheeless, C. R.: The salvage of the reproductive potential of women with anomalous development of the mullerian ducts: 1869–1968–2068. Amer. J. Obstet. Gynec., *104:* 348, 1969.

Manuel, M. D., Katayama, K. P., and Jones, H. W., Jr.: The age of occurrence of gonadal tumors in intersex patients with a Y chromosome. Amer. J. Obstet. Gynec. (In press.)

McIndoe, A.: Discussion on treatment of congenital absence of vagina with emphasis on long term results. Proc. Roy. Soc. Med., *52:* 952, 1959.

McKusick, V. A., Bauer, L., Koap, C. E., and Scott, B.: Hydrometrocolpos as a simply inherited malformation. J. A. M. A., *189:* 813, 1964.

Milet, R. G., Plunkett, E. R., and Carr, D. H.: Gonadal dysgenesis with XX-isochromosome constitution and abnormal thyroid patterns. Acta Endocr., *54:* 609–617, 1967.

Money, J., Hampson, J. G., and Hampson, J. I.: Hermaphroditism; recommendations concerning assignment of sex, change of sex and psychologic management. Bull. Johns Hopkins Hosp., *97:* 284, 1955.

Park, I. J., Aimakhu, V. E. and Jones, H. W., Jr.: An etiologic and pathogenetic classification of male hermaphroditism. Amer. J. Obstet. Gynec. (In press.)

Turner, H. H.: Syndrome of infantilism, congenital webbed neck, and cubitus valgus. Endocrinology, *23:* 566, 1938.

van Niekerk, W. A.: *True Hermaphroditism.* Harper & Row, Hagerstown, Md., 1974.

Wharton, L. R.: Two cases of supernumerary ovary and one of accessory ovary with an analysis of previously recorded cases. Amer. J. Obstet. Gynec., *78:* 1101, 1959.

Wilkins, L. W., Jones, H. W., Jr., Holman, G. H., and Stempfel, R. S., Jr.: Masculinization of the female fetus associated with administration of oral and intramuscular progestins during gestation; nonadrenal female pseudohermaphrodism. J. Clin. Endocr., *18:* 559, 1958.

chapter *9*

Diseases of the Vulva

DEVELOPMENTAL ABNORMALITIES

For the most part these consist of ambiguous external genitalia associated with chromosomal or hormonal aberrations, *e.g.,* the clitoral hypertrophy of congenital adneral hyperplasia and cloacal atypicalities in the mosaic. These and variations in hymeneal perforations are discussed in other chapters. The "double vulva" has been discribed but is one of the rarest of all anomalies.

VULVAR DERMATITIS

The vulvar skin, of ectodermal origin, may be the site of any and all of the common dermatologic diseases. Furthermore, it is subjected to a great variety of local irritants—vaginal discharges, menstrual fluids, urine and feces, as well as the secretion from the skin glands. As a final insult, these secretions are retained by tight, synthetic underwear, girdles, panty hose and "slacks." Consequently, in the treatment of any vulvar irritation it is imperative to instruct the patient carefully as to local measures that should be instigated, regardless of the basic pathologic process. These include the use of loose cotton underclothing; the removal of undergarments that retain secretions in the anogenital area; the employment of drying agents (non-perfumed powder); the elimination of potentially irritating local agents (*e.g.,* hygiene sprays, topical anesthetic agents, perfumed soaps, etc.) to which the tender vulvar skin may be sensitive; and a careful perineal toilet.

Intertrigo is common in the interlabial and crural folds as in any area where moist folds of integument are constantly opposed. In the initial phases, the skin is erythematous; and later often demonstrates linear fissuring. Finally there is thickening and cracking of the lichenified, hyperkeratotic skin. In this stage the erroneous diagnosis of "leukoplakia" may be entertained when in truth the process is simply chronic dermatitis with hyperkeratosis.

Seborrhoea and Seborrhoeic Dermatitis. As with intertrigo, the excessive secretion of the sebaceous glands onto both labial folds produces an irritation which in the later stages demonstrates crushing and scaling of the skin. The resultant chronic dermatitis is pruritic as are most such lesions.

Neurodermatitis has become a "waste basket," since any chronic irritative condition which does not seem to fall into a specific category may be labelled "neurodermatitis" since the patient is "nervous." Actually in the face of a constant pruritic process it would be remarkable if the patient did not demonstrate irritability and tenseness. In many instances, a careful history and examination will reveal the precipitating feature, and a diagnosis of "atopic dermatitis" would not only be more realistic but would assist the patient in preventing recurrences. The use of topical anesthetic agents, hygiene sprays, perfumed soaps or powders, strong detergents, and a host of other local irritants may be uncovered with a careful history. This process may obviously become persistent and result in the *chronic exzematoid* lesion which again is often labelled as neuradermatitis.

Psoriasis is uncommon on the vulva, and is usually associated with the classic, round or ovoid patches with linear excoriations and "silver" scales. Correct diagnosis will lead to more appropriate therapy, and these are discussed at length in more detailed texts. Suffice it to say, as noted above, it is important to instruct the patient to eliminate potential irritants to which she may have reacted; to keep the area as dry as possible with "baby powder" mixed with a little cornstarch; to use antipruritic creams or lotions, *not ointments* (usually a hydrocortisone); and to eliminate tight, "non-breathing" synthetic underclothing. Antihistamines may be helpful initially. A *warning* about the use of hydrocortisone - it may cause underlying fibrosis and eventually add to the basic problem, thus it is best employed in the acute situation and sparingly thereafter.

Fungus infections may be primary on the vulva or secondary to an associated vaginitis; in either case pruritus is the common symptom (Plate 9.1). Similarly yeast may present as a "vulvitis" with the development of thrushlike patches on the external genitalia. Either of these mycotic infections may be associated with diabetes and its characteristic "beefy-red" vulva (Plate 9.2).

As the vagina is frequently involved with such agents there is an irritating discharge which adds to the patient's discomfort and pruritus. Both the diabetes and the associated infectious process must be treated simultaneously and persistently if good results are to be obtained. The recognition of the combined etiologies depends obviously on careful urinalysis and blood sugar evaluations, and the demonstration of the offending organisms in vaginal smears and upon culture of the discharge on Nickerson's or Sabourauds' media. The former common therapy with 1 per cent aqueous solution of gentian violet has largely been superceded by the use of such fungicides as Sporostacin and Mycostatin because of the frequent irritation and staining which resulted from the gentian violet therapy. It should be appreciated that these infections not uncommonly follow the use of systemic antibiotics. (See Chapter 10.)

Similarly trichomonas and postmenopausal vaginitis may produce a severe vulvar edema, erythema, and concomitant pruritus. Thorough inspection of the vaginal canal and the secretions generally reveals the correct diagnosis. (See Chapter 10.)

CIRCULATORY DISEASES

Among circulatory disturbances involving the vulva, varices are perhaps the most common. They affect especially the labia majora, and are more prominent unilaterally. Since the pampiniform plexus of veins is primarily involved, a varicocele, such as that so commonly seen in the male, may develop. A common cause of such venous distention is intrapelvic pressure from pregnancy or large tumors; however no specific etiological agent can be recognized in most cases. As with varicose veins elsewhere, they distend with blood when the patient stands and tend to empty and become smaller when she lies down. The varices may become extremely large and may even rupture, with resultant bleeding (Fig. 9.1). Most commonly, however, the dilated veins appear as multiple small purplish elevations which simulate and are often mistaken for hemangiomata.

Edema of the vulva may be the result

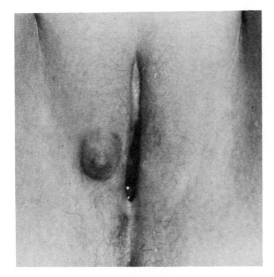

9.1. Large solitary varix on right vulva

of intrapelvic pressure from large tumors, marked ascites, or metastatic tumor in the regional lymph nodes. More often it is due to local inflammatory lesions. Even furunculosis or the secondarily infected herpetic lesions may lead to significant degrees of vulvar edema due to the dependent position or the external genitalia and the opportunity for distention in the loose adipose tissue of the majora. Inflammatory or parasitic blockage of the vulvar lymphatics may cause "elephantiasis" most dramatically recognized in lymphogranuloma venereum. The edema of pregnancy is undoubtedly related to temporary lymphostasis resulting from pressure phenomena; nevertheless, local or diffuse swelling may be due to abnormal activity of the apocrine glands which are closely related embryologically to the secretory elements of the breast. It must be noted that since the vulva is in the "milk line," normal breast tissue may be found in this area. Finally lymphoedema may result from chronic debilitating disease such as anemia, multiple sclerosis, Krohn's disease, etc.

INFLAMMATIONS

Gonorrheal Vulvovaginitis

This is described under "Vaginitis" in Chapter 10.

DISEASES OF THE VESTIBULAR GLANDS

Since Bartholin's gland is commonly classed as one of the constituent structures of the vulva, a discussion of its diseases and those associated with the minor vestibular glands is properly included in this chapter. The lesions of these gland are either inflammatory or neoplastic, the former extremely common, the latter very rare.

It should be appreciated that there are minor vestibular glands, as well as the major or "Bartholin's gland," which surround the outlet and may be involved in the same variety of pathologic processes as those commonly associated with the Bartholin structures.

Inflammation (Bartholin Adenitis)

Historically, in the majority of cases the causative organism has been the Gonococcus. There is no question, however, that other organisms, such as the colon bacillus, the pyogenes, etc., may at times be the primary agents.

In the acute stage the major and most prominent gland becomes turgid, swollen, and painful, and a purulent exudate can be expressed from the duct by gentle pressure or may issue from it spontaneously. Abscess is a common sequel, manifesting itself by fluctuation and the associated edema may produce enormous swelling of the entire labium (Fig. 9.2).

Treatment. The treatment should consist of bed rest, sufficient analgesics to relieve the pain, local thermotherapy (ice pack or hot sitz baths) and antibacterial therapy. When abscess formation is evident, incision with drainage affords immediate relief. Marsupialization of the sac in the recurrent case may be attempted but is usually not successful at this stage due to the associated induration and edema.

Chronic Bartholinitis

Chronic bartholinitis (properly Bartholin adenitis) may persist for many years. A history of an initial acute attack may or may not be elicited. The only clinical evidence of the disease is the presence of a small nodular swelling, pal-

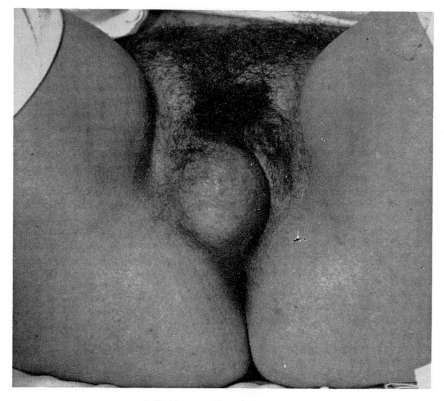

9.2. Abscess of Bartholin's gland

pable deep beneath the posterior portion of the labium majus. The patient is frequently unaware of the existence of such a nodule. The course of chronic bartholinitis may be punctuated by acute exacerbations, and, in the chronic cases, as a result of occlusion of either the main duct or one of its subdivisions, cysts of Bartholin's duct commonly develop and may undergo suppuration with abscess formation.

The pathological changes in chronic Bartholin adenitis are those characteristic of any chronic inflammation. Normally the main duct is lined by transitional epithelium, whereas a single layer of flattened cells lines the smaller branches. Severe inflammation may destroy all epithelium; however, the mucus secreting acini are almost always demonstrable in the deeper tissues (Fig. 9.3).

Treatment. No therapy is necessary for the asymptomatic chronically infected Bartholin gland or cyst. Simple marsupialization is quite efficacious for the

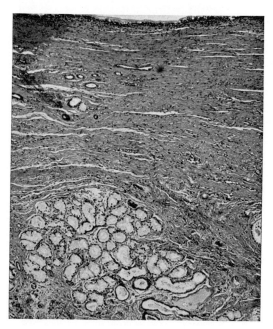

9.3. Microscopic picture of Bartholin's gland cyst, lined with flattened layer of transitional epithelium (*above*) and with gland tissue in wall (*below*).

uncomplicated cysts; however, when recurrent infection has been the problem it is necessary to remove not only the cyst but the entire infected gland. This is important because the inflammatory process involves the deep-lying lobules of the gland, and incomplete removal may be followed by recurrences of cyst or abscess.

HIDRADENITIS

Special consideration should be given to the infections which involve the apocrine system since they are unique to the areas which contain these specialized glands. The disease so commonly seen in the axilla and associated with local irritations is replicated in the vulva (Fig. 9.4). As is the axilla, suppuration may take place, often misdiagnozed as folliculitis, and lead to extensive tissue destruction, draining sinuses and lymphoedema, thus, on the vulva, simulating lymphopathia. In the mild case of recurrent pustule formation, the disease process may be modified by the use of oral contraceptives which reduce the secretion of these spe-

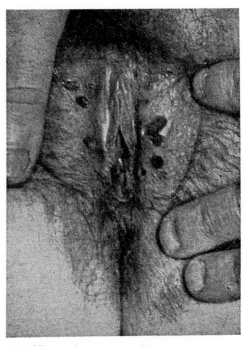

9.5. Ulcus vulvae acutum; Lipschutz ulcer.

cialized, cyclically functioning glands. Similarly the intense pruritus associated with the chronic stage, known as *Fox-Fordyce disease,* may be reduced strikingly with the use of such agents. In the later stage, the vulva is dotted with fine, slightly elevated papules often mistaken for infected sebaceous glands.

Finally in the patient with extensive suppurative disease, it may be necessary to perform wide, debriding surgery in an effort to stem the destructive process which has, on occasion, led to total vulvectomy and skin grafting.

ULCERATIVE LESIONS

Simple Acute Ulcer (Lipschutz) " Nonspecific Factitious and Aphthous Ulcers"

This rather nebulous condition may affect either the vulva or the lower vagina, the latter being more frequent. The ulcers may be single or multiple. They appear as shallow, rounded, or oval lesions (Fig. 9.5) which produce only slight local discomfort and which are readily amenable to simple antiseptic treatment. The causative agent

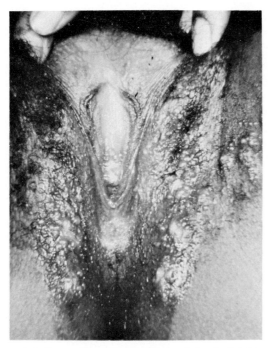

9.4. Suppurative hidradenitis involving both labia majora and crural folds.

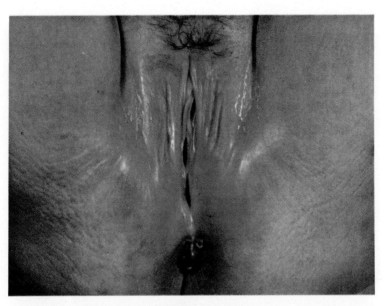

Plate 9.1. Diabetic vulvitis often associated with mycotic infection

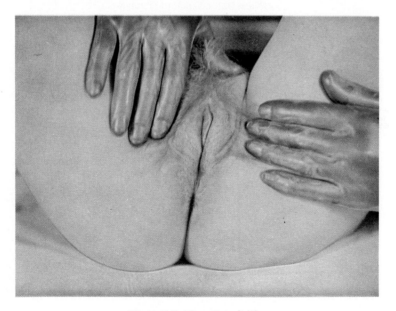

Plate 9.2. Mycotic vulvitis

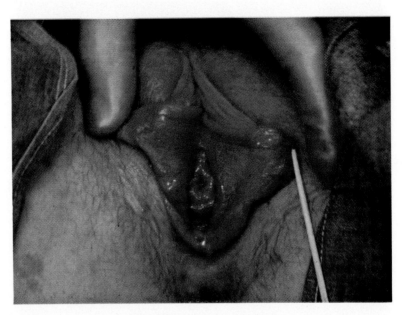

Plate 9.3. Chancroid of vulva

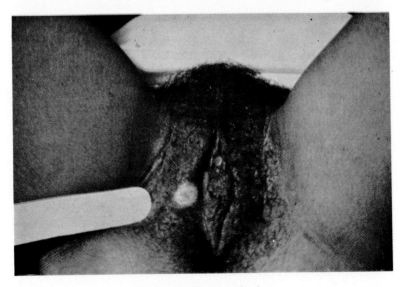

Plate 9.4. Chancre of vulva

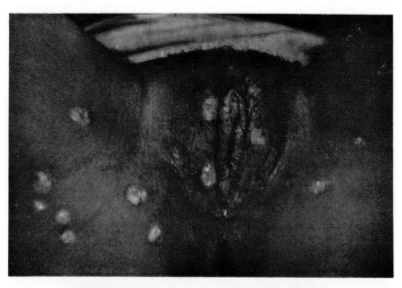

Plate 9.5. Condylomata lata of vulva and perineum

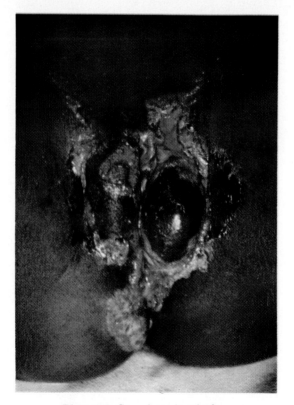

Plate 9.6. Granuloma inquinale

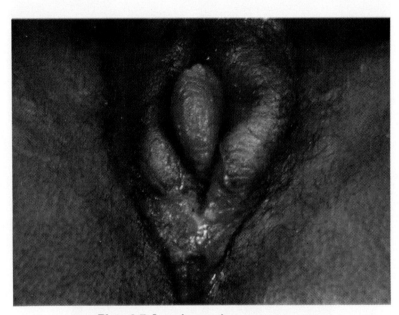

Plate 9.7. Lymphogranuloma venereum

has been said to be Bacillus crassus, a normal inhabitant of the vagina; however, it seems unlikely that this is true. It is more feasible to accept these lesions as aphthous, due possibly to Vincent's-type organisms or more nonspecific varieties. Suggestion has been made that such lesions may result from systemic disease such as lupus.

Finally factitious ulcers have been noted at the outlet and are often self-induced, thus associated with psychogenic disorders.

CHANCROID (SOFT CHANCRE, ULCUS MOLLE)

This lesion belongs to the group of venereal infections transmitted by coitus. The etiological agent is *Haemophilus ducreyi* which can be demonstrated in scrapings made from the base of the shallow ulcerations. The initial lesion presents as a small papule or pustule (Plate 9.3) which appears within two or three days of exposure, and progresses to ulceration but little induration. The lesion may affect any part of the vulva. When the labia are involved, there is often marked local edema. Characteristically this ulcerative lesion is painful at the onset, thus differing from the majority of the other so-called "venereal diseases." Inguinal adenitis is frequent, but the infected glands rarely show a tendency to suppurate.

Diagnosis. The diagnosis of chancroid is based on the history of exposure, the short latent period of usually two to four days, the clinical characteristics of the ulcer as described above, especially the painful nature of the primary lesion, the usual absence of induration, and the demonstration of the Ducrey bacillus in smears or scrapings from the ulcer.

Treatment. The treatment of chancroid is, with few exceptions, eminently satisfactory. Reliance is placed on meticulous cleanliness and the use of local antiseptics and sulfonamides, together with chloromycetin, achromycin or other antibiotics, with as yet no complete unanimity as to which is the most effective.

SYPHILLIS

(1) *Chancre.* This, the initial lesion of syphilis, is observed less commonly in women than in men. Chancre is recognized much more frequently on the vulva than in the vagina or cervix, probably because of the greater frequency in the former area of small abrasions which offer portals of entry to the spirochete and because the vaginal and cervical lesions are rarely visible or definitive. The lesion does not appear until three of four weeks after exposure. In many cases the initial lesion undoubtedly is overlooked due to its transient nature and minimal symptomatology.

The vulvar chancre is apt to be smaller and less prominent than its counterpart in the male, but otherwise its appearance is quite similar. It presents as a rounded or ovoid ulcer with raised, indurated edges and a depressed center (Plate 9.4). The surface is reddish or reddish brown. It appears usually on the labium majus, in which case there may be considerable surrounding edema. There is marked associated inguinal lymphadenitis. The initial lesion usually regresses spontaneously in four to six weeks.

It must be emphasized that any ulcerative lesion, regardless of its apparent noncharacteristic appearance, must be suspect and thoroughly studied prior to any therapy. In recent years many superficially excoriated bizarre lesions on both external genitalia and perirectal areas have proved to be "dark-field positive."

Diagnosis. The diagnosis of syphilis in this primary stage is dependent upon the demonstration of the spirochete in the lesion. The surface of the lesion is gently wiped with gauze moistened in normal saline solution, care being taken not to start bleeding. By firmly squeezing the lesion, droplets of lymph may be made to exude, and, if positive, examination of this transudate by the dark-field technique will reveal the characteristic spirochetes. *Treponema pallidum* may readily be recognized by the cork-screw-like activity particularly well demonstrated by the fluorescent technique. Various serological tests may not be positive at this primary stage.

(2) *Secondary Lesions-Condyloma Latum.* The typical secondary lesion observed in the vulvar area is the condyloma latum, which often occurs simultaneously with the cutaneous macules or papules characterizing the secondary stage. The typical syphilitic condylomas are slightly raised, round or oval, plateau-like lesions of various sizes, and often occur in clusters (Plate 9.5). The edges are slightly indurated, the surface is moist, and covered with a grayish necrotic exudate. The condylomas not only cover the vulva, but extend to the surrounding perineum, the inner side of the upper thighs, and the buttocks. Again there is marked lymphadenitis.

The microscopic examination is made by the same technique as described for the initial lesion. In this stage, corroborative evidence for the existence of syphilis can be obtained from blood tests, which by this time are routinely positive.

The common treatment is seven to eight million units of penicillin given over a period of five to seven days. The longer therapy is wise in an effort to prevent the Herxheimer reaction, particularly in the treatment of the secondary stage, since the titers are frequently higher than in the primary stage. Terramycin or similar antibiotics may be used in the patient sensitive to penicillin. Only cleanliness is necessary locally. Unfortunately, due generally to poor reporting of initial lesions and consequent inadequate social service follow-up of contacts, there has been a steady increase in primary syphilis in many areas since 1955.

(3) *Tertiary Syphilis-Gumma and Syphilitic Ulcer.* Although the characteristic tertiary syphilitic lesion is the gumma, and although this may occur on the vulva, its tendency to necrosis and ulceration is so great that the most common tertiary lesion is the syphilitic ulcer. The latter appears as a large, sluggish, necrotic ulceration which may cause much surrounding induration and edema, and which may produce fistulas between the vagina and rectum. In some cases the

hypertrophic changes are pseudoneoplastic, and must be distinguished from lymphogranuloma inguinale or carcinoma. Such lesions are rarely seen today.

Ulcers due to Tuberculosis or Carcinoma of Vulva

(See under appropriate sections.)

Granuloma Inguinale

This "venereal disease," transmitted usually by coitus, presents primarily as single or multiple small ulcerations affecting the vulva and adjacent perineum. It is found especially in the tropics and the southern section of the U.S. It is of interest that granuloma may at times affect various extragenital sites, particularly the skin and bone.

The incubation period of this disease varies widely from a few days to several months. It usually begins as a small papular lesion on one of the labia minora or in the inguinal region, followed, in a few weeks, by ulceration which tends to assume a characteristic serpiginous form. The surface is reddish and granular and there is a considerable seropurulent exudate (Plate 9.6). By contrast with some of the other chronic ulcerative vulvar le-

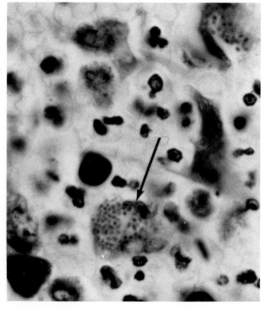

9.6. Donovan inclusions on smear or tissue specimen from acute or subacute lesion of granuloma inguinale.

sions, the lesions of granuloma tend to remain superficial, but in some cases they may become deep and destructive, probably as a result of secondary infection. Inguinal lymphadenopathy with suppuration rarely occurs.

The microscopic picture of the disease is characterized by an initial stage of subcutaneous infiltration with plasma cells, leukocytes, and large mononuclear cells, after which typical granulation tissue is formed. Especially characteristic are the so-called granuloma cells, which are large mononuclear clear cells with foamy, vasuolated cytoplasm. There is now general agreement that the disease can be transmitted by the Donovan inclusion, variously felt to be viral, bacterial (the Donovan virus or bacillus), or protozoal (Fig. 9.6). This can be demonstrated in smears from 60 to 80 per cent of the lesions and can be stained in tissues by the methods of Wright and Giemsa in 100 per cent of the cases (von Haam), during the acute and subacute stages of the disease. Greenblatt, Baldwin, and Dienst have reported the experimental production of the disease by the injection of an exudate containing only the Donovan inclusions. The latter are described as small encapsulated bodies resembling a "closed safety pin" as the result of the bipolar staining of the inclusions. Occasionally they are not encapsulated. In various southern clinics, a proportion of cases of vulvar carcinoma have been found to have been produced by granulomatous disease (Saltzstein, Woodruff and Novak, Collins and his co-workers, and others) (Fig. 9.7).

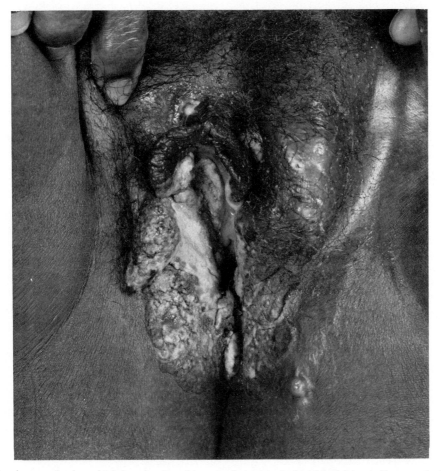

9.7. Carcinoma of vulva which has developed in granuloma inguinale (right labium). Donovan bodies were readily demonstrable.

Diagnosis. The diagnosis is made from the characteristic picture of the superficial granular inguinal lesion, together with the microscopic demonstration of the Donovan bodies. The lesion is generally more superficial and less painful than chancroid, in which the causative Ducrey bacillus may be found on smear examination. Carcinoma and tuberculosis can be excluded by microscopic examination of excised tissue specimens, although usually this is not necessary.

Syphilis does not often produce lesions which resemble those of granuloma; however, as noted previously, all such ulcers must be studied by dark-field examination and serological test. Finally, lymphogranuloma inguinale must be stressed as the disease which may present the greatest difficulty in its differentiation from granuloma. The former, however, is characterized by the frequent occurrence of subcutaneous suppurative foci, commonly diagnosed as acute, ulcerative, inguinale lymphadenitis, and which, in the later stages are characterized by cicatricial stricture of the rectum or urethra. The absence of Donovan bodies in the smear and the positive Frei test obtained in lymphogranuloma, will aid in establishing the diagnosis, but will, unfortunately, not be definitive. Clinical judgment, including biopsy, is the most important element in the study of such disease entities.

Treatment. In former years the treatment of granuloma consisted of the intravenous administration of antimony (tartar emetic) or Fuadin. Antibiotics have superseded the heavy metals as effective therapeutic agents and usually 10 gm. of chloromycetin, either 1 g. q.d. for 10 days or 2 g. per day for 5 days, will result in complete regression of the local lesion. Other "mycins" have also proven to be effective therapeutic agents in the acute stage. In the chronic stages such therapy is less effective, and surgery may be necessary if the lesion is localized enough to permit removal. Extragenital dermatological, osseous, and ophthalamological manifestations of granuloma inguinale have been reported and may prove fatal.

Lymphopathia Venereum (Lymphogranuloma)

The disease begins, after an incubation period of usually only a few days, as an initial ulcerative lesion in the vagina, on the cervix, or on the external genitalia. The initial papule or pustule quickly disappears and is almost always overlooked. It is followed, however, by the appearance of inguinal suppuration or bubo formation. The condition seems to be essentially a disease of the lymphatics and/or associated with hypertrophic changes, lymphedema, and draining sinuses (Fig. 9.8).

If the ulcerative process dominates the picture, a large, ragged ulcer may be produced, surrounded by fibrous induration and edema (Plate 9.7). On the other hand, when the hypertrophic process predominates, marked lymphedema with fibrocystic proliferation and leathery thickening of the skin produce a characteristic elephantiasis similar to the condition resulting from filariasis. (Fig. 9.9). As with granuloma, extragenital lesions, particularly in the bowel and meninges have been reported. During the stage of bubo formation constitutional symptoms such as fever and malaise are commonly seen.

Mention has already been made in the preceding section that carcinoma has oc-

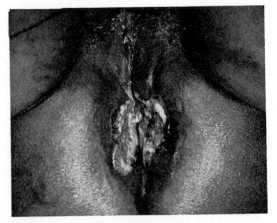

9.8. Carcinoma which has developed in lymphogranuloma venereum of vulva and vagina, extending up rectovaginal septum. In this case a 10-year salvage was achieved by vulvectomy plus posterior exenteration.

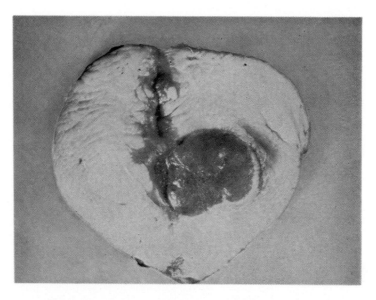

Plate 9.8. Carcinoma of vulva after excision by vulvectomy

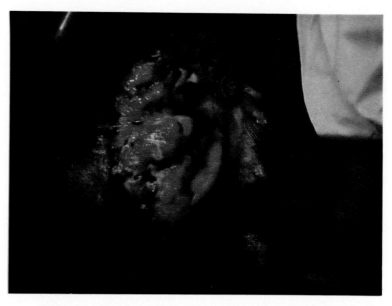

Plate 9.9. Carcinoma of vulva in black woman 45 years of age

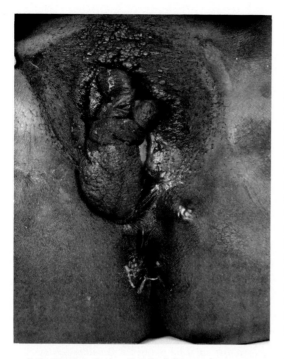

9.9. Elephantiasis of right labia and over mons with draining sinuses in left perineal and perirectal areas.

casionally developed on the basis of either preexisting lymphopathia or granuloma (Fig. 9.8).

Diagnosis. Microscopically, the chief features are an extensive inflammatory reaction with focal micro-abscess formation. The latter produce the common "draining sinuses" (Fig. 9.9). Endothelial proliferation with pseudotubercle formation is often characterized by central collections of polymorphonuclear cells rather than a "giant cell." The most striking feature is the proliferation and distortion of the epithelial rete pegs (pseudoepitheliomatous hyperplasia) (Fig. 9.10). Spread of the infecting agent through the lymphatics, with extensive inflammation and cicatrization of the endopelvic tissues results in rectal and urethral strictures as well as fenestration of the vulvar structures characteristic of the later stages of the disease.

The cause of lymphogranuloma is one of the largest known filterable viruses. The diagnosis may be made by means of the Frei test, consisting of a positive

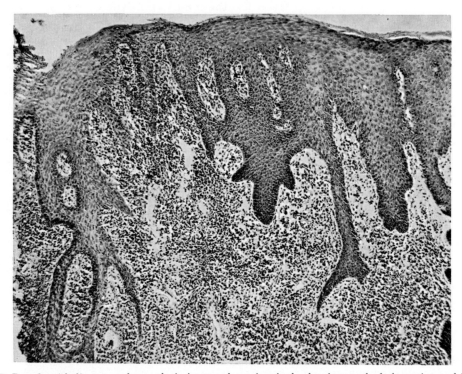

9.10. Pseudoepitheliomatous hyperplasia in granuloma inguinale showing marked elongation and irregularity of rete pegs suggesting anaplasia.

cutaneous response obtained after injection of an antigen, prepared from the sterilized pus of the buboes, or from the brain of the virus-infected mouse. Unfortunately the test is persistently positive and the acute lesion may be of another origin. The differentiation from granuloma has already been discussed in the previous section.

Treatment. Recently very satisfactory and at times striking results have been reported from sulfa therapy and even more from the antibiotics. Chloromycetin, streptomycin, and achromycin have all been used. The former, for example, can be given in doses of from 250 to 500 mg. four times a day for 5 to 10 days. Penicillin has been used effectively in many cases.

Surgical treatment is still occasionally necessary as in the excision of the enormous masses sometimes seen with elephantiasis. In the treatment of rectal strictures, colostomy may be required. With all granulomatous disease multiple biopsy should be performed to exclude concomitant malignancy.

Virus Diseases

Among the many viruses that may attack the vulvar integument, the condyloma or wart virus and the herpes simplex (HSV) Type II are, at present, by far the most prevalent. The agents of molluscum contagiosum and undoubtedly other varieties of virus including that of lymphogranuloma venereum are probably extremely common but infrequently diagnosed.

Herpes Simplex (HSV)

Herpetic infections are probably one of the most common if not the most common afflictions of the external genitalia. Nevertheless, the diagnosis is often not made since the initial vesicle is generally asymptomatic and the small, serpinginous superficial ulcerations are not recognized as the residuae of the ruptured and often secondarily infected lesions (Figs. 9.11 and 9.12). The latter ulcerations are often dramatic with extensive involvement of both labia, marked edema, and tender,

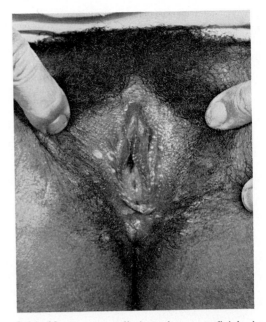

9.11. Numerous small, irregular, superficial ulcerations scattered over the inner surfaces of labia majora and adjacent perineum. Small vesicles could also be found in the immediate area.

enlarged inguinal lymph nodes. In view of the foregoing picture, care must be taken to rule out syphilis and granulomatous diseases before instituting therapy.

The vagina and cervix may be simultaneously affected, but again the lesions are by no means diagnostic. Nevertheless, vaginal and vulvar smears may demonstrate the presence of the typical intranuclear inclusions most strikingly visualized in the multinucleate cell. Titers for herpes antibodies may be of value in differential diagnosis. However, the infections are so common that as high as 30 to 40 of any population may demonstrate positive reactions. In spite of the helpful diagnostic pictures and laboratory studies, a majority of herpetic infections undoubtedly go undiagnosed in view of the minimal symptomatology and the consequent infrequency with which the patient seeks aid.

Pain is the most common complaint of the patient with vulva herpes. On occasions, discomfort, fever and malaise may be severe enough to demand hospitalization. Treatment of the secondarily

It must be recalled that although the acute disease probably produces only transient discomfort to the host, there is an additional worry during pregnancy at the time of delivery. Although the danger of infecting the newborn when an acute disease in the vulvovaginal area exists at the time of delivery may be minimal, nevertheless, that possibility should be kept in mind and cesarean section should be considered. (See Chapter 10.)

Molluscum Contagiosum

This viral infection is probably more common than generally appreciated since it rarely if ever produces symptoms except for a mild local irritation. The lesions are usually less than 1 cm. in diameter and have a slightly umbilicated center.

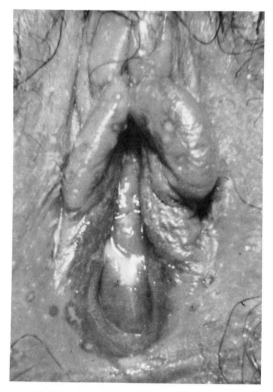

9.12. Small serpiginous superficial ulcerations and edema of herpes (HSV) infection.

infected vesicles with bed rest, local heat, chemotherapeutic agents (such as sulfonamide creams), and Burrow's solution (aluminum acetate) to reduce the edema produce much relief. Occasionally, hospitalization for 24 to 48 hours is necessary to allow for concentrated therapy and rest. Unfortunately, antiviral agents such as Herplex, Stoxil, and the thiosemicarbazones are of little value after the vesicular stage. Most recently the use of tricyclic dyes such as 1% neutral red or 0.1 per cent proflavin applied to the lesions after the vesicles are or have been opened, has afforded more effective therapy. The virus absorbs the dye and is inactivated by exposure of the area to direct light. The use of a fluorescent lamp or simply a 100–150 watt incandescent bulb for 10 minutes with a repeat treatment in 18–24 hours has been effective in alleviating the symptoms of 60 to 75% of patients.

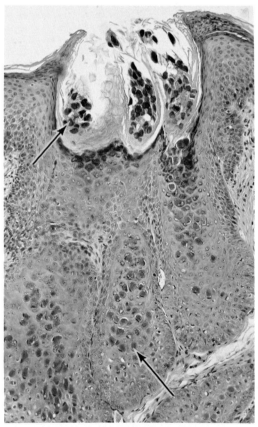

9.13. Molluscum contagiosum showing intranuclear inclusions (molluscum bodies) both at base and at surface (*arrows*) of the umbilication.

Treatment is accomplished by mere evacuation of the "waxy" core. Biopsy reveals the classic "molluscum bodies" which are intranuclear inclusions (Fig. 9.13). For discussion of condylomata accuminata see "Benign Tumors.")

WHITE LESIONS OF THE VULVA

Gross white appearance of the vulvar skin may be due to two general types of change namely: (1) absence or loss of pigment and (2) increased keratinization (hyperkeratosis).

Classification of White Lesions

I. Depigmentation—leukoderma or
   vitiligo
II. Hyperkeratosis
    A. Chronic infections
    B. Begnign tumors
    C. Dystrophies
       1. Lichen sclerosus
       2. Hyperplasia
          a. Typical
          b. Atypical
       3. Mixed (combination of 1 and 2)
    D. Carcinoma in situ
    E. Invasive cancer.

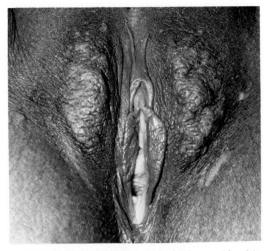

9.15. Chronic dermatitis with thick, grayish-white change, showing microscopic picture similar to Fig. 9.14 or "hypertrophic leukoplakia."

Absence of Pigment or Depigmentation

Leukoderma (congenital absence of pigment) appears most commonly in the late first or early second decade of life. There are rarely any symptoms associated with this condition, and it is usually found at various other areas of the body. Vitiligo, acquired loss of ligment, is commonly associated with chronic infection. Trauma, *e.g.*, the scarring relative to x-ray burn, may produce similar depigmentation (Fig. 9.14).

Increased Keratinization (Hyperkeratosis)

Chronic Infection

The end result of chronic infection may be scarring, especially in those cases of the granulomatous diseases; however, the common dermatitides (eczamatoid, neuro, seborrhoeic, etc.) frequently demonstrate thickening of the skin with whitish change (Fig. 9.15). The edges of these lesions are often elevated with striking keratosis and linear excoriations. Obviously, the latter description fits that of gross "leukoplakia" and unfortunately the microscopic appearance also demonstrates the histologic characteristics suggested in most texts as typical of leukoplakia. Nevertheless, such changes are also

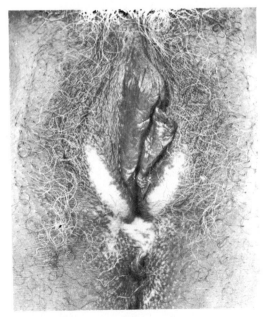

9.14. Vitiligo; loss of pigment due to chronic irritation.

typical of those seen with any chronic infection and have essentially no malignant potential.

Benign Tumors

Any of the papillomatous or verrucous lesions, in the chronic stages, may demonstrate areas of hyperkeratosis and whitish change.

Dystrophies

Controversy as to the pathogenesis, clinical course, and particularly the malignant potential of these so-called primary hyperkeratotic lesions, frequently described as the leukoplakias, has been a continuing issue in the study of vulvar disease. Schwimmer in 1877 first applied the term leukoplakia to a whitish, premalignant, hyperkeratotic lesion of the buccal mucous membrane. Later, Breisky in 1885 described a similar lesion on the vulva; however, microscopically the picture was that of a thinning of the epithelium and collagenization of the underlying

tissue, commonly referred to as "lichen sclerosus et atrophicus." Later Taussig described three developmental stages of the disease which he termed "chronic atrophic vulvitis": (1) erythema, edema, excoriation and dryness, associated with the microscopic finding of minimal hyperkeratosis, acanthosis, and mild inflammatory infiltrate; (2) thickening, with flattening of the folds and whitish change in the skin (Fig. 9.16), microscopically demonstrating epithelial hypertrophy in addition to increased hyperkeratosis, acanthosis, and round cell infiltrate (Fig. 9.17); and (3) cracking of the parchment-like skin with superficial ulceration and whitish or bluish white discoloration, now microscopically showing hyperkeratosis, epithelial thinning, and dermal collagenization (atrophic leukoplakia) (Fig. 9.18). The author recognized little, if any, difference in the malignant potential between the atrophic and hypertrophic stages. In addition to these proposed progressive changes. Taussig recognized a

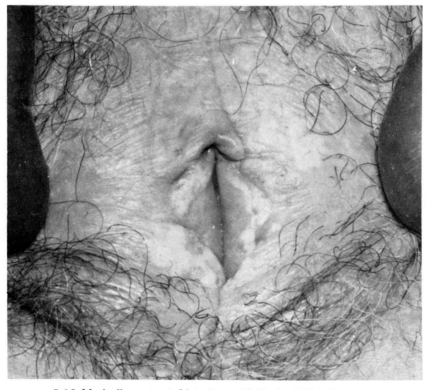

9.16. Markedly contracted introitus, with "leukoplakic" changes

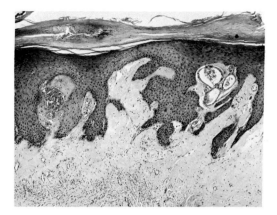

9.17. Hyperplastic alterations. Irregular rete pegs with collagenization of dermis, hyperkeratosis.

primary "simple kraurosis" or shriveling, evidenced by constriction or stenosis of the vaginal outlet. This was considered to be a nonleukoplakic change, although, constriction admittedly could develop as the final result of "chronic atrophic" or "leukoplakic vulvitis." Bonney, in general, agreed with Taussig's concept, although he did recognize a fourth, or quiescent, stage during which the malignant potential was essentially nonexistent.

The many terms that have been applied to these primary hyperkeratoses need some interpretation.

Leukoplakia has been used to describe a variety of whitish lesions since th term could be applied to any "white patch."

Thus since it has been so widely and poorly used, such descriptive terms as applied to specific disease for a designation which would relay information as to the degree of anaplastic activity to the clinician. Consequently the general term of *dystrophy* has been used in an effort to develop a more clinicopathologic significant terminology. As noted in the classification of "White Lesions", these alterations are divided into these with a thin parchment-like appearance (lichen sclerosus) and those covered with a thick layer of keratin and associated with epithelial proliferations. Not infrequently the two varieties are appreciated in the same vulva.

Lichen Sclerosus. Lichen sclerosus applies to a skin lesion which begins as a small bluish white papule. Frequently coalescence of these papules produces a picture of diffuse whitish change over the entire vulva and perianal region (Fig. 9.19). In its terminal stage there is loss of the subcutaneous tissue with flattening of the labial folds and constriction of the outlet. The term "kraurosis" has been used to describe these terminal changes as if this were a specific disease. Actually kraurosis is simply a descriptive term meaning "shrinkage." The microscopic pictures of atrophic leukoplakia, lichen sclerosus et atrophicus, and kraurosis are similar.

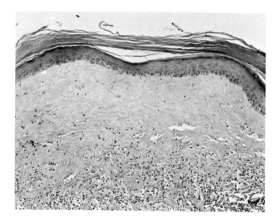

9.18. Lichen sclerosis with hyperkeratosis, thin epithelial layer, dermal collagenization, and inflammatory infiltrate.

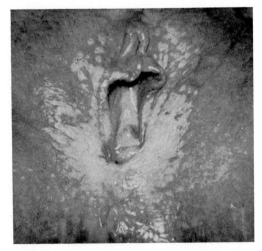

9.19. Lichen sclerosus in 56-year-old female showing isolated lesions with confluence at fourchette.

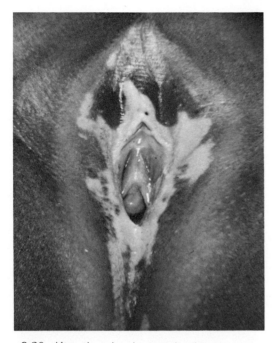

9.20. Alterations in pigmentation in seven-year-old child. Biopsy shows picture compatible with lichen sclerosus, but gross changes simulate leukoderma.

Lichen sclerosus commonly appears in the early postmenopausal years. Nevertheless, similar patterns may be seen prepuberal (Fig. 9.20), and at any time during the menstruating years. Interestingly, these lesions initially are essentially asymptomatic and may remain so unless the collagenization becomes extensive. Similar lesions are frequently seen in other areas such as beneath the breasts and the lower abdomen.

Although the term atrophy has been applied to these lesions, certain studies have indicated that the thinned epithelium is not metabolically inactive. Clark *et al.* noted that the uptake of radioactive phosphorus is as great in these atrophic lesions as in the carcinoma in situ. Similar findings have been recognized in our laboratory with the use of other methodologies. Although metabolic activity cannot be correlated directly with anaplasia, the changes do not justify the designation of atrophy. Furthermore, these lesions must be followed carefully as carcinoma can develop in this context

(Fig. 9.21). It is important to remember that any irritative lesion may become malignant although the thickened, elevated, hyperkeratotic type seems to be more prone to anaplastic alteration. Of major importance in the study and therapy of the lesions are the regular biopsy of suspicious, focal areas of hyperkeratosis or superficial ulceration, and the elimination of scratching with the use of antipruitics, particularly hydrocortisones and antihistamines, intravaginal estrogens postmenopausal, the treatment of specific vaginitis, the removal of local irritating agents, and if necessary some variety of nerve block. Plastic procedures to increase the caliber of outlet are often necessary to eliminate the dyspareunia and allow for satisfactory coitus. Vulvectomy is of importance only if anaplastic changes are noted in the tissue study.

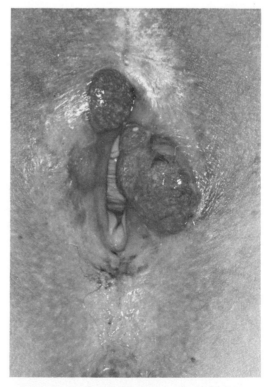

9.21. Carcinoma beginning in "atrophic" area. Patient had had partial excision of a lesion showing atypical hyperplasia and lichen scherosus (mixed dystrophy) 4 years prior to the appearance of gross cancer.

Hyperplasia. The term "hyperplasia" denotes an increase in the number of normal cellular elements in a specific situation. Thus in the endometrium the term is used to describe an increase in the cells of the glandular epithelium and the stroma. More specifically, to the term hyperplasia is added the designations typical or atypical to connote the degree of proliferation and its malignant potential. So should it be for the vulva. Consequently these terms have been applied to the general designation of "dystrophy" in order to assist the clinician in his evaluation and treatment of the specific case.

Obviously in order to make such interpretation *biopsy must be taken.* The importance of this procedure cannot be overemphasized. The instruments which seem most effective are the Keyes punch and the biopsy can be performed under local anesthesia. (Fig. 9.22).

The malignant potential of hyperplastic lesions obviously depends on the degree of cellular aberration. Particularly significant is the abnormal maturation of the epithelial cells in the basal layer. It should go without saying that the more active the therapy in elimination of local epithelial alterations including pruritus, the less the possibility of the development of neoplasia.

Finally it must be recognized that carcinoma-in-situ (Fig. 9.23) and invasive

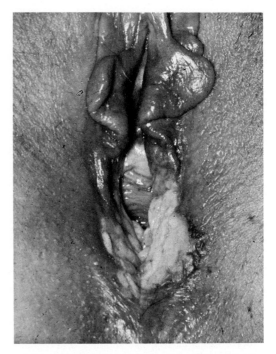

9.23. White, hyperkeratotic lesion occupying the area of the fourchette. Biopsy shows cancer in situ.

cancer can and frequently do appear as whitish lesions. As a consequence any hyperkeratotic area must be biopsied and followed carefully. Again therapy for the common symptomatology is imperative.

Pruritus Vulvae

This term, in the past, has been used as if it designated a specific disease entity. Obviously, however, pruritis describes only the symptom of "itching." As noted previously, almost all of the common dermatitides and local irritants produce itching since it is primarily due to an inflammatory reaction about the underlying nerves. A variety of vaginal infections produce a "reactive dermatitis" with its concomitant pruritus. Systemic diseases associated with itching as well as gross alterations such as lymphedema have been described earlier. Thus the term "pruritus vulvae" becomes a description of a symptom and should *not* be used to identify a disease entity.

The various treatments have been outlined earlier in the chapter. Basically these consist of establishing a specific diagnosis, if at all possible, eliminating

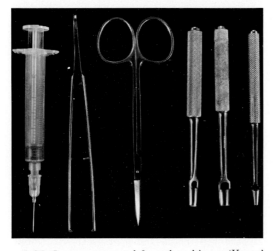

9.22. Instruments used for vulvar biopsy (Keyes' punches to the right)

local irritants, removal of tight-fitting clothing (non-absorbant synthetics, panty-hose, girdles, etc.), use of antipruritic agents such as the hydrocortisone *creams* and *Eurax* on a short term basis, and a careful follow up to determine the results of therapy and to prevent the development of a chronic, hyperplastic disease.

The use of local hormone preparations, specifically hydrocortisones, has been noted above. However, both estrogen and androgens have been proposed as therapy for certain specific conditions. It must be stated that although local estrogenic creams thicken the vaginal epithelium (see Chapter 10), they thin and soften the integument and are not helpful in the treatment of pruritus. Nevertheless, if the patient is postmenopausal, the elimination of the "weepy" thin discharge from the thin vaginal epithelium by the use of intravaginal estrogen is an important adjunctive therapy.

Conversely local testosterone preparations are most effective in the treatment of the pruritus associated with the thin vulvar skin of the patient with lichen sclerosus. Testosterone thickens the skin, improves the nutrition of the tissues, and eliminates or modifies the pruritis in a majority of such cases. A 1 or 2 per cent preparation used twice a day for a week and then every day for 6 weeks is the generally prescribed routine of therapy. Following this regime, if successful, the agent should be used at intervals, possibly 1 to 2 times a week to maintain the local reaction. It should also be noted that the troublesome symptom of "vulvar burning" may be treated in this manner.

Alcohol Injection. The injection of 95% alcohol subcutaneously by the technique recommended by Stone for puruitus ani has been employed also for puruitus vulvae, and it is undoubtedly helpful. This procedure should only be used in chronic conditions when medications have failed. Unfortunately, it may be followed by sloughing in the vulvar or anal region. Only 0.1 cc. of 95% or absolute alcohol is injected beneath the dermis, needle punctures situated about 1 cm. apart. An anesthetic is required, but

the resulting relief may continue for months. Various plans of incising the labia with undercutting and disruption of the sensory nerves have been suggested by Mering but it is important to evaluate each case very critically as the author suggests. Such procedures have the value of preserving normal anatomy. Vulvectomy should be performed only if biopsies demonstrate definite premalignant changes.

Whatever the type of therapy, abolition of the scratch reflex seems desirable, for it is possible that repeated mechanical trauma may be the stimulus that leads to carcinoma.

BENIGN TUMORS OF THE VULVA

Cystic
1. Bartholin duct cyst.
2. Sebaceous or inclusion cysts.
3. Mucinous cyst.
4. Wolffian duct cyst.
5. Cyst of canal of Nuck.
6. Endometriosis.

Solid
1. Fibroma.
2. Lipoma.
3. Verrucous lesions (condyloma acuminatum).
4. Angioma.
5. Hidradenoma.
6. Granular cell myoblastoma.
7. Nevus.

Cystic

Bartholin's Duct Cysts

These have been discussed under "Diseases of Bartholin's Glands," in this chapter.

Sebaceous or Inclusion Cysts

These result from inflammatory blockage of the ducts of sebaceous glands, and are usually of small size (Fig 9.24). They are most commonly on the inner surfaces of the labia majora and minora. They contain a cheesy, sebaceous material and are prone to suppuration, with the formation of small furuncle-like abscesses. If very small and asympto-

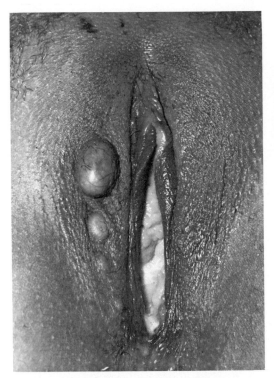

9.24. Inclusion cysts on right labium majus (usually the result of sebaceous gland infection).

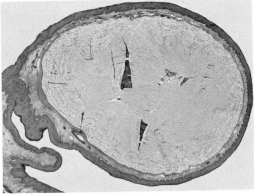

9.25. Mucinous cyst pedunculated at outlet.

matic, no treatment is necessary, but if they are sufficiently large to be annoying, or if they are recurrently infected, simple excision under local anesthesia is indicated.

In the infectious stage, the cavity has no specific lining but instead is filled with polymorphonuclear and foreign body giant cells. In the chronic stage, the cavity is lined by stratified epithelium and thus is classified as an "inclusion" cyst.

Mucinous Cysts

Occasionally noted near the urethra or inner surfaces of the labia minora, mucinous cysts are probably of embryonic origin. The time of separation of the cloaca by the urorectal fold into urogenital sinus and rectum, elements, originally destined to be rectal endoderm, may be displaced toward the urogenital side and subsequently develop into cystic structures of various sizes, often pedunculated. Nevertheless, as noted by Friedrich and Wilkinson, most of the small cysts which appear at the outlet are mucinous,

and probably represent dilation of the minor vestibular glands. (Fig. 9.25).

Wolffian Duct Cysts

These mesonephric remnants rarely appear on the vulva, but if they attain any size, they may project at the outlet.

Cyst of the Canal of Nuck (Hydrocele)

The round ligament inserts into the labium major and carries with it an investment of the peritoneum. The latter is usually firmly attached to its ligament, but may at any point be divorced from its attachment and fluid may accumulate

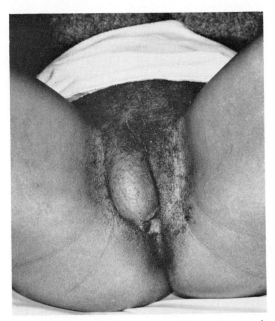

9.26. Hydrocele of the canal of Nuck. Aspirated and then the scar removed.

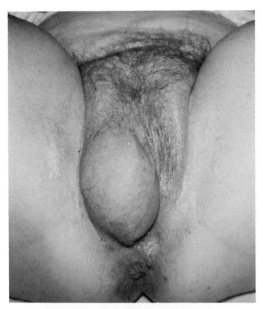

9.27. Fibroma, right labium majus

forming a cystic dilation (Fig. 9.26). Such may present in the labium at the point of insertion and corresponds to the hydrocele in the male.

Endometriosis

Implants of endometrium in the vulva are rare and are most commonly seen in the region of the Bartholin gland suggesting possible implantation at the time of surgery or drainage of a cyst or abscess. Cyclic recurrence of a painful nodule should suggest this possible diagnosis.

Solid

Fibroma

Fibromas arise from the fibrous tissue of the vulva, and are usually of small or moderate size (Fig. 9.27). They tend to become pedunculated, especially if large

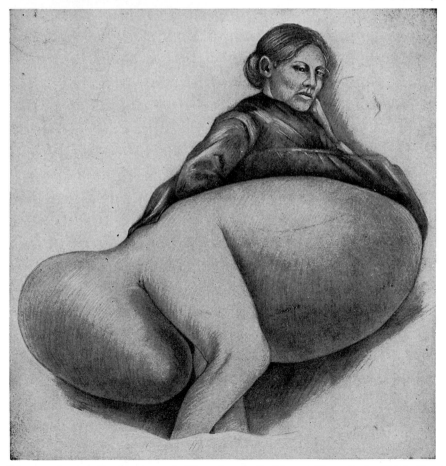

9.28. Fibroma of vulva (Buckner's case). (From Lynch, F. W., and Maxwell, A.: *Pelvic Neoplasms.* D. Appleton & Company, New York, 1922.)

and lymphadenomatous, and the pedicle may become so long that the growth dangles between the limbs like a pendulum. As a matter of fact, tumors of this sort have sometimes reached almost unbelievable size, the classical case reported by Buckner (1851) attaining a weight of 268 pounds (Fig. 9.28). The microscopic structure is that of fibrous tissue, usually light textured and edematous, resembling myxomatous tissue. In some tumors there is an admixture of smooth and striated muscle elements. Treatment is of course surgical.

Lipoma

In spite of the considerable amount of adipose tissue in the vulva, especially in the labia majora, lipoma is rare. It has the same clinical characteristics as those described for fibroma of vulvar origin, and the distinction is not always possible until microscopic examination. Both lipoma and the soft, nonpedunculated fibroma must be differentiated from the spongy varicocele. Such tumors are easily excised.

Verrucous Lesions

The most common form of vulvar verruca is that designated as condyloma acuminatum, to be distinguished from condyloma latum, the secondary syphilitic lesion in the vulva. Pathologically the condyloma acuminatum has a tree-like structure, with a central core of connective tissue covered with a hyperplastic epithelium characterized by elongated rete pegs (acanthosis) and superficial parakeratosis. The stroma is edematous and infiltrated with chronic inflammatory cells. The acuminate warts are often loosely spoken of as venereal warts. Since they are of viral origin, transmission by coitus is the common mode of infection.

Clinically condylomata acuminata appear in the form of warty growths of various sizes which are usually multiple and which are discretely scattered over the vulva, the adjacent perineum, buttocks, and inner thighs. (Fig. 9.29). They are also found in the lower vagina, and

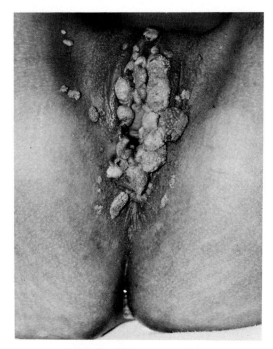

9.29. Condylomata acuminata

more rarely in the upper vagina and even on the cervix.

When numerous, they tend to become confluent, forming large clusters. They undergo pronounced hypertrophy during pregnancy, sometimes forming huge cauliflower masses which may even offer obstacles to vaginal delivery. Actually, many may regress spontaneously postpartum if removal is not necessary during pregnancy. Rarely, malignancy may develop in such lesions.

Topical applications of 20 per cent podophyllin in tincture of benzoin is quite effective in the treatment of the smaller lesions. To avoid a chemical burn, care must be taken to wash off the treated area within a few hours after application. Topical and systemic sulfonamides have been used effectively by some observers. Surgical excision or fulguration may be necessary for larger lesions. More recently topical 5 FU (fluorucacil) has been used with effectiveness in some cases.

Angioma

Although angiomata are rare, the congenital type occasionally cause problems

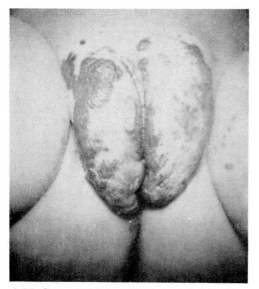

9.30. Congenital hemangiomata on both labia, appearing at two months of age and at one year it was much reduced without treatment.

due to irritations of diapers, urine, and feces. It is important to remember that most of these congenital types regress as the child grows (Fig. 9.30), and therapy should not be instituted unless absolutely necessary.

Hidradenoma

Although this is a rare lesion, it is of some importance because it is occasionally mistaken for adenocarcinoma microscopically (Fig. 9.31). The lesion arises from the vulvar sweat glands, and with rare exceptions it is benign. Clinically it appears as a small nodule usually raised above the surrounding surface, and having a fibroma-like appearance and consistency (Fig. 9.32). In some cases the overlying skin may be reddened, granular, or ulcerated. In such cases there may be slight bleeding. Most frequently there are no symptoms, although occasionally itching is present. The usual location of the lesion is on the inner surface of the labia majora, but it may be on the labia minora or the adjacent perineum. The treatment consists of simple excision. Only a rare malignancy was reported in the review of Chung and Greene.

Supernumerary breast tissue may be found on the vulva and microscopically simulates the apocrine adenoma since the breast is a modified apocrine gland.

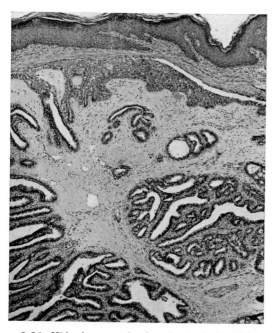

9.31. Hidradenoma of vulva. A rare lesion which may be mistaken for adenocarcinoma.

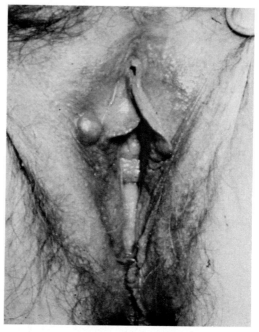

9.32. Gross appearance of hidradenoma of vulva.

Granular Cell Myoblastoma

This rather uncommon tumor, composed of irregular clumps of large pale staining cells with eosinophilic cytoplasmic granules, is most commonly noted in the tongue, but has been recorded at many sites. Although called myoblastoma, the tumor is felt to arise from the myelin sheath of the nerve. Of interest is the pseudo-epitheliomatous change in the overlying epithelium suggesting and occasionally mistaken for epidermoid cancer (Fig. 9.33).

Nevus

The nevus is an important lesion on the vulva since although the vulvar skin makes up only 1 per cent of the entire body surface, 7 to 10 per cent of malignant melanoma in the female occur on the external genitalia. This may be due to the many irritants which affect this area as well as the fact that junction activity is common in the vulvar nevus. Of particular significance is the flat, expanding pigmented lesion (Fig. 9.34). Such lesions should be excised with a wide margin without biopsy.

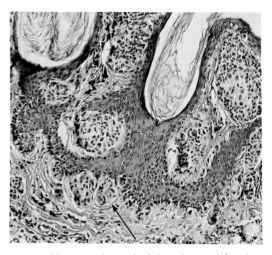

9.34. Nevus with marked junction activity (*arrow*).

CARCINOMA OF THE VULVA

The most important of vulvar tumors is carcinoma, the third most common of all

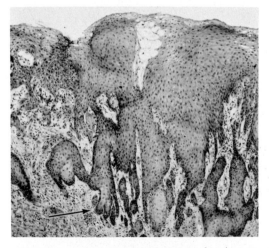

9.33. Granular cell myoblastoma showing extensive pseudoepitheliomatous hyperplasia simulating cancer. *Arrow* points to the underlying "granular" cells which lead to the correct diagnosis.

primary pelvic cancers, being exceeded in frequency only by uterine (cervix and corpus) and ovarian cancer. Vulvar cancer accounts for 3 to 4 per cent of all primary malignancies of the genital canal.

Carcinoma *in situ* of the vulva is a definite entity, although far less common than its counterpart on the cervix. Intraepithelial cancer of the vulva has the same relationships as the comparable cervical disease in its tendency to exist at the periphery of invasive cancer or to precede true infiltative cancer. Indeed, some of the patterns of the so-called atypical hyperplasias bear the same relation to early cancer that atypical cervical epithelium does to cervical intraepithelial cancer. By definition intraepithelial cervical cancer connotes full thickness replacement of the lining epithelium by undifferentiated abnormal cells, often of basal type; and similarly, intraepithelial cancer of the vulva shows abnormality of the lining epithelium with increased mitotic activity (Fig. 9.35). However, vulvar cancer is characteristically spinal in type, and some degree of differentiation of the component cells is often found despite undeniable intraepithelial anaplasia. It is important, however, to recognize that a pure cytological type of *in situ* vulvar cancer is as rare as a similar pure lesion in the

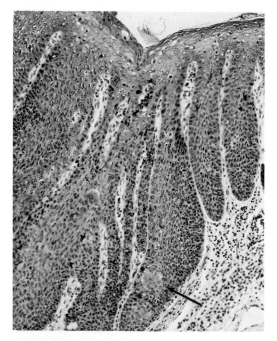

9.35. Microscopic of carcinoma in situ with intraepithelial pearl formation and abnormal nuclear figures.

cervix. A variety of terms such as Bowen's disease, erythroplasia of Quyrat, etc., have been used to describe types of in situ cancer, but basically the microscopic pictures are not sufficiently distinctive to be specific. Grossly the anaplasias may appear as reddened, pigmented, whitish or slightly elevated lesions and are commonly multicentric in origin.

With the apparent increase in the incidence of carcinoma-in-situ of the vulva has come the realization that certain lesions, histologically neoplastic, may in fact be reversible if only observed particularly, as noted by Friedrich, the alterations develop during pregnancy. Thus it is obvious that, since many are now noted in young women under 30 years of age, conservative therapy is in order.

Treatment in general demands wide local excision if only a solitary lesion is present and simple vulvectomy for the patient with multicentric foci. It is imperative that the vulva and adjacent perineum, vagina and cervix be thoroughly inspected, not only prior to

any therapy, but also in the *follow up* periods. Chemotherapy has been effective in certain instances.

Paget's disease of the vulva is a specific form of *in situ* cancer characterized grossly by a reddish lesion interspersed with white epithelial islands (Fig. 9.36) and microscopically by the large pale "Paget" cells. Whereas the similar lesion of the breast is usually associated with an underlying carcinoma, such is rare on the vulva.

Invasive carcinoma is preeminently a disease of elderly women, the incidence being highest in the seventh decade. The exception occurs in those cases preceded by granulomatous disease where the average age is about 40 years as noted by Salztein, Collins, and Alexander. The disease begins on any part of the vulva. The most common histological type is squamous-cell carcinoma. In all locations the cancer is of the squamous cell or epidermoid varieties (Fig. 9.37), except in primary carcinoma of Bartholin's gland which may be either adenocarcinoma

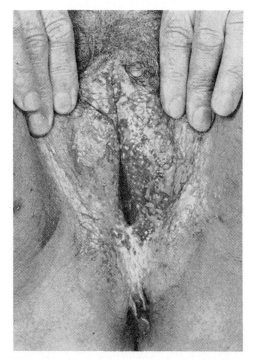

9.36. Paget's disease of the vulva. (Dark areas are red in color, and white "leukoplakoid" area are as seen).

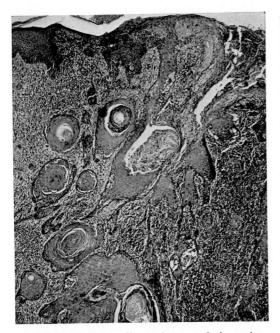

9.37. Squamous cell carcinoma of the vulva showing classic "pearl formation."

latter is not invariably present. In many instances, however, there is a history of long standing pruritus antedating the appearance of carcinoma. As the ulceration and infiltration extend, the pain increases, and in the advanced cases it may be persistent and intolerable unless controlled by narcotics.

Not uncommonly there is an unfortunate delay of one and a half to two years between the appearance of symptoms and diagnosis of the disease. Much of this delay is due to reluctance of the older patient to seek medical consultation; however, in about one-third of the cases the physician is at fault as noted by Howson and Montgomery. In the early stage the patient suffers very little discomfort, and the lesion may seem, even to the physician, a rather unimpressive one unless he is familiar with its potentialities. Biopsy and microscopic examination are of decisive importance, and they should never be omitted when a

(cribriform), transitional, or epidermoid in character. In such instances a hard stony mass can be felt in the region of the gland.

The gross appearance may be whitish, ulcerated, or granulomatous depending on the primary lesion (Plates 9.8, 9). As noted previously several authors have reported the premalignant nature of the granulomatous and hyperplastic lesions.

Basal cell carcinoma is rare and appears as on the skin elsewhere as a superficial ulcer with "rolled" edges. Microscopically the cells "drop" from the basal layer of the epithelium and seem to invade the underlying tissue, however local excision results in a cure (Fig 9.38).

In the usual forms of vulvar cancer, the initial lesion becomes steadily larger, with increasing induration, ulceration, and surrounding edema. If neglected, the destruction may involve most of the vulvar structure. Metastatic involvement of the superficial and deep inguinal and femoral glands soon develops, and the richness of the lymphatic communications leads to early contralateral nodal involvement.

The symptoms in the early stage are apt to be very slight, consisting only of slight soreness and itching, although the

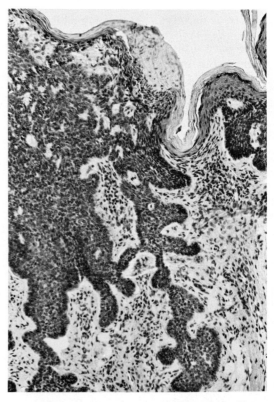

9.38. Basal cell carcinoma showing the uniform basal cells "dropping" into the underlying tissue.

chronic ulcerative vulvar lesion is observed, particularly in elderly women. Upon this diagnostic procedure one must depend for the differentiation from other ulcerative lesions, such as tertiary syphilis, or lymphogranuloma venereum.

Prophylaxis is of considerable importance, for it has been noted that both hyperplastic and various granulomatous or other irritative lesions are frequently precursors of cancer. Fortunately, these generally cause intense pruritus and discomfort which lead to the request for medical attention, but haphazard use of various ointments, lotions, and sprays can only be condemned if biopsy of any suspicious lesion is not performed.

Treatment of Vulvar Cancer

The primary treatment for carcinoma of the vulva is surgery. Vulvectomy is sufficient in those instances of in situ disease; however, thorough study of the removed tissue must be carried out to eliminate invasion. Radical vulvectomy with inguinal and femoral lymphade-

nectomy is mandatory for invasive cancer. There is considerable difference of opinion as to how extensive the surgery should be. The presence of palpable nodes should not be the criterion, because in one-third of the cases nodal enlargement is not due to cancer but to infection. Likewise in one third of the cases in which there is metastatic disease to the nodes, the nodes are not clinically enlarged.

Way emphasizes that vulvectomy must be so extensive as to disallow primary closure; and although most authorities do not concur with this thesis, they agree that radical removal of the vulva is the essential part of a surgical approach to this disease. The value of lymphadenectomy is argued, but, as noted by Green *et al.,* radical vulvectomy with extensive lymphadenectomy does result in an increased five-year salvage.

A one-stage vulvectomy and bilateral lymphadenectomy is accepted by most students as the procedure of choice (Fig. 9.39). Removal of, rather than under-

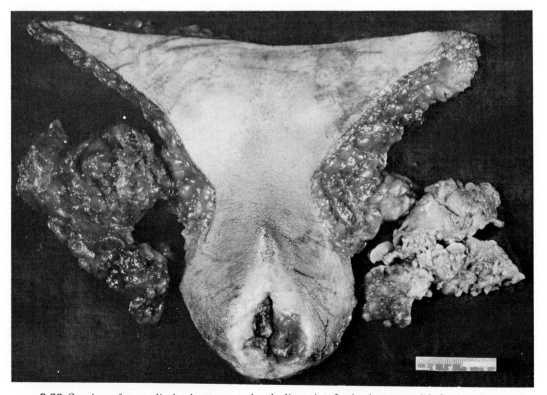

9.39. Specimen from radical vulvectomy and node dissection. Lesion is seen on right lower vulva.

mining, the skin has resulted in better primary healing. The New Orleans approach (Collins *et al.*) is more radical with an extended lymphadenectomy and freely performs exenteration if adjacent organs (vagina, urethra, or rectum) are involved without extrapelvic metastases. McKelvey, believing that complete excision of the local disease is paramount to salvage, feels that vulvectomy with superficial node dissection (one-stage under local anesthesia) is adequate.

Collins has also pointed out that curability roughly parallels the extent of the lesion when seen, and he notes 3 cm. as the critical size below which cure is usual and, above which, unlikely. A five-year salvage of all patients should approximate 50% if adequate surgery is carried out. X-ray therapy is felt to be rarely indicated by most authors; however, more recently there has been a resurgence of interest in radiation therapy and with new techniques excellent results have been reported in the treatment of extensive disease.

Although ultraradical surgery may seem an unjustifiably extensive approach for the age group usually affected and results in a rare salvage if the high nodes are involved, nevertheless such operative therapy is generally accepted as the therapeutic approach of choice. The lesion is slow to metastasize and usually does so in a superficial fashion. Wide local invasion and extension often precedes lymphatic or hematogenous dissemination. Such a disease process obviously deserves a wide local radical excision with some form of bilateral lymphadenectomy. The frequent crossover of lymphatics from one to the other side demands bilateral operation.

Classification of Vulvar Cancer

The International Federation of Gynecology and Obstetrics (FIGO) has recently accepted the TNM terminology for pelvic neoplasia and has developed the classification for vulvar cancer as shown in Table 9.1. This terminology is quite cumbersome and the simpler classification of the neoplasm into 4 stages is more applicable.

Table 9.1

FIGO Classification of Carcinoma of the Vulva

TNM classification and clinical staging of carcinoma of the vulva. (Adopted in 1970, to be used from January 1, 1971.)

T—Primary Tumor

T1	Tumor confined to the vulva—2 cm. or less in larger diameter
T2	Tumor confined to the vulva—more than 2 cm. in diameter
T3	Tumor of any size with adjacent spread to the urethra and/or perineum and/or the anus.
T4	Tumor of any size infiltrating the bladder mucosa and/or the rectum mucosa or both, including the upper part of the urethral mucosa and/or fixed to the bone.

Clinical Stage Groups

Stage I			Stage II		
T1	N0	M0	T2	N0	M0
T1	N1	M0	T2	N1	M0

Stage III			Stage IV		
T3	N0	M0	T1	N3	M0
T3	N1	M0	T2	N3	M0
T3	N2	M0	T3	N3	M0
T1	N2	M0	T4	N0	M0
T2	N2	M0	T4	N1	M0
			T4	N2	M0
			T4	N3	M0

All other conditions containing M1a or M1b.

N—Regional Lymph Nodes

N0	No nodes palpable.
N1	Nodes palpable in either groin, not enlarged, mobile (not clinically suspicious of neoplasm).
N2	Nodes palpable in either one or both groins, enlarged, firm and mobile (clinically suspicious of neoplasm).
N3	Fixed or ulcerated nodes.

M—Distance Metastases

M0	No clinical metastases.
M1a	Palpable deep pelvic lymph nodes.
M1b	Other distant metastases.

Other Vulvar Malignancies

Sarcoma of the vulva is exceedingly rare, only about 30 cases having been reported. Malignant melanoma is also rare; however, it is the second most common malignancy in the vulvar area. As in other parts of the body, its origin is usually in pigmented moles. Its tendency to widespread dissemination is well known, and a fatal termination is common. Symmonds has reported improved results with early and radical surgery.

URETHRA

Although the urethra is technically not part of the genital canal, the diseases that affect the area commonly involve the genitalia. Urethral infection is often gonococcal, the vulvovaginal glands and cervix being other frequent sites of involvement. Actually the urethra may be the primary organ invaded by the gonococcus, however, the symptoms are usually very transient. Residua may remain in the urethral glands or Skene's ducts.

Many other organisms also involve the posterior portion of the urethra, as well as of the trigone. The clinician must be mindful of the possibility that the suburethral gland infection may result in the formation of a diverticulum. This may be the cause of a recurrent cystitis. Palpation of the urethra may reveal a saclike outpouching from which pus can be "milked out," through the urethral meatus. Occasionally endoscopic examinations with urethrographic studies, as suggested by Davis and Cian, are necessary.

Although surgical excision of a diverticulum is the preferred treatment, simple urethritis, either acute or chronic, is frequently amenable to alkalinization of the urine and to the administration of sulfonamides or antibiotics. More helpful, particularly in the low grade, chronic infections, is the topical application of 2 to 5% silver nitrate. If the immediately adjacent Skene's glands are involved, as indicated by expression of pus on palpation, they may be easily fulgurated.

A real but frequently overlooked entity is the postmenopausal senile or atrophic urethritis (Fig. 9.40). This frequently occurs in conjuction with a similar type of vaginitis as a sequel to estrogen depri-

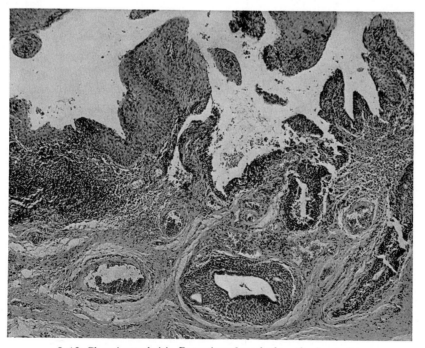

9.40. Chronic urethritis. Resection of marked urethral eversion

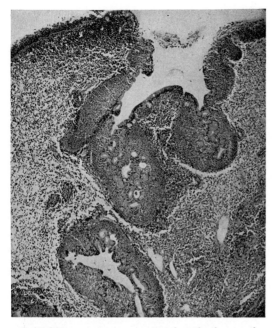

9.41. Microscopic appearance of urethral caruncle of papillomatous type.

vation. There is a reddening of the meatus as edema and prolapse of the urethral mucosal lining occur, and the resultant appearance is much like a urethral caruncle. Local pain, terminal burning on urination, strangury, and even hematuria may occur, but prompt remission and relief are achieved by estrogen therapy. Local estrogenic creams or suppositories usually afford more rapid relief of symptoms than does systemic therapy. Fulguration, the preferred treatment for a caruncle, is not necessary in this form of urethral disease.

Benign tumors are uncommon, the most frequent being the caruncle (Fig. 9.41). This small, reddish pedunculated lesion is occasionally tender and may bleed. Fulguration after biopsy is the treatment of choice.

The urethra may be the site of other pathological entities, such as stricture or fistula (frequently postirradiation or postoperative), granulomatous infection by lymphopathia or granuloma inguinale, prolapsed mucosa, and even carcinoma. Carcinoma is rare and carries a poor prognosis, less than 50%. Treatment is

generally radiation, as indicated by Brack and Farber, but occasionally radical surgical procedures are performed particularly in the radio resistant lesion.

REFERENCES

Abell, M. R.: Hyperplastic lesions of the vulva. J. Ark. Med. Soc., 53: 249, 1966.

Alexander, L. J., and Shields, T. L.: Squamous cell carcinoma of vulva secondary to granuloma inguinale. Arch. Derm., 67: 395, 1953.

Anderson, N. P.: Hidradenoma of vulva. Arch. Derm. Syph., 62: 873, 1950.

Barclay, D. L., and Collins, C. G.: Intraepithelial cancer of vulva. Amer. J. Obstet. Gynec., 86: 95, 1963.

Birch, H. W., and Sondag, D. R.: Granular cell myoblastoma of the vulva. Obstet. Gynec., 18: 443, 1961.

Brack, C. B., and Dickson, R. J.: Carcinoma of the female urethra. Amer. J. Roentgen., 79: 472, 1958.

Brack, C. B., and Guild, H. G.: Urethral obstruction in the female child. Amer. J. Obstet. Gynec., 76: 1105, 1958.

Buckingham, H. C., and McClure, J. H.: Reticulum cell sarcoma of vulva. Obstet. Gynec., 6: 121, 1955.

Chung, J. T., and Greene, R. R.: Hidradenoma of vulva. Amer. J. Obstet. Gynec., 75: 310, 1958.

Clark, D. G. Zumoff, B, Brunschwig, A., and Hellman, L.: Preferential uptake of phosphate by premalignant and malignant lesions of the vulva. Cancer, 13: 775, 1960.

Cockerell, E. G., Knox, J. M., and Rogers, S. F.: Lichen sclerosus et atrophicus. Obstet. Gynec., 15: 554, 1960.

Collins, C. G., Borman, R. G., McMahon, B., and Avent, J. C.: Vulvectomy for benign disease. Amer. J. Obstet. Gynec., 76: 363, 1958.

Collins, C. G., Hansen, L. H., and Theriot, E.: Clinical stain for use in selecting biopsy sites in patients with vulvar disease. Obstet. Gynec., 28: 158, 1966.

Collins, C. G., Kushner, J., Lewis, G. N., and LaPointe, R.: Noninvasive malignancy of the vulva. Obstet. Gynec., 6: 339, 1955.

Cosbie, W. G.: Treatment of carcinoma of the vulva. Amer. J. Obstet. Gynec., 63: 251, 1952.

Davis, H. J., and Cian, L. G.: Positive pressure urethrography; a new diagnostic study. J. Urol., 75: 753, 1956.

Dennis, E. J., Hester, L. H., Jr., and Wilson, L. A.: Primary carcinoma of Bartholin's glands. Obstet. Gynec., 6: 291, 1955.

Douglas, C. P.: Lymphangioma venereum and granuloma inguinale of the vulva. J. Obstet. Gynaec. Brit. Comm., 69: 871, 1962.

Eichner, E.: Adenoid cystic carcinoma of the Bartholin gland. Obstet. Gynec., 21: 608, 1963.

Falk, H. C., and Hyman, A. B.: Diagnosis and treatment of pruritus vulvae. Clin. Obstet. Gynec., 2: 461, 1959.

Friedrich, E. G., and Wilkinson, E. J.: Mucous cysts of the vulvar vestibule. Obstet. Gynec., 42: 407, 1974.

Friedrich, E. G.: Reversible vulvar atypia. Obstet. Gynec., 39: 173, 1972.

Gardiner, S. H., Stout, F. E., Arbogast, J. L., and Huber, C. D.: Intraepithelial carcinoma of the vulva. Amer. J. Obstet. Gynec., 65: 515, 1953.

Green, T. H., Ulfelder, H., and Meigs, J. V.: Epidermoid carcinoma of the vulva. Amer. J. Obstet. Gynec., 75: 834, 1958.

Greenblatt, R. B., Baldwin, K. R., and Dienst, R. B.: Minor veneral diseases. Clin. Obstet. Gynec., 2: 549, 1959.

Herndon, E. G.: Leukoplakic vulvitis and its relationship to the development of carcinoma of vulva. J. Bowman Gray Sch. Med., 4: 35, 1946.

Hester, L. J.: Granuloma venereum of cervix and vulva. Amer. J. Obstet. Gynec., *62:* 312, 1951.

Howson, J. V., and Montgomery, T. L.: Delay period in diagnosis of genital cancer. Amer. J. Obstet. Gynec., *57:* 1098, 1949.

Huber, C. P., Gardiner, S. H., and Michael, A.: Paget's disease of vulva. Amer. J. Obstet. Gynec., *62:* 778, 1951.

Huffman, J. W.: Detailed anatomy of paraurethral ducts in adult human female. Amer. J. Obstet. Gynec., *55:* 86, 1948.

Hutsfield, D. C.: Genital strains of herpes simplex virus. Brit. J. Vener. Dis., *43:* 48, 1967.

Hyman, A. B., and Falk, H. C.: White lesions of the vulva. Obstet. Gynec. *12:* 407, 1958.

Issacs, J. H., and Topek, N. H.: Carcinoma of the vulva. Amer. J. Obstet. Gynec., *73:* 1277, 1957.

Jeffcoate, T. N. A.: Dermatology of vulva. J. Obstet. Gynaec. Brit. Comm., *69:* 888, 1962.

Josey, W. E., Nahmias, A. J., Naib, Z. M. *et al.:* Genital herpes simplex infection in the female. Amer. J. Obstet. Gynec., *96:* 493, 1966.

Kanter, A. E., and Strean, B. J.: Melanoma of the vulva. Obstet. Gynec., *12:* 516, 1958.

Knight, R. V.: Bowen's disease. Amer. J. Obstet. Gynec., *6:* 514, 1943.

Lacy, G. R.: Hydradenoma and hydradenoid carcinoma of vulva. Amer. J. Obstet. Gynec., *51:* 268, 1945.

Lang, W. R.: Genital infections in female children. Clin. Obstet. Gynec., *2:* 428, 1959.

Langley, I. I., Hertig, A. T., and Smith, G. van S.: Relation of leucoplakic vulvitis to squamous carcinoma of vulva. Amer. J. Obstet. Gynec., *62:* 167, 1951.

Lipschutz, B.: Ulcus Vulvae acutum. In *Jadassohn's Handbuch der Haut-und Geschlechtskrankheiten.* Julius Springer, Berlin, 1927.

Marcus, S. L.: Basal cell and basal-squamous cell carcinomas of the vulva. Amer. J. Obstet. Gynec., *79:* 461, 1960.

Marcus, S. L.: Multiple squamous cell carcinomas involving the cervix, vagina and vulva. Amer. J. Obstet. Gynec., *80:* 802, 1960.

Masterson, J. G., and Goss, A. S.: Carcinoma of Bartholin gland. Amer. J. Obstet. Gynec., *69:* 1323, 1955.

Matthews, D.: Marsupialization of Bartholin's cysts. J. Obstet. Gynaec. Brit. Comm., *73:* 1010, 1966.

McKelvey, J. L.: Carcinoma of vulva. Obstet. Gynec., *5:* 452, 1955.

Mering, J. H.: A surgical approach to intractable pruritus vulvae. Amer. J. Obstet. Gynec., *64:* 619, 1952.

Miller, N. F., Riley, G. M., and Stanley, M.: Leukoplakia vulvae. Amer. J. Obstet. Gynec., *64:* 768, 1952.

Newman, B., and Cromen, J. K.: Multicentric origin of carcinomas of the female anogenital tract. Surg. Gynec. Obstet., *108:* 273, 1959.

Nolan, J. F.: Carcinoma of the vulva. Amer. J. Obstet. Gynec., *78:* 833, 1959.

Novak, E., and Novak, E. R.: *Gynecologic and Obstetric Pathology,* ed. 7, W. B. Saunders Company, Philadelphia, 1974.

Novak, E., and Stevenson, R. F.: Sweat gland tumors of vulva, benign (hidradenoma) and malignant (adenocarcinoma). Amer. J. Obstet. Gynec., *50:* 641, 1945.

Plachta, A., and Speer, F. D.: Apocrine gland adenocarcinoma and extra-mammary Paget's disease of the vulva. Cancer, *7:* 910, 1954.

Purola, E., and Widholm, O.: Primary carcinoma of Bartholin's gland. Acta Obstet. Gynec. Scand., *45:* 205, 1966.

Rainey, R.: Association of lymphogranuloma inguinale and cancer. Surgery, *34:* 221, 1954.

Rubin, A.: Granular cell myoblastoma of the vulva. Amer. J. Obstet. Gynec. *77:* 292, 1959.

Saltzstein, S. L., Woodruff, J. D., and Novak, E. R.: Postgranulomatous carcinoma of the vulva. Obstet. Gynec., *7:* 80, 1956.

Siegler, A. M., and Greene, H. J.: Basal-cell carcinoma of vulva. Amer. J. Obstet. Gynec., *62:* 1219, 1951.

Stening, M., and Elliott, P.: Primary carcinoma of the vulva, with special reference to leukoplakia. J. Obstet. Gynaec. Brit. Comm., *66:* 897, 1959.

Symmonds, R. E., Pratt, J. H. and Dockerty, M. B.: Melanoma of the vulva. Obstet. Gynec., *15:* 543, 1960.

Taussig, F.: *Diseases of Vulva.* D. Appleton-Century Company, New York, 1921.

Taussig, F.: Leukoplakic vulvitis and cancer of the vulva. Amer. J. Obstet. Gynec., *18:* 472, 1929.

Taussig, F.: Cancer of the vulva. Amer. J. Obstet. Gynec., *40:* 764, 1940.

Taylor, C. W.: Dermatology of the vulva. J. Obstet. Gynaec. Brit. Comm., *69:* 881, 1962.

Thomas, W. A.: Clinical study of granuloma inguinale with a routine for the diagnosis of lesions of the vulva. Amer. J. Obstet. Gynec., *61:* 790, 1951.

Tomskey, G. C., Vickery, G. W., and Getzoff, P. L.: Successful treatment of granuloma inguinale, with special reference to use of podophyllin. J. Urol., *48:* 401, 1942.

Ulfelder, H.: Radical vulvectomy with bilateral inguinal, femoral and iliac node resection. Amer. J. Obstet. Gynec., *78:* 1074, 1959.

Wallace, H. J., Vulva leukoplakia. J. Obstet. Gynaec. Brit. Comm., *69:* 865, 1962.

Way, S.: *Malignant Disease of the Female Genital Tract,* Blakiston Company, Division of McGraw-Hill Book Company, Inc., New York, 1951.

Way, S.: Carcinoma of the vulva. Amer. J. Obstet. Gynec., *79:* 692, 1960.

Way, S., and Hennigan, M.: Late results of extended radical vulvectomy for carcinoma of vulva. J. Obstet. Gynaec. Brit. Comm., *73:* 594, 1966.

Wharton, L. R., and Everett, H. S.: Primary malignant Bartholin gland tumors. Obstet. Gynec. Survey, *6:* 1, 1951.

Woodruff, J. D.: Paget's disease of the vulva. Obstet. Gynec., *5:* 175, 1955.

Woodruff, J. D.: Premalignant lesions of the vulva. In *Treatment of Cancer and Allied Diseases,* edited by G. Pack and I. Ariel, Paul B. Hoeber, Inc., New York, 1962.

Woodruff, J. D., and Brack, C. B.: Unusual malignancies of vulvourethal region. Obstet. Gynec., *12:* 677, 1958.

Woodruff, J. D., and Hildebrandt, E. E.: Carcinoma in situ of the vulva. Obstet. Gynec., *12:* 414, 1958.

Woodruff, J. D., and Richardson, E. H. Jr.: Malignant vulvar Paget's disease. Obstet. Gynec., *10:* 10, 1957.

Woodruff, J. D., and Williams, T. J.: Multiple sites of anaplastic change in the lower genital system. Amer. J. Obstet. Gynec., *85:* 724, 1963.

Woodruff, J. D., Julian, C. G., Puray, T., Mermut, S., and Katayama, P.: The contemporary challenge of carcinoma-in-situ of the vulva. Amer. J. Obstet. Gynec., *115:* 677, 1973.

chapter 10

Diseases of the Vagina

VAGINITIS

Vaginal infections are among the more common problems which challenge the gynecologist. It is difficult for the clinician to be enthusiastic about such patients, for, although the patient has a most valid and disturbing complaint, the infection is rarely of serious import, is often difficult to eradicate and frequently recurrent. Since the histology of the vagina varies at different age periods, it is not strange that certain infections are characteristic of these specific eras. During reproductive life, for example, the vaginal epithelium is many cell layers thick. This fact, together with the absence of glands, makes gonorrheal infection very rare as compared to its incidence in the young child. In the latter, the Gonococcus finds a fertile field in the thin prepuberal vaginal epithelium. Again, in the postmenopausal phase of life, there is atrophy of the vaginal wall, so that various organisms, including the Gonococcus, are common invaders.

The normal flora of the vagina includes many organisms, Streptococcus, Staphylococcus, Döderlein's bacillus, the diphtheroids and not infrequently fungi.

Nevertheless, the full scope of the vaginal flora remains an unsolved puzzle. It seems clear that the bacillus of Döderlein, a normal inhabitant, plays an important role in maintaining the acidity which characterizes the normal vaginal secretion. This acidity is due to the presence of lactic acid formed from the splitting of the glycogen present in the vaginal epithelial cells. The pH of the normal vaginal secretion averages from 4.5 to 5.

Causes

A variety of agents are involved in the production of vaginal infections. During the menstrual years, the most frequent offenders are *Trichomonas vaginalis*, the Monilia or Candida, *Haemophilus vaginalis*, and herpes virus. In the prepubertal and postmenopausal years, the thin vaginal epithelium is easily infected by a variety of agents, including the Gonococcus and many nonspecific organisms.

As with the vulva, certain systemic diseases may predispose to vulvovaginitis. In the diabetic, monilial infections affect the epithelia of the entire area. The obvious question must be raised, namely, does a high concentration of sugar in the urine predispose to this problem? One must question this concept, although possibly the growth of these agents may be enhanced by the medium. Nevertheless, it seems more likely that the patient has less resistance to the infection as is true with infection elsewhere in the body. In debilitating states, particularly cardiovascular disease, the vagina may be the site of "bleb" formation characteristic of vaginitis emphysematosa. This interesting alteration in the subepithelial tissues is most commonly seen in pregnancy and often associated with trichomoniasis. In the infant, the acute exanthematous diseases may be found both in the vagina and on the vulva, the most frequent offender probably being chicken pox. Foreign bodies are a particular hazard during early childhood when various agents may be introduced into the vagina without knowledge of the parents. The rather purulent vaginitis which may result goes unnoticed unless the physician is aware of the possibility. On other occasions, pessaries, inserted in the treatment of prolapse and not changed periodically, may produce a severe reactive vaginitis and deep fissures may result with the embedding of the agent in the vaginal mucosa. A variety of douches are present on the market and, as one might expect, they may produce reactions in certain individuals who are sensitive to the ingredients. This is particularly true when the agent contains high quantities of chlorine or caustics.

Symptoms and Signs

The primary symptom of vaginitis is a discharge commonly called leukorrhea. It must be appreciated that during the normal cycle there are well-known variations in this discharge, depending on the time in the cycle at which the woman is observed. During the pre- and postmenstrual days, the "flow" is often milky and may appear as small, white clumps of "material." Conversely, at midcycle, the prominent cervical mucus component becomes dominant and the

discharge is thick and mucilaginous. Obviously, the patient may be apprehensive that an infection is present and should be reassured as to the normalcy of these patterns.

With most vaginal infections, in addition to the discharge, the patient commonly complains of vulvar irritation and itching which symptoms are especially prominent on urination. The latter may lead the patient and the physician into the erroneous diagnosis of cystitis or urethritis, particularly if only a voided specimen is studied. The importance of a "clean catch" urine and thorough examination is obvious.

Investigation usually reveals that the vaginal mucosal is extremely erythematous and congested, as is the epithelium of the introitus, the urethral meatus and often the vulvo-perianal areas. Differential points in diagnosis between the varieties of infections will be dealt with under the discussion of the specific disease.

Nonspecific Vaginitis

In the past, this has been a common designation for the vaginal infection for which there appears to be no definable infecting agent. At present, it would seem only realistic that the diagnosis of "nonspecific vaginitis" should be relegated to those reactions occurring in the prepubertal and postmenopausal years during which the thin vaginal epithelium is quite susceptible to a variety of irritative phenomena, as well as the Gonococcus and many nonspecific infective agents. Conversely, during the menstrual years, the mature vaginal epithelium resists the inroads of these nonspecific bacteria as well as the Gonococcus, and every effort should be made to arrive at a specific cause for the vaginitis. Appreciating the innocuous nature of most vaginal infections, it is a great temptation to suggest that the problem is nonspecific and prescribe some rather general cleansing or antibiotic agent. Nevertheless, all too commonly these measures are not helpful in the treatment of the specific disease and, in certain instances, may even prolong the process or delay more definitive therapy. With present sophisticated techniques for study of any disease process, an epitaph should be written for the diagnosis of nonspecific vaginitis during the menstrual years. Obviously, the correct therapeutic agent for specific infective agent will lead to better results.

Even in the cases of nonspecific vaginitis occurring in children, speculum examination is important if the "nonspecific infection" does not respond to local or systemic therapy. In such instances, endoscopic investigation of the vaginal canal by means of such instruments, as the "Kelly cystoscope," foreign bodies and even neoplastic disease, specifically sarcoma botryoides, may be ruled out.

Treatment

Obviously the treatment of "nonspecific" vaginitis entails first a thorough study to rule out a "specific." Certainly, during the menstrual years, careful investigation of the vaginal preparation and the use of available cultural techniques will demonstrate one of the agents noted above and thus make the therapy more effective. Cleansing, hot water douches are an adjunct to any local or systemic treatment, appreciating that they should not be employed immediately after the use of intravaginal medications. Chemical agents in the douche may produce local reactions and are rarely if ever therapeutic.

The true nonspecific vaginitis of the prepubertal or postmenopausal patient is best treated with the use of local estrogen. These agents thicken the thin stratified epithelium of these periods of life, and in most instances will spontaneously effect a "cure." Particularly in the postmenopausal years, it is important to instruct the patient to continue with a maintenance program of treatment indefinitely, possibly the insertion of the local agent once a week, in order to prevent recurrence of the problem.

Trichomonas Vaginitis

Although the organism known as the *Trichomonas vaginalis* was described by Donne as far back as 1836, its importance as the etiological factor in a frequent and troublesome form of vaginitis was not appreciated until recent years. As a matter of fact, there are still some who believe that without the presence of certain pathogenic bacteria, the trichomonas alone cannot produce vaginal inflammation.

Incidence

The infection is extremely common. In a report of 5712 obstetrical and gynecological patients examined routinely for the Trichomonas, Peterson states that 24.6% of the smears were positive. Bland and Goldstein, and others, have shown that the infection is exceedingly common in pregnant women. Many asymptomatic patients may harbor the organisms as noted by an unpublished study of 100 consecutive patients visiting the outpatient department at The Johns Hopkins Hospital in whom trichomonads were found in approximately two-thirds of the vaginal preparations. These patients may serve as carriers and thus become a source of infection in the male.

Symptoms

The chief manifestation of trichomonas vaginitis is leukorrhea, almost invariably associated with vaginal soreness, burning, and itching. As might be expected, dyspareunia is a common complaint. Although involvement of the urethra and/or the vulvovaginal glands is not commonly demonstrated, nevertheless, burning on urination and at the vaginal outlet create associated problems.

Speculum examination commonly reveals a pool of thin, greenish-yellow, foamy or bubbly discharge in the dependent vaginal fornix. The mucus membrane is diffusely reddened and the posterior fornix often presents a granular or strawberry-like appearance which is almost pathognomonic. Small petechial erosions are seen on the epithelium of the vagina and portio of the cervix (Plate 10.1).

Diagnosis

The diagnosis is made by demonstration of the Trichomonas. The

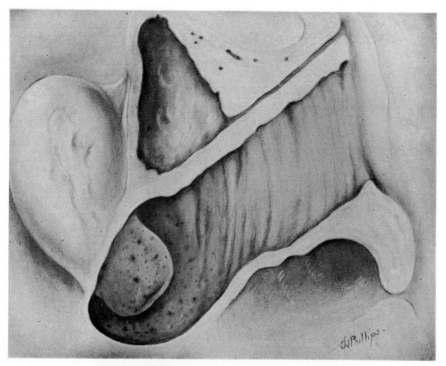

Plate 10.1. *Trichomonas vaginalis* vaginitis. (From Davis, C. H. (Editor): *Gynecology and Obstetrics*. W. F. Prior Company, Inc., Hagerstown, Maryland, 1933.)

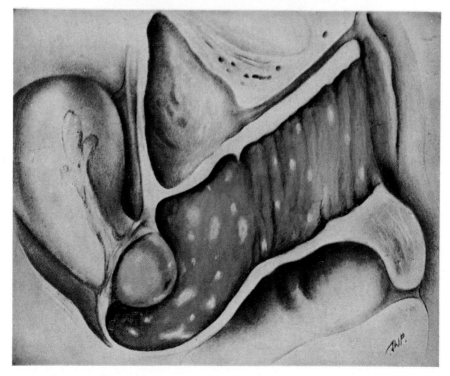

Plate 10.2. Thrush vaginitis during pregnancy. (From Davis, C. H. (Editor): *Gynecology and Obstetrics*. W. F. Prior Company, Inc., Hagerstown, Maryland, 1933.)

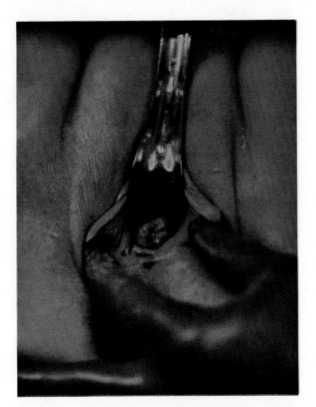

Plate 10.3. A rather extensive carcinoma of posterior wall of vagina

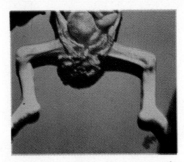

Plate 10.4 Autopsy specimen of sarcoma botryoides in a 2-year-old child.

patient is cautioned to take no douche on the day of examination. A bivalve speculum is introduced without the use of a lubricant, as this destroys the activity of the parasite. A drop of pus is taken and a smear is then made on a warm slide, using normal saline solution to dilute the pus and to avoid too rapid drying out of the smear. A cover glass may be used, but is not essential.

The slide is examined under moderately high power, part of the illumination being cut off. The organisms, when present, are readily recognizable as motile, pear-shaped parasites, with long flagellae at the narrow end, and with an undulating cell membrane. They are intermediate in size between the ordinary pus cells and the pavement epithelial cells which are found in practically all vaginal smears. The active movements of the flagellae are readily seen, but must be distinguished from sperm (Fig. 10.1).

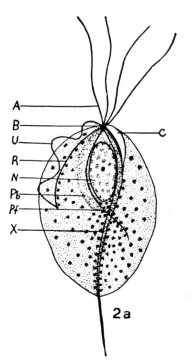

10.1. Trichomonas vaginalis. *A*, four anterior flagella; *B*, blepharoplast; *U*, undulating membrane; *R*, chromatic basal rod; *N*, nucleus; *Pb*, parabasal body; *Pf*, parabasal fibril; *X* cytostome. (From Davis, C. H. (Editor): *Gynecology and Obstetrics*. W. F. Prior Company, Inc., Hagerstown, Maryland, 1933.)

Methods of Infection

The source of vaginal infection with trichomonas has been discussed ad infinitum and possible contaminations from the rectum, bath water, towels, and a variety of instruments have been considered as potential sources of the infection. Nevertheless, at present, the evidence that the organisms are transmitted through coitus is convincing.

Treatment

In view of the frequency of the infection and of recurrences, a tremendous variety of therapies have been proposed. Basically, these have been designed to increase the acidity of the vagina, appreciating that, with the normal pH of 4.5 to 5, the trichomonas does not survive. Preparations promoting the growth of lactobacilli (Butabs) and acidifying agents such as picric acid suppositories have been used over the years with various degrees of success dependent largely on the patient's activity with the cleansing agent. Agents which are toxic to the trichomonas such as systemic antimony and arsenicals such as carbarsone, acetarsone and Devegan enjoyed some degrees of success in the past as has the local agent Tricofuron.

In recent years, metronidazide or Flagyl has proven to be a most effective trichomonacide. The usual dosage is 250 mg. three times a day by mouth for 10 days. It should go without saying that since this disease is transmitted by sexual contact, the partner or partners must be treated with the patient, particularly if recurrences develop. Certainly, there is no possibility of eliminating any venereal disease without treatment of the source.

Treatment in Pregnancy

As already mentioned, trichomonas infection is extremely common in pregnant women. At the present moment, there is no evidence that Flagyl will produce any abnormality in the fetus. Nevertheless, it has generally been proposed that this agent not be used during the first three months of pregnancy. As a result, it is more common to use a variety of local agents during this period of time along with cleanliness and protection of the patient during coitus. The condom probably is as satisfactory as any agent to accomplish this result. The methods of treatment are essentially the same as in the nonpregnant condition, and they can be carried out with safety until the last month of pregnancy, when they should be discontinued. The discontinuance of douches as early as possible seems advisable.

Mycotic Vaginitis (Fungous or Monilial Vaginitis)

As with trichomonas infection, the frequency and importance of the mycotic form has been recognized only in recent years. Hesseltine states that about 10% of nonpregnant women who complain of vaginal discharge harbor fungi of the yeast group, and that in about one-third of pregnant women such fungi are to be found in the vagina, although only a small proportion have symptoms sufficiently troublesome to seek medical relief. The vulvovaginal inflammation so often seen in diabetes is usually due to the presence of fungi which thrive in the presence of the carbohydrate-rich environment characterizing that disease. It is most common in postmenopausal women.

The organisms responsible for this type of infection are fungi of the yeast group, similar to those which so often produce thrush in the oral cavity of the infant. There is still some confusion as to nomenclature, and various names are applied to the causative organism, *viz., Monilia albicans, Saccharomyces albicans, Oidium albicans,* but it is usually believed that the *Candida albicans* is the one most commonly involved.

Symptoms

The disease is characterized by a discharge which varies between a thin watery to a thick purulent character, pruritus which may be intense, local irritation, and marked reddening of the entire vaginal or vulvovaginal mucous membrane. In addition, there are often thrushlike patches on the vagina, vulva, or both (Plate 10.2). When the vulva is extensively involved, its surface may show large whitish or graying areas of the aphthous deposit, and itching may be exceedingly distressing, so that scratch marks are often present.

Diagnosis

Although the above described clinical picture should at once suggest the probability of the mycotic etiology, the diagnosis is made positive by microscopic demonstration of the fungi. A smear is made from the exudate, and this is stained with the Gram stain. The fungi appear in the form of long threadlike fibers or mycelia, to which are attached the tiny buds or conidia. For confirmation, the organism may be cultured on Sabouraud's or Nickerson's medium (Fig. 10.2).

Methods of Infection

As with Trichomonas, the mode of contamination is rarely clearly explainable, although it seems certain that dissemination is by means of the hands, towels, coitus, clothing, bath water, or instruments. The organism grows readily in moist atmospheres and at a pH of more than 5. Thus the Lactobacillus is almost routinely absent in smear with Monilia. Furthermore, the use of systemic or local antibiotics promote the growth of this agent since the normal flora of the vagina is often destroyed by these medications.

Treatment

Gentian violet has been the most commonly used agent over the years and had become almost "specific" for such infections. It is still a most effective but messy agent; side reactions are not uncommon; however, particularly at the introitus some denudation of the epithelium may occur with rather severe soreness and irritation. More recently, various fungicides have been introduced into the market and Mycostatin has proven to be one of the more effective agents. It should be appreciated that in general the treatment of monilial infections is not complete under three months since recurrences pre- or postmenstrually

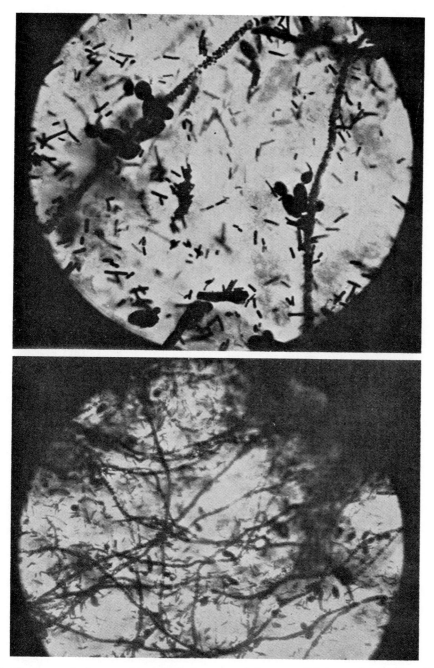

10.2. Monilia in a vaginal smear. *Above,* high-dry power; *below,* mycelial forms with budding elements as well as other organisms (oil immersion). (From Plass, E. D.: In *Gynecology and Obstetrics,* edited by C. H. Davis. W. F. Prior Company, Inc., Hagerstown, Maryland, 1933.)

are frequent in view of the alterations in the pH of the vagina. It is recommended that the agent be used through at least three cycles and on a most rigid program during the intermenstrual period, possibly once to twice a week. Mycolog cream is effective to reduce the local reactive vulvar irritation and itching. Candeptin has also been an effective agent in the treatment of the persistent or recurrent problems.

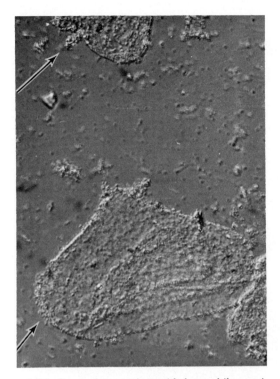

10.3. Smear from patient with hemophilus vaginalis vaginitis. Note the absence of lactobaccili and the paucity of pus cells. *Arrows* denote the accumulation of organisms at the edge of the epithelial cell—"clue" cells.

Haemophilus vaginalis Vaginitis

This agent as a sole or contributory cause to vaginitis has been noted by Gardner and Dukes (1955), Brewer, Halpern, and Thomas (1957), and others. Culture is taken with the use of Casman's blood agar medium as well as thioglycolate broth. The organism may be grown and identified. Possibly the most important diagnostic test is the simple vaginal smear. In the usual preparation, the common organisms may be appreciated, particularly the Lactobacillus. In the preparation from the patient with Haemophilus infection, the lactobacilli are almost routinely absent and number of other organisms are reduced greatly as are the numbers of "pus cells." The Haemophilus, being a nonmotile, short gram-negative bacillus, agglutinates to the epithelial cells to form the so-called "clue cells." In the preparation, these groups of cells are noted along the epithelial border in large or small nests, almost appearing as "whiskers." Careful survey of the slide will make the diagnosis in a majority of cases (Fig. 10.3).

In cases of haemophilus infection, the patient usually complains of an offensive discharge with little or no discomfort or itching. Inspection of the vagina frequently reveals local evidence of infection in the epithelium and a very slight creamy discharge. In view of the absence of any dramatic physical signs such as noted with the trichomonas or mycotic infections, it becomes imperative to make a careful study of the smear for the classic organism and the "clue" cells.

Treatment

Haemophilus vaginalis vaginitis commonly responds to local therapy with sulfonamides. Triple sulfa cream used over a protracted period of time, at least three to four weeks, will frequently give relief of the symptoms. Conversely, about one-half of the cases seem to resist this therapy. Terramycin suppositories have been used effectively, particularly by Gardner and his colleagues, although, as noted by Brewer, there may be a resultant mycotic infection. Sterisil vaginal jell has been recommended by some observers. In a majority of cases, however, triple sulfa cream intravaginally and ampicillin, 500 mg. q. 6 hours for 5 days, will give usually excellent results. Since *Haemophilus vaginalis* vaginitis is classified as a venereal disease, all contacts of the patient must be treated in order to prevent recurrences.

Herpetic Vaginitis

Herpetic infections of the vulva are well documented and recent years have seen a tremendous increase both in the frequency of the disease and the diagnosed cases. The part that such infections may play in the development of cervical neoplasia has furthered interest in the disease process. A final concern has been the possibility that delivery of the fetus through an infected "birth canal" may lead to viremia in the newborn with a variety of complications developing therefrom, including neonatal death.

In spite of these advances in knowledge of the disease entity, little attention has been paid to the vaginal lesion. Nevertheless there are those investigators who feel that Type II herpes simplex viral infections of the vaginal and cervical epithelia are as common, if not more so, than those of the vulvar skin.

There are commonly no symptoms related directly to the vaginal lesions of herpes, although a nonspecific discharge may be present. Nevertheless close inspection of the vagina in such cases, particularly those who have vulvar herpes, will reveal numerous tiny, serpiginous ulcerations classic of those present on the vulva. On rare occasions deeper, phagadenic ulcers may develop.

The diagnosis is usually made by thorough inspection of the vagina in the patient who has vulvar lesions. The vaginal smear may demonstrate the presence of acidophilic nuclear inclusions since herpes is a DNA virus. The more dramatic "multinucleate" cell, also containing intranuclear material, is less commonly noted.

Basically the disease is transmitted by sexual contact, thus the patient's partner may also have evidence of such lesions on the foreskin or glans penis. The incubation period may be as short as 48 to 72 hours, thus contacts can usually be established.

Treatment for the vaginal lesions is difficult due to inaccessibility of light for use of the tricyclic dyes which have been generally effective in treatment of the vulvar disease. Furthermore the lesions are seldom symptomatic. Nevertheless it is important to make the diagnosis in view of the danger to the fetus should the patient be pregnant. With a positive diagnosis, cesarean section should be considered as the safest route for delivery of the child. Finally, careful follow-up is important if this disease is found to be related to the future development of neoplasia in the lower genital canal.

Gonorrheal Vulvovaginitis in Children

Although the histological structure of the adult vagina, with its many layers of squamous epithelium and its lack of glands, protects it from the attacks of the Gonococcus, this is not true of the immature vagina of the young child, with its thin mucous membrane covered with only a few layers of epithelial cells. Gonorrheal vaginitis, while not common in recent years, should always be considered in the differential diagnosis of the child with vaginitis.

Mode of Infection

The disease is spread through contact with infected persons, often other children. Although the method of spread can by proper investigation be explained in some cases, in many others this may be altogether impossible. In institutions like school, hospitals, or children's homes, the disease used to assume epidemic proportions. In a certain proportion of cases the infection is caused by rape, often incited by the superstition still prevalent among ignorant men that coitus with a child will cure gonorrhea.

Symptoms

The chief and often the only symptom is persistent vaginal discharge, producing a soiling of the child's clothing. There is apt to be considerable local irritation, which may at times lead to masturbation. The course of the disease if untreated is extremely chronic, with alternation of periods of remission and exacerbation, but the tendency is to disappearance of the vaginal inflammation and discharge with the onset of puberty.

Diagnosis

There is no question that many errors of diagnosis occur through failure to recognize the fact that causes other than the Gonococcus may be responsible for vaginal discharges in children. Among these may be mentioned pinworms, foreign bodies, and infection with such organisms as the *Micrococcus catarrhalis,* Streptococcus, or colon bacillus. The criteria for diagnosis are the microscopic demonstration of the Gonococcus, and a positive culture. The finding of the typical coffee bean, gram-negative organisms within the cells (intracellular) is essential for diagnosis. Greenhill states that "there must be more than 10 typical gram-negative diplococci intracellularly in the same slide and two or more within the same cell" in order to permit of positive diagnosis.

Treatment

Until 1933 there were few diseases with as poor a "cure record" as gonorrheal vulvovaginitis of children. Protracted treatment with local antiseptics, such as silver nitrate, Argyrol, or Mercurochrome, was commonly employed, with notoriously unsatisfactory results. The introduction of the estrogenic plan of treatment in 1933 has been replaced by intramuscular or even oral penicillin for three to four days. Results are uniformly good with either method.

Postmenopausal Vaginitis

The atrophy of the vaginal mucosa which takes place normally at the time of the menopause makes it very prone to infection. Frequently tiny superficial areas of granulation or ulceration develop, giving rise to slight vaginal staining. In seeking for the cause of slight postmenopausal bleeding, senile vaginitis, like the corresponding condition in the cervix and corpus uteri, must be borne in mind as a not infrequent one. The most characteristic symptoms, however, are discharge, itching, burning, and soreness in the vaginal region. The discharge is usually rather thin, and it may, as already mentioned, be blood tinged. In later stages there may be contraction of the vaginal lumen, with dyspareunia or complete inability to carry on marital relations.

Treatment

Here again estrogenic therapy is often invoked with benefit, and this should be local unless there is some other reason for oral administration. Vaginal suppositories of stilbestrol (0.5 mg.) or some form of estrogenic vaginal cream, used two to three times per week, will usually relieve the symptoms promptly. It should be appreciated that treatment must be continued, possibly at weekly intervals, if recurrences are to be avoided. On rare occasions, local estrogen therapy may produce uterine bleeding, an undesirable occurrence because of the concern about endometrial proliferation. Nevertheless, this is a rare complication to the local variety of estrogen therapy.

Ulcerations

There are undoubtedly many causes for vaginal ulcerations. However, one of the "nonspecific" alterations occurs in the patient with a total prolapse. In this situation the vaginal epithelium (Fig. 10.4) is frequently keratinized and skin-like with superficial and deep ulcerations result from the decubitus situation. Furthermore, atypical cytologic findings are often associated with this condition.

For the local pruritus and irritation, one may resort to any of the measures described in the section on pruritus vulvae (Chapter 9).

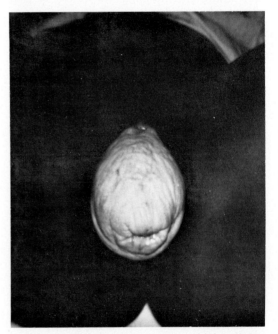

10.4. Total prolapse of the vagina with keratinization of the vaginal epithelium.

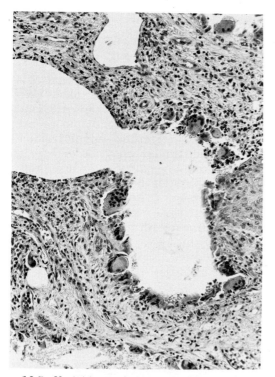

10.5. Vaginitis emphysematosa. Note the giant cell lining the gas-filled space.

Emphysematous Vaginitis

Vaginitis emphysematosa is a rare condition. It has been recognized during pregnancy and with heart failure. It is characterized by the appearance of bleb-like, gas-filled cysts in the submucous layers of the upper vagina. There have been various hypotheses as to the source and type but the only positive finding is the presence of carbon dioxide. Foreign body giant cells are found in the walls of the cavities (Fig. 10.5).

Since the alterations seen with vaginitis emphysematosa are usually associated with other infections, primarily trichomonas, treatment should be directed at the specific disease.

NEOPLASMS OF THE VAGINA

These, as usual, fall into two categories, namely; cystic or solid. Aside from a few rare cases produced by distention of an anomalous blind ureter or of a rudimentary unfused Müllerian duct, cysts of the vagina arise in one of two ways.

Inclusion Cysts

These cysts, occurring at the lower end of the vagina and usually on the posterior surface, arise from inclusion beneath the surface of tags of mucosa resulting from perineal lacerations or from imperfect denudation in the course of surgical repair of the perineum. Such bits of mucosa become encysted, although the cysts are always small, rarely exceeding a few centimeters in diameter. Occasionally such cysts are found at the apex of the vagina post-hysterectomy in the region of the scar (Fig. 10.6). They are lined by a stratified squamous epithelium and the content is usually cheesy (Fig. 10.7).

Gartner Duct Cysts

These arise from the vestigial remains of the Wolffian canals, which, as the so-called Gartner ducts, course along the outer anterior aspect of the vaginal canal. The resulting cysts may be small, or they may become so large as to bulge from the vaginal outlet (Fig. 10.8). They are generally located on the anterolateral aspect of the canal, as already mentioned. Microscopically they are lined with a varying type of epithelium, cuboidal or

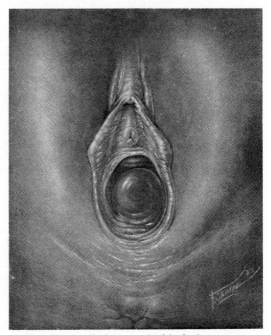

10.6. Unusually large vaginal inclusion cyst.

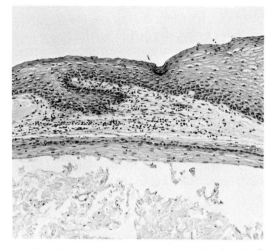

10.7. Microscopic appearance of wall of vaginal inclusion cyst (*below*); skin surface *above*.

columnar, ciliated or nonciliated, and sometimes stratisfied (Fig. 10.9).

Solid Tumors

The most common of the solid tumors is *the acuminate wart.* These have been described extensively in Chapter 9, and most cases of vaginal condylomata are associated with similar vulvar lesions. The vaginal tumors may become exuberant during pregnancy and cause problems with bleeding during delivery, thus cesarian section must be considered in cases of extensive involvement. Furthermore, treatment with podophyllin, so successful on the vulva, may be associated with extensive slough and resultant systemic collapse. Thus this variety of

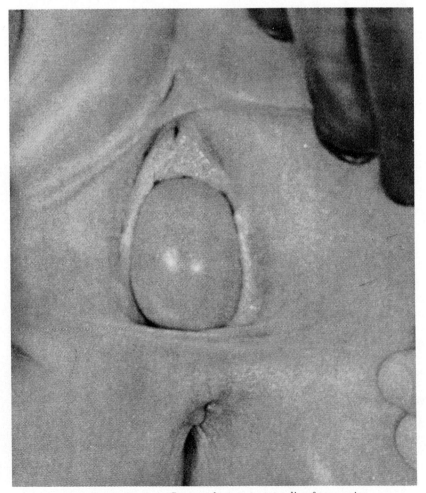

10.8. Unusually large Gartner duct cyst protruding from vagina

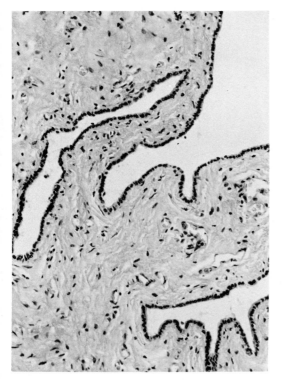

10.9. Low flat epithelium noted often in meso-nephric (Gartner) cyst of vagina.

therapy is not recommended for vaginal warts. Generally it is wiser to treat with sulfonamides and remove the larger lesions surgically.

Endometriosis may on rare occasions occur as a diffuse process and simulate adenosis. More commonly it penetrates through the cul-de-sac of Douglas and may appear as an area of subepithelial nodularity or as an irregular hemorrhagic mass (Figs. 10.10, 11). Treatment follows the general pattern of that described for endometriosis elsewhere in the pelvis. Positive biopsy diagnosis is obviously of importance prior to the institution of any therapy.

The benign solid tumors include the *fibromyoma* and *leiomyoma.* The latter may represent a subserous uterine tumor which has developed extraperitoneally, divorced itself from the fundus, and is finding its way outside.

Adenosis vaginae is demonstrated by roughened areas in which mucus-secreting glands are found microscopically (Fig. 10.12). Congenital hydrocolpos or hematocolpos must always be borne in mind.

Aside from the occasional large growth, there are usually no symptoms produced by the benign vaginal growth, which are generally found accidentally or because they can be felt by the patient. These neoplasms are properly treated by surgical excision.

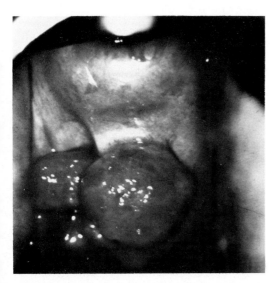

10.10. Endometriosis penetrating through the cul-de-sac. (From Novak, E. R., and Woodruff, J. D.: *Gynecologic and Obstetric Pathology,* W. B. Saunders Company, Philadelphia, 1974.)

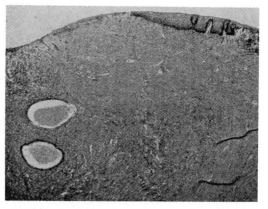

10.11. Endometriosis of vagina produced by penetration to vagina of endometriosis of rectovaginal septum.

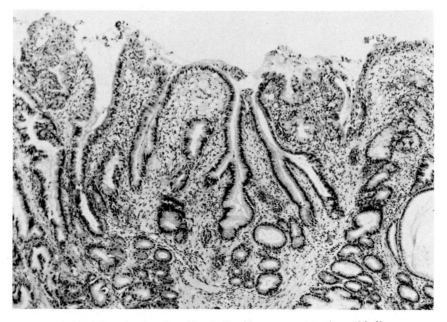

10.12. Adenosis of vagina. Glands lined by mucus-secreting epithelium

A rare form of ulcerative lesion may occur in the lateral fornices of the vagina, in association with adenomatous changes in the Wolffian or mesonephric duct vestiges located in this portion of the vagina. Biopsy of such a lesion, which may be clinically suspicious of cancer, will show in the base of the ulcer the acinous or tubular elements derived from the mesonephric duct. A few of these cases were found in the group reported by Novak, Woodruff, and Novak.

Adenosis Vaginae

An unusual finding in the examination of the vagina, clinically or pathologically, a decade ago, Sandberg has, nevertheless, commented on its frequent occurrence in normal adults. More recently, adenosis has taken on new clinico-pathologic significance with the discovery of an unique malignancy developing in young women whose mothers received estrogens, usually synthetic, during pregnancy. Admittedly this "mesonephroid" tumor has been described previously in both the ovary and the lower genital canal; however, the recent increase in incidence suggests a developmental patho-physiologic altera-tion that is unique. The possibility that the administration of estrogens during the earliest stages of development of the urogenital canal might alter the point of junction between the urogenital and paramesonephric systems and eventually place the zone of transformation lower in the vaginal canal now seems a logical explanation for the development of adenosis. Studies by Herbst and others suggest that the unique mesonephroid or clear cell carcinoma is of paramesonephroid origin and is the result of abnormal placement of these tissues which normally are found above the squamocolumnar junction, *i.e.*, the region of the external cervical os (Fig. 10.13). At present approximately 150 "clear cell mesonephroid" carcinomas have been accumulated by a special registry (Fig. 10.14). The number of patients at risk is presently unknown but probably is well over one million. The incidence of this unique malignancy arising in such situations must be very low and thus, at present, it would seem wise to carefully observe such patients at risk, but perform no ablative surgery because of the difficulty in delineating the extent of the con-

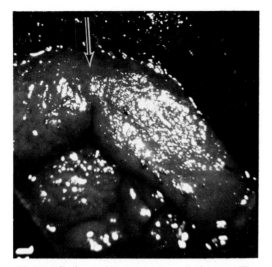

10.13. "Cockscomb" appearance of adenosis. The *arrow* is not at the squamocolumnar junction of the ovary, but well out on the vagina. Vagina is stained with iodine to demonstrate the transition.

dition and the hazards of complications to the nearby bladder and rectum. Future problems may arise at the many new "transition zones" created by the glandular elements in the normally squamous epithelial-lined vagina, and these transformation zones may represent future areas at risk. As Mattingly and Stafl have pointed out, these patients with adenosis may develop "epidermoid carcinoma" at any of the many transitional zones existing between the vaginal, stratified epithelium and the endocervical, *i.e.,* the mucus-secreting elements.

The 150 or more cases of "clear cell" or mesonephroid carcinoma of vagina have been described in young women, generally between the ages of 13 and 25 years, and they have been largely asymptomatic.

It is too early to develop a plan for routine study and treatment of the patient at risk, however, as noted above, most students are suggesting careful observation. Cytologic studies should be carried out regularly but have not been of great assistance in diagnosing the premalignant changes at present. Colposcopy offers another diagnostic technique which could be particularly helpful in the diagnosis of atypical vascular patterns at the transformation zone as noted by Stafl.

Appreciating the fact that the mesonephroid lesions are developing at pu-

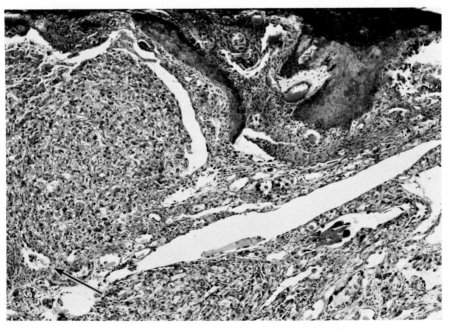

10.14. Vaginal adenocarcinoma arising in adenosis. Clear cell and "hobnail" components, the latter at the *arrow.*

berty when the elements are first exposed to the stimulating effects of estrogen, Herbst has suggested the use of vaginal suppositories of progesterone to modify the growth pattern of the paramesonephric epithelium. It is too early to determine the effectiveness of this therapy; more recent evidence indicates that the results are equivocal.

MALIGNANT TUMORS

Primary vaginal neoplasia is rare, accounting for about 0.5 per cent of all primary malignancy arising in the genital canal.

Clinical Features

Primary carcinoma is usually found in the patient in the early 6th decade of life. Obviously this figure excludes the adenocarcinoma noted above which is found in the young woman.

The primary symptom is, as with cervical cancer, a bloody discharge. Late symptoms are the presence of a protruding mass and pain, the latter usually due to extension of the tumor.

The lesion occurs most commonly on anterior or posterior vaults. It is grossly either exfoliative and friable or ulcerative. Obviously there is early invasion of the bladder, the rectum, or adjacent cervix. Lesions involving the cervix are generally classified as primary cervical lesions regardless of the apparent differential in size.

Pathology

Squamous cell carcinoma comprises approximately 92-95% of all primary vaginal neoplasia. The remainder of the lesions are adenocarcinoma, sarcoma or melanoma, but all are extremely rare. The lesions may be well differentiated (Fig. 10.15) or more epidermoid in nature (Fig. 10.16).

Treatment

Radiation therapy is the treatment of choice in most clinics. If surgery is employed, the procedure is usually extensive involving removal of the uterus, vagina and either adjacent bladder or rectum or both with the formation of urinary or

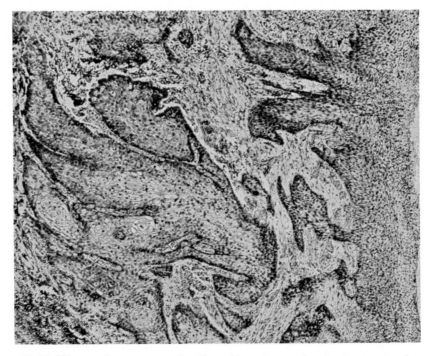

10.15. Microscopic appearance of epidermoid carcinoma of vagina (mature type).

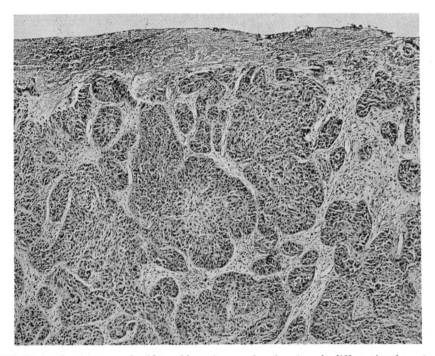

10.16. Another instance of epidermoid carcinoma of vagina, (poorly differentiated type).

bowel diversions. Prognosis obviously depends on the extent of the disease, thus salvage rates vary with the International Federation of Gynecology and Obstetrics (FIGO) staging of the disease (Table 10.1).

Carcinoma-in-situ

As with invasive, carcinoma-in-situ of the vagina is rare. Of interest has been the appearance of such lesions in conjunction with an apparent "regional response to a carcinogen." Thus the in-situ disease of the vagina is often found with or subsequent to the discovery of cervical or vulvar neoplasia and is not uncommonly multicentric. Thus in the follow-up of any malignancy in the adjacent area, the vagina should be inspected thoroughly for evidences of malignant alterations.

Therapy has consisted largely of either surgery or irradiation. The former should be total vaginectomy with the formation of a neo-vagina by skin graft in the sexually active woman. Irradiation is obviously less of a procedure; however, it offers the disadvantage of constriction of the vagina and radiation alterations in the cytologic preparation, thus confusing interpretation. Most recently local chemotherapeutic agents have been used with some degree of success. Longer follow-up is necessary before accurate evaluation of these methodologies is available.

Secondary Carcinoma

This is common, chiefly because of the frequency with which carcinoma of the cervix extends to the surrounding vaginal wall. Adenocarcinoma of the corpus in its later stages may metastasize to the vagina, as may chorionepithelioma, and also carcinoma of distant organs.

Sarcoma

Sarcoma is infrequent but may occur at any age. An interesting but very rare type is the grapelike variety, sarcoma botryoides (Figs. 10.17, 18). This highly malignant lesion was described by Spiegelberg as far back as 1879 as "sarcoma colli uteri hydropicum papillare." The tumor arises from the proliferating

Table 10.1

FIGO Classification of Vaginal Cancer

Preinvasive Carcinoma of the Vagina

Stage 0	Carcinoma in situ, intraepithelial carcinoma.

Invasive Carcinoma of the Vagina

Stage I	The carcinoma is limited to the vaginal wall.
Stage II	The carcinoma has involved the subvaginal tissue but has not extended on to the pelvic wall.
Stage III	The carcinoma has extended on to the pelvic wall.
Stage IV	The carcinoma has extended beyond the true pelvis or has involved the mucosa of the bladder or rectum; however, bullous edema as such does not permit one to classify a case as Stage IV.

Cases should be classified as carcinoma of the vagina when the primary site of the growth is in the vagina. A growth that involves the cervix should be classified as carcinoma of the cervix.

A growth that has extended to the vulva should be classified as carcinoma of the vulva. A growth that is limited to the urethra should be classified as carcinoma of the urethra.

---

tension to the cervix, uterus, parametrium, and abdomen. The disease is almost uniformly fatal; irradiation affords at best only temporary palliation (Figs. 10.19, 20).

The study by Daniel points out the multicentric origin of this disease with polyps springing up at various levels of the vagina. This emphasizes the necessity of total vaginectomy plus radical hysterectomy as a minimal surgical approach to this disease, and a handful of five-year survivors are noted.

Few lethal tumors present such an innocuous microscopic pattern as may sarcoma botryoides. The squamous epithelium may be lifted up into multiple edematous papillae by subepithelial accumulations of fusiform tumor cells. Sometimes these are rather sparse, and since the individual cells themselves are not overly forbidding it is easy to see why a diagnosis of "benign vaginal poly" is made, resulting in an unfortunate delay in treatment. There was in Daniel's series a complete absence of such mesenchymal structures as cartilage or gland elements as are noted frequently in uterine mixed mesodermal tumors, although striated tumor cells were seen on occasion.

Melanoma

Rarely melanoma may arise primarily in the vagina. As one might expect, the

stroma of the growing tip of the "Müllerian Tubercle" and is thus closely akin to uterine mixed mesodermal tumors. There is often close histological resemblance to uterine mixed mesodermal sarcoma despite the different origin.

From a clinical standpoint this type of sarcoma occurs almost exclusively in infants, although a few young adults having a typical botryoid tumor are reported. Actually several cases have been reported in newborns. The characteristic grapelike mass of pinkish, edematous polyps protruding from the vagina is almost pathognomonic. In advanced stages, the whole vagina may be filled, with ex-

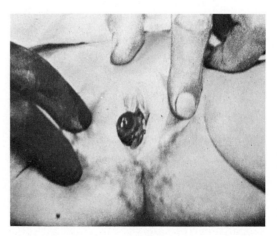

10.17. Polypoid sarcoma extruding from introitus

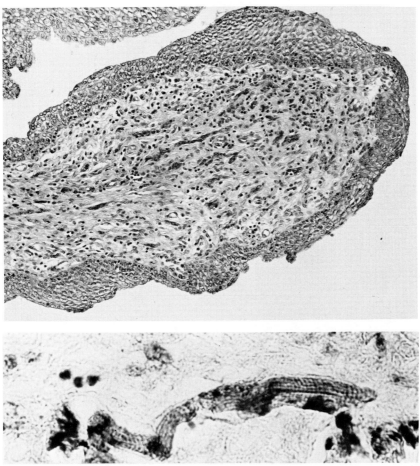

10.18. Composite: (*upper*) Low power illustration of sarcoma botryoides showing polypoid nature of the lesion; (*lower*) characteristic rhabdomyoblast. (Courtesy of Dr. W. W. Daniel, New York.)

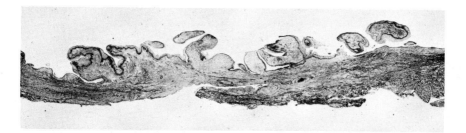

10.19. Low power photomicrograph of a section of the vagina from a patient with sarcoma botryoides illustrating the origin of this tumor from multiple foci (H & E, × 15). *From* Daniel, W. W., Koss, L. G., and Brunschwig, A., Sarcoma botryoides of the vagina, Cancer, *12:* 74, 1959.

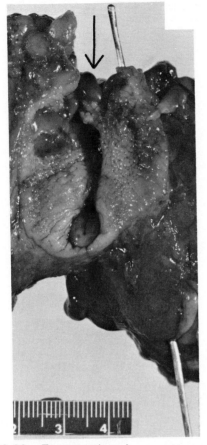

10.20. Extenteration in recent sarcoma botyroides. Rectum with probe, *right*; bladder, *left*; and uterus, *center*. Note multipolypoid-origin tumor (cervix and vagina).

prognosis is poor and preinvasive disease is rarely diagnosed.

REFERENCES

Abel, S.: Diagnosis and treatment of vaginitis, GP, *4:* 35, 1951.

Allen, E., and Butler, S.: Studies of origin and treatment of recurrent trichomonas vaginitis. Amer. J. Obstet. Gynec., *51:* 387, 1946.

Amolsch, A. L.: Mixed mesodermal tumors of uterus and vagina, with report of 6 cases. Amer. J. Cancer, *37:* 435, 1929.

Arronet, G. H., Latour, M. P. A., and Tremblay, P. C.: Primary carcinoma of the vagina. Amer. J. Obstet. Gynec., *79:* 445, 1960.

Bivens, M. D.: Primary carcinoma of vagina—a report of 46 cases. Amer. J. Obstet. Gynec., *65:* 390, 1953.

Boatwright, D. C., and Moore, V.: Suburethral diverticula in the female. J. Urol. *89:* 581, 1963.

Brack, C. B., Merritt, R. I., and Dickson, R. J.: Primary carcinoma of the vagina. Obstet. Gynec., *12:* 104, 1958.

Brewer, J. I., Halpern, B., and Thomas, G.: Hemophilus vaginalis vaginitis. Amer. J. Obstet. Gynec., *74:* 834, 1957.

Burch, T. A., Rees, C. W., and Reardon, L.: Diagnosis of *Trichomonas vaginalis* vaginitis. Amer. J. Obstet. Gynec., *77:* 309, 1959.

Butler, B. C., and Beakley, J. W.: Bacterial flora in vaginitis. Amer. J. Obstet. Gynec., *79:* 432, 1960.

Copenhaven, E. H., Salzman, F. A., and Wright, K. A.: Carcinoma in situ of the vagina. Amer. J. Obstet. Gynec., *89:* 962, 1964.

Daniel, W. W., Koss, L. G., and Brunschwig, A.: Sarcoma botyroides of the vagina. Cancer, 12: 74, 1959.

Duckett, H. C., Davis, C. D., and McCall, J. B.: Sarcoma botyroides. Obstet. Gynec., *10:* 517, 1957.

Duncan, A. S., and Fahmy, E. C.: Sarcoma botyroides of the vagina and cervix in children. J. Obstet. Gynaec. Brit. Comm., *60:* 87, 1953.

Gardner, H. L.: Trichomoniasis. Obstet. Gynec., *19:* 279, 1962.

Gardner, H. L., Dukes, C. D., and Damper, T. K.: Prevalence of vaginitis; study in incidence. Amer. J. Obstet. Gynec., *73:* 1080, 1957.

Gardner, H. L., and Dukes, C. D.: *Hemophilus vaginalis* vaginitis. Amer. J. Obstet. Gynec., *69:* 962, 1955.

Gardner, H. L., and Fernet, P.: Etiology of vaginitis emphaysematosa. Amer. J. Obstet. Gynec., *88:* 680, 1964.

Gardner, H. L., and Kaufman, R. H.: *Benign Diseases of the Vulva and Vagina,* C. V. Mosby Co., St. Louis, 1969.

Gray, L. A., and Barnes, M. L.: Vaginitis in women—diagnosis and treatment. Amer. J. Obstet. Gynec., *92:* 125, 1965.

Hesseltine, H. C.: Vulval and vaginal mycosis and trichomoniasis. Amer. J. Obstet. Gynec., *40:* 641, 1940.

Herbst, A. L., and Scully, R. E.: Adenocarcinoma of the vagina in adolescence. Cancer, *25:* 745, 1970.

Herbst, A. L., Green, T. H., Jr., and Ulfelder, H.: Primary carcinoma of the vagina—an analysis of 68 cases. Amer. J. Obstet. Gynec., *106:* 210, 1970.

Herbst, A. H., Robboy, S. J., MacDonald, G. J., and Scully, R. E.: The effects of local progesterone or stilbestrol-associated vaginal adenosis. Amer. J. Obstet. Gynec., *118:* 607, 1974.

Kaiser, I. H.: Primary carcinoma of vagina. Cancer, *5:* 1146, 1952.

Kessel, J. F., and Gafford, J. A.: Observations on pathology of trichomonas vaginitis and on vaginal implants with *Trichomonas vaginalis* and *Trichomonas intestinalis.* Amer. J. Obstet. Gynec., *39:* 1005, 1940.

Lang, W. R.: Premenarchal vaginitis. Obstet. Gynec., *13:* 723, 1959.

Laufe, L. E., and Bernstein, E. D.: Primary malignant melanoma of the vagina. Obstet. Gynec., *37:* 148, 1971.

Marcus, S. L.: Muüllerian mixed sarcoma (sarcoma botryoides) of the cervix. Obstet. Gynec., *15:* 47, 1960.

McGoogan, L. S.: The treatment of vaginitis. Clin. Obstet. Gynec., *2:* 450, 1959.

McVay, L. V., Evans, L., and Sprunt, D. H.: New method of treatment of *Trichomonas vaginalis.* Surg. Gynec. Obstet., *99:* 177, 1954.

Merrill, J. A., and Bencer, W. T.: Primary carcinoma of the vagina. Obstet. Gynec., *11:* 3, 1958.

Novak, E., Woodruff, J. D., and Novak, E. R.: Probable mesonephric origin of certain genital tumors. Amer. J. Obstet. Gynec., *68:* 1222, 1954.

Ober, W. B., and Edgcomb, J. H.: Sarcoma botyroides in the female urogenital tract. Cancer, *7:* 75, 1954.

Pace, H. R., and Schantz, S. I.: Nystatin (Mycostatin) in treatment of monilial and non-monilial vaginitis. J. A. M. A., *162:* 268, 1956.

Reich, W. J., Nechtow, M. J., Zaworsky, B., and Adams, A. P.: Investigation and management of the patient with vaginal discharge. Clin. Obstet. Gynec., 2: 441, 1959.

Russ, J. D., and Collins, C. G.: Treatment of prepuberal vulvovaginitis, with new synthetic estrogen (diethylstilbestrol); preliminary report. J. A. M. A., 114: 2446, 1940.

Rutledge, F.: Cancer of the vagina. Amer. J. Obstet. Gynec., 97: 635, 1967.

Searle, G. C.: Symposium on Flagyl. Research, 56: 26, 1964.

Sheets, J. L., Dockerty, M. B., Decker, D. G., and Welch, J. S.: Primary epithelial malignancy in the vagina. Amer. J. Obstet. Gynec., 89: 121, 1964.

Stafl, A., Mattingly, R. F., Foley, D. V. and Fetherston, W. C.: Clinical diagnosis of vaginal adenosis. Obstet. Gynec., 43: 118, 1974.

Studdiford, W. E.: Vaginal lesions of adenomatous origin. Amer. J. Obstet. Gynec. 73: 641, 1957.

Thomas, H. H.: Candidal vulvovaginitis. Obstet. Gynec., 9: 163, 1957.

Westerhout, F. C., Hodgman, J. E., Anderson, G. V., and Sack, R. A.: Congenital hydrocolpos. Amer. J. Obstet. Gynec., 89: 957, 1964.

Woodruff, J. D., and Williams, T. J. Multiple sites of change in the lower genital system. Amer. J. Obstet. Gynec., 85: 724, 1963.

chapter 11

Cervicitis and Cervical Polyp

Inflammation of the cervix uteri, or cervicitis, may be either acute or chronic, and may involve the portio, the endocervix, or, more frequently, both. The etiology of cervicitis is usually bacterial, the organisms concerned being the gonococcus, or any one of a number of other bacteria which are normal inhabitants of the genital canal or which are introduced from the outside. In this latter group the various strains of streptococci are most important. Viral, protozoal and fungal infestation may also occur. The gonococcus is almost always introduced through coitus, but the nongonorrheal variety of infection is not easy to explain except on the somewhat meaningless general basis of a relative *increased pathogenicity of the genital flora* in relation to the adjacent tissues, especially in the presence of recent or previous *trauma* of some sort.

Most important in the nongonorrheal group is *childbirth* with commonly associated trauma and minute lacerations of the cervix which become secondarily infected. In certain serious forms of infection, especially in the case of septic abortion, the portal of entry is the cervix, whence it spreads to other pelvic structures by way of the lymphatics (lymphangitis and perilymphangitis) and veins (phlebitis and periphlebitis) of the broad ligaments. More frequently the infection is of a milder form, and entrenches itself in chronic form in the cervix, which has frequently suffered some degree of laceration. Here it may persist for many years, its only symptom usually being a persistent leukorrhea.

ACUTE CERVICITIS

Pathology

In the acute stage, which clinically is seen in most typical form in acute gonorrheal infection, the cervix is reddened, congested, and somewhat swollen, while from the canal there escapes a profuse, purulent exudate, sometimes white and sometimes yellowish. *Microscopically,* this phase is characterized by intense polymorphonuclear infiltration of the mucosa and immediately underlying tissue, hyperemia, and more or less edema. The gland lumina may be distended with an exudate consisting of large numbers of dead leukocytes, desquamated epithelial cells, and mucus.

Clinical Symptoms

By far the most constant and usually the only symptom of cervicitis is *leukorrhea*. In the acute stage this is purulent, and in the gonorrheal type, especially where there is associated urethritis, there may be much vaginal and urinary irritability, suggesting cystitis. During this stage the infection is very active, and in the gonorrheal cases, if no antibiotic has been given, the causative organisms can be readily found in large numbers in the purulent discharge. There may be an associated acute infection of the urethra, Skene's ducts, or vulvovaginal glands, but there are frequent exceptions to this. There may even be a slight elevation of body temperature, with a sensation of congestion in the vaginal region, combined with urinary irritability and burning if there is an associated urethritis.

Acute cervicitis is seldom seen as an isolated condition. Most often it is seen in patients who also have an acute infection of other segments of the generative tract, especially of the fallopian tubes.

Diagnosis

The diagnosis of acute cervicitis must be made by inspection of the cervix by means of a speculum. The cervix, on exposure, will be seen to be congested and perhaps swollen, while from the cervical canal a whitish or yellowish purulent discharge is seen to exude, and, in virulent cases, literally to pour from the canal. The os may be surrounded by a reddish, granular halo. The epithelium of the *pars vaginalis* may present tiny abrasion-like areas, due to the macerating effect of the discharge. Gonococcal smears and cultures are often positive in this stage of the disease (Plate 11.1). Realistically, acute gonorrheal cervicitis is rarely diagnosed until there is adnexal involvement. However, routine cultures for gonococci taken from the cervices of asymptomatic women coming to the outpatient department at Johns Hopkins have showed that about 5 per cent were positive and apparently represented recovery of organisms from asymptomatic carriers.

Treatment

Antibiotics have become the most important part of the therapy of acute cervicitis of the gonorrheal variety. Penicillin is the drug to be preferred, since the gonococcus is one of the organisms against which penicillin has been most highly effective, although certain drug-resistant strains seem to be on the increase. The general principles and the dosages are more fully discussed in the chapter, "Pelvic Inflammatory Disease."

CHRONIC CERVICITIS

This is perhaps the most common of all gynecological lesions, and is, along with vaginitis, the most frequent cause of leukorrhea. While it may represent a residual phase of gonorrheal infection, it is even more frequently due to infection by any of the other organisms found in the vagina, especially streptococci and staphylococci, which ascend to involve an injured cervix. With the continuing improvement in obstetrical care, the incidence of symptomatic, chronic cervicitis is constantly decreasing.

Pathology

The chronic stage is characterized grossly by any one of a number of pathological pictures, *viz.:*

(1) The cervix is quite normal in appearance on its vaginal surface, but the endocervix is thickened and produces a whitish pus.

(2) The anatomical cervical os is surrounded by a reddish area which may vary in diameter from a centimeter or so to several centimeters. Within this, or without it also, the vaginal surface may show a number of small or large *retention cysts* of the cervical glands (Nabothian cysts). These may be translucent when they contain a clear mucus, or they may appear as opaque whitish blebs when the content is a viscid pus (Plate 11.5).

(3) When the cervix has been deeply lacerated, as is often the case, it is likely

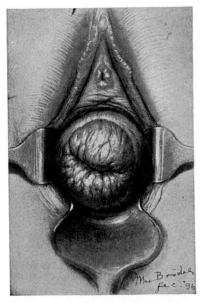

11.1. A classical sketch by Max Brödel of the cervix of a young girl with the squamocolumnar junction located well out in the vaginal portion of the cervix, in part due to a laceration of the cervix in childbirth.

to be large and hypertrophic, sometimes enormously so. Under such conditions the infected and swollen mucous membrane lining the canal often rolls out, much like the lining of a sleeve which is too long for the cloth. (Fig. 11.1). This rolling out may be seen even without laceration, but it is with the latter that the most pronounced examples are seen, to the extent that early cancer may be simulated. The differentiation of cancer from cervicitis by the naked eye is often impossible (Plate 11.6).

Microscopic. The microscopic picture of chronic cervicitis is that of chronic inflammation, with round cell infiltration, often intense, not only in the mucous membrane, but usually invading the deeper structure of the cervix as well (Fig. 11.2). Especially interesting are the changes which take place in the zone between the endocervical mucosa and the original squamous epithelium of the portio vaginalis of the cervix. Because of the congenital location of the squamocolumnar junction or under the

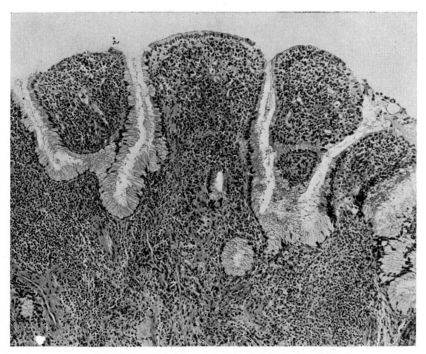

11.2. Microscopic appearance of chronic cervicitis

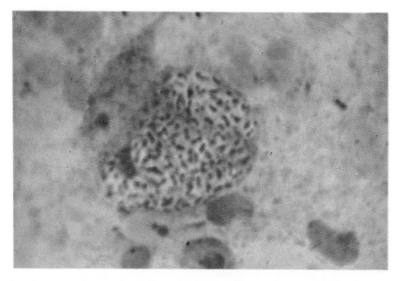

Plate 11.1. Microscopic appearance of gonococci in leukocyte of cervical smear

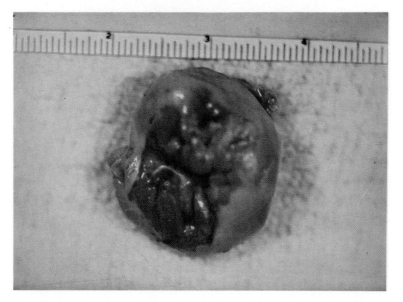

Plate 11.2. A cervix showing a bilateral laceration and columnar epithelium abnormally located on the vaginal portion of the cervix.

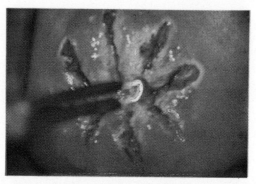

Plate 11.3. Appearance of cervix just after radial electrocauterization. Complete healing usually requires six to eight weeks.

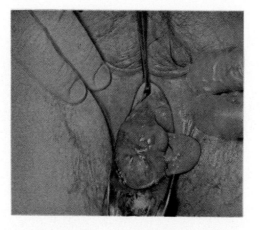

Plate 11.4. Huge bilobed benign cervical polyp presenting at introitus.

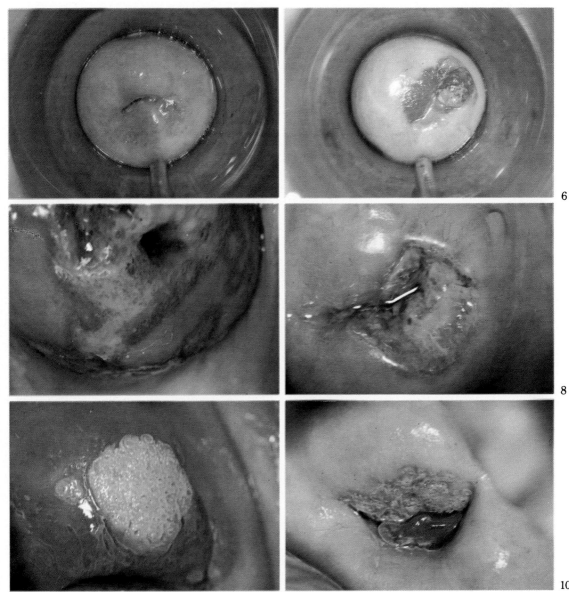

Plate 11.5–10

Plate 11.5. The projections on the anterior and posterior lips of the cervix are Nabothian cysts. They are covered by squamous epithelium, and on palpation are much firmer than the surrounding cervix. The epithelium over them is sometimes so thin that the Nabothian cysts are translucent and appear bluish.

Plate 11.6. Cervicitis or cancer? Biopsy showed epidermoid cancer. This is a stage 1D.

Plate 11.7. Acute herpetic infection of the cervix (courtesy of Dr. A. Stafl).

Plate 11.8. A primary luetic ulcer of the cervix. This lesion is essentially asymptomatic and it is rare to see one (courtesy of Dr. A. Stafl).

Plate 11.9. Condyloma acuminatum of the cervix (courtesy of Dr. A. Stafl).

Plate 11.10. A typical cervical polyp peeking through the cervical canal (courtesy of Dr. A. Stafl).

influence of inflammation a proliferative excursion of the cylindrical epithelium beyond the os takes place, this epithelium retaining its gland-forming tendency, so that glands are found far beyond the os. With recession of the process, a squamous metaplastic process takes place or the squamous epithelium flows back, often blocking the glands and forming *retention cysts.*

The so-called *squamous metaplasia* or *epidermidization,* which is frequently seen with chronic cervicitis or in cervical polyps, is produced during the healing stage.

The replacement of the columnar epithelium by squamous epithelium has been the subject of much study and has great significance in the histogenesis of epidermoid carcinoma (see Chapter 12, where it is discussed in some detail). At this point it is only necessary to be familiar with the reparative process and to be aware that its histologic appearance at times may suggest neoplasms to the inexperienced. In a thorough study, De Alvarez *et al.* have discussed this problem completely. According to their view, the basal layers of the squamous epithelium have a tendency to push downward into the deeper tissue on the scaffolding of the glands which they encounter. The invading epithelium may often be seen forming a layer beneath the cervical epithelium of the glands (Fig. 11.3). It may proliferate luxuriantly, blotting out the cervical epithelium and producing solid or almost solid nests of epithelium far beneath the surface, and *thus mimicking carcinoma* (Figs. 11.4, 11.5). It can be distinguished from the latter by the fact that the epithelial invasion takes place on the framework of the glands and that the invading epithelium lacks the cell characteristics of malignancy.

In a number of papers, Fluhmann also has presented the results of his studies of the reparative process.

In the first place, he noted that there was a marked variation in the relation-

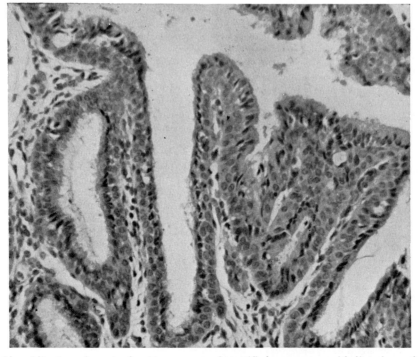

11.3. Epidermidization of cervix showing creepers of stratified squamous epithelium beneath the cylindrical cells.

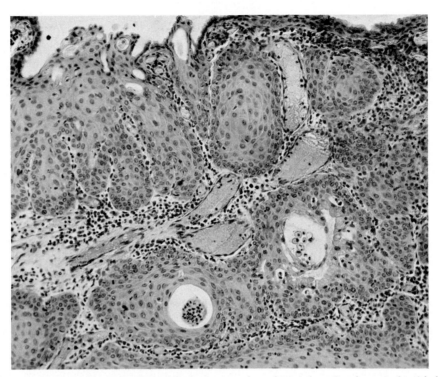

11.4. More extensive epidermidization with almost complete obstruction of endocervical epithelium and glands.

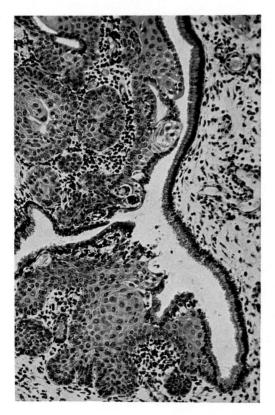

ship between fully differentiated squamous and columnar epithelia in different specimens and in different segments of the same specimen. An abrupt squamocolumnar junction was noted in only 29 per cent of the sections and in 71 per cent there was a zone of transition between the original squamous and columnar epithelia.

The transitional zone varied from a fraction of a millimeter to 10 mm. in width and, within this area, there was a zone of intense infiltration with leukocytes. The epithelium in this zone was composed of cells which, according to Fluhmann, were of groups of immature cells evolving into squamous epithelium. These are the areas of "squamous metaplasia" or "epidermidization." Along with most authors, Fluhmann concluded that the squamocolumnar junction was not a static structure, but that the epithelium was constantly undergoing repair and

11.5. Benign epidermidization of cervix. Note how squamous cells undermine columnar epithelium.

regeneration after destruction by trauma or infection.

There is general agreement on the histopathological picture, as just enumerated, but there is no general agreement on the cell or tissue of origin for the regenerating squamous epithelium. A number of authors, including Fluhmann, have thought that a "reserve" or "indifferent cell" perhaps derived from the columnar cells was the source of the new squamous epithelium by a process called by Fluhmann prosoplasia, and by others squamous metaplasia. A number of others have found it unnecessary to make the cervix the only known exception to the well recognized process of healing as it occurs elsewhere in the body, whereby squamous epithelium, in this case of the cervix, will regenerate from the healthy edges of the original squamous epithelium.

As mentioned above, these matters, as related to the histogenesis of epidermoid carcinoma of the cervix, are further discussed in some detail in the chapter on that subject.

Symptoms

In the chronic stages of the disease the prominent and sometimes only symptom in most cases is persistent *leukorrhea.* The discharge may be thick, viscid, and like white of egg, but it is often mucopurulent in character. Where the cervix is quite vascular, slight *staining* may occur after coitus.

Focal infections of cervical origin may occur, but they are far less frequent than from foci of the teeth or tonsils, probably because of the usually good drainage from the cervical canal. However, the cervix should be taken into consideration in seeking for an explanation for arthritis, neuritis, and muscular pains of obscure origin, although our current ideas are that this will rarely be of assistance.

Lower abdominal discomfort and dyspareunia caused by motion of the cervix may be eliminated by the successful treatment of chronic cervicitis. Such symptoms seem to be due to a focus of infection in the cervix with pelvic lymphangitis.

Diagnosis

Speculum examination of the cervix usually reveals evidences of changes in the *pars vaginalis,* as has already been discussed. Occasionally the chronic infection may involve the endocervical mucosa alone, so that the diagnosis is based upon the presence of a thick, glairy exudate in conjunction with a normal appearing portio. One must be aware that the early degrees of cervical malignancy show no gross abnormality; occasionally an infected hypertrophic cervix appears more ominous than an early malignancy.

In some cases the vascularity or the proliferative tendency is so marked as to lead to the definite *suspicion of cancer.* Examination by colposcopy can be extraordinarily helpful but only *biopsy* or *cytological smears* or both can make the differentiation. It is in this group of chronic inflammatory lesions of the cervix that we have our greatest field for detecting the earliest stages of cancer. Furthermore, it is this group of chronic inflammatory and irritative lesions of the cervix which are believed to be so important as *predisposing factors in the development of cancer,* so that their eradication is rather generally accepted as carrying with it at least a measure of prophylactic value.

Treatment

In former years the treatment of chronic cervicitis consisted in the *application of such antiseptic or caustic chemicals* as tincture of iodine, Mercurochrome, Merthiolate, and many others. Silver nitrate has always been a most popular substance, being used in a strength of from 5 to 10 per cent. Such local applications are quite ineffective.

Systemic therapy with antibiotics is sometimes useful and worth trying, especially in cases of infertility when the infected cervix seems to produce mucus hostile to sperm. In general, however, physical destruction of the infected abnormal epithelium is in vogue.

Cauterization (Fig. 11.6). It is remarkable to observe the transformation in the appearance of the cervix after healing has been completed following

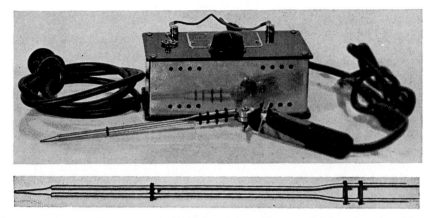

11.6. Cautery apparatus. *Top,* cautery knife of the type used in cauterization of cervix, with a convenient office type of cautery and transformer. *Bottom,* a good type of cautery blade for cervical cauterization.

cauterization. A large, hypertrophic, and spongy cervix not infrequently is transformed into one scarcely distinguishable from a nulliparous cervix.

The cervix is exposed by means of a bivalve speculum and in the best possible light. The vagina and the cervical canal are thoroughly cleared of all exudate, and it should be emphasized to the patient that no anesthetic is required, the cervix being comparatively insensitive to heat. Tenacula should be avoided if possible, as traction on the cervix does cause some pain. The simple method illustrated in Figure 11.7 is of value in protecting the vaginal walls from burning, especially if they are redundant.

The cautery tip should be heated to a dull cherry-red, and strokes of the blade made in a more or less radial fashion about the cervical canal. When the canal is small, it should not be entered by the cautery tip, but when widely patulous, shallow strokes may be carried into the infected and often everted mucosa of the canal. In most cases the cauterization is carried out entirely outside the canal. The danger of invading the cervical canal with the cautery lies in the possibility of cervical stricture, a not infrequent complication (Plate 11.3).

The cauterization produces an ugly, grayish green slough which ordinarily comes away in about two weeks, followed by granulation and later firm cicatrization. Complete healing ordinarily requires

seven or eight weeks, and during this time topical applications of antiseptic creams and jellies are used by some. Inspection at one and two months is sufficient. The patient is instructed to take daily douches (the type is immaterial) to wash away the discharge and so add to the patient's comfort. She should abstain from coitus for about two weeks.

The doctor should not fail to warn the patient that slight bleeding may appear at any time during the first few weeks after cauterization, as otherwise she might be

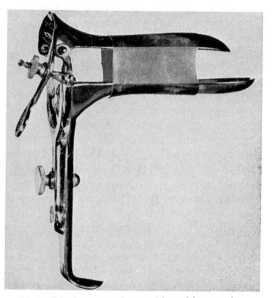

11.7. Bivalve speculum with rubber casing to protect vaginal wall during cauterization.

unduly alarmed. At times the bleeding may be rather free, necessitating rest in bed for a day or two, and occasionally application of a pack.

Cryotherapy. Cervical probes, using liquid nitrogen, as well as other methods of freezing, have been used to destroy the infected areas. The tissue repair, after necrosis by freezing, is not unlike that following destruction by heat. Posttreatment discharge, bleeding, discomfort, etc. are essentially the same as after cauterization. Healing is usually complete within eight weeks. The destruction of the tissue may be more precise with freezing than with heat, and the visible posttreatment inflammatory reaction may be somewhat less. The end result is essentially the same, but the apparatus is less portable and more expensive than a heat cautery.

Conization. Although destruction by heat or cold is the simplest, most effective, and most generally applicable method of treatment of chronic cervicitis, extensive endocervicitis with profuse discharge but a normal appearing portio may be treated by means of the conization technique of Hyams. By this method the entire mucous membrane of the canal is coned out by means of a high frequency electrode. Light anesthesia and hospital admission are standard, because of the possibility of bleeding, but secondary hemorrhage may occur a week or so later.

Such surgical procedures as tracheloplasty (Sturmdorf) have been rightfully almost completely abandoned, although diagnostic "sharp" conization is highly useful in evaluating certain cases suspected of invasive cervical cancer.

VIRAL CERVICITIS

Infection of the generative tract by viruses and allied organisms has become more frequently recognized. The infection of the cervix is to be considered only a part of a more general infection of the generative tract. However, the cervix seems to serve as a focus for asymptomatic carriers of these organisms, at least in some instances.

Herpes progenitalis has long been used to designate herpetic lesions of the external genitalia. Josey *et al.* have described the variegated manifestations which may consist of edema, vesicles, ulcers and, in extreme cases, granulomatous lesions. These lesions may involve the cervix as part of the more general involvement (Plate 11.7, Fig. 11.8). Herpetic infection of the upper generative tract does not seem to have been observed.

The clinical manifestation of the lesion in the cervix is self-limited and endures no more than 2 to 3 weeks. However, in some instances the manifestations in the vulva, vagina and cervix are quite severe and accompanied by considerable local discomfort and fever in the range of 103 or 104°F. No specific therapy is known.

The diagnosis is based on the history, the gross appearance of the lesion and specific changes in exfoliated vaginal and cervical cells (see chapter on cytology). Josey *et al.* collected considerable evidence to indicate that genital herpetic infection is venereally transmitted.

T-mycoplasma and *mycoplasma*

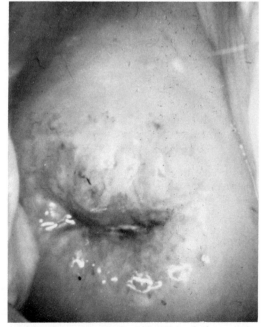

11.8. Acute herpetic infection of the cervix. (Courtesy of Dr. W. Josey.)

hominis have been implicated in genital infections in women, including acute infections of the fallopian tubes. Chronic, non-symptomatic infection of the cervix apparently can exist for McCormack *et al.* showed that positive cultures could be obtained in 65% of asymptomatic women. There seems to be no specific gross clinical manifestation of mycoplasmic infection of the cervix.

GRANULOMA INGUINALE AND OTHER NON-BACTERIAL LESIONS OF THE CERVIX

Although this disease was formerly considered to occur only on the vulva and perineum, it is now known, chiefly as a result of the studies of Pund and Greenblatt, that it may occur in the cervix or, for that matter, in such extragenital sites as the face and mouth. Although cervical granuloma is rare, it at times enters into diagnostic conflict with carcinoma, especially as in later stages it presents an exuberant growth not unlike that of cauliflower cancer. The differential diagnosis from the latter is made by demonstration of the Donovan bodies, which is not always easy, as well as by absence of the characteristic carcinoma histology. Streptomycin is highly effective in the treatment of the disease, as are most of the other antibiotics except penicillin. *Lymphopathia venereum* rarely involves the cervix. Although syphilis must often involve the cervix, it is rare to see a primary lesion (Plate 11.8).

TUBERCULOUS CERVICITIS

This is an uncommon lesion, and is, with a few exceptions, secondary to tuberculous infection in the tubes and uterus, although it may be contracted through coitus. It may bring about a hyperplastic or ulcerative lesion which grossly *can be mistaken for the far more common carcinoma* of the cervix (Figs. 11.9, 10). The microscopic appearance is that of tuberculosis elsewhere, with characteristic tubercles, giant cells, and epithelioid cells (Fig. 11.11). No characteristic *symptoms* are produced, although a mucopurulent discharge is commonly noted. The *diag-*

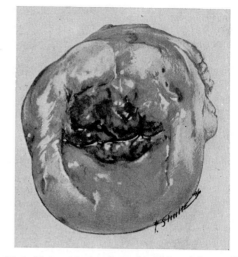

11.9. Tuberculosis of cervix. This might readily be mistaken for carcinoma unless biopsy is done. (Courtesy of Dr. C. N. Stevenson.)

nosis is not difficult if biopsy is resorted to, although grossly the usual clinical impression in such cases is of malignancy because of the far greater incidence of the latter. (See chapter on "Tuberculosis of Female Generative Organs."

CONDYLOMA ACUMINATUM

Condylomata generally involve the external genitalia, are much less common in the vagina and are a relatively uncommon finding in the cervix. However, we have seen a good many instances, including a group in pregnancy, when they appear to be somewhat disproportionately common. When large, excision or fulguration is preferable to podophyllin therapy (Fig. 11.12).

There are some who distinguish condyloma from *papilloma,* chiefly on the basis of the specific etiology of the former, but this is not likely to be demonstrable. Pathologically, it seems difficult to make any worthwhile distinction between the two lesions. For a discussion of the differing viewpoints held the reader may be referred to the papers of Marsh, Goforth, and Greene and Peckham (Plate 11.9).

CERVICAL POLYP

Cervical polyps are generally pedunculated tumors which usually arise from the

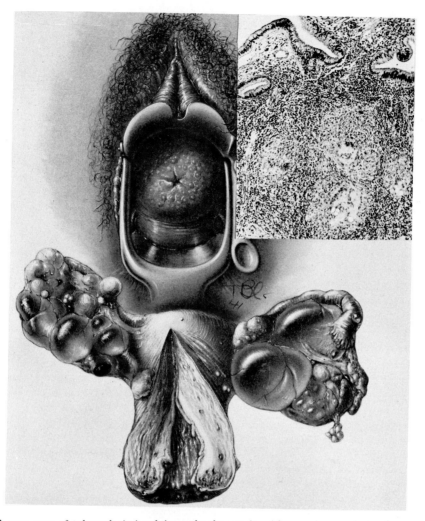

11.10. A rare case of tuberculosis involving only the cervix with no microscopic involvement of tubes. (Courtesy of Dr. E. Henricksen, Los Angeles, California.)

intracervical mucosa, but which may at times spring from the external or vaginal surface of the cervix. In recording a 4 per cent incidence of polyps among nearly 25,000 obstetrical and gynecological specimens Farrar and Nedoss found only rare instances of origin from the pars vaginalis (ectocervix). They are single or multiple, usually of bright red color, and of rather fragile, spongy structure. Clinically they present as small bright red growths which peep or protrude from the cervical canal (Plate 11.10). Although generally very small, they may reach a diameter of several centimeters, and the pedicle may be so elongated that the polyp protrudes from the vaginal orifice.

Rarely does a polyp reach such large size as portrayed in Plate 11.4. In the much less common variety which arises from the external surface of the cervix, the polyp is of firmer structure and paler appearance. Such growths may reach a diameter of many centimeters, and the pedicle may be as thick as the little finger.

The *histological structure* of the cervical polyp is in general that of the mucosa from which it springs. In the most common variety, therefore, the microscope reveals a covering epithelium made up of a single layer of the very tall cylindrical cells which characterize the normal endocervix, the typical cervical glands,

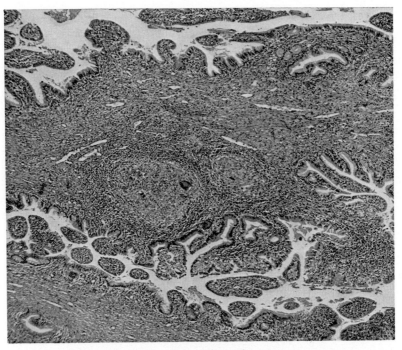

11.11. Tuberculosis of cervix

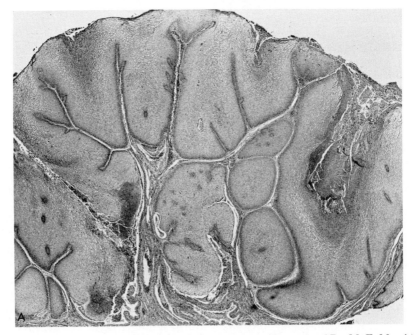

11.12. Condyloma acuminatum on cervix in pregnancy. (Courtesy of Dr. M. E. Marsh).

and a stroma of light connective tissue which often shows much edema and round cell infiltration (Fig. 11.13). Not infrequently there is ulceration of the tip of the polyp which, with the vascular congestion, explains the bleeding which such tumors may cause (Fig. 11.14).

Many cervical polyps originating in the endocervix will show extensive squamous metaplasia, which with superimposed infection, may mimic early cancer. Squamous cell cancer may originate in such a polyp but this is extremely rare.

Symptoms

Cervical polyps are frequently revealed in the course of routine examinations for other indications, and they often cause no symptoms when very small. As a rule, however, the larger polyps produce intermenstrual staining and the contact type of bleeding, which occurs especially after coitus. Straining efforts, as in defecation, may likewise cause slight bleeding. It will be seen, therefore, that the symptoms are exactly the same as one sees in the early stages of cervical cancer,

and the examiner will often breathe a sigh of relief if a cervical polyp is revealed as the ostensible cause of the bleeding.

Diagnosis

Although palpation of the cervix will readily reveal the larger growths, it is remarkable how elusive the smaller ones may be to the examining finger. Inspection of the cervix through a bivalve speculum should always be a part of the examination, and it will often reveal small polyps which have been missed by palpation. It is important to stress that the finding of cervical polyps should not close one's eyes to the possibility of other more serious causes of the bleeding in any particular case, especially if the bleeding is rather free, since such free bleeding is relatively rare with the smaller polyps.

Treatment

Removal of the polyps is indicated, and this is a simple procedure. Where the polyp is fairly large and the pedicle easily demonstrable, it can be twisted off, and the base touched up with a cautery point.

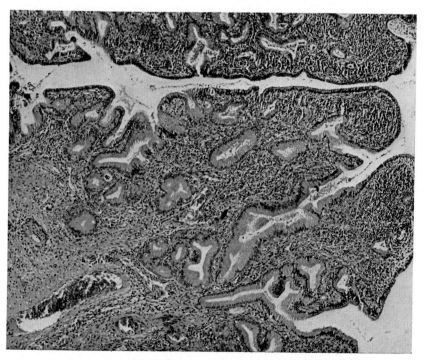

11.13. Structure of cervical polyp

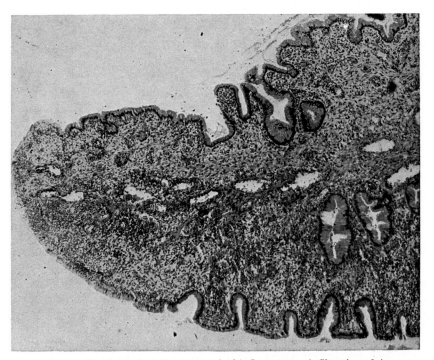

11.14. Cervical polyp showing marked inflammatory infiltration of tip

If they are multiple, and the canal appears to be crowded with them, it is best to dilate and curette the canal very thoroughly. Malignant degeneration is rare but recurrence rather common. Pathological study of the polyp and adjacent cervix should be routine.

REFERENCES

Adams, J. I., and Packer, H.: Granuloma inguinale of the cervix. Southern Med. J., *48:* 27, 1955.

Curtis, A. H.: Stricture of uterine cervix. J.A.M.A., *98:* 861, 1932.

De Alvarez, R. R., Figge, D. C., Brown, D. V., and May, K. J.: Long range studies of the biologic behavior of the human uterine cervix. II. Histology, cytology, and clinical course of cervical disease. III. Squamous metaplasia. Amer. J. Obstet. Gynec., *74:* 769, 1957; *75:* 945, 1958.

Farrar, H. K., Jr., and Nedoss, B. R.: Benign tumors of uterine cervix. Amer. J. Obstet. Gynec., *81:* 124, 1961.

Fluhmann, C. F.: The nature and development of the so-called glands of the cervix uteri. Amer. J. Obstet. Gynec., *74:* 753, 1957.

Fluhmann, C. F.: The glandular structures of the cervix uteri during pregnancy. Amer. J. Obstet. Gynec., *78:* 990, 1959.

Fluhmann, C. F.: The squamocolumnar transitional zone of the cervix uteri. Obstet. Gynec., *14:* 133, 1959.

Fluhmann, C. F.: The histogenesis of acquired erosions of the cervix uteri. Amer. J. Obstet. Gynec., *82:* 970, 1961.

Fluhmann, C. F.: *The Cervix Uteri and Its Diseases.* W. B. Saunders Company, Philadelphia, 1961.

Fluhmann, C. F., and Dickmann, Z.: Glandular structures of the cervix. Obstet. Gynec., *11:* 543, 1958.

Goforth, J. L.: Polyps and papillomas of cervix. Texas J. Med., *49:* 78, 1953.

Goodall, J. R., and Power, R. M. H.: Pathology and treatment of inflammatory diseases of cervix. Amer. J. Obstet. Gynec., *33:* 1050, 1937.

Greene, R. R., and Peckham, B. M.: Squamous papillomas of cervix. Amer. J. Obstet. Gynec., *67:* 883, 1954.

Hofmesiter, F. J., and Gorthey, R. L.: Benign lesions of cervix. Obstet. Gynec., *5:* 504, 1955.

Holden, F. C.: Treatment of cervicitis, particularly by cautery and operation. Amer. J. Obstet. Gynec., *16:* 624, 1928.

Hyams, M. N.: Conization of uterine cervix. Amer. J. Obstet. Gynec., *25:* 653, 1933.

Johnson, D. G.: Infections of the cervix. Clin. Obstet. Gynec., *2:* 476, 1959.

Josey, W. E., Nahmias, A. J., and Naib, Z. M.: The epidemiology of type 2 (genital) herpes simplex virus infection. Obstet. Gynec. Survey, *27:* 295, 1972.

Josey, W. E., Nahmias, A. J., Naib, Z. M., Ucley, E. M., McKenzie, W. M., and Coleman, M. D.: Genital herpes simplex infections in females. Amer. J. Obstet. Gynec., *96:* 493, 1966.

Kistner, R. W., and Hertig, A. T.: Papillomas of uterine cervix—their malignant potentiality. Obstet. Gynec., *6:* 147, 1955.

Kleegman, S. J.: Office treatment of pathologic cervix. Amer. J. Surg., *38:* 294, 1940.

Lang, W. R. (Editor): Symposium on benign lesions of the cervix. Clin. Obstet. Gynec., *6:* 265, 1963.

Marsh, M. R.: Papilloma of cervix. Amer. J. Obstet. Gynec., *64:* 281, 1952.

Martzloff, K. H.: Diseases of cervix uteri. In *Practice of Surgery,* edited by D. Lewis, Vol. 10, Ch. 14. W. F. Prior Company, Hagerstown, Md. 1940.

McCormack, W. M., Rankin, J. S., and Lee, Y. H.: Localization of genital mycoplasma in women. Amer. J. Obstet. Gynec., *126:* 920, 1972.

Motyloff, L.: Epidermoid heteroplasia (heterologous epidermoid differentiation) of basal cells of endometrium versus squamous-cell metaplasia. Amer. J. Obstet. Gynec., *60:* 1240, 1950.

Novak, E.: Pathological diagnosis of early cervical and corporeal cancer, with special reference to differentiation from pseudomalignant inflammatory lesions. Amer. J. Obstet. Gynec., *18:* 449. 1929.

Ostergard, D. R., Townsend, D. E., and Hirose, F. M.: Treatment of chronic cervicitis by cryotherapy. Amer. J. Obstet. Gynec., *102:* 426, 1968.

Pommerenke, W. T., and Viergiver, E.: Cyclic variations in viscosity of cervical mucus. Amer. J. Obstet. Gynec., *51:* 192, 1946.

Pund, E. R., and Greenblatt, R. B.: Granuloma venereum of cervix. J.A.M.A., *108:* 1401, 1937.

Raferty, A., and Payne, W. S.: Condyloma accuminatum of cervix. Obstet. Gynec., *4:* 581, 1954.

Roblee, M. A.: On the etiology of cervicitis. Amer. J. Obstet. Gynec., *35:* 1039, 1938.

Stevenson, C. S.: Tuberculosis of cervix, with report of so-called primary case. Amer. J. Obstet. Gynec., *36:* 1017, 1938.

Woodruff, J. D., and Peterson, W. F.: Condylomata accuminata of the cervix. Amer. J. Obstet. Gynec., *15:* 1354, 1958.

Zondek, B., and Rozin, S.: Cervical mucus arborization. Obstet. Gynec., *3:* 463, 1954.

chapter *12*

Carcinoma of the Cervix

Carcinoma of the cervix uteri is probably the most important of all diseases with which the gynecologist must contend, because of its great frequency and its extreme gravity to the individual patient. Although breast cancer is more frequent, cervical cancer is more lethal; more than 10,000 women in the United States succumb annually to this form of genital malignancy.

More is known about the natural history of epidermoid carcinoma of the cervix than about any other cancer. Invasive symptomatic cancer may develop from the normal epithelium by a slow process which consumes many years. From the time of appearance of intraepithelial carcinoma, which is now generally considered as carcinoma in the true sense of the word, until invasion of surrounding connective tissue by the malignant tissue, 10 or more years may elapse. Even before full blown intraepithelial carcinoma certain microscopic changes in the epithelium have been considered by some authors as precancerous in nature. If these atypical findings be considered as the first step to malignancy, 15 or more years may elapse from initiation of the first changes to

death from untreated epidermoid cancer of the cervix.

INCIDENCE

The death rate from cancer of the cervix is impossible to state with great accuracy as it is only in recent years that cancer of the cervix has been separated from cancer of the uterus (entire) in the list of official causes of death. However, the National Office of Vital Statistics annually gives a rate of about 10 per 100,000.

Of much greater significance are the various incidence studies which have been carried out on population groups under the auspices of the United States Public Health Service. For example, Haenszel and Hillhouse report an age-adjusted incidence rate for invasive cancer of 14.9 per 100,000 for the total female population in New York City. The rates varied for the different social and ethnic groups from a low of 3.6 per 100,000 for Jewish women to a high of 97.6 per 100,000 for Puerto Rican women. Negro women had a rate of 47.8 per 100,000, and other white women of 13.5 per 100,000. The rates naturally vary with age of the population and with the stage of the cancer.

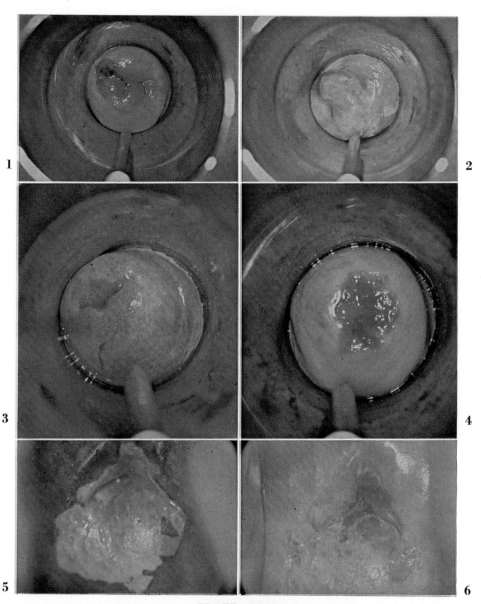

PLATE 12.1–6

Plate 12.1. An abnormal appearing cervix. Biopsy showed chronic cervicitis.

Plate 12.2. This cervix may be described as showing leukoplakia, which is a clinical term. Biopsy showed only chronic cervicitis.

Plate 12.3. A rather normal appearing cervix. Biopsy showed intraepithelial carcinoma.

Plate 12.4. A grossly abnormal cervix, but a diagnosis on appearance alone is not possible. Biopsy showed intraepithelial carcinoma.

Plate 12.5. A low power colposcopic view of a cervix showing a positive Schiller's test. The unstained area is to be considered suspicious of malignancy. Biopsy proved this area to be intraepithelial cancer. The Schiller test may be used without the colposcope. (Courtesy of Dr. Hugh Davis.)

Plate 12.6. A low power colposcopic view of the same cervix shown in 12.5 before the application of the iodine solution. The prominent capillary network and the ground glass mosaic appearance are suspicious features. Biopsy proved to be intraepithelial cancer. (Courtesy of Dr. Hugh Davis.)

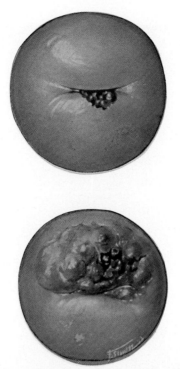

Plate 12.7. Clinical appearance of epidermoid carcinoma in early (*top*) and moderately advanced (*bottom*) stages.

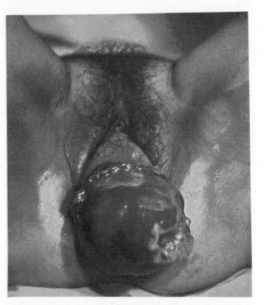

Plate 12.8. Carcinoma (at 3 o'clock) developing with prolapse, a rather rare occurrence. (Case of Dr. Diaz-Bazan, from Novak, E., and Novak, E. R.: *Gynecologic and Obstetric Pathology.* W. B. Saunders, Company, Philadelphia, 1958.)

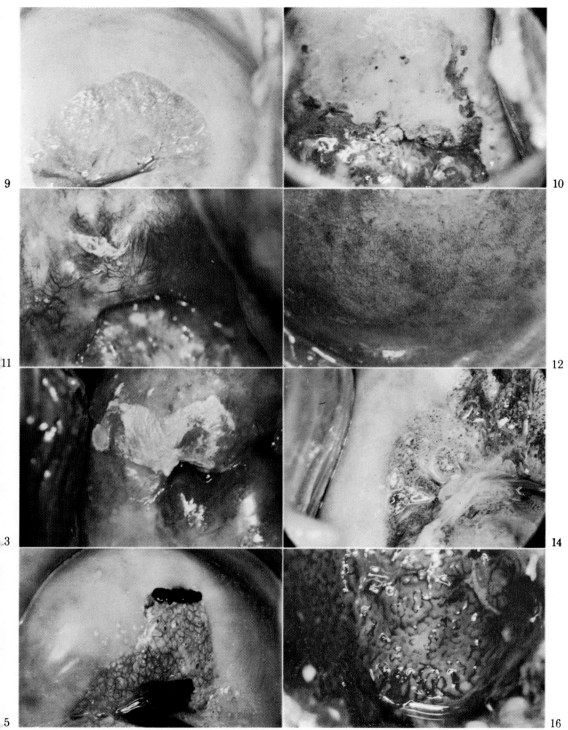

9 10

11 12

3 14

5 16

PLATE 12.9–16

Plate 12.9. Columnar epithelium. Sharp border between columnar and squamous epithelium. Note grape-like structure of the columnar epithelium.

Plate 12.10. Typical transformation zone. Islands of columnar epithelium remain between squamous epithelium. Several openings are visible.

Plate 12.11. Transformation zone. Nabothian cysts in the centre of the picture. Rich vascularity, normal branching of the vessels.

Plate 12.12. Cervicitis. Red stippling dots diffusely evident on the entire cervix, associated with acute trichomonas infestation.

Plate 12.13. Leukoplakia. Biopsy showed moderate squamous atypia.

Plate 12.14. Atypical transformation zone. Papillary punctation. Sharp bordered focal lesion. Directed biopsy showed intraepithelial carcinoma.

Plate 12.15. Mosaic. Sharp bordered focal lesion, blue strips mark the area selected for the directed biopsy, which showed intraepithelial carcinoma.

Plate 12.16. Highly atypical vessels, hairpin capillaries. Biopsy showed invasive carcinoma.

Several screening studies of asymptomatic women have given *prevalence* rates very much higher than the *incidence* rates just quoted. For example, Davis and many others have found rates in excess of 1,000 per 100,000 for intraepithelial cancer among age 30 to 45. The extraordinary high figures are understandable when it is realized that the *prevalence* (disease existing at any given time) rates include all those cases which will remain undiscovered due to the death of the individual from other causes, and all those cases which will become invasive and, therefore, symptomatic in future years, whereas the *incidence* figures given above by definition include only those cases which have become symptomatic in the year in question. Such comparative figures represent one line of evidence supporting the view that intraepithelial cancer exists for many years before invasion.

Many recent publications have stated a changing ratio of cervical to endometrial cancer which formerly was quoted in the ratio of six or eight to one. Webb, Margolis, and Traut noted that in their own clinic (California) cervical carcinoma was only three times as common as the fundal variety, and Tweeddale found that in Lincoln, Nebraska, there was an actual preponderance of the corporeal disease. One must, although accepting the validity of their reports, consider how patient selection in a hospital may flavor the statistics. Novak and VillaSanta have found that at the Johns Hopkins Hospital the ratio of cervical to endometrial cancer was 6.7 to 1, or if intraepithelial carcinoma was excluded, 5.8 to 1. At another local hospital a few miles away, the ratio was 1.2 to 1 or 1.1 to 1, respectively. This disparity is quite easily reconciled if one considers that the Hopkins patient load comprises a considerable proportion of black ward women; at the other the patient load is almost exclusively white and private in nature.

ETIOLOGICAL FACTORS

In a biological sense the cause of carcinoma of the cervix, like the cause of all cancer, is unknown. However, certain circumstances are so closely associated with it that they may be regarded as etiological factors.

There have been many efforts devoted to studying the diverse economic and sociological factors that may contribute to the varied incidence of cervical cancer. All are agreed that cervical cancer is relatively rare in the Jewish woman, and Wynder *et al.* indicate that its occurrence is about one-eighth as common as in similar groups of gentiles. In a review, based on the large material of Mount Sinai Hospital in New York City, Rothman and his co-workers found that carcinoma of the cervix was nine times as frequent in non-Jewish women as in Jewish women. On the other hand, the two groups showed no significant difference as regards the incidence of endometrial cancer. Similar notations have been made by others, *e.g.*, Tennis and Oalmann.

The low incidence of cervical cancer among Jewish women has led to the suspicion that coitus with an uncircumcised male might act in some way as a causal influence, with poor penile hygiene and resultant smegma being particularly suspected, as noted by Fischer. Indeed Heins, Dennis, and Pratt-Thomas have noted the development of cervical cancer in certain strains of mice subjected to stimulation by human smegma for at least 14 months. Wynder *et al.* have published an extensive review on the importance of varied extraneous factors, and are forced to conclude that carcinogenesis can be regarded only as a result of many exogenous and endogenous stimuli. Such factors as mixed sexual partners, incomplete circumcision, and lack of adherence to the Mosaic doctrine which forbids intercourse for one full week after menstruation must always be considered. However, Jones and his co-workers have detected no significant difference in cervical cancer, irrespective of the state of circumcision of the male partner. In a comprehensive report from the University of Madras, Rewell has found the incidence of cervical cancer to be the same among Moslems (males circumcised) and Hindus (males uncircumcised). The supposed relationship between circumcision and cervical cancer was critically studied by Lilienfeld and Graham who showed there was a 34.4 per cent disagreement between the statement of 213 male partners about their own circumcision and the actual situation of the foreskin as revealed by examination. All in all, there is little except supposition to support this supposed etiological relationship.

On the other hand, within the past decade some half dozen major studies have examined the relationship between coitus or marriage and cervical cancer. All studies agree that cervical cancer risk is increased by early marriage or by first coitus at early ages. Rotkin has studied the matter and his results seem to indicate that the ages 15 to 20 are the susceptible period when first and subsequent intercourse predisposes to subsequent cancer. The mean latency period between first intercourse and the detection of cancer was about 30 years. To emphasize the factors stressed by many as resulting from economic poverty, for example, early intercourse, marriage, and pregnancy, Rewell also notes that in India where usually girls marry between the ages of 14 and 15 years, cervical cancer is found about 10 years earlier than the usually stipulated age.

The impression has been held for many years that the childbearing woman is far more prone to cervical cancer than the unmarried one. Unquestionably, the most impressive evidence on this point was set forth in the study by Gagnon, who in a review of the histories and death certificates of no less than 13,000 Canadian nuns, was unable to find a single case of cervical cancer. On the other hand, a subsequent study by Towne of an equal number of celibate women revealed six cases of carcinoma of the cervix, although even this finding represents an extremely low incidence. Wide acquaintance of our own with certain Catholic hospitals, and of many doctors with similar religious affiliations, had revealed not a single such case until finally one did occur. The nun so afflicted, however, was from a certain Mother House which accepts wayward young girls, and direct questioning of this unfortunate although cooperative young woman revealed that her early life had been anything but virginal.

Thus, it is very likely that childbearing *per se* is not the important etiological event, but rather it is sexual exposure. In this sense, epidermoid carcinoma of the cervix may be regarded as a venereal disease.

Epidemiological studies have implicated a variety of other circumstances which are associated with low or high risk for carcinoma of the cervix. For example, a table from a paper by Clyde E. Martin lists several such characteristics (Table 12.1). Epidemiological evidence is essentially and largely circumstantial. As such, common sense must be used in interpreting the information. Thus, the information listed in the Table is quite interesting and informative, but it is quite another thing to settle upon one or more of these characteristics as the cause of the disease. The point being made is brought out in a paper on the relation of tobacco to carcinoma of the cervix by Tokuhata. His conclusions are interesting: "The results indicate that there was a significant association between the use of snuff and/or chewing tobacco, and cancer of the female genitalia, and that cigarettes were not related to the disease under study." Interestingly enough, serious consideration was given to whether snuff and chewing tobacco might have had something to do with the cause. Is it to be believed that snuff and chewing tobacco are etiological agents? No more than it is to be believed that attending religious services of itself will prevent it, as might be implied from the information in Table 12.1.

The epidemiological evidence has, as has been emphasized, implicated early sexual exposure especially with multiple partners as an important etiological factor. This has naturally led to the suspicion that an infective agent may be involved. At one time or another, the commonly associated trichomonas has been under suspicion.

Of more current interest has been the

Table 12.1*

Groups of Women Found to be at Relatively Low and High Risk of Cervical Cancer

Low Risk Groups	High Risk Groups
Moslem women (Kmet *et al.*, 1963; Wynder *et al.*, 1954)	Puerto Rican women (Haenszel and Hillhouse, 1959)
Amish women†	Mexican immigrant women (Haenszel, 1961; Slate and Merritt, 1962)
Jewish women (Haenszel and Hillhouse, 1959; Kennaway, 1948)	Negro women (Haenszel and Hillhouse, 1959)
Seventh-Day Adventist women (Lemon *et al.*, 1964; Wynder *et al.*, 1959)	Inmates of a women's prison (Pereyra, 1961)
Irish immigrant women (Haenszel, 1961)	Prostitutes (Røjel, 1953)
Italian immigrant women (Haenszel, 1961)	Venereal disease clinic patients (Greene *et al.*, 1965)
Protestant and Catholic women who regularly attend religious services (Naguib *et al.*, 1966)	Protestant and Catholic women who rarely or never attend religious services (Naguib *et al.* 1966)
Women of high economic status (Dorn and Cutler, 1959)	Women of low economic status (Dorn and Cutler, 1959)
Rural women (Levin *et al.*, 1960)	Urban women (Levin *et al.*, 1960)

* From Martin, C. E.: Amer. J. Public Health, *57*: 803, 1967.

† Unpublished data compiled by Mr. Kenneth Polen, Pomerene Memorial Hospital, Millersburg, Ohio; courtesy of Dr. Harold E. Cross, Johns Hopkins School of Medicine (Feb.), 1966. One in situ and one invasive carcinoma of the squamous cell type were discovered in the course of obtaining smears from about 1,900 Amish women, as of January, 1966—a rate considerably lower than that found among non-Amish women utilizing the same hospital.

relation of herpes simplex virus type 2 with epidermoid cervical cancer. Josey *et al.* reviewed the evidence which seemed to clearly indicate that the epidemiological pattern of herpes simplex virus type 2 infection was that of a venereally transmitted disease. Furthermore, a number of investigators, including Josey *et al.* and Rawles *et al.*, reported on the high prevalence of antibodies to herpes type 2 virus in the serum of women with cancer of the cervix. However, the association is far from straightforward. For example, in the Rawles *et al.* series, 83% of patients with cancer had antibodies, while 20% of controls who were free from cancer also had antibodies. Additionally, the isolation of the herpes type 2 virus from cervical cancer cells has been quite fickle.

Aurelian, using a very sensitive assay technique, found a 100 per cent positive antibody reaction to herpes type 2 virus in the serum of patients with cervical cancer but also found a 67 per cent positive reaction in matched controls. More interesting are the data of Aurelian *et al.* using as an antigen a crude extract of previously uninfected cervical epithelial cells incubated for 4 hours with herpes virus type 2. Antibodies to this antigen were present in the serum of 90 per cent of patients with invasive cancer, but in only 10 per cent of matched controls. The data suggest that the virus was somehow altered by its contact with the epithelial cells in such a way to make an antigen which was more highly specific.

Therefore, at this moment, it appears that herpes virus type 2 is clearly associated with cancer of the cervix, but if the relation is one of cause and effect, there are as yet additional unidentified factors or circumstances which must be operational to make for an etiological association.

PATHOLOGICAL TYPES

There are two principal pathological types of cervical cancer, corresponding to one or another of the two types of epithelium found in the cervix. It will be recalled that the epithelium covering the external or vaginal surface of the *pars vaginalis* of the cervix is of the stratified squamous variety, continuous with the stratified squamous epithelium of the vagina. Corresponding to this type of cervical epithelium is the *squamous cell or epidermoid carcinoma*. On the other hand, from the cylindric epithelium of the cervical canal arises the cylindric cell carcinoma, which assumes a gland pattern in its growth, and which is therefore designated as *adenocarcinoma* of the cervix. Of these two varieties, the first is many times more common than the other. Both varieties are definitely more malignant than carcinoma of the uterine body. There is little to choose between the two forms of cervical carcinoma as to malignancy, although adenocarcinoma, partly because of its frequently insidious origin within the canal, perhaps offers the more unfavorable prognosis (Fig. 12.1).

Some tumors have been found to have both adenomatous and squamous cell components and are referred to as *adenosquamous carcinoma* of the cervix. It is thought that such a finding is explainable by metaplasia of the cell type into the other. Such tumors seem to carry a more serious prognosis than either pure squamous cell tumors or adenocarcinoma.

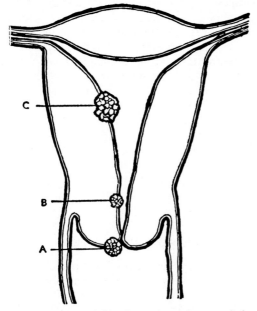

12.1. Types and locations of carcinoma of the uterus. *A,* epidermoid carcinoma of cervix; *B,* adenocarcinoma of cervix; *C,* adenocarcinoma of corpus uteri.

Sarcomas of the uterine cervix are found infrequently. The excessively rare *sarcoma botryoides* may occasionally involve the cervix, but as noted previously, in most cases primary development occurs in the vagina.

GROSS PATHOLOGY

Preclinical Stage

There are no distinctive pathological changes which help to identify an intraepithelial carcinoma of the cervix on gross inspection. In fact, some examples of chronic cervicitis present a more abnormal appearance than a cervix with intraepithelial carcinoma (Plates 12.1–4).

Early Stage

In its early clinical stage cervical cancer presents most often as a small lesion at or near the external os, *i.e.,* at the junction of the two types of cervical epithelium. It appears as a small, hardened, granular area, which to the palpating finger is often slightly raised above the surrounding surface. On speculum examination the surface of the area is granular or slightly elevated and bleeds on slight touch. Sometimes the surface may even in this early stage be covered with a fine papillary outgrowth. The surrounding cervix may be normal, but more frequently is the seat of chronic inflammatory disease, with often a laceration from a preceding childbirth (Plate 12.7).

Indeed, as with intraepithelial carcinoma, it should be emphasized that it is frequently impossible to make a visual distinction between early invasive cancer and such benign lesions as so-called erosions and eversions.

Moderately Advanced Stage

From its original site the cancer spreads until it involves the whole or the greater portion of one lip of the cervix, or portions of both lips. As it grows, it exhibits one of two chief characteristics. The papillary tendency may be dominant, the growth being chiefly above the surface, so that the lesion takes the form of the so-called cauliflower growth. This constitutes the *everting or exophytic* variety. On the other hand, there may be little or no surface growth, the lesion extending into the cervical tissues, producing a very hard, sometimes almost stony induration, although practically always there is some ulceration. To this type of lesion the designation of *inverting* or *endophytic* is applied. The infiltration of the growth may already involve the adjoining vaginal fornix, and the broad ligaments may, or may not, show infiltration.

Advanced Stage

In its late stages the progress of the cancerous process brings about increasing destruction of the cervix, which may be replaced by an excavated ulcerating cavity with ragged, friable walls, so that free bleeding is caused by any but the gentlest examination. The vaginal walls adjoining the cervix are hard and indurated by the cancerous infiltration, and the broad ligaments show extensive infiltration, not only as a result of cancer extension, but also as a result of inflammatory infiltration secondary to the septic ulcerative lesion in the cervix (Figs. 12.2 and 12.3).

Where the growth is chiefly exophytic, a huge cauliflower mass is formed which may almost fill the vagina. In this variety there may be surprisingly little gross infil-

tration of the adjoining tissues even when the cervical growth is very large.

The further progress of the disease is one of advancing involvement and destruction, producing more and more broad ligament infiltration, with blockage of one or both ureters, and not infrequently involving the bladder or rectum, and with often the production of fistulous openings between either of these organs and the vagina.

Distant Metastasis

In advanced degrees of disease metastatic involvement of practically any organ may occur, and liver, lung, brain, and other areas have occasionally been listed as sites of spread. Much more frequent, as noted by Henriksen and more recently by de Alvarez, is the high incidence of extrapelvic lymphatic spread, which, may occur in approximately 35 per cent of autopsy specimens.

For many years it has been known that tumor cells can be detected in the blood stream, especially after some kind of trauma to the tumor. In any case, the finding of malignant cells in vascular channels does not necessarily indicate that clinical metastases will occur; therefore, this has little prognostic value in the untreated or treated patient. Some kind of host resistance or sensitivity must

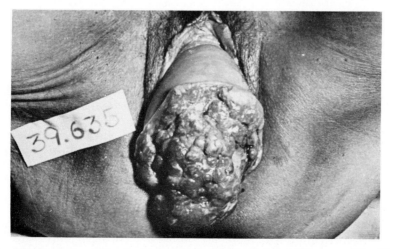

12.2. Epidermoid carcinoma of cervix developing in prolapsed uterus. (Courtesy of Dr. Diaz-Bazan, San Salvador.)

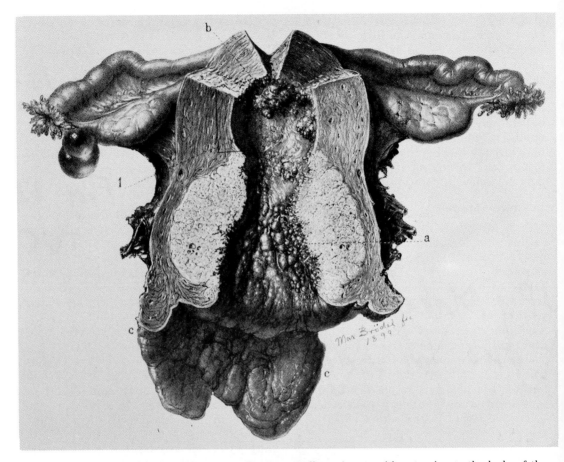

12.3. Advanced carcinoma of the cervix. Squamous-cell carcinoma with extension to the body of the uterus. A classical drawing by Max Brödel made in 1899 showing what would now be considered a very advanced carcinoma of the cervix. The uterus has been opened posteriorly. The growth is sharply defined and has invaded the uterine walls to a depth of more than 1 cm. The mucosa in the upper portion of the uterine cavity in some places has been invaded by tumor, but the uterus and tubes are basically normal. Such a large barrel lesion of the cervix is fortunately now rarely seen in this advanced state. Great progress in the early diagnosis and treatment of this disease has been made in the last several decades. (From Cullen, T. S.: *Cancer of the Uterus,* D. Appleton and Company, 1900.)

exist to determine whether the circulating cells can grow and form a metastatic focus, but it would seem that a transitory shower of tumor cells into the blood stream is not rare in many neoplastic diseases.

MICROSCOPIC PATHOLOGY OF EPIDERMOID CARCINOMA

Intraepithelial Carcinoma

As was previously mentioned, more is known about the natural history of epidermoid carcinoma of the cervix than about the course of any other cancer. In spite of this, the exact cell of origin remains in doubt. For many years there seemed no reason to think other than that epidermoid carcinoma arose from the squamous epithelium of the portio vaginalis of the cervix.

One of the significant findings in very early microscopic carcinoma is the constancy of its origin at the squamous columnar junction. Furthermore, many workers have been impressed by the importance of the transitional zone between the squamous and columnar epithelium.

These and other reasons have given rise to the theory of origin from the so-called reserve cell or subcylindrical cell.

In order to understand the various proposed sites of origin of carcinoma in situ it is first necessary to define clearly the histological zones of the cervix, to distinguish these zones from the anatomical areas of the cervix, and to understand the various histological processes whereby squamous epithelium comes to lie on the surface of endocervical stroma. Figure 12.4 is a schematic presentation of (1) the histological zones, (2) the anatomical areas with reference to the histological zones, (3) the various normal histological findings in the area of the squamocolumnar junction, and (4) the sites of origin of carcinoma in situ proposed by various investigators.

There are three histological zones: the portio vaginalis (histological portio), the transitional zone, and the endocervix. The histological portio is defined as cervical stroma without glands covered by squamous epithelium (Fig. 12.4). Thus, portio epithelium indicates squamous epithelium of the histological portio. The transitional zone lies between the histological portio and the endocervix (Fig. 12.4, III and IV) and consists of endocervical stroma with glands covered with some form of squamous epithelium. Other authors arbitrarily designate a portion of the endocervix abutting the histological portio as the transitional zone (Fig. 12.4, I and II). The histological endocervix consists of endocervical stroma containing glands with surface and glandular epithelium of columnar cells (Fig. 12.4).

The anatomical areas are considered to be (1) the portio vaginalis, and (2) the endocervix. The anatomical portio is that portion of the cervix lying external to the external os, the surface of which is visualized by the clinician with a bivalve speculum; this includes, not only the squamous epithelium and subepithelial stroma, but also the columnar epithelium and glandular stroma within the area everted by laceration of the original external os and within a clinical erosion. The endocervix is that portion of the

cervix that cannot be visualized by the clinician, lying above the external os and below the internal os.

The relationship between the histological zones and the anatomical areas varies; it depends on the position of the external os with reference to the histological zones. Thus, if the external os lies at *arrow 2* in Fig. 12.4, the anatomical portio consists of the histological portio in

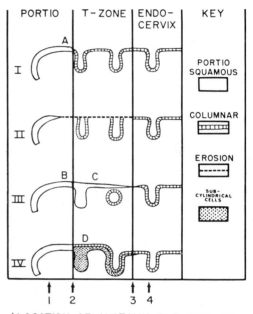

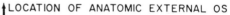

12.4. Schematic drawing of the histological zones, with reference to the position of the anatomical external os, depicting the various types of squamocolumnar junction and the cellular sites of origin of carcinoma in situ. The histological zones are the portio, transitional zone, and endocervix. The anatomic areas are the portio (*to the left of any given arrow*) and the endocervix (*to the right of any given arrow*). The four types of squamocolumnar junction are: *I*, normal; *II*, pathological erosion; *III*, portio squamous epithelial component of erosion healing; and *IV*, subcylindrical cell reserve metaplasia. The four possible cellular sites of origin of carcinoma in situ are: *A*, basal cells of the portio epithelium; *B*, basal cells of the portio epithelium at the margin of an old pathological erosion; *C*, basal cells of the portio epithelial component of erosion healing; and *D*, subcylindrical reserve cells within the transitional zone. (From Johnson, L. D., Easterday, C. L., Gore, H., and Hertig, A. T.: The histogenesis of carcinoma in situ of the uterine cervix. Cancer, *17:* 213, 1964.)

all four variations of the squamocolumnar junction and the anatomical endocervix consists of the histological endocervix (Fig. 12.4, I and II) and of the transitional zone and histological endocervix (Fig. 12.4, III and IV). If the external os lies at *arrow 3* in Fig. 12.4, the anatomical portio consists of the histological portio and histological endocervix (Fig. 12.4, I and II) and of the histological portio and histological transitional zone (Fig. 12.4, II and IV); if it is at *arrow 4,* the anatomical portio consists of the histological portio, histological transitional zone, and histological endocervix (Fig. 12.4, I to IV). If the external os lies at *arrow 1* (as it frequently does in postmenopausal women) the anatomical portio consists of the histological portio but the anatomical endocervix consists of the histological portio and histological endocervix (Fig. 12.4, I and II) or of the histological portio, histological transition zone, and histological endocervix (Fig. 12.4, III and IV). In the majority of cervices of women of the childbearing age the external os lies at *arrow 3* or *4* of Fig. 12.4. Thus, the cervical atypias frequently found in the transitional zone are wholly or partially on the anatomical portio. Once these relationships are understood, it is seen that the cellular origin of precancerous lesions is unrelated to the anatomical area in which the lesion is found.

The normal squamocolumnar junction, in which the normal histological portio abuts the normal histological endocervix, is illustrated in Fig. 12.4, I. In women of the childbearing age, this rarely occurs.

A pathological erosion of the histological portio and adjacent endocervix is shown in Fig. 12.4, II. A pathological erosion is an area in which the surface epithelium has been lost and the denuded stroma is inflamed. The pathological or true erosion must be distinguished from the clinical erosion in which there is a reddened area about the external os. The clinical erosion may be caused be eversion of the endocervix, metaplastic or anaplastic squamous epithelium, squamous epithelium in the process of healing a pathological erosion, or an unhealed pathological erosion.

Figure 12.4, III depicts squamous epithelium within the transitional zone that is morphologically indistinguishable from the squamous epithelium of the histological portio and that is not only contiguous to, but continuous with, the portio epithelium. The origin of this type of epithelium is controversial.

The four cellular sites of origin of carcinoma in situ that have been proposed are indicated by *A, B, C,* and *D* in Fig. 12.4. *A* indicates the basal cells of the histological portio epithelium; *B,* the basal cells of the histological portio epithelium at the margin of an old pathological erosion; *C,* the basal cells of the portio epithelial component involved in erosion healing; and *D,* the subcylindrical cells of the endocervix adjacent to the histological portio.

It has been proposed that carcinoma in situ may sometimes arise in the subcylindrical cells of the endocervix adjacent to the histological portio (Fig. 12.4 *D*). This supposition is based on several pieces of evidence: (1) the resemblance of the cytological features and the morphological pattern of growth of some forms of carcinoma in situ to subcylindrical cell metaplasia; (2) atypical and anaplastic subcylindrical cells in areas contiguous to the carcinoma in situ; (3) the most frequent occurrence of carcinoma in situ in the transitional zone over endocervical portio exclusively; and (4) the sharp vertical line of demarcation between carcinoma in situ and the normal squamous epithelium.

The high association of carcinoma in situ with anaplasia and subcylindrical cell anaplasia suggests that carcinoma in situ may be preceded by one or both of these lesions. The site of the carcinoma in situ, often surrounded by anaplasia, suggests that the carcinoma in situ arose within the field of anaplasia. Furthermore, the position of the anaplasia and carcinoma in situ with subcylindrical cell anaplasia at the periphery further suggests that either or both of these lesions may be preceded by subcylindrical cell anaplasia.

It was proposed by Johnson *et al.* that the histogenesis of invasive cancer occurs most frequently as shown schematically in Figure 12.5. This scheme is an ex-

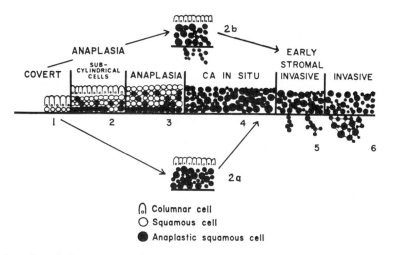

12.5. Evolution of cervical carcinoma. This is an extension of Fluhmann's schematic drawing of the evolution of cervical carcinoma. *Parts 1, 2, 3, 4,* and *2a* are potential neoplastic fields; they may regress or progress to invasive cancer. (From Johnson, L. D., Easterday, C. L., Gore, H., and Hertig, A.: The histogenesis of carcinoma in situ of the uterine cervix. Cancer, *17:* 213, 1964.)

tension of Fluhmann's drawing of the evolution of cervical cancer. A covert potential cancerous field is in the subcylindrical cells of the endocervix, in the transitional zone (Fig. 12.5, Part 1). These cells, with unknown stimuli, proliferate in an abnormal way to form anaplastic subcylindrical cells (Fig. 12.5, Part 2). Perhaps the most common evolution occurs from anaplasia (Fig. 12.5, Part 3) which gradually develops into carcinoma in situ (Fig. 12.5, Part 4), which in turn minimally invades the stroma (Fig. 12.5, Part 5) and ultimately develops into clinically invasive cancer (Fig. 12.5, Part 6). Alternatively, however, there may be a faster evolution (perhaps with an increased dose of carcinogen or an increased response from the host) whereby subcylindrical cell anaplasia is converted directly into carcinoma in situ (Fig. 12.5, Part 2a) or even converted in a relatively short period of time into early stromal invasion (Fig. 12.5, Part 2b).

As was indicated above, not all observers agree with the subcylindrical cell concept. There are at least two problems: (1) the general difficulty of establishing the origin of cell lines by microscopic technique, and (2) the necessity of calling upon an indifferent cell in the adult to provide a cell of origin for a tumor.

The difficulty of establishing the cell or tissue by microscopic technique is well known and has plagued descriptive embryology to this day. While the technique has been extraordinarily helpful and is the basis for most of our embryological understanding, we need only to recall the difficulties in establishing the origin of the vagina, or the origin of the primary and secondary sex cords of the ovary, or, indeed, the origin of the primitive germ cell, which was argued for years, to realize that tissues of origin are established only with great difficulty by microscopic techniques.

The necessity of calling upon an undifferentiated cell in the adult to furnish the site of origin for a tumor is partly related to the problem of the preceding paragraph. Robert Meyer saw the cells now called subcylindrical cells but thought that they were isolated basal cells of the squamous epithelium, isolated by the process of erosion and attempted repair. The use of the undifferentiated subcylindrical cell is quite a different concept from the discarded Cohnheim theory, but it is now customary to think of tumors as arising in adult differentiated tissues. For example, we do not think of tumors of the lung, stomach, adrenals, or whatever site, as coming from some type of undifferentiated cell, but rather of coming from the adult differentiated cell of the tissue of origin. And so, on theoretical grounds, the evidence is not clear that we need to resort to a modification of the Cohnheim theory to explain these matters.

Many workers do not subscribe to the sub-cylindrical cell concept but to a concept of metaplasia of the columnar cells. This view was well summarized by Stafl and Mattingly. According to this view, held by many who are trained colposcopists, the columnar epithelium, established on the ectocervix during fetal development in approximately 70 per cent of fetuses, is exposed to the vaginal environment and, after puberty, the columnar epithelium is stimulated to the development of squamous metaplasia. It has been suggested that the change in the vaginal pH, from an alkaline to an acid state, triggers this change. Subsequently, the physiological metaplasia of columnar

epithelium may progress to complete stratification, or be altered to produce dysplastic or neoplastic changes (Fig. 12.6). The period of early squamous metaplasia is a most critical event for the potential risk of cellular transformation and for the development of cervical neoplasia.

In the absence of a mutagen in the vagina at the time of early metaplasia, normal squamous metaplasia and maturation of the epithelium occurs. This process produces a normal transformation zone and has no abnormal colposcopic lesion. The biologic result of this normal metaplastic process is the production of a well-differentiated squamous epithelium. Should a mutagen be present in the vagina during this early process of squamous metaplasia, transformation of the epithelium toward pre-malignant changes may occur. This altered metaplastic process can be recognized colposcopically by the presence of an abnormal col-

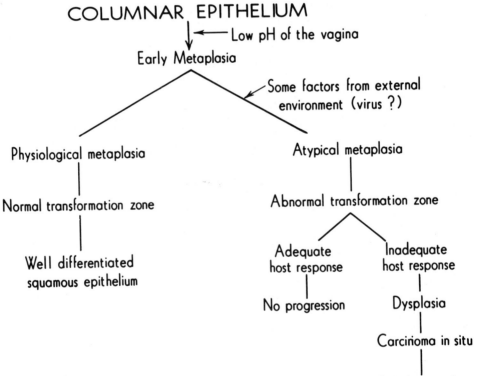

12.6. Diagram of alternate pathways of metaplastic sequence from columnar cells. (From Stafl, A., and Mattingly, R. F.: Vaginal adenosis—a precancerous lesion, Amer. J. Obstet. Gynec., *120:* 666, 1974.)

poscopic lesion, *i.e.,* white epithelium, mosaic pattern, punctation, etc. Although the etiologic agent remains undetermined at the present time, the important aspect is that the mutagenic agent must be present at a very specific time in the life cycle of a specific cell to produce neoplastic transformation. For columnar epithelium, the specific time for this biologic event is during the beginning of squamous metaplasia when the activated columnar cells are susceptible to this transformation process. When this atypical metaplastic process occurs, an abnormal colposcopic lesion develops which may, in some cases, progress to dysplasia, carcinoma in situ or invasive cancer.

Thus, it is impossible at this time to state with assurance the exact cell of origin of epidermoid carcinoma of the cervix. However, there is impressive evidence that the tumor does arise from a single cell rather than from multiple sites. For example, Park *et al.* and Townsend, using women who were heterozygous for the A and B form of glucose 6-phosphate dehydrogenase, found that cancer tissue had only the A or B form. Since the locus of this enzyme is on the X chromosome, the result can be explained by the development of the tumor mass from a single cell which was active for one or the other form of this enzyme.

Carcinoma in situ has been classically defined as a microscopic pattern in which the full thickness of the lining squamous epithelium *must be completely replaced* by undifferentiated abnormal cells morphologically indistinguishable from cancer, although most pathologists agree that some stratification of the superficial epithelium may present with abnormal maturation and dedifferentiation of the underlying epithelium as in the "spray carcinoma," as described by Schiller. Although abnormal epithelial cells generally resemble the basal cell, Woodruff and Mattingly point out that atypical spinal cells may likewise replace the normal epithelial surface. In any case, these cells are uniformly immature and atypical, and there is complete loss of the usual

process of orderly maturation. However, there is no break through the basement membrane into the stroma or the lymphatics. Extension into the glands may occur as this abnormal epithelium creeps into the gland lumina, but there is no extension beyond. Glandular extension rather than invasion is completely compatible with an intraepithelial form of disease (Figs. 12.7–9).

Diagnosis of *early degrees of stromal invasion* is difficult, for buds of tumor may completely replace glands in the absence of true invasion. If the framework of the gland is well preserved and smooth, there is no invasion. If the outline is grayed and hazy, possibly there is beginning stromal invasion (Fig. 12.10).

One must not infer, then, that the *diagnosis of intraepithelial cancer* is simple and clear-cut; on the contrary, it may be one of the most complex and difficult which the pathologist must make. Squamous metaplasia, tangential cuts, condylomata, and other patterns may be misleading, but unquestionably the most confusing pictures are those due to varying degrees of epithelial hyperactivity and atypia. The partial replacement of the covering epithelium by immature undifferentiated basal cells does not warrant a diagnosis of in situ cancer *unless* there is *complete* absence of stratification and lack of mature cells.

These incomplete degrees of aberration of the epithelium are variously designated as *atypical cervical epithelium, atypia, basal cell hyperplasia, dysplasia,* or *hyperactivity,* and many other terms. Their significance is not completely understood, but it would appear that major degrees may either antedate or exist at the periphery of intraepithelial and invasive cancer, thereby exhibiting the same relationship to intraepithelial cancer that this latter lesion does to invasive cancer. On the other hand, minor degrees of these cervical changes appear to be of little significance, for they are frequently transient and likely to be associated with cervical infection or irritation.

A term formerly often applied to abnormal cervical architecture, the

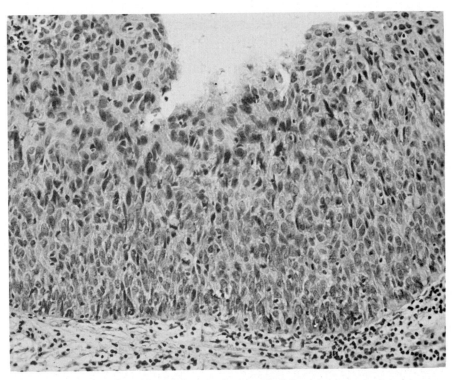

12.7. Carcinoma in situ (intraepithelial carcinoma)

leukoplakia of Hinselmann, with his four-grade rubric pattern, has been rather generally discarded. Actually, leukoplakia is a clinical term denoting various types of whitish plaquelike areas, but neither this nor any other clinical picture is characteristic of intraepithelial cancer or basal cell hyperactivity, which may exist in an innocuous appearing cervix (Figs. 12.11, 12).

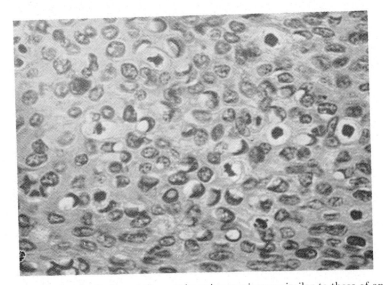

12.8. High power picture of cell changes in a preinvasive carcinoma similar to those of an invasive carcinoma.

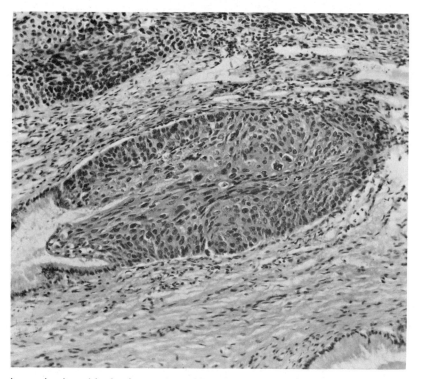

12.9. Carcinoma in situ with gland extension, although this in itself is not considered indicative of histological invasiveness.

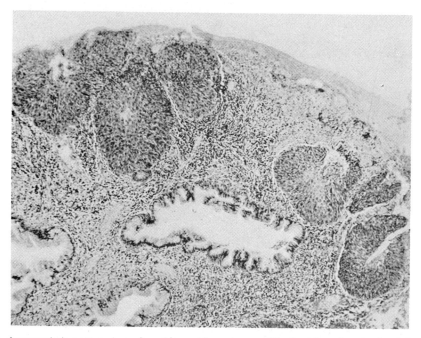

12.10. A characteristic pattern in early epidermoid carcinoma. Whether there is only glandular extension or early stromal invasion is a difficult diagnosis.

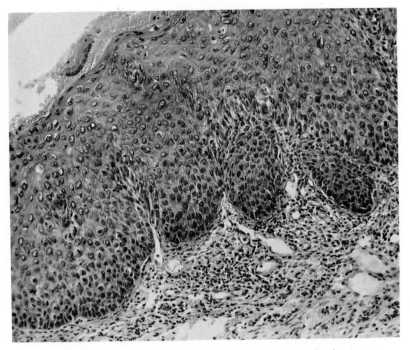

12.11. Rather marked dysplasia but not carcinoma in situ

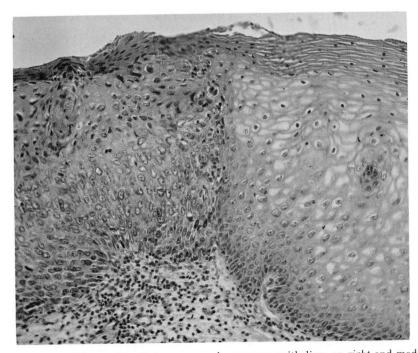

12.12. Definite line of demarcation between normal squamous epithelium on *right* and moderate atypia on *left*.

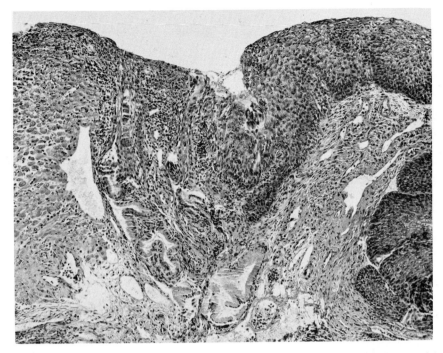

12.13. "Pregnant" cervix; decidual reaction to *left* and markedly atypical epithelium to *right.*

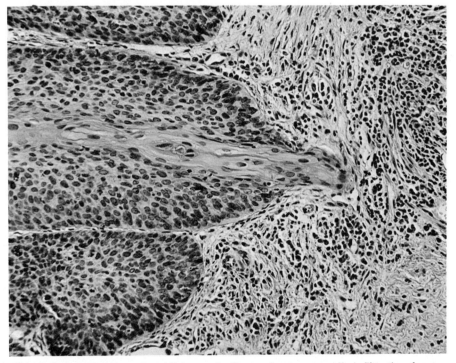

12.14. Microinvasive carcinoma. In addition to the finger of squamous cells infiltrating the stroma from the epithelium, there were nests of tumor cells deeper in the tissue (H & E × 200). (From Jones *et al.,* Obstet. Gynec., *30:* 790, 1967.)

To lend further confusion to an already confused subject, increasing numbers of cases of marked degrees of atypia, and even of intraepithelial cancer, have been reported as undergoing complete regression (Wespi and others). A certain number of these lesions have been noted in pregnant women and some still believe that pregnancy can produce changes in the cervix that may be histologically indistinguishable from cancer but which may regress with termination of pregnancy. At this writing, however, most of us agree with Green, and his associates, who emphasize that, irrespective of a concomitant pregnancy, the microscopic pattern of true intraepithelial cancer is indicative of a real preinvasive cancer. In other words, the pregnancy is merely incidental; however, there is rarely need for haste, and the pregnancy may be allowed to progress to term under careful observation with final evaluation of the problem postpartum (Fig. 12.13).

It may be that an examination of the chromosomes from atypical epithelium will help to determine its neoplastic status. It has been established in a number of laboratories that acquired chromosomal aneuploidy is always, or at least almost always, found in intraepithelial and invasive epidermoid cancer of the cervix, when a direct squash technique is used (Figs. 12.14–16).

Applying the same technique to samples of cervical atypia, Jones *et al.* found aneuploid chromosomes in over one-third of a small group of samples of atypia (Figs. 12.17–19). In the remaining atypias, the chromosomes were either normal or difficult to obtain, exactly as is the situation in non-neoplastic epithelium, which may suggest that acquired chromosomal aneuploidy is the first de-

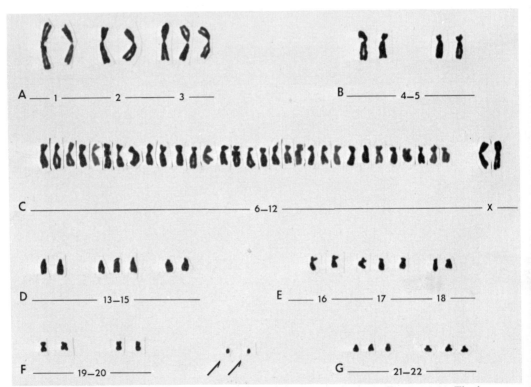

12.15. Chromosomes obtained by a direct squash from the tissue shown in Figure 12.14. The karyotype shows a cell with 70 chromosomes with two additional marker chromosomes indicated by the *arrow.* Such chromosomes may be obtained from no other lesion except carcinoma. (From Jones *et al.,* Obstet. Gynec., *30:* 790, 1967.)

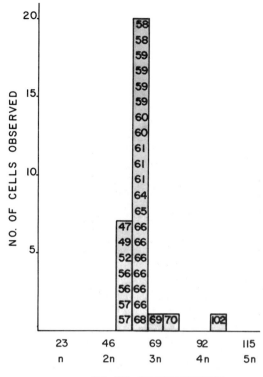

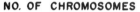

NO. OF CHROMOSOMES

12.16. Histogram showing the distribution of cells analyzed from the case shown in Figure 12.14. Each figure in the bar graph represents the number of chromosomes found in a single cell. (From Jones *et al.*, Obstet. Gynec., *30:* 790, 1967.)

terminable change in the recognition of carcinoma.

Invasive Carcinoma

As with carcinoma elsewhere, the microscopic diagnosis of invasive carcinoma of the cervix is based on two chief characteristics: (1) an abnormal pattern or architecture, and (2) abnormalities in the constituent cells.

(1) Whereas in the normal epithelial surface the epithelial cells are sharply demarcated from the stroma by the basement membrane, in cancer the latter is broken through, so that the epithelium pushes into the stroma, at first in small buds, but later in the form of long columns which grow deep into the stroma much as the roots of a tree grow down into the soil. In all but the earliest phases, therefore, a reasonably certain diagnosis can usually be made with the low power alone, as this suffices to reveal the disorderly and illegitimate invasion of the stroma by the epithelium. It is this invasiveness, with the dissemination of cells by the lymphatics, which is responsible for the characteristics traditionally associated with malignancy, such as local infiltration, metastasis, and recurrence after incomplete removal.

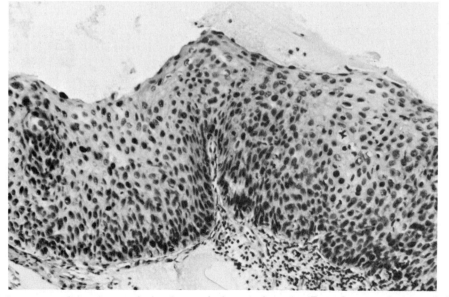

12.17. Low power photomicrograph showing marked cervical atypia. (From Jones *et al.*, Amer. J. Obstet., Gynec., *102:* 624, 1968.)

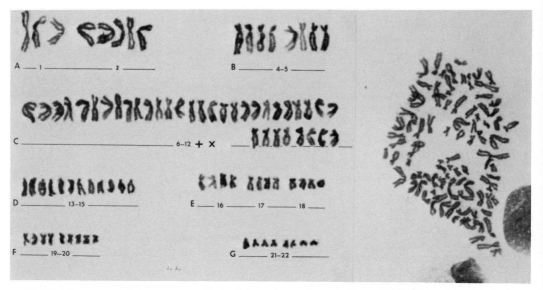

12.18. A karyotype of chromosomes obtained from tissue shown in Figure 12.17 (From Jones *et al.*, Amer. J. Obstet. Gynec., *102:* 624, 1968.)

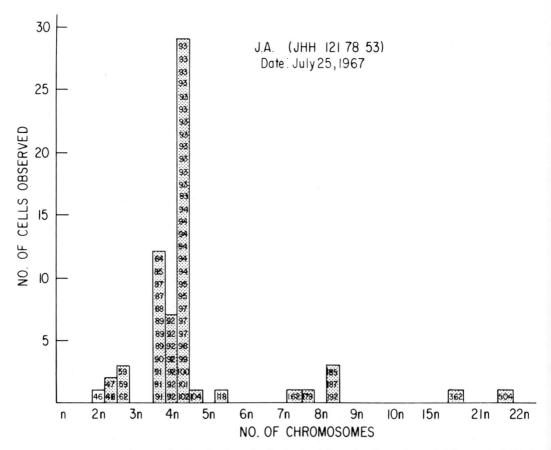

12.19. A histogram showing the distribution of cells obtained from the tissue shown in Figure 12.17. Each figure in the bar graph represents the number of chromosomes in a particular cell. Chromosomes from this patient with atypia are indistinguishable from chromosomes obtained from patients with intraepithelial or invasive epidermoid carcinoma of the cervix. (From Jones *et al.*, Amer. J. Obstet. Gynec., *102:* 624, 1968.)

(2) Whereas the normal epithelium is made up of cells of adult, differentiated type, that of cancer shows varying degrees of immaturity and unripeness. Histologically this is indicated by such features as disparity in the size of cells and nuclei, hyperchromatosis, mitoses, either normal or abnormal, and karyorrhexis.

Our own laboratory recognizes but doubts the usage of the histological classification proposed by Martzloff. According to this, growths made up dominantly of highly differentiated cells resembling those of the prickle cell layer are designated as the *spinal cell* group, making up approximately 15 per cent of the total; at the other extreme, the type in which the constituent cells resemble the basal layers of the epithelium, or even more the spindle cells of fat tissue, is spoken of as the *basal* or *spindle cell* variety, seen in only about 10 per cent of the cases. The large intermediate group, with transitional cell characteristics, makes up the largest proportion, about 75 per cent of all (Figs. 12.20–22).

Perhaps even more popular is the plan of designating various numerical groups or grades, as suggested by Broders. In Grade I the dedifferentiation is least, in Grade IV most extreme, with Grades II and III between.

The significance of such plans of classification lies in the accepted fact that, generally speaking, the clinical malignancy of a tumor parallels the degree of unripeness of its cells. On the other hand, it must be remembered that the greater the degree of unripeness of the cells, the more favorable their response to radiotherapy. There are exceptions to both these rules, however, although from the standpoint of prognosis *the stage of the disease is much more important than is the cell type.*

Again, it must be recalled that most cases do not exhibit a pure cell type, that biopsy does not always give an accurate picture, and that individual pathologists will differ about the grouping of certain cases. For this reason the determination of the cell type is not as important as

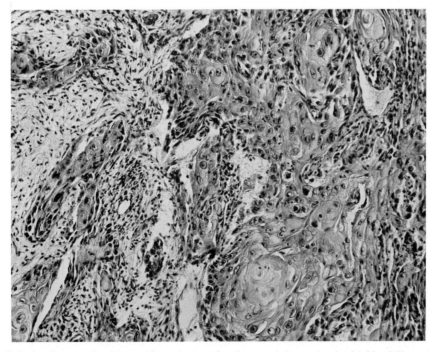

12.20. Spinal cell type of epidermoid carcinoma showing pearl formation by highly differentiated cells, but many anaplastic forms are obvious.

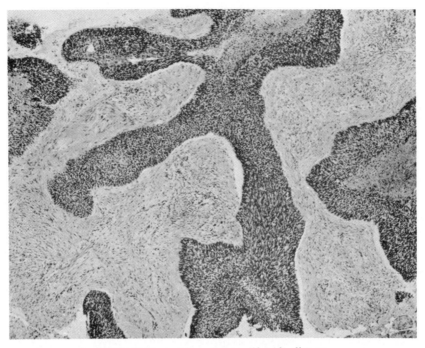

12.21. Epidermoid carcinoma of basal cell type

might at first thought seem, although spinal cell malignancies of the cervix were at one time regarded as being notoriously radioresistant.

The elapsed time from cervical atypia to invasive cancer is of considerable importance and has been studied by a number of workers. From an historical point of view one of the first reasons for suspecting the prolonged duration of intraepithelial carcinoma was the great difference in the average age of women

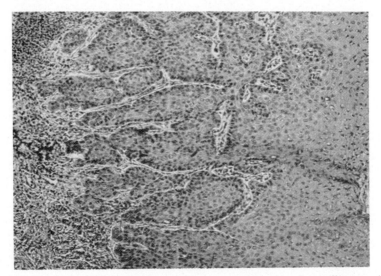

12.22. A very early and small epidermoid carcinoma measuring only a few millimeters in diameter, but showing the same characteristics of cell change and invasive pattern found in much later lesions. This is a transitional cell lesion.

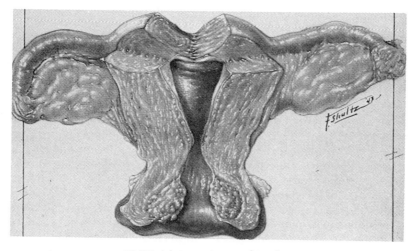

12.23. Adenocarcinoma of cervix

with intraepithelial cancer as contrasted with invasive cancer. For example, McKay, Hertig, and Younge noted a mean age of 48 years for invasive cancer, 38 years for intraepithelial cancer, and 34.9 years for atypical hyperplasia. Many other workers have similar statistics. Dunn, in a study of data from the population screening of 53,585 women, concluded that intraepithelial carcinoma lasted about five years but that three or four additional years elapsed after pathological invasion before the onset of symptoms. The practical and fortunate point is that there is an opportunity of several years duration during which the diagnosis of the disease may be made in its very curable stage.

ADENOCARCINOMA OF CERVIX

As has already been said, cervical adenocarcinoma is much the least common of the three forms of uterine carcinoma, being only from one-fifteenth to one-twentieth as common as the epidermoid cervical variety. While it usually begins within the cervical canal, the initial lesion may appear at or near the external os, and in the later stages it may form a large vegetative growth presenting on the vaginal surface of the cervix. More characteristically, however, the growth produces increasing involvement of the cervix and adjoining tissues without extensive external lesions on the vaginal surface (Figs. 12.23, 24).

Microscopically it is characterized by the atypical gland pattern so distinctive of adenocarcinoma, in striking contrast with

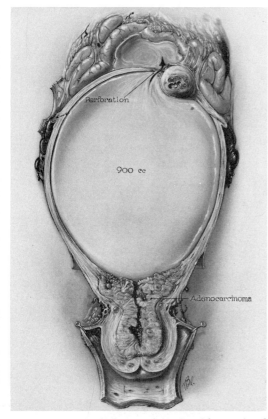

12.24. Adenocarcinoma of cervix with associated pyometra and perforation. (Courtesy of Dr. Erle Henricksen, Los Angeles, California.)

the orderly distribution and appearance of the normal cervical glands. In some cases the departure from normal is moderate, in others the abnormal gland pattern is intricate and highly atypical. The same variations in degree apply to the cell changes. In some adenocarcinomas the gland epithelium may be for the most part of one cell thickness, and many of the cells may still retain the mature columnar shape of normal cervical epithelium. In others the gland epithelium may be many layers thick, and may even fill the lumina so completely that in individual areas the carcinoma may appear to be of the solid epidermoid variety (Figs. 12.25, 26).

On the basis of such variations in the same family of tumors, systems of *histological gradation* have become popular, the one most commonly employed being that suggested by Broders. The least undifferentiated variety is Grade I (often mucinous); the most undifferentiated type is Grade IV, with Grades II and III as intervening varieties.

Adenocanthoma of the cervix may occur as a primary disease or, more frequently, by direct extension from the corpus (see "Carcinoma of the Endometrium," in Chapter 15). We prefer to confine the term "adenoacanthoma" only to *malignant* adenomatous disease with associated *benign* squamous metaplasia which may confuse the picture but in no way alters the prognosis. It is unfortunate that some writers use this term to signify a mixed epidermoid adenocarcinoma. With this dual malignancy, a very different process than our interpretation of adenoacanthoma is present. The term *adenoepithelioma*, as proposed by Way, seems more appropriate and much less confusing.

When adenocarcinoma or adenoacanthoma is found in the cervix it is

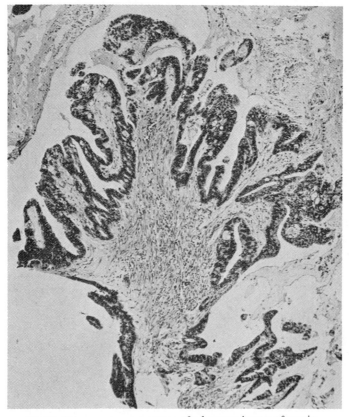

12.25. Microscopic appearance of adenocarcinoma of cervix

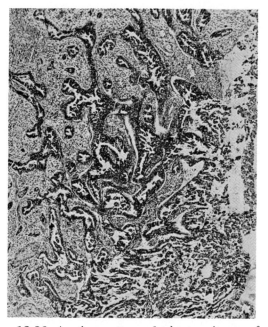

12.26. Another pattern of adenocarcinoma of cervix.

important to know if it is primary or secondary to endometrial tumor. Differential curettage of the endocervix and uterine cavity is frequently helpful. If it seems likely that the cervix is the primary site of the adenocarcinoma, our policy is to treat as epidermoid cancer. Should the cervical adenocarcinoma be secondary to fundal disease, we irradiate both cervix and endometrium and later perform a hysterectomy.

A rare variety of cervical adenocarcinoma has its *origin from the tubular or glandlike mesonephric vestiges* which may at times be noted deep in the cervical structure, as described in Chapter 1. The adenocarcinoma arising from these elements may show no connection with the endocervix, and microscopically it may be characterized by a rather tubular pattern. Carcinomas of the cervix which occur in children are exclusively of this variety.

CARCINOMA OF CERVICAL STUMP

With the contemporary use of total hysterectomy, this is becoming an increasingly less common gynecological problem, although it is by no means rare to see such cases today. In close to 50 per cent of patients with malignancy of the cervical stump the disease is detected less than a year after subtotal hysterectomy, making it appear probable that the cancer was present at the time of the incomplete and inadequately studied hysterectomy. Routine preoperative biopsy or smear of all cases where only a subtotal operation seems possible (as is very rarely necessary) or similar routine study of a preserved cervix might lead to detection of this "coincidental cancer."

Cancer of the stump has acquired a reputation for being unusually difficult to treat and attended by a poor prognosis. In our experience this stigma is not deserved if treatment is modified to fit the individual (see "Treatment"). Salvage is just as good, and complications no more frequent. Actually it seems that the woman who has had a subtotal operation with a resultant surgical menopause is much more apt to seek medical advice if bleeding occurs than the complacent woman of 45 who interprets any menstrual irregularity as being due to change of life. Cervical stump cancer may be epidermoid or adenocarcinoma in type, and obviously the prognosis will vary as to the histological pattern and degree of disease.

CLINICAL CHARACTERISTICS OF CERVICAL CARCINOMA

As was mentioned previously, the mean age of patients with symptomatic cancer of the cervix is about 48 years. In contrast, patients with intraepithelial carcinoma average 38 years of age. Intraepithelial carcinoma is basically asymptomatic. However, clinical studies of patients with this condition usually result in the listing of a series of symptoms, most of which are coincidental. For example, Younge, Hertig, and Armstrong reported that 46 per cent of 135 patients had absolutely no symptoms, 24 per cent complained of leukorrhea and 30 per cent had abnormal bleeding of some kind.

Pain is not a symptom of cervical carcinoma until the late stages of the disease. Ignorance of this fact is one of the most important obstacles in the campaign for the early recognition of cancer. In the majority of cases the first symptom is *bleeding*, although this is usually slight. Characteristically, it is of intermenstrual type if the patient is still within the reproductive years. It is apt to be noted after coitus, severe exertion, or the straining of defecation. The "contact" bleeding following coitus or simple pelvic examination is especially characteristic. Unfortunately, in some cases bleeding does not occur until the disease has obtained a fairly good foothold and extended into the lymphatics, so that even an alert and intelligent patient may be doomed before the appearance of symptoms. In the intracervical forms of cancer, moreover, bleeding is apt to be later in appearance, because of the more protected position of the lesion.

Abnormal discharge, usually rather watery, may at times be noted even before the appearance of the bleeding, especially with adenocarcinoma. As the disease advances, both *bleeding and discharge* become more persistent and profuse, and the increasing ulceration and secondary infection make the discharge increasingly offensive. Other symptoms, such as *bladder irritability*, may arise from involvement of the vesicovaginal septum with corresponding *rectal discomfort* from posterior extension. Heavy, aching *pain* is now usually a prominent symptom and may become severe as the disease advances. Persistent lumbosacral pain, especially when accompanied by lymphedema of the leg, is a very serious prognostic sign. Fistulas into the bladder or rectum may develop, adding tremendously to the patient's misery. Increasing lateral infiltration obstructs the ureters, and *uremia is the terminal cause of death* in perhaps the largest proportion of cases.

DIAGNOSIS OF CERVICAL CANCER

Recent years have witnessed a complete revision in our methods of evaluating office patients as regards the diagnosis of uterine cancer, especially cervical. Indeed, previous editions of this text stressed the importance of a careful questioning for contact bleeding, the gross appearance of the cervix, the value of palpation, and certain other methods which must now be regarded as of purely secondary status.

Exfoliative Cytology

The development of an *accurate cytological method* for assessing asymptomatic women with a completely normal appearing cervix has led to the diagnosis of many cases of early cancer long before symptomatology or overt pathological abnormalities are apparent. If routine smears cannot be carried out on all patients, certainly every parous woman over 30 is entitled to a cancer smear, which is inexpensive and which we sincerely tell patients is the best investment they can make.

Nevertheless, a thorough history as regards intermenstrual bleeding should be taken, and careful palpation of the cervix and speculum examination should be carried out. Where there is a typical cancer present or even a definite but merely suspicious lesion, biopsy should be performed *in addition* to vaginal smear, for the two diagnostic methods should never be regarded as antagonistic, but rather as highly complementary. Actually, cytological methods may not permit diagnosis of a badly ulcerated clinical cancer due to bizarre inflammatory changes in the exfoliated cells, and likewise four-quadrant biopsy may miss a very early lesion. At this writing, however, there is practically no woman who should die of cervical cancer if she develops early habits of a check-up at the hands of a reputable, well qualified gynecologist. The technique and results of cytopathology will be discussed more fully in Chapter 36. Let it be made clear, however, that there is no skilled gynecological pathologist who can clinically interpret such cervical abnormalities as leukoplakia, polyp, or erosion nearly as accurately as biopsy or smear; indeed, carcinoma in situ may be found in conjunction with cervical epithelium that appears normal.

In addition to the use of the cytological examination for individual patients, the technique has wide application in population screening. Shelby County, Tennessee, Washington County, Maryland, Frederiksberg Borough, Copenhagen, and the Province of British Columbia have been especially studied by this method. In 1962 Fidler *et al.* were able to report that over one-third of the female population of British Columbia over 20 years of age had been screened, as a result of which the incidence of invasive carcinoma had dropped by 30.6 per cent in a period of six years.

Repeat screening in Frederiksberg Borough of Copenhagen has been carried out since 1962. In 1973, Gad and Koch reported on the fourth screen. The data show that from the first screening through the fourth, a span of some 11 years, the yield of invasive cancer fell from 4 per thousand to 0. In situ carcinoma fell from 8.6 per thousand to 0.3 per thousand, and suspicious smears from atypia and the like from 31 per thousand to 3 per thousand.

Such figures point out the extreme usefulness of population screening but also emphasize the false negativity problem associated with the cytologic method. The constant diminution of rates displayed by the Copenhagen studies and, indeed, by many other studies with successive screenings, indicate this false negativity problem, for if no positive cases penetrated the first screening, the yield from subsequent screenings would not diminish with each screening but would level off immediately after the first screening to a level indicative of the development of new cases.

Very few laboratories of cytopathology are aware of their false negative rate for the simple reason that patients with negative smears are normally not followed in any systematic way. However, it is possible to calculate false negative rates from data from repeat screenings, and several studies, as for example that of Silbar and Woodruff, have developed

false negative rates in other ways. From these and other studies, it turns out that exfoliative cytology has an inherent false negative rate of about 20 per cent.

This by no means indicates that exfoliative cytology is not an extremely useful procedure, but it does mean that gynecologists must be aware of this problem in the application of the cytologic method. The false negativity problem is one of the principal reasons for advising screening on an annual basis but, if a patient has two or, even better, three negative screens over a period of 3 years or so, the slow evolution of cancer of the cervix suggests that a subsequent smear need not be done on an annual basis but could be put off for a period of 3 or 4 or even 5 years.

From a theoretical point of view, the widespread community use of a cytological examination at appropriate intervals could control death from this disease by finding it in its early and curable stage. The actuality, as contrasted with the potentiality for control of cancer of the cervix by cytological screening has now come into sharp focus. There was a time, after the development of this cytological method, when it seemed as if the problem of cervical cancer would be solved by providing cytological facilities, by announcing their availability, and by sitting back and waiting for all women to do the necessary and sensible thing of seeking an examination through the channels they normally used for their regular medical service. It now seems quite clear that it was naive to expect effective widespread community control of cancer of the cervix by this approach.

This is not to say that a closed population of women cannot provide protection for itself by this method, and there are a number of reports from private patient groups which substantiate this. For example, Tilden and Nishimura described a cytological screening program among private patients which has been in operation since 1948. As time has gone along and the repeat smears have increased, the rate of discovery has fallen off substantially as the carcinomas in the population are weeded out. Although this approach is not undesirable, it is to be noted that in terms of community control and total energy expended in relation to total cancers found, it is a somewhat ineffective and inefficient technique. A study by Kashgarian *et al.* of the public awareness of uterine cytology in the Memphis, Shelby County, Tennessee, program showed that, even among those who were once motivated by community propaganda to seek an original smear, after a five-year period, the very considerable and prolonged propaganda effort had left but about one-fifth of the total population motivated to seek continuing annual examinations even when there was no direct cost to the examinee.

Therefore, the primary problem in community control of cervical cancer is not one of technique and facilities, but rather of community organization and motivation.

Schiller Test

This simple measure is based on the fact that cancer epithelium contains no glycogen and hence does not take up iodine like the normally glycogen-rich epithelium of cervix or vagina. Thus, application of iodine solution (Gram or Lugol) may show normal epithelium in deep mahogany color, whereas cancer areas are unstained and present in sharp distinction (Plate 12.5).

Unfortunately, trauma and various benign inflammatory processes may likewise lead to a "positive Schiller test," and more liberal use of smear and biopsy has to a certain extent limited its employment. However, it has a definite value, especially where smears are positive and biopsies inconclusive; or, should smears become positive after hysterectomy for an in situ cancer, it points out logical targets for biopsy.

Colposcopy

The colposcope is an instrument by which the cervix may be visualized in bright light under 10 to 40× magnification. The examination technique is rapid, requiring almost the same time as inspection of the cervix with the naked eye. After securing cytological specimens, the cervix may be cleansed with a cotton sponge, the colposcope focused and the entire cervix carefully scanned, first with normal illumination and then with a green filter to improve visualization of the vascular pattern. The cervix is then further cleansed with a 3 per cent acetic acid solution, which provides better differentiation of the columnar epithelium and the squamocolumnar junction. Then the cervix may also be stained by Schiller's solution to delineate glycogen negative areas.

Colposcopic findings may be divided into several categories. Using the terminology adopted by the American Society of Colposcopy and Colpomicroscopy, the following patterns may be seen.

Normal Colposcopic Findings:
1. Original squamous epithelium
2. Columnar epithelium (ectopy)
3. Typical transformation zone

Abnormal Colposcopic Findings:
1. Atypical transformation zone
   A. White epithelium
   B. Punctation
   C. Mosaic
   D. Leukoplakia
   E. Abnormal blood vessels
2. Suspect invasive cancer

Unsatisfactory Colposcopy

Other Colposcopic Findings:
   Vaginocervicitis
   True erosion
   Atrophic epithelium
   Condyloma, papilloma, etc.,
   Etc., etc.

Normal Colposcopic Findings

1. **Original Squamous Epithelium** is a smooth, pink and featureless epithelium originally established on the cervix and vagina. There are no remnants of columnar epithelium identified, such as mucous secreting epithelium, cleft openings, or Nabothian cysts (Plate 12.9).

2. **Columnar Epithelium** is a single layer mucus producing tall epithelium, which extends between the

endometrium cranially and either the original squamous epithelium or the metaplastic epithelium caudally. Area covered with columnar epithelium has irregular surface with long stromal papillae and deep clefts. In the colposcope after acetic acid test has a typical grapelike structure. Columnar epithelium may be present in the endocervix, on the portio or even in the vagina (Plate 12.9).

3. **Transformation Zone** is the area between original squamous epithelium and columnar epithelium in which metaplastic epithelium in varying degrees of maturity is identified. Components of a normal transformation zone may be islands of columnar epithelium surrounded by metaplastic squamous epithelium, "gland openings," and Nabothian cysts. In normal transformation zones there are no colposcopic findings suggestive of cervical neoplasia (Plate 12.10).

Abnormal Colposcopic Findings

1. **Atypical Transformation Zone.** A transformation zone in which there are colposcopic findings suggestive of cervical neoplasia.

   A. *White epithelium*—a focal abnormal colposcopic pattern seen after acetic acid test. The white epithelium is a transient phenomenon which is seen in the area of increased nuclear density.

   B. *Punctation*—a focal abnormal colposcopic pattern in which the capillaries appear as a stippled pattern (Plate 12.14).

   C. *Mosaic*—a focal abnormal colposcopic lesion in which the tissue has a mosaic pattern. The fields of mosaic are separated by reddish borders (Plate 12.15).

   D. *Leukoplakia*—a focal colposcopic pattern in which hyperkeratosis or parakeratosis is present and appears as an elevated whitened plaque. This whitened plaque is identified before the application of acetic acid. At times, leukoplakia may be identified outside the transformation zone (Plate 12.13).

   E. *Abnormal blood vessels*—a focal abnormal colposcopic pattern in which the blood vessel pattern appears not as punctation, mosaic, or as delicately branching vessels, but rather as irregular vessels with abrupt courses appearing as commas, corkscrew capillaries, or spaghetti-like forms (Plate 12.16).

2. **Suspect Frank Invasive Cancer.** Colposcopically obvious invasive cancer which is not evident on clinical examination.

Unsatisfactory Colposcopic Findings

Cases where the squamocolumnar junction cannot be visualized.

Other Colposcopic Findings

Vaginocervicitis—is a diffuse colposcopic pattern of hyperemia in which the blood vessels may appear in a diffuse stippled pattern similar to the vascular pattern in punctation.

True Erosion—is an area denuded of epithelium usually by trauma.

Atrophic Epithelium—is an estrogen deprived squamous epithelium in which the vascular pattern is more readily identified due to the relative thinness of the overlying squamous epithelium.

Condyloma, Papilloma—are exophytic lesions which might be inside or outside of the transformation zone.

There are many studies comparing the diagnostic accuracy of colposcopy and cytology. The results depend principally on the experience of the authors with each technique. Using both methods improves the diagnostic accuracy, because the advantages of both methods complement each other. The main disadvantage of colposcopy is that it is possible to examine only the visible part of the cervix. Therefore, if the squamocolumnar junction cannot be visualized, the colposcopic examination is unsatisfactory and it is necessary to rely on cytology only. This situation exists in about 15 per cent of premenopausal women. On the other hand, cytology suffers from the disadvantage that it does not indicate precisely where the suspect cells arise from the cervix. By colposcopy it is usually possible to localize the suspect area, to evaluate its size and severity, and to take directed biopsies to establish the histological diagnosis. Correlation of the cytological, colposcopic, and histological findings permits more rational patient management than reliance on any single methodology.

Although colposcopy was developed by Hinselmann in 1925 and has been widely used in Europe and in South America for the diagnosis of lesions on the cervix, the technique has been slower to gain popularity in the United States, probably because of the earlier development of diagnostic facilities for cytology. In recent years, cytological techniques have become so refined that more and more problems are presented in finding small suspect areas on the cervix for clinical investigation. Blind biopsies in cases with suspect or positive cytology and with no target lesion can result in false-negative histological diagnosis. On the other hand, to proceed directly to conization on the basis of a single suspect cytological specimen leads to large numbers of unnecessary conizations, which are not without morbidity. Much to be preferred is the use of the colposcope to direct the site for biopsy. With the discovery of earlier and earlier lesions during routine and population screen, the colposcope is assuming an increasingly important place in the sophisticated management of patients with abnormal cytology, although earlier editions of this text have deprecated its value.

Colpomicroscopy

The colpomicroscope gives a higher magnification than the colposcope. The cervical epithelium is vitally stained by Meyer hematoxylin or Toluidine blue and the surface histology of the cervical epithelium may be observed. Because the field of view is limited and the depth of focus poor, the method is rather tedious and not as popular as a routine procedure.

Biopsy

Our own preference is to supplement smear with a colposcopically directed biopsy whenever the smear is other than negative or if there is a suspect pattern by colposcopy. It should be apparent that the pathologist can assay only the material presented to him, and it is paramount to obtain adequate bits of tissue, although biopsy may sometimes be technically difficult.

In the event a trained colposcopist is not available, the technique of *multiple punch biopsy*, with 2 bites of the forceps at 12 and 6 o'clock—the most frequent sites of beginning neoplasia—or with bites of the forceps at 12, 3, 6, and 9 o'clock of the cervical circumference at the squamocolumnar junction, has been widely adopted.

For this purpose a cervical biopsy punch of the Gaylord type (Fig. 12.27) may be used, although several other biopsy forceps are available.

What has been said above does not apply to the more advanced cases, in which a section from any part of a bit of tissue excised from any part of the gross lesion will show cancer, and usually nothing but cancer. Even in the most advanced cases, biopsy is advisable in order to determine

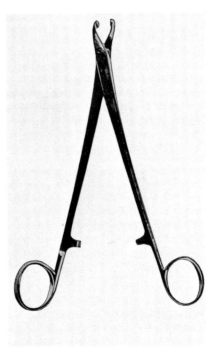

12.27. Cervical biopsy punch

the exact pathological type of the lesion and also to eliminate the rare case in which such lesions as cervical tuberculosis may simulate the gross picture of cancer.

Although there has been much discussion as to the *possible danger* of disseminating cancer by the performance of biopsy, the evidence on this point is very dubious. From a practical standpoint it may be said that even if there were any very convincing evidence of such a risk in cervical biopsy, it would quite surely be far less than that of delay in deciding as to the nature of suspicious lesions, or delay in confirming a doubtful or positive smear. Although we have the greatest respect for cytological methods, it is rare that treatment is actually instituted before confirmatory biopsies are obtained.

Conization of the Cervix

When there is no gross lesion visible on the cervix, it has been suggested by a number of authors that conization of the cervix for diagnostic purposes should be the next step after a doubtful or a positive smear. Such a conization is often referred to as a cold conization in distinction to a hot conization which is done with the electrocautery and results in charred tissue unsuitable for pathological examination. A cold conization is simply done with a sharp knife. However, as already indicated, our own preference in further investigation of a patient with a doubtful or positive smear with no gross lesion is for a colposcopic examination and a directed biopsy. However, in about 15 per cent of patients, the squamocolumnar junction is not visible because it is within the endocervical canal. In this circumstance or when for any other reason a good colposcopic view of the cervix cannot be obtained, cold diagnostic conization is a necessary and useful procedure. Conization is useful, not only in establishing a diagnosis of cancer in situ, but, sometimes, including the possibility of invasion, for it must constantly be borne in mind that carcinoma in situ may exist at the periphery of true invasive cancer.

From a laboratory standpoint, the two chief injunctions are (1) to be sure that the tissue is excised in such a way as to reveal the endocervical mucous membrane as well as the squamous epithelium of the portio vaginalis and the necessary underlying stroma and glands, and (2) to cut a sufficient number of blocks and sections at various levels to be sure that a small area of intraepithelial carcinoma is not overlooked. The first of these precautions seems self-evident, as the pathologist can thus evaluate not only the in situ but the early invasive potentialities. As to the second point, it should be emphasized that a pathological report based on a single section may lead to a serious error in diagnosis in these very early stages of cancer.

Since the institution of more or less routine colposcopy at the Johns Hopkins Hospital, the use of diagnostic conization has greatly diminished. In patients who are pregnant, it has been practically eliminated and is carried out in only about 15 per cent of patients who were having it done a few years ago.

In the event that conization is necessary, an immediate frozen section in a cryostat is a very useful procedure, for it allows a definitive diagnosis to be made at once. In this way, if further treatment is necessary it may be carried out without delay while the patient is under the same anesthesia.

CLINICAL CLASSIFICATION OF CERVICAL CANCER

It is obvious that for comparative study of the statistical reports of the results of treatment there must be some part of standard to indicate the clinical stage of the disease. Various systems of classification have been devised, none being perfect (League of Nations, Schmitz, American College of Surgeons). A step in the right direction was made at the International Federation of Gynecology and Obstetrics at its meeting in New York in May 1951, through the segregation of carcinoma in situ as a special group (Stage 0). This International Classification has been widely endorsed and adopted. It is the classification used in the

"*Annual Report of the Results of Treatment in Carcinoma of the Uterus*" published under the patronage of the International Federation of Gynecology and Obstetrics. The classification as revised in 1973 is as follows.

Stage O. Carcinoma in situ: also known as preinvasive carcinoma, intraepithelial carcinoma and similar conditions.

Stage I. The carcinoma is strictly confined to the cervix (extension to the corpus should be disregarded).

Stage Ia. Microinvasion.

Stage Ib. All other cases of Stage I.

Stage II. The carcinoma extends beyond the cervix, but has not reached the pelvic wall. The carcinoma involves the vagina, but not the lower third.

Subgrouping of Stage II cases into *IIa* (no parametrial involvement) and *IIb* (parametrial involvement) is recommended.

Stage III. The carcinoma has reached the pelvic wall. (On rectal examination no "cancer-free" space is found between it and the pelvic wall.) The carcinoma involves the lower third of the vagina. Hydronephrosis or a non-functioning kidney is present.

Stage IV. The carcinoma has extended beyond the true pelvis or has involved the mucosa of the bladder or rectum.

Stage IVa. Involvement of the bladder or rectum.

Stage IVb. Extension beyond the true pelvis.

A case should be allotted to Stage Ia only following microscopic diagnosis of the earliest stromal invasion performed before planned treatment. Stage Ia represents that group of cases of carcinoma of the cervix which can only be diagnosed microscopically following biopsy. They have often been called microcarcinoma. In the remainder of Stage I cases a clinical diagnosis will be possible.

A patient with a growth fixed to the pelvic wall by a short and indurated but not nodular parametrium should be allotted to Stage II. It is impossible at clinical examination to decide whether a smooth and indurated parametrium is truly cancerous or only inflammatory. Therefore, the case should be placed in Stage III only if the parametrium is nodular out on the pelvic wall where the growth itself extends out on the pelvic wall.

The presence of a bullous edema or a growth bulging into the bladder or the rectum does not permit consignment of a case to Stage IV unless the invasion of the bladder is proved by biopsy. Ridges and furrows into the bladder wall should only be interpreted as signs of involvement if they remain fixed to the growth at examination, thus bearing out that the carcinoma has invaded the submocosa of the bladder.

The above classification is a clinical estimation of extent of disease and according to the rules of the International Federation a change in classification is not to be made after therapy is initiated. Doctors Meigs and Brunschwig have suggested an additional classification for patients treated primarily by surgery. It is as follows.

Class O. Carcinoma in situ, also known as preinvasive carcinoma, intraepithelial carcinoma, microcarcinoma.

Class A. The carcinoma is strictly confined to the cervix.

Class Ao. After a positive biopsy of infiltrating carcinoma, no tumor is found in the cervix in the surgical specimen.

Class B. The carcinoma extends from the cervix to involve the vagina, except lower third. The carcinoma extends into the corpus. The carcinoma may involve the upper vagina and corpus. Vaginal or uterine extension or both may be by direct spread or be metastatic.

Class C. The carcinoma has involved paracervical or paravaginal tissue or both by direct extension or by lymphatic vessels, or in nodes within such tissues. Vaginal metastases or direct extension or both into the lower third of the vagina.

Class D. Lymph vessel and node involvement beyond paracervical and paravaginal regions. This includes all lymphatic vessels or nodes or both in the true pelvis, except as described in Class C. Metastasis to the ovary or tube.

Class E. The carcinoma has penetrated to the serosa, musculature, or mucosa of the bladder, colon, or rectum.

Class F. The carcinoma involves the pelvic wall (fascia, muscle, bone, or sacral plexus, or both).

Either or both of the above classifications are very useful in reporting end results of treatment and the workup of no patient is complete until the stage of the disease is determined and recorded.

TREATMENT OF INTRAEPITHELIAL CARCINOMA

Cancer in situ is a comparatively recently accepted entity, and it is not surprising that the exact treatment is not completely standardized. On one point there is agreement, that therapy be surgical rather than by irradiation. Unquestionably radiotherapy would cure all but the few resistant cases, but would also induce the menopause in these frequently young (average age 38 years) women, where it seems that conservation of ovarian function is attended by no appreciable risk. In addition, radiotherapy will not allow microscopic confirmation of any removed tissue and, regardless of how intensive the preoperative study may be, there is always some lingering doubt as to whether invasive cancer may be present in some area.

It would seem to us that for the average case acceptable surgery should be total hysterectomy, including excision of an appropriate segment of vaginal cuff with preservation of one or both ovaries in the young woman. The hysterectomy may be done abdominally or vaginally. Careful preoperative examination by colposcopy and by the Schiller test will delineate the extent of the lesion and dictate some variation in the amount of vaginal cuff which must be removed.

Conization, cauterization or freezing can be used as an alternate to hysterectomy if careful examination of the cervix has clearly delineated the extent of the lesion, and the limits of the lesion are modest.

Therapeutic conization has been used much longer than the other two simple methods and was first used as an alternate to hysterectomy with a view to preserving fertility. Many studies in the 1950's and early 1960's, prior to the widespread use of colposcopy to carefully delineate the limits of the lesion, showed that conization failed to cure the patient in about 20% of patients as judged by a persistent positive smear after conization, or by residual tumor in hysterectomized specimens. More contemporary studies, for example that of Krieger *et al.*, have shown a somewhat lesser incidence (9%) of residual disease after conization due to more careful preoperative examination of the cervix and due no doubt to the lesser extent of lesions now being found by contemporary methods of case finding.

One of the advantages of conization is the preservation of fertility. However, the conization itself may adversely affect reproductive function, MacVicar and Willocks followed some 632 patients who had been previously conized. They found a fertility rate of 64% but, among those who became pregnant, 24% had a miscarriage or premature labor. Another study by Kullander and Sjöberg showed an excellent post-conization fertility rate of about 83%, but again there was an abortion and premature delivery rate of 21%.

The treatment of cervical atypia and intraepithelial carcinoma by cauterization or freezing is a more recent development and has the great advantage of being possible on an outpatient basis.

Long term results are not available from either of these methods but, as judged by persistent positive smears after treatment, Wilbanks *et al.* found that with cauterization atypia was cured in 84% of patients.

There have been many advocates of cryosurgery for cervical intraepithelial neoplasia. Creasman *et al.* reported on the persistence of tumor in hysterectomized specimens in 75 patients with biopsy proved carcinoma in situ or severe dysplasia. With a double freeze, 82% of the specimens showed no residual tumor but, if a single freeze was used, there was a

48% persistence of tumor in the specimen removed after freezing.

There has been much controversy, some of it heated, over the relative merits of cauterization and freezing. However, on the basis of published data, an interesting comparative study by Miller and Elstein concluded "no difference was shown in either symptomatic cure rates or an objective measurements of cure."

In summary, the present evidence seems to indicate that for definitive therapy and with less concern for follow-up, a hysterectomy, either abdominal or vaginal, remains the method of choice. However, for lesions of limited extent, or where the preservation of fertility is of surpassing importance, conization, cauterization or freezing can be used as an alternate method, provided both the patient and physician are prepared to follow the patient for a prolonged period of time and are prepared to resort to hysterectomy in the event residual disease is demonstrated.

TREATMENT OF CLINICAL CANCER

Irradiation

This can be utilized for any stage of disease and is applicable for the very obese, the elderly, or the poor medical risk.

The end results from radiation vary considerably from clinic to clinic depending upon clinical material, technique, and intangible factors. Perhaps the best idea of what can be accomplished by this modality is obtained from the combined figures from over 100 clinics published in the "Annual Report." Thus, for the five-year period 1959 to 1963 as reported in the 15th edition, the end results from 67,493 patients are available. The recovery rates for Stages I, II, III, and IV were 77.4, 56.3, 31.7, and 9.1 per cent, respectively. The over-all recovery rate for these stages combined was 52.2 per cent.

Over the years the recovery rates as reported in the "Annual Report" have gradually improved. For example in 1941 the over-all rate was 30.9 per cent and this has gradually improved to the most recent 52.2 per cent. The improvement has resulted partly from a shift of clinical material into earlier stages and partly from improved results by stage.

To understand the logic of radiation therapy, it is helpful to bear in mind a few elementary principles of radiation physics.

For many years radium-226 has been a dependable source of radiation energy for the treatment of gynecological cancer. During spontaneous disintegration, radium-226, which in equilibrium has a half-life of 1,622 years, gives off α, β, and γ rays, but, with the filtration of the container capsules, the α and β rays are effectively screened out so that only γ rays of energy between 0.18 and 2.19 million electron volts (Mev.) are available and used for therapeutic purposes. It is to be recalled that the higher the Mev., the shorter the wave length and the greater the penetrability which is inversely proportional to the wave length. Thus, it is to be noted that radium has a spectrum of penetrability of its effective γ radiation.

More recently, cesium-137 has tended to supplant radium because, as a by-product of nuclear fission, it is less expensive and has the great advantage of admitting only a γ ray which is of uniform energy and penetrability of 0.66 Mev. This ray is satisfactory for therapeutic purposes and the absence of rays of higher energy, as from radium, makes cesium, relative to radium, safer to use in that there is less danger to nursing and other personnel from the very high energy penetrating rays of radium. Cesium-137 has a half-life of 29.6 years so that the sources must be recalibrated every six months to assure accurate dosage. Amounts of cesium are expressed in milligram equivalents meaning, thereby, the amount of cesium equivalent in radiation to that number of milligrams of radium.

Radiation is generally measured in *rads* which is defined as the absorbed dose of radiation which is accompanied by the liberation of 100 ergs of energy per gram of absorbing material, and it is very important to recall in planning therapy as well as protection, that the intensity of radiation varies inversely with the square of the distance between the point source of the energy and the point of its effect.

In discussing dosage, as related to carcinoma of the cervix, one other technical matter must be kept in mind. In order to express dosage in the cervix and the pelvic lymph nodes, Todd and Meredith a number of years ago, proposed that dosage be related to two theoretical points, *viz. A*, defined as 2 cm. lateral to the axis of the uterine canal and 2 cm. above the vaginal fornix, and *B*, 3 cm. lateral to *A* (Fig. 12.28). It was the intention of Todd and Meredith that the dosage at point *A* would represent a convenient method of expressing the dosage received by the primary carcinoma located in the cervix, and it was their intention that the dosage received at point *B* would represent the dosage received in the lymph-bearing area which is so often involved in carcinoma.

Many techniques of irradiation for cancer of the cervix have been described. At the present time at the Johns Hopkins Hospital, the standard treatment consists of two cesium-137 applications to the cervix, supplemented by external cobalt therapy.

The Fletcher after-loading applicator is currently the instrument of choice (Fig. 12.29) in our clinic except when (1) the vaginal vault is too small to use the smallest Fletcher ovoids, *i.e.*, there is less than a 1 cm. gap between the ovoids when the applicator is in position or (2) the vaginal wall lesion extends beyond the upper one-third of the vagina. In these instances, a special lucite plaque to hold the cesium sources is utilized.

The applicator is inserted under general anesthesia in the operating room. After insertion into the uterus and to the upper vagina, the applicator is held in place by packing the vagina with a gauze pack (Fig. 12.30). An indwelling catheter is placed in the bladder and, after this is done, inactive (dummy) sources identical in size to the active cesium sources are inserted into the intrauterine tandem and into the ovoids for the purpose of taking

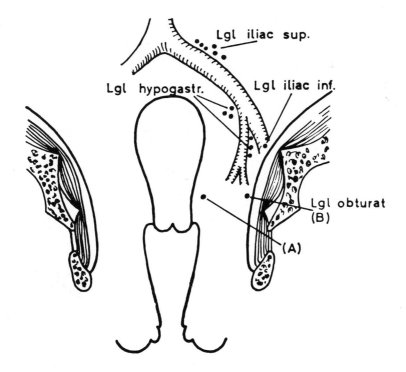

12.28. Irradiation targets, points A and B.

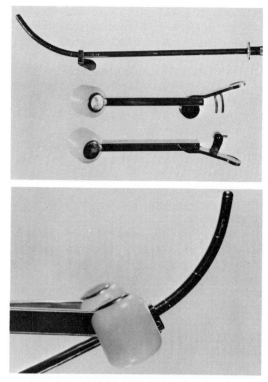

12.29. (*top*) Photograph of the components of a Fletcher after-loading cesium applicator. (*bottom*) The various components assembled.

dosimetry films. Roentgenological examinations anteroposteriorly and laterally, using polaroid films, are taken and examined immediately to insure that the applicators are properly positioned and, if they are not, they are adjusted as

necessary (Fig. 12.31). When the application is judged to be satisfactory, the patient is removed from the operating room to an area which is shielded to protect others from radiation and where the correct sources of cesium are introduced into the applicator. The applicator is loaded in the tandem either with one, two, or three cesium tubes, depending upon the size of the applicator it was possible to introduce, and the vaginal ovoids are loaded each with a single tube of 15, 20, or 25 mg. equivalents of cesium, depending upon the size of the ovoids used. The dose delivered per hour of exposure with the various combinations of loadings which are possible in an individual case may be read from a suitable table (Table 12.2).

The total desirable dose at point *A* is 6,000 to 6,500 rads including both of the cesium applications which are made at two-week intervals and the cobalt-60 external beam therapy. If cesium can contribute this total dose to point *A*, the midline of the patient is shielded during external beam therapy so that no further radiation is contributed by the external therapy to the region of the cervix. If the cesium contributes less than the desired dosage to point *A*, the midline is not shielded from the cobalt therapy until the desired dosage is reached at point *A*.

The total dose to point *B* is a minimum of 5,000 to 5,500 rads with combined cesium and external beam therapy.

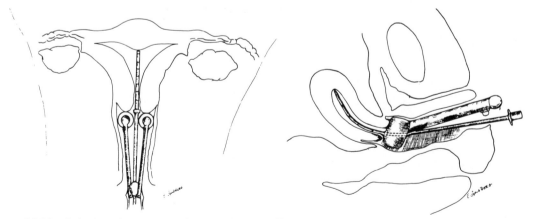

12.30. (*Left*) Anterior, posterior drawing showing a Fletcher Applicator in place. (*Right*) Lateral drawing of a Fletcher Applicator in place.

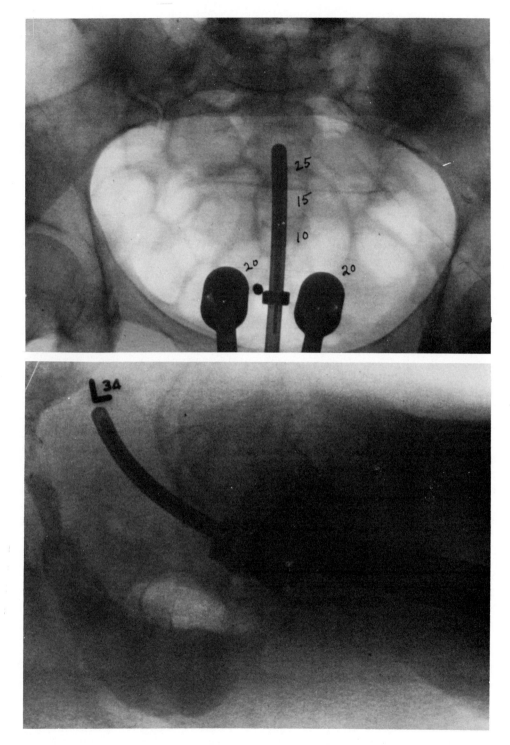

12.31. (*top*) An anterior posterior roentgenogram showing a satisfactory application of the tandem and ovoids in a patient with carcinoma of the cervix. The numbers are the milligrams of radium equivalents of cesium in the tandem and ovoids. (*bottom*) A lateral view of a satisfactory cesium application. A small amount of barium has been introduced in the rectum to show its location.

Table 12.2

Radiation Dosage: Fletcher Applicator

Uterine Loading	Vaginal Loading	Point A	Point B	Time for 3000 Rads Point A
		rads/hr.	*rads/hr.*	
25	Large 25 + 25	72	22	42
15	Medium 20 + 20	70	20	43
10	Small 15 + 15	67	18	45
20	Large 25 + 25	65	19	46
10	Medium 20 + 20	64	17	47
	Small 15 + 15	61	15	49
25	Large 25 + 25	59	17	51*
	Medium 20 + 20	57	16	52.5
	Small 15 + 15	54	14	55.5

* Maximal application time 50 hr. Use supplementary Co⁶⁰ to Point A to compensate for lower cesium dose.

It is hoped to deliver about 3,000 rads to point A at the first cesium treatment and an equal amount of radiation with the second cesium treatment two weeks after the first. About one week after the second treatment, external cobalt-60 therapy is started and the treatment consists of approximately 3,500 rads to the mid pelvis, although this latter dosage will depend upon the dosage delivered by the cesium at point B and the final dosage determination is made by delivering sufficient external therapy to have point B receive from 5,000 to 5,500 rads. The necessary dosage with cobalt-60 therapy usually requires about three weeks in divided daily doses and the midpelvic treatment dosage in rads may be read from a standard table and depends on the particular therapy machine and the thickness of the patient.

The maximal dose which the rectum can safely tolerate is about 5,000 to 5,500 rads from total combined treatment at any point. At the time of the cesium application, a rectal dosimeter is used to determine the amount of radiation being received by the rectal mucosa. The maximal vaginal wall dose should not exceed 15,000 rads.

If, for any reason, cesium cannot be used as an initial therapy, a split course of external cobalt therapy to the whole pelvis may be used. The first course will deliver 2,500 rads to the midpelvis in about 2 and one-half weeks. This will be followed by an interval of about two weeks when a second course of 2,000 rads will be delivered in about two weeks. After a second rest period of two weeks, the third and final course of about 2,000 rads will be administered in two weeks.

In many cases after the first or second course of external therapy there will be considerable improvement in the cervix so that local cesium applications become possible. In that event the cesium applicator is introduced for one or two treatments with the doses adjusted to achieve the desired number of rads to points A and B as enumerated above. This reversal of order of the internal and external components of treatment is particularly useful with the so-called "barrel" lesion and other bulky tumors of the cervix.

Cesium application is generally contraindicated in the presence of serious pelvic infection. Thus, if pyometra is encountered when the cervix is dilated, the course of radiation is usually started with cobalt-60 beam therapy followed with cesium application when possible. In the event there are inflammatory adnexal masses, these should be surgically removed before instituting radiation therapy.

Special mention may be made of the effect of radiation on lymph node metastasis, since this has been widely discussed. Information on this point must be deduced from the average lymph node involvement in various stages of the disease as compared with involvement after radiation. Morton *et al.* have compiled the reported incidence of lymph node involvement by stage as follows: State I, 16.5 per cent; Stage II, 31.9 per cent; and Stage III, 46.7 per cent. Figures for involvement after radiation vary considerably but most reported series show figures considerably below these so that it may be considered that radiotherapy is effective in destroying cancer metastasis in at least some patients.

Morton *et al.* found that the average incidence of lymph node involvement postradiation was about 10 per cent in Stage I and about 10 per cent in Stage II. It may be estimated, therefore, that about one-third of the patients with positive lymph nodes have them sterilized by radiation.

Lymphangiography has been used to ascertain the presence of metastases in lymph nodes (Fig. 12.32), but the technique is not completely reliable.

Indeed, the Sloane Hospital group (Gray, Gusberg, and Guttman) feel that supervoltage irradiation is so effective that lymphadenectomy should never be employed as an adjunct to radical irradiation. Not only is this form of x-ray destructive to cancerous lymph nodes, but in addition it is not attended by the high morbidity rate associated with lymph node dissection. Above all complications the authors specify postoperative pelvic lymphocyst, in which there may be sufficient retroperitoneal collection of lymphatic fluid to seriously compromise the function of the urinary tract, the large vessels, etc. Rutledge and Fletcher, from the M. D. Anderson Hospital, also question routine lymphadenectomy after irradiation, while pointing out the cancerocidal nature of irradiation therapy to the pelvis.

Despite all precautions, it is inevitable that irradiation should have some complications. Many women notice varying degrees of bladder irritability, diarrhea, and rectal bleeding during and after therapy, but in most cases these are transitory and short-lived. Far more distressing and troublesome are the bowel or bladder fistulas that may occur at any stage after treatment, even in the complete absence of cancer. It must be borne in mind that the initial ulcerative and destructive effect of irradiation is replaced by a later stage of marked scarification and fibrosis. An endarteritis may occur with gradual obliteration of the blood supply, with rectal or vesical fistula the result. Because the fistula is a direct result of tissue ischemia and impaired circulation, surgical repair is sometimes extremely difficult as the devitalized ne-

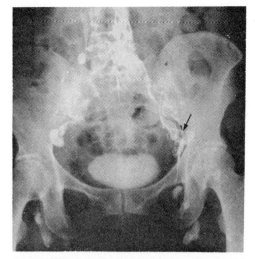

12.32. External lymphangiogram obtained by intralymphatic injection. This shows malignant invasion of left external iliac lymph nodes verified at laparotomy. (From Pattillo, R. A., Foley, D. V., and Mattingly, R. F.: Internal pelvic lymphography. Amer. J. Obstet. Gynec. *88:* 110, 1964.)

crotic tissue simply will not heal. In the absence of cancer, however, even these patients may be helped to lead a comfortable if not ideal existence by such procedures as colpocleisis, colostomy, or ureteral transplantation, as noted by Dean and Taylor. Every clinic must expect a certain percentage of fistulas or else the salvage will be poor. It is just not technically possible to deliver effectively cancerocidal doses to cervix and parametrium without occasionally damaging adjacent structures. In addition, it seems probable that certain individuals are unduly sensitive to irradiation and, where this seems likely after the first application, further dosage should be decreased. In cancer of the cervical stump it is likewise important to diminish the radium dosage; the fundus usually acts as a type of screen and, if this is absent, severe irradiation damage may occur.

Surgery

The resurgence of surgery as a primary treatment for cancer of the cervix is directly attributable to such medical advances as improved anesthesia, well equipped blood banks, antibiotic drugs, etc., which have made it possible to perform extensive, radical surgery with minimal operative mortality. Surgical proponents feel that irradiation has little effect on the pelvic lymph nodes, which can, however, be removed by surgery. Furthermore, it is argued, certain types of cervical cancer are resistant to irradiation and show no response to radiation therapy. The surgeons also argue that removal of the uterus prevents local recurrence and that operation avoids irradiation complications.

For example, it may prove that adenosquamous carcinoma of the cervix is best treated by surgery, but adequate information is not available to be sure of this point.

Meigs and others suggested the routine use of an improved radical Wertheim hysterectomy and pelvic lymphadenectomy in medically fit women with Stage I and early Stage II lesions. There is no question but that a skilled operator can perform this procedure with negligible mortality, but even in expert hands there is appreciable morbidity.

Unfortunately, there are few clinics where all patients with Stage I and Stage II disease are treated by surgery. Thus, surgical series are selected and end results must be interpreted with this in mind. Just as with radiation, surgical results vary greatly from institution to institution probably due to the degree of patient selection. Nevertheless, the five-year figures quoted below for abdominal radical hysterectomy and lymphadenectomy (Wertheim) may be considered representative. Liu and Meigs reported that for Stage I, they obtained a 74 per cent recovery rate in 116 patients and for Stage II 57 per cent for 49 patients. Parsons, Cesare, and Friedell reported 78 per cent recovery rate for Stage I, 85 per cent for Stage IIa, and 45 per cent for Stage IIb in a relatively small selected series. Welch, Pratt, and Symmonds reported 85.7 per cent for Stage I and 80 per cent for Stage II, again with a selected series. It is regrettable that there is no compilation of very large numbers of patients or a true alternate treatment series so that a comparison with the end results from radiation may be made.

Some clinics, primarily European, have advocated the radical vaginal hysterectomy (Schauta) for cancer of the cervix. Navratil reported an 83.3 per cent survival rate for 294 patients with Stage I and 51.7 per cent for 203 patients with Stage II. With this operation, no lymphadenectomy is routinely done and postoperative radiation to the lymph nodes is ordinarily carried out.

The curability of lymph node metastasis by surgery has received special attention just as it has with radiation. There is no doubt that lymph node involvement is of ominous prognostic significance. Nevertheless, all authors are able to report some curability with lymph node involvement. For example, Liu and Meigs with a 74 per cent over-all survival rate for Stage I, cured but 5 of 14 patients who had lymph node involvement. Other authors report similar figures.

On the other hand, Rauscher and Spurny reported the relative cure rates for 315 patients, 158 of whom had hysterectomy without lymphadenectomy and 157 of whom had hysterectomy with lymphadenectomy. The cure rates for Stages I and II combined were 75.04 and 75.79 per cent, respectively.

Surgical therapy, like radiation, is associated with complications principally to the urinary tract. Ureteral or vesical fistulas may occur in up to 10 per cent of patients.

In the 1970's, many clinics are using the selective approach to the identification of patients for surgical therapy.

Stage Ia, *i.e.*, microinvasive carcinoma, represents a special situation in this regard. A number of studies, such as those by Frick *et al.* and Ng and Reagan, have demonstrated that microinvasion up to 5 mm is practically never associated with lymph node metastases. For this reason, a simple hysterectomy, either vaginal or abdominal, as for intraepithelial carcinoma of the cervix, is used at Johns Hopkins and many other institutions for this stage of the disease, almost regardless of any other factors.

At our clinic, it is the current practice to use a wide hysterectomy and lymphadenectomy for all medically fit patients with Stage Ib lesions (Fig. 12.33) and early IIa lesions. Such patients must be relatively young, thin and have no serious other medical condition. In application, this means that about 75% of patients with Stage Ib lesions and fewer IIa lesions are being submitted to radical surgery.

Combined Irradiation and Surgery

It is our feeling that this should not be a routine form of treatment, and for two different reasons. First, there is no doubt that irradiation, by virtue of its tendency to cause increased vascularity, edema, and scarring, makes subsequent surgery more difficult, with a resultant increase in complicating fistula. Of even more importance, however, is the tendency of surgery to undo one of the most important and vital irradiation effects. In addition to an immediately destructive and lethal effect on cancer, both radium and x-ray lead to later fibrosis and scarring that may entrap and hold in check microscopically viable-appearing tumor cells. Surgery tends to cut across and break down these fibrotic barriers with dissemination of malignant cells into lymphatic and vascular channels, and we have observed this apparent sequence in more than one instance. However, Stevenson, Carter *et al.*, and others have reported encouraging results by utilizing combined irradiation and surgery. In a small series of Stage I and early Stage II lesions, their resultant 85 per cent five-year salvage rate seems impressive, but it must be realized that the series is very highly selected. Furthermore, statistical results from a series of patients so treated have not shown any augmentation over results from surgery or irradiation for comparable stages of disease.

TREATMENT OF RADIORESISTANT CANCER

A certain small percentage (probably less than 5 per cent) of cervical cancer is completely resistant to standard amounts of irradiation, and the clinician will be alerted to this by a consistently positive biopsy. Actually, even in patients ultimately cured, biopsies may remain

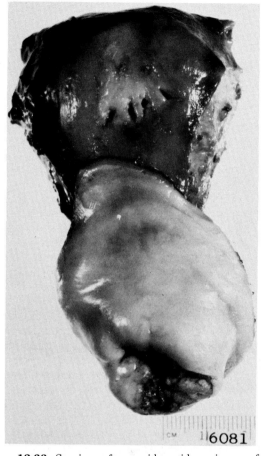

12.33. Specimen from epidermoid carcinoma of the cervix clinical Stage Ib. Note the very large vaginal cuff and the fact that the tubes and ovaries were not removed. In operations for Stage Ia and Ib about one-half of the patients, depending on the age, have the tubes and ovaries left in situ.

positive for several weeks following completion of therapy, but experience suggests that persistence of tumor more than 8 to 10 weeks posttherapy indicates failure of response.

Evaluation of postirradiation biopsies is an exceedingly difficult and sometimes impossible task. Novak has indicated that degenerative changes closely mimic neoplastic ones, and at certain times it is impossible to distinguish viable from nonviable tumor cells. Yet this is of paramount importance, and where biopsies are equivocal it is sometimes desirable to perform conization to establish failure of response to irradiation. Although some British feel that sequential biopsies during and after therapy are helpful in formulating a prognosis, we are frequently dissatisfied with them as a means of early detection of radioresistance.

Although much time and effort have been spent in devising tests for radioresistance, none of these has practical value and at the present time an estimation of radiation response by clinical examination remains still the best method.

There are only two indications for surgery in the conservative clinic that utilizes only irradiation as standard therapy. The first of these is the detection of *radioresistance* and, if this can be detected early, while the disease is localized, the prognosis is that much better. The second is *late recurrence after complete adequate irradiation.* Experience has shown that once a postirradiation recurrence has appeared, no further amounts of radiotherapy will be effective.

We would emphasize the extreme difficulty as well as importance of making a diagnosis of resistant or recurrent lesion. Where cervical biopsy or smear is unequivocally positive this is simple, but where this clue is absent the problem is formidable. A high index of suspicion should be reserved for increasing radiating backache, pelvic pain with induration, dilatation of the urinary tract, leg or vulvar edema, etc. However, even earlier diagnosis should be striven for if there is to be any hope for successful surgery in the face of radioresistance. Although premature unfounded suspicion should not mandate radical complicated surgery, nevertheless, the patient who does poorly following radiation generally will show a recurrent or resistant tumor even though proof may be difficult to obtain. We favor hospital admission, with examination under anesthesia, conization, and curettage as well as cytological studies, pyelography, and other x-ray study.

Biopsy of the parametria represents a special problem and opportunity, as the main uncertainty in recurrence of carcinoma of the cervix is not in the cervix but in the parametria. The difficulty is that when one can be reasonably sure of trouble by palpation, the horse is often out of the barn. Theoretically needle biopsy of the parametria should help, but in our own clinic the use of the Vim-Silverman needle through the years has been only moderately successful and has been used only spasmodically. However, El-Minawi and Perez-Mesa, reporting from the Missouri State Cancer Hospital, have more encouraging results and, indeed, their results are quite impressive. Overall, 28 of 51 specimens proved to be positive, and 23 of 51 negative with only 5 of the latter being false negative, as judged by subsequent events. Thus, the use of such information, when the biopsy is positive, might be extremely helpful. Perhaps the Vim-Silverman biopsy of the parametria should be used more often than it has been in the past.

If there should be positive or even suggestive evidence of radioresistance or recurrence, some operative procedure may be considered, but Burns and Brack pointed out that this is generally performed too late. The surgery can depend on the extent of the disease when resistance or recurrence is noted. If early, a *radical hysterectomy with pelvic lymphadenectomy may be utilized,* but this in insufficient for advanced degrees of disease. Ultraradical surgery, as proposed by Brunschwig, is sometimes a lifesaving procedure in these circumstances. The procedure of *complete pelvic exenteration* involves removal of all pelvic organs, bladder, and rectum, and transplantation of the ureters into an exteriorized colon or ileal segment as well as removal of the pelvic lymph nodes. It is very doubtful that the use of this heroic procedure for purely palliative purposes is indicated.

Less radical procedures can be utilized where the rectum is free of disease, so that only the bladder and pelvic organs need be removed along with ureteral transplantation. This so-called *anterior exenteration* is greatly to be preferred to the total operation if the extent of disease permits its use.

Where the rectum is involved but the bladder is free of disease, a *posterior exenteration* can be utilized which, of course, leaves the patient with a colostomy. Either one of these partial exenterations is utilized by most clinics on occasional selected and qualified patients with less distaste than for the complete operation. All of these show a not inconsiderable mortality and morbidity even if done by trained gynecologists. With recurrent or resistant irradiated cancer, one must admit that there is no other chance for cure than by surgery.

Where partial exenteration or a radical Wertheim operation is feasible, the results are worthwhile, as indicated by the reports of Thompson and Brack from our own clinic, Brunschwig, Douglas, Schmitz, and others. Alexander Brunschwig has certainly had the largest experience in the surgical treatment of recurrent or persistent cervical cancer. In 1967, he reported on 901 patients with an additional diagnosis of recurrent or persistent cervical cancer but some of whom were recurrent after attempted cures by surgery. Pathological examination after surgery revealed that 138 cases or 14 per cent did not actually have cancer, but had extensive radiation reaction. Of the 583 patients in whom cancer was proved to be present, 52 per cent were subjected to surgery in an attempt to cure. There were 125 patients who had operations that were less than exenterations, and thus had preserved normal urinary and fecal functions. The five-year survival among these was 50 patients or 40 per cent. There were 318 patients with disease so advanced that total or partial pelvic exenteration was necessary. Among these, 56 survived for five or more years, a cure rate of 17.6 per cent. In the exenteration group, the surgical mortality was 17 per cent, whereas in the patients who had less than an exenteration, it was but 2.4 per cent.

With accumulated experience there is a tendency away from less than exenteration of recurrent lesions because of the difficulty in identifying the extent of disease during operation. This view is justified by the declining mortality and morbidity with the ultra-radical procedure.

The prognosis for patients with positive lymph nodes after irradiation is exceedingly serious. In Brunschwig's series just mentioned, of 98 cases of radiation failure with positive lymph nodes in the removed specimens, 6 per cent survived five years. In view of the fact that there is a substantial increase in surgical morbidity associated with the lymph node dissection, it is a moot point as to whether lymphadenectomy in patients who have previously been treated by radiation is a desirable procedure. Presence of lymph node involvement at this point is apparently an indication of a biologically bad tumor and if the nodes *are* involved, are they an absolute barrier to malignant cells, and is it not likely that tumor has spread beyond the nodal borders so that no form of lymphadenectomy will be beneficial? Because of our belief in this tenet, plus the increased morbidity as opposed to the beneficial results of therapy, we cannot help but feel that routine lymphadenectomy in radical surgery after radiation is merely a gesture.

TREATMENT OF CERVICAL CANCER IN PREGNANCY

This must of necessity vary in different cases, depending chiefly on the stage of the disease and the stage of pregnancy at which the cancer is recognized, although there are often other factors to be considered, such as the religious beliefs of the patient and her family. Fortunately, cancer of the cervix in the pregnant woman is relatively rare.

If careful study of the cervix, by the methods recorded in the section on diagnosis, indicates that the disease is intraepithelial, the pregnancy may be allowed to go to term with the treatment of the cervix deferred until after delivery. For more advanced cancer the disease should be treated without regard to the pregnancy except in rare circumstances after the fifth month of gestation.

In general, if the cancer is recognized in the early stages of pregnancy, the disease is treated without regard to the pregnancy. Thus, for Ib and early IIa cases, radical surgery may be used. For other

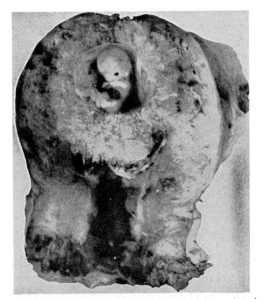

12.34. Epidermoid carcinoma of cervix associated with pregnancy of 6 to 8 weeks.

stage of the disease and the personal predilection of the clinician. In later stages, one can wait a short time for viability, or, if this has been reached, deliver the baby by the abdominal route, followed usually by irradiation. There are various modifications of this general plan which may be indicated in individual cases, but the prime motive is to treat the cancer with disregard of the pregnancy, although occasional individualization is practiced. The results by stage are somewhat inferior to those obtained in the nonpregnant (Figs. 12.34, 35).

THE TREATMENT OF PATIENTS WITH HOPELESS CANCER

Based on the collected statistics of the annual report, about one-half of all patients with stages I–IV are cured. This means that about one-half are not cured, and it becomes the responsibility of the physician to see that these patients have sympathetic and responsible attention.

Death from cancer of the cervix is most often due to uremia secondary to ureteral obstruction. Infection, hemorrhage, and

stages irradiation is the best plan. Spontaneous abortion usually follows. Others prefer to do therapeutic abortion or hysterotomy, followed by either irradiation or radical operation, depending upon the

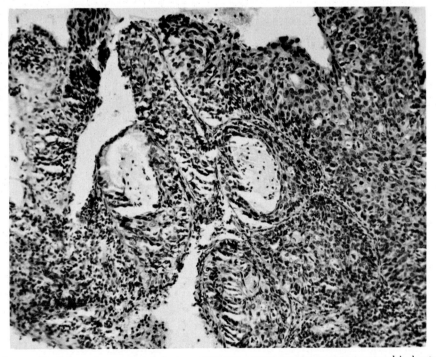

12.35. Intraepithelial carcinoma found during pregnancy; same pattern postpartum and in hysterectomy specimen.

malnutrition are also involved. In some patients, pain is the most troublesome symptom to combat.

Systemic or regional chemotherapy has been disappointing for most patients with epidermoid carcinoma of the cervix. However, modest improvement is sometimes noted, and Smith *et al.* reported 19 per cent objective response in 107 patients treated with cyclophosphamide, which they found to be the safest and most easily administered chemotherapeutic agent among many which they tried. Although no cures were noted and doubtful prolongation of life was obtained, the patients reported an improved sense of well being and required less narcotics.

Hormones are ineffective as might be anticipated from the fact that carcinoma of the cervix is not hormone dependent. However, steriods with an anabolic effect, *e.g.*, testosterone, are frequently helpful in improving appetite and nutrition.

As noted above relief of pain is often the most serious problem. Characteristically, the pain may begin in the sacroiliac region from infiltration of the pelvic lymph nodes with resultant pressure on the nerves to the legs. Such pain radiating down the leg, and especially when accompanied by a swollen extremity, is an exceedingly serious prognostic situation. For any patient with localized pain and a predicted life span of more than three or four months, some consideration should be given to a chordotomy, if liberal use of narcotics is ineffective.

REFERENCES

Annual Report on the Results of Treatment in *Carcinoma of the Uterus,* Vol. 14. Stockholm, 1967.

Aurelian, L.: Varions and antigens of herpes type 2 in cervical carcinoma. Cancer Res., *33:* 1548, 1973.

Boyd, J. R., Royle, D., Fidler, H. K., and Boyes, D. A.: Conservative management of in situ carcinoma of the cervix. Amer. J. Obstet. Gynec., *85:* 322, 1963.

Boyd, J. T., and Doll, R.: A study of the aetiology of carcinoma of the cervix uteri. Brit. J. Cancer, *18:* 419, 1964.

Brack, C. B., Everett, H. S., and Dickson, R.: Irradiation therapy for carcinoma of the cervix; its effect upon the urinary tract. Obstet. Gynec., *7:* 196, 1956.

Broders, A. C.: Grading of carcinoma. Minnesota Med., *8:* 726, 1925.

Brunschwig, A.: Complete excision of pelvic viscera for advanced carcinoma; a one-stage abdominoperineal operation with end colostomy and bilateral ureteral implantation into the colon above the colostomy. Cancer, *1:* 177, 1948.

Brunschwig, A.: Surgical treatment of stage I cancer of the cervix. Cancer, *13:* 34, 1960.

Brunschwig, A.: Surgical treatment of carcinoma of the cervix, recurrent after irradiation of the combination of irradiation and surgery. Amer. J. Roentgen., *99:* 365, 1967.

Burns, B. C., and Brack, C. B.: Prognostic factors in radioresistant cervical cancer. Obstet. Gynec., *16:* 1, 1960.

Carter, B., Parker, R. T., Thomas, W. L., Creadick, R. N., Peete, C., Cherny, W. B., and Williams, J. B.: Follow-up of patients with cancer of cervix treated by radical hysterectomy and radical pelvic lymphadenectomy. Amer. J. Obstet. Gynec., *76:* 1099, 1958.

Creasman, W. T., Weed, Jr., J. C., Curry, S. L., Johnston, W. W., and Parker, R. T.: Efficacy of cryosurgical treatment of severe cervical intraepithelial neoplasia. Obstet. Gynec., *41:* 501, 1973.

de Alvarez, R. R.: The sites of metastasis in carcinoma of the cervix. Western J. Surg., *61:* 623, 1953.

Dean, R. E., and Taylor, E. S.: Surgical treatment of complications resulting from irradiation therapy of cervical cancer. Amer. J. Obstet. Gynec., *19:* 34, 1960.

Diaz-Bazan, N.: Prolapso uterino y cancer del Cuello. Arch. Col. Med. El Salvador, *5:* 15, 1952.

Douglas, R. G., and Sweeney, J. H.: Exenteration operations in advanced pelvic cancer. Amer. J. Obstet. Gynec., *73:* 1169, 1957.

Dunn, J. E., Jr.: Preliminary findings of the Memphis-Shelby County uterine cancer study and their interpretations. Amer. J. Public Health, *48:* 861, 1958.

El-Minawi, M. R., and Perz-Mesa, C. M.: Parametrial needle biopsy follow-up of cervical cancer. Int. J. Obstet. Gynec., *12:* 1, 1974.

Enterline, E. T., Arvan, D. A., and Davis, R. E.: The predictability of residual carcinoma in situ from study of cervical cones. Amer. J. Obstet. Gynec., *85:* 940, 1963.

Epperson, J. W. W., Hellman, L. M., Galvin, G. A., and Busby, T.: Morphologic changes in cervix during pregnancy, including intraepithelial carcinoma. Amer. J. Obstet. Gynec., *61:* 50, 1951.

Fidler, H. K., Boyes, D. A., Aversperg, N., and Lock, D. R.: The cytology program in British Columbia. Canad. Med. Ass. J., *86:* 779, 1962.

Fischer, R.: Possible role of smegma in etiology of squamous cell carcinoma of cervix. Obstet. Gynec. Survey, *8:* 232, 1953.

Fluhmann, C. F.: Carcinoma in situ and the transitional zone of the cervix uteri. Obstet. Gynec., *16:* 424, 1960.

Frick, II, H. C., Janovski, N. A., Gusberg, S. B., and Taylor, Jr., H. C.: Early invasive cancer of the cervix. Amer. J. Obstet. Gynec., *85:* 926, 1963.

Gad, C., and Koch, F.: Population screening for cervical carcinoma in Fredriksberg Borough. Results of second and third rescreenings, 1966–1972. Danish Med. Bull., *20:* 141, 1973.

Gagnon, F.: Contribution to study of etiology and prevention of cancer of cervix of uterus. Amer. J. Obstet. Gynec., *60:* 516, 1950.

Galvin, G. A., Jones, H. W., and Te Linde, R. W.: Clinical relationship of carcinoma in situ and invasive carcinoma of the cervix. J.A.M.A., *149:* 744, 1952.

Galvin, G. A., Jones, H. W., and Te Linde, R. W.: Significance of basal cell hyperactivity in cervical biopsies. Amer. J. Obstet. Gynec., *70:* 808, 1955.

Gilliam, A. G.: Fertility and cancer of the breast and of the uterine cervix. Comparisons between rates of pregnancy in women with cancer at these and other sites. J. Nat. Cancer Inst., *12:* 287, 1951.

Gray, M. J., Gusberg, S. B., and Guttman, R.: Pelvic lymph

node dissection following radiotherapy. Amer. J. Obstet. Gynec., 76: 629, 1958.

Greene, R. R., and Peckham, B. M.: Preinvasive cancer of the cervix, and pregnancy. Amer. J. Obstet. Gynec., 75: 551, 1958.

Greene, R. R., Peckham, B. M., Chung, J. T., Bayly, M. A., Benaron, H. B. W., Carrow, L. A., and Gardner, G. H.: Preinvasive carcinoma of cervix during pregnancy. Surg. Gynec. Obstet., 96: 71, 1953.

Haenszel, W., and Hillhouse, M.: Uterine cancer morbidity in New York City and its relation to the pattern of regional variation within the United States. J. Nat. Cancer Inst., 22: 1157, 1959.

Heins, H. C., Jr., Dennis, E. J., and Pratt-Thomas, H. R.: Possible role of smegma in carcinoma of the cervix. Amer. J. Obstet. Gynec., 76: 726, 1958.

Henriksen, E.: The lymphatic spread of carcinoma of the cervix and body of the uterus. Amer. J. Obstet. Gynec., 58: 924, 1949.

Hertig, A. T., and Younge, P. A.: What is cancer in situ of the cervix? Is it the preinvasive form of true carcinoma? Amer. J. Obstet. Gynec., 64: 807, 1952.

Hinselmann, H.: Davis and Carter Gynec. and Obstet. 3: Ch. 4. W. F. Pryor Co., Hagerstown, Md.

Johnson, L. D., Easterday, C. L., Gore, H., and Hertig, A. T.: The histogenesis of carcinoma in situ of the uterine cervix. Cancer, 17: 213, 1964.

Jones, E. G., McDonald, I., and Brestlow, L.: Epidemiologic factors in carcinoma of the cervix. Amer. J. Obstet. Gynec., 76: 1, 1958.

Jones, H. W., Jr., Galvin, G. A., and Te Linde, R. W.: Intraepithelial carcinoma of cervix and its clinical implications. Int. Abstr. Surg., 92: 521, 1951.

Jones, H. W., Jr., Katayama, K. P., Stafl, A., and Davis, H. J.: The chromosomes of cervical atypia, carcinoma in situ and invasive carcinoma of the cervix. Obstet. Gynec., 30: 790, 1967.

Jones, H. W., Jr., Davis, H. J., Frost, J. K., Park, I.-J., Salimi, R., Tseng, P.-Y., and Woodruff, J. D.: The value of the assay of chromosomes in the diagnosis of cervical neoplasia. Amer. J. Obstet. Gynec., 102: 624, 1968.

Josey, W. E., Nahmias, A. J., and Naib, Z. M.: The epidemiology of type 2 (genital) herpes simplex virus infection. Obstet. Gynec. Surv., 27: 295, 1972.

Josey, W. E., Nahmias, A. J., Naib, Z. M., Utley, P. M., McKenzie, W. J., and Coleman, M. T.: Genital herpes simplex infection in the female. Amer. J. Obstet. Gynec., 96: 493, 1966.

Kashgarian, M., Erickson, C. C., Dunn, J. J. E., Jr., and Sprunt, D. H.: A survey of public awareness of uterine cytology in Memphis-Shelby County. Acta Cytol., 10: 11, 1966.

Kottmaier, H. L.: Current treatment of carcinoma of the cervix. Amer. J. Obstet. Gynec., 76: 243, 1958.

Krieger, J. S., and McCormack, L. J.: Graded treatment for in situ carcinoma of the uterine cervix. Amer. J. Obstet. Gynec., 101: 171, 1968.

Kullander, S., and Sjööberg, Nils-Otto: Treatment of carcinoma in situ of the cervix uteri by conization. Acta Obstet. Gynec Scand., 50: 153, 1971.

Lilienfeld, A. M., and Graham, S.: Validity of determining circumcision status by questionnaires as related to epidemiological studies of cancer of the cervix. J. Nat. Cancer Inst., 21: 713, 1958.

Liu, W., and Meigs, J. V.: Radical hysterectomy and pelvic lymphadenectomy. Amer. J. Obstet. Gynec., 69: 1, 1955.

Lombard, H. L., and Potter, E. A.: Epidemiological aspects of cancer of the cervix. Cancer, 3: 960, 1950.

MacVicar, J., and Willocks, J.: The effect of diathermy conization of the cervix on subsequent fertility, pregnancy and delivery. J. Obstet. Gynaec. Brit. Comm., 75: 355, 1968.

Martin, C. E.: Marital and coital factors in cervical cancer. Amer. J. Public Health, 57: 803, 1967.

Martzloff, K. H.: Carcinoma of the cervix uteri. Bull. Hopkins Hosp., 40: 960, 1927.

McKay, D. G., Hertig, A. T., and Younge, P. A.: Carcinoma in situ. J. Int. Coll. Surg., 21: 212, 1954.

McKelvey, J. L., Stenstrom, K. W., and Gillam, J. S.: Results of experimental therapy of carcinoma of cervix. Amer. J. Obstet. Gynec., 58: 896, 1949.

Meigs, J. V.: Surgical Treatment of Cancer of the Cervix. Grune & Stratton, Inc., New York, 1954.

Meigs, J. V.: Radical hysterectomy with bilateral pelvic-lymph-node dissection for cancer of the uterine cervix. Clin. Obstet. Gynec., 1: 1029, 1958.

Meigs, J. V., and Brunschwig, A.: Proposed classification for cases of cancer of the cervix treated by surgery. Amer. J. Obstet. Gynec., 64: 413, 1952.

Meyer, R.: Basis of histologic diagnosis of cervical carcinoma, and similar lesions. Surg. Gynec. Obstet., 73: 14, 1941.

Miller, J. F., and Elstein, M.: A comparison of electrocautery and cryocautery for the treatment of cervical erosions and chronic cervicitis. J. Obstet. Gynaec. Brit. Comm., 86: 58, 1973.

Morton, D. G., Lagasse, L. D., Moore, J. C., Jacobs, M., and Amromin, G.: Pelvic lymphnodectomy following radiation in cervical carcinoma. Amer. J. Obstet. Gynec., 88: 932, 1964.

Murphy, D. P.: Heredity in Uterine Cancer. Harvard University Press, Cambridge, 1952.

Navratil, E.: Indications and results of the Schauta-Amreich operation with and without postoperative roentgen treatment in epidermoid carcinoma of the cervix of the uterus. Amer. J. Obstet. Gynec., 86: 141, 1963.

Ng, A. B. P., and Reagan, J. W.: Microinvasive carcinoma of the uterine cervix. Amer. J. Clin. Path., 52: 511, 1969.

Novak, E. R.: Radioresistant cervical cancer. Obstet. Gynec., 4: 251, 1954.

Novak, E. R., and VillaSanta, U.: Factors influencing the ratio of uterine cancer in a community. J.A.M.A., 174: 1395, 1960.

Park, I. J., and Jones, H. W., Jr.: Glucose 6-phosphate dehydrogenase and the histogenesis of epidermoid carcinoma of the cervix. Amer. J. Obstet. Gynec., 102: 106, 1968.

Parsons, L., Cesare, F., and Friedell, G. H.: Primary surgical treatment of invasive cancer of the cervix. Surg. Gynec. Obstet., 109: 279, 1959.

Pattillo, R. A., Foley, D. V., and Mattingly, R. F.: Internal pelvic lymphography. Amer. J. Obstet. Gynec., 88: 110, 1964.

Petersen, O.: Spontaneous course of cervical precancerous conditions. Amer. J. Obstet. Gynec., 73: 1063, 1957.

Rauscher, H., and Spurny, J.: Results with the radical Wertheim operation with and without obligatory lymphadenectomy. Geburtsh. Frauenheilk., 19: 651, 1959.

Rawles, W. E., Thompkins, W. A. F., Figueroam, E., and Melnick, J. L.: Herpes virus type 2 association with carcinoma of the cervix. Science, 151: 1255, 1968.

Rewell, R. E.: Population structure and apparent incidence of cancer; a study of endometrial carcinoma in England and South India. J. Obstet. Gynaec. Brit. Comm., 65: 590, 1958.

Rothman, A.: Carcinoma of cervix in Jewish women. Amer. J. Obstet. Gynec., 62: 160, 1951.

Rotkin, I. D.: Relation of adolescent coitus to cervical cancer risk. J.A.M.A., 179: 110. 1962.

Rotkin, I. D.: A comparison review of key epidemiological studies in cervical cancer related to current searches for transmissible agents. Cancer Res., 33: 1353, 1973.

Rutledge, F. N., and Fletcher, G. H.: Lymphadenectomy after supervoltage irradiation. Amer. J. Obstet. Gynec., 76: 321, 1958.

Schiller, W.: Untersuchungen zur Entstehung der Ge-schivulste. I. Collumcarcinom des Uterus. Virchow. Arch. Path. Anat., 263: 279, 1927.

Schmitz, H. E., Smith, C. J., Foley, D. V., and Schack, C. B.: Evaluation of surgical procedures employed following the failure of irradiation therapy in cancer of the cervix. Amer. J. Obstet. Gynec., 74: 1165, 1957.

Schmitz, R. L., Schmitz, H. E., Smith, C. J., and Molitor, J. J.: Details of pelvic exenteration evolved during an experience with 75 cases. Amer. J. Obstet. Gynec., 80: 43, 1960.

Silbar, E. L., and Woodruff, J. D.: Evaluation of biopsy, cone and hysterectomy sequence in intraepithelial carcinoma of the cervix. Obstet. Gynec., 27: 89, 1966.

Smith, J. P., Rutledge, F., Burns, B. C., Jr., and Soffar, S.: Systemic chemotherapy for carcinoma of the cervix. Amer. J. Obstet. Gynec., 97: 800, 1967.

Sparkes, R. S., Boluda, M. C., and Towsend, D. E.: Detection of glucose 6-phosphate dehydrogenase by fluorescence after cellulose acetate electrophoresis. Anal. Biochem., 30: 289, 1969.

Stafl, A., and Mattingly, R. A.: Vaginal adenosis—a precancerous lesion. Amer. J. Obstet. Gynec., 120: 666, 1974.

Stephenson, J. H., and Grace, W. J.: Life stress and cancer of the cervix. Psychosom. Med., 16: 287, 1954.

Stern, E., and Dixon, W. J.: Cancer of the cervix: A biometric approach to etiology. Cancer, 14: 153, 1961.

Stevenson, C. S.: Treatment of carcinoma of the cervix with full irradiation therapy followed by radical pelvic surgery. Amer. J. Obstet. Gynec., 75: 888, 1958.

Tennis, M., and Oalmann, M. C.: Carcinoma of the cervix; an epidemiologic study. J.A.M.A., 174: 155, 1960.

Terris, M., and Oalmann, M. C.: Carcinoma of the cervix. J.A.M.A., 174: 1847, 1960.

Thompson, J. D., and Brack, C. B.: Radical surgery for radioresistant cancer. Obstet. Gynec., 10: 676, 1957.

Thornton, W. N., Fox, C. H., and Smith, D. E.: Relationship of the squamo-columnar junction and the endocervical glands to the site of origin of carcinoma of the cervix. Amer. J. Obstet. Gynec., 78: 1060. 1959.

Tilden, I. L., and Nishimura, J. K.: Detection of cervical cancer by cytologic screening: Periods 1948–53 and 1958–63. Pacif. Med. Surg., 74: 53, 1966.

Todd, M. C., and Meredith, W. J.: The treatment of cancer of the uterine cervix. Brit. J. Radiol., 11: 809, 1938.

Todd, M. C., and Meredith, W. J.: Treatment of cancer of the cervix uteri. A revised "Manchester Method." Brit. J. Radiol., 26: 252, 1953.

Tokuhata, G. K.: Tobacco and cancer of the genitalia among married women. Amer. J. Public Health, 57: 830, May 1967.

Towne, J. E.: Carcinoma of cervix in nulliparous and celibate women. Amer. J. Obstet. Gynec., 69: 606, 1955.

Tweeddale, D. N., Gorthey, R. L., Harvey, H. E., and Tanner, F. H.: Cervical versus endometrial carcinoma; relative incidence. Obstet. Gynec., 2: 623, 1953.

Way, S.: Malignant Disease of the Female Genital Tract, Blakiston Company, Division of McGraw-Hill Book Company, Inc., New York, 1951.

Webb, G. A., Margolis, A. J., and Traut, H. F.: Adenocarcinoma of the endometrium; evaluation of factors influencing prognosis and outline of plan of therapy based on these factors. Western J. Surg., 63: 407, 1955.

Welch, J. S., Pratt, J. H., and Symmonds, R. E.: The Wertheim hysterectomy for squamous cell carcinoma of the uterine cervix. Thirty years' experience at the Mayo Clinic. Amer. J. Obstet. Gynec., 51: 978, 1961.

Wespi, H.: Early Carcinoma of the Uterine Cervix. Grune & Stratton, Inc., New York, 1949.

Wilbanks, G. D., Creasman, W. T., Kaufmann, L. A., and Parker, R. T.: Treatment of cervical dysplasia with electrocautery and tetracycline suppositories. Amer. J. Obstet. Gynec., 117: 460, 1973.

Woodruff, J. D., and Mattingly, R. F.: Epithelial changes preceding spinal cell carcinoma of cervix uteri. Amer. J. Obstet. Gynec., 77: 977, 1959.

Wynder, E. L., Cornfield, J., Schroff, P. O., and Doraiswami, K. R.: A study of environmental factors in carcinoma of the cervix. Amer. J. Obstet. Gynec., 68: 1016, 1954.

Younge, P. A., Hertig, A. T., and Armstrong, D.: A study of 135 cases of carcinoma in situ of cervix at Free Hospital for Women. Amer. J. Obstet. Gynec., 58: 867, 1949.

chapter 13

Relaxations, Incontinence, Fistulas, and Malpositions

STRUCTURE OF THE VAGINAL OUTLET

The pelvic floor, closing the outlet of the pelvis, is made up of a number of muscular and fascial structures which are pierced by the rectum, vagina, and urethra as these canals pass to the exterior of the body. The most important of the muscles is the levator ani, which forms a broad muscular sheet, concave above and convex below, and which extends like a diaphragm from one side of the pelvis to the other. It consists of a pubic portion which arises from the pubic bone anteriorly, and passes backward to encircle the rectum, whereas the iliac portion arises from the so-called white line of the pelvis and passes downward to meet its fellow of the opposite side in the midline, extending to the tip of the coccyx behind. Most of its fibers pass behind the rectum and, according to the majority of anatomists, few or no fibers pass between the vagina and the rectum.

Even more important in the support of the pelvic organs is the fascia. The superior or pelvic fascia covers the upper surface of the muscular diaphragm, extending from the white line of the pelvis on one side to that of the other, and giving off fascial coverings to the vaginal and rectal canals as they pass through the pelvic floor.

The inferior or external pelvic fascia, found beneath the levator diaphragm, is divisible into two parts, one *anterior* and one *posterior* to a line between the tuberosities of the ischia. The posterior covers the under surface of the levator muscles, whereas the anterior constitutes the so-called urogenital diaphragm or inferior triangular ligament. This is a dense fascial sheet which fills in the triangle formed by the pubic arch, the rami, and a line drawn between the two tuberosities. It is composed of a superficial and a deep layer. The superficial perineal muscles are placed superficial to the urogenital diaphragm, but the deeper group, with other important structures, is situated in the space between the two layers (Figs. 13.1–13.3).

LACERATIONS OF THE PERINEUM

These are best subdivided into those of the *incomplete* and *complete* varieties. In the former, the laceration does not involve

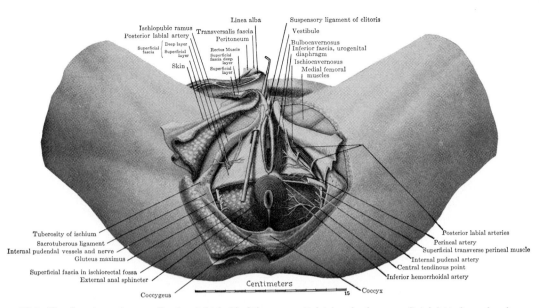

13.1. The female perineum. On the right half of the urogenital triangle the superficial fatty layer has been turned aside to display the deep layer of the superficial fascia; the latter, on the left half, has been reflected to show the contents of the superficial perineal compartment. (From Anson, B. J.: in *A Textbook of Gynecology,* Ed. 6, edited by A. H. Curtis and J. W. Huffman, W. B. Saunders Company, Philadelphia, 1950.)

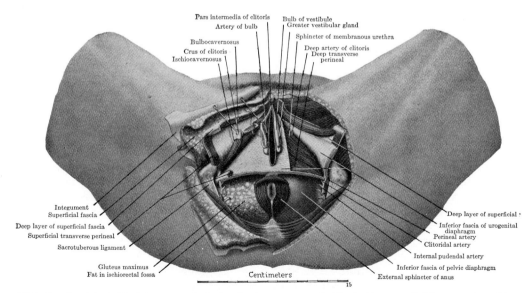

13.2. On the right half of the urogenital triangle the cavernous bodies in the superficial compartment have been exposed by partial removal of the superficial perineal muscles; on the left, the inferior fascia of the urogenital diaphragm has been reflected to show the musculature in the deep perineal compartment. In the anal triangle, on the left side, the superficial (fatty) tissue has been removed from the ischiorectal fossa. (From Anson, B. J.: in *A Textbook of Gynecology,* Ed. 6, edited by A. H. Curtis and J. W. Huffman, W. B. Saunders Company, Philadelphia, 1950.)

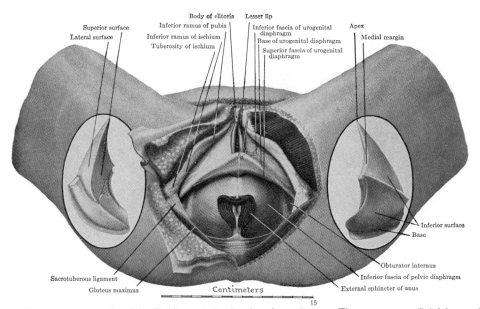

13.3. The urogenital and pelvic diaphragms in the female perineum. The more superficial layers have been removed to show the urogenital diaphragm; the latter has been drawn forward, revealing the anterior continuation of the ischiorectal fossa, the superior boundary of which is the pelvic diaphragm. *Inserts:* upper and lower aspects of plaster cast of the left ischiorectal fossa showing the extent and shape of the space. (From Anson, B. J.: in *A Textbook of Gynecology*, Ed. 6, edited by A. H. Curtis and J. W. Huffman, W. B. Saunders Company, Philadelphia, 1950.)

the sphincter ani, whereas in the latter this muscle is partly or completely torn. Incomplete tears are sometimes subdivided into those of *first* and *second degree*, according to their extent, the complete variety being considered as of the *third degree*. In the overwhelming majority of cases, *lacerations of the genital canal* are due to childbirth, often complicated, but other forms of trauma, such as coitus, attempted rape, or external violence may at times be responsible.

The significance of perineal laceration depends upon its extent and upon the structures involved by the laceration. The importance of proper *immediate repair* of lacerations as a part of the management of labor need scarcely be emphasized. Median tears are much less likely to produce subsequent relaxation than are the lateral or sulcal lacerations. The latter often produce injuries of the fascial and muscular tissues of the perineum, whereas even complete median tears may be associated with little or no relaxation. In other cases, however, the median tear may be combined with extensive injury or

relaxation of the levator muscle and the perineal fascial supports, with extensive vaginal relaxation as a result.

CERVICAL LACERATIONS

Cervical lacerations are frequent findings in the woman who has had complicated labors. Lacerations may be slight or deep with extension into the vaginal fornices or even into the base of the broad ligament. They may be unilateral, bilateral, or stellate (Fig. 13.4). On occasion such lacerations heal well with no residua except a rather rigid fibrous scar with only minimal inflammation. More commonly, however, there is superimposed infection which leads to varying degrees of cervicitis. The swollen, mucous surfaces are extruded out of the endocervical canal, producing the picture spoken of as *eversion,* a frequent and characteristic finding with deep bilateral tears. Due to the infection and edema there may be marked hypertrophy of either or both lips of the cervix. Where concomitant inflammation is extreme, a more forbidding ap-

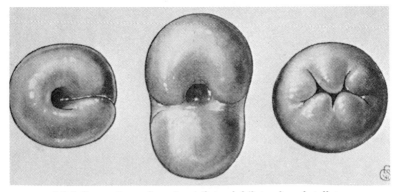

13.4. Lacerations of cervix, unilateral, bilateral, and stellate

pearance may be found than in many early malignant conditions.

Although there is no difficulty as a rule in making a gross diagnosis of cancer in advanced lesions, it is frankly impossible to make any distinction between certain Stage I cervical cancers, and various benign, everted, and hypertrophic cervices. Cytology, colposcopy and biopsy must be resorted to for diagnosis. However, there is very suggestive evidence that persistent chronic infection of the cervix may be of importance in the later development of carcinoma; therefore, every effort should be made to minimize the infectious process. The importance of herpes virus type 2 in the causation of cervical cancer has been noted in previous chapters.

Treatment of the lacerated infected cervix is directed primarily at the secondary inflammatory changes, and this usually involves cauterization or conization as described in Chapter 11. It is remarkable how a big, boggy, badly infected cervix can be converted into a fairly normal appearing organ by such simple office procedures as cauterization. It is generally agreed that cryosurgery is no more effective. Such operations as tracheloplasty or cervical amputations of one sort or another were formerly rather popular, but are rarely found in the modern day operative schedule.

RELAXATION OF THE VAGINAL OUTLET (RVO)

A relaxed vaginal outlet is usually a sequel to mere overstretching of the perineal supporting tissues, generally as a result of previous parturition. Although the actual damage usually occurs in the childbearing era, it may not become manifest until the fifth or sixth decade, when generalized muscular atony and loss of elastic tissue are superimposed. Varying degrees of perineal laceration may be apparent (Fig. 13.5), but even without visible evidence there may be extensive submucosal laceration and division of the muscular and fascial supports.

Cystocele and *rectocele* (Figs. 13.6, 7) are frequent concomitants as may be *prolapse,* and actually these three generally occur in association with one or the other being predominant. *Cystocele* occurs as a result of a defect in the pubocervical fascial plane which supports the bladder anteriorly, and as this increases it tends to permit the bladder to sag down below and beyond the uterus, and, in extreme degrees, out the vagina. If the defective fascia involves the urethra, this too tends to drop downward with the production of a *urethrocele,* although this may of course occur independently of cystocele. *Rectocele* is the result of a very similar mechanism involving an attenuated pararectal fascia. With it there may be associated an abnormally deep posterior peritoneal pouch, which may be drawn farther downward along the anterior surface of the rectum. There may thus be formed a long peritoneal hernial sac, often containing loops of small intestine (*enterocele*) as well as rectum. *Prolapse* will be discussed more fully under "Malpositions."

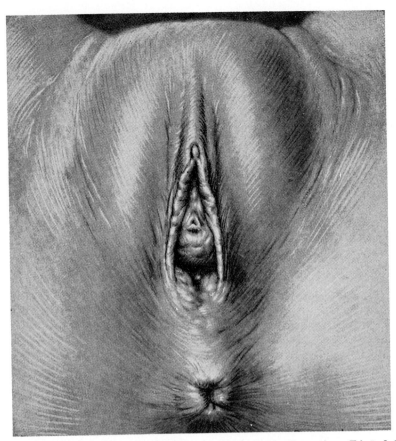

13.5. Relaxed outlet (incomplete laceration). (From Anspach, B. M.: *Gynecology,* Ed. 5. J. B. Lippincott Company, Philadelphia, 1934.)

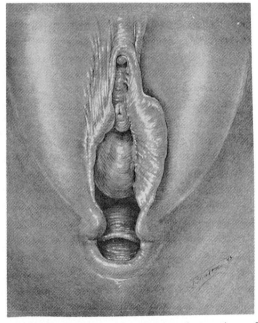

13.6. Complete (3rd degree) laceration of perineum showing also large cystocele.

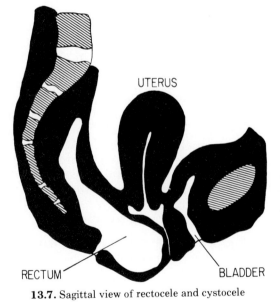

13.7. Sagittal view of rectocele and cystocele

UTERUS

RECTUM

BLADDER

SYMPTOMS OF GENITAL RELAXATION

Even extensive relaxation of the outlet may be entirely symptomless, whereas in other cases there is a complaint of *pressure and heaviness in the vaginal region,* especially after prolonged standing. The patient not infrequently describes her symptoms as a sensation of "everything dropping out." There may be some *bearing-down discomfort in the lower abdomen,* and *backache.* However, troublesome backache should always lead to a search for such more frequent causes as abnormalities of the back itself.

Where relaxation is associated with *complete perineal laceration,* at least partial *fecal incontinence* is produced. In the latter, the patient may have fairly good control, but if the stools are rather loose, distressing incontinence develops.

Although moderate *cystocele* often causes no symptoms, the more marked degrees bring about increasing *difficulty in emptying the bladder.* In extreme cases the patient may be unable to void unless the bladder is first pushed back in the vagina with the finger. In the more marked cases, the bladder may contain much residual urine, and *cystitis* is almost always the result, with the possibility of ascending infection. There is, therefore, a complaint of *increased frequency of urination,* with perhaps *tenesmus,* the symptoms being most troublesome during the day, and improved by night or when the patient is in the recumbent position. *Incontinence of urine* is frequent (see page 298), and this *incontinence* is usually of the *stress* variety, with escape of urine on coughing, laughing, sneezing, or other muscular effort. Although stress incontinence may occur with cystocele or urethrocele, it may occur with no obvious relaxation and from many causes.

Rectocele, like cystocele, may produce few symptoms, but where the protruding rectal pouch is large (Fig. 13.8), there may be a deflection of feces into the pouch, with increasing *difficulty of defecation* and *constipation,* because of the impaired overstretched rectal wall. *Hemorrhoids* frequently develop, adding

to the patient's discomfort. Finally, in cases associated with *prolapse of the uterus,* there is added the strain of symptoms characterizing the latter, especially the discomfort produced by the *protrusion* of the uterus, bladder, and rectum.

Diagnosis

The simpler *relaxations of the vagina* are usually evident, even on simple inspection, from the gaping appearance of the orifice and the separation of the anterior and posterior vaginal walls, normally in juxtaposition. Where there has been extensive laceration, scar tissue may be plainly visible, either in the midline or in one or both sulci. When the examining fingers are introduced, and the patient is asked to strain down, one can at once note the *absence of the resistance of the muscles* surrounding the lower vagina.

Cystocele and rectocele, when large, may be at once visible on inspection, but often they recede when the patient is lying flat. It is always important to ask the patient to strain, this bringing out the cystocele and rectocele so that their extent can be seen. The presence of *urethrocele* is indicated by marked bulging just below the urethral orifice. This must be distinguished from a suburethral diverticulum.

The demonstration of a *rectocele* can be made more striking by introducing a finger into the rectum and pushing it upward and forward into the rectal pouch. By thrusting the finger forward, the anterior rectal wall can be hooked outward from the vagina, the rectovaginal septum being exceedingly thin and atrophic in such cases. On occasion it may be difficult to distinguish between a high rectocele and enterocele; a light of some kind placed up the rectum will suggest an *enterocele,* if there is no observed vaginal transillumination (Altchek).

When *complete laceration* exists, there is often a deep midline cleft from the posterior vaginal margin through the perineum into the rectum, and sometimes extending upward into the anterior rectal wall. Under such circumstances, the rectal mucosa is commonly everted,

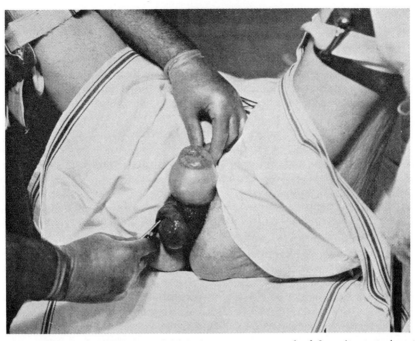

13.8. Unusually extensive birth injury in which the rectum was avulsed from its posterior attachments. The patient had had complete incontinence of feces for 30 years. It was possible to repair this injury at a single operation, with resulting satisfactory bowel control.

presenting as a bright red spongy area. Even when the anus seems intact, the sphincter may have been injured. Here, as in the case of the vagina, a demonstration of the adequacy or inadequacy of the sphincter control may be made by asking the patient to "draw in" on a finger inserted into the anus.

Stress Incontinence

The diagnosis of *stress incontinence* is not always easy, for urgency due to infection, leakage from fistulas, and other modes of urinary loss are sometimes difficult to exclude. A good history is of course paramount. Various methods of elevating the vaginal wall by two fingers (Bonney test) or Allis clamps (Marchetti test) tend to prevent loss of urine on straining. Urinalysis, cystoscopy, cystometric studies, and urethrocystograms with or without a metallic bead chain as advised by Hodgkinson and Green are occasionally necessary.

The uncertain mechanism of incontinence has resulted in many different types of treatment as indicated in the review by Green, and an earlier symposium edited by Lund fully treats the complicated subject of urinary incontinence. *Loss of the urethrovesical angle* as indicated by the excellent chain cystometic studies of Green is presumed to be the usual factor in producing stress incontinence; restoration of this by various surgical procedures seems the keynote for successful correction.

Most women, especially if they have borne children, will occasionally experience trivial degrees of urinary loss which needs no treatment. When the patient is in the childbearing age, and when she is anxious for further pregnancies, the conservative plan is always advisable with the more moderate degrees of relaxation, and when symptoms are absent or slight, as they so often are, plastic correction can be deferred until after the completion of childbearing in a large proportion of cases. Occasionally the "perineometer" will encourage development of muscles of the bladder neck so that stress incontinence is markedly improved.

It is not the intent of this text to discuss the myriad of operative procedures devised for the correction of urinary incontinence for another one appears every month or two in specialty journals. Where there are significant degrees of incontinence, however, some type of operative intervention becomes necessary, and a wide variety of procedures have been suggested. Where there is a demonstrable *cystourethrocele,* anterior repair with a Kelly plication is the rule. With recurrence or without relaxation, some variation of the strap procedure (Goebell-Stoeckel) or vesicourethral suspension (Marshall-Marchetti) is usually performed. Of particular merit is the "Pereyra procedure," a simple atraumatic operation especially for the poor risk patient.

Treatment

Correction of any of these forms of genital relaxation is possible only by surgical procedures, but in a large proportion of cases operations may be deferred for long periods of time, and in the less pronounced cases they may be avoided altogether. Jeffcoate points out the frequency of dyspareunia, if injudicious, too snug, posterior repair is utilized. Indeed, even if an adequate vagina is preserved in the menstrual era, postmenopausal atrophy superimposed on a vagina of borderline caliber may lead to distressing dyspareunia. Our own tendency is to avoid posterior repair in the younger woman unless there are major degrees of relaxation.

Reparative Surgery

When any type of vaginal plastic procedure is contemplated, the rational gynecologist will at once consider the possibility of *vaginal hysterectomy* with appropriate repair. As to the age-old question, "Isn't she too young?" the informed gynecologist will reply that only a rare woman is "too young" for hysterectomy if she has completed her family. Admittedly, one stroke of lightning could wipe out that family with the woman unable to have more children, but this is certainly a pessimistic approach to life in general. Nevertheless, the conscientious gynecologist will discuss this possibility with the patient and her husband.

Many multiparous 30-year-old women have a 50-year-old pelvis. In most instances they are sufficiently intelligent to appreciate that hysterectomy will be followed only by cessation of the menstrual period, and by no further pregnancies, and that ovarian function will continue. Consequently removal of the symptomatic prolapsed uterus should result in no psychological problems, particularly when it is pointed out that some 8–10,000 women annually succumb to uterine cancer. This is particularly valid if concomitant repair is done, for unless the uterus is removed, and if the woman should become pregnant again, even the most proficient repair might be impaired by vaginal delivery.

It has already been indicated that tubal ligation is rapidly becoming an archaic procedure (Chapter 5), which preserves the functionless uterus that may well become the site of myoma, cancer, and other forms of pathology. Indeed tubal ligation except in the immediate postpartum or poor risk patient hardly seems a justifiable operation, although admittedly morbidity is low. Hysterectomy, usually by the vaginal route, has generally superceded this procedure as an elective method of sterilization, especially where there are even minor asymptomatic disease, such as cystocele, rectocele, or prolapse. By the same token uterine suspension is rarely carried out in this era in the multiparous individual who desires no further pregnancies, and it is generally reserved for the youthful individual. Today suspension is usually performed only as part of a conservative procedure for endometriosis.

Above all, it should be emphasized that pelvic repair is an elective procedure, which should generally be deferred until after the desire for children has been satisfied. On occasion judicious use of pessaries may obviate the necessity for any operative intervention until the family has been completed, at which time, irrespective of age, definitive surgery can be accomplished. There is nothing urgent about cystocele, rectocele, or prolapse, and only if these are symptomatic should surgery be contemplated. Where, however, there is frank protrusion out of the introitus with chafing and ulceration of the mucosa, bleeding is inevitable, and this degree of prolapse, although otherwise asymptomatic, should mandate surgical treatment.

FISTULAS

Genital Fistulas

A genital fistula is an abnormal communication between some part of the genital canal, on the one hand, and either the urinary or intestinal tract or both.

Etiology

By far the most common cause of genital fistulas in past years was *obstetrical trauma,* especially in cases of prolonged and difficult labor. In such cases the fistula is due to necrosis and sloughing of the genital canal, usually the vagina, and also of the wall of the subjacent viscus, generally the bladder. The *improper use of forceps* likewise adds to the incidence of such fistulas. The great improvement in obstetrical management which has occurred in recent years has lessened the frequency of fistulas due to this group of causes.

On the other hand, the development of major *surgery* and the widespread *employment of radium* for many gynecological indications have led to a not inconsiderable incidence of genital fistulas. The majority of fistulas seen nowadays are the result of injury to the bladder, ureter, or rectum in the course of operations, particularly radical hysterectomy, or they result from necrosis and sloughing produced by the application of radium. Other causes are the *destruction of tissue* by *malignant tumors, ulceration due to foreign bodies,* especially vaginal pessaries, and occasionally, *cystocele repair.*

It is obvious to any gynecological surgeon that urinary fistula may occur after a very simple uncomplicated case where the best standards of medical practice have been observed. Unfortunately, such cases represent a significant proportion of medicolegal problems today, and it may be difficult to explain the occurrence to an unsympathetic jury. Presumably some patients may seemingly be "poor healers," and since there is always some trauma to the bladder or bowel with either vaginal or abdominal hysterectomy, a fistula may ensue despite acceptable technique.

Urinary Fistulas

Even the most accomplished gynecological surgeon will at one time or another inadvertently damage the urinary tract, and Graber, O'Rourke, and McElrath have indicated that serious injury (accidental laceration) of the bladder occurs in almost 2 per cent of the hysterectomies. Complications are minimized if the damage is recognized, but serious problems (as fistula) may ensue if the injury is not noted. The causative factors and treatment of bladder damage are well summarized. The authors quote Mengert's apt remark, "It is no sin to cut into the bladder; the sin is not recognize it." The abnormal communication may involve various portions of the urinary and genital canals. The following are the chief varieties: (1) vesicovaginal, (2) urethrovaginal, (3) ureterovaginal, and (4) combinations thereof.

Of these the most frequent variety is the *vesicovaginal.* This possesses a special historic interest, since the first successful repair of this type by Sims in 1855 laid the foundation of gynecology as a specialty. Although a relatively common condition in a preceding generation, it is today among the less frequently encountered gynecological conditions, although a few cases have followed in the wake of certain types of operation and radiotherapy, as already mentioned. The fistulous communication between the bladder and the vagina may be of such tiny size that it is difficult to demonstrate, or it may involve destruction of the whole base of the bladder, not infrequently extending to the urethra below or the ureter above (Fig. 13.9).

The locations of the other types of fistula are indicated by their designations

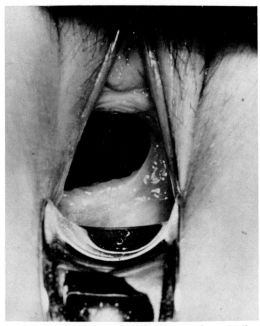

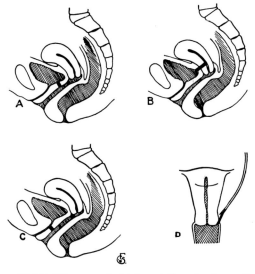

13.10. Diagram of chief varieties of urinary fistula. *A,* vesicovaginal; *B,* vesicouterine; *C,* urethrovagina; *D,* ureterovaginal.

13.9. Large vesicovaginal fistula cured surgically. (Courtesy of Dr. Albert Brown, Wilmington, N. C.)

and they are depicted in the accompanying diagrams (Figs. 13.10, 11) so that they need not be described in detail. The *ureterovaginal* merits special mention, because it is the type most often resulting from accidental injury to the ureter during the operation of hysterectomy, especially where radical surgery for malignant disease is being performed. Actually, even in the best clinics a 5 to 10% complication of urinary fistula had been routine in conjunction with radical

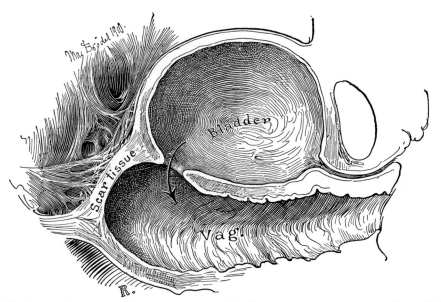

13.11. Vesicovaginal fistula resulting from injury to bladder during panhysterectomy. (From Kelly, H. A., and Burnam, C. F.: *Diseases of Kidneys, Ureters and Bladder.* Appleton-Century-Crofts, Inc., New York, 1922).

Wertheim hysterectomy although improved techniques in recent years have led to a decreased incidence. *Urethrovaginal* fistulas are more likely to be sequelae of anterior repair and plication or excision of a suburethral diverticulum than an obstetrical injury (Gray).

Symptoms

The characteristic symptom is *leakage of urine from the vagina.* This, with small fistulas, may be only in the form of a slight dribble, more noticeable in some postures than others. In other cases, the flow of urine is constant and profuse, and none may be voided through the meatus in such cases. The distress of the patient is increased by the *irritation of the vagina, vulva, and perineum* produced by such constant leakage, to say nothing of the unpleasant *ammoniacal odor.* Unless meticulous cleansing be observed, phosphatic incrustations may develop about the fistula, thus further adding to the local irritation. It is easy to understand how such a condition as fistula, especially when this is large, limits the patient's activities and makes her a social recluse, with nervousness, irritability, insomnia, and depression as natural sequelae.

Diagnosis

The diagnosis of urinary fistula is usually comparatively simple although varying amounts of the usual postoperative vaginal discharge may confuse the issue. In any case it is not always so easy to determine the exact location and nature of the fistula. Leakage of urine may be the result of extreme relaxation of the vesical sphincter, without a fistula. When this occurs after difficult delivery or after operation, it may make one apprehensive that a fistula exists. With simple *sphincter atony* the leakage is apt to be intermittent and it often occurs only after such straining efforts as coughing, sneezing, or laughing.

Vesicovaginal fistula presents no difficulty in diagnosis unless it is very small or unless it is in an inaccessible location high up in the vagina, where it may be concealed by extensive cicatricial deposits following operation. In the ordinary case the fistula can be readily seen when the patient is examined in the knee-chest position, which gives an excellent view of the whole anterior vaginal wall and fornix. For that matter, the larger fistulas are readily palpated by the finger in the vagina. The smaller, more inaccessible fistulas can be demonstrated by filling the bladder with *methylene-blue colored sterile water* and observing the escape of the bluish fluid from the abnormal opening. Cystoscopic examination, preferably by the Kelly air distention method, often gives valuable information as to the location of the fistula and its relation to the ureters.

In the not infrequent *ureterovaginal* fistula the demonstration of urinary leakage from within the vagina and the elimination of a vesical source by such simple methods as have been described leave little doubt as to the existence of leakage from the ureter. This should be verified by more intensive urological study, often including intravenous or retrograde pyelograms or both.

Treatment

Small fistulas, unless produced by malignant disease, occasionally close spontaneously, and this may often be facilitated by postural treatment, limitation of fluids, urinary antiseptics, and the employment of a retention catheter. Such a happy outcome, however, is *not* the rule, and surgical treatment must almost always be resorted to. The operation must be adapted to the indications of the particular case, but the well versed gynecologist will probably prefer a vaginal to a transvesical approach. Without detailing the operative methods which may be called for, suffice it to say that by the utilization of such principles as partial closure of the vagina (Latzko), or free mobilization of the bladder, there are few cases in which the trained operator cannot effect cure (Blaikley). If the defect is near the trigone, it may be wise to catheterize the ureters preoperatively. The postradiation fistulas tend to heal very poorly because of the impaired blood supply, unlike the surgical and obstetrical defects;

estrogen suppositories may be helpful. On occasion diversion of the urinary tract may be necessary.

A cardinal rule, frequently overlooked, is the *desirability* of waiting four to six months after injury before attempting any kind of reparative procedure. This delay is not easy to justify to the patient, but sufficient time must be allowed for subsidence of edema and induration if there is to be any chance of a successful surgical outcome. Where there is evidence of severe upper tract damage nephrostomy is preferable to premature attempts to restore lower urinary tract integrity. Collins has recently suggested cortisone to minimize fibrosis and speed up the time needed before repair. Local palliative measures and antibiotics are also used preoperatively.

Vaginal Fecal Fistula

Rectovaginal fistula is by far the most common form of vaginal fecal fistula. The possible *causes* are in the main the same as those concerned in the etiology of urinary fistula, namely, irradiation, obstetrical trauma, and surgery (especially vaginal). The operations which are most apt to be followed by the development of such a fistula are vaginal puncture for pelvic abscess, perineorrhaphy, and hemorrhoidectomy. Lymphogranuloma inguinale is another possible cause. Much less frequently the fecal fistula may involve the sigmoid colon, or small intestine, the usual cause being malignancy, diverticulitis, or operations upon either the pelvic organs or the intestine, although *posterior colpotomy* for a postoperative infected pelvic hematoma seems a frequent agent in the causation of vaginal fecal fistulas.

A rectovaginal fistula may be very tiny, producing only occasional escape of gas or fecal matter from the vagina, and even this may be noted only when the stools are soft or liquid, as after purgatives. Such small fistulas may close spontaneously. In the larger fistulas, the lot of the patient may be made distressing by continuous leakage of fecal material, with resulting irritation and a constantly offensive odor. The *treatment* is surgical,

the operation being done by the vaginal route in the rectovaginal type. Occasionally, temporary colostomy is advisable to permit the badly infected tissues to undergo some preliminary improvement as regards healing properties.

Abdominal procedures are required for the closure of vaginal fistulas involving other parts of the intestinal tract; rarely suction ("sump") drainage will close a high fistula but will often minimize autodigestion of the adjacent tissues. The site of the intestinal component of the fistula should be ascertained by barium and other studies; obviously, a colostomy would be valueless for an ileovaginal fistula, and this type of defect warrants prompt surgery without a prolonged waiting period. Bowel "prep" should be routine.

MALPOSITIONS

Normal Position of Uterus

Normally the uterus occupies a position in the pelvic cavity between the bladder anteriorly and the rectum posteriorly. The long axis of the uterus is in the nearly horizontal plane, and forms an approximate right angle with the long axis of the vagina. The easy mobility of the uterus is an important characteristic, as can be noted in pelvic examinations of normal women. Under abnormal conditions it is greatly restricted, as when the uterus is fixed by surrounding inflammatory disease.

Normal Supports of the Uterus

The normal position of the uterus is maintained by three factors.

(1) The Pelvic Floor. The fascial planes of the pelvic floor are inserted at about the level of the internal os, the strongest band being the fasciomuscular condensation in the base of the broad ligament, constituting the so-called ligament of Mackenrodt or *cardinal* ligament.

(2) The Uterine Ligaments. Of these the most important in the support of the uterus are the *broad* and the *uterosacral* ligaments. This is true particularly because in the base of the former is the fascial condensation above alluded to as the cardinal ligament, whereas the uterosacral ligament likewise includes a strong fascial band stretching backward to the junction of the second and third sacral vertebrae. The round ligaments, formerly spoken of picturesquely as exerting a guy-rope function on the fundus, are now looked upon as having little supporting function except perhaps during pregnancy, when they become thick and hypertrophic, and may even, as some believe, help to direct the presenting part of the child downward toward the pelvic canal during labor. In the nonpregnant uterus, their laxity and their circuitous course make it difficult to believe that they can have a supporting function, although they may become extremely hypertrophic when there is an enlarged myomatous uterus.

(3) Intraabdominal Pressure. Normally this considerable force is directed upon the posterior surface of the uterus, driving it downward and forward, and thus tending to accentuate the normal position of the organ. Intestinal loops are, so to speak, deflected into the posterior cul-de-sac, and are not normally found between the uterus and bladder. The same intraabdominal force can become a power for evil if the uterus is displaced backward, as it is then exerted on the anterior uterine surface, tending to crowd the uterus farther backward and downward.

Displacements of the Uterus

Anteflexion can be most simply defined as a bending forward of the uterus, which involves chiefly the body. The anteflexed uterus often shows some degree of hypoplasia, although most often of rather slight degree. *Anteversion* needs no treatment. Hypoplasia in the degree suggesting a really infantile uterus often responds to the stimulus of the estrogenic hormone.

Of far greater importance to the gynecologist than the anterior displacements are the *retrodisplacements*. These may be either *congenital or acquired,* the latter

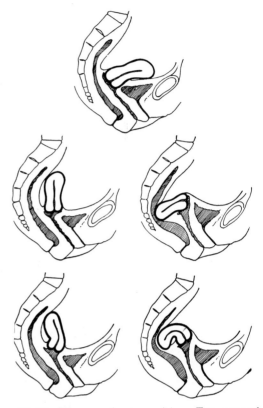

13.12. Degrees of retroposition. *Top,* normal position of uterus; *center left,* slight retroversion; *center right,* marked retroversion; *bottom left,* slight retroflexion; *bottom right,* marked retroflexion.

being the more important, especially when complicated by other pelvic lesions, such as pelvic inflammatory disease or endometriosis.

Types and Degrees (Fig. 13.12)

Retroversion refers to the retrodisplacement in which the uterus is tilted backward on its transverse axis to a greater or lesser degree. When comparatively slight, so that the fundus is about vertical or pointing no farther back than the sacral promontory, the retroversion is spoken of as of *first degree.* When the fundus is within the hollow of the sacrum but not below the level of the cervix, the designation of *second degree* is commonly used. Finally, when the uterus is so far back that the fundus is below the level of the cervix, the retroversion is *third degree.*

Retroflexion, simply defined, is a bending backward of the uterus, *i.e.,* of the body upon the cervix. The latter may still be directed normally downward and backward, but more frequently has tilted downward and forward (erect position of the woman) toward the symphysis as the fundus falls backward.

Causes

The causes of retrodisplacements of the uterus may be grouped as follows.

(1) Congenital. Retrodisplacement of one type or another is frequently observed in the uteri of fetuses or very young children. This condition often persists into adult life, probably as a result of certain developmental deficiencies.

(2) Acquired. Retrodisplacement of a previously normally placed uterus may occur from a number of causes, the most important of which may be grouped as follows.

(a) Puerperal. This group embraces a considerable number of possible factors which may develop following full term and especially complicated delivery, or, much less frequently, miscarriage. After parturition, the uterus is large and soft during the period of involution. Increased stress and strain on the supporting ligaments may lead to so much attenuation that when the uterus does involute, the overstretched ligaments can no longer maintain it in the normal anterior position.

Much more important are injuries of the supporting structures, especially the fascial structures of the pelvic floor. When these are injured or when they are overstretched, the cervix drops forward and downward, tending to swing more and more into the long axis of the vagina. Once this process has started, it tends to continue, the fundus falling backward, after which the intraabdominal pressure tends to futher accentuate the backward displacement. It is easy to understand, therefore, why some degree of descensus of the uterus is seen in almost all cases of acquired retrodisplacement.

(b) Adnexal Disease. The complicated form of retroflexion is as a rule associated with adnexal disease, either inflammatory or endometriosis. The sequence may be in the order of retrodisplacement followed later by adnexitis or endometriosis, or *vice versa.* In either case the retrodisplaced fundus, instead of being free and movable, is adherent to other structures. especially the adnexa or the rectum, or both.

(c) Neoplasms. The effect of pelvic neoplasms of one sort or another in producing retrodisplacements is a mechanical one. For example, a large myoma developing in the anterior wall of the uterus will tend to push the uterus backward, whereas certain ovarian tumors impacted deep in the cul-de-sac may, by pushing the cervix far forward, cause backward displacement of the corpus.

(d) Trauma. The question of whether acute displacement can occur as a result of trauma is not infrequently of medicolegal importance. The protected position of the uterus, and the nature of its support, makes it difficult to believe that any but the most severe trauma could bring about displacement. The generally accepted opinion is that such acute traumatic displacement can occur, but that it is exceedingly rare. However, the burden of medicolegal proof rests on the certainty that trauma has led to retrodisplacement, bleeding, and abortion.

Symptoms

Simple uncomplicated retrodisplacements of the uterus are often entirely symptomless, although dysmenorrhea and *backache* may be noted. Certainly every gynecologist, in the course of routine examinations, encounters innumerable cases of even marked retrodisplacement in which not the slightest menstrual cramps, backache, or any other symptom has been complained of which might be linked up with the displacement. Even when backache is a symptom, it is often due to other causes than the position of the uterus.

Backache. One of the most frequent complaints found in any gynecological practice is backache, for the average woman with such a problem will immediately make the diagnosis that "her womb is out of place." Far more often, of course, the difficulties are due to musculoligamentous or osseous ailments of the back itself, and are in the realm of what most practicing gynecologists refer to as an *"orthopedic backache," i.e.,* they require orthopedic consultation. Arthritis, a ruptured disc, and many other entities may be causative factors.

BACKACHE DUE TO PELVIC CAUSE

Retrodisplacement *may* be associated with backache, especially when there is a marked retroflexion producing a boggy, edematous fundus. Frequently, there is some degree of concomitant prolapse, and in either case the backache may be accentuated around the menses or when the patient has been on her feet a great deal. The mechanics of the forces of gravity tend to further aggravate the anatomical deformity, and this seems more logical than the so-called generalized "pelvic congestion" phenomenon. Endometriosis and pelvic inflammatory disease frequently are associated with a backache, in part as a result of a fixed retroversion, but in part because of turgor of the adherent pelvic structures. Large posterior tumors may be painful by virtue of pressure or impingement on the sacral plexus.

A very ominous type of backache may occur with certain pelvic malignancies, especially *carcinoma of the cervix.* It is not unlike the type of backache associated with a herniated disc, but in the cancer patient, treated or otherwise, it is generally the harbinger of involvement of the iliac nodes. Enlargement of these may ensue, even before obvious lymphedema, with irritation of the sciatic nerve trunks and severe pain radiating down the back of the leg. In the patient treated for carcinoma of the cervix this is often the first sign of recurrence before nodes are palpable. Pyelograms, lymphangiograms, and x-rays of the spine should be obtained, but even if these appear normal, the gynecologist will keep his fingers crossed when this typically suggestive symptom appears. Unfortunately, he is

not yet justified in making a diagnosis of recurrent malignancy; when he is able, the patient has generally passed beyond the stage of salvageability (Chapter 12).

Our own experience has been that simple congenital retrodisplacements have little or no tendency to cause backache. In the acquired type, however, in which the uterus is often heavy, subinvoluted, and edematous, *premenstrual backache* and *dysmenorrhea* are often produced and may occasionally be relieved by suspension of the uterus after trial by pessary.

Menstrual disorders may or may not be present. A prolonged flow with protracted, tarry staining of odoriferous nature is often noticed and seems quite in keeping with a retroflexion that opposes the forces of gravity. Should the cervix be pointing toward the symphysis, it is obvious that *infertility* might be incurred.

If *pregnancy* occurs in a retrodisplaced uterus, there seems to be general agreement that the hazard of miscarriage is slightly increased. This is not the usual occurrence, because even a markedly retroflexed pregnant uterus will ordinarily, before the end of the third month, lift itself above the pelvic brim into the abdomen. In some cases of marked retroflexion, especially if the uterus is adherent, the enlarging uterus is crowded more and more into the hollow of the sacrum, where it is *incarcerated,* with miscarriage as the usual result. If the pregnancy should continue, *sacculation* (a diffuse ballooning of part of the uterine wall) may ensue as indicated by Fadel and Misenheimer. It will be seen, therefore, that the management of retroflexion combined with pregnancy calls for special supervision and for occasional use of a pessary through the first trimester.

After the menopause, women with uncorrected retrodisplacements ordinarily experience marked mitigation in symptoms, as a result of the lessened congestion, the abolition of menstruation and the general shrinkage of the organs.

The so-called *Allen-Masters* syndrome is characterized by painful laceration of the posterior leaf of the broad ligament, a retroverted uterus, and an abnormally mobile cervix (according to the authors). Frankly, we suspect such patients with this syndrome may have the same psychic overlay as occurs in such other pelvic disorders as "chronic pelvic congestion."

Diagnosis

The symptoms of retroposition are of little value in diagnosis. Certainly the mere existence of backache is anything but characteristic, contrary to the lay view. Careful elimination of postural, spinal, and other causes is essential before one is justified in attributing backache to a retrodisplacement, as noted previously.

Pelvic examination is necessary for diagnosis, and this is usually easy (Fig. 13.13). The cardinal points are as follows.

(1) The cervix usually points toward the symphysis, instead of downward and toward the sacrum.

(2) The fundus cannot be felt anteriorly, where it should be placed, but it can be palpated posteriorly. When bimanual examination is difficult because of obesity or extreme abdominal rigidity, the diagnosis is often possible from internal palpation alone. By the usual methods of bimanual palpation, one not only determines the position of the uterus, but also its size and its degree of movability. A part of such an examination is to determine the presence of complicating pelvic pathology, such as adnexitis or tumors. In virgins the examination must be made *per* rectum, and even in married women vaginorectal examination may yield worthwhile information. Occasionally anesthesia may be required for satisfactory evaluation.

Differential Diagnosis

Although the diagnosis is usually easy enough, there are certain cases in which it may be exceedingly difficult, even if the conditions for palpation are satisfactory. A *myoma of the posterior wall* may be difficult to distinguish from a retroflexed fundus, whereas, on the other hand, a sharply retroflexed fundus may feel like a myoma. A firm *inflammatory mass densely adherent to the posterior wall* may likewise simulate a retroflexed uterus. A *pregnant retroflexed fundus*

may even be mistaken for an ovarian cyst, and various other possibilities for error may be encountered. In the occasional case where differentiation is important, it may be necessary, under strict aseptic preparations, to insert a uterine sound in order to determine the position of the uterus. It need scarcely be said that this is not to be done when there is any suspicion of pregnancy. On occasion, even the best gynecologist cannot properly evaluate pelvic masses and distinguish myomas from endometriosis from inflammatory disease from retroflexed normal uteri, etc.

Treatment

Postural. The use of the knee-chest position is advocated by many, both in prophylaxis and in the management of cases which respond to bimanual replacement, as well as in the uncomplicated cases in which satisfactory replacement and vaginal pessaries are not possible. There is some difference of opinion as to its value, but we believe it to be useful in many cases, especially postpartum. As soon as a woman assumes the knee-chest posture, and air distends the vagina, a freely movable uterus falls toward the front. The maintenance of the normal position is often made more certain by instructing the patient to assume the knee-chest position three or four times a day for a period of five minutes at a time. (See Fig. 13.14.) The indications for a *pessary* will be discussed in a subsequent portion of this chapter.

Suspension Operations

Suspension operations should never be contemplated unless a preliminary trial by pessary has been carried out. If a pessary should anatomically replace a retroposed uterus with complete relief of symptoms, it is significant. If removal of the pessary is followed by a subsequent retrodisplacement, with a return of the previously alleviated symptoms, this might suggest that the patient is a suitable candidate for suspension. Failure to improve after *proper* application of a pessary should of course contraindicate uterine suspension, and it should be mandatory that *trial of a pessary should*

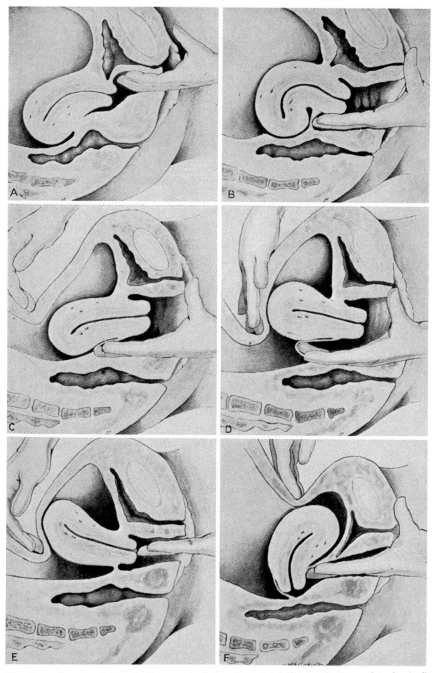

13.13. The three degrees of retrodisplacement of the uterus and the touch signs of each. *A,* first degree, corpus out of reach of examining fingers, both above and below; *B,* second degree, vaginal fingers feel posterior surface of corpus uteri extending directly back; *C,* third degree, vaginal fingers impinge on corpus uteri turned down into the posterior cul-de-sac; *D,* grasping the fundus through the abdominal wall and pushing it upward with internal finger; *E,* further replacement by pushing backward and upward on cervix; *F,* continuing this maneuver to full replacement. (From Crossen, H. S., and Crossen, R. J.: *Diseases of Women.* C. V. Mosby Company, St. Louis, 1935.)

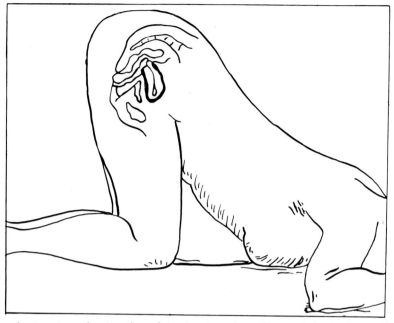

13.14. Knee-chest posture showing the pelvic structures in outline and the tendency of the uterus to gravitate forward.

precede any operation for retroposition unless, of course, the uterus is fixed posteriorly.

Although there is some difference of opinion, most gynecologists feel that an occasional suspension operation is indicated in the correction of *infertility.* As Tompkins has pointed out, this is justifiable only when the uterus cannot be maintained anteriorly by a pessary, when all the usual sterility tests have been performed and found normal, and when there has been a two-year span of infertility after all minor defects have been corrected.

Prolapse of the Uterus (Descensus Uteri)

This is an extremely common condition, being far more frequent in elderly than in young patients. This is explained by the increasing laxity and atony of the muscular and fascial structures in later life. The effects of childbirth injuries may thus make themselves evident, in the form of uterine prolapse, many years after the last pregnancy. Pregnancy in a prolapsed uterus may lead to numerous complications as noted by Piver and Spezia.

The important factor in the mechanism of prolapse is undoubtedly injury or overstretching of the pelvic floor, and especially of the cardinal ligaments (Mackenrodt) in the bases of the broad ligaments. Combined with this there is usually extensive injury to the perineal structures, producing marked vaginal relaxation, and also frequent injury to the fascia of the anterior or posterior vaginal walls, with the production of cystocele or rectocele. Usually, various combinations of these conditions are seen, although at times little or no cystocele or rectocele is associated with the prolapse. Occasional cases are seen, for that matter, in women who have never borne children, and in these the prolapse apparently represents a hernia of the uterus through a defect in the pelvic fascial floor. When the cervix of the prolapsed uterus, usually pointing in the axis of the vagina because of the associated retrodisplacement, is well within the vaginal orifice, the prolapse is spoken of as of *first degree.* In prolapse of *second degree,* the cervix is at or near the introitus. Finally, when the cervix protrudes well beyond the vaginal orifice, the prolapse is of *third degree (procidentia uteri).* Complete prolapse of the posthysterectomy (abdominal or vaginal) vagina may occur and is often difficult to repair if a functioning vagina is desired, as noted by Lee and Symmonds.

Pathology

Aside from the prolapse of the uterus, and the frequently associated cystocele or rectocele, there are other possible pathological sequelae of this condition. Ulceration *(decubitus ulcer)* of the cervix not infrequently occurs (Plate 13.1), as a result of friction against the patient's thighs, her clothing, or the protective napkins which many of these patients wear. *Hypertrophy* of the cervix is another frequent concomitant, this portion of the uterus being often enormously elongated but may occur without prolapse, even in the nulliparous woman, apparently as a congenital malformation.

When the relaxation is marked, there may be complete inversion of the vagina (Fig. 13.15), the canal being literally turned inside out. The drying effect of the air produces a skinlike thickening of the vaginal mucosa, with ulceration and bleeding. In addition, marked degrees of prolapse and cystocele may lead to angulation of the ureter at the urethrovesical junction, with significant degrees of upper tract dilatation. Pyelograms should be routine with complete procidentia.

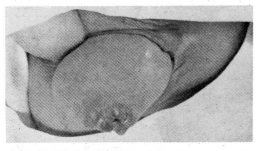

13.15. Complete inversion of vagina with cystocele, rectocele, and enterocele. (Note ulceration of cervix.)

Cervical Cancer with Prolapse

This combination is considered very rare so that relatively few cases are encountered in gynecological literature. Diaz-Bazan reports an astounding number of cases from El Salvador, which amount to almost 20 per cent of all cases in the world literature, and since he has been good enough to send us pictures and microscopic sections, we can testify to the accuracy of his findings (Fig. 13.16).

El Salvador certainly has relatively low standards of living, but they do not differ materially from other adjacent Central American countries where combined procidentia and cervical cancer are rare. Other factors must operate, and we would agree with Diaz-Bazan that the high incidence in El Salvador deserves investigation.

Symptoms of Prolapse

As with other forms of uterine displacement, there are marked individual differences in the symptomatology. Even the most complete prolapse may be associated with no symptoms except for the discomfort produced by the mechanical protrusion of the uterus. In most cases, however, there is likely to be some degree of bearing down and heaviness in the lower abdomen and some backache, both of these being probably due to traction on the uterine ligaments and the venous congestion produced by the prolapse. Cystocele and rectocele are often associated and productive of their respective symptoms (Fig. 13.17).

Diagnosis

The diagnosis is usually simple, and, as a matter of fact, the usual complaint of the patient when she presents herself is that she has "falling of the womb." Although the history of difficult or instrumental labors is suggestive, it is of no great value in diagnosis, which must be made from pelvic examination.

Inspection will, in many cases, reveal the prolapse at once, if this is of the complete type. In such cases the cervix, even with the patient lying down, protrudes beyond the outlet, often occupying a

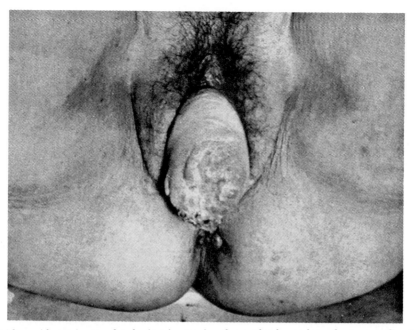

13.16. Epidermoid carcinoma developing in cervix of completely prolapsed uterus. (Courtesy of Dr. Narcisco Diaz-Bazan, San Salvador).

position between a soft boggy cystocele anteriorly and a pouchlike protrusion of the rectocele posteriorly, should these coexist. When massive degrees of prolapse, cystocele, rectocele, and enterocele are present, there may be such a mass of bulging, billowy mucosa presenting at the introitus that it is sometimes difficult to be certain of "how much of what type of relaxation is present." Marked edema and sometimes partial strangulation may occur.

Even in cases of complete prolapse, however, the protrusion usually recedes when the patient lies down, whereas in first or second degree prolapse no external protrusion exists. In such cases the patient is asked to strain, this bringing the cervix far down into the vagina and perhaps beyond the introitus. The same straining effort will ordinarily reveal the cystocele and rectocele, should they be present. In the complete variety, if straining does not restore the protrusion,

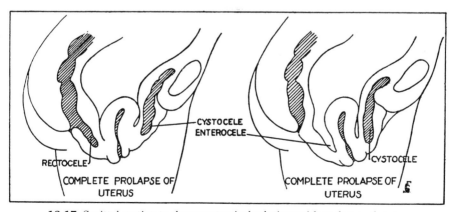

13.17. Sagittal section to show anatomical relations with prolapse of uterus

gentle traction on the cervix with a light tenaculum will usually do so.

Differential Diagnosis

The chief source of error is to mistake for prolapse the *simple hypertrophy of the cervix* which is seen at times, even with little or no vaginal relaxation. The cervix may become so elongated as to present at or beyond the introitus. Careful examination, however, will show that the cervical elongation is all below the cervicovaginal junction, and that the latter is still high up in the vaginal canal. Cystocele and rectocele are usually not present. Remarkable degrees of *vaginal prolapse* or *inversion* may exist with only minor degrees of cystocele, rectocele, or uterine prolapse.

Treatment

Among the factors which influence the management of this condition are the patient's age, marital status, and general health, on the one hand; and on the other, the degree of the prolapse and the presence or absence of any associated pathological conditions. Emge and Durfee have surveyed the evolution of the treatment of prolapse.

Surgical. This is best deferred until the family has been completed, for further pregnancy, even over an adequately repaired pelvic floor, will often undo the best surgical results. Although many operations have been devised for the correction of prolapse, 99% of such cases are satisfactorily handled by any one of the following procedures (along with appropriate repairs).

(1) Vaginal Hysterectomy (see Chapter 5). This is suitable for all but the most massive degrees of prolapse and, if combined with adequate anterior or posterior repair, gives excellent results. It furthermore removes the usual site of later cancers, tumors, or bleeding, and is obviously sterilizing. It should be stressed that abdominal hysterectomy and suspension of the vaginal vault from above is *not* the proper operation for prolapse; removal from below with adequate building up of the weakened and attenuated structures is the only feasible surgical approach. The *composite operation* which preserves the uterine isthmus while removing fundus and cervix has won no wide support.

Although most vaginal procedures are uncomplicated, there may be problems such as massive intraperitoneal hemorrhage or severe vaginal bleeding. When this occurs, prompt reoperation is indicated, and if resuture of the bleeding area is difficult because of the proximity of the ureter, ligation of the hypogastric arteries is an alternate solution. (See Chapter 5.)

(2) Manchester Operation. Although this is the usual English manner of surgically correcting any degree of prolapse, American gynecologists seem to utilize this procedure primarily for the lesser degrees of prolapse, especially in association with a large cystocele. Curettage to exclude malignancy should precede the operation, and it should rarely be done in the childbearing era, for cervical amputation (although not included in the original Manchester procedure) seems an integral part of the operation. The *Watkins* procedure is rarely utilized today; on occasion it may be useful in the elderly poor-risk woman. Pregnancy after either of the procedures is apt to be complicated and should suggest cesarean section.

(3) Colpocleisis (Le Fort Operation). Occasional cases of massive procidentia, often failures by other procedures, require closing the vagina. Obviously, this operation is performed only in the elderly spinster or widow, although various modifications allow partial vaginal function. Colpocleisis is generally easily and quickly performed and may, of course, be preceded by vaginal hysterectomy. This type of surgery should be a last resort, but is almost infallable if properly performed. Stress incontinence may be incurred if approximation of the vaginal walls includes the region of the bladder neck.

Nonsurgical. There are a few elderly women who are poor operative risks and have a limited life span, and these represent the main indication for pessary treatment. With modern anesthesia (local, block, and low spinal), such easily performed procedures as the Le Fort operation are usually preferred; but there is a small number of cases in which operation is not feasible or desirable. Pessaries are utilized for such women, but these have certain definite unpleasant aspects, as will be discussed.

The Vaginal Pessary

Because of the safety of modern-day surgery, various vaginal plastic and other reparative procedures are performed with relative impunity. At the same time it should be recalled that the old fashioned pessary still plays a role in the treatment of current gynecological conditions. It is no panacea, for it frequently leads to leukorrhea despite daily douches, and frequent removal and cleansing are necessary. An improperly fitted, too large pessary may induce urinary retention, whereas a pessary that is too small may slip out. Lastly, there are a few women who, because of individual structural deviations, just cannot be satisfactorily fitted with any of the standard types of pessary.

Indications

The two main indications for employment of a pessary are *prolapse* and *retrodisplacement,* in certain cases only and under certain conditions.

For the patient who is not a candidate for surgery, a *ring pessary* is probably most suitable, for it tends to take up slack in the vagina as well as form a kind of cradle under the cervix. Hard rubber or plastic is preferable to the soft rubber, "doughnut" type of pessary, which becomes foul rapidly and leads to leukorrhea, ulceration, and bleeding. As to the size of the pessary, individualization is necessary, for it must be large enough to stay in and small enough to allow for removal and cleansing. Too tight a pessary can cause severe ulceration.

Retrodisplacement. Asymptomatic retropositions require no treatment, but when a patient with either a congenital or postpartum backward displacement of the uterus complains of cramps, rectal or back pressure, or prolonged dribbling menstruation, a pessary deserves consideration. It is important to emphasize that the uterus must first be manually restored to its normal anterior position, for a pessary, merely shoved in, accomplishes nothing. Sometimes the uterus, even when it is free, is boggy and tender, so that light anesthesia may be necessary for proper application of the pessary.

As a general rule the *Smith-Hodge* or *Findley folding pessary* (in which a small segment at each end is of soft rubber for easier insertion) is preferable (Fig. 13.18). After the fundus is pushed upward by combined pressure in the posterior fornix, along with downward and backward pressure on the cervix, the pessary is applied (Fig. 13.19). The pessary should fit snugly with its front end up under the pubic arch; but if this is too snug, retention of urine may follow because of

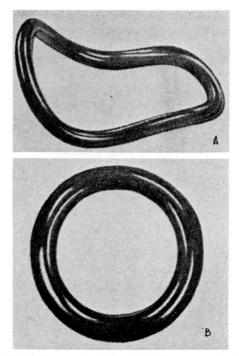

13.18. Types of pessary for ordinary use. *A,* the Smith-Hodge pessary especially valuable in the treatment of retrodisplacements *B,* the ordinary ring pessary of hard rubber employed especially in cases of prolapse.

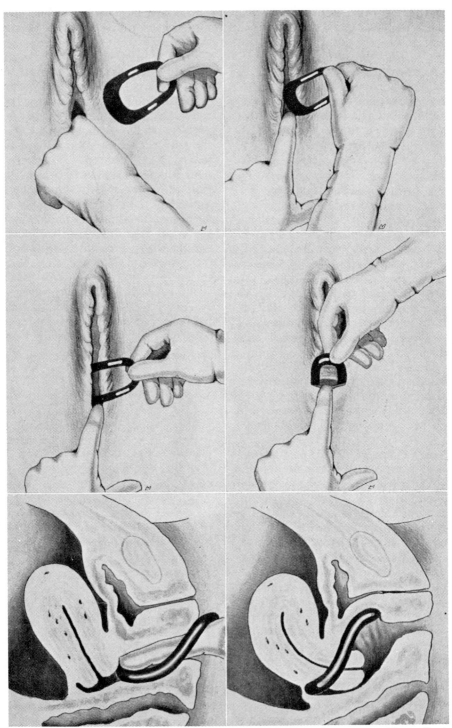

13.19. Diagram showing the successive steps in the introduction of a pessary. (From Davis, C. H. (Editor): *Gynecology and Obstetrics.* W. F. Prior Company, Inc., Hagerstown, Md. 1933.)

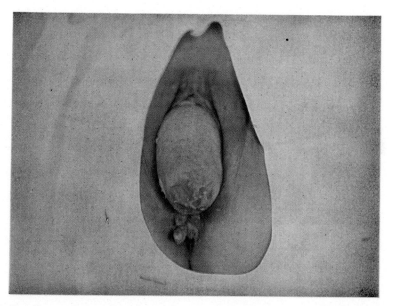

Plate 13.1. Complete prolapse of uterus with large cystocele. Note the superficial ulceration of the cervix, and also the rather large hemorrhoidal tags.

suburethral pressure. The back end encompasses the cervix, and fits snugly against the posterior fornix and uterosacral ligaments, and it is probably the latter leverage that maintains the replaced uterus in its normal position. A hard rubber pessary, if immersed in hot water, can be easily molded to fit the specific anatomy of the individual patient.

Contraindications and Complications of Pessaries

(1) A fixed retroposition such as may occur with inflammatory disease or endometriosis is a contraindication, for if the uterus cannot be mobilized anteriorly, a pessary will be worthless.

(2) Marked outlet relaxation with cystocele and rectocele frequently leads to such atonic tissues that a pessary does no good. Although prolapse and retrodisplacement frequently coexist, they are still amenable to pessary treatment, but an appropriate pessary may not be easy to find except by much "trial and error."

(3) Severe vaginitis or cervical infection militate against usage of a pessary. Despite daily douches and occasional (every six or eight weeks) removal of the instrument for cleansing, long continued wearing of a pessary is invariably followed by some irritative trauma to the vaginal epithelium, especially where there is a pasty-thin postmenopausal vagina. Actually, the neglected pessary may become encrusted and literally burrow its way into the submucosal tissues; indeed, in past generations frequent use of a special instrument (the "pessariotome") was necessary to cut the pessary out.

(4) A publication by a British colleague is actually entitled "The Dangerous Vaginal Pessary," and refers to 13 patients, all of whom had serious pelvic complications following prolonged usage of a pessary. Primary cancer, severe infections, fistulas, etc., are recorded. Indeed, of eight cases of primary vaginal cancer, six women had worn a pessary for many years. Although not a valid reason for discontinuance of the application of a pessary, the gynecologist should be wary of undue prolonged irritation, and consider biopsy where there is suspicious cytopathology.

Practical Use of Pessaries

The rational clinician will use pessaries infrequently, but they are of extreme service in the following groups of cases.

(1) In the occasional elderly, bad medical risk.

(2) In the immediate postpartum woman with a boggy, retroflexed uterus. A properly applied pessary will permit the attenuated ligaments to "take up slack" so that after a few months the instrument may be removed, and the uterus may stay anterior. Routine use of the so-called "knee-chest" exercises are also helpful.

(3) In the habitual aborter, where the uterus falls back and can actually become incarcerated in the pelvis. If the pessary is worn until the uterus becomes large enough to rise above the pelvic brim, it can then be safely removed.

(4) As a therapeutic test to determine whether suspension operation is indicated. As noted earlier, the conscientious gynecologist would prefer to avoid any surgery until the family has been completed, after which he is free to perform such definitive surgery as vaginal hysterectomy and repair. There are, however, occasional young women with marked retropositions who have bitter complaints, and it should be mandatory that the first step is application of a pessary. If this is followed by relief of symptoms, which later recur after removal of the pessary, it would seem likely that the faulty position of the uterus is the cause of the symptoms. Patients so tested will generally profit by a suspension operation, and it is a shame that this procedure, so helpful in properly selected cases, has acquired a bad name as a result of indiscriminate usage. A pessary is not a good long term investment in the young woman, and is useful primarily as a therapeutic test or in any case as a temporary stop-gap pending more appropriate treatment.

As indicated, we believe that Smith-Hodge and ring pessaries, both of which may be obtained in various sizes, are all that the average doctor needs for this type of therapy. Although pessaries are employed only occasionally, they still have very definite indications, particularly where operation would be attended by considerable risk. As Bantock remarked in 1905, "I am not aware that there is on record a single case in which a woman has lost her life through the use, or even the abuse, of a vaginal pessary."

REFERENCES

Allen, W. M., and Masters, W. H.: Traumatic laceration of uterine supports. Amer. J. Obstet. Gynec., 70: 500, 1955.

Altchek, A.: Diagnosis of enterocele by negative intrarectal transillumination. Obstet. Gynec., 26: 636, 1965.

Bader, W. F. (Editor): Vaginal relaxation. Clin. Obstet. Gynec., 15: 1033, 1972.

Beecham, C. T. (Editor): Complications of gynecologic surgery. Clin. Obstet. Gynec., 5: 501, 1962.

Beecham, C. T., and Beecham, J. B.: Vaginal repair with fascia lata. Obstet. Gynec., 42: 542, 1973.

Birnbaum, S. J.: Prolapsed vagina. Amer. J. Obstet. Gynec., 115: 411, 1973.

Blaikley, J. B.: Colpocleises for difficult vesicovaginal and rectovaginal fistulas. Amer. J. Obstet. Gynec., 91: 589, 1964.

Boronow, R. C.: Radiation-induced vaginal fistulas. Amer. J. Obstet. Gynec., 109: 1, 1971.

Boronow, R. C., and Rutledge, R.: Vesico-vaginal fistula, radiation and gynecological cancer. Amer. J. Obstet. Gynec., 111: 85, 1971.

Calame, R. J.: Ureterovaginal fistula as a complication of radical pelvic surgery. Arch. Surg., 94: 876, 1967.

Carter, B., Palumbo, L., Creadick, R. N., and Ross, R. A.: Vesicovaginal fistula. Amer. J. Obstet. Gynec., 63: 479, 1952.

Collins, C. G., and Jones, F. B.: Preoperative cortisone for vaginal fistulae. Obstet. Gynec., 9: 533 1957.

Collins, C., et al.: Early repair vesico-vaginal fistula. Amer. J. Obstet. Gynec., 111: 524, 1971.

Diaz-Bazan, N.: Cervical carcinoma with procidentia in El Salvador. Obstet. Gynec., 23: 281, 1964.

Emge, L. A., and Durnfee, R. B.: Pelvic organ prolapse: four thousand years of treatment. Clin. Obstet. Gynec., 9: 997, 1966.

Everett, H. S., and Mattingly, R. F.: Urinary tract injuries as a result of pelvic surgery. Amer. J. Obstet. Gynec., 71: 503, 1956.

Fadel, H. E., and Misemhimer, H. R.: Incarceration of the introverted gravid uterus with sacculation. Obstet. Gynec., 43: 46, 1974.

Falk, H. C.: Prevention of vesicovaginal fistula in hysterectomy for benign disease. Obstet. Gynec., 29: 65, 1967.

Given, F. T.: Recto-vaginal fistula. Amer. J. Obstet. Gynec., 108: 41, 1971.

Graber, E. R., O'Rourke, J. J., and McElrath, T.: Iatrogenic bladder damage during hysterectomy. Obstet. Gynec., 23: 267, 1964.

Gray, L. A.: Place of vaginal hysterectomy in gynecologic surgery. Western J. Surg., 67: 153, 1959.

Gray, L. A.: Prolapse of uterus and vagina. Postgrad. Med., 30: 207, 1961.

Gray, L. A.: Urethrovaginal fistulas. Amer. J. Obstet. Gynec., 101: 28, 1968.

Green, T. H.: Development of a plan for the diagnosis and treatment of urinary stress incontinence. Amer. J. Obstet. Gynec., 83: 632, 1962.

Green, T. H.: The problem of urinary stress incontinence in the female: an appraisal of its current status. Obstet. Gynec. Survey., 23: 603, 1968.

Harrow, B. R.: Conservative and surgical management of operative bladder injuries. Obstet. Gynec., 33: 852, 1969.

Hesselberg, E.: Cancer of the cervix associated with procidentia. South Afric. J. Obstet. Gynec., 46: 589, 1963.

Hodgkinson, C. P.: Stress incontinence 1970. Amer. J. Obstet. Gynec., 108: 1141, 1970.

Hodgkinson, C. P., Doub, H. P., and Kelly, W. T.: Urethrocystograms: metallic bead chain technique. Clin. Obstet. Gynec., 1: 668, 1958.

Hodgkinson, C. P., and Kelly, W. T.: Urinary stress incontinence in the female. Obstet. Gynec., 10: 493, 1957.

Jeffcoate, T. N. A.: Posterior colpoperineorrhaphy. Amer. J. Obstet. Gynec., 77: 490, 1959.

Jeffcoate, T. N. A., and Francis, W. J. A.: Urgency incontinence in the female. Amer. J. Obstet. Gynec., 94: 604, 1966.

Kelly, H. A.: Operative Gynecology. Appleton-Century-Crofts, Inc., New York, 1928.

Kinzel, G. E.: Enterocele: study of 265 cases. Amer. J. Obstet. Gynec., 81: 1166, 1961.

Lapides, J.: Cystometry. J. A. M. A., 201: 124, 1967.

Latzko, W.: Postoperative vesicovaginal fistulas. Amer. J. Surg., 58: 211, 1942.

Lee, R. A., and Symmonds, R. E.: Uretero-vaginal fistula. Amer. J. Obstet. Gynec., 109: 1032, 1971.

Lee, R. A., and Symmonds, R. E.: Repair of posthysterectomy vault prolapse. Amer. J. Obstet. Gynec., 112: 953, 1972.

Lund, C. J. (Editor): Symposium on urinary incontinence in the female. Clin. Obstet. Gynec., 6: 125, 1963.

Marchetti, A. A., Marshall, V. F., and Shultis, L. D.: Simple vesicourethral suspension. Amer. J. Obstet. Gynec., 74: 57, 1957.

McCall, M. L.: Posterior culdoplasty. Obstet. Gynec., 10: 595, 1957.

Mengert, W. F.: Vesicovaginal fistula; principles of closure. Amer. J. Obstet. Gynec., 84: 1213, 1962.

Moir, J. C.: The gauze-hammock operation: a modified Aldridge sling procedure. J. Obstet. Gynaec. Brit. Comm., 75: 1, 1968.

Moir, J. C.: "Circumferential" vesicovaginal fistulae. J. Obstet. Gynec., India, 15: 441, 1965.

Moir, J. C.: Injuries of bladder. Amer. J. Obstet. Gynec., 82: 124, 1961.

Moir, J. C.: The Vesicovaginal Fistula. Balliere, Tindall, & Cox, London, 1961.

Nichols, R. H.: Surgery for enterocele. Obstet. Gynec., 40: 257, 1972.

Parks, J.: Section of urethral wall for correction of urethrovaginal fistulas and urethra diverticula. Amer. J. Obstet. Gynec., 93: 683, 1965.

Pereyra, A. J., and Lebherz, T. B.: Combined urethrovesical suspension and vagino-urethroplasty for correction of urinary stress incontinence. Obstet. Gynec., 30: 537, 1967.

Piven, M. S., and Spezia, J.: Obstet. Gynec., 32: 765, 1968.

Porges, R. F.: Classification of pelvic relaxations. Surg. Gynec. Obstet., 117: 769, 1963.

Portnuff, J. C., and Ballon, S. C.: Pererya procedure. Amer. J. Obstet. Gynec., 115: 411, 1973.

Reich, W. J., and Nechtow, M. J.: Ligation of internal iliac (hypogastric) arteries; life-saving procedure for uncontrollable gynecological and obstetrical hemorrhage. J. Internat. Coll. Surgeons, 36: 157, 1961.

Ridley, J. H.: Colpocleisis operation. Amer. J. Obstet. Gynec., 113: 1114, 1972.

Russell, J. K.: The dangerous vaginal pessary. J. Obstet Gynaec. Brit. Comm., *69:* 405, 1962.

Russell, C. S.: Management of vesico-vaginal fistula. Int. J. Obstet. Gynec., *8:* 1, 1970.

Siegel, P., and Mengert, W. F.: Internal iliac ligations in obstetrics and gynecology. J. A. M. A., *178:* 1059, 1961.

Skjaeraasen, J. S.: Stress incontinence. Acta Obstet. Gynec. Scandi., *48:* 575, 1969.

Symmonds, R. E., and Pratt, J. H.: Vaginal prolapse following hysterectomy. Amer. J. Obstet. Gynec., *79:* 899, 1960.

Taylor, E. S., and Droegemueller, W.: Repair of urinary vaginal fistulas. Obstet. Gynec., *30:* 674, 1967.

TeLinde, R. W. and Mattingly, R. F.: *Operative Gyne-cology,* Ed. 4. J. B. Lippincott Company, Philadelphia, 1970.

TeLinde, R. W.: Prolapse of the uterus and allied conditions (an evaluation). Amer. J. Obstet. Gynec., *94:* 444, 1966.

Tompkins, P.: In defense of suspension of the uterus in treatment of infertility. Fertil. Steril., *7:* 317. 1956.

Uhlenhuth, S., and Nolley, G. W.: Vaginal fascia, a myth. Obstet. Gynec., *10:* 349, 1957.

Wharton, L. R., Jr., and TeLinde, R. W.: An evaluation of fascial sling operation for urinary incontinence in female patients. J. Urol., *82:* 76, 1959.

Zeigerman, J. H., Stahlgren, L., and Tulsky, E. G.: Sigmoidovaginal fistulas. Amer. J. Obstet. Gynec., *88:* 1003, 1964.

chapter 14

Hyperplasia of the Endometrium and Endometrial Polyps

HYPERPLASIA

The condition designated as *hyperplasia* of the endometrium was, at one time, rather distinctively correlated with *functional uterine bleeding,* and this association is frequent but far from invariable. Actually, (*dys*)-*functional* bleeding is purely a clinical term, and endometrial hyperplasia a pathological classification. Although the latter represents the chief cause of functional bleeding, this may occur from any type of endometrium.

In the postmenopausal woman, hyperplasia is usually a result of hormone therapy. Where there is no history of this, an ovarian or adrenal source seems likely.

Histological Pattern

The histological pattern of hyperplasia in the menstrual years is produced by *persistent estrogen stimulation in the absence of progesterone.* This implies that it is associated with an *anovulatory* type

of cycle. A single follicle may fail to rupture, but continue to grow and to function beyond the usual ovulation period, so that an abnormal growth effect is produced upon the endometrium. In other cases of anovulatory menstruation, a group of follicles continues to mature to various levels and to produce estrogen, with a pronounced growth effect.

The *characteristic changes in the ovary,* therefore, are an absence of functioning corpora lutea, and the presence of either a single, persistent, functioning follicle or a considerable group of smaller, functionally active follicles. In the latter case, the ovaries may be grossly cystic, but the small cysts are lined with an intact granulosa. There is a thick cortex with no or rare evidence of a recent corpus luteum and, indeed, there may be a close resemblance to the so-called Stein-Leventhal ovary. Where a single large follicle appears to dominate the picture, it may present clinically as a follicle cyst of considerable size, although there is a well preserved granulosa-theca zone and an active estrogenic function.

The factor which checks the growth and continued function of the follicles is believed to be an inhibition of the anterior pituitary gonadotrophins by increased amounts of estrogen (the "feedback" mechanism), resulting in withdrawal of the stimulus to follicle growth, rapid regression due to withdrawal of estrogen, and thereby a bleeding phase. The important role of the hypothalamic luteinizing hormone-release factor (LRF) has been discussed in Chapter 2.

Microscopic Appearance of Hyperplasia. This, in the frank case, is extremely distinctive. The most characteristic feature is the gland pattern, which is commonly spoken of as the *Swiss-cheese type* (Figs. 14.1, 2), because of the disparity in size of the gland lumina. Some are large and cystic, whereas others, perhaps in the same microscopic field, are small in caliber. The epithelium is cuboidal or columnar, with heavily stained nuclei, and in the small glands it may even show some stratification. The stroma is abundant and hyperplastic, so that an endometrial sarcoma may be simulated (Fig. 14.3). Mitoses are numerous in the epithelium, and not infrequent in the stroma. The epithelium shows an *absence of the secretory activity* produced by progesterone, since the secretion of the latter is absent. The finding of ciliated tubal-like epithelium is not at all uncommon in endometrial hyperplasia (Fig. 14.9).

Squamous Metaplasia (Acanthosis)

It is by no means rare to find *squamous metaplasia or acanthosis* in conjunction with endometrial hyperplasia and various other benign conditions of the endometrium, although it may be associated with adenocarcinoma as a malignant adenoacanthoma. In such cases, however, it is the glandular element that determines the malignant potential, for the squamous cells are well differentiated and quite benign.

Squamous metaplasia of the endometrium may be a sequel of chronic infection, radium, any long-standing irritant such as intrauterine contraceptive devices (IUD) or foreign bodies, various

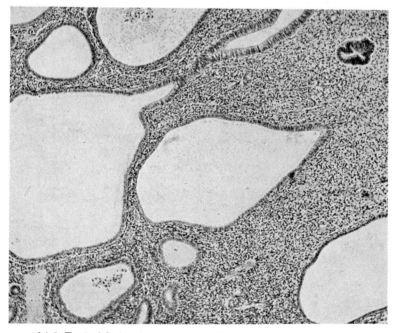

14.1. Typical Swiss-cheese pattern of hyperplasia of endometrium

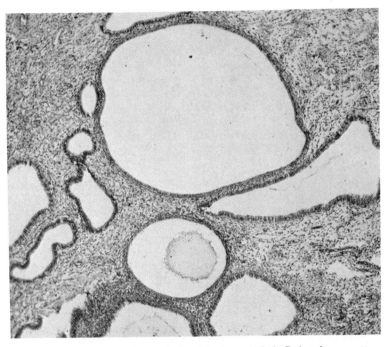

14.2. Another example of hyperplasia with characteristic Swiss-cheese pattern

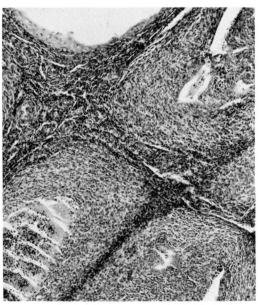

14.3. Markedly proliferative stroma with endometrial hyperplasia.

14.4. Syncytial bud of squamous cells seemingly arising by metaplasia of the lining epithelium.

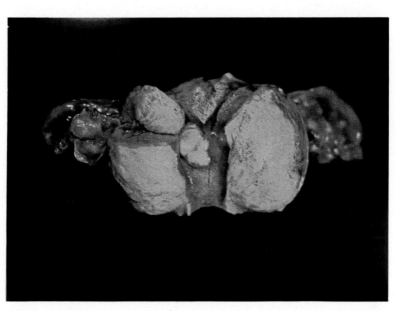

Plate 14.1. Endometrial polyp of moderate size (previous amputation cervix)

hormonal stimuli, vitamin A deficiency, as well as other causes. Many believe that the source of the squamous cell is an indifferent reserve cell at the epithelial-stromal border even if such a cell has never been demonstrated. However, it seems that a mature epithelial cell can be converted into a squamous cell, for we have seen all types of seeming transition between the lining epithelium and a mature squamous cell with frank pearl formation (Fig. 14.4).

On occasion, the whole endometrial surface may be converted into a stratified squamous surface, the so-called "icthyosis uteri." Malignant degeneration may occur with the production of the rare primary epidermoid cancer of the endometrium, or combined adenosquamous lesions may occur.

Squamous cells in the endometrium are not indicative of any malignant trend as long as the epithelioid cells are mature and well developed, but one must be certain that the associated glandular pattern is benign. If this is true, the clinician may relax, for Bomze and Friedman have offered additional assurance that en-

dometrial acanthosis is not itself a harbinger of malignancy. Nevertheless, one might rightfully be concerned about a chronic long-standing irritant to the endometrium, such as an IUD, for this might ultimately lead not only to metaplasia but neoplasia (Ober *et al.*).

Focal Hyperplasia

Occasionally patches of hyperplastic endometrium may be found in conjunction with a general secretory reaction. It must be borne in mind that the basalis endometrium is not responsive to the biphasic hormonal stimulus. Where an intact endometrium is available for study as in a hysterectomy specimen, one often finds that there are occasionally patches of superficial immature basal tissue that have not acquired the capacity of response to progesterone and hence exhibit a proliferative or hyperplastic pattern despite a biphasic cycle (Fig. 14.5).

Gross Appearance of the Endometrium. This is variable; in some cases it may be enormously thickened and polypoid, so that the large amounts removed by curettage may lead the sur-

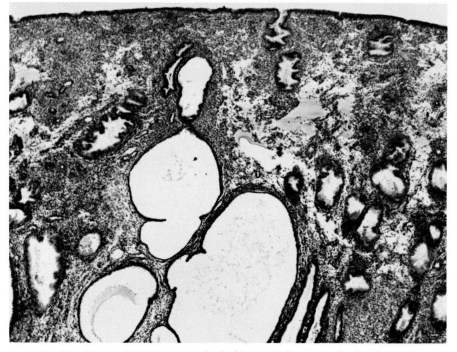

14.5. "Focal hyperplasia" in center flanked by typical progestational endometrium

geon to assume the likelihood of cancer. In such cases, the polypoid overgrowth presents a sharp line of demarcation at the internal os from the cervical mucosa (Figs. 14.6, 7), which lacks the responsiveness of the endometrium to the estrogenic hormone. In other cases, and with the same microscopic pattern, the endometrium is of normal thickness, or it may even be thinner than normal.

Proliferative (Atypical) Hyperplasia

In a majority of cases the microscopic pattern of hyperplasia is a frankly benign one. In a small proportion, however, markedly proliferative and adenomatous pictures are produced, sometimes diffusely involving the whole endometrium but more often only certain focal areas, and these may well be mistaken for cancer. The percentage of these doubtful cases, however, is very small. When there is serious doubt, the safe plan is that expressed in the dictum of Halban, "Nich Karzinom, aber besser heraus!" (Not carcinoma, but better out!) In the milder degrees of proliferative overactivity, however, there is rarely any difficulty in excluding malignancy, and conservative treatment is indicated (Fig. 14.8.). The differential diagnosis and relationship of atypical hyperplasia and endometrial adenocarcinoma is discussed in Chapter 15, with consideration of estrogen as a causative agent.

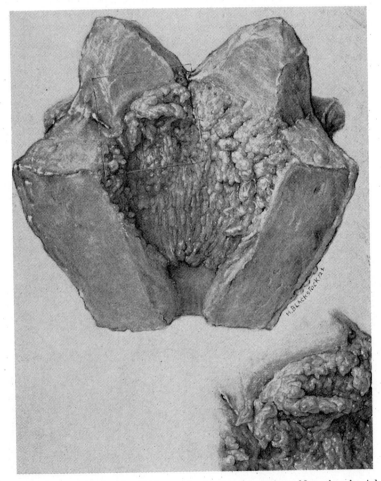

14.6. Gross appearance of benign polypoid hyperplasia of endometrium. Note the physiological line of demarcation at the internal os.

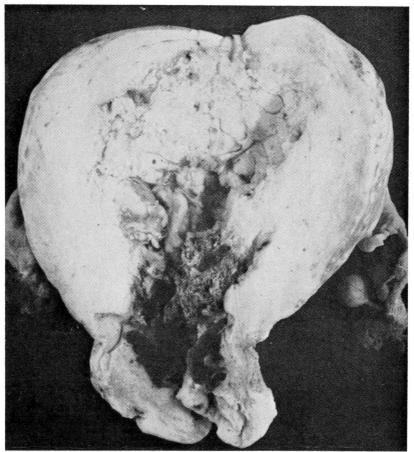

14.7. Marked polypoid hyperplasia (histologically benign) following prolonged estrogen therapy. (Courtesy of Dr. Derek Tacchio, New Castle, England.)

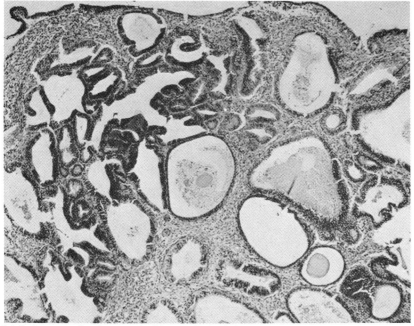

14.8. An example of an atypical hyperplasia (*left*) with associated cystic hyperplasia

Differentiation of Progestational and Hyperplastic Endometrium

McKay *et al.* have carried out extensive studies on endometrial histochemistry in normal, atrophic, hyperplastic (cystic and adenomatous), and malignant tissues. Ribonucleoprotein, acid and alkaline phosphatase, and glycogen content were studied by appropriate stains. For details, the reader is referred to their publications, but in essence this work suggested that the earlier stages of endometrial cancer showed a progestational pattern. This would, of course, help to explain certain secretory changes that seem to occur in low grade adenocarcinoma, but is difficult to reconcile with the frequent postmenopausal status of the patient. It is likewise difficult to reconcile with the presumed estrogen role in certain hyperplasias and possibly adenocarcinoma unless we assume an altered metabolic background, "a long continued estrogen plus progesterone stimulation." The possibility of convertability of the steroids at either the site of production or the end organ is currently generally accepted.

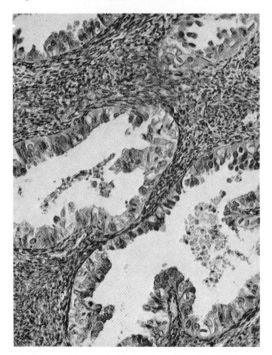

14.9. Areas of pale-staining tubal epithelium may occasionally be seen with hyperplasia.

Whatever the mechanism, it may on occasion be extremely difficult to distinguish between certain progestational endometria and various forms of proliferative hyperplasia. Both exhibit abundant evidence of secretory activity, considerable infolding and intraluminal tufting by tall pale-staining cells, and extensive proliferation of the glands. Both may justifiably be called a secretory endometrium, but this does not necessarily imply that ovulation has occurred.

The report of a "secretory" endometrium in a woman over 50 years of age, especially if there is abnormal bleeding, should suggest that the patient may be anovulatory (although this is not absolute). If a well developed decidual-like stroma is present, there is considerable support for recent ovulation and progesterone influence. If not, one must consider an atypical hyperplasia, especially if there are associated areas of the benign cystic ("Swiss cheese") variety. This matter of distinction is of more than academic importance, for these proliferative endometrial patterns seem to be a *precursor to adenocarcinoma,* or coexist in conjunction with a true malignancy.

A study by Novak in 1970 would make it seem that ovulation may occur in the woman beyond 50 years with some frequency despite the rarity of pregnancies in that age group. We suspect that Figure 14.10 represents a true postovulation endometrium despite the age and a seemingly monophasic temperature chart. The marked edema, vascularity, and decidual changes strongly suggest a progesterone stimulus which is not found in the stroma of patients with postmenopausal hyperplasia. (Contrast with Fig. 15.12 *left.*)

Postmenopausal Hyperplasia

It is now well known that the urine of postmenopausal women, even many years beyond the menopause, may, show the presence of estrogenic hormone. The source of this is not known, although there is considerable evidence for the adrenal cortex as a probable source of the hormone. Studies of our own, utilizing his-

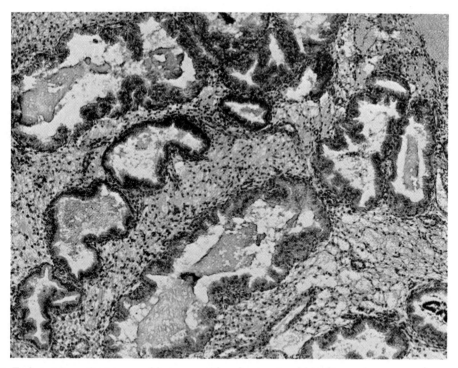

14.10. Endometrium of a 54-year-old woman with only occasional bleeding and a presumed monophasic temperature chart. The stromal pattern suggests ovulation (contrast Fig. 15.12 *left*).

tochemical techniques, would suggest frequent steroidal function of hilus cells as well as by ovarian stromal cells (both estrogenic and androgenic).

There is some evidence, however, that hyperplastic ovarian stromal cells not only look like, but act like, theca cells in an ability to secrete estrogen, even in the postmenopausal era. Scully has previously commented on certain ovarian stromal cells which are enzymatically active (EASC) and a presumed source of steroidogenesis in ovaries at all ages. Plotz *et al.* have utilized radio-active substrates to substantiate enzyme activity in the postmenopausal ovary. They also found estrogens less commonly than androgens, but postulate that conversion to estrogens may occur at such extra-ovarian sources as adrenal or various peripheral tissues. This must be regarded as a real possibility in view of the ability of the castrate adrenalectomized woman to convert radio-active testosterone into estrone and estradiol. Indeed, recent studies suggest that androstenedione is the major steroid

produced but may then be converted into various estrogenic substances.

However, Bulbrook and Greenwood have found estrogen in the urine of women with breast cancer who have had oophorectomy, adrenalectomy, and hypophysectomy. What this might evolve from is speculative, but cholesterol intake in the diet must be suspect with possible conversion into estrogens and androgens. Indeed it was years after this speculation by us that cholesterol was first noted as an intermediate biosynthetic product in androgen or estrogen formation. It is not surprising, therefore, that hyperplasia, formerly looked upon as exclusively a lesion of reproductive life, may at times be found in women far beyond the menopause, and that it may occasionally cause postmenopausal bleeding.

Novak and Yui have found postmenopausal hyperplasia in association with adenocarcinoma in at least 25% of cases. There is suggestive evidence that, in the menopausal and postmenopausal woman, hyperplasia, especially proliferative, may progress to adenocarcinoma. The hyperplasia of reproductive life, on the other hand, appears to have little relation to the development of cancer. A study of postmenopausal endometria by Novak and Richardson revealed the frequent occurrence of active and even hyperplastic endometria in women at times many years after the menopause.

No present day discussion of this topic would be complete without calling attention to the fact that hyperplasia of the endometrium, sometimes of the atypical variety, is often the result of *excessive and prolonged administration of estrogens* in the treatment of menopausal symptoms (see Chapter 15).

Management of Hyperplasia

Endometrial hyperplasia in the menstrual era is usually an innocuous and self-limited process which frequently reverts to normal following curettage. Where hyperplasia is constantly recurrent in the aging endometrium, in general or in a polyp, it is somewhat more ominous in respect to the later development of fundal adenocarcinoma, especially if the woman concerned is in the menopausal age bracket. Indeed we are convinced that recurrent hyperplasia, especially if it is *increasingly* atypical or proliferative does not warrant conservatism because of the higher incidence of subsequent endometrial cancer. The continued pattern of a sustained stimulus (probably estrogen) suggests that hysterectomy is a well warranted prophylaxis against the advent of carcinoma of the endometrium.

Cause of Bleeding in Hyperplasia

The hormonal factors in the bleeding, as already discussed, are brought about by the reciprocal interplay of the pituitary and ovaries. As for local factors, Schröder believes that these consist of small localized areas of necrobiosis, from which the blood has its source (Fig. 14.11). Others, although conceding the presence of such small areas of necrosis, do not believe that these are sufficient to explain the frequently profuse hemorrhage, and are inclined to attribute the chief role to changes in the blood vessels, with increased permeability of their walls. Sippe describes various sinus-like vascular channels with a rather super-

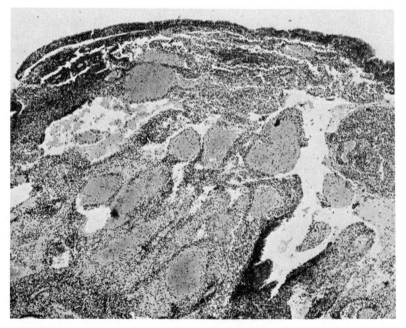

14.11. Thromboses in an area of necrobiosis in hyperplasia of endometrium

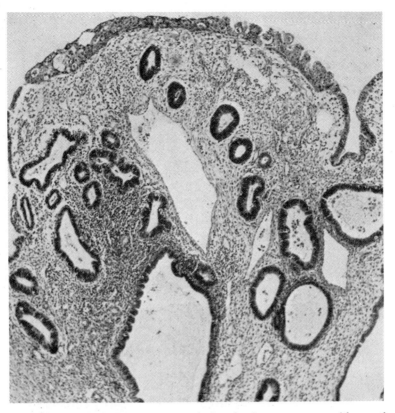

14.12. So-called epidermization or squamous metaplasia, a benign process, seen either on the surface or in the glands in occasional cases of hyperplasia.

ficial position that may be the source of profuse bleeding.

Depolymerization

It might seem that when implantation does not occur, a complex series of endometrial enzymatic activities lead to bleeding. Due to combined estrogen-progesterone action, various hydrolytic enzymes are manufactured and stored in the endometrial cells. Estrogens seem responsible for the production of certain acid mucopolysaccharides (AMPS) and deposition of the stromal ground substances due to polymerization. Progesterone stimulation prevents further AMPS synthesis with resultant depolymerization of the ground substance. In the absence of pregnancy there is a decrease in progesterone, and the lysosomal membrane breaks down with hydrolysis and endometrial slough.

This would seem a logical explanation for not only ovulatory but anovulatory menstruation. The role of prostaglandin is poorly understood.

Clinical Characteristics and Treatment

These are fully discussed in Chapter 31, "Functional Bleeding."

ENDOMETRIAL POLYPS

The term polyp is a clinical one, referring to tumors attached by a stem or pedicle. Thus a polypoid tumor within the uterus may be a myoma, carcinoma, or sarcoma, or it might be made up of retained placental tissue (placental polyp). The common *endometrial polyp* is made up of endometrial tissue. Such polyps may be single or multiple, small, or large enough to fill the uterine cavity. The pedicle may become so long that the growth projects beyond the cervix, and, in rare cases, beyond the vaginal introitus.

Incidence

It is difficult to quote an incidence for endometrial polyps, for unquestionably many are removed piecemeal at the time of curettage and not recognized. On other occasions a prominent vascular core is suggestive.

Microscopic Structure

The microscopic structure of these polyps is like that of the endometrium from which they spring, with some qualification on the basis of the *functional* or *nonfunctional* type of the constituent epithelium. In some polyps the endometrial tissue shows a *functional* cyclical response paralleling that of the general uterine mucosa. When the latter exhibits a progestational picture, for example, so does the endometrium of the polyp.

In a far larger proportion of cases, however, the polyp is made up of an *immature or unripe* type of endometrium like that seen in the basalis, and not responsive to progesterone. Such polyps, therefore, show a proliferative picture,

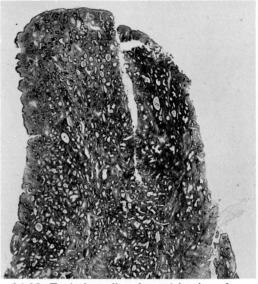

14.13. Typical small endometrial polyp of non-functioning type.

with often a typical Swiss-cheese hyperplasia pattern, at all phases of the menstrual cycle, even when the surrounding endometrium is in a progestational phase. Schröder's concept of an

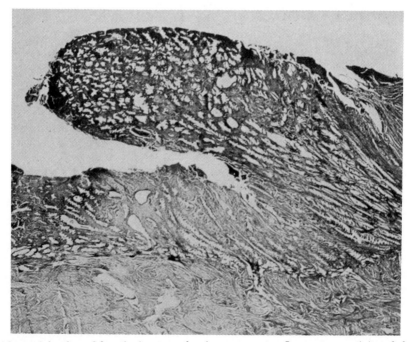

14.14. Endometrial polyp of functioning type showing premenstruaL secretory activity of glands similar to that in surrounding endometrium.

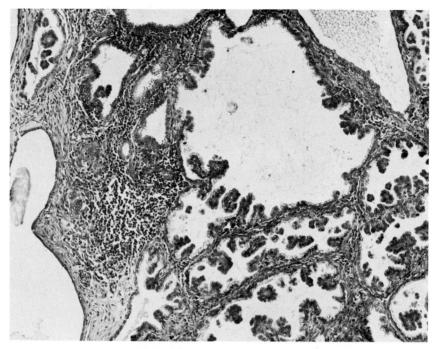

14.15. Proliferative hyperplasia in a polyp

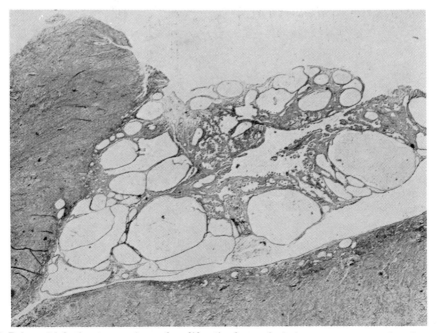

14.16. Polyp with both retrogressive and proliferative hyperplasia in a postmenopausal patient.

origin from the basalis portion of the endometrium with a surrounding mantle of more superficial and responsive tissue seems particularly rational.

Clinical Characteristics

Unless they become large enough to protrude from the cervix, or unless secondary degenerative or ulcerative changes develop, endometrial polyps are apt to be entirely asymptomatic, although the constituent immature endometrium may lead to various types of abnormal bleeding. As a matter of fact a proportion are not discovered until uteri removed for other indications are opened, whereas others are brought away in the course of curettage for diagnostic or other indications.

In the larger polyps or those which obtrude into the cervical or vaginal canals, *bleeding* is almost always a symptom, because of the secondary ulcerative changes which develop. As a rule it is of metrorrhagic type and moderate degree, but, in some cases, it may be quite profuse. Through interference with the blood supply in the pedicle, the larger polyps may undergo necrosis and sloughing, with the production of an offensive discharge as well as bleeding.

Premalignant Potentialities of Endometrial Polyp

It has generally been assumed that endometrial polyps have little tendency to be associated with or to evolve into fundal adenocarcinoma, and there seems little doubt that this view is correct as regards women during menstrual life. In the menopausal and postmenopausal eras, however, there would seem to be considerable question as to whether such lesions can be regarded with complete equanimity. A study by Peterson and Novak would indicate that polyps in postmenopausal women must be regarded with a certain degree of suspicion, because of associated malignancy, although the polyp itself rarely undergoes malignant degeneration (0.5 to 1%). More recent work by Wolfe and Mackles would seem to confirm our impressions that

polyps in the climacteric must be viewed with certain misgivings.

Indeed, analysis of some 1100 polyps in our clinic revealed that 10 to 15% were *associated* with malignancy in postmenopausal women. Of particular interest were those polyps which exhibited an active hyperplasia after cessation of menstrual life. These appeared to represent a focal patchy form of hyperplasia which deserves the same consideration as a diffuse postmenopausal hyperplasia (discussed in this chapter). Adenomatous or recurrent atypical polypoid lesions should not be viewed too conservatively, for they may be associated with or be forerunners of endometrial cancer.

Treatment

The polyps which manifest themselves by protrusion through the cervical canal are readily diagnosed, although it is not

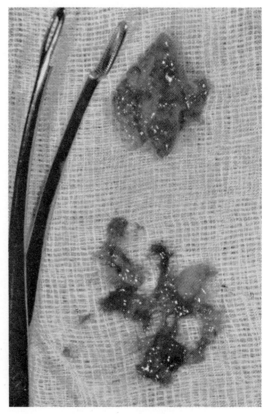

14.17. Polyp forceps

always easy to be sure whether they spring from the cervix or from the endometrium. The distinction is not usually of practical importance, as the method of treatment is the same for both types. For the endometrial growths, especially those of larger size, the cervix should be dilated and the growth removed, followed by curettage, to make sure that other small polyps are not present. It is wise to follow any curettage with the introduction of a long narrow forceps (Fig. 14.17) to "fish around" for a possibly overlooked polyp. This may easily happen despite the most thorough uterine scraping.

REFERENCES

Baggish, M. S., and Woodruff, J. D.: The occurrence of squamous epithelium in the endometrium. Obstet. Gynec. Survey, *22:* 69, 1967.

Bomze, E. J., and Friedman, N. B.: Squamous metaplasia and adenoacanthosis of the endometrium. Obstet. Gynec., *30:* 619, 1967.

Brown, J. B., Kellan, R. and Matthew, G. D.: Preliminary observations on urinary oestrogen excretion in certain gynecological disorders. Obstet. Gynaec. Brit. Cwlth. *68:* 668, 1961.

Bulbrook, R. D., and Greenwood, F. C.: Persistence of urinary estrogen excretion after oophorectory and adrenalectomy. Brit. Med. J., *1:* 662, 1957.

Bulbrook, R. D., and Greenwood, F. C.: Effects of hypophysectomy on urinary estrogen in breast cancer. Brit. Med. J., *1:* 666, 1957.

Campbell, P. E., and Barter, R. A.: Significance of atypical endometrial hyperplasia. J. Obstet. Gynaec. Brit. Comm.,*66:* 668, 1961.

Chamlian, D. L., and Taylor, H. B.: Endometrial hyperplasia in young women. Obstet. Gynec., *36:* 659, 1970.

Cope, E.: Management of abnormal bleeding. Brit. Med. J., *2:* 700, 1971.

Israel, R., Mishell, D. R., and Labudovich, M.: Mechanism of uterine bleeding. Clin. Obstet. Gynec., *13:* 386, 1972.

Israel, S. L., and Weber, L. L.: Postmenopausal uterine bleeding. Obstet. Gynec., *7:* 286, 1956.

Lambeth, S. S., and Kinter, E. P.: Endometrial hyperplasia. Obstet. Gynec., *5:* 692, 1955.

Larson, J. A.: Estrogens and endometrial carcinoma. Obstet. Gynec., *3:* 1, 1954.

McBride, J. M.: Premenopausal cystic hyperplasia and endometrial carcinoma. J. Obstet. Gynaec. Brit. Comm., *66:* 288, 1959.

McKay, D. G., Hertig, A. T., Bardawil, W. A., and Velardo, J. T.: Histochemical observations on endometrium. II. Abnormal endometrium. Obstet. Gynec., *8:* 140, 1956.

McLennan, C. E.: Current concepts of prolonged or irregular menstrual shedding. Am. J. Obstet. Gynec. *64:* 988, 1952.

Novak, E., and Richardson, E. H., Jr.: Proliferative changes in senile endometrium. Amer. J. Obstet. Gynec., *42:* 564, 1941.

Novak, E., and Rutledge, F.: Atypical proliferative hyperplasia of endometrium. Amer. J. Obstet. Gynec., *55:* 46, 1948.

Novak, E., and Yui, E.: Relation of hyperplasia to adenocarcinoma of uterus. Amer. J. Obstet. Gynec., *32:* 674, 1936.

Novak, E. R.: Relationship of endometrial hyperine bleeding. Surg. Gynec. Obstet., *106:* 321, plasia and adenocarcinoma of the uterine fundus. J.A.M.A., *154:* 217, 1954.

Novak, E. R.: Postmenopausal endometrial hyperplasia. Amer. J. Obstet. Gynec., *71:* 1312, 1956.

Novak, E. R.: Ovulation after fifty. Obstet. Gynec., *36:* 903, 1970.

Ober, W. B., Sobrero, A. J., Korman, R., and Gold, S.: Endometrial morphology and polyethylene intrauterine devices; a study of 200 endometrial biopsies. Obstet. Gynec., *32:* 782, 1968.

Overstreet, E. W.: Clinical aspects of endometrial polyps. Surg. Clin. N. Amer., *42:* 1013, 1962.

Peterson, W. F., and Novak, E. R.: Endometrial polyps. Obstet. Gynec., *8:* 40, 1956.

Randall, C. L., Birtsch, P. K., and Harkins, L. L.: Ovarian function after the menopause. Amer. J. Obstet. Gynec., *74:* 719, 1957.

Randall, L. M.: Management of dysfunctional uterine bleeding during adolescence. J. Louisiana Med. Soc., *110:* 160, 1958.

Roddick, J. W., and Greene, R. R.: Endometrial changes and ovarian morphology. Amer. J. Obstet. Gynec., *75:* 235, 1958.

Schröder, R.: Endometrial hyperplasia in relation to genital function. Amer. J. Obstet. Gynec., *68:* 294, 1954.

Scommegna, A., and Dmowski, W. P.: Dysfunctional uterine bleeding. Clin. Obstet. Gynec., *16:* 221, 1973.

Scott, R. B.: The elusive endometrial polyp. Obstet. Gynec., *1:* 125, 1953.

Scully, R. E., and Cohen, R. B.: Oxidative-enzyme activity in normal and pathological human ovaries. Obstet. Gynec., *24:* 667, 1964.

Shearman, R. P.: Progress in the investigation and treatment of anovulation. Amer. J. Obstet. Gynec., *103:* 444, 1968.

Sippe, G.: Endometrial hyperplasia and uterine bleeding. J. Obstet. Gynaec. Brit. Comm., *69:* 1015, 1962.

Sobrina, L. G., and Kase, N.: Endocrinologic aspects of dysfunctional uterine bleeding. Clin. Obstet. Gynec., *13:* 400, 1970.

Taylor, H. C.: Endometrial hyperplasia and carcinoma of body of uterus. Amer. J. Obstet. Gynec., *23:* 309, 1932.

Wall, J. A., and Jacobs, W. M.: Dysfunctional uterine bleeding in the premenopausal and menopausal years. Amer. J. Obstet. Gynec., *74:* 985, 1957.

Wall, J. A., Franklin, R. R., and Kaufman, R. H.: Reversal of benign and malignant endometrial changes with chlomiphene. Amer. J. Obstet. Gynec., *88:* 1072, 1964.

Wallach, E. E. (Editor): Dysfunctional uterine bleeding. Clin. Obstet. Gynec., *13:* 363, 1972.

Wentz, W. B.: Treatment of persistent endometrial hyperplasia by progestins. Amer. J. Obstet. Gynec., *95:* 999, 1966.

Wolfe, S. A., and Mackles, A.: Malignant lesions arising from benign endometrial polyps. Obstet. Gynec., *20:* 542, 1963.

chapter 15

Adenocarcinoma of the Corpus Uteri

Ninety-five per cent of all fundal malignancies consist of endometrial adenocarcinoma which is much more frequent than adenocarcinoma of the cervix, but less common than epidermoid cervical cancer. In past years it was felt that fundal adenocarcinoma was only one-fifth or one-sixth as frequent as squamous cell cancer of the cervix, but more recent observations suggest that adenocarcinoma is increasing in incidence, particularly in communities where there is a high proportion of white private patients.

As indicated earlier by Novak and Villa Santa, a hospital having a large number of poor socio-economic patients will have a high ratio of cervical cancer, whereas corpus cancer increases with a restricted white clientele. Obviously, geographical, racial, and ethnic status are influential factors and deserve careful evaluation; however, the *increased life expectancy* of the American female probably allows more endometrial malignancies to develop while increasing cytopathological recognition of cervical atypias has led to a marked decrease in invasive disease of the cervix. Indeed, in certain areas the ratio of endometrial and cervical malignancy is even.

Endometrial cancer is characteristically a disease of the aging woman, and with the average female life span increased to nearly 75 years, it follows that more women are living long enough to develop this disease, which is most common in the aging postmenopausal patient. The *average age of 57 years* is a full decade later than with cervical cancer.

Gross Pathology

Adenocarcinoma may arise from any portion of the uterus, and may present in either of two chief forms, which, however, are not always sharply separable.

Diffuse Form. In the so-called diffuse form a large portion of, or perhaps the entire, endometrial surface is involved in the growth, which appears as a fungoid overgrowth, with surface ulceration and necrosis. In the advanced stages the muscular wall may show extensive involvement, with penetration to the serosa, forming nodules on the surface. On the other hand, even extensive surface involvement may be associated with little or no demonstrable infiltration of the deeper layers. With more diffuse disease the myometrial involvement causes marked increase in the size of the uterus. The *size of the uterus* has been used as the chief criterion in certain clinical classifications of the disease, although associated myomata or adenomyosis might create a very erroneous impression. Today other methods of classification are being utilized.

Circumscribed Form. There are certain cases in which adenocarcinoma, irrespective of the stage of the disease, appears to be limited to a comparatively small area of the endometrium, despite extensive invasion of the musculature. As a matter of fact, in certain early forms the cancer may present as a small polypoid growth. In such cases, the curette may remove all traces of the disease, so that examination of the uterus, after its removal, may show no evidence of the cancerous process. This should not invalidate the diagnosis. (See Fig. 15.1.)

Clinical Classification of Endometrial Carcinoma

The most *important* single factor in formulating a prognosis for endometrial cancer is the extent of the disease, and *secondarily* the microscopic appearance (degree of differentiation) of the tumor.

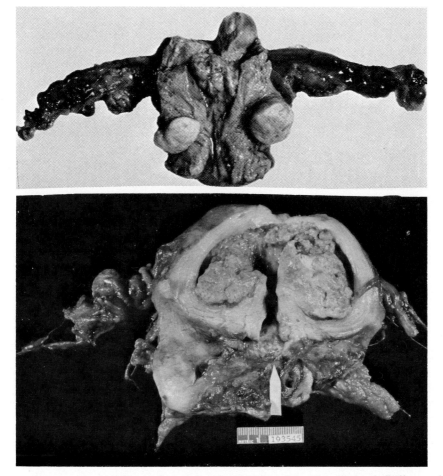

15.1 (*top*). Circumscribed endometrial cancer with coincidental myoma. (*bottom*). Diffuse endometrial adenocarcinoma in patient irradiated for cervical cancer five years earlier (note cervix completely missing).

The two often but not invariably parallel one another.

The International Federation of Gynecology and Obstetrics (FIGO) and subsequently the American College of Obstetrics and Gynecology have recommended that *carcinoma of the endometrial corpus* be staged thusly:

Stage 0, histological findings suspicious of malignancy, but not proven;

Stage 1, the carcinoma is confined to the corpus;

Stage 1a, The length of the uterine cavity is 8 cm. or less;

Stage 1b, The length of the uterine cavity is more than 8 cm.

Stage 1 cases should be further qualified as to whether they are highly *differentiated* adenomatous carcinomas; differentiated but with partly solid areas (*intermediate*); or predominantly solid or *undifferentiated* carcinomas.

Stage 2, the carcinoma has involved the corpus and the cervix;

Stage 3, the carcinoma has extended outside the uterus, but not outside the true pelvis;

Stage 4, the carcinoma has extended outside the true pelvis or has obviously involved the mucosa of the bladder or rectum.

This is a logical if not ideal method of classification, but allows too much latitude in Stage 1, for lesions confined to the endometrium are close to 100% curable, whereas major degrees of myometrial involvement markedly impair salvage. Because, however, it has been recommended by such an august organization, it has been generally accepted. The size of the uterus hardly seems the answer, for concomitant diseases as myomata or adenomyosis are not rare, and one may find a large uterus with only minor degrees of cancer.

Carcinoma corporis et endocervicis is the suggested terminology where the presence of tumor in both locales makes it impossible to assign a primary site. Fractional curettage of the endocervix first, and then corpus, with tumor in both may indicate the likely primary source, and histological niceties may suggest an endometrial origin (if there is acanthosis) or an endocervical origin (if mucus-forming). Treatment of carcinoma of corpus and cervix is less satisfactory and incompletely standardized.

Where microscopically indistinguishable cancer involves ovary and endometrium, the term *carcinoma uteri et ovarii* has been proposed. This combination of endometrial and gonadal tumors occurs with some frequency, and on occasion it is impossible to ascertain which is the primary, or if there are two lesions. Uterine and ovarian carcinoma may indicate endometrium stimulated to malignancy in a normal and ectopic locale; the prognosis is much better than metastatic disease as noted in Chapter 25.

The American Joint Committee for Cancer Staging has advocated qualification of any tumor by such terms as T (primary tumor), N (lymph node involvement) and M (metastases); all of these are qualified numerically according to the extent. Although recognizing a need for standardization, we dislike having such a cumbersome and impractical classification applied to uterine malignancy, and it is not utilized in this chapter.

Microscopic Diagnosis

Histological gradation of cancer is the other factor involved in classifying adenocarcinomas. The microscopic diagnosis is made on the basis of two chief criteria, *viz.*

(1) The Pattern or Architecture. Whereas in the normal endometrium at any phase of menstrual or postmenstrual life the gland pattern is a uniform one, in adenocarcinoma there is marked departure from this orderly arrangement of the glands, which show not only a marked increase in number, but also varying degrees of atypicality, with such adenomatous hyperplasia as to obliterate the intervening stroma ("back-to-back" crowding), papillary formation due to increasing stratification, and such cell proliferation as to obliterate the gland pattern (Fig. 15.2).

(2) Individual Cell Changes. In adenocarcinoma, the cells show varying degrees of immaturity and dedifferentia-

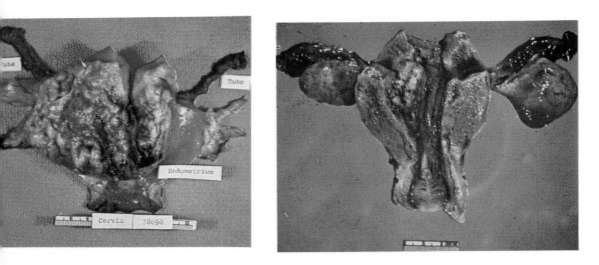

Plate 15.1. *Left,* diffuse extensive cancer extending through myometrium; *right,* polypoid adenocarcinoma associated with corpus luteum.

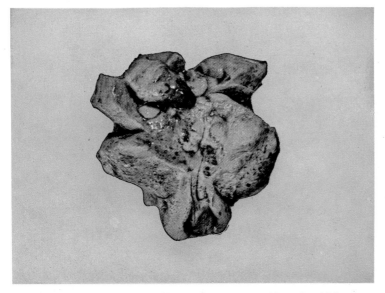

Plate 15.2. Fundal cancer after estrogen therapy for 11 years. Note the thick myometrium with endometrial proliferation and the polypoid adenocarcinoma at left cornu.

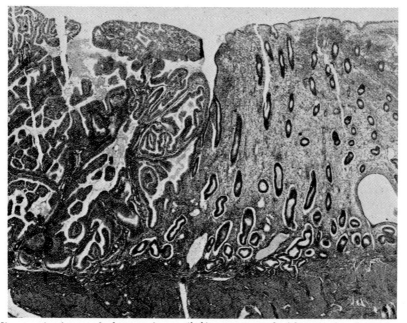

15.2. Microscopic picture of adenocarcinoma (*left*) as contrasted with normal endometrium (*right*).

tion with abnormal pleomorphic nuclei; many of the latter show hyperchromatosis, abnormal mitotic activity, and other evidences of anaplasia. Various degenerative changes with the production of lipoid-like and "foam" cells may be found, producing a mesonephroma-like pattern (Fig. 15.11).

Differential Microscopic Diagnosis

Although the microscopic diagnosis of adenocarcinoma is often simple, there may be considerable difficulty in distinguishing certain *atypical, proliferative, or adenomatous varieties of hyperplasia* which have been described in Chapter 14. Where the atypical changes are of mild degree the differentiation is simple enough. When the lesion is a very adenomatous one, with marked epithelial proliferation, the simulation of low grade carcinoma is so perfect that pathologists will differ in their diagnostic interpretation.

In any form of hyperplasia mitoses are present, often in large numbers, so that these are not helpful in the microscopic differentiation. In the lower grade adenocarcinomas, there is little dedifferentiation of the epithelial cells, whereas in either the benign or malignant lesion the epithelial layer may be stratified. Actually, a proportion of adenocarcinomas will show only minimal or no invasion of the myometrium. Indeed, there is usually far more invasion of the muscle in the entirely benign adenomyosis than is seen in many adenocarcinomas.

Cytogenetic studies of the normal and abnormal endometrium have been performed by such students as Stanley and Kirkland, who indicate a marked difference from the aneuploidy generally noted in cervical and ovarian malignancy. Indeed, there is a marked similarity between the karyotype of the normal endometrium (diploid) and adenocarcinoma ("pseudo" diploid). It is difficult to comprehend the full significance of these excellent and well controlled studies, which differ somewhat from the findings of Katayama and Jones, who indicate both diploidy and aneuploidy.

Endometrial Adenocarcinoma "in Situ"

This term has considerable vogue in current gynecological parlance and literature, and we deplore its wide usage for all kinds of minor deviation from typical endometrial hyperplasia. Although cervical cancer in situ has certain definite diagnostic requirements, such as full thickness replacement of the lining epithelium by abnormal, undifferentiated, basal cells, there are no such rigid criteria for a definition of adenocarcinoma in situ of the endometrium. Although cognizant of what such an excellent gynecological pathologist as Hertig means to imply by the appellation, we dislike it, for it has stimulated a too frequent improper diagnosis of "in situ adenocarcinoma." Often the lesion in question is simple cystic glandular hyperplasia; occasionally normal secretory patterns are suspect, and these can present a problem. There is the common intraluminal tufting and budding by tall, pale-staining secretory or pseudo-secretory cells (Figs. 15.3). In many instances it appears that this intraglandular secretion represents mucin rather than glycogen. Salm has pointed out that this occurs in the normal endometrium or well differentiated carcinomas.

The FIGO classification of adenocarcinoma Stage 0 might include such patterns as shown in Figure 15.3 (which we suspect

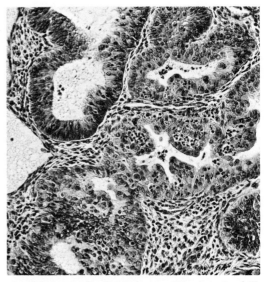

15.4. Marked adenomatous ("back-to-back") crowding with beginning stratication and proliferation of lining epithelium with small papillae.

is benign though atypical) and Figure 15.4 (which we would call malignant). This might serve to illustrate the extreme difficulty in evaluating these border-line lesions. Whether it is justifiable to

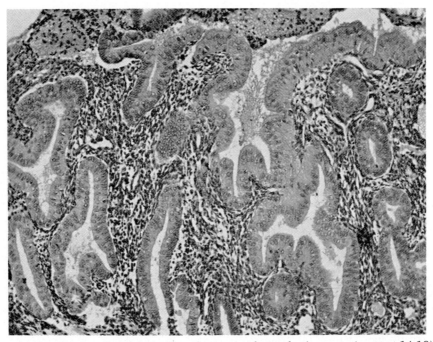

15.3. Atypical adenomatous hyperplasia. Note the compact hyperplastic stroma (contrast **14.10**) although a glandular pattern is similar.

designate a lesion as malignant, even ICO, if the microscopic pattern is only suspicious, is a moot point.

The clinically malignant nature of the true adenocarcinoma, as indicated by its extension to lymphatic glands, is proof that its cells do actually break through the basement membrane, and in certain cases this penetration is easily demonstrable, as well as its extension to the muscularis. It thus appears that there is a whole series of gradations, a species of histological stepping stones, between atypical hyperplasia and adenocarcinoma, and there is no sure criterion as to the point at which the lesion assumes actually malignant characteristics. In the doubtful group the safe clinical plan is to treat them as potential cancer, which is usually easy in that most such patients are in the peri-menopausal era and have completed their family.

PROLIFERATIVE HYPERPLASIA IN THE YOUNG WOMAN

Younger women are afflicted only occasionally, but these represent a greater problem. If the diagnosis is not 100% certain following curettage it would seem that another confirmatory curettage several months later is warranted before any definitive therapy, and with no real risk to the patient. Jackson and Dockerty have indicated the frequent finding of low grade adenoacanthoma with clinical and pathological findings in the ovary suggesting a Stein-Leventhal syndrome. This unquestionably occurs, and we are cognizant of at least a dozen of our own or referred cases, although Stein himself has never seen such a coincidence in 25 years of experience. Perhaps his diligence in treating this problem early has prevented this sequel, and prompt treatment of this syndrome might be considered a form of prophylaxis against endometrial adenocarcinoma (Fig. 15.5).

Kaufman, Abbott, and Wall suggested in past years that varied forms of abnormal endometrium are associated with the Stein-Leventhal ovary. The pattern is frequently proliferative or hyperplastic, occasionally adenomatous, but wedge resection of the ovary is often followed by reversion to normal. Today, however, a thorough trial with *clomiphene* might be suggested, for the above authors, Kistner, and many others have indicated that markedly atypical endometria, and possibly early adenocarcinoma, will revert if ovulation can be incurred.

Progesterone therapy may likewise prove valuable in treating certain atypical

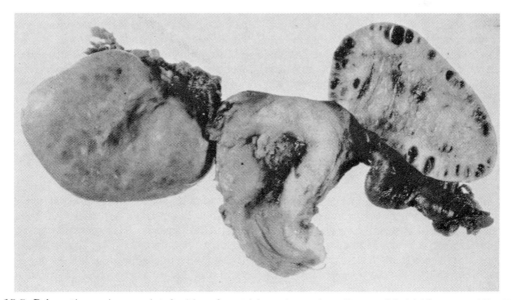

15.5. Polycystic ovaries associated with endometrial carcinoma in a 15-year-old girl (Courtesy of Dr. R. Greenblatt, Augusta, Georgia).

endometria even where there is no apparent polycystic ovarian disease. Indeed there have been a certain number of cases of presumed early adenocarcinoma successfully treated by progesterone with subsequent pregnancy (O'Neill). However, there have also been a few cases of endometrial cancer in conjunction with an intrauterine pregnancy (Karlen *et al.*).

Histological Grading of Adenocarcinoma

In keeping with the accepted rule that the greater the degree of immaturity and dedifferentiation of the cells the greater the clinical malignancy of the tumor, systems of grading these tumors have been suggested by various authors. According to this, four grades are distinguished. In Grade I, the least malignant, the proportion of dedifferentiated cells is relatively small, not exceeding 25%. In this type the atypicality of the gland pattern is not nearly so marked as in the more malignant grades (Fig. 15.6). This variety is often spoken of as *adenoma malignum.* At the other extreme, Grade IV, malignant cells are present in 75 to 100%.

Along with increasing cell dedifferentiation there is progressive loss of the rather delicate adenomatous pattern seen in Figure 15.8 (*top*) due to proliferation of the epithelial lining cell. As this stratification continues there may be obliteration of the glandular pattern with little resemblance to an adenocarcinoma so that the lesion mimics an epidermoid or an undifferentiated carcinoma. However, examination of other areas may suggest glandular acini, indicating an advanced Grade IV adenocarcinoma.

In our own laboratory, we arbitrarily assign four histological gradations to endometrial adenocarcinoma, but actually, such qualifying terms as "differentiated, intermediate, and undifferentiated" are of equal service in histologically grading adenocarcinoma; indeed, this is the histologic classification suggested by FIGO. It seems quite apparent that microscopic grade generally parallels myometrial invasion and ultimate prognosis in many cases. In other words, a *well differentiated tumor is much less apt to invade or metastasize,* and should offer a much better prognosis.

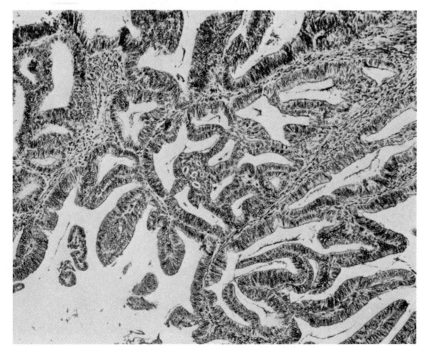

15.6. Well differentiated adenocarcinoma

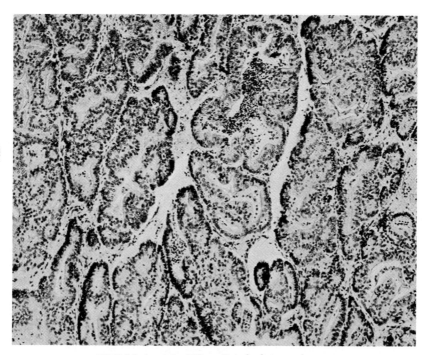

15.7. Moderately differentiated adenocarcinoma

Adenoacanthoma of Uterus (Fig. 15.9)

This specific variant of endometrial adenocarcinoma is characterized by the presence of many squamous cells, filling the gland lumina and/or lining and replacing the surface endometrium. The squamous cells are well differentiated, generally uniform, and obviously benign; where this acanthosis occurs with adenocarcinoma, the lesion is malignant, although not because of the squamous cells. It is the *glandular component* that is decisive, and indeed this same squamous metaplasia may occur with benign endometrial hyperplasia, in which event the lesion is benign.

The source of these squamous cells is generally presumed to be certain indifferent or reserve cells lying at the epithelial stromal border, although Novak and Nally in their study of uterine adenocanthosis speculate about the possibility of a direct metaplasia from the adult endometrial lining cell. Although metaplasia of an adult cell is generally not accepted, our study seemed to indicate all intermediate transition forms from lining epithelium to a mature squa-

mous cell with frank pearl formation. However, majority opinion favors a reserve cell origin, although these indifferent cells are not demonstrable.

In any case the finding of squamous cells in the endometrium is not normal, but may occur with such diverse causes as chronic infection, foreign bodies such as an IUCD, irradiation, vitamin A deficiency, hormonal stimulus, or neoplasm. Where acanthosis is extensive with adenocarcinoma, it has often led to the erroneous diagnosis of a mixed squamous cell and endometrial cancer. Although this entity may occur as an *adenosquamous* malignancy, the epidermoid cells show obvious evidence of malignant change with nuclear abnormalities, mitotic activity, pleomorphism, etc., a striking contrast to the uniform often spinal differentiation seen in benign acanthosis.

Our own study suggests that adenoacanthoma is seen in less than 10% of endometrial adenocarcinoma and is relatively benign due to the disproportionate frequency of acanthosis in the early better differentiated forms of adenocarcinoma,

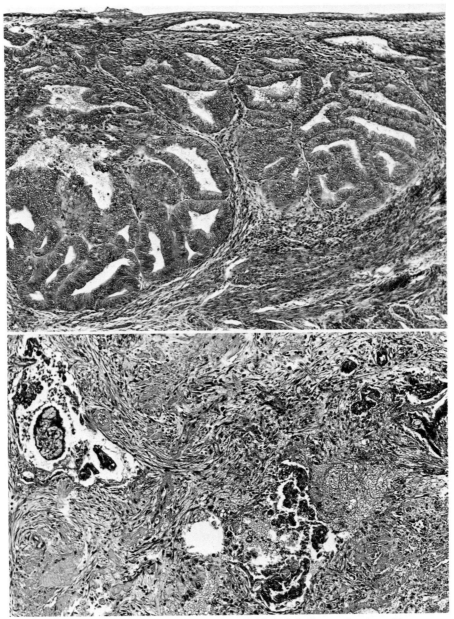

15.8 (*top*). Tiny well differentiated adenocarcinoma, an incidental finding at the time of hysterectomy for myomata. (*bottom*). Lymphatic metastases in ovaries removed in above case. It is extremely rare to find extension of a superficial well differentiated tumor.

yet certain authors indicate it represents more than one-third of endometrial malignancies (Tweedale, 43.7%; Charles, 37.1%) and suggest a decreased salvage. Renning and Javert, 35.9%). Certainly we have seen occasional cases of uterine adenoacanthoma which have extended or metastasized and ultimately proved fatal, but these are exceptional, and it is our belief that this lesion is certainly no more, if as, malignant as endometrial cancer in general. This conforms with the recent study by Silverberg, Bolin, and Degiongi, who note an 83 per cent 5-year survival with adenoacanthoma, 56% with adenocarcinoma, and 35% for adenosqua-

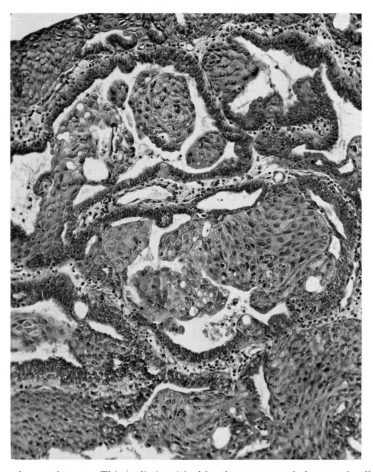

15.9. Adenoacanthoma of uterus. This is distinguished by the presence of plaques of well differentiated, obviously benign, squamous cells in association with adenocarcinoma.

mous lesions where both adenoid and squamous components are malignant. Like us, they feel that the capability for benign acanthosis is of good prognostic import. Badib *et al.* imply that adenoacanthoma behaves like any adenocarcinoma of corresponding grade and stage.

One explanation for the divergent impressions is that many so-called adenoacanthomas are in reality cases of advanced adenocarcinoma where there is such edema and distortion of the proliferating tumor cell that they simulate squamous cells. These, of course, are generally advanced histological degrees of tumor where a poor prognosis should be expected. Where true well differentiated acanthosis presents, it is most likely to be associated with the histologically well dif-

ferentiated noninvasive cancer, and as a group, adenoacanthoma should be regarded as a relatively favorable type of malignancy with salvage at least that of corresponding grades of endometrial cancer, despite many pessimistic reports. Lastly, certain series of adenoacanthomas reported with an unfavorable prognosis often include adenosquamous cancer (Morrison).

Epidermoid carcinoma may invade the endometrium but is usually secondary to cervical disease which may on occasion arise high in the endocervical canal and involve or completely replace the endometrium and tubal epithelium. Only rarely does epidermoid cancer arise primarily in the corpus, without cervical disease, as noted by White *et al.*

Adenoepidermoid and squamous cancer, where there is definite malignancy of both the squamous and glandular components, are reportedly more commonly of cervical origin, but may arise in the uterus (Fig. 15.10). The most likely source would seem to be malignant degeneration of the generally benign squamous cells in adenoacanthoma.

Mesonephroma of the Endometrium

On occasion one may encounter the classic pattern of a mesonephroma arising from the endometrium in the absence of any other primary source in the ovary, vagina, or elsewhere. The clear-cell pattern seems to predominate, but the papillary tubular pattern lined by a flat peglike epithelium as described by Schiller may be seen on occasion. Villa Santa has reported four such cases, including one of his own (Fig. 15.11), and Rutledge has added another. We have seen several classic endometrial mesonephroma in our laboratory.

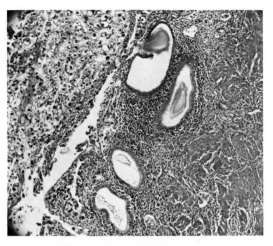

15.11. Typical hyperplasia and adenocarcinoma to *right*, clear-cell mesonephroma to *left* (no other pelvic tumor). (Courtesy of Dr. Umberto Villa Santa, Baltimore, Maryland.)

Since the vestigial remnants of the mesonephric duct do not occur in the endometrium, one may of course theorize about a possible aberrant location for these embryonic remnants. We can also speculate about various degenerative (fatty) and metaplastic change. On the other hand Scully (Chapter 25) expresses belief that ovarian mesonephromas arise from endometriosis, and are of paramesonephric rather than mesonephric origin, and the finding of an occasional endometrial mesonephroma would serve to support this concept.

The association of vaginal adenocarcinoma and adenosis in the daughters of women treated by stilbestrol when pregnant might offer further support as indicated in Chapter 10. At the present, however, we are more or less open minded about these possibilities, and are inclined to wonder if certain morphologically similar tumors may not have different methods of origin.

Relationship of Endometrial Hyperplasia to Adenocarcinoma

Although it seems probable that myomata and adenomyosis are rather frequent concomitants of fundal cancer, there is no definite evidence that these have more than a casual relationship, al-

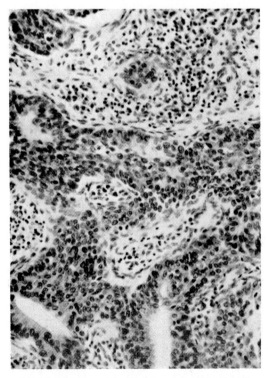

15.10. Adenoepidermoid carcinoma showing "gland" pattern below but almost solid area elsewhere.

though estrogen would seem a possible common denominator. Similarly, endometrial hyperplasia *during the menstrual era* appears of no particular import and often seems to be a rather transient and self-limited affair.

On the other hand, hyperplasia *around and after the menopause,* especially where it is recurrent and assumes an adenomatous proliferative pattern (Fig. 15.12), is considerably more worrisome: (1) Such atypical microscopic varieties may be encountered as to make differentiation from early neoplasm utterly impossible, even though some extremely adenomatous patterns may be completely benign and followed by no malignant trends. It is important to emphasize that these equivocal histological architectures may be a sequel to exogenous estrogen (frequently given without indication or discrimination) or may be spontaneous. (2) Adenocarcinoma is frequently preceded by these intensely hyperplastic patterns, which may occur during either the menstrual or postmenopausal era. In the latter instance, one may only conjecture as to the source of estrogen, which is known to be the usual stimulus to hyperplasia. The adrenal gland has been proved capable of estrogen production, but in recent years there has been considerable speculation about the function of the postmenopausal ovary. Some feel that hyperplastic stromal cells (morphologically indistinguishable from theca cells and often taking up fat avidly) may be a source of estrogen despite disagreement by Roddick and Greene. In any case, numerous publications have stressed the frequency with which corpus cancer is preceded by an atypical endometrial hyperplasia.

Since estrogen is the normal stimulus to endometrial hyperplasia, and since estrogen therapy has been observed to produce hyperplastic patterns indistinguishable from adenocarcinoma, it is only logical that this steroid has been under considerable suspicion as a possible factor in the evolution of fundal cancer. Admittedly there is not final proof that estrogens are carcinogenic, although we find it difficult to accept statements (Wilson) "that estrogen and progesterone are prophylactic to breast and genital cancer to an unknown degree." Wilson enlarges on his point by advocating that women be kept "endocrine rich and thereby cancer poor" by elimination of the menopause. Lifelong cyclic therapy with periodic shedding of the endometrium is advocated as a prophylaxis against endometrial cancer. We would urge all readers to be cautious before accepting this astonishingly different approach to reality.

The review by Andrews affords additional evidence as to the possible role of estrogen in the etiology of endometrial cancer. Of equal importance, however, is the belated admission by a senior

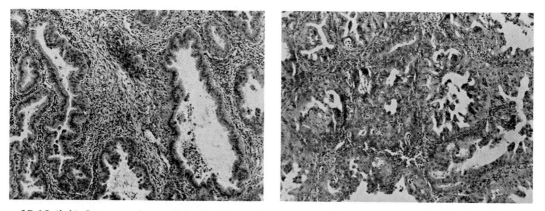

15.12 (*left*). Interpreted as proliferative hyperplasia at age 50; x-ray induction of menopause instituted. (*right*). Evolvement of frank adenocarcinoma seven years later.

statesman, Dr. L. A. Emge that "I, for one, believe that such hazards as long-term estrogenization in the postmenopausal woman are real and deserve serious consideration." If a critical gynecologist of this stature could make such a statement, it behooves all of us to be attentive.

Estrogen must be regarded as possibly carcinogenic because of many different observations, no one of which is conclusive; but *in toto* they seem highly suggestive. These may only be summarized as follows.

Animal Experiments. It had been impossible to produce adenocarcinoma in experimental animals by huge doses of estrogens; however, Meissner, Sommers, and Sherman have been able to produce in certain strains of rabbit unequivocal adenocarcinoma which, even after cessation of the steroid, went on to metastasize and kill the animal. Earlier attempts of our own, utilizing stilbestrol in the hamster, produced a markedly adenomatous pattern along with an aseptic pyometra, an almost inevitable sequel in animals treated with protracted estrogens.

Late Menopause. Repeated observations have noted that postmenopausal women with adenocarcinoma have a history of a protracted late menopause and, since anovulation at this era is common, the opportunity for prolonged unopposed estrogen is present. This deserves reevaluation, for most clinicians believe that today's woman is apt to menstruate and ovulate longer.

"Bloody Menopause." In patients who develop adenocarcinoma in later life there is a high incidence of perimenopausal bleeding, necessitating curettage, which shows hyperplasia or an anovulatory pattern in a high percentage of cases. (See Fig. 15.12.)

Castration. Repeated observations have noted the rarity of endometrial cancer following bilateral oophorectomy, a not uncommon procedure until recent years. The study by Cianfrani reporting 12 cases of cancer developing after castration might seem to negate this thesis

but the reader must recall the frequent difficulty in ablating all ovarian tissue in certain cases (pelvic inflammatory disease, endometriosis, etc.) or the confusion in microscopically diagnosing early cases.

Hoffmeister and Vandrak have also recorded endomentrial adenocarcinoma in castrates, either surgical or postirradiation, and Shay *et al.* report a case with gonadal agenesis; obviously there are, however, extra-ovarian sources of steroid function.

Feminizing Ovarian Tumors. Many granulosa-theca cell tumors which are capable of estrogen production have been frequently noted as coexisting with endometrial cancer in a much higher ratio than the laws of chance would allow. This frequent association (15 to 25% in most series) has been called the "spontaneous biological experiment" and would seem to afford a real basis for concepts of estrogen as a profound proliferative stimulus.

Estrogen Therapy. There have been numerous cases reported with the sequence of prolonged estrogen therapy and later adenocarcinoma and, although no one can state positively that this is a matter of cause and effect, discriminating gynecologists are rather reluctant to utilize prolonged unopposed estrogens. Of particular interest in certain of these cases is the finding of all degrees of endometrial proliferation up to frank adenocarcinoma in the same specimen. Gusberg and Hall note 23 patients in a 20-year span who had received exogenous estrogens for over a year.

Even more suggestive is the series reported by Cutler *et al.,* which concerns patients with gonadal dysgenesis, treated by estrogens, generally stilbestrol, who subsequently developed endometrial adenocarcinoma after a varying period of years. They record three cases of their own to add to three previous reports in the literature. The duration of estrogen therapy was anywhere from 4 to 20 years. More recently a similar case, which we have had the opportunity of reviewing, has been reported by Wilkerson. Closely related is the report by Reid and Shirley

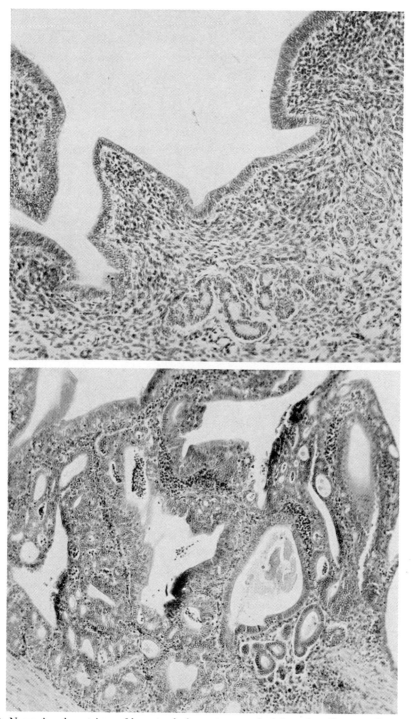

15.13 (*top*). Normal endometrium of hamster before estrogen administration. (*bottom*). Endometrium of hamster after long course of estrogen. (Courtesy of Dr. R. A. Bacon, Department of Anatomy, Johns Hopkins Medical School, Baltimore, Maryland.)

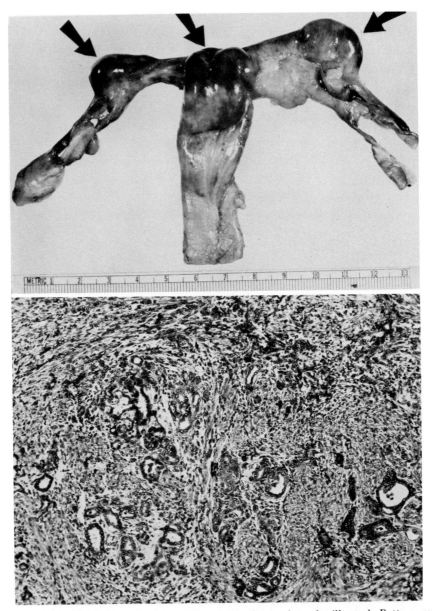

15.14. *Top,* tumor nodules in bicornuate rabbit uterus after prolonged stilbestrol. *Bottom,* microscopic cancer. The cancer depicted in the lower figure metastasized and led to death even after cessation of the steroid stimulation. (Courtesy of Dr. Sheldon Sommers, Bostom, Massachusetts.)

of a woman with Sheehan's syndrome who developed adenocarcinoma after prolonged stilbestrol therapy.

Association of Hyperplasia and Adenocarcinoma. This association was first noted by Taylor in 1932 and Novak and Yui in 1936, and there has been considerable confirmation by more recent authors. Not only may adenocarcinoma coexist with hyperplasia, but it is not infrequently preceded by it around the menopausal era. Extremely atypical proliferative degrees of hyperplasia may be found, and indeed all variants of simple and adenomatous hyperplasia may be found along with adenocarcinoma.

Postmenopausal Hyperplasia. Hyperplasia in the menstrual era rarely

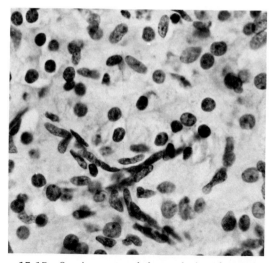

15.15. Ovarian stromal hyperplasia (thecosis). Stromal cells enlarged, polyhedral, and identical to theca-lutein cell, an estrogen-secreting agent.

has any dire sequelae and is often a transient innocuous process unlike hyperplasia in the climacteric woman. An earlier publication by Novak points out the similarities between women with *postmenopausal* hyperplasia and malignant adenocarcinoma in regard to such

features as obesity, hypertension, diabetes, nulliparity, prolonged menstruation, bloody menopause, etc., all of which have been repeatedly noted as occurring commonly with adenocarcinoma. Indeed it is hard to avoid the impression that postmenopausal hyperplasia and adenocarcinoma are mere variants of a similar generalized metabolic or endocrine process with carcinoma an exaggerated and extreme end-stage if there is a continuance of the stimulus (perhaps *estrogen*) although Dunn *et al.* disagree with this tenet.

Association with Stein-Leventhal Syndrome. This has already been alluded to on page 337, and we have seen this association on occasion. Obviously the pertinent factor is the absence of ovulation and progesterone secretion by the S-L ovary, which leads to prolonged unopposed stimulation of the endometrium by the estrogenic hormone.

The high incidence of ovarian stromal hyperplasia in association with endometrial endocarcinoma has been noted by Woll *et al.*, Novak and Mohler, and more recently by Marcus who has reviewed the literature and discussed the

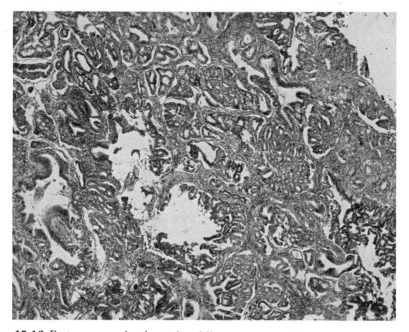

15.16. Postmenopausal endometrium following long-standing estrogen therapy

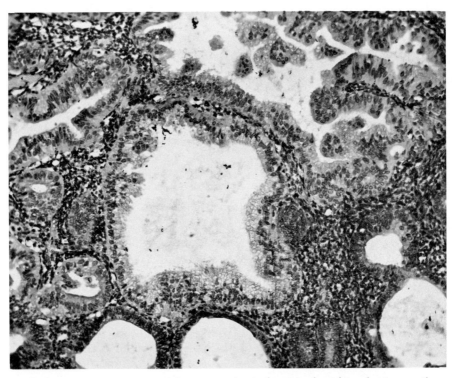

15.17. Endometrium of postmenopausal woman who had received prolonged estrogen therapy with resultant bleeding. Repetition of curettage six weeks later showed normal senile endometrium with complete regression of the atypical hyperplasia after stoppage of estrogens. (Courtesy of Dr. D. Dickson, Santa Barbara, California.)

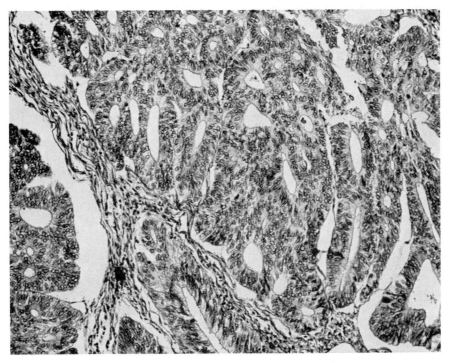

15.18. High power of more proliferative areas in polyp depicted in Plate 15.1

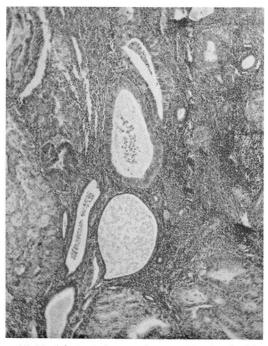

15.19. Adenocarcinoma of uterus associated with postmenopausal hyperplasia.

pros and cons of this controversial subject. Sherman and Woolf, however, are more concerned with hyperplasia of the hilus cells and their production of a bisexual steroid ("sexagen") that may induce adenocarcinoma. During the menstrual era the function of the hilus cell is suppressed by the ovarian hormones; with impaired postmenopausal gonadal function and increased follicle-stimulating hormone (FSH) there is stimulation of the hilus cells with production of a steriod (estrogenic) that incites later adenocarcinoma. If there is incomplete suppression during the menstrual era, the hilus cell may manufacture an androgenic steroid that provokes the Stein-Leventhal picture.

The later study by Varga and Henriksen would seem to question the validity of the above concept. They note marked variation in LH excretion, and no significant response to progesterone therapy in patients with endometrial cancer or a control group.

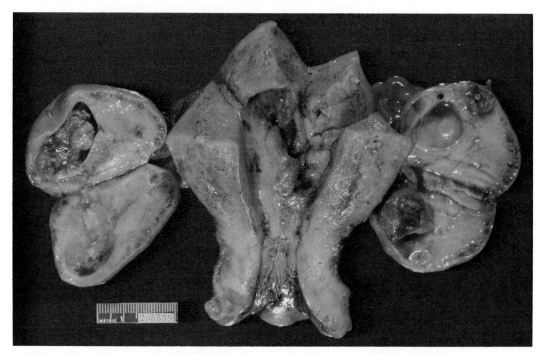

15.20. Polypoid endometrial adenocarcinoma with Stein-Leventhal ovaries and incidental bilateral dermoids.

One must be cognizant of the occasional young women who develop adenocarcinoma in the face of a biphasic cycle with obvious evidence of ovulation. The pathologist, however, frequently finds patches of hyperplasia in association with a generally progestational endometrium, and it is felt that these foci represent unripe undifferentiated endometrium which may be incapable of response to progesterone and thereby subject to *protracted unopposed estrogen stimulation* (Fig. 15.21). These areas may occur in a polyp or in the endometrium, but show a common incapability of response to progesterone. This would seem a very logical answer to those who deride the "estrogen theory" by quoting small groups of women with adenocarcinoma associated with a corpus luteum or a generally secretory endometrium or both. Carcinoma in the young ovulating woman seems a different and infrequent type of adenocarcinoma, and the usual variety would make it difficult to discount the important role of estrogen. Genetic predisposition to cancer is likewise of considerable import.

We have seen several cases such as a 29-year-old para II, who had been on "the pills" for three years. Although most of the endometrium showed a profound secretory effect, focal adenocarcinoma was present, possibly due to a localized lack of response to progesterone and resultant stimulation by the estrogen component (Fig. 15.22). Birth control pills cannot be advocated as routine "replacement therapy" of the menopause, for this reason as well as the added expense.

Clinical Characteristics

More than the two-thirds of all cases occur in women beyond the menopause, the proportion being roughly 75% postmenopausal, 15% perimenopausal,

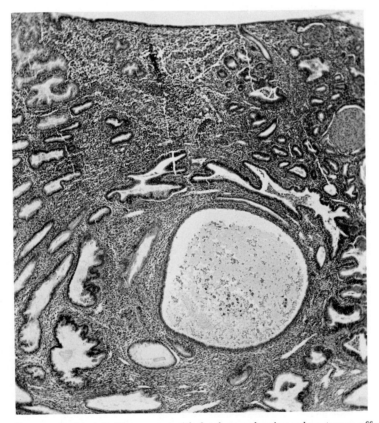

15.21. Generally progestational (*left*) response with focal area showing only estrogen effect. (Note benign squamous metaplasia on *right*.)

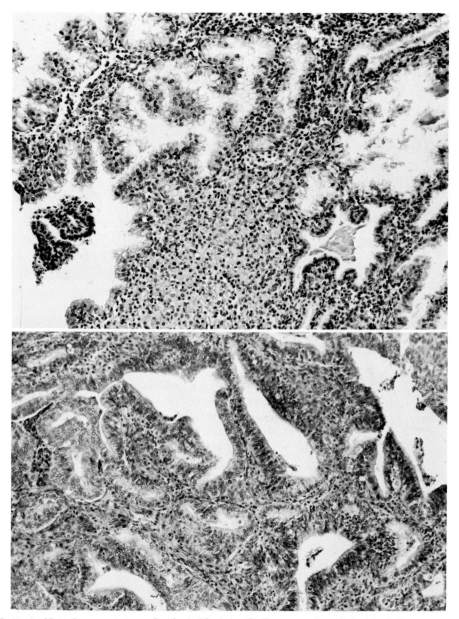

15.22 (*top*). Note hypersecretory glands (with Arias-Stella pattern) and decidual-like appearance of stroma. (*bottom*). Marked adenomatous pattern compatible with early adenocarcinoma.

and 10% still menstruating, according to compiled reports. Obesity, hypertension, diabetes, and a history of previous curettage are frequent concomitants. There is often a history of sterility or poor fertility. The question of whether an irradiation menopause is a causative factor is speculative, despite much suggestive evidence that irradiation in general must be regarded as under some suspicion as far as the genesis of certain malignancy is concerned (Novak and Woodruff).

The only important symptom is *abnormal bleeding*, commonly postmenopausal. In the case of women still in the menstruating age, *menorrhagia* is frequently observed. Next to bleeding, the most significant symptom is an *abnormal discharge*, at first watery, but soon admixed with blood. As with cancer

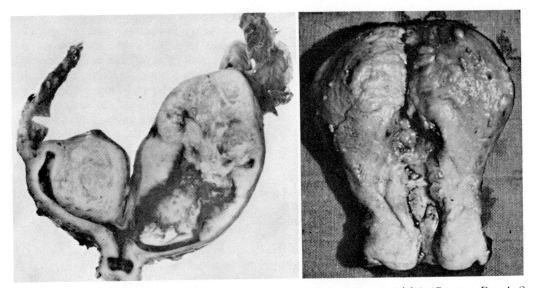

15.23 (*left*). Bicornuate uterus with adenomyosis (*left*) and adenocarcinoma (*right*). (Courtesy Drs. A. S. Duncan and A. H. John, Cardiff, Wales.) (*right*). Endometrial adenocarcinoma with diffuse adenomyosis. (From Emge, L.: Elusive adenomyosis of the uterus, Amer. J. Obstet. Gynec., *83:* 1541, 1962, C. V. Mosby Co., Publishers.)

elsewhere, *pain* is not a symptom until the later invasive stages of the disease. The same statement can be made with reference to *loss of weight* and *general debility,* although *anemia* may become marked if there is any pronounced blood loss.

On occasion there may be no abnormal bleeding, but pressure symptoms due to a uterus massively distended by blood which cannot escape due to some obstruction in the lower genital tract. Arrata and Zarou find that about one-third of their cases of postmenopausal hematometra are due to an endometrial carcinoma.

Diagnosis

The first thought of every physician when confronted with a case of *postmenopausal bleeding* should concern cancer of the uterus, either of the cervix or of the body. Cervical cancer can usually be eliminated by careful inspection and office smears and biopsy.

Assuming, however, that a cervical or vaginal source for the bleeding can be eliminated, an intrauterine source may be safely assumed. As a matter of fact, it is often possible to observe a blood-stained discharge or a trickle of blood es-

caping from the cervical canal. Even then, it is by no means certain that adenocarcinoma exists, this being found in less than 10% of all cases of postmenopausal bleeding. Other possible causes are benign polyps or hyperplasia (often estrogen induced), submucous myoma, or senile vaginitis.

A few women cannot establish whether bleeding is urinary or vaginal in origin, and the gynecologist should be aware of the fact that certain bladder tumors may produce only intermittent hematuria. A Tampax, if inserted overnight, will show staining near the string if the bleeding is urinary but in the back if there is a vaginal source. Endometrial biopsy may be performed; if this is positive, the diagnosis is established, but, if negative, cancer cannot be excluded.

There is only one decisive way to make the diagnosis, and *dilatation and curettage* should be standard procedure. Aspiration or lavage of the endometrial cavity do not approach the efficacy of curettage. No facts exist that curettage leads to metastases although there may be a temporary rise of tumor cells in the blood stream. Vaginal cytology with maturation index (MI) should never be neglected although its accuracy in detecting endometrial cancer perhaps approaches only 80 to 85%. There is frequently a shift to the right which suggests estrogen hyperactivity.

If curettage yields only extremely scant tissue from the uterine cavity, it is probable that cancer will not be found on microscopic examination, but Beutler, Dockerty, and Randall have noted that adenocarcinoma in conjunction with an atrophic endometrium is often missed. If abundant tissue is brought away, and the uterus is enlarged, the gynecologist will be suspicious especially if the woman is well beyond the menopause, and if the removed tissue is polypoid, necrotic, and friable.

When the patient is still in the menstruating age, the significance of abundant curettings is much less, for such a finding is frequent with such conditions as benign hyperplasia and unsuspected incomplete abortion, to mention only the most important.

The polypoid tissue obtained in some cases of hyperplasia may easily mislead the inexperienced, but the distinction can often be made with reasonable certainty with the naked eye from the firmness of the polypoid growth, the smoothness of the covering mucosa, and the absence of the necrosis and friability which would ordinarily be found in an adenocarcinoma yielding a corresponding amount of tissue.

The Gravlee Jet Wash has been highly recommended by many observers, and we concur with their impressions that it seems to be a reliable method of detecting endometrial lesions. In the average good risk patient, however, we still prefer a complete dilatation and curettage. Not only does it seem more accurate, but it possesses the other advantage of an opportunity to allow examination under anesthesia. On such occasions even the most astute gynecologist may detect pathology, which is not noted in the office, particularly in an apprehensive, uncooperative patient.

Extension of Adenocarcinoma

This is the most favorable type of uterine cancer by virtue of its frequent

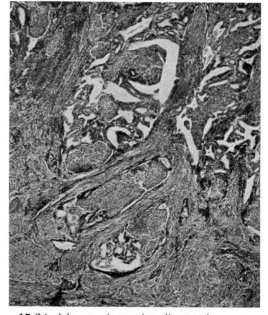

15.24. Adenocarcinoma invading uterine musculature.

tendency to remain confined to the surface. Myometrial extension may occur, and increased degrees impair the prognosis. Ovarian involvement by tubal or lymphatic extension is evident in 10% of our own cases. Vaginal, especially suburethral, tumor was frequent in the pre-irradiation days. A review by Boutselis, Ullery, and Bain confirms the relative infrequency of vaginal metastasis in irradiated patients, and Ingersoll has carried out a more recent study. The prognosis where the vagina is involved is poor, perhaps because this type of lesion is generally quite undifferentiated.

Gland Involvement

Different studies regarding gland involvement show considerable variation. Javert's 28% must be regarded as an extreme degree of nodal involvement. Some authors note a considerably lower figure, although if the cervix shows extension of endometrial cancer, nodal involvement is proportionately more frequent. Such patients are suggested as candidates for Wertheim hysterectomy despite medical complications, unless one believes (as we do) that the deep pelvic

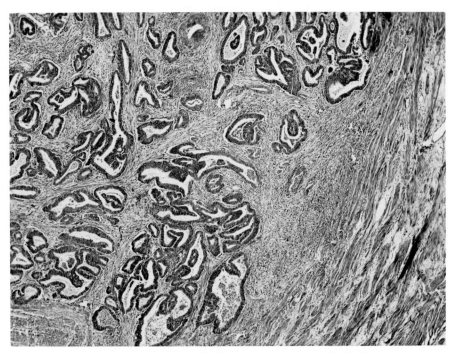

15.25. Adenocarcinoma with tubal extension (tubal wall at right).

nodes are responsive to external irradiation.

Much more logical is Beck and Latour's negative approach as to the value of pelvic lymphadenectomy. In studying 36 cases of endometrial cancer coming to autopsy they conclusively show that where there is deep myometrial invasion or pelvic lymph node involvement, there is a high (over 90%) association of extrapelvic metastasis. Thus, why increase morbidity by lymphadenectomy if it is of minimal value, as would appear to be the case in most series.

In advanced cases the peritoneum may be the seat of implantation. The cancerous disease may, especially in growths involving the lower part of the corpus, extend into the *cervix,* and metastasis or extension to the *vagina* may occur. Carcinoma involving the corpus and endocervix has a worse prognosis and is a distinct entity requiring special treatment such as irradiation to corpus and cervix (Thompson and Graham) or radical surgery. *Distant metastases* to such locations as the liver or lungs may likewise be noted

in the later stages, as may any form of extracorporeal extension.

In attempting evaluation of metastatic disease, one must be cognizant of Bailar's observations that almost 5% of women with endometrial cancer had another extrauterine malignancy. Breast cancer is much more frequent, and lower bowel lesions are disproportionately common.

Treatment

One of the most controversial points is the method by which endometrial cancer should usually be treated. All are agreed that a small proportion of women have such serious medical handicaps that they cannot tolerate major surgery, and irradiation therapy alone must be utilized. Most are likewise agreed that where the preliminary curettings are scant and of low grade activity, and the uterus is small and free, simple total hysterectomy and adnexectomy will probably suffice. However, the prognosis decreases where extrauterine extension or significant myometrial involvement has occurred, and these are factors which do not always become apparent until after laparotomy. Three main approaches to the treatment of corpus cancer are utilized which may be merely summarized as follows.

(1) Irradiation. There are very few American gynecologists who would prefer this as the sole means of therapy in the medically fit patient, although it has been the usual method of treatment in many areas. No one would deny that there is a certain salvage, in the nature of 33%, and in the poor risk woman or the one who for various reasons has a limited life expectancy, it deserves consideration, as it does in the treatment of vaginal recurrences. External irradiation plus some means of radium therapy, preferably by the Heyman multiple capsules, rather than a simple tandem, are employed. A vaginal source seems to be of value in minimizing recurrence in that area.

(2) Surgery. Few would question that the operation of total hysterectomy and adnexectomy is the most important part of the usual therapy of corpus cancer, a disease frequently characterized merely by surface extension, minor degrees of myometrial involvement, and rare nodal spread. The abdominal approach is routine, although Pratt, Symmonds, and Welch advocate a vaginal hysterectomy, which we utilize only in the occasional poor risk, obese patients. Certain excellent American gynecologists utilize surgery alone, and this is the usual form of therapy by many European gynecologists. Preliminary suture of the cervix is the rule in unirradiated patients to militate against manipulation leading to vaginal recurrence.

(3) Irradiation plus Surgery. Dispassionate observers seem uniform in agreeing that for all stages of fundal adenocarcinoma, a combined treatment gives the best results, while admitting that if there is still localized disease, irradiation is not necessary. Yet it is impossible to state dogmatically what the extent of the disease may be from prehysterectomy examination and evaluation of the curettings.

As to just why irradiation should be so effective, there is considerable speculation, for in many independent observations the removed uterus has evidenced a significant (over 50%) evidence of tumor. Histologically, the criteria for what is *viable* tumor are extremely tenuous, and one must conclude that, although irradiation may not obliterate all neoplasm, it creates an environment designed to make subsequent implantation and extension less likely.

However, it is difficult to argue with many well constructed statistics dealing with patients treated (1) by surgery alone and (2) by combined therapy, with a 15 per cent difference in favor of the latter method of treatment. Actually the results are even more impressive, for the more favorable patients are treated surgically, with irradiation an adjuvant only if the lesion is found to be more advanced.

The usual plan was to allow an interval of about six weeks between irradiation and surgery—enough time for the edema and vascularity to subside without permitting the tumor to spread. Decker has suggested earlier surgery with the logical argument that, once delivered, the irradiation effect will persist, and Johnson has utilized this "single admission" approach with equal salvage and no adverse effects. Although we have utilized this in only a few cases, with no major complications, the patients have occasionally had a markedly adhesive vaginitis (due to surgery plus irradiation effect) so that subsequent postoperative examinations were difficult. Above all, this short interval between irradiation and surgery might allow insufficient time for fibrosis and scarring of the lymphatics, and lead to dissemination of the tumor at the time of hysterectomy.

There would seem to be obvious difference of opinion as to the type and sequence of the combined irradiation-surgical approach. In past years our own policy was to utilize intracavitary radium and after a six week interim to perform surgery, but we have modified this approach. A recent study by Shah and Greene has reviewed the treatment of endometrial adenocarcinoma, and has come to the same conclusions as those by Graham and Frick *et al.* little matter whether the irradiation is administered pre- or postoperative so long as some form of irradiation is utilized. Vaginal vault recurrence is minimized if some source of *vaginal applicator* is utilized one to two weeks posthysterectomy, if there is early myometrial involvement.

Our current format is to proceed to surgery, after which the extent of the disease can then be assessed with certainty (as opposed to the preoperative radium era). If there is extensive myometrial invasion or vascular spread, postoperative cobalt it utilized along with 3–4000 rads from a vaginal source during the same hospital admission. Complications of this have been minimal, and we are anticipating a close to 75 per cent salvage with this routine. Regardless of the method of administration, it would seem apparent that irradiation improves the 5-year salvage in all cases of endometrial adenocarcinoma, although surgery alone seems adequate when there is a small, free uterus and hysterectomy reveals a well differentiated tumor confined to the endometrium without evidence of vascular spread. Frick *et al.* confirm this by finding no increased salvage in stage I cases, but better results and less vaginal recurrence with adjuvant radiotherapy in more advanced disease.

Hormone and Chemotherapy

That endometrial adenocarcinoma may be an estrogen dependent tumor seems probable, and since estrogen and progesterone sometimes seem synergistic, there have been an increasing number of studies advocating the use of *progesterone* in treating certain cases of endometrial neoplasm. Although the results are perhaps not as spectacular as those obtained with methotrexate therapy for trophoblastic lesions, they represent a valuable contribution in the increasingly successful attempts at treating cancer in a systemic fashion (Fig. 15.26).

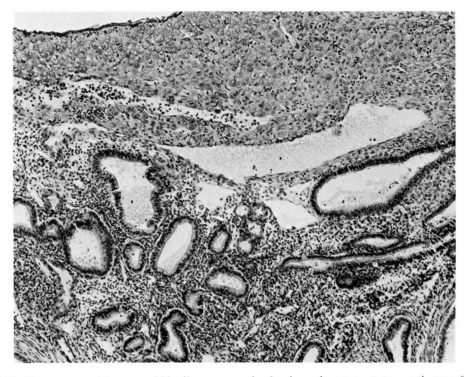

15.26. Uterus removed because of bleeding one month after large-dosage progesterone therapy for well differentiated adenocarcinoma. Marked decidual response above with remaining glands seemingly normal.

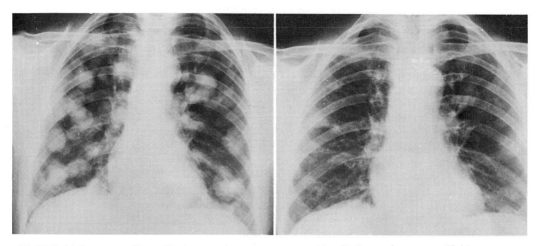

15.27 (*left*). Recurrent Stage II adenocarcinoma one year postirradiation and surgery with biopsy-proven metastasis. (*right*). X-ray eight months later after large dose progesterone. Patient now has complete six-year remission. (Courtesy of Dr. P. A. Nilsen, Oslo, Norway.)

Progesterone

(1) Therapy of Advanced and Recurrent Treated Tumor. Kelly and Baker, Kennedy, Mussey, and Varga'and Henricksen have been enthusiastic about prolonged remission (up to two years) in approximately one-third of the patients treated. Most responsive were those women who had prolonged symptoms before initial surgical and irradiation therapy and a sustained interval before recurrence; *i.e.,* a slow-growing tumor. Treatment consisted of no less than 750 mg. of intramuscular progesterone (Delalutin) per week, and patients have been maintained on such therapy in decreasing dosage more or less indefinitely. Our own limited experience would suggest that endocrine therapy is less effective in treating local recurrence than metastatic disease; we have had several satisfactory results in treating biopsy proven pulmonary recurrences as well as several disappointing results where there was pelvic disease (Fig. 15.27). Oral progesterone (megestrol acetate) is available and Wait advocates 40 mg. daily for at least two months; we prefer indefinite small dose therapy.

Estrogen Receptors

Various reports by Jensen and others have indicated that end organ targets of estrogen contain certain protein macromolecules that bind estradiol; *i.e., estrogen receptors.* These can be detected and measured by various radiological techniques, as noted by Rubin *et al.,* and seemingly indicate which tumors of the endometrium and breast are hormone dependent. Thus it might be possible to predict which uterine cancer might respond to progesterone therapy or if mastectomy has been carried out for breast cancer, the possibility of adjuvant oophorectomy and/or adrenalectomy might be considered.

Specific estradiol binding has been noted in many cases of endometrial cancer, and such tumors might respond to hormones more favorably than those with a predominence of estrone. Gusberg notes that there is less estriol as compared to estrone in conjunction with endometrial carcinoma, and speculates that estriol might evert a protective action against the advent of the malignant disease. Apparently the precursory hormone is $\Delta 4$-androstenedione which is converted primarily to estrone. It should be noted that this work on estrogen receptors is in its infancy but seems eminently promising.

While it would seem that a majority of cases of endometrial cancer is estrogen dependent (or induced), in some instances some other cause must be considered. On occasion vaginal or endometrial atrophy with a low urinary estrogen is observed.

(2) Treatment of Markedly Adenomatous Hyperplasia. Kistner and Wall *et al.* have been successful in causing disappearance of a markedly atypical endometrial pattern and possibly adenocarcinoma after large dosage of progesterone for many months. Curettage after prolonged progesterone therapy generally reveals almost total absence of the glands ("glandular exhaustion") and a marked decidual reaction of the stroma (Fig. 15.26). At this writing it is impossible to say dogmatically as to how long treatment should be continued and what should be expected following cessation of the progesterone. Prolonged large dosage progesterone is an expensive method of therapy, and it would seem to us that there is a very limited sphere of practical application. In the younger patient, clomiphene appears to be a more precise method of treatment; in the older parous individual, hysterectomy is more definitive where there is real doubt as to whether the endometrium is benign or malignant. Perhaps the medically unfit patient who is postmenopausal is a likely candidate for progesterone therapy if the endometrial pattern is equivocal.

Salvage

There is nothing more difficult than assessing the salvage of adenocarcinoma as reported by different clinics using different and often varied methods of treatment. One great drawback is the fact that some clinics report and treat as early adenocarcinoma many cases of what we believe to be merely benign proliferative hyperplasia, and the reader must be mindful of this possibility in evaluating statistics.

Where only the endometrium is involved, surgery alone or in conjunction with irradiation should afford close to 100% salvage. Where the superficial myometrium is involved, the salvage begins to decrease in proportion to the degree of myometrial involvement, but even where this is widespread, salvage should be upwards of 50%. Where extrau-

terine extension or metastasis occurs, salvage becomes markedly decreased (10% or less). A recent report by Gusberg and his associates summarizes most studies. Among 1383 women treated by hysterectomy alone, the cure rate was 64%; where preoperative radium was utilized in 1146 patients, the figure was over 76%. Such statistics on large series make it difficult to belittle the importance of irradiation. Obviously endometrial cancer is a more favorable disease than the cervical variety, although Miller believes that we are overly enthusiastic in assessing results.

REFERENCES

Anderson, D. G.: Management of advanced endometrial carcinoma with methoxy progesterone acetate (Provera). Amer. J. Obstet. Gynec., *92:* 87, 1963.

Andrews, W. C.: Estrogen and endometrial carcinoma. Obstet. Gynec. Survey, *16:* 747, 1961.

Annual Report on the Results of Treatment in Carcinoma of the Uterus, Vol. 15. Stockholm, 1973.

Arneson, A. N.: Longterm follow-up observations in corporeal cancer. Amer. J. Roentgen., *91:* 3, 1964.

Arrata, W. S., and Zarou, G. S.: Postmenopausal hematometra. Amer. J. Obstet. Gynec., *85:* 959, 1963.

Badib, A. C., *et al.*: Biologic behavior of adenoacanthoma of the endometrium. Amer. J. Obstet. Gynec., *106:* 205, 1970.

Bailar, J. C.: Miltiple tumors with uterine cancer. Cancer, *16:* 842, 1963.

Bamford, D. S., and Wagman, H.: Radium menopause: long term follow-up. J. Obstet. Gynaec. Brit. Commonw., *79:* 82, 1972.

Barber, K. W., Jr., Dockerty, M. B., and Pratt, J. H.: A clinicopathologic study of surgically treated carcinoma of the endometrium with nodal metastases. Surg. Gynec. Obstet., *115:* 568, 1962.

Beck, R. P., Latour, J. P. A., and Bourne, H. B.: Treatment of endometrial carcinoma reassessed. Amer. J. Obstet. Gynec., *88:* 178, 1964.

Bengsjo, P., and Wilson, P. A.: Carcinoma of the endometrium. Amer. J. Obstet. Gynec., *95:* 496, 1966.

Bettinger, H. F.: Hyperplasia and carcinoma of the endometrium. Amer. J. Obstet. Gynec., *109:* 194, 1971.

Beutler, H. K., Dockerty, M. B., and Randall, L. M.: Precancerous lesions of the endometrium. Amer. J. Obstet. Gynec., *86:* 433, 1963.

Boronow, R. C.: A fresh look at corpus cancer. Obstet. Gynec., *42:* 448, 1973.

Bouteselis, J. G., Ullery, J. C., and Bain, J.: Vaginal metastases following treatment of endometrial carcinoma. Obstet. Gynec., *21:* 622, 1963.

Chanen, W.: A clinical and pathological study of adenoacanthoma of the uterine body. J. Obstet. Gynaec. Brit. Comm., *67:* 287, 1960.

Charles, D.: Endometrial adenoacanthoma. Cancer, *18:* 737, 1965.

Charles, D., Bell, E. T., Loraine, J. A., and Harkness, R. A.: Endometrial cancer—endocrinological and clinical studies. Amer. J. Obstet. Gynec., *91:* 1050, 1965.

Cianfrani, T.: Endometrial cancer after bilateral oophorectomy. Amer. J. Obstet. Gynec., *69:* 64, 1955.

Cutler, B. S. *et al.*: Endometrial carcinoma after stilbestrol therapy in gonadal dysgenesis. New Eng. J. Med., *287:* 628, 1972.

Dockerty, M. B., Lovelady, S., and Foust, G. T., Jr.: Carcinoma of corpus uteri in young women. Amer. J. Obstet. Gynec., *61:* 966, 1951.

Doran, T. A., and Thompson, D. W.: Malignant cells in the peripheral blood of patients with endometrial cancer. Amer. J. Obstet. Gynec., *94:* 985, 1966.

Dunn, L. J., Merchant, J. A., Bradbury, J. T., and Stone, D. B.: Glucose findings in carcinoma of endometrium. Arch. Intern. Med., *121:* 246, 1968.

Emge, L. A.: The estrogen-cancer hypothesis in reference to protracted estrogen substitution. Obstet. Gynec., *20:* 915, 1962.

Frick, H. C., et al.: Carcinoma of the endometrium. Amer. J. Obstet. Gynec., *115:* 663, 1973.

Gore, H., and Hertig, A. T.: Carcinoma in situ of the endometrium. Amer. J. Obstet. Gynec., *94:* 134, 1966.

Graham, J.: Endometrial adenocarcinoma: Value of preoperative or postoperative treatment. Obstet. Gynec., *35:* 513, 1970.

Gravlee, L. C., Jr.: Jet irrigation for diagnosis of endometrial adenocarcinoma. Obstet. Gynec., *45:* 168, 1969.

Gray, L. A., and Barnes, M. L.: Histogenesis of endometrial cancer. Ann. Surg., *159:* 976, 1964.

Gray, P. H., Anderson, C. T., Jr., and Munnell, E. W.: Endometrial adenocarcinoma and ovarian genesis. Obstet. Gynec., *315:* 513, 1971.

Greene, J. W.: Feminizing mesenchymomas and endometrial carcinoma. Amer. J. Obstet. Gynec., *74:* 31, 1957.

Geisler, H. E., Huber, C. P., and Rogers, S.: Carcinoma of endometrium in premenopausal women. Amer. J. Obstet. Gynec., *104:* 657, 1969.

Gusberg, S. B.: The problem of staging endometrial cancer. Obstet. Gynec., *28:* 305, 1966.

Gusberg, S. B.: Dysfunctional and neoplastic: clinical investigation in endometrial carcinoma. Amer. J. Obstet. Gynec., *116:* 175, 1973.

Gusberg, S. B., and Hall, R. E.: Precursors of corpus cancer. IV. Adenomatous hyperplasia as stage O carcinoma of the endometrium. Amer. J. Obstet. Gynec., *87:* 662, 1963.

Gusberg, S. B., and Yannopoulos, D.: Therapeutic decisions in corpus cancer. Amer. J. Obstet. Gynec., *88:* 157, 1963.

Harris, H. R.: Foam cells in the stroma of carcinoma of the body of the uterus. J. Clin. Path., *11:* 19, 1958.

Hausknecht, R. V., and Gusberg, S. B.: Estrogen metabolism in endometrial carcinoma. Amer. J. Obstet. Gynec., *116:* 981, 1973.

Hertig, A. T., and Sommers, S. C.: Genesis of endometrial carcinoma. I. Study of prior biopsies. Cancer, *2:* 946, 1949.

Hoffmeister, F. J., and Vondrak, B. F.: Endometrial cancer after castration. Amer. J. Obstet. Gynec., *107:* 1099, 1970.

Ingersoll, F. M.: Vaginal recurrence of corpus cancer. Amer. J. Surg., *121:* 473, 1971.

Jackson, R. L., and Dockerty, M. B.: Stein-Leventhal syndrome and endometrial cancer. Amer. J. Obstet. Gynec., *73:* 161, 1957.

Jensen et al: *Steroid Dynamics.* Academic Press, New York, 1966.

Johnson, F. L.: Adenocarcinoma of the endometrium. Obstet. Gynec., *27:* 622, 1966.

Jones, W. E., et al.: Adenocarcinoma of the endometrium. Amer. J. Obstet. Gynec., *113:* 549, 1972.

Karlen, J. R., Sternberg, L. B., and Abbott, J. N.: Carcinoma of the endometrium coexisting with pregnancy. Obstet. Gynec., *40:* 334, 1972.

Katayama, K. P., and Jones, H. W.: Chromosomes of

atypical hyperplasia and carcinoma of the endometrium. Amer. J. Obstet. Gynec., *97:* 978, 1967.

Kaufman, R. H., Abbott, J. P., and Wall, J. A.: The endometrium before and after wedge resection of the ovaries in the Stein-Leventhal syndrome. Amer. J. Obstet. Gynec. *77:* 1271, 1959.

Kistner, R. W.: The effects of progestational agents on hyperplasia and carcinoma in situ of the endometrium. Int. J. Gynec. Obstet., *8:* 561, 1970.

Kistner, R. W., Gore, H., and Hertig, A. T.: Carcinoma of endometrium; a preventable disease. Amer. J. Obstet. Gynec., *95:* 1011, 1966.

Kottmeier, H. L.: Carcinoma of the corpus uteri; diagnosis and therapy. Amer. J. Obstet. Gynec., *78:* 1127, 1959.

Malkasian, G. D., Jr., et al.: Progesterone treatment of recurrent endometrial carcinoma. Amer. J. Obstet. Gynec., *110:* 15, 1971.

Marcus, C. C.: Ovarian cortical stromal hyperplasia and carcinoma of the endometrium. Obstet. Gynec., *21:* 175, 1963.

McBride, J. M.: Premenopausal cystic hyperplasia and endometrial hyperplasia. J. Obstet. Gynaec. Brit. Comm., *66:* 288, 1959.

McGarrity, K. A., and Scott, G. C.: A review of cancer of the corpus uteri in New South Wales. J. Obstet. Gynaec. Brit. Comm., *75:* 14, 1968.

Meissner, W. A., Sommers, S. C., and Sherman, G.: Endometrial hyperplasia, endometrial carcinoma and endometriosis produced experimentally by estrogen. Cancer, *10:* 500, 1957.

Montgomery, J. B., Land, W. R., Farrell, D. M., and Hahn, G. A.: End results in adenocarcinoma of the endometrium managed by preoperative irradiation. Amer. J. Obstet. Gynec., *80:* 972, 1960.

Morrison, D. L.: Adenoacanthoma of the uterine body. J. Obstet. Gynec. Brit. Comm., *73:* 605, 1966.

Morrow, C. P., DiSaia, P. J., and Townsend, D. E.: Current management of endometrial carcinoma. Obstet. Gynec., *42:* 399, 1973.

Mussey, E., and Malkasian, G. D.: Progesterone treatment of recurrent carcinoma of the endometrium. Amer. J. Obstet. Gynec., *94:* 786, 1966.

Ng, A. B. P., and Reagan, J. W.: Incidence and prognosis of endometrial carcinoma by histological grade and extent. Obstet. Gynec., *35:* 437, 1970.

Nilsen, P. A.: Hormonal treatment of recurrent endometrial carcinoma. J. Obstet. Gynaec. Brit. Comm., *75:* 99, 1968.

Nolan, J. F., Donough, M. E., and Anson, J. H.: The value of preoperative radiation therapy in Stage I of the uterine corpus. Amer. J. Obstet. Gynec., *98:* 663, 1967.

Novak, E. R.: Postmenopausal endometrial hyperplasia. Amer. J. Obstet. Gynec., *71:* 1312, 1956.

Novak, E. R., and Mohler, D. I.: Ovarian stromal changes in endometrial cancer. Amer. J. Obstet. Gynec., *65:* 1099, 1953.

Novak, E. R., and Nalley, W. B.: Uterine adenoacanthoma. Obstet. Gynec., *10:* 396, 1957.

Novak, E. R., and Villa Santa, U.: Factors influencing the ratio of uterine cancer. J. A. M. A., *174:* 1395, 1960.

Novak, E. R., and Woodruff, J. D.: Postirradiation malignancy. Amer. J. Obstet. Gynec., *77:* 667, 1959.

Novak, E. R., Goldberg, B., Jones, G. S., O'Toole, R. V.: Enzyme histochemistry of the menopausal ovary associated with normal and abnormal endometrium. Amer. J. Obstet. Gynec., *93:* 669, 1965.

Novak, E., and Yui, E.: Relation of endometrial hyperplasia to adenocarcinoma of the uterus. Amer. J. Obstet. Gynec., *32:* 674, 1936.

O'Neill R. T.: Pregnancy following hormonal therapy for adenocarcinoma of the endometrium. Amer. J. Obstet. Gynec., *108:* 318, 1970.

Porter, J. E.: Cancer of corpus uteri in premenopausal siblings. Obstet. Gynec., 28: 675, 1966.

Pratt, J. H., Symmonds, R. E., and Welch, J. S.: Vaginal hysterectomy for carcinoma of the fundus. Amer. J. Obstet. Gynec., 88: 1063, 1964.

Price, J. J., Hahn, G. A., and Donough, M. E.: Vaginal involvement in endometrial carcinoma. Amer. J. Obstet. Gynec., 91: 1060, 1965.

Reid, D. E., and Shirley, R. L.: Endometrial adenocarcinoma associated with Sheehan's syndrome and stilbestrol therapy. Amer. J. Obstet. Gynec., 119: 264, 1974.

Renning, E. L., and Javert, C. T.: Analysis of a series of cases of carcinoma of the endometrium treated by radium and operation. Amer. J. Obstet. Gynec., 88: 171, 1964.

Ritchie, D. E.: The vaginal maturation index and endometrial carcinoma. Amer. J. Obstet. Gynec., 91: 578, 1965.

Roddick, J. W., and Greene, R. R.: Ovarian stromal hyperplasia and endometrial cancer. Amer. J. Obstet. Gynec., 75: 1015, 1958.

Rubin, B. L.: Estrogen dependence of endometrial carcinoma. Amer. J. Obstet. Gynec., 114: 660, 1972.

Rutledge, F. N., Tan, S. K., and Fletcher, G. H.: Vaginal metastases from adenocarcinoma of corpus uteri. Amer. J. Obstet. Gynec., 75: 167, 1958.

Sall, S., and Calanog, A.: Steroid excretion in the postmenopause. Amer. J. Obstet. Gynec., 114: 153, 1972.

Sall, S., Sonnenblick, B., and Stone, N. L.: Factors affecting survival with endometrial carcinoma. Amer. J. Obstet. Gynec., 107: 116, 1970.

Salm, R.: Mucin production of normal and abnormal endometrium. Arch. Path., 73: 42, 1962.

Schmitz, H. E., Smith, C. J., and Fetherston, W. C.: The effect of preoperative irradiation on adenocarcinoma of the uterus. Amer. J. Obstet. Gynec., 78: 1048, 1959.

Schwartz, A. E., and Brunschwig, A.: Radical panhysterectomy and pelvic node excision for carcinoma of corpus uteri. Surg. Gynec. Obstet., 105: 675, 1957.

Shah, C. A., and Greene, T. J. Jr.: Evaluation of current management of endometrial carcinoma. Obstet. Gynec., 39: 500, 1972.

Shaw, W., and Dasteur, B.: Association of certain ovarian cells with endometrial cancer. Brit. Med. J., 2: 113, 1949.

Sherman, A. I.: Progesterone caproate in treatment of endometrial cancer. Obstet. Gynec., 28: 309, 1966.

Sherman, A. I., and Woolf, R. B.: Endocrine basis for endometrial carcinoma. Amer. J. Obstet. Gynec., 77: 233, 1959.

Silverberg, S. G., Bolin, M. G., and De Giorgi, L. S.: Adenoacanthoma and mixed adenosquamous carcinoma of the endometrium. Cancer, 30: 1307, 1972.

Smith, J. P., Rutledge, F., and Soffan, S. W.: Progestins in the treatment of endometrial adenocarcinoma. Amer. J. Obstet. Gynec., 94: 977, 1966.

Speert, H.: Corpus cancer; clinical, pathological, and etiological aspects. Cancer, 1: 584, 1948.

Stallworthy, J. A.: Surgery of endometrial cancer in the Bonney tradition. Ann. Roy. Coll. Surg. Engl., 48: 293, 1971.

Stander, R. W.: Irradiation castration. Obstet. Gynec., 10: 223, 1957.

Stanley, M. A., and Kirkland, J. A.: Cytogenetic studies of endometrial carcinoma. Amer. J. Obstet. Gynec., 102: 1070, 1968.

Steiner, G. J., Kistner, R. W., and Craig, J. M.: Histological effects of progestins on hyperplasia and carcinoma in situ of the endometrium. Metabolism, 14: 356, 1965.

Taki, I., Lyima, M., Doi, T., Vetsuki, Y., and Mori, M.: Histochemistry of hydrolytic and oxidative enzymes in human and experimentally induced adenocarcinoma of the endometrium. Amer. J. Obstet. Gynec., 94: 36, 1966.

Tatra, G., Jahoda, E., and Feigl, W.: Endometrial carcinoma. Gynaek., 94: 1351, 1972.

Thompson, N. J., and Graham, J. B.: Carcinoma of corpus and endocervix. Obstet. Gynec., 24: 144, 1964.

Tweeddale, D. M., Early, L. S., and Goodsitt, E. S.: Endometrial adenoacanthoma. Obstet. Gynec., 23: 611, 1964.

Varga, A., and Henricksen, E.: Urinary excretion assays of pituitary luteinizing hormone (LH) related to endometrial cancer. Obstet. Gynec., 22: 129, 1963.

Villa Santa, U.: Tumors of mesonephric origin in the female genital tract. Amer. J. Obstet. Gynec., 89: 680, 1964.

Wade, M. E., Kohorn, E. I., and Morris J. McL.: Adenocarcinoma of the endometrium. Amer. J. Obstet. Gynec., 99: 869, 1967.

Wahhas, W. A., Lund, C. J., and Rudolph, J. H.: Carcinoma of the corpus uteri. Obstet. Gynec., 37: 564, 1971.

Wait, R. B.: Megestrol acetate in advanced endometrial cancer. Obstet. Gynec., 41: 129, 1973.

Wall, J. A., Franklin, R. R., and Kaufman, R. H.: Reversal of benign and malignant endometrial changes with clomiphene. Amer. J. Obstet. Gynec., 88: 1072, 1964.

Wall, J. A., Franklin, R. R., Kaufman, R. H., and Kaplan, R. H.: The effects of clomiphene citrate on the endometrium. Amer. J. Obstet. Gynec., 93: 842, 1965.

White, A. J., Buchsbaum, H. S., and Macasset, M. A.: Primary squamous cell carcinoma of the endometrium. Obstet. Gynec., 41: 912, 1973.

Wilkinson, E. J., et al.: Turner's syndrome with endometrial carcinoma and stilbestrol therapy. Obstet. Gynec., 42: 193, 1973.

Wilson, R. A.: The roles of estrogen and progesterone in breast and genital cancer. J. A. M. A., 182: 101, 1962.

Woll, E., Hertig, A. T., Smith, G. V. and Johnson, L. C.: Ovary in endometrial carcinoma. Amer. J. Obstet. Gynec., 56: 617, 1948.

chapter 16

Myoma of the Uterus

General Characteristics

By far the most common tumor of the uterus is the myoma. It is estimated that fully 20 per cent of all women over 35 years of age harbor uterine *myomas*, although frequently without symptoms. For unknown reasons the incidence of myoma is much higher in the black than the white race, especially between the ages of 30 and 45, although Barber and Graber note a case in an 11-year-old female. New tumors rarely develop after the menopause, and already existing growths diminish in size, although they do not always disappear. Postmenopausal increase in size is almost always indicative of secondary degeneration, and should lead to the suspicion of sarcomatous change.

Myomas are frequently spoken of as *fibroids*, but are of muscle cell origin and not derived from fibrous tissue elements. The term *fibroid* is now so thoroughly entrenched in popular use that it would be difficult to dislodge, and the terms are used more or less interchangeably. Myomas of the uterus may be single or, more frequently, multiple. They may be of microscopic size, or of mammoth proportions, weighing over 100 pounds (Fig. 16.1). They are of dense structure, well

encapsulated, and form small or large nodules which can be peeled out from the surrounding muscular wall of the uterus. On cutting into such a tumor its surface is seen to be of a glistening white color, with a characteristic whorl-like trabeculation (Fig. 16.2), so that is stands out in sharp contrast to the surrounding muscularis.

Location

The location of the tumors may be *cervical* or *corporeal*, the former being much less common. When they reach very large size they impinge on the bladder and may bring about urinary retention through blockage of the urethra. Such large cervical tumors not infrequently become impacted in the pelvic cavity, and the technical difficulty in their removal is apt to be much greater than with the more movable tumors of the corpus uteri.

Types

From the standpoint of their position as regards the various layers of the uterine wall, myomas are divisible into three groups (Fig. 16.2).

Submucous tumors (Figs. 16.3–16.6), developing just beneath the endometrium, push the latter before them as they grow.

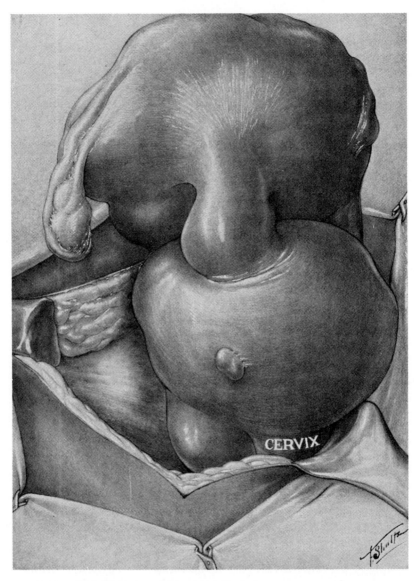

16.1. Bizarre cervical myoma displacing corpus upward

They constitute about 5% of all myomas, but are much more likely than either of the other varieties to cause profuse bleeding and require hysterectomy, even though small. Their presence can usually be detected by feeling the curette "bump" over the protruding surface, although they are generally too firmly embedded to be removed by the curette. The hazard of sarcomatous degeneration is likewise greater with this group. The covering mucous membrane becomes thin, atrophic, and ulcerated.

Although some submucous tumors, even of large size, are sessile (Fig. 16.3), others become pedunculated as a result of the expulsive action of the uterine muscle and may protrude from the cervix (Fig. 16.4) or even from the vagina. The surface of these *pedunculated submucous* tumors frequently becomes ulcerated, infected, and even infarcted.

Interstitial or *intramural* myomas are situated in the muscular wall, with no close propinquity to either the mucosa or serosa. When large or multiple, they cause

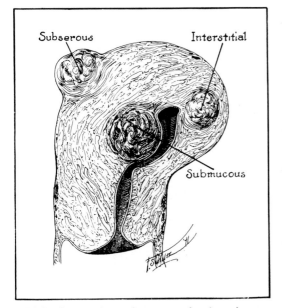

16.2. Cut surface of myoma showing characteristic whorl-like appearance.

Often subserous tumors grow out between the folds of the broad ligament (*intraligamentary*) even impinging on the ureter and iliac vessels, and sometimes giving rise to difficult problems in diagnosis and operative treatment.

In some such cases the tumor receives more and more blood supply from the omental vessels and less and less from the uterine vessels. Gradually the tumor may be weaned away from the uterus entirely, the pedicle becoming thinner and thinner and finally disappearing. Such *parasitic* myomas are rare, but may present interesting diagnostic problems.

Microscopic Structure

The characteristic histological picture of myoma is that of spindle muscle cells arranged in an interlacing or whorl-like pattern (Fig. 16.7). The cells are uniform in size, if one makes allowance for the different angles at which they are cut, and there is a variable amount of connective tissue. There is no definite capsule about the myomatous elements, but they are usually sharply marked off from the surrounding uterine musculature by a pseudocapsule of light areolar tissue. "Mast cells," presumably containing heparin, are often present in the myometrium and should not be interpreted as neoplastic or giant cells (Fox and Abel).

marked uterine enlargement and a nodular contour and consistency.

Subserous or *subperitoneal* tumors, like the submucous, may be sessile pedunculated. On occasion large veins overlying the surface of the fibroid may rupture with massive intraperitoneal bleeding; Saidi has tabulated 26 cases, a few of which have occurred during pregnancy.

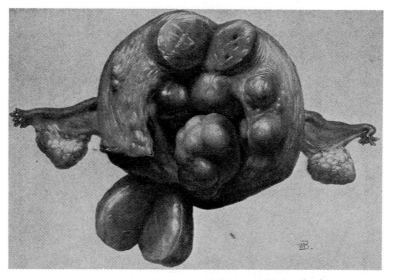

16.3. Gross appearance of myoma, chiefly interstitial and submucous

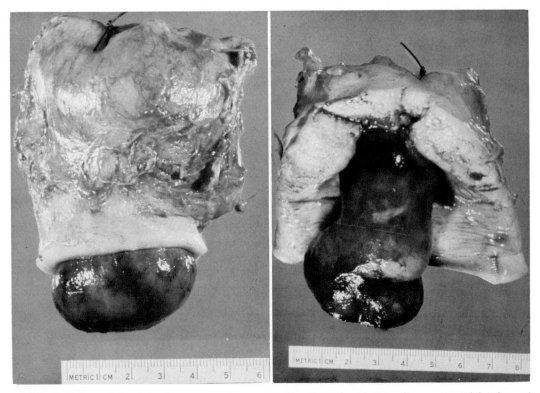

16.4. (*left*) Large infarcted submucous myoma protruding through and distending cervix. (*right*) Opened uterus. Thick sessile base would have made vaginal removal difficult.

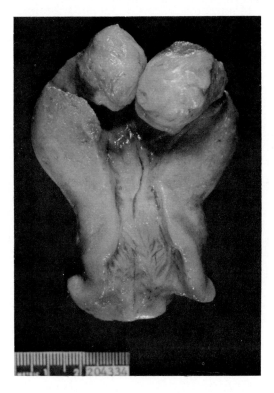

Intravenous Leiomyomatosis

One may rarely find *intravenous* extension of benign myomatous tumor into the pelvic veins. In discussing this infrequent occurrence, Harper and Scully note the difficulty in distinguishing this from certain malignant processes as (endometrial) sarcoma or stromatosis, but indicate a favorable prognosis. Boyce and Buddhev, Ariel and Trinidad, and Edwards *et al.* describe benign but metastasizing myoma and review the literature; it would seem difficult to exclude the possibility of sarcoma in some area of the tumors despite the extensive studies by the authors to establish this fact. Taubert *et al.* describe *leiomyomatosis peritonealis disseminata, i.e.,* histologically benign myomatous implants in the omentum and peritoneum. Two of their three patients were pregnant, and this might suggest an endocrine stimulus (as in Lipschütz's animal experiments).

16.5. Solitary submucous myoma

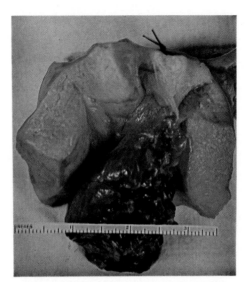

Plate 16.1. Sloughing submucous myoma

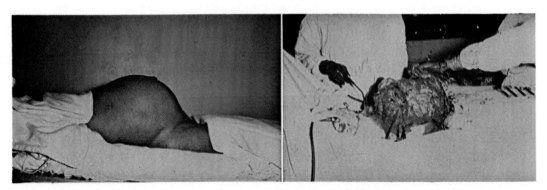

Plate 16.2. *Left*, gross distortion of abdomen in 110-pound patient by otherwise asymptomatic myoma. *Right*, part of 30-pound tumor as viewed at operation, some being deep in pelvis.

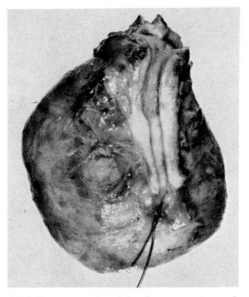

16.6. Large myoma arising from posterior surface of cervix (end of probe at cervix).

All of the patients remained well postoperative, further proof of the benign nature of this process.

Secondary Changes in Myoma

(1) **Hyaline Degeneration.** This, the most common of all secondary changes, is seen to some degree in almost all myomas, except those of very tiny size. The hyaline change may involve broad areas of the tumor, or it may occur in long intercommunicating strands and columns which appear to tease apart the muscle bundles (Figs. 16.8–16.10). Whether the so-called "plexiform tumorlet" as noted by Larbig et al., Buddinger and Greene, and most recently Patchevsky, is a tumor of stromal origin or a form of hyaline degeneration seems uncertain.

(2) **Cystic Degeneration** (Fig. 16.11). The tendency of hyaline degeneration is toward liquefaction, and in extreme cases practically all of the original tumor is thus involved, being converted into a large cystic cavity. The clinical impression may thus simulate pregnancy or an ovarian cyst. Extreme edema and engorgement of the lymphatics may occur and simulate a lymphangiomatous pattern.

(3) **Calcification.** This is especially likely to occur where there is some circulatory disturbance, as in the myomas of old women. Where extreme, the myoma may be converted into a hard, stony mass, the "wombstone" of the older writers. Preoperative flat plate may reveal

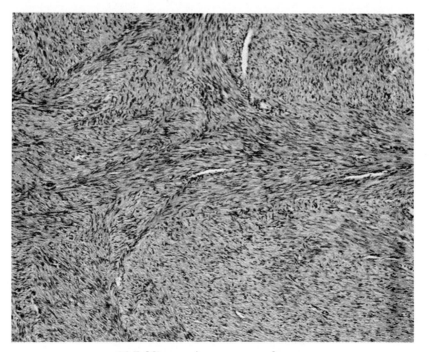

16.7. Microscopic appearance of myoma

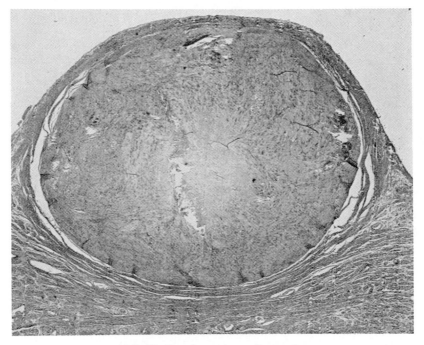

16.8. Hyaline change in small myoma

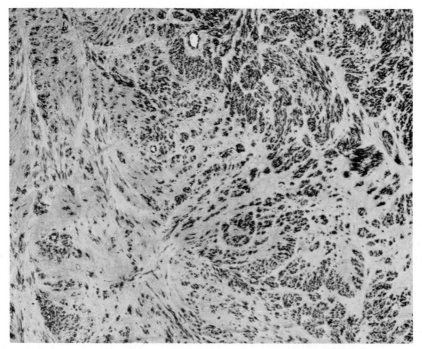

16.9. Hyaline degeneration of myoma (microscopic)

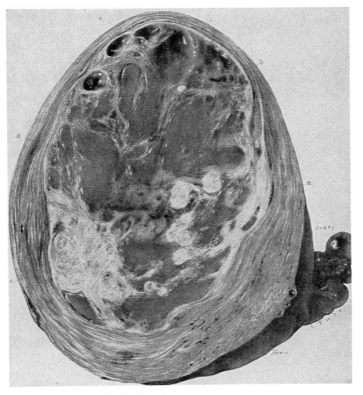

16.10. Hyaline degeneration of myoma

multiple foci of calcium deposits (Fig. 16.12).

(4) Infection and Suppuration. This is most common in the submucous variety of myoma, which is so prone to thinning and ulceration of the overlying mucosa, thus giving access to organisms from the uterine canal.

(5) Necrosis (Fig. 16.13). This is commonly due to impairment of the blood

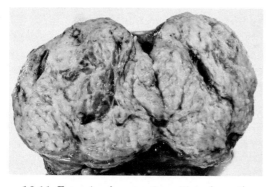

16.11. Extensive degeneration with early cystic changes

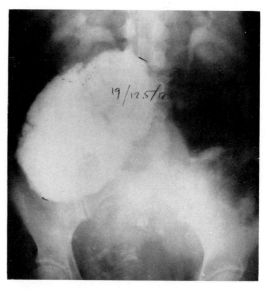

16.12. Large calcified myomatous tumor as visualized by intravenous pyelogram.

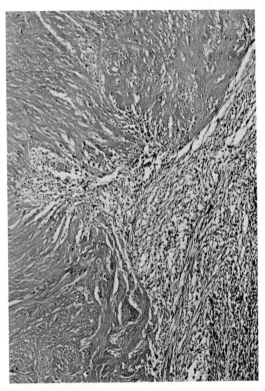

16.13. Margin of myoma undergoing necrosis.

supply or to severe infection. Pedunculated tumors may become necrotic through torsion of the pedicle. An interesting form of necrosis is the so-called *carneous* or *red degeneration*, seen most often but not always in association with pregnancy. Its cause is not definitely known, although many believe it to be explained by an aseptic degeneration associated with hemolysis or a local tissue ischemia.

(6) Fatty Degeneration. This is rare, but may occur with advanced hyaline degeneration. In other cases, large areas of genuine fat in the substance of a myoma are probably due to the fact that the tumor is of mixed variety.

(7) Sarcomatous Degeneration. This important type of change is discussed in Chapter 18, "Sarcoma of the Uterus," but is so rare, as not to influence the usual management of myomata. Even less common is metastasis to a myoma by a distant malignancy noted by Banooni.

Etiology and Histogenesis

Nothing definite is known as to the etiology of uterine myomas, although it is established that they are of muscle histogenesis. Most investigators accept Meyer's view that the source is not from mature muscle elements, but from immature cells.

Evidence for a possible role of the *ovarian hormones* in the causation of uterine myoma is far from convincing. No explanation has been suggested as to why they occur in some women and not in others, since estrogen is produced in practically all women. Furthermore, a good many women with myomas ovulate, producing progesterone, supposedly more or less antiestrogenic and antitumorigenic. Therefor, replacement therapy by estrogen in the postmenopausal individual with known myomata should warrant due consideration.

The experimental production of fibroid tumors has been reported by a number of observers but, with one or two exceptions, these artificially produced tumors do not resemble the common form of uterine myoma either histologically or in their topographical distribution. Especially provocative has been the work of Lipschütz, who utilized estrogens to produce fibromatous tumors in guinea pigs, not only on the surface of the uterus but also in various extragenital locations throughout the abdomen. This fibromatogenic effect of estrogen could be prevented by the simultaneous administration of progesterone or testosterone propionate.

Symptoms and Physical Signs

The presence of myoma does not necessarily produce any symptoms, and every practitioner knows that even large growths may be entirely symptomless.

Palpable Mass. In a considerable proportion of cases the patient is impelled to seek advice because she or her physician has noticed a lump in the lower abdomen or, in the case of large tumors, a general enlargement of the abdomen.

Bleeding. The main symptom, not always present, characteristic of fibroids is excessive or prolonged menstruation. One must always be on the alert for an associated lesion, such as adenocarcinoma, polyp, or a functional factor, for *hyperplasia* is frequently associated with myomata.

The myoma most likely to cause bleeding is the submucous as a result of ruptured venules in the endometrium. Farrer-Brown *et al.* likewise feel that venous stasis with mechanical obstruction due to the tumor mass may produce bleeding. Interstital growths may produce menstrual excess, the mechanism in such cases being an interference with uterine contractility. Subserous growths do not generally produce abnormal hemorrhage.

Pain. Pain is not a characteristic symptom of myoma, although it is often present. Concomitant pelvic inflammatory disease or endometriosis, as well as various genitourinary or gastrointestinal causes of pain must be considered (Fig. 16.14). The most frequent form seen with the larger tumors is a *sensation of weight* and *bearing-down* or *dysmenorrhea.*

The development of pain and tenderness in large, previously painless myomas is generally due to circulatory disturbances, with perhaps local necrosis, or to inflammatory change, with adhesions to structures such as the omentum or intestine. In the rare cases in which pedunculated subserous myomas undergo torsion of the pedicle, the pain may be acute, and accompanied by nausea and vomiting. Finally, in very large growths, or in those firmly impacted in the pelvis, pain may be the result of pressure upon nerve trunks, with radiation to the back and lower extremities.

Pressure Effects. The larger myomas impinge on the bladder, producing *irritability, increased frequency of urination*, and possibly *dysuria*. When impacted in the pelvis they may bring about *retention of urine* through blockage of the urethra. *Hydroureteronephrosis* may ensue, along with a real possibility of damage to the urinary tract at operation. The pressure effects upon the rectum are less conspicuous, although *constipation* and occasionally *pain on defecation* may

be produced. Very large growths into the upper abdomen may produce *digestive disturbances*, and in extreme cases pressure upon the vena cava or iliac veins may even cause *edema* of the lower extremities.

Secondary Symptoms

Anemia with *weakness, lassitude, headache,* and *shortness of breath* may occur. There was formerly much discussion of the so-called *"fibroid heart,"* referring to a form of myocardial degeneration supposedly characteristically associated with uterine myoma. It is now generally agreed that no such specific cardiac condition exists. A few cases of erythrocytosis have been attributed to myomata which are generally large (Rothman and Rennard; Spurlin *et al.*).

Myoma and Pregnancy

There is a considerable difference of opinion as to the role of myoma in the production of infertility. No one would doubt that even very large myomata are perfectly compatible with uncomplicated pregnancy and normal delivery. On the other hand, most students, such as the late Isadore Rubin, feel strongly that fibroids may on occasion be a factor in impairing fertility, and consequently mandate myomectomy, *after other causes for sterility are excluded.*

The incidence of pregnancy following myomectomy is 25 to 40%, far higher than nonoperated sterile women might achieve, even after prolonged marital relationships. The size, number, and location of fibroids in relation to the cornua and endometrial cavities are obvious variables so that no guarantee can be given to any woman in whom myomectomy is contemplated. Rubin suggests that it be considered "an alternative to hysterectomy in order to improve the chances of parenthood," and a more recent review by Ingersoll summarizes the indications for and results with myomectomy.

A patient should never be promised myomectomy before operation; the surgeon may find it desirable or even

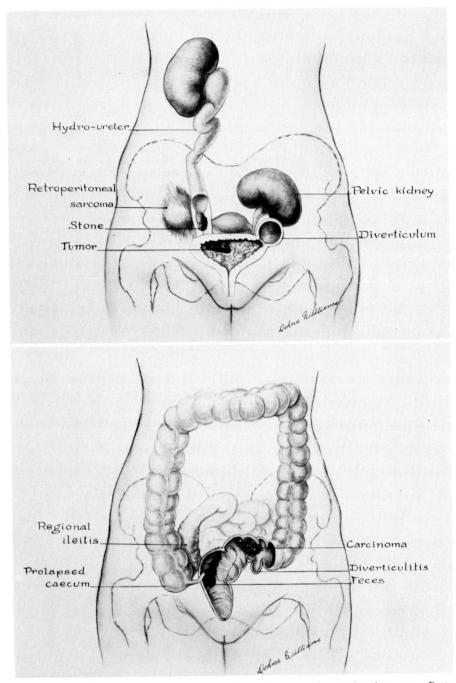

16.14. *Top,* urinary disorders leading to lower abdominal pain with associated myoma. *Bottom,* gastrointestinal causes of pain which may coexist with myoma.

necessary to remove the uterus, because of excessive bleeding. The careful clinician will assure the woman that he is cognizant of her wishes and will do his best to abide by them, but the ultimate decision must be his. He should likewise point out that myomectomy will not assure pregnancy, and there is a definite possibility, 25 to 35% (Brown, A. L., *et al.,* and Brown, J. M., *et al.*) that subsequent hysterectomy may be required. If, however, within that interim a pregnancy or two should intervene, most women will gladly accept a second operation. In addition to producing infertility, myomas may be a factor in causing a disproportionately high incidence of abortion, generally in the *first trimester*. In the *second trimester* pain and tenderness may occur in a previously asymptomatic myoma, with fever, leukocytosis, and development of a surgically acute abdomen. This is generally due to *carneous (red) degeneration*, a curious phenomenon of pregnancy which is probably related to impaired or inadequate circulation in the fibroid, although other degenerative changes or causes of an acute abdomen must be considered. Should expectant conservative treatment not avail, exploration with myomectomy is reluctantly carried out. Curiously enough most of these surgically treated women do not go into labor or bleed, and such bland behavior may occur even when the uterine cavity is entered. Nevertheless, many obstetricians will give large doses of prophylactic progesterone. Similarly, many will later elect cesarean section, although it is our own opinion that myomectomy itself would not always contraindicate delivery from below.

In the *third trimester* and at delivery a fibroid may cause premature bleeding, uterine inertia, or mechanical blockage to normal passage through the birth canal. Postpartum hemorrhage due to an atonic uterus and infection of the endometrium and adjacent myoma is more common after vaginal delivery. Casarean section with hysterectomy is performed frequently these days, and is probably easier and preferable to multiple myomectomy when procreative desires are complete. Total hysterectomy immediately following cesarean section is generally simple for the well trained gynecologist. Although the tissues are quite vascular, planes of cleavage are extraordinarily good. At operation the cervix is so soft that it is difficult to feel within the vagina; if a subtotal hysterectomy is first accomplished, the operator's finger can then be placed down into the endocervical canal, allowing for easy identification and removal of the cervix.

The clinician should recall, however, that small myomas may increase remarkably in size during the course of pregnancy, and yet regress when it is terminated. Whether this is due to an increased hormonal stimulus or simply to a better blood supply is uncertain, although the latter seems likely. Full consideration of the temporary but evanescent growth of fibroids should precede any final decision to perform hysterectomy at the time of cesarean section.

Physical Signs

Abdominal Palpation. In some cases a presumptive diagnosis of uterine myoma can be made by palpating the tumor through the abdominal wall, especially when the latter is not too obese. Such tumors are hard, generally of irregular nodular contour, movable unless so large that they fill most of the abdomen, and not tender.

Bimanual Pelvic Examination. In many cases the diagnosis of myoma is extremely easy, especially when bowel and bladder are empty. One or more nodular outgrowths on the uterine surface can be felt between the examining fingers within the vagina and the external hand. The problem, however, is not always so simple, and examination under anesthesia is occasionally necessary. In obese or highly nervous women, where the uterus is hard to outline, it may be difficult to determine whether a firm globular mass felt behind the cervix is a myoma of the posterior wall or merely a rather large retroflexed fundus. Again, when a firm, solid mass is felt laterally, it is not always easy to decide between a pedunculated subserous myoma and a solid tumor of the ovary. Adnexal masses, either inflammatory or neoplastic, may be so firmly adherent to the uterus that they may simulate uterine myoma. Where there is any question that the intrapelvic tumor is ovarian rather than uterine in origin, laparotomy should be performed because of the dismal nature of many ovarian lesions.

One of the most important diagnostic

problems presented to the gynecologist is to differentiate between myoma and early pregnancy, or to decide whether or not pregnancy exists in an obviously myomatous uterus. Nowadays the problem has been much simplified because of the accuracy of even early "quick" pregnancy tests, and it is desirable to obtain such tests whenever there is any suspicion of pregnancy; however, even the most astute clinician may on rare occasion find that a presumed "pelvic tumor" will be a pregnant uterus. Sonograms may be of considerable assistance.

The submucous variety of myoma presents special difficulties in diagnosis; being concealed within the uterus, they may show no appreciable enlargement or irregularity. In such cases *diagnostic curettage* is indicated in an effort to determine the cause of the patient's bleeding, which may be due to any one of a number of causes, such as submucous myoma, incomplete abortion, polyp, adenocarcinoma, or to a functional factor. The diagnosis is often made by noting the curette to "bump over" a protruding intracavitary nodule which is too firmly embedded to be removed, unlike the usual polyp. We feel that the use of hysteroscopy or hysterograms are unnecessary.

Myometrial Hypertrophy

The condition of an enlarged symmetrical uterus (in the absence of adenomyosis) has been in a sense a "dumping ground," dignified by such nomenclature as *"fibrosis uteri, chronic subinvolution, chronic passive congestion,* etc." Although in rare instances the terminology may represent an attempt by an overenthusiastic surgeon to sneak a normal parous uterus by an alert tissue committee, we believe that on occasion the grossly but diffusely enlarged uterus may represent a valid symptom-producing entity which Lewis, Lee, and Easler have chosen to speak of as *myometrial hypertrophy.*

They arbitrarily utilize a weight of more than 120 gm. as a diagnostic index, and point out that the increased size is merely a sequel to smooth muscle hypertrophy. It is suggested that over 5% of uteri removed warrant this designation which is associated with excessive menstrual bleeding. Although the authors seem loath to assign a cause-effect basis, it would seem that the mere increase in size of the uterus might be expected to incur more profuse periods, aided in part by an overstretched if hypertrophic myometrium that might be incompetent and unable to exhibit adequate contraction, so that the periods are prolonged and heavy. Certainly any uterus weighing more than 200 gm. should be considered abnormally large. Even if there is no demonstrable lesion, the pathologist should not be critical of the surgeon who removes a uterus in which abnormal bleeding persists after several curettages and trials of hormone therapy.

TREATMENT

(1) Expectant Treatment with Periodic Examination

Not all myomas call for surgery, but since they all present some potentiality for subsequent problems, an expectant plan of treatment should always be combined with the advice that periodic examination be sought at regular six-month intervals. When menstrual function ceases, a myoma rarely causes difficulty, often involuting. Thus, in the immediately premenopausal woman simple observation is all the treatment that an only slightly symptomatic myoma warrants. In every case age, procreative desires, the likelihood of an incipient menopause, etc., should be factors to consider, even when symptoms suggest surgery.

We feel it unwise, however, to allow even an asymptomatic myoma to grow larger than a 12- to 14-week pregnancy, particularly when the woman is young and the tumor has a long time to grow, or when there is evidence of rapid growth. Very large myomas can be difficult surgical problems, and when ultimate hysterectomy seems inevitable, it is best performed before the possibility of operative complications is increased.

In the postmenopausal era, a myomatous uterus is rarely symptomatic. However, any postclimacteric growth of a myoma suggests either sarcomatous change or the possibility that the supposed uterine tumor is really ovarian; in either case exploration is indicated.

(2) Radiotherapy

In this era of improved surgical techniques, an irradiation menopause is utilized only in bad risk patients. The fibroid must be smaller than a three-month pregnancy, not submucous, not associated with inflammatory disease, or impinging on the rectum. Today's gynecologist will find rare indications for an irradiation menopause, much preferring hysterectomy.

An important preliminary to radiation is *diagnostic curettage*, and microscopic examination of the endometrium. *The mere fact that a patient with uterine myomata has abnormal bleeding is no proof that the myoma is the cause of the bleeding*, which may be due to malignant intrauterine disease (Fig. 16.15). Indeed, there is some controversy as to whether an irradiation menopause may incite endometrial cancer in the postmenopausal era. Obviously radiotherapy should be avoided in the young woman lest an artificial menopause is produced.

In discussing *radiotherapy* in the treatment of uterine myoma, reference is made to both radium and deep x-ray therapy, both of which are effective. Radium has the advantage of requiring only a single treatment, and this can often be applied at the time of the diagnostic curettage. As for ultimate results, our experience has been that these are just as satisfactory with the use of deep x-ray, although termination of the bleeding is not so rapid. Brinkley and Haybittle find a significant increase in pelvic cancer mortality in patients who have had an irradiation induction of the menopause, as noted earlier.

(3) Surgical Treatment

Myomectomy has its great field in the removal of tumors in cases where the preservation of reproductiveness is of importance. However, there are disad-

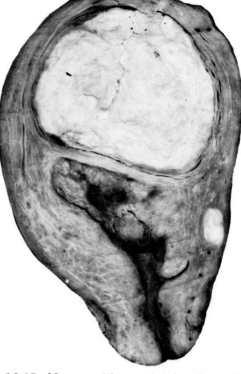

16.15. Myoma with associated endometrial cancer. (Courtesy of Prof. Robert J. Kellar, Edinburgh.)

vantages to be considered, such as the development of extensive adhesions, the weakening of the uterine wall produced by the removal of large tumors, and subsequent tumor formation. Lock has summarized the indications and techniques of myomectomy. Myomectomy should always be preceded by diagnostic curettage if there has been abnormal bleeding, as the latter may be due to an intrauterine lesion, like adenocarcinoma, and not to the myoma.

On the other hand, in the presence of large and numerous myomatous nodules, the chances for the patient to bear children are so slight, and the risks of subsequent trouble so real, that *hysterectomy* is unquestionably the wiser procedure. When *hysterectomy* is performed upon women still in the menstruating age, there is no question as to the *advisability of leaving one or both ovaries*. In preventing development of a precipitate menopause, there is considerable evidence that the postmenopausal ovary is not to be regarded as a functionless, useless organ. In discussing pathology found in postsurgical preserved ovaries, Randall *et al.* indicate that there is a certain risk of subsequent neoplasm, but conservation of ovarian tissue is worth the risk, even where the previous operation was done for ovarian disease (see Chapter 5).

The qualified gynecologist will of course perform total hysterectomy in something more than 95% of all cases. The realistic clinician will admit, however, that an occasional case, complicated by extensive inflammatory disease or endometriosis, is best treated by a subtotal operation. He should be praised rather than criticized for his discrimination, and we do not instruct our residents to *always* perform a complete operation in the face of medical or other complicating factors. Where conservation of the cervical stump seems likely, preoperative smear and biopsy are mandatory.

REFERENCES

Abithol, M. M.: Submucous fibroids complicating pregnancy labor, and delivery. Obstet. Gynec., *10:* 529, 1957.

Ariel, I. M., and Trinidad, S.: Pulmonary metastases from a uterine "leiomyoma." Amer. J. Obstet. Gynec., *94:* 110, 1966.

Banooni, F., Labes, J., and Goodman, P. A.: Uterine leiomyoma containing metastatic breast carcinoma. Amer. J. Obst. Gynec., *111:* 427, 1971.

Barber, J. R. K., and Graber, E. A.: Gynecological tumors in childhood and adolescence. Obstet. Gynec. Survey, *28:* 357, 1973.

Barter, R. H., and Parks, J.: Myoma uteri associated with pregnancy. Clin. Obstet. Gynec., *1:* 519, 1958.

Boyce, C. R., and Buddhev, H. N.: Pregnancy complicated by metastasizing leiomyoma. Obstet. Gynec. *42:* 252, 1973.

Brinkley, D., and Haybittle, J. L.: Late effects of artificial menopause by x-radiation. Brit. J. Radiol., *42:* 519, 1969.

Brown, A. L., Chamberlain, R. W., and TeLinde, R. W.: Myomectomy, Amer. J. Obstet. Gynec., *71:* 759, 1956.

Brown, J. M., Malkasian, G. D., and Symmonds, R. E.: Abdominal myomectomy. Amer. J. Obstet. Gynec., *99:* 126, 1967.

Buddinger, J. M., and Greene, R. R.: A distinctive myometrial tumor of undetermined origin. Cancer, *17:* 1155, 1964.

Edwards, D. L., and Peacock, J. F.: Intravenous leiomyomatosis of the uterus. Obstet. Gynec., *27:* 176, 1966.

Everett, H. S.: Effect of uterine myomas on the urinary tract. Clin. Obstet. Gynec., *1:* 429, 1958.

Farrer-Brown, G., Beilby, J. O. W., and Tarbit, M. H.: Vascular patterns in myomatous uteri. J. Obstet. Gynaec. Brit. Comm. *77:* 917, 1970;, Venous changes in the endometrium of myomatous uteri. Obstet. Gynec. *38:* 743, 1971.

Fox, J. E., and Abell, M. R.: Mast cells in uterine myometrium and leiomyomatous neoplasms. Amer. J. Obstet. Gynec., *91:* 413, 1965.

Faulkner, R. L.: Red degeneration of myomas. Amer. J. Obstet. Gynec., *53:* 474, 1947.

Gerbie, A. B., Greene, R. R., and Reis, R. A.: Heteroplastic bone and cartilage in the female genital tract. Obstet. Gynec., *11:* 573, 1958.

Harper, R. S., and Scully, R. E.: Intravenous leiomyomatosis of the uterus. Obstet. Gynec., *18:* 519, 1961.

Henriksen, E.: Lipoma of uterus; report of 3 cases. Western J. Surg., *60:* 609, 1952.

Ingersoll, F. M.: Myomectomy and fertility. Fertil. Steril., *14:* 596, 1963.

Kelly, H. A., and Cullen, T. S.: *Myomata of the Uterus.* W. B. Saunders Company, Philadelphia, 1909.

Kimbrough, R. A.: General considerations in the treatment of myoma uteri. Clin. Obstet. Gynec., *1:* 437, 1958.

Larbig, C. G., *et al.*: Plexiform tumorlets of endometrial stromal origin. Amer. J. Clin. Path., *44:* 32, 1965.

Lardaro, H. H.: Extensive myomectomy. Amer. J. Obstet. Gynec,, *79:* 43, 1960.

Lewis, P. L., Lee, A. B. H., and Easler, R. E.: Myometrial hypertrophy. Amer. J. Obstet. Gynec., *84:* 1032, 1962.

Lipschütz, A.: *Steroid Hormones and Tumors,* Ed. 1. The Williams and Wilkins Company, Baltimore, 1950.

Lock, F. R.: Multiple myomectomy. Amer. J. Obstet. Gynec., *104:* 642, 1969.

Meyer, R.: Die pathologische Anatomie der Gerbarmutter. In *Handbuch der spezielle pathologische Anatomie und Histologie,* edited by F. Henke and O. Lubarsch, Vol. 7, Part 1. Julius Springer, Berlin, 1930.

Novak, E. R.: Benign and malignant changes in uterine myomas. Clin. Obstet. Gynec., *1:* 421, 1958.

Patchevsky, A. S.: Plexiform tumorlet of the uterus. Obstet. Gynec., *35:* 592, 1970.

Pedowitz, P., Felmus, L. B., and Grayzel, D. M.: Vascular tumors of uterus. I. Benign vascular tumors. II. Malignant vascular tumors. Amer. J. Obstet. Gynec., *69:* 1291, 1309, 1955.

Pedowitz, P., Felmus, L. B., and Grayzel, D. M.: Vascular tumors of the uterus. Amer. J. Obstet. Gynec., *71:* 1256, 1956.

Randall, C. L., Hall, D. W., and Armenia, C. S.: Pathology in the preserved ovary after unilateral oophorectomy. Amer. J. Obstet. Gynec., *84:* 1233, 1962.

Rothman, D., and Rennard, M.: Myoma-erythrocytosis syndrome. Obstet. Gynec., *21:* 102, 1962.

Rubin, I. C.: Uterine fibromyomas and sterility. Clin. Obstet. Gynec., *1:* 501, 1958.

Sabbagh, M. L.: Lipoma of the uterus. Obstet. Gynec., *4:* 399, 1954.

Saidi, F., Constable, J. D., and Ulfelder, H.: Massive intraperitoneal hemorrhage due to uterine fibroids. Amer. J. Obstet. Gynec., *82:* 367, 1961.

Sampson, J. A.: Blood supply of uterine myomata. Surg. Gynec. Obstet., *14:* 215, 1912.

Schwartz, O.: Benign diffuse enlargement of the uterus. Amer. J. Obstet. Gynec., *61:* 902, 1951.

Spurlin, G. W., *et al.*: Uterine myomas and erythrocytosis. Obstet. Gynec., *40:* 646, 1972.

Stearns, H. C., and Sneeden, V. D.: Observations on the clinical and pathological aspects of the pelvic congestion syndrome. Amer. J. Obstet. Gynec., *94:* 718, 1966.

Taubert, H. D., Wissner, S. E., and Haskins, A. L.: Leiomyomatosis peritonealis disseminata. Obstet. Gynec., *25:* 561, 1965.

Wright, C. J. E.: Solitary malignant lymphoma of the uterus. Amer. J. Obstet. Gynec., *117:* 114, 1973.

chapter 17

Adenomyosis
of the Uterus

Adenomyosis of the uterus is characterized by histologically benign invasion of the uterine musculature by the endometrium, which normally is found lining only the uterine cavity. There are many points of similarity between adenomyosis and pelvic endometriosis, although adenomyosis characteristically affects the 40-year-old, parous woman, and endometriosis the younger infertile patient. In both, however, there is ectopic growth of endometrial tissue. For that matter, adenomyosis was at one time spoken of as *endometriosis interna,* to distinguish it from *endometriosis externa* or pelvic endometriosis.

It is true that in some locations definite tumor masses may occur which are made up of muscle tissue and endometrium, and to these the term *adenomyoma* is more properly applied. Such tumor nodules not infrequently develop on the round and uterosacral ligaments, but as a rule the process is too diffuse to be considered as a discrete tumor. With adenomyosis of the uterus we apparently deal with an exaggerated growth activity of the endometrium, which pushes down into the underlying muscle. With this endometrial invasion is combined a marked, generalized overgrowth of the muscle elements.

Incidence

Bird *et al.* record a 61.5% incidence of adenomyosis in 200 consecutive hysterectomies, an excessive figure compared to such studies as those of Molitar (8.8%). However, nearly one-half of his cases occurred less than one low power field below the basal endometrium—even if these are deleted the resultant figure of 38.5% seems much greater than the incidence usually quoted in the literature (10–20%).

Pathology

The enlargement of the uterus produced by adenomyosis is a diffuse one, and not nodular, as in the case of myoma. There is often enormous thickening of the uterine wall, usually asymmetrical, the posterior wall being usually more extensively involved than the anterior (Fig. 17.1). Never, however, does the uterus reach the large proportions seen in many cases of myoma, rarely being larger than

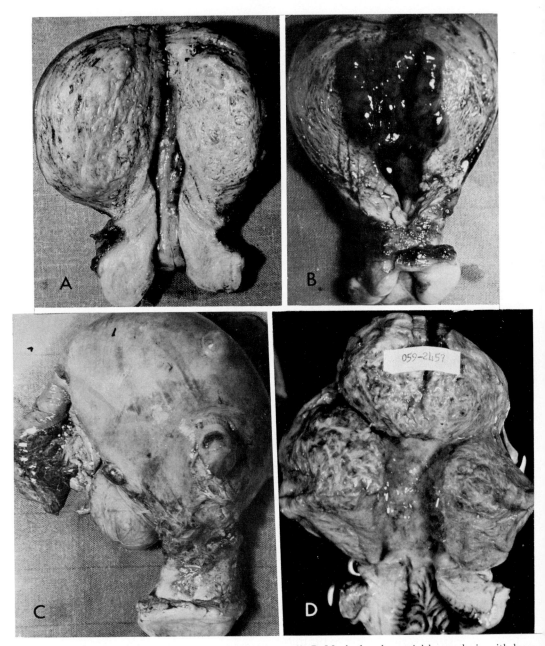

17.1. *A,* Extensive adenomyosis of posterior uterine wall. *B,* Marked endometrial hyperplasia with large uterus although no significant adenomyosis. *C,* Adenomyosis and myomas. *D,* Extensive diffuse adenomyosis extending into cervix. (Courtesy of Emge, L.: Elusive adenomyosis of the uterus, Amer. J. Obstet. Gynec., *83:* 1541, 1962, C. V. Mosby Co., Publishers.)

a grapefruit. It should not be forgotten, however, that myoma and adenomyosis often coexist.

The distinctive *microscopic* characteristic is the presence of islands of typical endometrial tissue scattered throughout the muscle, often far beneath the endometrial surface, and sometimes extending to the peritoneal surface. The endometrial glands in the ectopic tissue are surrounded by typical endometrial stromal cells. Occasionally the endometrium is of *functioning type,* menstruating just as does the normal surface endometrium. In such cases collections of chocolate-colored menstrual blood are seen throughout the wall, constituting miniature uterine cavities (Fig. 17.2).

More frequently the endometrium is of the immature, *nonfunctioning type,* often presenting a typical Swiss-cheese hyperplasia pattern (Fig. 17.3). When the endometrium penetrates to the peritoneum, it may continue to propagate itself, sometimes producing extensive pelvic endometriosis. In such cases, the uterus is often densely adherent to the rectum and other surrounding organs. The muscle tissue shows marked hyperplasia, with a whorl-like tendency not unlike that seen in myoma. Pregnancy may bring about decidual changes (Fig. 17.4) in the invading endometrium quite like those noted in the uterine mucosa proper.

Sandberg and Cohn have indicated that superficial adenomyosis rarely shows decidual changes whereas this is relatively frequent in the more extreme degrees of myometrial invasion (Fig. 17.5). The most

logical explanation is that continued growth has allowed the aberrant endometrium to mature and achieve the faculty of progesterone response, and indeed this is one of several possibilities noted by the authors.

It would thus seem that adenomyosis may be compared to an inverting polyp, composed of a mature responsive form of endometrium or more often an immature juvenile tissue completely incapable of response to progesterone. Hyperplasia in conjunction with a biphasic cycle is common, but, *adenocarcinoma* developing in these aberrant islands has been reported on only a few occasions (Novak and Woodruff). Perhaps this origin is more common than appreciated. Extension of any malignant spread of adenomyosis would almost certainly traverse up the lines of least resistance, the glandular channels, and involve the endometrial surface (Fig. 17.6). Symptoms such as bleeding would often be produced only at this time, but when hysterectomy is finally accomplished the pathological diagnosis is "endometrial adenocarcinoma

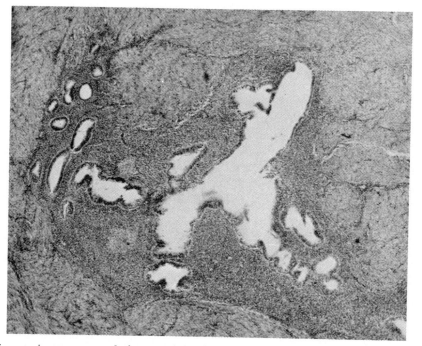

17.2. Microscopic appearance of adenomyosis in which the invading endometrium is of functioning (secretory) type.

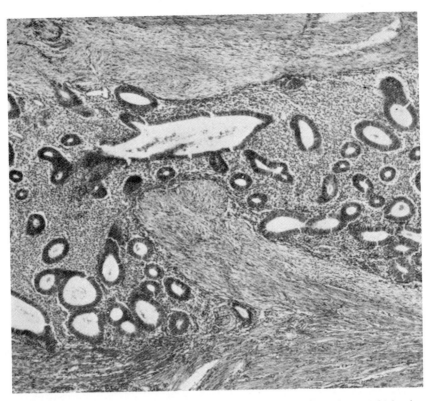

17.3. Adenomyosis showing a nonfunctioning hyperplasia-like endometrial island

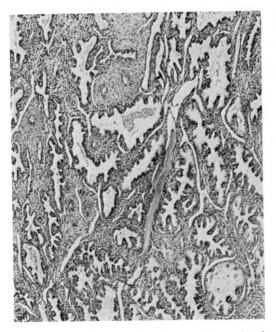

17.4. Decidual changes in adenomyosis associated with pregnancy.

with myometrial extension." For a review, the reader is referred to the article by Colman and Rosenthal.

In any case, a frequent and difficult problem to the pathologist is distinction between well differentiated endometrial adenocarcinoma with early invasion and superficial malignancy with associated adenomyosis. If however, there is no observed evidence of direct invasion with reaction on the part of the invaded myometrium or if the ectopic endometrium is obviously better differentiated than the surface adenocarcinoma, it is probable that there is merely associated adenomyosis.

The most outstanding critique of *adenomyosis* is that by Emge, who discusses the history, etiology, and symptomatology of the disease. He further comments on the concurrence of adenomyosis and endometrial malignancy. Perhaps the most intriguing aspect of his study is the frequency of adenomyosis at

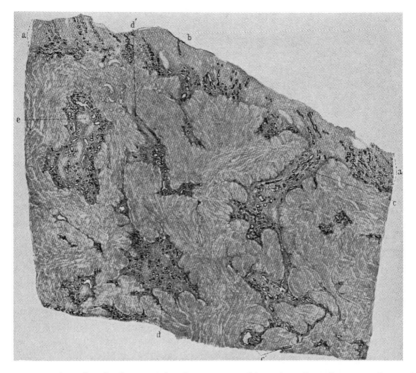

17.5. Low power section of wall of uterus showing manner of invasion of uterine musculature by endometrium.

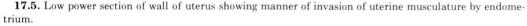

the time of hysterectomy for fibroids (52%), endometriosis (69%), unselected hysterectomies (29%), corpus cancer (33%), and in uteri removed at autopsy (53.7%). Obviously the range of co-associations with other lesions is wide. In discussing the diagnostic approach to adenomyosis, Emge points out the suggestive importance of associated endometrial hyperplasia which is frequently but not inevitably found in conjunction with adenomyosis. Seemingly this is an estrogen-dependent disease process.

Histogenesis

The histogenesis of aberrant endometrium was formerly widely discussed, but it is now clearly established, as a result of the work of Cullen and others, that it has its source from downward growth of the surface endometrium. Histological studies often show direct continuity of the deep islands with the surface mucosa, although the over-growth of muscle elements may nip off the connecting endometrial

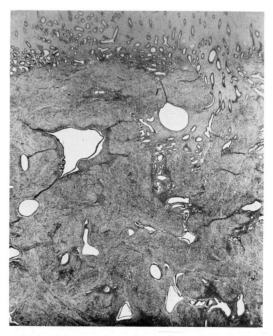

17.6. Showing how glands of basal endometrium push down into uterine muscle in case of adenomyosis.

process. Endometrial islands should be noted at least one HPF (high-power field) below the level of the basal layer to warrant the diagnosis of *adenomyosis*.

Clinical Characteristics of Adenomyosis

The two most frequent symptoms are *menorrhagia* and *dysmenorrhea*, generally increasingly severe in the older (fifth decade) woman who has borne children. The former may be partly explained by the increased amount of endometrium, but is often due to the ovarian dysfunction so frequently associated. The dysmenorrhea, is typically of colicky nature, due to the painful contractions of the uterine muscle, induced by the menstrual swelling of the endometrial islands. When pelvic endometriosis is present, it often involves the uterosacral ligaments, and the menstrual swelling of the endometrium in the region produces *pain* referred to the rectum or the lower sacral region. Where endometriosis is present there may be some intermenstrual discomfort, but this is not nearly as characteristic as the menstrual symptoms.

Novak and De Lima indicate that pelvic endometriosis and adenomyosis coexist with relative frequency. Benson states that pelvic endometriosis occurs in only 13% of cases of adenomyosis; he also adds that surface endometrial hyperplasia is a rare accompaniment which differs from Emge's findings and our own impressions.

Diagnosis

Although the diagnosis is not usually made until after pathological examination, there is a group of cases in which at least a strongly presumptive diagnosis can be made clinically. When one finds a moderately and diffusely enlarged uterus firmly fixed in the pelvis, with one or more small nodules palpable in the region of the uterosacral ligaments, and when these findings are combined with menorrhagia and a colicky dysmenorrhea referred to the rectum or lower sacral or coccygeal regions in a parous woman, there will be little doubt of the presence of adenomyosis probably combined with endometriosis. In a proportion of cases, however, pelvic endometriosis does not coexist, and preoperative diagnosis is often not possible. A symmetrically enlarged uterus with the proved absence of pregnancy in a 40-year-old woman with increasing dysmenorrhea and menorrhagia should be highly suggestive of adenomyosis.

Treatment

Because, like myoma, this disease is usually dependent on continued ovarian function, minor symptoms in the premenopausal woman require only palliative treatment. Where symptoms are extreme, however, the proper treatment is surgical; in many cases the operation is performed on the incorrect diagnosis of myoma, pelvic inflammatory disease, or a combination of the two. Hysterectomy is indicated, the fate of the ovaries being decided on the basis of such factors as the age of the patient and the presence or absence of ovarian or general pelvic endometriosis.

Stromal Adenomyosis or Endometriosis

Robertson *et al.* have called attention to a form of adenomyosis in which the invading tissue is altogether stromal, with no gland elements, and which some clinicians designate as *stromatosis*, although a better designation would seem to be *stromal endometriosis* or *adenomyosis*. Although such stromal invasion occurs, it is relatively rare, and it should not be assumed unless the study of many sections demonstrates an actual absence of glands. Various authors speak of benign and malignant forms, but the latter is better looked upon as akin to a low grade endometrial sarcoma (see Chapter 18, "Sarcoma of the Uterus").

Publications on the subject of this lesion, frequently referred to as *stromatosis*, have clarified many of its pathological and clinical characteristics, although its comparative rarity suggests the need for only a short discussion. It has been suggested that there are three categories of cases, with all intermediate gra-

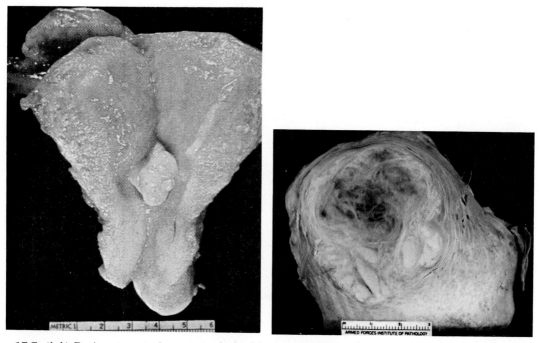

17.7. (*left*) Benign stromatosis; compare lack of invasion with that shown in **17.9.** (Courtesy of Dr. D. Nichols, Buffalo, New York.) (*right*). Cut surface of a uterus containing a stromal tumor with a pushing margin. Note the circumscription and lack of infiltration of myometrium at the periphery of the tumor. (Courtesy of Norris, H. J., and Taylor, H. B.: Mesenchymal tumors of the uterus. I. A clinical and pathological study of 53 endometrial stromal tumors. Cancer, *19:* 755, 1966.)

dations. (1) The simplest is identical with ordinary adenomyosis except that the invading endometrium is made up entirely of stroma, with no glands. It is clinically entirely benign (Fig. 17.7). (2) In this group the endometrial stroma invades not only the musculature but may also exhibit endolymphatic and intravascular penetrativeness, growing in a rubbery, wormlike fashion into both lymphatics and veins (Figs. 17.7, 8). It may thus become at least locally invasive, pushing into the broad ligaments, but it has no tendency to distant metastases. According to Henderson, cases of this kind can often be temporarily cured even if the removal of tumor tissue is not altogether complete, although death may occur from local extension. (3) The definitely malignant group, speaking histologically, is also malignant clinically (Fig. 17.9). For this reason, we prefer to classify such cases as *endometrial sar-*

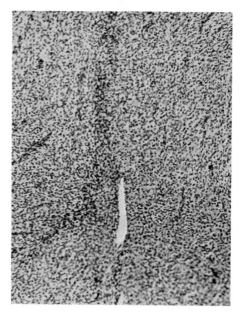

17.8. Stromal adenomyosis. The invading stroma in this case showing malignant characteristics.

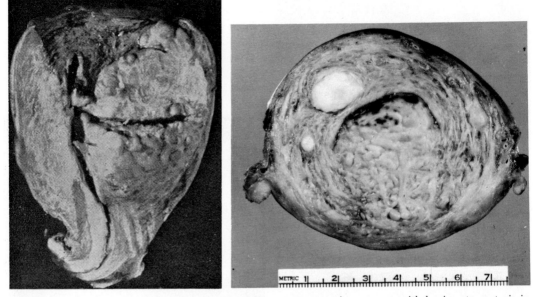

17.9 (*left*). Gross appearance of uterus with malignant stromatosis; compare with benign stromatosis in **17.7**. (Courtesy of Harper Hospital, Detroit.) (*right*). Cross section of a uterus containing a stromal tumor with infiltrating margins (endolymphatic stromal myosis). There is poor circumscription and poorly defined extensions of the tumor bulge above the cut tumor, infiltrate the myometrium, and obliterate the endometrial cavity. (Courtesy of Norris, H. J., and Taylor, H. B.: Mesenchymal tumors of the uterus. I. A clinical and pathological study of 53 endometrial stromal tumors. Cancer, *19:* 755, 1966.)

coma, in spite of the fact that the morphological characteristics of the sarcoma cells are remindful of the stroma from which they arise. The histological differences between these three types are exceedingly tenuous, and there is considerable logic in accepting only benign stromatosis or a malignant type which is a low grade variant of endometrial sarcoma.

In an excellent and comprehensive study of 53 endometrial stromal tumors, Norris and Taylor reach similar conclusions. They distinguish between stromal nodules (tumors with *pushing margins*) (Fig. 17.7 *right*) and lacking the capacity to infiltrate myometrium, extend beyond the uterus, or metastasize. None of 18 patients with the benign stromal tumors died or had recurrence of the disease.

As opposed to the above, they describe endolymphatic stromal myosis and stromal sarcoma as tumors with *infiltrating margins* (Fig. 17.9 *right*) and with the capacity to invade lymphatics and veins, extend beyond the uterus, and

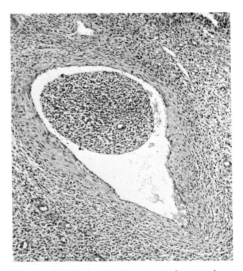

17.10. Endolymphatic stromal myosis surrounding and within a vein (the circumferential muscle layer identifies the vessel as a vein). The major portion of the tumor growth is outside the vein. (Courtesy of Norris, H. J., and Taylor, H. B.: Mesenchymal tumors of the uterus. I. A clinical and pathological study of 53 endometrial stromal tumors. Cancer, *19:* 755, 1966.)

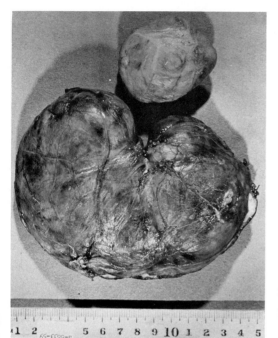

17.11. Intraligamentary hemangiopericytoma (*below*) with myoma. (Courtesy of Dr. Albert Brown, Wilmington, N.C.).

metastasize (Fig. 17.10). Patients with this malignant form of stromatosis had close to a 50% possibility of recurrence or death. There was, however, a marked difference between the behavior of lesions with less than 10 mitotic figures per high power field (endolymphatic stromal myosis) and those with more than 10 mitotic figures per high power field (stromal sarcoma). Of the latter group only four of 15 patients (26%) were free of their disease. The patients with endolymphatic stromal myosis showed a much slower progression of their disease and a much better prognosis, 53% being free of disease, 31% living with the disease, and only one patient (5%) dying of the disease after 12 years (11% of patients died of other causes).

Although these lesions arising from the endometrial stroma are not common, one would presume that some beneficial effects might be expected from progesterone therapy as in the case of some endometrial cancers and such cases have been described by Pellillo (see Chapter 18) and Baggish and Woodruff.

Hemangiopericytoma

On occasion the pathologist may encounter difficulty in distinguishing between stromal endometriosis and *hemangiopericytoma,* a vascular lesion closely related to a glomus tumor (Fig. 17.11). Histologically, it is characterized by a concentric arrangement of pericytes around capillaries, but such special stains as Massons, silver, and reticulum are often necessary. Grossly one may find a tumor much like a vascular myoma, generally unlike the wormlike buds of stromatosis. Hemangiopericytoma is generally regarded as a low grade (20 to 25%) malignant tumor.

REFERENCES

Baggish, M. S., and Woodruff, J. D.: Uterine stromatosis. Obstet. Gynec., *40:* 487, 1972.

Benson, R. C., and Smeeden, V. D.: Adenomyosis; a reappraisal of symptomatology. Amer. J. Obstet. Gynec., *76:* 1044, 1958.

Bird, C. C., McElin, T. W., and Menalo-Estrella, P.: The elusive adenomyosis of the uterus—revisited. Amer. J. Obstet. Gynec., *112:* 583, 1972.

Coleman, H. I., and Rosenthal, A. H.: Carcinoma developing in areas of adenomyosis. Obstet. Gynec., *14:* 342, 1959.

Cope, E.: Adenocarcinoma of the endometrium with malignant stromatosis. J. Obstet. Gynaec. Brit. Comm., *65:* 58, 1958.

Cullen, T. S.: *Adenomyoma of Uterus.* W. B. Saunders Company, Philadelphia, 1908.

Cullen, T. S.: Distribution of adenomyomata containing uterine mucosa. Arch. Surg., *1:* 215, 1920.

Emge, L. A.: Elusive adenomyosis of uterus; its historic past and its present state of recognition. Amer. J. Obstet. Gynec., *83:* 1541, 1962.

Giammalvo, J. T., and Kaplan, K.: Endometriosis interna and endometrial carcinoma. Amer. J. Obstet. Gynec., *75:* 161, 1958.

Goldfarb, S., Richart, R. M., and Ogaki, T.: Nuclear DNA content in endolymphatic stromal myosis. Amer. J. Obstet. Gynec., *106:* 524, 1970.

Green, R. R., Gerbie, A. B., and Eckman, T. R.: Hemangiopericytoma of the uterus. Amer. J. Obstet. Gynec., *106:* 1020, 1970.

Henderson, D. N.: Endolymphatic stromal myosis. Amer. J. Obstet. Gynec., *52:* 1000, 1946.

Hunter, W. C., and Lattig, G. J.: Stromal endometriosis and uterine adenomyosis. Amer. J. Obstet. Gynec., *75:* 258, 1958.

Kinshen, E. J., Nattolin, F., and Benirschke, K.: Uterine hemangiopericytoma in a 19-year-old girl. Obstet. Gynec., *40:* 652, 1972.

Kistner, R. W.: Endometriosis and adenomyosis. In Davis: *Gynecology and Obstetrics,* Vol. II, Chapter 43. Harper & Rowe, Hagerstown, Md., 1968.

Koss, L. G., Spiro, D. H., and Bronschwig, A.: Endometrial stromal sarcoma. Surg. Gynec. Obstet., *121:* 531, 1965.

Kumar, D., and Anderson, W.: Malignancy in endometriosis interna. J. Obstet. Gynaec. Brit. Comm., *65:* 435, 1958.

Molitor, J. J.: Adenomyosis. Amer. J. Obstet. Gynec., *110:* 275, 1971.

GYNECOLOGY

Norris, H. J. and Taylor, H. B., Jr.: Mesenchymal tumors of the uterus. I. A clinical and pathological study at 53 endometrial stromal tumors. Cancer, *19:* 755, 1966.

Norris, H. J., and Taylor, H. B., Jr.: Postirradiation sarcomas of the uterus. Obstet. Gynec., *26:* 689, 1965.

Novak, E., and De Lima, O. A.: A correlative study of adenomyosis and pelvic endometriosis, with special reference to the hormonal reaction of ectopic endometrium. Amer. J. Obstet. Gynec., *56:* 634, 1958.

Novak, E. R. and Woodruff, J. D.: Postirradiation malignancy of the pelvic organs. Amer. J. Obstet. Gynec., *77:* 667, 1959.

Park, W. W.: Stromatosis. J. Obstet. Gynaec. Brit. Comm., *56:* 755, 1952.

Pedowitz, P., Felmus, L. B., and Grayzel, D. M.: Vascular tumors of the uterus. Amer. J. Obstet. Gynec., *69:* 1291, 1955.

Pedowitz, P., Felmus, L. B., and Grayzel, D. M.: Benign vascular tumors. Amer. J. Obstet. Gynec., *69:* 1309, 1955.

Robertson, T. B., Hunter, W. C., Larson, C. P., and Snyder, G. A. C.: Benign and malignant stromal endometriosis. Amer. J. Clin. Path., *12:* 1, 1942.

Sandberg, E. C., and Cohn, F.: Adenomyosis in the gravid uterus at term. Amer. J. Obstet. Gynec., *84:* 1457, 1962.

Scott, R. B.: Adenomyosis and adenomyoma. Clin. Obstet. Gynec., *1:* 413, 1958.

Stearns, H. C.: Study of stromal endometriosis. Amer. J. Obstet. Gynec., *75:* 603, 1958.

Stout, A. P.: Hemangiopericytoma. Cancer, *2:* 1027, 1949.

Winkelman, J., and Robinson, R.: Adenocarcinoma of endometrium involving adenomyosis. Cancer, *19:* .901, 1966.

chapter 18

Sarcoma of the Uterus

Sarcoma of the uterus is far less common than carcinoma; however, any precise statistics are difficult to assemble, for many clinics designate as low grade sarcomas what others might consider as merely cellular myomas. Obviously, this discrepancy affects not only salvage but also the incidence. In an early study from our own laboratory sarcomas constituted less than 5 per cent of all uterine malignant tumors, and we suspect this is the approximate ratio at the present time. Although uncommon, it is a rather serious lesion because of its tendency to spread via the blood stream, so that lung and liver metastases as well as local invasion are common.

Pathology and Classification

It is now generally accepted that sarcoma of the uterus may arise from any of the connective tissue elements of the uterine structure, and that it may be of myogenic origin as well. Thus it may arise from the myometrium (Fig. 18.1), endometrium, blood vessels, or a myoma. Whether any lesion should be categorized as a leiomyosarcoma (of smooth muscle origin) or fibromyosarcoma (of connective tissue variety) seems of purely academic interest as compared to whether it is ma-lignant or benign. Such designations as round, spindle, mixed, or other are purely descriptive.

Ober, among others, has attempted to classify sarcoma on a histogenetic basis, and he proposes the following scheme (which is presented here only in outline form).

(1) Leiomyosarcoma
(2) Mesenchymal sarcoma
    (a) Pure homologous as endometrial sarcoma
    (b) Pure heterologous as rhabdomyosarcoma
    (c) Mixed homologous as carcinosarcoma
    (d) Mixed heterologous as carcinosarcoma plus other heterologous elements
(3) Blood vessel sarcomas
(4) Lymphomas
(5) Unclassified
(6) Metastatic

There are numerous subclassifications which are not necessary for a simple workable means of dividing these lesions. It is often difficult enough to distinguish them from various epithelial tumors without specific regard to their precise histogenesis.

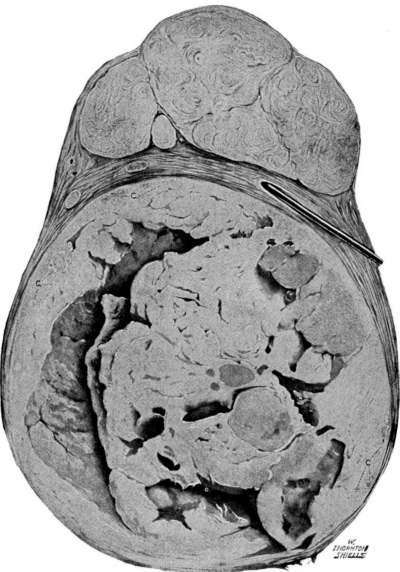

18.1. Sarcoma of body of uterus. (From Kelly, H. A.: *Operative Gynecology*. Appleton-Century-Crofts, Inc., New York, 1928.)

LEIOMYOSARCOMA

Although *leiomyosarcoma* is a very infrequent complication of myoma, in the nature of 0.2% or less (Thornton and Carter, Corscaden and Singh, and Montague *et al.*), the prevalence of myomata still makes this the most common form of uterine sarcoma. Because of the rarity of malignant degeneration, however, the clinician tends to disregard this in his treatment of myomata. *Sudden ac-celerated growth* of a previously static tumor or *postmenopausal enlargement* will always suggest the possibility of sarcoma, and indicate surgery despite any symptoms; actually most cases will ultimately show only degenerative changes, but the clinician cannot afford to procrastinate.

The diagnosis of this particular lesion is rarely made preoperatively, because the symptoms and physical findings are attributed to the myomata; indeed, surgery itself only rarely affords a clue, for in many instances the malignant change will involve only the central area of the tumor so that the surface is not abnormal. On occasion the myoma may be somewhat softer, cytic, and yellowish, and thus quite different from the firm nodular consistency usually found.

If the tumor is cut open after its removal, one will find an absence of the symmetrically whorled white, firm, surface. Instead there is apt to be a softer yellowish consistency, or when necrotic changes are marked, a more pultaceous appearance with cystic and hemorrhagic degeneration. Although this may represent merely degenerative phenomena, it should impel the surgeon to increase the scope of his operation; i.e., removal of, rather than ovarian conservation, hysterectomy rather than myomectomy, etc.

With reference to the much discussed question of the *incidence* of sarcomatous changes in myomas, the wide discrepancy of figures quoted suggests that there is incomplete uniformity in recognition of the histological criteria of malignancy. The most common error is to mistake very cellular but benign myomas for spindle cell sarcoma, so that in some series an incidence of 10% malignancy is reported. It would seem that mere cellularity in the absence of increased mitoses and abnormal and giant cells should not warrant the diagnosis of even a "low-grade sarcoma." Such is not the rule, however, and this might account for the high incidence of sarcoma in some clinics, as well as a high salvage, for these lesions rarely cause difficulties in the patient's subsequent course.

Microscopic Pattern

At least two mitotic figures per high power field should be encountered before considering a diagnosis of sarcoma. Montague *et al.*, note that with two to five mitoses per high power field, the five-year salvage exceeds 75%; with six to ten mitoses, salvage drops to less than 40%, and is negligible where there are more than 10/HPF. The salvage of over 50% is much more encouraging than other figures, although the series is small.

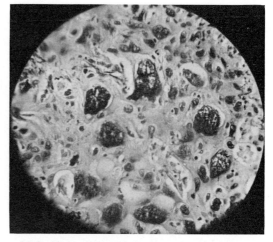

18.2. Note abnormal forms and mitotic figures which are of extreme importance in assesing the malignancy of sarcoma. (Courtesy of Dr. N. Diaz-Bazan, San Salvador.)

Mitotic activity (Fig. 18.2), giant cell formation (Fig. 18.3), and increasing degrees of pleomorphism (Figs. 18.4,5) are frequent in leiomyosarcoma, and often offer a distinctive contrast to the orderly

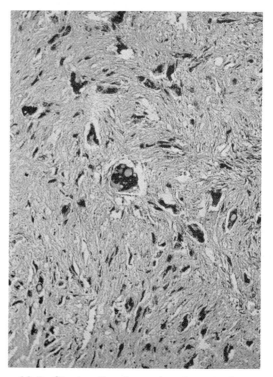

18.3. Giant cells of symplasmic type due to degenerative process.

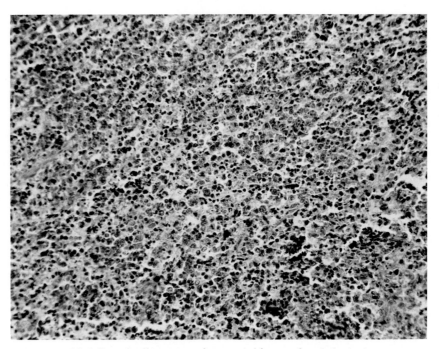

18.4. Round cell sarcoma of uterus (with secondary infection)

pattern of myoma from which the malignancy may have arisen. Nevertheless, it is not always easy to be sure whether or not sarcoma is secondary to benign myoma. The mere presence of myomas does not justify this assumption and, moreover, it must be remembered that sarcoma may arise as a rather nodular growth which might simulate a myoma. On the other hand, when a sarcoma is found developing in the interior of a myoma in which one can still find abundant evidence of the original benign tumor, the origin from such a tumor seems clear. In the late stages of the disease, however, such aids in determining the origin of the tumor are not available, and one can only speculate.

In an early series at the Hopkins, it was considered that in 66.1%, the sarcoma was secondary in myomas. This gives an incidence of 0.56% of sarcomatous degeneration in the 6981 myomas encountered in our earlier clinic material, a figure somewhat lower than the 1.2% of Kelly and Cullen in prior study from the same laboratory. Certainly, however, the incidence would seem less than 1% according to accrued statistics, but one must

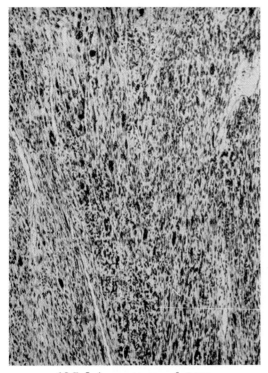

18.5. Leiomyosarcoma of uterus

always be mindful of "what constitutes a sarcoma."

Such interpretation obviously dictates the salvage; for example, an article by Radman and Korman notes 17 of 19 patients alive following treatment for sarcoma. It would seem that their cases must include certain lesions of low grade activity, or else other figures as the report of 100% fatality by Bartsich, Bowe, and Moore are extremely pessimistic. However, they utilize such criteria as myometrial or blood vessel invasion and marked anaplasia. The usual salvage lies in the 25 to 50% bracket, although Corscaden and Singh, in reporting at most a 0.13% incidence of malignant change in myomas, indicate that salvage with true sarcoma is very low. In a group of 41 women who had all their treatment at the Mayo Clinic, Aaro and Dockerty note a surprisingly high 46% five-year survival. It is likewise apparent from their study that mitosis count in a frequently helpful method of assessing the prognosis.

Silverberg indicates that cellular atypia rather than mitosis count is the most important prognostic factor. He likewise suggests that when the sarcoma is confined to the myoma, the results should be favorable; we are in complete agreement if there is no vascular invasion.

MESENCHYMAL SARCOMA

This variety of uterine malignancy is usually diagnosed preoperatively since it arises from the endometrium, and causes bleeding which necessitates curettage.

Endometrial sarcoma is less common, but more malignant than leiomyosarcoma and salvage is probably in the nature of 25%. There is, however, a real difficulty in evaluating published statistics in that some clinics include certain cases of what others would interpret as benign stromatosis, hemangiopericytoma, etc.

Microscopically endometrial sarcoma (Fig. 18.6) shows a marked proliferation of the stromal elements, with progressive loss of the endometrial glands. Marked nuclear hyperchromatosis, mitotic activity, and pleomorphism are present.

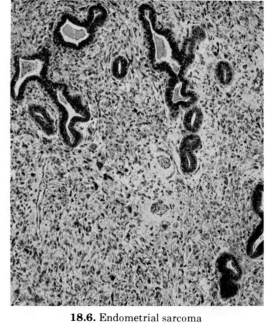

18.6. Endometrial sarcoma

The tumor *grossly* presents a polypoid architecture (Fig. 18.7) like a cervical polyp. However, benign polyps are generally smoother and less friable than these endometrial lesions, which histologically show complete overgrowth of a proliferative stroma although an infrequent abnormal gland may be found. On occasion both connective tissue and epithelium are stimulated to malignancy with the development of a *carcinosarcoma*. This should be regarded merely as a variant of endometrial sarcoma, and is composed only of *homologous* elements (in contrast to the mixed mesodermal sarcoma). Williams and Woodruff have discussed its relationship to benign polyp and endometrial adenocarcinoma.

There are all degrees of histological and clinical malignancy with endometrial sarcoma. As noted earlier, it may be very difficult to make a distinction between this and the locally invasive but nonmetastasizing *stromal endometriosis*, or *stromatosis* (see Chapter 17) which may be a rather completely benign process or locally malignant with venous and lymphatic extension but rarely distant metastasis. (The rare hemangiopericytoma may histologically be a

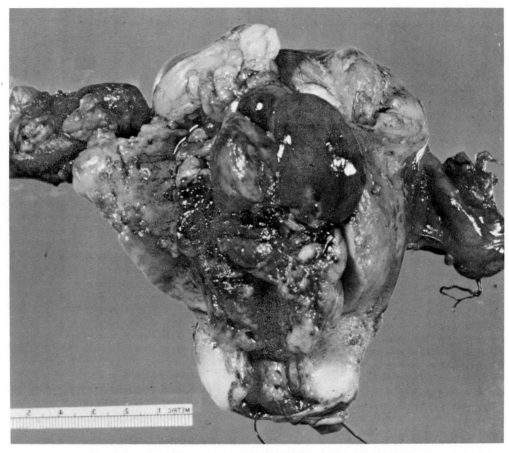

18.7. Multipolypoid lesion may extend down cervix and present in vagina

very difficult diagnostic problem.) More malignant degrees of stromal endometriosis or adenomyosis (*stromatosis*) merge imperceptibly into the patterns of an endometrial sarcoma, as noted by Symmonds and Dockerty, and Ober and Tovell. One should recall that there are certain benign epithelial-stromal tumors such as the rare papillary adenofibromas reported by Vellios.

Mixed mesodermal tumors are stromal sarcomas that also contain such *heterologous* elements as bone, cartilage, and striated muscle (Fig. 18.8). Williams and Woodruff point out the considerable confusion as to their nature and histogenesis, but today it is generally accepted that the foreign elements arise from a simple metaplasia of the common stem cell of the stroma. Norris *et al.* suggest that the presence of cartilage is a good prognostic sign. Baggish suggests that there is no point in making a distinction between carcinosarcoma and mixed mesodermal tumors and that we consider these as simple variants of endometrial sarcoma.

Taylor has reemphasized that all of the elements are of stromal (Müllerian) origin, with abnormal differentiation being responsible for the component bone and cartilage formation. With this current view we are in complete accord. The frequency of *preceding irradiation* has been noted in most reports of these tumors and in reviewing 400 reported cases Williams and Woodruff observed this in one-third. A recent case in association with bilateral thecoma has been reported by Laurian and Monroe. The prognosis is poor with

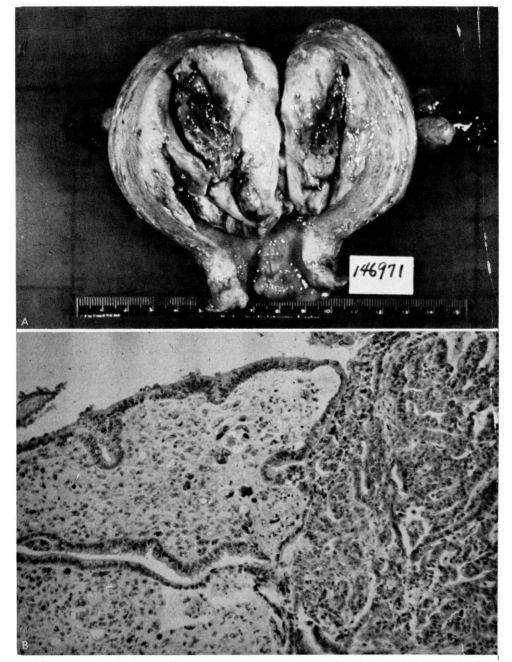

18.8. Mixed mesodermal tumor. *Top*, gross pathology characterized by polypoid lesions arising from endometrial surfaces. *Bottom*, histologically, various sarcomatous and carcinoid elements of mesodermal origin
may be noted.

frequent metastases to distant parts of the
body as well as the regional nodes, and
Taylor has noted only six survivors in 40
patients studied, Norris *et al.* record 19%
salvage.

Certain of these lesions seem to involve
the cervix and vagina even in adults.
There seems a close kinship between
these and the *sarcoma botryoides* of
vagina and cervix, seen primarily in

children, although the histogenesis is not necessarily the same (see Chapter on Vagina).

MURAL SARCOMA

These may at times arise as nodular and fairly circumscribed tumors, so that it may be difficult to be sure whether or not the tumor was preceded by a benign myoma. More often, however, they are much more diffuse in their growth so that they may produce a fairly uniform enlargement of the uterus, which may even resemble an early pregnancy. The same thing is true of the diffuse varieties arising from the endometrial stroma. These myometrial and endometrial lesions are rare.

LYMPHOMAS

The various lymphoid malignancies are rare in the uterus, but still more commonly found than in the ovary. Ober and Tovell have noted occasional cases of lymphosarcoma which present primarily in the uterus with no apparent evidence of this disease in other areas of the body and, more recently, Wright has recorded a "solitary malignant lymphoma." Leukemoid deposits may likewise involve the genital tract, but generally in connection with an extensive spread or infiltrates so that the prognosis is very poor. In any case the outcome with any pelvic lymphoma is guarded.

Clinical Characteristics

The disease most frequently affects women during the middle period of life, our own series showing the highest incidence during the fifth decade. Most authors agree that the prognosis is better in the younger rather than the postmenopausal patient. Any portion of the uterus may be the seat of the tumor, although the body is far more frequently involved than is the cervix. The greater frequency of corporeal as compared with cervical myomas will no doubt explain in part at least the prediction of sarcoma for the corpus uteri.

The *symptomatology* is not distinctive, and is usually that of myoma in which most sarcomas arise. The diagnosis is not made until operation, or even more frequently, not until the pathological examination. *Abnormal bleeding* may be entirely absent, especially when the endometrium is not involved. On the other hand, it may be of great significance, especially when it occurs after the menopause, and particularly when in these postmenopausal cases the uterus is the seat of presumably myomatous enlargement. In younger women there may be either menstrual excess or intermenstrual bleeding, or both. Needless to say the hemorrhage is in any event only suggestive of possible malignancy, and carcinoma will be found more frequently to be its cause than sarcoma.

Certain tumors arise *retroperitoneally* and, although they are generally not of pelvic origin, must be considered in differential diagnosis. Clinically they may present as a pelvic mass of considerable size with no associated menstrual abnormality. Pratt has pointed out the surgical difficulties with these lesions which are usually lymphomas or sarcomas.

Abnormal discharge is common, but *pain* is usual only in advanced disease, along with *anemia, cachexia,* and *weakness. Rapid increase in the size of myomatous tumors*, especially when associated with bleeding, should likewise suggest the possibility of sacoma. Although recurrence and metastases with a fatal outcome are usually rapid, there are such exceptions as that noted by Drake and Dobben. They report a case with probable recurrence 18 years after complete operation and recovery, and their publication, with microscopic sections, would seem to suggest that it is a recurrent rather than a new malignancy.

Extension of the disease is by direct continuity (Fig. 18.9), by the blood stream, and less commonly by the lymphatics. The hematogenous route is most important in metastasis, which therefore is more characteristically systematic rather than regional. Among the organs most frequently involved are the lungs and liver. Chest x-ray is routine when uterine sarcoma is diagnosed.

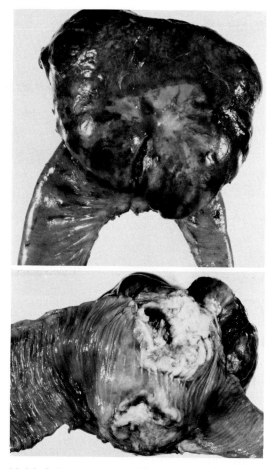

18.9A. Leiomyosarcoma with extension to bowel. **B.** Above with invasion bowel lumen.

Treatment

Because of the difficulties of diagnosis, the treatment of sarcoma is often a matter of expediency rather than of deliberate planning. Surgery has been, and still is, the backbone of treatment, especially as so large a proportion of sarcomas are not discovered until operation for supposed myoma, or until the laboratory examination of such supposedly benign tumors. The possibility of *sarcomatous change* in *myomas* must always be borne in mind by the surgeon, and it is a wise precaution to cut into the tumor masses as soon as the uterus is removed, for a presumptive diagnosis of sarcoma can sometimes be made from the gross appearance of the cut surface.

Occasionally sarcoma is found after myomectomy has been performed or, more frequently in earlier days, when subtotal hysterectomy was the operation of choice, yet many patients were cured with no further treatment. It would seem that the patient's salvation was due to the fact that many of the sarcomas developing in myomas are comparatively early and of a relatively low degree of malignancy, *i.e.*, cellular myoma. When endometrial sarcoma is diagnosed preoperatively by curettage it is treated like adenocarcinoma, *i.e.*, hysterectomy with possible subsequent irradiation. This type of lesion seems more radiosensitive than leiomyosarcoma. The recent case report by Pellillo in which a pulmonary metastasis from a recurrent "proliferative stromatosis" underwent a two-year remission following *large dosage progesterone therapy* suggests that this hormone may be effective in certain cases where the malignancy involves not only the adenomatous but also the stromal portion of the endometrium.

Even the most extensive surgery and the most complete radiotherapy will fail to curse the more malignant types of sarcoma when these have reached an advanced stage, as they unfortunately often do, before the patient comes to operation. These advanced cases are poor operative risks as a result of such factors as extreme anemia, cachexia, and early extension and metastasis. The preferable plan to treatment is hysterectomy followed by irradiation, although there is considerable question as to how effective deep x-ray may be, especially with leiomyosarcoma. Chemotherapy is generally ineffectual (Malkasian *et al.*), although more recently Hoovis has obtained a one-year remission of metastatic endometrial sarcoma with cyclophosphamide.

REFERENCES

Aaro, L. A., and Dockerty, M. B.: Leiomyosarcoma of the uterus. Amer. J. Obstet. Gynec., 77: 1187, 1959.

Aaro, L. A., Symmonds, R. E., and Dockerty, M. B.: Sarcoma of the uterus. Amer. J. Obstet. Gynec., 94: 101, 1966.

Baggish, M. S.: Mesenchymal tumors of the uterus. Clin. Obstet. Gynec., 17: 51, 1974.

Bartsich, E. G., O'Leary, J. A., and Moore, J. G.: Carcinosarcoma of the uterus. Obstet. Gynec., 30: 518, 1967.

Bartsich, E. G., Bowe, E. T., and Moore, J. G.: Leiomyosarcoma of the uterus. Obstet. Gynec., *32:* 101, 1968.

Carleton, C. C., and Williamson, J. W.: Osteogenic sarcoma of the uterus. Arch. Path., *20:* 121, 378, 1961.

Chuang, J. T., Van Velder, D. J., and Graham, J. B.: Carcinoma and mixed mesoderal tumors of the uterus. Obstet. Gynec., *35:* 769, 1970.

Cope, E.: Adenocarcinoma of the endometrium with malignant stromatosis. J. Obstet. Gynaec. Brit. Comm., *65:* 58, 1958.

Corscaden, J. A., and Singh, B. P.: Leiomyosarcoma of uterus. Amer. J. Obstet. Gynec., *75:* 149, 1958.

Crawford, E. J., and Tucker, W.: Sarcoma of the uterus. Amer. J. Obstet. Gynec., *77:* 286, 1959.

Donkers, B., Kazzas, B. A., and Meijening, W.: Rhabdomyosarcoma of the corpus uteri. Amer. J. Obstet. Gynec., *114:* 1025, 1972.

Drake, E. T., and Dobben, G. D.: Leiomyosarcoma of the uterus with unusual metastasis. J.A.M.A. *170:* 1294, 1959.

Giarratona, R. C., and Slate, T. A.: Sarcomas of the uterus. Obstet. Gynec., *38:* 472, 1971.

Hahn, G. A.: Gynecologic considerations in malignant lymphoma. Amer. J. Obstet. Gynec., *75:* 673, 1958.

Hall, J. E.: Leiomyosarcoma of the uterus. Obstet. Gynec., *38:* 629, 1971.

Hoovis, M. L.: Response of endometrial sarcoma to cyclophosphamide. Amer. J. Obstet. Gynec., *108,* 117, 1970.

Hughesdon, P. E., and Cocks, D. P.: Endometrial sarcoma complicating cystic hyperplasia. J. Obstet. Gynaec. Brit. Comm., *62:* 567, 1955.

Hunter, W. C.: Benign and malignant (sarcoma) stromal endometriosis. Surgery, *34:* 258, 1953.

Hunter, W. C., Nohlgren, J. S., and Lancefield, S. M.: Stromal endometriosis or endometrial sarcoma. Amer. J. Obstet. Gynec., *72:* 1072, 1956.

Jensen, P. A., Dockerty, M. B., Symmonds, R. E., and Wilson, R. B.: Endometrioid sarcoma ("stromal endometriosis") Amer. J. Obstet. Gynec., *95:* 79, 1966.

Kelly, H. A., and Cullen, T. S.: *Myomata of the Uterus.* W. B. Saunders Company, Philadelphia, 1909.

Koss, L. G., Spiro, R. H., and Bronschwig, A.: Endometrial sarcoma. Surg. Gynec. Obstet., *121:* 531, 1965.

Laurain, A. R., and Monroe, T. C.: Mixed mesodermal sarcoma of the corpus uteri with associated bilateral thecoma. Amer. J. Obstet. Gynec., *78:* 613, 1959.

Malkasian, G. D., Jr., Mussey, E., Decker, D. G., and Johnson, C. E.: Chemotherapy of gynecologic sarcomas. Cancer Chemother. Rep., *51:* 507, 1967.

Montague, A., Schwarz, D. P., and Woodruff, J. D.: Leiomyosarcoma originating in myoma. Amer. J. Obstet. Gynec., *92:* 421, 1965.

Norris, H. J. Roth, E., and Taylor, H. B.: Mesenchymal tumors of the uterus. II. A clinical and pathological study of 31 mixed mesodermal tumors. Obstet. Gynec., *28:* 57, 1966.

Ober, W. B.: Uterine sarcomas; histogenesis and taxonomy. Ann. N.Y. Acad. Sci., *75:* 568, 1959.

Ober, W. B., and Tovell, H. M.: Mesenchymal sarcomas of the uterus. Amer. J. Obstet. Gynec., *77:* 246, 1959.

Ober, W. B., and Tovell, H. M.: Malignant lymphomas of the uterus. Bull. Sloane Hosp., *5:* 65, 1959.

Pellillo, D.: Proliferative stromatosis of the uterus with pulmonary metastases. Obstet. Gynec., *31:* 33, 1968.

Piven, M. S., *et al.:* Embryonal rhabdomyosarcoma. Obstet. Gynec., *42:* 522, 1973.

Pratt, J. H.: Some surgical considerations of retroperitoneal tumors. Amer. J. Obstet. Gynec., *87:* 956, 1963.

Radman, H. M., and Korman, W.: Sarcoma of the uterus. Amer. J. Obstet. Gynec., *78:* 604, 1959.

Retikas, D. G. Hodkgin's sarcoma of the cervix. Amer. J. Obstet. Gynec., *80:* 1104, 1960.

Rubin, A.: Histogenesis of carcinosarcoma of the uterus. Amer. J. Obstet. Gynec., *77:* 269, 1959.

Schiffer, M. A., and Mackles, A.: Stromal endometriosis. Obstet. Gynec., *7:* 531, 1956.

Silverberg, S. G.: Leiomyosarcoma of the uterus. Obstet. Gynec., *38:* 613, 1971.

Stearns, H. C., and Sneeden, V. D.: Leiomyosarcoma of the uterus. Amer. J. Obstet. Gynec., *95:* 374, 1966.

Symmonds, R. E., and Dockerty, M. B.: Sarcoma and sarcoma-like proliferations of the endometrial stroma. Surg. Gynec. Obstet., *100:* 232, 322, 1955.

Symmonds, R. E., Dockerty, M. B., and Pratt, J. H.: Sarcoma and sarcoma-like proliferation of the endometrial stroma. Amer. J. Obstet. Gynec., *73:* 1054, 1957.

Taylor, C. W.: Mixed mesodermal tumors of the female genital tract. J. Obstet. Gynaec. Brit. Comm., *65:* 177, 1958.

Vellios, F., Ng, A. B. P., and Reagan, J. W.: Papillary adenofibroma of the uterus. Amer. J. Clin. Path., *60:* 543, 1973.

Webb, G. A.: Uterine sarcoma. Obstet. Gynec., *6:* 38, 1955.

Williams, T. J., and Woodruff, J. D.: Similarities in malignant mixed mesenchymal tumors of the endometrium. Obstet. Gynec. Survey, *17:* 1, 1962.

Wright, C. J. E.: Solitary malignant lymphoma uterus. Amer. J. Obstet. Gynec., *117:* 114, 1973.

chapter 19

Pelvic Infection

ACUTE PELVIC INFLAMMATORY DISEASE

Pelvic inflammatory disease is usually secondary to upward migration of various bacteria introduced at a lower level, although in its incipient form there may be remarkably little in the way of symptomatology. In any case, the course of the disease is dependent on the strain and virulence of the particular organisms involved, as well as individual body resistance to the offending bacteria. Although in most cases the tubes seem to bear the primary impact of the infectious process, there is a strong tendency for extension to the ovaries and pelvic peritoneum as a result of the propinquity of these structures to the uterus and tubes, and the intimacy of the lymphatic and vascular supply of all the pelvic organs (Fig. 19.1).

Thus, the syndrome of genital infection is frequently a composite one, produced by various degrees of tubal involvement, with or without extension to the ovaries and pelvic peritoneum. As a rule, the uterus itself is more or less immune to the inflammatory impact, for although there may be a very definite pathological involvement of the endometrial surface, this contributes little to the general symptomatology. This composite clinical syndrome is usually designated as *pelvic inflammatory disease,* and although there are many exceptions, the usual tendency is to begin with a rather acute episode, followed by either complete resolution or else gradual subsidence into a more chronic process characterized by not infrequent acute or subacute resurgence.

Etiology

From an etiological as well as from a clinical standpoint, one may distinguish three basic types of pelvic inflammatory disease.

(1) Gonorrheal, due to infection by the Gonococcus, and comprising the largest proportion, about 60% of all cases, although recent studies by Lukasik find the Gonococcus much less frequent than intestinal bacilli in tubal cultures. This should not imply any decrease in gonorrheal disease, for frequently culture is negative in cases of undoubted gonococcal tubo-ovarian abscess.

(2) Pyogenic, due to infection by any one of a number of organisms, most frequently the Streptococcus (aerobic or anaerobic), Staphylococcus, *Escherichia coli,* etc. It is this variety of infection which is chiefly concerned in the frequent

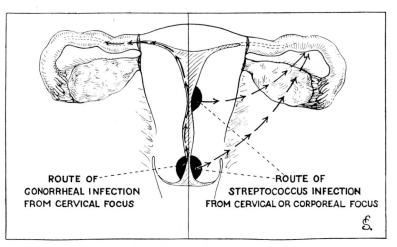

19.1. Two chief routes of pelvic infection

cases of puerperal, postabortive, and postoperative infection.

(3) Tuberculous, the result of infection by the tubercle bacillus, and embracing approximately 5% of the cases of pelvic inflammatory disease in areas where poverty and malnutrition abound. This form of pelvic infection is of chronic nature, and is discussed in Chapter 20.

(4) Such rare entities as *actinomycosis, schistosomiasis,* and other rare *tropical infections* do not seem to warrant extensive discussion.

Gonorrheal Type

Incidence

Gonorrhea seems to be increasing in incidence and currently represents a problem afflicting all social strata, particularly in large urban areas. If routine cultures are obtained as part of a screening program in asymptomatic women, as many as 5%, even among private patients, may be found to harbor a gonococcal infection.

Pathology

The immediate focus in most cases of infection of the upper genital tract is gonorrheal involvement of the cervix, urethra, rectum, or any mucus membrane. In many instances the infection seems to be self-limiting, with spontaneous resolution within two weeks, al-

though this does not imply a cure, and many such women may be asymptomatic carriers of the disease.

In a certain number of cases, however, possibly in the nature of 10 per cent, upper genital tract involvement may occur as the organisms make their way by surface invasion along the endometrium to the tube, and often beyond this to the peritoneum and ovary. It is only when there is tubal spread of the disease that the characteristic symptoms of pelvic inflammatory disease become apparent.

Acute Endometritis of Gonorrheal Type

This form is encountered rather rarely in the pathological laboratory, inasmuch as both curettage and hysterectomy are usually contraindicated in the course of acute gonorrheal infections. It is characterized grossly by edema and hyperemia of the mucosa, and microscopically by edema and infiltration by large numbers of polymorphonuclear leukocytes. Its tendency is toward spontaneous resolution, because of the usually good drainage of the uterine canal, and even more because of the monthly desquamation of menstruation with gradual attenuation in each cycle. Whether the endometrium itself destroys the gonococcal pathogen by some type of immunological reaction, as has been suggested, seems highly uncertain; however,

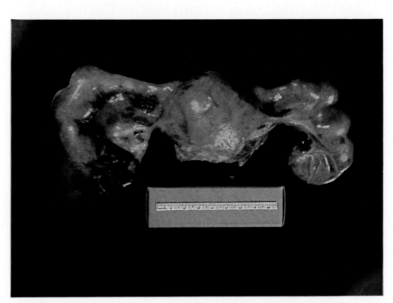

Plate 19.1. Typical appearance of chronic salpingitis (cervix removed separately)

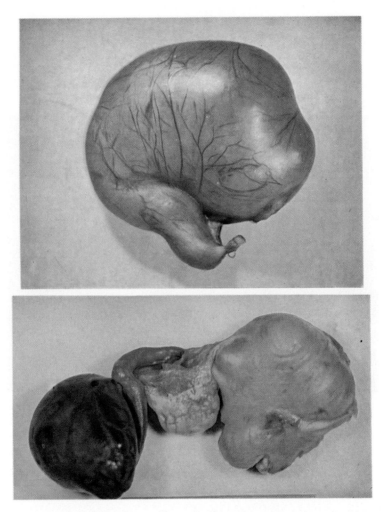

Plate 19.2. *Top,* large thin-walled hydrosalpinx. *Bottom,* moderate-sized hydrosalpinx which has undergone torsion in its distal portion.

there is often scant evidence of endometritis despite extensive chronic tubal or tubo-ovarian infection.

Acute Salpingitis

This may be an almost immediate sequel of acute gonorrheal infection of the lower genital tract, or it may not occur until long afterward, perhaps many months or even years after the original infection. Because the organisms reach the tube by way of the mucous membrane, it is not surprising that the latter is the primary site of the pathological changes. It becomes edematous and soon gives forth an exudate which, except in the mildest cases, is purulent. This type of involvement is unfortunate for the patient, in that distention and later occlusion of the tube so frequently occurs, with sterility a common sequel. The exudate may escape from the still open end of the tube, producing *acute pelvic peritonitis* and sometimes *pelvic abscess.*

The inflammatory process is rarely limited to the endosalpinx alone, the whole tube being swollen, hyperemic, and reddened. Occlusion of the fimbriated orifice or of other parts of the lumen may occur, with the production of a *pyosalpinx,* although this is more often encountered in an acute exacerbation of the chronic form. *Pelvic abscess* may result from bacterial invasion or even escape of purulent exudate into the pelvis. Finally, and most frequently, the subsidence of the acute infection leaves a residue of chronic salpingitis of one form or another (Plate 9.1).

The *microscopic characteristics* of acute gonorrheal salpingitis are like those of acute inflammation in general. The chief features are infiltration with polymorphonuclear leukocytes, hyperemia, and edema (Fig. 19.2). In the milder cases the epithelium may be intact (Fig. 19.3), but in the more severe forms it shows degeneration and often is lost over considerable areas, with frequent involvement of the muscular and serous coat.

A very important characteristic of acute gonorrheal salpingitis, and one which has a great bearing on the practical treatment of such cases, is the tendency of the infecting organisms to disappear within a

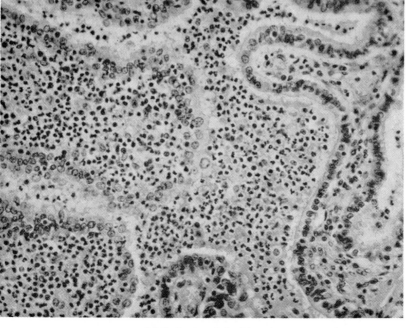

19.2. Acute salpingitis

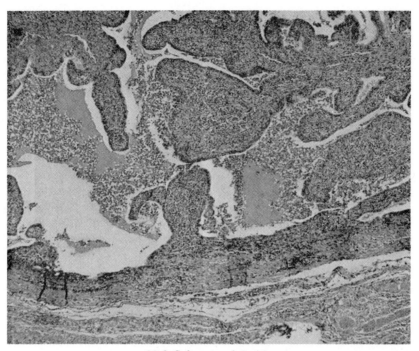

19.3. Subacute salpingitis

short time, ordinarily about 10 days, so that culture is often sterile. Desultory antibiotic treatment may further confuse the issue, as has been confirmed by Blinick.

In discussing the current status of gonorrhea, Simpson and Brown deplore the efficacy of past methods in detection and treatment. They suggest that the use of fluorescent antibody technique, as noted by Deacon, will disclose that a considerable number of promiscuous although asymptomatic women may harbor the gonococcus. While the gram stain is extremely helpful, it is not always possible to have facilities available to perform this. Fortunately, however, various culture methods (Thayer-Martin, Transgrow, etc.) have been devised. They seem to be accurate and convenient provided there is no undue delay, heat, or drying.

Septic or Pyogenic Type

The pyogenic form of acute salpingitis usually follows *childbirth* or *abortion,* the latter especially of the criminal type, but may be a sequel to any type of pelvic surgery, often vaginal hysterectomy. The infecting organism, generally the Strepto-coccus or Staphylococcus, reaches the tube by a route quite different from that followed by the Gonococcus (Fig. 19.1), and the resulting changes in the tube are likewise quite different from those described for the gonorrheal variety. From portals of entry in the lower genital canal, usually the cervix, the organisms are disseminated outward through the veins and lymphatics of the broad ligaments. *Thrombophlebitis* and *lymphangitis* with cellulitis and even abscess of the broad ligaments are frequent results.

It might be appropriate to note that Fathalla (Egypt) and Sarma (India) have tabulated a list of exotic diseases which may cause infection in the gravid or normal woman. Kala-azar, bilharziasis, malaria, and other diseases rarely seen in this country deserve consideration in various pelvic disorders seen in certain tropical areas, as does schistosomiasis (Bachany *et al.*).

Acute Endometritis (Fig. 19.4)

In the milder forms of infection, the endometrium may be merely hyperemic and edematous, but in the more virulent infections, it may show extensive necrosis. With this one also finds in most cases degenerated villi and decidual tissue, and not infrequently extensive hemorrhage and thrombosis. On occasion a postabortal infection may be due to the *Clostridium welchii,* and women harboring this organism may be critically ill with general sepsis, shock, and renal failure. Massive antibiotics and such heroic measures as dialysis or an artificial kidney may not suffice; Rabinowitz *et al.* suggest the desirability of hysterectomy, and in a small group of cases this seemed to produce better results, especially if combined with a massive dosage of drugs.

Acute Parametritis and Salpingitis

There may be extreme induration and thickening of the parametrium (*parametritis*) so that the resultant tubal involvement is in essence a peri- rather than an endosalpingitis. The infection reaches the tube from the outside, so to speak, and this explains why the resulting salpingitis is of interstitial type, with little or no involvement of the mucosa. The cross section of such a tube characteristically shows an enormously thickened and infiltrated mesosalpinx, with great thickening of the tubal wall, but with a lumen which is quite normal and which is lined by an almost intact mucosa.

This is in sharp contrast to the *gonorrheal* form, in which the destructive force of the infection is vented upon the mucosa primarily, with frequent occlusion of the lumen and subsequent sterility. Obstruction at the fimbriated ends of the tube may lead to enormous purulent distention of the tube (pyosalpinx (Fig. 19.5)) as noted earlier. On the other hand, the prognosis as to childbearing following *pyogenic* infection of the tubes is much better, and one not infrequently observes later pregnancies in cases of extensive pelvic inflammation of the pyogenic type.

The *microscopic picture* of acute pyogenic salpingitis, as might be expected, is that of a normal or only slightly infiltrated mucosa, with great thickening of the muscularis as a result of edema and

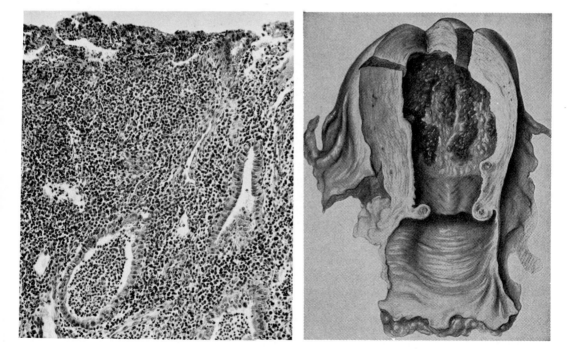

19.4. (*left*) Acute endometritis. Note the purulent exudate in the glands. (*right*) Acute necrotic endometritis. (From Watson, B. P.: In *Obstetrics and Gynecology,* edited by A. H. Curtis. W. B. Saunders Company, Philadelphia, 1933.)

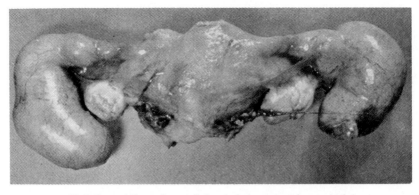

19.5. Large bilateral pyosalpinx (cervix removed separately)

leukocytic infiltration, along with some degree of acute fibrinous peritonitis of the tubal serosa.

Acute Oophoritis

The ovary not infrequently participates in acute pelvic inflammatory processes, because of its proximity to the tube. However, one only rarely observes oophoritis except in association with salpingitis, whereas, on the other hand, the ovary is frequently uninvolved even in the presence of severe tubal inflammation, either acute or chronic. The fact remains, however, that acute oophoritis, and even ovarian abscess, is at times found as a part of acute pelvic inflammatory disease, although abscesses are also often seen in association with longstanding chronic inflammation. Pelvic abscesses are often tubo-ovarian, representing the merging of tubal and ovarian cavities. *Ovarian abscess* with normal tubes is occasionally seen as a sequel to posthysterectomy infection which apparently spreads along lymphatic routes. Wilson and Black point out that this most commonly follows vaginal hysterectomy.

Acute Pelvic Peritonitis

In either the gonorrheal or pyogenic forms of infection acute pelvic peritonitis is a common concomitant. This manifests itself most frequently in the form of serous or fibrinous exudates with early development of adhesions between any of the adjoining pelvic structures, or between these and the small intestine, sigmoid, or rectum.

As a result of exudation of infected material from the tube, or perhaps more frequently through the virulence of the peritoneal infection itself, *pelvic abscess* frequently results. It is not always easy to distinguish clinically between large abscesses within the tube or ovary (tubo-ovarian abscesses) and the extratubal variety, in which the pus is situated in the pelvic cavity proper, generally in the cul-de-sac, in which case its upper wall is usually formed by the matted and adherent intestinal coils. The usual location of the pelvic abscess in the region of the cul-de-sac points the way to its easy evacuation by incision through the posterior vaginal vault (*posterior colpotomy*). Occasionally this is utilized in the postsurgical patient in whom there has been persistent slight bleeding; this may localize in the cul-de-sac and, if secondarily infected, may form an infected pelvic hematocele, amenable to drainage.

Symptoms and Signs
Gonorrheal Form

The gonorrheal form may follow this infection in the lower genital canal, or at times its nature can be assumed if there is a history of recent gonorrheal infection in the marital partner. In many cases, the acute symptoms appear during or immediately after a menstrual period due to greater vulnerability of the uterine cavity to gonorrheal invasion at the time of menstrual desquamation. Severe *pain* in the pelvic and lower abdominal region, *muscular rigidity,* and *tenderness, ab-*

dominal distention, *nausea and vomiting, fever, leukocytosis, rapid pulse,* with considerable *prostration* in the severe cases, are the common symptoms. The fever may reach 103° or even higher, with a marked leukocytosis, increased pulse rate, and evidence of a pelvic peritonitis.

Pelvic Examination. This may be difficult and unsatisfactory, because of the patient's pain, tenderness, and rigidity. When the uterus can be outlined, it is apt to be rather fixed, and efforts to move it by manipulation of the cervix cause much pain. There is extreme bilateral tenderness, but no definite mass or enlargement of the adnexa can be made out. When the fever and pelvic pain persist, accompanied often by rectal pressure and pain, examination may reveal increasing induration, with later fluctuation and even bulging, in the region of the cul-de-sac, at times extending into the sides of the pelvis and perhaps downward along the posterior vaginal wall to a level which may be considerably lower than the cervix. Such findings leave no doubt as to the presence of a *pelvic abscess.*

Postpartum and Postabortive Types

In these cases the patient is often very weak and septic, with evidence of local trauma in the perineum and vagina, so that much gentleness is necessary in the examination, ideally performed with sterile technique. The cervix is apt to be lacerated and infected, especially if the pelvic infection follows full term delivery. The uterus is large and incompletely involuted, whereas in early criminal abortions, it is only slightly enlarged. Even gentle manipulation of the uterus may be quite painful. One must always be cognizant of the possibility of uterine perforation and other trauma associated with criminal abortion. Thrombophlebitis is a frequent complication (Fig. 19.7 and Fig. 19.8).

Where the infection has invaded the broad ligaments the latter may be enormously thickened and infiltrated (*broad ligament cellulitis*). When broad ligament abscesses are present, as they often are at a later stage, the lateral masses are even large. In some cases,

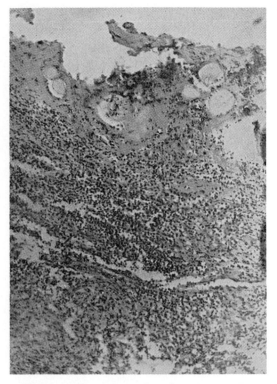

19.6. Acute puerperal endometritis. (From Watson, B. P.: In *Obstetrics and Gynecology,* edited by A. H. Curtis, W. B. Saunders Co., Philadelphia, 1933.)

however, the broad ligaments show little involvement, and the enlarged and inflamed adnexa may be palpated as irregular, tender masses in the sides of the pelvis. Marked thickening, infiltration, and tenderness of the broad and uterosacral ligaments is a frequent manifestation of the *parametritis* so commonly present.

Infection following IUD

In the last decade the intrauterine device (IUD) has gained wide acceptance in all parts of the world. Various adverse results have been noted, as will be indicated in succeeding chapters. Indeed, an earlier study by Scott has recorded at least 10 deaths primarily due to pelvic inflammation, peritonitis, and other complications. Actually it is difficult to be sure of how many cases of pelvic inflammation following insertion of an IUD are actually associated with the device or represent merely a flare up of a pre-

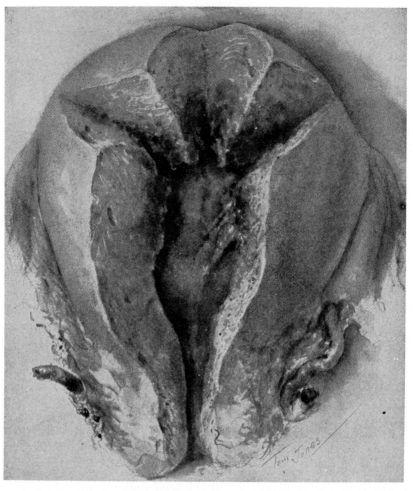

19.7. Acute postabortive infection. Uterus large and edematous. Necrosis of uterine wall at placental site. Remnant of retained placental tissue. Bilateral thrombosis of uterine veins. (From Danforth, D. W.: In *Obstetrics and Gynecology,* edited by A. H. Curtis. W. B. Saunders Company, Philadelphia, 1933.)

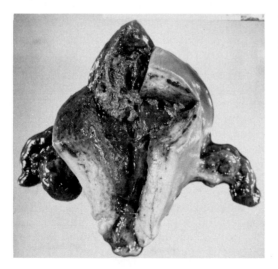

19.8. Gas-gangrene (postabortal) complicated by complete renal shutdown.

existing pelvic inflammatory disease. Infection seems most fulminating if pregnancy occurs with certain IUDs in place.

That insertion of an IUD may produce pelvic inflammation seems likely, particularly where there is a severe cervicitis, so that bacterial contamination of the uterine cavity may be produced in its insertion. Mishell and Moyer, however, point out that when an inflammatory disease occurs more than a month after insertion of an IUD it seems unlikely that the IUD should be incriminated as the cause of the problem. Many individuals feel that general pelvic infection associated with insertion of an IUD does not seem particularly common. Personal experience based on endometria reviewed in our pathology laboratory of patients who wore an IUD, seems to indicate that there is always an inflammatory reaction present (Figs. 19.9, 19.10). It has, however, been suggested that the culture is almost uniformly sterile, and this might imply merely some type of antigen-antibody immune reaction. Nevertheless in this community a number of gynecologists have certain reservations about the use of the IUD because of the possibility of infection as well as other complications. Indeed, because of a number of serious and even fatal infections associated with pregnancy and an IUD, a certain type of device has been withdrawn from the market.

Diagnosis

Gonorrheal Infection

A history of gonorrhea in either the patient or her husband is of great value in diagnosis, but this is lacking in the great majority of cases. The occurrence of

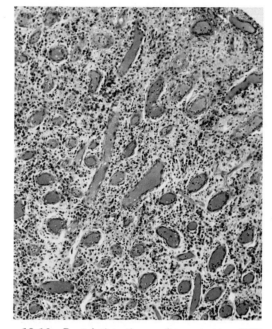

19.10. Granulation tissue after extensive IUD contraception. This involves full thickness endometrium (cavity above).

severe lower abdominal pain, usually bilateral, during or just after menstruation, with lower abdominal tenderness and rigidity, moderate tympanites, fever, often nausea and vomiting, rapid pulse, leukocytosis, leukorrhea, and marked pelvic tenderness on bimanual examination, will usually suffice to make the diagnosis reasonably certain. When acute cervicitis or urethritis is present, gonococci are occasionally demonstrable in the discharges. Culture will be decisive.

Pyogenic Infection

Here the history of onset following delivery or abortion is of obvious importance, but postabortal patients are often reluctant to even admit the possibility of pregnancy although in this era of "abortion on demand," the woman may be more honest and accurate. The symptomatology is similar to that described for the gonorrheal group except that in the more virulent cases, usually of streptococcal type, the systemic reaction is more acute. The symptoms may manifest themselves within six or eight hours or not for a number of days

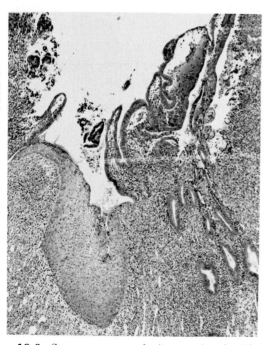

19.9. Squamous metaplasia associated with prolonged usage of IUD.

following the delivery or abortion. There is a tendency to localization in the pelvis, with often a residue in the form of a large pelvic inflammatory mass or a broad ligament cellulitis or abscess. Thrombophlebitis with septic emboli may occur. Unlike the gonorrheal cases, the fever in cases of this group is apt to persist, dragging along for weeks. The importance of blood cultures, both aerobic and anaerobic, cannot be too strongly emphasized.

Many clinicians feel that evacuation of the necrotic uterine contents will decrease the fever much sooner and thus avoid prolonged hospitalization. Massive dosage of antibiotics for less than 24 hours is followed by (suction) curettage, a procedure undreamed of for the febrile patient heretofore. Yet preliminary results indicate no ill effects, and make possible great financial and time saving to the patient. Considerable care must be exercised not to perforate the soft edematous uterus, with added injury to bowel or bladder.

Differential Diagnosis

Acute Appendicitis

Although the initial pain in acute appendicitis may be diffuse, it soon tends to localize in the McBurney area. There is only slight fever, with a leukocytosis which in proportion to the fever is much higher than with pelvic inflammation. The problem is more difficult and sometimes impossible in the case of a perforative appendicitis with peritonitis. Under such conditions the abdominal pain, tenderness, and rigidity, like that of acute pelvic inflammation, involve the whole lower abdominal zone. Moreover, fever may be quite high and the pulse rapid. Although pelvic examination may show some tenderness even in cases of appendiceal peritonitis, it is rarely as clearcut and pronounced as in the severe case of acute pelvic inflammation, while in some cases of the latter definite adnexal enlargement, or possibly even a pelvic abscess, may be palpable. In the occasional case where it is impossible to distinguish between an acute salpingitis

and appendicitis, laporotomy and appendectomy seems advisable, with subsequent antibiotic therapy.

Acute Pyelitis

Although the kidneys are situated far above the pelvic level, the fact remains that severe acute pyelitis can at times produce a clinical picture not unlike that of acute pelvic inflammatory disease. The pain of pyelitis usually involves chiefly the upper abdominal zone, although sometimes it is general over the entire abdomen. Palpation over the kidney region may show marked tenderness in the costovertebral angle. With pyelitis there may be a high fever and some pain, but patients do not appear as ill or distressed as with salpingitis or appendicitis.

As a rule the abdominal pain of pyelitis is preceded or accompanied by pain in the lumbar region, radiating along the flanks, and there is likely to be increased frequency of urination, with some dysuria and tenesmus, although in a surprising proportion of cases such symptoms are not elicited. Of obvious importance is microscopic examination of the catheterized urine, which in pyelitis is likely to reveal large numbers of pus cells, often in clumps. Because of edema and ureteral blockage with poor drainage, however, the urine may be entirely negative for considerable periods of time.

Rupture or Torsion of Ovarian Cyst and/or Tube

The symptomatology and clinical picture of twisted or ruptured ovarian cyst is discussed at some length in subsequent pages. At the same time it should be realized that the tube alone or both the tube and ovary may undergo torsion (Fig. 19.11). Such an accident may occur with a diseased tube and Diamant has described 4 cases of hydrosalpinx in which torsion has occurred (Plate 19.2). At the same time it may occur with intrinsically normal adnexa, and in their separate texts Woodruff and Pauerstein, and Huffman have described such sequelae. It is most prone to occur in the

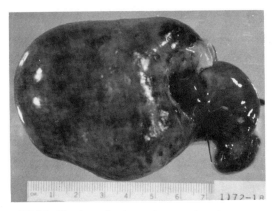

19.11. Torsion of tube and ovary (cystic corpus luteum of pregnancy).

youthful pregnant individual, but has also been described in the postmenopausal individual by Powell *et al.* The etiology is uncertain, but undue activity has been suggested as a possible factor by some authors. Considerable care should be exercised in the operative management of such cases for simple untwisting of the adnexa might conceivably release thrombi, with a potentially disastrous outcome.

In our own experience adnexal torsion seems most likely to occur in the posthysterectomy female, at which time the preserved adnexae were not firmly suspended and were permitted to dangle rather loosely from the infundibulopelvic ligament. The woman with a twisted adnexae is apt to have rather marked degrees of abdominal pain and distention, although as a rule there is not the increased leukocytosis or fever that one finds with inflammatory disease. In certain instances the symptomatology must be minimal. On occasion the gynecologist views a patient at the time of operation where one adnexa is missing without prior surgery. The explanation is probably not congenital absence but more likely a torsion at some time with resultant gangrene, atrophy, and ultimately disappearance of the tube. A rather recent example of this was a 22-year-old girl recently operated on because of asymptomatic endometriosis. About 4 years previously she has been seen be-

cause of a possible appendicitis, but surgery had not been performed. At subsequent laparotomy for the endometriosis it was seen that there was only a nubbin of right tube left, and apparently the earlier acute episode had represented torsion of the right adnexa with subsequent almost complete disappearance.

A number of other diseases may cause difficulty. Diagnosis of such other problems as endometriosis, ectopic pregnancy, etc., will be discussed in the appropriate chapters.

Treatment

Bed rest, adequate fluids, analgesics, etc., are obvious necessities in the treatment of acute pelvic inflammatory disease. It is likewise our feeling that heat in any form increases comfort and promotes resolution of the inflammatory process, and douches or sitz baths are utilized except in the extremely ill patient. Pelvic diathermy seems an expensive and cumbersome means of achieving the same effect, and this is rarely used.

Gonorrheal Inflammatory Disease

A large variety of antibiotics is effective in treating the disease, and optimal therapy would depend on the result of the cervical culture and sensitivity test which should never be neglected. Until this is available, however, something like one million units of penicillin plus 1 gm. of streptomycin should be administered daily, or else large dosage of one of the broad spectrum antibiotics. The study by Lucas *et al.* suggests that tetracycline is 20% more effective than even very large doses of penicillin, and Mead and Louria have summarized the use of the respective antibiotics in pelvic infection. The suggested therapy of both gonorrhea and syphilis in this community is tabulated in Tables 19.1, 2. A diagnosis of gonorrhea should make the clinician wary of possible syphilis.

With pelvic peritonitis, there may be profound degrees of abdominal distention due to an adynamic or *paralytic ileus,* and judicious use of a tube is important. Frequent x-rays are indicated, and one

Table 19.1

Recommended Treatment Schedules for Gonorrhea—March 1972 (USDHEW)

For *Neisseria gonorrhoeae* infection the preferred drug is penicillin G or ampicillin. Physicians are cautioned to use no less than the recommended doses of antibiotics.

FOR TREATMENT OF UNCOMPLICATED GONORRHEA
(URETHRAL, CERVICAL, PHARYNGEAL, OR RECTAL)

Parenteral—Men or Women—Aqueous procaine penicillin G, 4.8 million units intramuscularly divided into at least two doses and injected at different sites at one visit, together with 1 gram of oral probenecid, preferably given at least 30 minutes prior to the injection.

OR

Oral—Men or Women—Ampicillin, 3.5 gm., with probenecid, 1 gm., administered simultaneously.
Treatment of contacts: Patients with known exposure to gonorrhea should receive the same treatment as those known to have gonorrhea.

WHEN PENICILLIN OR AMPICILLIN IS CONTRAINDICATED,*
OR WHEN THE ABOVE SCHEDULES ARE INEFFECTIVE

Parenteral—Men—Spectinomycin, 2 gm., in one intramuscular injection.
　　　　　　Women—Spectinomycin, 4 gm., in one intramuscular injection.
Oral—Men or Women—Tetracycline HCl, 1.5 gm. initially, followed by 0.5 gm. four times a day for 4 days, a total dosage of 9 gm. Other tetracyclines are not more effective.

FOLLOW-UP

It is desirable that follow-up urethral cultures be obtained from males 7 days after completion of treatment; it is desirable that cervical and rectal cultures be obtained from females 7–14 days after completion of treatment.

COMPLICATIONS

Although treatment of complications (gonococcal salpingitis, bacteremia, arthritis, etc.) must be individualized, repeated large parenteral doses of aqueous crystalline penicillin G have been shown to be effective. The efficacy of alternative antibiotic regimens is unproven. Postgonococcal urethritis can be treated with tetracycline, 0.5 gm, orally four times a day for at least 7 days.

---

must remember that a true *mechanical obstruction* may occur. However, astute evaluation of the clinical findings and interpretation of the x-rays will generally make the distinction, although on occasion this is admittedly not easy.

Surgery is best avoided during the acute phase of inflammatory disease, and should be reserved primarily for recurrent disease in a chronic phase or when there is failure to respond to therapy. When a spiking temperature persists and examination discloses a soft, fluctuant mass dissecting down the rectovaginal septum one should suspect the development of a pelvic abscess. *Posterior colpotomy* with suitable drainage often produces dramatic results, but one must make certain the abscess is sufficiently low and fluctuant before attempting pelvic puncture.

A *ruptured tubo-ovarian abscess* must always be considered if there is a sudden deterioration of the patient with the development of severe shock, tachycardia, and hyperpyrexia. The disappearance of a previously known adnexal mass is of considerable diagnostic importance. A ruptured tubo-ovarian abscess warrants prompt surgical exploration with complete pelvic "clean-out" much preferable to a unilateral adnexectomy, as indicated by earlier work by Vermeeren and Te

Linde. Pedowitz and Bloomfield note 100% mortality in the early days of conservative therapy as opposed to a figure of 4% or less where more radical surgery plus massive antibiotic therapy was utilized. Mickal *et al.* likewise stress the desirability of aggressive therapy.

Kaplan *et al.* advise laparotomy for the tubo-ovarian abscess that does not respond promptly to adequate conservative therapy. Admittedly there is a slightly higher morbidity due primarily to gastrointestinal injury, but this must be balanced against the otherwise prolonged disability and increased hospital expenses

plus the possibility of some subsequent rupture of the abscess. Tubo-ovarian abcesses may occur in pregnancy (Hunt).

Pyogenic (Post-Abortal) Infection

Again the treatment should be conservative and large dosages of appropriate antibiotics should be utilized after culture and sensitivity tests have been obtained. Although it is permissible to remove any loose placental fragments lying in the cervical os, complete (suction) curettage is best deferred. Blood transfusions are utilized as needed, and fibrinogen determinations obtained. Oxytocics are

Table 19.2

Treatment and Post-Treatment Observation Schedule for Syphilis

Diagnosis	Treatment	Post-Treatment Observation
Primary syphilis Secondary syphilis Relapsing syphilis (clinical or serological) Early latent syphilis	2,400,000 units of Bicillin I.M. (one injection)	Once a month for 3 months; then every 3 months thereafter for the first year.
Early congenital syphilis (from infancy up to 2 years of age)	1,200,000 units of Bicillin, I.M. (one injection)	Same as for primary syphilis.
Late latent syphilis (negative spinal fluid) Late congenital syphilis, *asymptomatic* (over 2 years of age and adults)	2,400,000 units of Bicillin, I.M. (one injection)	Every 6 months for first year following completion of treatment.
Syphilis in pregnancy	According to stage of syphilis	As indicated by diagnosis. If there has never been a spinal fluid examination, should have same 3 months after delivery.
Prophylactic treatment for syphilis	2,400,000 units of Bicillin, I.M. (one injection)	Return in 3 months.
Treatment of Patients Who Are Allergic To Penicillin		
Syphilis—all stages except late and in pregnancy		Tetracycline 0.5 gm. orally 4 times a day for 15 days.
Late syphilis (neurosyphilis, cardiovascular, osseous, gumma, etc.)		Tetracycline 0.5 gm. orally 4 times a day for 20 days.
Syphilis in pregnancy		Erythromycin 0.5 gm. orally 4 times a day for 20 days.

administered where there is bleeding. Where pelvic thrombophlebitis is suspected, anticoagulant therapy should be considered (Schulman).

If bleeding is profuse, however, (suction) curettage must be performed with the greatest care to avoid perforation of the softened, edematous uterus. This is ideally postponed until there is evidence of a favorable response to antibiotic therapy. In some instances especially of the streptococcus variety most common after criminal abortions, examination may show enormous thickening and infiltration of the broad ligments. A continued septic course may indicate the presence of a broad ligament abscess which is too high to be drained by colpotomy and is best treated by a gridiron type of incision just above Pouparts ligament with extra-peritoneal drainage.

There will still be the occasional patient who does not respond to conservative therapy, and will remain critically ill with a high spiking fever. Repeat blood cultures are important because of the possibility of an incipient gram-negative bacteremia and severe endotoxic shock. In such instances, laparotomy with complete "clean-out" and adequate drainage may be a life-saving measure along with transfusions, massive amounts of antibiotics, and appropriate vasopressors. The possibility of ovarian vein thrombophlebitis must be recognized, and heparin theapy should be considered.

Pyometra

Where there is any blockage of the canal, as may occur particularly with senile changes in the cervix or upper vagina, pus may accumulate, with the formation of a pyometra (Fig. 19.12). This is particularly common with a *uterine malignancy*, especially after irradiation, and is *not* a sequel to acute endometritis in the usual young woman. Whiteley and Hamlett believe that the association of pyometra and malignancy has been overestimated and note only 14%. Where pyometra persists, they recommend hysterectomy. It is our belief that many cases follow simple senile cervical stenosis which is amenable to periodic dilatation along with estrogen suppositories.

Despite the massive accumulation of

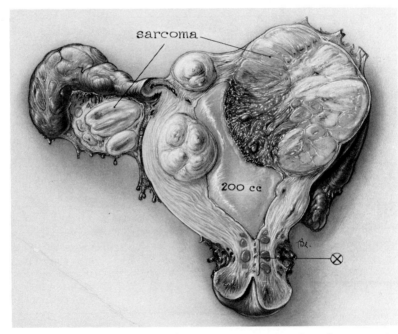

19.12. Cervical stenosis with degenerating submucous myosarcoma and resultant pyometra. (Courtesy of Dr. Erle Henricksen, Los Angeles, California.)

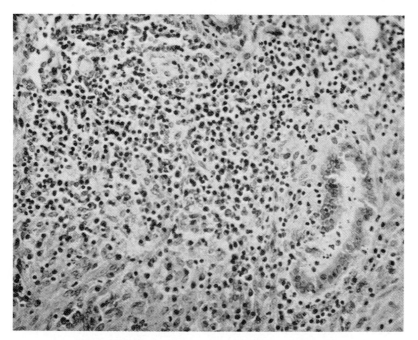

19.13. Microscopic appearance of chronic endometritis

pus, there may be little systemic reaction. Misdiagnosis is rather frequent, for the overdistended softened uterus suggests an ovarian cyst. Culture is frequently reported as sterile; however, anaerobic studies have not been performed routinely in many cases.

CHRONIC INFLAMMATORY DISEASE

Even a single attack of acute pelvic inflammation used to leave some residue of chronic disease with repeated reinfection and exacerbations. The peritoneal involvement was indicated by the development of pelvic adhesions involving the uterus, tubes, and ovaries. Currently, it would appear that the newer antibiotics may completely cure salpingitis without the usual residue of "closed tubes" and sterility. Unquestionably, this is a factor in the increased birth rate of the "ghetto patient."

Chronic Endometritis

This is a relatively common lesion, although much less than once believed. Even in the presence of extensive chronic adnexitis, the endometrium may be entirely normal, due to the usually good drainage of the uterine canal, and the monthly desquamation of menstruation. As the endometritis becomes chronic it is attenuated with each menstrual desquamation, so that after two or three cycles the endometrium is rather completely purged of its infection. Reinfections from the cervix, however, are very frequent.

The *microscopic characteristics* of chronic salpingitis are similar to those of chronic inflammation elsewhere. The chief feature is a more or less extensive infiltration with round or plasma cells (Fig. 19.13). Vasudeva *et al.* and Nolan and Osborne stress the importance of the latter in establishing a diagnosis.

One of the most common forms of chronic endometritis is the *postabortal*, although it may occur in conjunction with an intrauterine contraceptive device, submucous myoma, etc. Retention of placental tissue is frequent after either full term delivery or abortion, especially the latter. Even in spontaneous abortion, the uterine cavity is soon invaded by organisms from the cervix and vagina, so that one may expect to find chronic endometritis in numerous cases of incomplete abortion in which operative removal

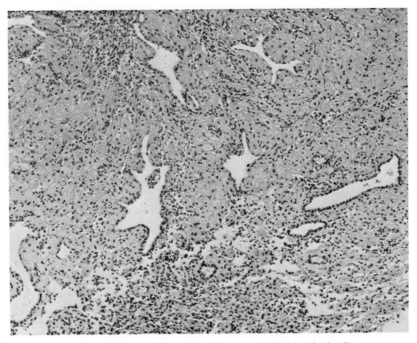

19.14. Chronic endometritis with large field of decidual cells

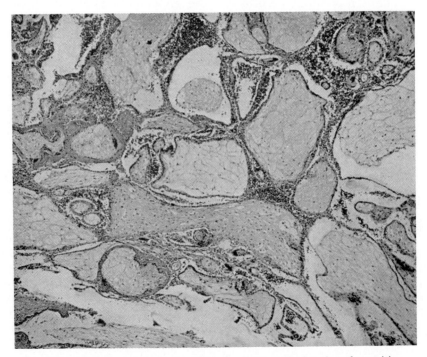

19.15. Degenerated chorionic villi in association with chronic endometritis

of the retained placental tissue is necessary. It is a good rule in all cases of chronic endometritis to examine the microscopic slides for chorionic villi and other evidences of recent pregnancy (Figs. 19.14, 15).

When villi are found they may be well preserved or they may show marked degeneration with fibrosis or hyalinization (ghost or shadow villi), at the same time retaining the characteristic two-cell lining of trophoblast. Not infrequently the retained villi may form a polypoid mass of grumous material firmly attached to the uterine wall. The finding of villi or trophoblastic cells is absolutely diagnostic of preceding pregnancy. Decidual cells are also often found, but since these are of maternal origin, they cannot be considered as decisive in diagnosis as trophoblastic elements, and they may at times be simulated by other cells. Some degree of myometritis may be a concomitant of endometritis.

Subinvolution of Uterus (Fig. 19.16)

Subinvolution of the uterus, as the term indicates, refers to the condition in which *postabortal involution* is incomplete. The term, however, is not merely a clinical one, for Schwarz and his coworkers, as well as other writers, have shown that it is characterized by distinctive histological changes. Whereas normally involution is complete in 8 or 10 weeks after delivery, the subinvoluted uterus may show, many months later, a persistent moderate enlargement and congestion, especially when it is retro-displaced, as it so commonly is. Unrelated is the syndrome of *"pelvic congestion"* as described by Taylor which seems to us to be a rather nebulous dumping ground for all kinds of vague psychosomatic problems, and a frequent excuse in attempting justification of questionable hysterectomies before tissue committees (see "Myometrial Hypertrophy," page 372).

The chief *microscopic* feature appears to be an increased amount of elastic tissue around the vessels and between the muscle bundles as a result of incompleteness of absorption of this tissue following delivery. Another characteristic finding is the formation of new blood vessels in the lumina of the degenerated and obliterated original vessels.

Chronic Salpingitis (Plate 19.1)

This may be present either in the form of a diffuse chronic inflammation of the tubal wall (chronic interstitial salpingitis; Fig. 19.17) or of certain sequelae of the inflammatory process, marked by overdistention of the tube with retained exudate (hydrosalpinx) or by various tubo-inflammatory cystic masses.

An interesting special variety of chronic salpingitis is the so-called *salpingitis isthmica nodosa* (Figs. 19.18, 19), in which the residue of a sustained chronic inflammatory process is limited chiefly to the isthmic portion of the tube. In such cases marked nodulation of the tubal isthmus is seen, the nodules being sometimes so large as to simulate small cornual fibroid tumors. The remainder of the tube may seem fairly normal, and the fimbriated end may be open.

Microscopic examination in such cases presents a curious picture, in that there may appear to be many small lumina instead of just one. The original isthmic lumen may or may not be still recognizable, but in addition to this, many

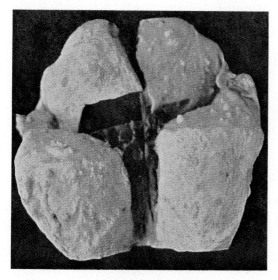

19.16. Gross picture of chronic subinvolution showing the thickness of the uterine wall and the bumpy appearance due to enlarged blood vessels.

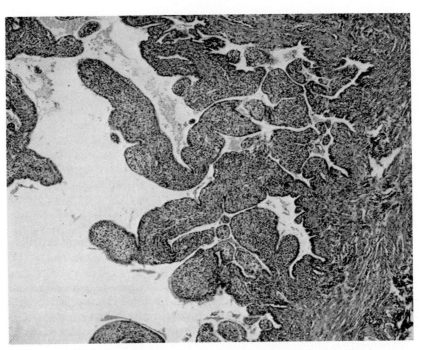

19.17. Microscopic appearance of chronic interstitial salpingitis

epithelium-lined glandlike cavities are scattered throughout the muscularis. Such cases are often mistaken for adenomyosis of the tube, but they differ from the latter in that the lining epithelium is tubal rather than uterine, that endometrial stroma is lacking, and that the muscle shows various degrees of round cell infiltration. Most evidence would suggest that long-standing inflammation and scarring leads to invagination and proliferation of the tubal epithelium, with the ultimate histological picture.

Hydrosalpinx

Gonorrheal infection especially is prone to cause inflammatory obstruction at various points in the tube, especially the

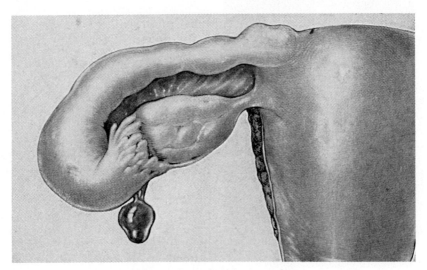

19.18. Salpingitis isthmica nodosa

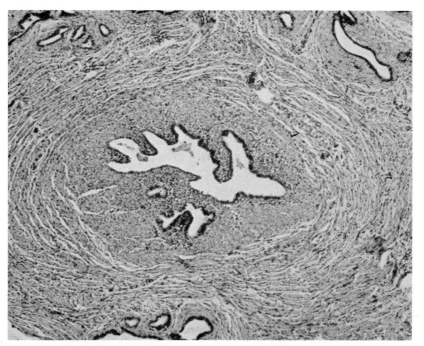

19.19. Microscopic appearance of salpingitis isthmica nodosa

uterine and fimbriated ends, and produce a *pyosalpinx,* and with absorption of the pus, a *hydrosalpinx* (Fig. 19.20); either may present as a large adherent mass frequently mistaken for an ovarian cyst.

Two types of *hydrosalpinx* are described, *simplex* and *follicularis.* In the former the lumen on cross section is seen to consist of a single thin-walled cavity. In the follicular variety, on the other hand, it is divided into a number of small compartments by trabeculae representing the fused tubal folds. In this variety, the overdistention of the lumen is preceded by a follicular salpingitis, in which this same matting together and fusion of adjacent folds takes place.

The *microscopic* appearance of *hydrosalpinx simplex* (Fig. 19.21) shows a clear cystic central cavity, with a flattened tubal mucosa whose folds have been ironed out and almost or entirely obliterated although, usually, an occasional small fold can be seen here and there. In *hydrosalpinx follicularis* (Fig. 19.22), as mentioned in the gross description, the distended lumen presents a multilocular appearance, each locule being a cross section of a gutter-like subdivision of the lumen.

Chronic Oophoritis and Perioophoritis

The ovaries may be extensively involved in chronic pelvic inflammatory disease, but on the whole much less frequently than the tubes. In most cases the ovarian involvement is secondary to that of the adjacent tube.

Perhaps the most frequent of all ovarian lesions in chronic pelvic inflammatory disease is *chronic perioophoritis,* which is practically always found when the ovarian substance is involved, and in addition is often present when the ovary itself is comparatively normal. The surface involvement of the ovary is expressed through the presence of adhesions of light or dense fibrous texture. The germinal epithelium often extends to the undersurface of such adhesions, producing slitlike or glandlike spaces (Fig. 19.23) which may be mistaken for endometriosis, especially as the epithelium often becomes cuboidal or cylindric as a result of the inflammatory stimulus.

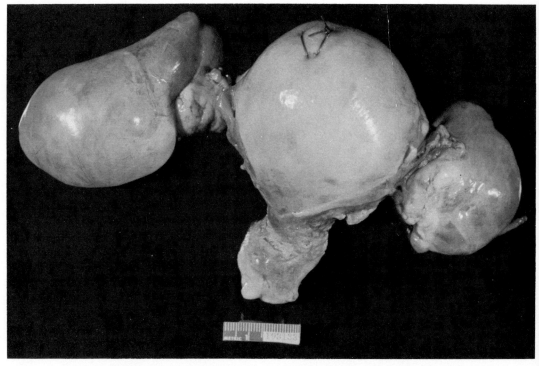

19.20. Bilateral hydrosalpinx, a probable end stage of pyosalpinx

Symptoms of Chronic Pelvic Inflammatory Disease

As a rule the symptoms develop gradually, although at any time the clinical course of chronic pelvic inflammatory disease may be punctuated by acute exacerbations.

Pain may be so severe as to incapacitate the patient, but in a surprisingly large proportion it is of moderate or mild degree, even in the presence of extensive pelvic pathology. It is expressed generally as a *bearing-down* or *aching discomfort in the lower abdominal quadrants and pelvic regions,* but it is sometimes described as sharp and severe. Rather characteristically the pain is exaggerated just before or during menstruation.

Backache and rectal discomfort or pressure are frequent complaints, explainable by the fact that the diseased adnexa impinge upon the back and rectum, to which they are not infrequently adherent. *Dysmenorrhea* is the most common of the menstrual symptoms, and it may be so severe as to

necessitate bed rest for a day or two each month. *Menorrhagia* is not uncommon, although rarely excessive, and *disturbances in menstrual rhythm* are also frequent, generally in the direction of a shortening of the intervals.

Sterility is an unfortunate feature of many cases, particularly those of gonorrheal type, this disease being one of the most important of all causes of childlessness. *Leukorrhea* of some degree is almost always noted. It is not due to the adnexal disease *per se,* but is the result of the chronic cervical infection so commonly associated. *Bladder irritability,* with increased frequency of urination, dysuria, or tenesmus, may be observed even when there is no associated inflammatory involvement of the bladder or urethra.

Diagnosis

When such symptoms as have been described develop following an acute attack of pelvic infection, the natural suspicion must be of chronic pelvic inflamma-

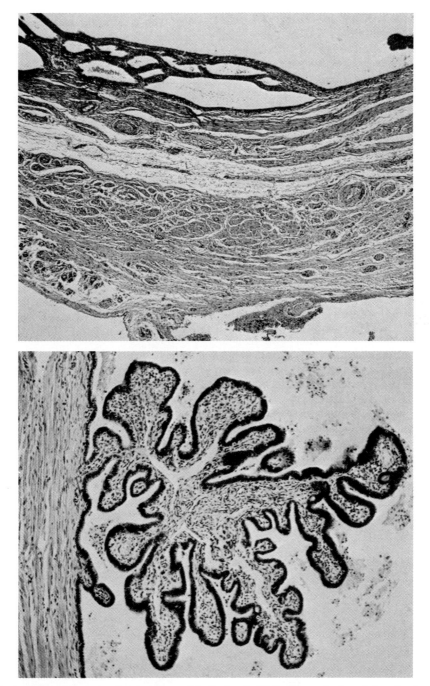

19.21 (*top*). Hydrosalpinx simplex (microscopic). (*bottom*). Wall of large hydrosalpinx simplex showing persistence of stunted tubal folds.

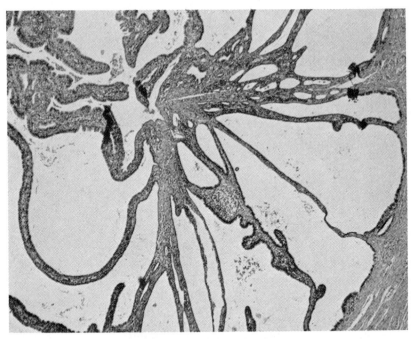

19.22. Hydrosalpinx follicularis

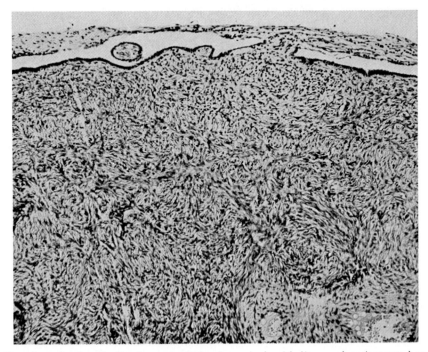

19.23. Chronic perioophoritis showing metaplasia of germinal epithelium and peritoneum beneath adhesions on surface of ovary.

tory disease. Even when no such history is obtainable, such an array of symptoms as those described in the previous section would be highly suggestive. One should remember that the Gonococcus does not respect social status.

More important than the history is the physical examination, and especially bimanual palpation of the pelvic organs. This reveals in the typical case a small or large, usually irregular, tender and rather fixed mass in both sides of the pelvis and sometimes filling the cul-de-sac. The uterus may be in normal position, but is often retroverted or retroflexed, and often much less movable than normally. Efforts to move it about by manipulation of the cervix or fundus may cause much pain, and drawing the cervix forward will also make the patient complain of pain, which not infrequently is referred to the rectum. The uterosacral ligaments are often thickened and sensitive, but not nodular as in endometriosis. Examination under anesthesia is frequently helpful, especially in the tense patient.

Differential Diagnosis

Among the pelvic conditions which may be mistaken for chronic pelvic inflammatory disease, and *vice versa,* is *ectopic pregnancy.* In the latter condition there is likely to be a history of slight delay in menstruation, followed by persistent slight bleeding of a "spotting" character. In pelvic inflammatory disease the menstrual rhythm is often not disturbed. With ectopic pregnancy the pain is likely to be colicky, severe, and one-sided, with not infrequently associated nausea and attacks of faintness. The latter are lacking in chronic pelvic inflammation, and the pain is most often bilateral and of heavy bearing-down or aching character. Pelvic examination in cases of tubal pregnancy shows a unilateral tender mass, with no tenderness in the opposite side. Laparoscopy or culdoscopy may be decisive, and these simple endoscopic methods of visualizing the pelvic organs are highly recommended in the study of many pelvic complaints.

Pelvic endometriosis is another con-dition which may be difficult to distinguish from chronic pelvic inflammatory disease. In either, there may be a history of pelvic pain, increasing dysmenorrhea, dyspareunia, and involuntary sterility; in either the pelvic examination may reveal the adnexa to be enlarged and adherent to the posterior surface of a retroplaced uterus. The presence of one or more nodules in the uterosacral ligaments is always highly suggestive of endometriosis, but this physical sign is often absent. Of circumstantial value is the fact that endometriosis is more likely to occur in the higher types of patient, whereas pelvic inflammatory disease is more apt to be seen in the dispensary group. In the presence of severe symptoms, surgery is likely to be indicated with either disease, so that failure to make an accurate preoperative diagnosis works no hardship on the patient.

Evaluation of tubal disease is often facilitated by examination under anesthesia along with curettage which may on occasion reveal a tuberculous disease. We likewise feel that a Rubin's test may be of assistance in the distinction of inflammatory disease and endometriosis, as does Sweeney.

Treatment

In women with large tubo-ovarian masses and with often a retrodisplaced uterus firmly fixed to the rectum, and with troublesome symptoms which can not be relieved by palliative measures, surgery is fully justified. This is true even in the case of younger women, especially when repeated tubal patency tests have shown the tubes to be closed. If pregnancy is to be denied such women, the next best thing is to restore them to health, as can be done in most cases by surgery.

It must also be remembered that women with chronic pelvic inflammatory disease must run the risk of acute exacerbations as a result of reinfection from the cervix or from an infected sex partner. Such is probably the usual explanation of exacerbations, rather than the assumption of a flare-up in a dormant tubal infection. Abdominal operation is usually contraindicated in the acute stage, and should ordinarily be deferred for a number of weeks after subsidence of the acute symptoms, if there is an adequate response to therapy.

On the whole, however, conservative treatment is indicated when the patient gets along quite comfortably, with perhaps no discomfort other than slight dysmenorrhea or occasional slight bearing-down in the pelvic region, or perhaps not even these symptoms. Even if the symptoms are pronounced, there is no urgency in recommending surgical treatment, and conservative treatment should be given a trial if one can be certain that an adnexal mass is not a true neoplasm.

This consists of such simple measures as enforcing a reasonable amount of rest, moderation in sexual intercourse, the eradication of any foci of infection in the cervix, urethra, or vulvovaginal glands, the avoidance insofar as possible of reinfection, and the use of hot douches or sitz baths. Some have advocated the use of some form of cortisone (for its antifibrotic effect) in conjunction with *antibiotics*.

When, on the other hand, the patient becomes increasingly miserable because of pain in the lower abdomen, severe dysmenorrhea, menstrual irregularities, and sometimes even a condition of semi-invalidism, elective operation is ordinarily indicated. In the same way, the nature and extent of the operation must be decided on an individual basis. In most cases, unfortunately, both tubes are involved and both must often be removed.

Even if both tubes are closed, some form of plastic operation such as salpingostomy, resection and tubouterine anastomosis, or cornual implantation of the ovaries is justified in the occasional case in which the woman is desperately anxious for motherhood, with full explanation of the very small percentage of successful results in such cases, probably not over about 10%.

Results with tuboplastic surgery following tubal sterilization are somewhat better, for one is not dealing with a basically diseased tube. Indeed operation on infected closed tubes may often restore patency but not the vital physiological and peristaltic action of the oviduct.

The matter of tubal occlusion and surgery is discussed in Chapter 29, but a few words seem appropriate here. Simple tubolysis gives much better results than actual tubal reconstructions, but the results are still rather discouraging. Associated hydrotubation with a corticosteroid and an anti-allergen has been recommended by some. Unfortunately, the results with tuboplastics have simply not improved enough to counterbalance the paucity of infants for adoption, a shortage caused by liberal abortion policies throughout much of this country.

In a recent study of plastic surgery between 1965 and 1972, Umezaki *et al.* record 39% pregnancy in 66 patients with the average pregnancy occurring about 3 years following surgery. The expectation of pregnancy followed indefinitely revealed a 50 per cent result: tubolysis, 66%; fimbrioplasty, 40%; anastomosis, 50%; cornual implantation, 38%; and multiple procedures, 21%.

When both tubes are so hopelessly involved that their removal is necessary, opinion is uniform that hysterectomy is advisable. There is no reason to preserve the uterus when pregnancy cannot ensue, but of course the woman should be advised as to what hysterectomy will entail, namely (1) no further pregnancy and (2) no subsequent menstruation. The true facts are apt to be very different from what she had heard in the beauty parlor or her bridge club. Only in the youthful, unrealistic woman who cannot be convinced of the unimportance of continued menstruation should the uterus be preserved. The *importance of conserving ovarian tissue* whenever possible cannot be too strongly emphasized. On the other hand, the availability of many oral hormones has seemingly minimized any ill effects incurred by castration.

Idiopathic Retroperitoneal Fibrosis

Idiopathic retroperitoneal fibrosis is placed in this chapter with certain misgivings, for it is by no means certain that this represents an inflammatory process. Actually it is a rather new entity in gynecological journals, and it is only in the last 20 years that this ill defined disease has been recognized by us, although such urologists as Ormond noted it earlier.

Clinically, the symptoms are rather vague, consisting primarily of nondescript pain with occasional nausea, anorexia, low grade fever, with urinary symptoms. Pelvic examination may suggest varying degrees of induration or the presence of a mass, and pyelography often shows bilateral ureteral obstruction with a tendency towards medial displacement of the ureters.

The cause is highly speculative; infections of various types including tuberculosis, collagen disorders, hypersensitivity reaction, and a host of other etiological factors have been suggested. In 1966, Graham reported 27 cases which occurred after methysergide maleate treatment for migraine headache. A vasculitis secondary to a drug sensitivity is proposed as a causative factor. Treatment has generally consisted of lysis of the obstructed ureter, occasionally with intraperitoneal fixation, although x-ray and cortisone have also been suggested as therapeutic measures.

REFERENCES

Bahany, C. M., Ovacia, Y., and Neri, A.: Schistosoma mansoni of the ovary. Amer. J. Obstet. Gynec., 98: 290, 1967.

Blinick, G.: Gonorrheal disease in the female. Clin. Obstet. Gynec., 2: 492, 1959.

Cavanagh, D., and Rao, P. S.: Septic (endotoxic) shock. Clin. Obstet. Gynec., 16: 25, 1973.

Cedena, D., et al.: Chronic endometritis. Obstet. Gynec., 41: 733, 1973.

Clark, D. O.: Gonorrhea: changing concepts in diagnosis and management. Clin. Obstet. Gynec., 16, 3, 1973.

Collins, C. G., and Jansen, F. W.: Treatment of pelvic abscess. Clin. Obstet. Gynec., 2: 512, 1959.

Deacon, W. E.: Fluorescent antibody tests for detection of gonococcus in women. Public Health Rep., 75: 125, 1960.

Decker, W. H., and Hall, W.: Treatment of abortions infected with Clostridium welchii. Amer. J. Obstet. Gynec., 95: 394, 1966.

Diamant, Y. Z., Aboulatia, Y., and Raz, S.: Torsion of hydrosalpinx. Int. Surg., 57: 303, 1972.

Fathalla, M. F.: Assuit Univ., Cairo, Egypt. Personal communication.

Franklin, E. W., Hevron, J. E., and Thompson, J. D.: Management of the pelvic abscess.

Girardet, R., and Enquist, I. F.: Differential diagnosis between appendicitis and acute pelvic inflammatory disease. Surg. Gynec. Obstet., 116: 212, 1963.

Goodmo, J. A., Jr., Cushner, I. M., and Molumphy, P. E.: Management of infected abortion: an analysis of 342 cases. Amer. J. Obstet. Gynec., 85: 16, 1963.

Goplerud, C. P., and White, C. A.: Postpartum infection. Obstet. Gynec., 25: 227, 1965.

Graham, J. R.: Fibrotic disorders associated with methysergide therapy for headache. New Eng. J. Med., 274: 359, 1966.

Hall, W. L., Sobel, A. L., Jones, C. P., and Parker, R. T.: Anaerobic postoperative pelvic infections. Obstet. Gynec., 30: 1, 1967.

Harrow, B. R., and Sloane, J. A.: Ideopathic retroperitoneal fibrosis. J.A.M.A., 182: 148, 1962.

Huffman, J. W.: Gynecology in Childhood and Adolescence. W. B. Saunders Co., Philadelphia, 1969.

Hunt, S. M., Kincheloe, B. W., and Schreier, P. C.: Tubo-ovarian abcess in pregnancy. Obstet. Gynec., 43: 57, 1974.

Hurtig, A.: Cortisone in obstetrics and gynecology. In Year Book of Obstetrics and Gynecology, 1963-1964, edited by J. P. Greenhill, p. 369. Year Book Medical Publishers, Inc., Chicago, 1964.

Josey, W., Hoch, W., Moon, E. C., and Thompson, J. D.: Analysis of 21 septic abortion deaths with special reference to the Schwartzman phenomenon. Obst. Gynec., 28: 335, 1965.

Kaplan, A. L., Jacobs, W. M., and Ehresman, J. B.: Aggressive management of pelvic abscess. Amer. J. Obstet. Gynec., 98: 482, 1967.

Lucas, J. B., Price, E. V., Thayer, J. D., and Schroeter, A.: Diagnosis and treatment of gonorrhea in the female. New Eng. J. Med., 276: 1454, 1967.

Lukasik, J.: A comparative evolution of the bacteriological flora of the uterine cervix and the fallopian tubes in cases of salpingitis. Amer. J. Obstet. Gynec., 87: 1028, 1963.

Mead, P. B., and Louria, D. B.: Antibiotics in pelvic infections. Clin. Obstet. Gynec., 12: 219, 1969.

Mickal, A., and Sellman, A. H.: Tubo-ovarian abscess. Clin. Obstet. Gynec., 12: 252, 1969.

Mickal, A., Sellman, A. H., and Beebe, J. L.: Ruptured tubo-ovarian abscess. Amer. J. Obstet. Gynec., 100: 432, 1968.

Mishell, D. R., and Moyer, D. L.: Association of pelvic inflammatory disease with the intrauterine device. Clin. Obstet. Gynec., 12: 179, 1969.

Moyer, D. L., and Mishell, D. R.: Reaction of human endometrium to intrauterine foreign body. Amer. J. Obstet. Gynec., 111: 66, 1971.

Mulligan, W. J.: Results of salpingostomy. Int. J. Fertil., 11: 424, 1966.

Nabel, W. A., and Lucas, W. E.: Management of tubo-ovarian abscess. Obstet. Gynec., 32: 382, 1968.

Nolan, G. H., and Osborne, N.: G. C.: infection in the female. Obstet. Gynec., 42: 156, 1973.

O'Brien, J. R., Arronet, G. H., and Eduljee, G. Y.: Operative Treatment of Fallopian Tube Pathology. Amer. J. Obstet. Gynec., 103: 520, 1969.

Ormond, J. K.: Bilateral ureteral obstruction due to envelopment and compression by an inflammatory retroperitoneal process. J. Urol., 59: 1072, 1948.

Pedowitz, P., and Bloomfield, R. D.: Ruptured adnexal abscess (tubo-ovarian) with generalized peritonitis. Amer. J. Obstet. Gynec., 88: 721, 1964.

Powell, J. L., Foley, G. P., and Llorens, A. S.: Fallopian tube torsion. Amer. J. Obstet. Gynec., 113: 115, 1972.

Rabinowitz, P., Schiffer, M. A., Pomerance, W., and Friedman, I. S.: Management of postabortal infections complicated by acute renal failure. Amer. J. Obstet. Gynec., 84: 780, 1962.

Rust, J. A., and Maas, H. E.: Pelvic retroperitoneal fibrosis with response to prednisolone. Amer. J. Obstet. Gynec., 98: 654, 1967.

Sarma, V.: Gynecologic and obstetric aspects of tropical diseases, Medioscope, *45:* 181, 1961.

Schuler, H.: Use of anticoagulants in suspected pelvic infection. Clin. Obstet. Gynec., *12:* 240, 1969.

Schwartz, O.: Benign diffuse enlargement of the uterus. Amer. J. Obstet. Gynec., *61:* 902, 1951.

Scott, R. B.: Critical illnesses and deaths associated with intrauterine devices. Obstet. Gynec., *31:* 322, 1968.

Schroeder, A. L., and Lucas, J. B.: Gonorrhea—diagnosis and treatment. Obstet. Gynec., *39:* 274, 1972.

Shapiro, L. H., *et al.*: One day oral ampicillin treatment of gonorrhea. Obstet. Gynec., *37:* 414, 1971.

Sweeney, W. J.: Pitfalls in present-day methods of evaluating tubal function. Fertil. Steril., *13:* 124, 1962.

Symmonds, R. E., Dahlin, D. C., and Engel, S.: Ideopathic retroperitoneal fibrosis. Obstet. Gynec., *18:* 591, 1961.

Taylor, H. C.: Pelvic pain based on vascular and autonomic nervous system disorder. Amer. J. Obstet. Gynec., *67:* 1177, 1954.

Umezaki, C., Katayama, P., and Jones, H. W.: Pregnancy rates after reconstructive surgery on the Fallopian tubes. Obstet. Gynec., *43:* 418, 1974.

Vasudeva, K., Thrasher, T. V., and Richart, R. M.: Chronic endometritis. Amer. J. Obstet. Gynec., *112:* 749, 1972.

Vermereen, J., and Te Linde, R. W.: Intraabdominal rupture of pelvic abscesses. Amer. J. Obstet. Gynec., *68:* 402, 1954.

Whiteley, P. F., and Hamlett, J. D.: Pyometra—a reappraisal. Amer. J. Obstet. Gynec., *109:* 108, 1971.

Willson, J. R., and Black, J. R.: Ovarian abscess. Amer. J. Obstet. Gynec., *90:* 34, 1964.

Willson, J. R., Ledger, W. J., and Andros, G. J.: The effect of an intrauterine contraceptive device on the histological pattern of the endometrium. Amer. J. Obstet. Gynec., *93:* 802, 1965.

Woodruff, J. D., and Pauerstein, C. J.: *The Fallopian Tube.* Williams & Wilkins, Baltimore, Md., 1969.

chapter 20

Genital Tuberculosis

With pelvic tuberculosis, there is almost uniformly initial pelvic involvement of the tubes, although there are rare cases of primary cervical tuberculosis in which the sexual partner has been thought to be the source of infection. With the exception of these few instances, in which infection is incurred by a male having tuberculous epididymitis, tubal involvement is almost 100% in the woman with pelvic tuberculosis (Table 20.1).

By the same token, peritonitis is almost always secondary to pelvic (tubal) tuberculosis, although it is often difficult to establish. Certainly involvement of the peritoneum without a real tuberculous endo- (not just peri-) salpingitis is unusual. With the routine pasteurization of milk and the disappearance of bovine tuberculosis, primary gastrointestinal acid-fast disease is rare, and the tubes seem to be the only logical focus for both pelvic and intraabdominal tuberculosis, at least in the United States.

Modes of Infection

In almost all cases tuberculous involvement of the female genitalia is secondary to extragenital tuberculosis, although it is rare to find that this lesion in currently active. Occasionally pelvic tuberculosis may be a part of a generalized miliary tuberculous disease, but we have been so impressed by the infrequent association of urinary and genital tuberculosis as to speculate as to whether involvement of one system may tend to immunize the other.

However, *pulmonary disease* is the usual *primary site* and the probable route of dissemination is almost certainly hematogenous. It is difficult to explain why the tubes usually receive the primary impact of this blood stream involvement. It is likewise difficult to understand how pelvic tuberculosis can occur in the absence of an active pulmonary lesion, unless we assume that a clinically undetected lung disease has undergone spontaneous resolution *after* there has been some type of bacteremia to which the tubes alone are singularly responsive. In any case chest x-ray usually shows evidence of only an old primary complex. Other extra-pulmonic sites may serve as a primary focus.

TUBERCULOSIS OF TUBES

As already stated, the tubes constitute the initial seat of genital tuberculosis in the overwhelming majority of cases, the

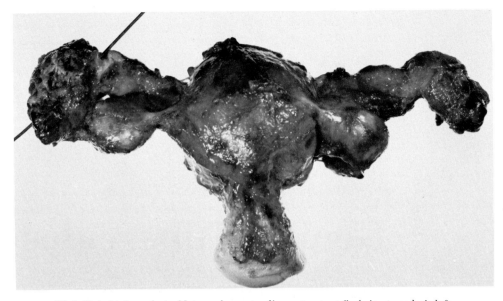

20.1. Tubal tuberculosis. Note probe protruding out patent fimbria at reader's left

bacilli reaching them by any one of the routes mentioned above. Tuberculous salpingitis is not rare and comprises approximately 5% of all cases of salpingitis in some areas of the world where disease and malnutrition are present, although it is much less common in this country. In earlier studies Schaefer noted an eight per cent incidence of genital disease in women dying of pulmonary tuberculosis.

Pathology

The *gross* appearance of the tuberculous tube varies in different cases, but as a rule is not different from that of the various forms of chronic gonorrheal salpingitis. The tube may resemble a

Table 20.1*

Frequency of Tuberculosis in Genital Organs

Organ	Per Cent
Tubes	90–100
Uterus	50–60
Ovaries	20–30
Cervix	5–15
Vagina	1

* Courtesy of Dr. Geo. Schaefer, New York.

pyosalpinx, occasionally hydrosalpinx, frequently chronic interstitial salpingitis, and not infrequently salpingitis isthmica nodosa. In the form associated with miliary tuberculous peritonitis, numerous tubercles may stud the surface, just as they do the pelvic peritoneal cavity. Far more frequently, however, no tubercles are visible externally, although they may be present in advanced stages of the hematogenous variety. Greenberg and others have called attention to the so-called tobacco-pouch or mail-pouch appearance of the fimbriated extremity, produced by the eversion of the fimbriae (see Figs. 20.1, 2). This is in contrast to the closed bulbous fimbriated extremity so characteristic of the gonorrheal variety. This feature, however, is by no means a constant one. As a matter of fact the diagnosis of tuberculous salpingitis is usually not made until microscopic examination has been carried out.

Microscopic. The microscopic diagnosis is easy in the frank, advanced case, but it may be difficult in the early phases of the disease or in the late reparative phase, which is not infrequently noted. Many blocks may have to be taken from various parts of the tube before the telltale evidence, in the form of tubercles and

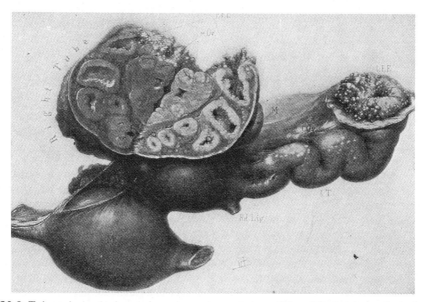

20.2. Tuberculosis of tubes and ovaries; note overted condition of fimbriated end of tube.

giant cells, can be demonstrated (Fig. 20.3). Acid-fast stains are more specific; even when these are negative, a positive culture may be obtained.

In the early stages one often finds a markedly proliferative, adenomatous-looking pattern in the folds. This should always excite suspicion, and it *should not be mistaken for adenocarcinoma*, as it has often been. In the more outspoken cases, one finds numerous tubercles, many with giant cells, and chronic inflammation. The tubercles may be limited to the mucosa, or they may be scattered

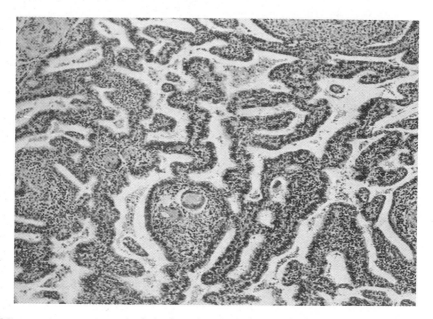

20.3. Microscopic appearance of tubal tuberculosis with typical tubercles and giant cells and marked proliferation of tubal folds.

throughout the muscularis and on the peritoneal coat. In advanced stages, extensive caseation is common.

The histological criteria noted above should suggest a tuberculous infection, but it must be realized that other diseases may produce a similar granulomatous process. These include various lesions such as fungus, sarcoid, syphilis, etc., and giant cells may occur because of foreign bodies—iodized oil introduced in the course of a hysterosalpingogram or starch granules on suture material from a previous operation. The final diagnosis lies in the demonstration of the acid-fast bacillus by means of appropriate stain or culture.

TUBERCULOSIS OF THE ENDOMETRIUM

As noted by Greenberg, this is always secondary to tubal involvement, occurring in about 50% of patients with tuberculous salpingitis, although Knauss, in performing bilateral salpingectomy, has found residual endometritis in 80% of all women. Most of these patients also had a tuberculous peritonitis, a further testimony to the high association of tubal and peritoneal disease. The presence of acid-fast endometritis is presumptive evidence of tubal disease, but the absence of tubercles in a removed endometrium by no means excludes a specific tuberculous adnexitis. In certain areas of the world where poverty and poor nutrition abound, sterility work-ups have disclosed an unsuspected tuberculous endometritis in nearly 5% of cases (but 20% in India), and such writers as Sharman conclude that latent tubal tuberculosis is a not infrequent factor in the production of sterility.

The *pathology* of tuberculous endometritis is characterized by the presence of typical tubercles with epithelioid and giant cells, involving the endometrium and occasional extension into the myometrium. In late stages there are extensive tubercles with many giant cells and varying degrees of caseation, but even in advanced disease there are no specific gross findings. Acid-fast culture of the endometrium is positive in less than 50% of all cases, and acid-fast stains are often unsuccessful. As a rule pelvic tuberculosis behaves like tuberculosis anywhere. While more common in the younger woman, tuberculous endometritis has been noted in postmenopausal patients by Schaefer *et al.* Bleeding was the presenting complaint.

TUBERCULOSIS OF THE OVARIES

This practically never occurs in the absence of tubal involvement, and when present, it generally consists of a rather marked perioophoritis rather than a real ovarian involvement. This tends to heal spontaneously following removal of the tube so that preservation of at least one ovary can generally be accomplished even in very extensive pelvic tuberculosis afflicting a young woman. The study by Francis would seem to confirm the desirability of ovarian conservation in the young woman.

TUBERCULOSIS OF THE CERVIX

This has already been discussed in Chapter 11. (See Fig. 20.4.)

TUBERCULOSIS OF VAGINA AND VULVA

Both of these lesions are extremely rare and, although the mode of infection is often difficult to determine, the majority appear to be secondary to disease higher in the genital tract. In a very few cases it appears probable that the male sexual partner has transmitted the lesion from any infected epididymis, seminal vesicles, etc.

As a rule tuberculosis of the vulva or vagina presents as a shaggy ulcerative lesion which may be difficult to distinguish from a luetic ulcer. On occasion it may assume a hypertrophic character which, as with tuberculous cervicitis, may be mistaken for a genuine carcinoma. Biopsy is generally decisive.

CLINICAL FEATURES OF PELVIC TUBERCULOSIS

There is nothing pathognomonic about *tuberculous salpingitis* to distinguish it

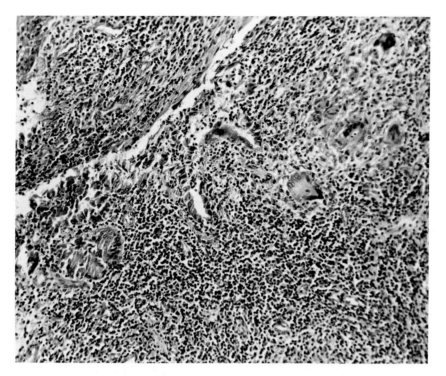

20.4. Typical tuberculosis involving the cervix (squamous epithelium, *upper left,* barely distinguishable).

from the much more common chronic gonococcal salpingitis, and, as a result of this similarity, preoperative diagnosis is rarely made. There are, however, a few features which should arouse suspicion that the adnexal involvement may be of acid-fast origin. Sutherland points out that a history of pulmonary, osseous, or miliary tuberculosis should be suggestive, although gonorrhea may of course coexist. The finding of adnexal inflammatory masses in virgins or women in whom other types of tubal infection can reasonably be excluded may likewise lead to a suspicion of tuberculous salpingitis (Fig. 20.5), especially if there is a tendency towards a persistent slight evening elevation of temperature, slight anemia, or tachycardia. Salpingitis which is refractory to the usual means of therapy should suggest tuberculosis, although this may not prove to be the case.

Tuberculous endometritis (Fig. 20.6) may occur without obvious tubal involvement, although it is a safe presumption that there is a primary adnexal disease. The symptomatology is not, however, in any way characteristic. There may be a persistent discharge, watery or pinkish, and there is a frequent tendency towards diminished or absent menstruation, although Brown, Gilbert, and Te Linde noticed this menstrual pattern only rarely. In the vast majority of cases, however, it is the symptoms of tubal involvement or sterility which direct the patient to seek medical attention.

SILENT PELVIC TUBERCULOSIS

In recent years there has been a considerable number of publications concerning the chance finding of endometrial tuberculosis in women with no other symptom or complaint than sterility. In such areas as Israel, Belgium, or Scotland, tuberculous endometritis has been noted in nearly 5% of all sterility work-ups, but this figure must be weighed against the poor sanitary and living conditions during the years in which these data were compiled. In the United States,

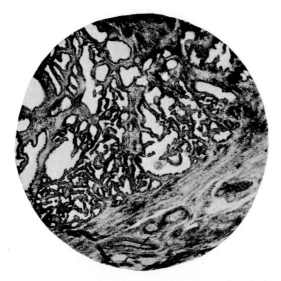

20.5. Adenoma-like proliferation of tubal epithelium seen in some cases of tubal tuberculosis. Even though no tubercles or giant cells are seen such a picture should make one highly suspicious of tuberculosis.

however, genital tuberculosis is much less frequent, possibly due to better living conditions. Israel found 0.09% of gynecological admissions and 0.15% of pathological specimens as being tuberculous in nature.

As noted previously, belief is rather uniform that endometrial involvement is nearly always secondary to diseased tubes; although the tubes are the primary pelvic focus, there is nevertheless insufficient disease to produce symptoms. In many instances the tubes may be patent, and ovulation is the rule. It is in this group of individuals, generally young and desirous of pregnancy, that modern methods of medical treatment have found their widest application.

TUBERCULOUS PERITONITIS

Although acid-fast infection of the pelvic peritoneum is frequently seen in association with tuberculous salpingitis, it is believed by some, notably the British, that tuberculous peritonitis may precede the genital disease or even exist in its absence. In most instances, however, tuberculous peritonitis is associated with tubal disease, generally of extensive nature, and tends to behave like other adnexal disease with the addition of ascites. Usually the pelvic peritoneum alone shows tuberculous seeding (along with that of the tubes), although the extrapelvic peritoneum is not involved.

Tuberculous peritonitis may present in several different forms. The *wet* variety may show extensive tubercle formation involving all visceral and parietal surfaces of the peritoneum but most marked in the pelvis. The omentum may be studded with nodules and be greatly thickened and indurated in a boardlike fashion. Ascites is the rule. It is frequently not generalized, but is likely to be composed of multiple sacs of ascitic fluid enclosed in loops of agglutinated intestine and omentum. Various types of masses and pseudomasses may be produced by these encysted fluid sacs, but there is generally additional free fluid.

The *dry* type of peritonitis is perhaps a later stage of the ascitic form, after there have been varying amounts of resorption

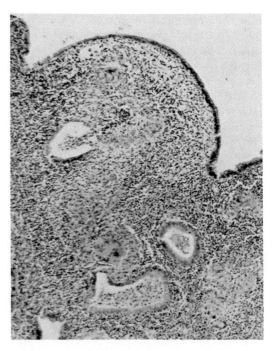

20.6. Tuberculous endometritis in a rather advanced stage with typical giant cells and tubercles.

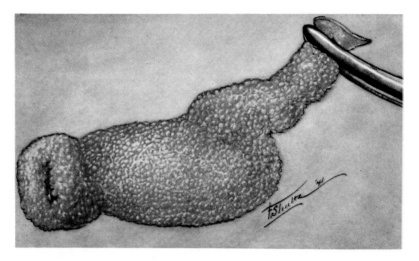

Plate 20.1. Tuberculosis of tube associated with tuberculous peritonitis

of the fluid. This fibroplastic form is characterized by only minor degrees of ascites, but there may be extensive adhesions and induration, with literal welding of pelvic and intestinal surfaces. Caseation, necrosis, and fistulas may occur.

All gradations between the ascitic (wet) and the adhesive (dry) types of peritoneal involvement may occur, and all types of confusing differential diagnoses may be simulated. Ascites of renal or cardiac origin must be distinguished, as must hepatic cirrhosis. Ovarian carcinomatosis is frequently suspected, especially where there is tuberculous adnexitis and abscess formation (see Fig. 20.7).

Clinical Course

Patients with tuberculous peritonitis may evidence no other symptom than abdominal swelling due to ascitic fluid. On the other hand, there may be profound systemic symptoms with high spiking fever, tachycardia, anorexia, and weight loss. In the fibroplastic form one may observe symptoms suggesting partial intestinal obstruction, such as obstipation, bloating, etc. If there is miliary or pulmonary tuberculosis, other symptoms may be added, so that diagnosis may be difficult.

The finding of ascites, however, in a young woman with no history of cardiorenal or hepatic difficulties, should make one suspect tuberculous peritonitis, especially if there is systemic and laboratory evidence of an inflammatory process. Palpation of tubal masses and the finding of a fixed uterus are often noted and, if this adnexal disease does not respond to the usual antibiotics and chemotherapy, a tuberculous etiology may be suspected.

DIAGNOSIS OF PELVIC TUBERCULOSIS

Many cases with acid-fast disease of the female generative organs are asymptomatic, and many more show only the diverse symptoms associated with any nonspecific inflammatory disease. Schaefer rightfully emphasizes the importance of being always suspicious of the possibility of the disease, particularly where there is a family history of tuberculosis or some proved extragenital manifestation. Infertility for which no other cause can be found, pelvic pain, general malaise, adnexal masses in virgins, and chronic refractory adnexal disease are by no means pathognomonic but might alert the wary examiner. Chest x-ray and tuberculin testing should not be neglected though of dubious value.

Where there is suspicion of the disease,

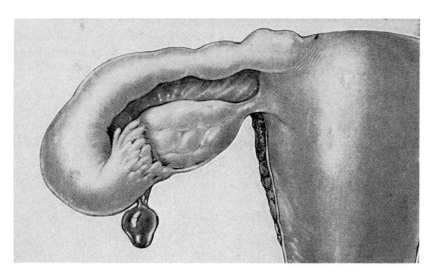

20.7. Wall of tuberculous abscess of ovary studded with conglomerate tubercles

we do not hesitate to perform a curettage, with full cognizance of the fact that only about 50% of those women having tubal disease also have tuberculous endometritis. In other words, the finding of endometrial tuberculosis clinches the diagnosis; failure to find the characteristic histological pattern in no way excludes the acid-fast bacillus. Bacteriological culture of menstrual blood or aspiration culture of the endometrial cavity may be obtained, but even more effective is direct culture and guinea pig inoculation with removed endometrium. We elect to perform curettage in the premenstrual phase of the cycle where possible, and it is of interest to note that even extensive amounts of pelvic tuberculosis rarely impair ovulation. The removed endometrium may be scanty but, if removed in the progestational phase of the cycle, rarely fails to show a secretory pattern even though it be riddled by tuberculosis. We have experienced no specific complications with curettage, although Schaefer mentions that some writers have raised the question of reactivating a latent lesion or of causing a hematogenous spread by such operative manipulation.

Siegler, Schaefer (Table 20.2), and others have emphasized the use of hysterosalpingography in establishing the diagnosis of acid-fast involvement of the tubes, and if a water-soluble medium is used there is probably little danger. Various x-ray changes may be noted, but interpretation of these changes are difficult and complex, so that there has been no uniform acceptance in the larger clinics. Laparoscopy may be informative if there are serosal tubercles.

The final diagnosis of pelvic tuberculosis is often not made until laparotomy is performed, and may not be apparent even at the operating table. Careful histological study is necessary and may require many blocks and many sections. Care must be taken to exclude various other granulomatous processes and foreign body giant cell reaction. Bilateral tubal involvement seems to be almost the uniform rule.

Sarcoidosis may involve the female genitalia and produce granulomatous le-

Table 20.2*

Order of Examination in Female Genital Tuberculosis

1. Family history
2. Plant history
3. Physical examination
4. Chest roentgenogram
5. Tuberculin test
6. Endometrial curettage
   a. Histologic examination
   b. Bacteriologic examination
7. Menstrual blood examination
8. Hysterosalpingogram
9. Laparotomy, culdoscopy

* Courtesy of Dr. Geo. Schaefer, New York.

sions similar to tuberculosis, although there is not, of course, bacteriological evidence of the tubercle bacillus. In addition, sarcoid frequently involves many other organs as indicated in the recent case report by Winslow and Funkhowsen. Various diseases as actinomycosis as well as schistosomiasis may produce a granulomatous appearance, as noted by Fathalla (Fig. 20.8).

TREATMENT

In past years the treatment of diagnosed pelvic tuberculosis was almost entirely surgical plus the usual regimen of rest, fresh air, good nutrition, etc. Recent advances in the fields of antibiotics and chemotherapy in the last 15 years have equipped us with a number of effective antituberculous drugs. At this writing there are several effective antituberculous drugs, but extensive work on the development of others is currently under way.

One must not infer that surgical procedures have been completely abandoned, for this is certainly not true. Schaefer advocates hysterectomy and bilateral salpingo-oophorectomy in the woman over forty after preoperative drug therapy. Chemotherapy alone is used only in those patients who have patent tubes, are desirous of further pregnancy, and have little or no discomfort. Persistent, painful adnexal masses, continued fever, and elevated sedimentation rate, ascites, and failure to respond to medical treatment are indications for a surgical rather than a medical treatment.

Medical Treatment

Of the main available drugs, the first to be used was *streptomycin,* and it is still widely utilized today if sensitivity tests indicate that the organism to be treated will respond. Streptomycin must be given intramuscularly, and initially 1 gm. daily is given. Dosage is gradually decreased to 1 gm. biweekly, and the patient may be maintained on this dosage for many months, or until toxicity is noted. This

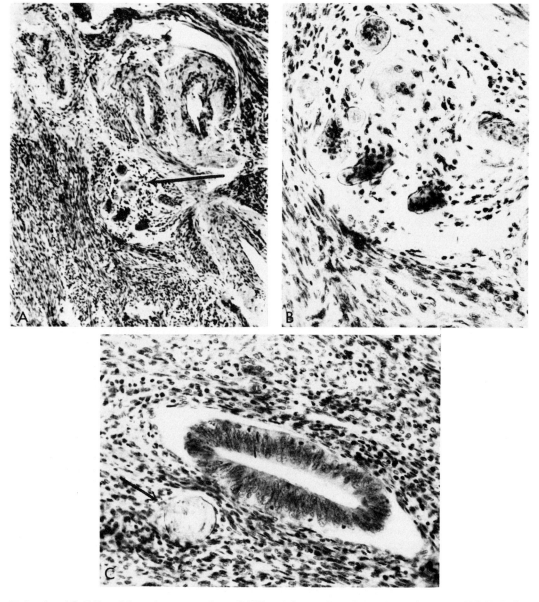

20.8 *A* and *B*, Bilharzial ova in myometrium. *C*, Bilharzial ovum in endometrium. (Courtesy of M. Fathalla, Assuit Univ., Cairo, Egypt.)

consists primarily of evidence of eighth nerve damage, both acoustic and cochlear branches being susceptible, with resultant deafness, vertigo, nausea, etc. These toxic effects are by no means universal and actually afflict only a few patients. However, once toxic effects appear, they are very slow to disappear even after cessation of the offending drug; therefore, the physician is wise to be alert for any incipient signs of toxicity.

Frequently utilized in conjunction with streptomycin has been *paraaminosalicylic acid* (PAS) which, although only mildly bactericidal, has seemed to enhance the effect of streptomycin. PAS must be taken orally and in large dosage, generally 3 gm. four times a day, but a great many patients have such severe gastrointestinal disorders as to mandate discontinuance of this drug. Profound anorexia, nausea, vomiting, and diarrhea can be expected in a considerable proportion of those patients taking PAS, so that this medication simply must be stopped.

A more recent addition to antituberculous chemotherapy has been *isonicotinic acid* (INH). This has the advantage of oral administration and in small doses has been considered to be nontoxic. Dosage has varied according to body weight, 5mg. per kg. of body weight, which generally approximates 300 to 400 mg. daily.

Thus, there are different drugs available for the medical treatment of tuberculosis of the female generative tract, although many new chemotherapeutic agents are becoming available. It would seem that no one drug is nearly as effective as a combination of any two, but any combination of two is just about as effective as any other. PAS and INH can of course be taken orally, but equally good results may be obtained by combinations of streptomycin and INH, which will of course obviate the unpleasant gastrointestinal disorders incurred by PAS although a twice weekly intramuscular injection is necessary. Currently, Sutherland suggests 1 gm. of streptomycin, 15 gm. of PAS, and 300 mg. of INH daily; after four months the streptomycin is dis-

continued, but the other two drugs are maintained for *18 months*. Various newer drugs seem forthcoming, notably *ethambutol* in doses of 15–25 mg./kg.; although occasional visual disturbances may occur, they are transitory.

Following diagnosis and medical treatment the patient must be kept under close observation. Pelvic tuberculosis is still a potentially serious disease, and miliary or various forms of extragenital tuberculosis can arise. If a patient has been treated because of a curettage-proved tuberculous endometritis, repeat curettage is in order every six months for several years. Should the endometritis persist or recede only to recur later, surgery is indicated.

Surgical Treatment

Persistent or recurrent endometritis is only one of several indications for surgical intervention. In a 1966 study of 419 cases of genital tract tuberculosis, Sutherland has found surgery indicated in 43 (over 10%). Prime indications are continuous or recurrent pain (26), persistent or developing adnexal masses (8), and recurring endometritis (8). We are in complete accord with Zummo, Sered, and Falls who feel that patients with the more advanced forms of pelvic disease are to be considered as candidates for surgery. Indications consist of adnexal masses, abscesses, prominent thickenings, and ascites, and with such tenets these authors are in full accord.

Indeed, if it can be determined that the tubes are closed or there is no desire for further pregnancy, there is little justification for prolonged medical therapy. Medical therapy should be reserved for those individuals who have patent tubes and are anxious for further pregnancies. The extensive review from Liverpool (Francis) would suggest a surgical approach where the tubes are occluded or where there is persistent extensive disease. Highly enlightening discussions by Schaefer and Sutherland clarify the indications for surgical treatment and emphasize the necessity of preoperative drug therapy. Schaefer states categorically that "cure of genital tuberculosis is achieved more quickly with surgery than with drugs alone."

Should a patient have extensive pelvic tuberculosis initially, closed tubes, persistent adnexal masses, or is over forty, it is probable that her interests are best served by operation. It must be understood that pelvic tuberculosis was formerly treated by surgery alone, and that these operations were often the most difficult a surgeon would be asked to perform. The tissues were edematous and friable, adhesions were multiple and cartilaginous, and the patients were often in poor general health. Morbidity was high in the days of surgical treatment alone for extensive tuberculosis, with a considerable proportion of such complications as fistulas, wound disruption, bowel obstruction, and even death.

It has been conclusively shown that preoperative chemotherapy will cause enough tissue improvement to make operation technically less difficult and fraught with fewer complications. Some combination, then, of drugs should precede surgery for several months at least; indeed, chemotherapy has been advocated for many months preoperative unless there is evidence of drug resistance. Our belief is that with extensive pelvic involvement, a prolonged course of drugs is desirable, but where there is a freely mobile uterus without adnexal masses (but with closed tubes and with biopsy proven acid-fast disease of the endometrium), only a token one week course of drugs is sufficient. Subsequent chemotherapy for another 18 months is usually recommended.

Opinion is uniform that total hysterectomy is desirable, with removal of the tubes and frequently both ovaries in case of extensive disease. Even where frank tuberculous abscesses are encountered with free spillage of the necrotic caseous contents, drainage is to be avoided because of the very real possibility of fistula formation. Although it is probable that conservation of an ovary might lead to no complications, in this era of effective oral hormones, complete operation seems preferable.

PREGNANCY AND TUBERCULOSIS

It has been noted that there is a rather large number of women, outwardly healthy and with no other complaint than infertility, who are found to have endometrial tuberculosis. Sharman estimates these comprise about 5% of all patients appearing at a Sterility Clinic, but he also believes that a much truer index of pelvic tuberculosis would be 10%, since the endometrium is involved in only about 50% of patients with tubal disease. Greenhill is inclined to feel that this figure is much higher than the likely incidence in the United States, and this certainly seems true today. Yet sporadic cases occur, such as the recent report by Ramos, Hibbard and Craig, in which a premature infant developed pulmonary tuberculosis several days postpartum as an apparent sequel to an unsuspected maternal tuberculous endometritis.

Once a diagnosis of tuberculous endometritis has been established in the young woman desiring pregnancy, how then shall she be handled? If there is no other contraindication to pregnancy such as closed tubes, if there are no palpable adnexal masses, fever, or ascites, and if the patient is cooperative, medical therapy is instituted, and such cases represent the main indication for drug therapy. It seems only fair to warn the woman that although her disease can be controlled in most instances, there may be exceptional drug-resistant cases which culminate in hysterectomy. At the same time she should be advised that the chances of a normal intrauterine pregnancy are relatively slim despite good medical response.

The woman is then placed on one of the plans for medical therapy and is curetted (with culture) about twice a year. Should there be no recurrence of endometrial tuberculosis and no palpable evidence of incipient adnexal masses or induration, there is no reason not to continue conservative management. Yet it is a mistake to think that the antituberculous drugs are a panacea, for resistant strains occur. It is likewise possible to obliterate the disease in the endometrium without really curing the primary site, the tubes.

Schaefer has critically analyzed cases of full term pregnancy following genital tuberculosis where such an analysis was possible. His careful critique makes it seem apparent that in many reported cases the initial diagnosis of tuberculosis was far from absolute, and without histological or culture proof of acid-fast disease. Schaefer states that "less than 100 of 7357 patients with genital tuberculosis have had full term intrauterine pregnancies. The exact number is difficult to ascertain." The author adds that in the infrequent cases of pregnancy following genital tuberculosis, the end result is usually an abortion or an ectopic pregnancy. He further emphasizes the failure of tubal plastic surgery after antituberculous therapy, and points out that extensive degrees of genital infection lead to permanent infertility. This scholarly review should emphasize the extreme infrequency of normal term pregnancy in the woman with treated pelvic tuberculosis, and the patient should be appraised of this fact before institution of therapy. The simultaneous occurrence of pregnancy and pelvic tuberculosis is rare today in this country. Older reviews took a serious view of this concurrence, but this should be modified in view of today's chemotherapeutic agents, as indicated by Schaefer.

An excellent review of the subject is that of Halbrecht, who reported his material from Israel where constant warfare, with resultant poor nutrition and hygiene, have made pelvic tuberculosis unusually common. Halbrecht notes the important role that drugs and antibiotics play in controlling tubal infection, but states that they cannot restore an injured endosalpinx to normal, nor can they eliminate cicatricial lesions that may alter the tubal lumen. One hundred patients with pelvic tuberculosis were treated, and of these a surprisingly high 20% conceived; 14 patients, however, had one

or more ectopic gestations, and three patients suffered a spontaneous abortion. Halbrecht states that "any pregnancy occurring after antibiotic treatment of genital tuberculosis demands watchful supervision, considering the fact that such a pregnancy has a four to one chance to be a tubal pregnancy or to end in miscarriage. This is especially true if the disease has reached the endometrial stage before the treatment was started." We would be somewhat skeptical of cortisone therapy with tubal occlusion following healed genital tract tuberculosis as noted by Halbrecht and various other authors.

Thus the chances of a normal child following medical treatment of tuberculosis are really minimal. The tendency is to treat young sterile patients conservatively, and with this policy we are in complete agreement, providing the tubes are patent. The knowledge that successful pregnancies have occurred (although few) following antituberculous treatment can frequently be a great morale builder for these young brides.

However, in other cases of unsuspected endometrial tuberculosis, diagnosed as a mere chance finding, medical treatment may be inadequate. Although it would seem that the endometrium itself may be rendered free of disease, the primary lesion in the tube is more deeply seated and much more difficult to eradicate. Actually, Schaefer found that, in cases in which healing of the endometrium and tubes apparently occurred following antituberculous therapy, the tubes if removed showed such extensive disorganization as to render them functionless.

In addition, there are strains of the tubercle bacillus that appear to be rather refractory to chemotherapy, and that, despite initial apparently successful response, may re-occur with the possibility of extrapelvic spread. There is reason for encouragement, however, since the advent of the antituberculous drugs. In a series of 28 patients during the years 1945 to 1947, treated by accepted procedures of that day, Zummo, Sered, and Falls found that within two years 18 women had died, four were alive, and six could not be traced. Brown, Gilbert, and Te Linde also noted a considerable mortality, especially among cases in which there was an evidence of a tuberculous peritonitis. Both groups of authors compare the poor results of earlier days with the excellent response of most treated patients in this era.

Despite the impression that tuberculosis is a vanishing disease, the astute practitioner will be wise to bear this possibility in mind when confronted by women with pelvic complaints or women who are concerned about a barren marriage. Pelvic tuberculosis must still be accepted as a potentially serious problem, despite the advances of the last two decades.

REFERENCES

Bobrow, M. L., Winkelstein, L. B., and Friedman, S.: Streptomycin in advanced pelvic tuberculosis. Obstet. Gynec., 8: 299, 1956.

Brown, A. B., Gilbert, C. R. A., and Te Linde, R. W.: Pelvic tuberculosis. Obstet. Gynec., 2: 476, 1953.

Earn, A. A.: Living births following drug therapy for infertility associated with genital tuberculosis. J. Obstet. Gynaec. Brit. Commonw., 65: 739, 1958.

Farrion, H. L., and Rathbun, L. S.: Pelvic actinomycosis. Amer. J. Obstet. Gynec., 103: 908, 1969.

Fathalla, M. S.: Assuit Univ., Cairo, Egypt. Personal communication.

Francis, W. J. A.: Female genital tuberculosis. J. Obstet. Gynaec. Brit. Commonw., 71: 418, 1964.

Govan, A. D. T.: Tuberculous endometritis. J. Path. Bact., 83: 363, 1962.

Greenberg, J. P.: Tuberculous salpingitis; a clinical study of 200 cases. Johns Hopkins Hosp. Rep., 21: 97, 1921.

Haines, M.: Genital tuberculosis in the female. J. Obstet. Gynaec. Brit. Comm., 59: 721, 1952.

Haines, M.: Tuberculous salpingitis. Amer. J. Obstet. Gynec., 75: 472, 1958.

Halbrecht, I.: Healed genital tuberculosis. Obstet. Gynec., 10: 73, 1957.

Halbrecht, I.: Latent genital tuberculosis in women; its early diagnosis and treatment. Tuberkulosearzt, 12: 712, 1958.

Halbrecht, I.: Cortisone in the treatment of tubal occlusion caused by healed genital tuberculosis. Fertil. Steril., 13: 371, 1962.

Henderson, N., Hankins, J., and Stitt, J. F.: Pelvic tuberculosis. Amer. J. Obstet. Gynec., 94: 630, 1966.

Israel, S. L., Roitman, H. B., and Clancy, C.: Infrequency of unsuspected endometrial tuberculosis. J. A. M. A., 183: 63, 1963.

Knauss, H. H.: Surgical treatment of genital and peritoneal tuberculosis in the female. Amer. J. Obstet. Gynec., 83: 73, 1962.

Nokes, J. M.: Extrauterine pregnancy and tuberculous salpingitis. Obstet. Gynec., 10: 206, 1957.

Patat, P.: Genital tuberculosis and pregnancy. Zbl. Gynaek., 84: 506, 1962.

Ramos, A. D., Hibbord, L. T., and Craig, J. R.: Congenital tuberculosis. Obstet. Gynec., 43: 61, 1974.

Rozin, S.: X-ray diagnosis of genital tuberculosis. J. Obstet. Gynaec. Brit. Comm., 59: 59, 1952.

Sant, M. V., and Limaye, S. S.: Tuberculous endometritis: Histologic study of 301 cases. J. Obstet. Gynec. India, 16: 205, 1966.

Schaefer, G.: Diagnosis and treatment of female tuberculosis. Clin. Obstet. Gynec., 2: 530, 1959.

Schaefer, G.: Pulmonary infections in pregnancy. Clin. Obstet. Gynec., 2: 639, 1959.

Schaefer, G.: Full term pregnancy following genital tuberculosis. Obstet. Gynec. Survey, 19: 81, 1964.

Schaefer, G.: Tuberculosis of the genital organs. Amer. J. Obstet. Gynec., 91: 714, 1965.

Schaefer, G.: Diagnosis and treatment of female genital tuberculosis. Int. Surg., 48: 240, 1967.

Schaefer, G.: Tuberculosis of the female genital tract. Clin. Obstet. Gynec., 13: 965, 1970.

Schaefer, G., Douglas, R. G., and Silverman, F.: A reevaluation of the management of pregnancy and tuberculosis. J. Obstet. Gynaec. Brit. Comm., 66: 990, 1959.

Schaefer, G., Marcus, R. S., and Kramer, E. E.: Postmenopausal endometrial tuberculosis. Amer. J. Obstet. Gynec., 112: 681, 1972.

Shapiro, W. J.: Pregnancy after pelvic tuberculosis. Obstet. Gynec., 12: 148, 1958.

Sharman, A.: Genital tuberculosis in the female. J. Obstet. Gynaec. Brit. Comm., 59: 740, 1952.

Siegler, A. M.: Tuberculosis of the uterine tubes. Obstet. Gynec., 6: 188, 1955.

Snaith, L. M., and Barnes, T.: Fertility in pelvic tuberculosis. Lancet, 1: 712, 1962.

Stallworthy, J.: Fertility and genital tuberculosis. Fertil. Steril., 14: 284, 1963.

Sutherland, A. M.: Streptomycin and PAS. J. Brit. Tuberc. Assn., 38: 46, 1957.

Sutherland, A. M.: Genital tuberculosis in women. Amer. J. Obstet. Gynec., 79: 486, 1960.

Sutherland, A. M.: Tuberculosis of the genital organs. Amer. J. Obstet. Gynec., 91: 717, 1965.

Sutherland, A. M.: The treatment of genital tuberculosis in women. Geneesk. Gids, 45: 20, 362; 21, 386, 1967.

Sutherland, A. M.: Genital tuberculosis in women. Bull. Sloane Hosp., 13: 127, 1967.

Winslow, R. C., and Funkhowsen, J. W.: Sarcoidosis of the female reproductive organs. Obstet. Gynec., 32: 285, 1968.

Zummo, B. P., Sered, H., and Falls, F. H.: Diagnosis and prognosis of female genital tuberculosis. Amer. J. Obstet. Gynec., 70: 34, 1955.

chapter 21

Tumors of the Tube, Parovarium, and Uterine Ligaments

CARCINOMA OF FALLOPIAN TUBE

Primary

The most important tumor of the tube is carcinoma, but it is extremely rare with only 724 cases having been reported in the review by Hurlbutt and Nelson. A more recent study by Momtazee and Kempson suggests that there are more than 800 reported cases. The incidence in collected hospital series varies between 1% (Hayden and Potter) and 0.1% (Green and Scully) of all genital malignancies; obviously many cases are not reported. The disease occurs usually in middle life, but may occur also in very old women. Not infrequently it is associated with various other diseases of the adnexa, such as chronic salpingitis or ovarian cyst. There are some who believe that chronic inflammation of the tube is an important predisposing factor, but there is no certainty on this point. As a matter of fact this seems unlikely in view of the extreme rarity of carcinoma as compared to the great frequency of chronic salpingitis.

Pathology. The pathology of primary tubal carcinoma is quite characteristic. Grossly the tube is enlarged, sometimes enormously. In the latter case it may resemble a huge pyosalpinx, which often is almost entirely free of adhesions to surrounding structures, and unlike pelvic inflammatory disease, the contralateral tube is often normal, although Sedlis notes bilateral tumors in 26%. In most cases the carcinoma arises in the outer or middle portion of the tube, and in the occasional very early case there may be only a small nodular enlargement at the involved area. Extension out the fimbriated end of the tube as well as lymphatic involvement are early sequelae (Fig. 21.1).

Microscopically the typical pattern is of a *papillary* growth pushing concentrically toward the lumen (Figs. 21.2 and 21.3), which in advanced cases is filled with the treelike growth, although there is little or no tendency to invasion through the muscularis to the serosa. A less common form of the papillary type is the *alveolar* variety, in which a gland pattern is simu-

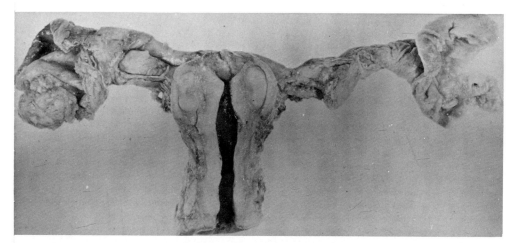

21.1. Carcinoma to *left*, note fungoid lesion extruding from fimbria; hydrosalpinx to *right*. (Courtesy of Dr. Albert Brown, Wilmington, N.C.)

lated by the fusion of the papillary folds. That very early "in situ" carcinomas of the tube exist is suggested by Ryan, and Pauerstein and Woodruff (Fig. 21.4).

Clinical Characteristics. The symptoms are not distinctive and in most cases they are so slight that the disease is well advanced before the patient seeks advice. Most frequent among the symptoms are postmenopausal bleeding, abnormal

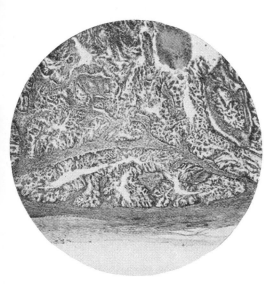

21.2. Characteristic concentric papillomatous growth pattern of the most common variety of primary tubal carcinoma; note the uninvolvement of the thin muscular coat.

discharge which may be watery or, more often, tinged with blood. Later symptoms are backache and sacral pain.

It is obvious that preoperative *diagnosis* will almost never be made since any palpable adnexal mass will properly be interpreted as a much more common ovarian tumor. Occasionally a profuse but sporadic serosanguineous vaginal discharge may occur, and if heed is given to this symptom of *hemohydrops tubae profluens*, an occasional preoperative diagnosis may be possible. The finding of cancer cells in the vaginal smear, with completely negative findings on biopsy of the cervix and uterine curettage, might be of value, and a few such cases have been reported.

Dodson *et al.* have recommended the following system of staging similar to the FIGO classification of ovarian tumors, and this seems a logical approach:

Stage I: Growth limited to the tube
  Stage Ia: Growth limited to one tube; no ascites
  Stage Ib: Growth limited to both tubes; no ascites
  Stage Ic: Growth limited to one or both tubes; ascites present with malignant cells in fluid
Stage II: Growth involving one or both tubes with pelvic extension
  Stage IIa: Extension and/or metastasis to the uterus or ovary

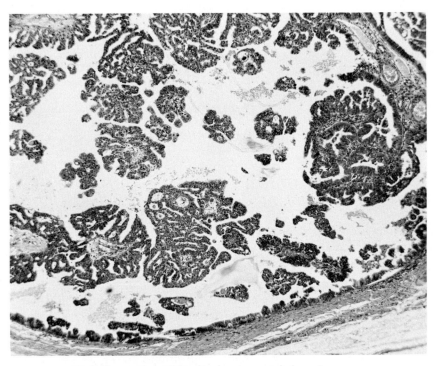

21.3. Very early, still localized, primary tubal carcinoma

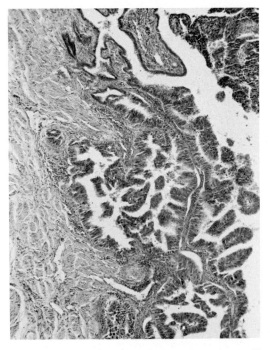

21.4. Early lesion showing origin from "normal" tubal epithelium above and adenomatous pattern in center.

Stage IIb: Extension to other pelvic tissues
Stage III: Growth involving one or both tubes with widespread intraperitoneal metastasis to abdomen
Stage IV: Growth involving one or both tubes with distant metastasis outside the peritoneal cavity

Treatment. The treatment consists of hysterectomy with bilateral removal of the adnexa. Postoperative radiation is ordinarily employed, but there is some question as to its value. Salvage is in the nature of 34% (Sedlis), 40% (Kneale *et al.*) to 45% (Hanton). The recent report by Boronow implies that chemotherapy may be helpful. If certain tumors of the tube (like the ovary) originate from the mesothelium, this would appear logical.

Secondary Carcinoma (Figs. 21.5,6)

Secondary carcinoma of the tube is far more frequent than the primary form, as might be expected from the position of the tube between the uterus and ovary, with both of which it is intimately linked up

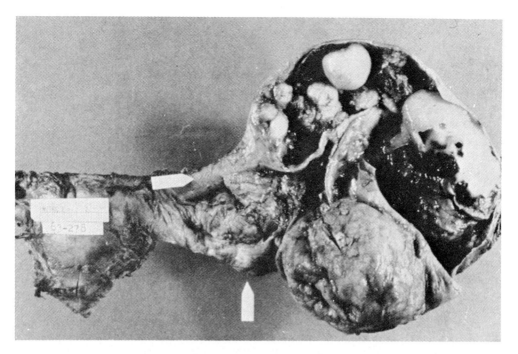

21.5. *Perpendicular arrow* designates normal ovary; *transverse arrow* points to hydrosalpinx merging into malignant tumor. (Courtesy of Dr. A. J. McQueeney, Santa Barbara, California.)

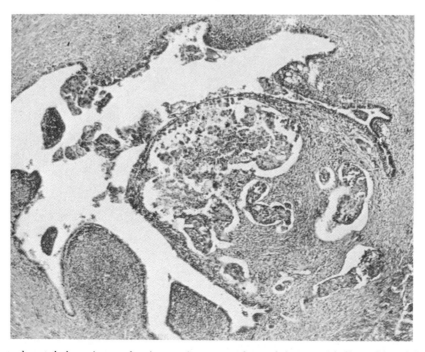

21.6. Secondary tubal carcinoma showing carcinoma area beneath intact epithelium although loss of latter would give impression of implantation of cancer on surface instead of spread by lymphatics.

from the standpoint of lymphatics, and in both of which carcinoma is frequent. There are some who believe that ovarian and even uterine carcinoma may produce secondary lesions in the tube through the implantation of cancer cells migrating through the tube, but it is probable that in most instances the lymphatic route is the responsible factor in the dissemination of the neoplasm.

OTHER TUMORS OF THE TUBE

Other tumors of the tube are rare, some exceedingly so. (Adeno)myoma, malignant mixed mesodermal tumors, primary chorionepithelioma following tubal pregnancy, sarcoma, fibroma, fibromyoma, and dermoid cysts have all been reported. With the exception of the first, itself uncommon, all are exceedingly rare, only 31 cases, for example, of sarcoma having been reported by Abrams, Kazal, and Hobbs. Any secondary or metastatic tumor may be noted.

Various *adenomatoid* tumors, probably mesothelial in type or originating from the remnants of the rete testis, are usually benign; although uncommon they are being recognized with more frequency. In a recent review, Grimes and Kornmesser record 31 cases of dermoid (benign teratomatous) cysts of the tube. Dede and Janovski record 13 cases of lipoma of the tube and speculate on the origin of this extremely unusual tubal neoplasm. We have recently viewed a hilus cell tumor from our own clinic.

PAROVARIAN CYSTS

In the mesosalpinx between the tube and ovary is situated the parovarium (epoophoron or organ of Rosenmüller) a vestigial structure corresponding to the sexual portion of the Wolffian body. Its chief duct is spoken of as Gartner's duct, the homologue of the vas deferens in the male. From the main duct a group of tiny tubules (tubules of Kobelt) extend toward and often into both the hilium of the ovary and the broad ligament border of the tube (Fig. 21.7).

Cysts may arise either from the main duct or from any of the accessory tubules, constituting the so-called parovarian

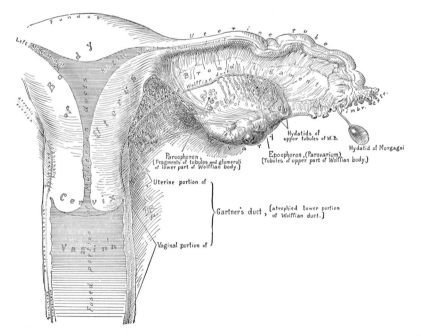

21.7. Relations of parovarian and Gartner's duct to pelvic organs. (From Cullen, T. S.: Bull. Johns Hopkins Hosp., 7:112, 1896.)

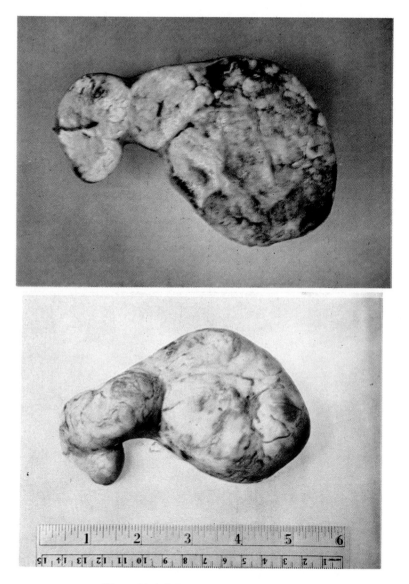

Plate 21.1. Primary carcinoma of tube

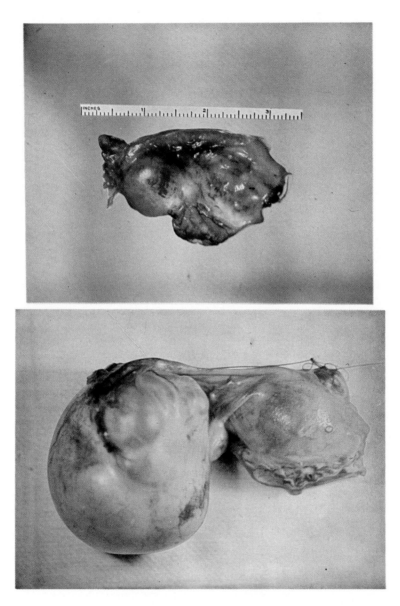

Plate 21.2. *Top*, small parovarian cyst; note its position between ovary and end of tube. *Bottom*, rather large parovarian cyst which might be mistaken for ovarian; note, however, the separateness of the ovary from the growth.

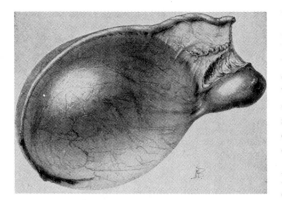

21.8. Large parovarian cyst

being intact and separate from the tumor, and the tube being stretched across the upper circumference of the cyst. The walls are very thin and the cavity contains a clear fluid. A papillomatous tendency is often noted on the inner wall of the cysts, more particularly in the smaller growths (Fig. 21.9). Microscopically the cyst is lined by a single layer of cuboidal or flat epithelium.

The symptoms of parovarian cyst are like those of the more common ovarian cysts, for which they are usually mistaken preoperatively. There is no tendency to malignancy, and treatment is surgical.

cysts. They may be very small, occurring as incidental findings in operations for other conditions. On the other hand, parovarian cysts may reach a very large size (Fig. 21.8), although rarely as large as many cysts of the ovary itself. They are usually easily recognizable as of parovarian origin by their position, the ovary

TUMORS OF THE ROUND LIGAMENTS

Like the uterus, the round ligaments are made up of smooth muscle. *Myoma* (Fig. 21.10) is therefore fairly common, presenting the same histological structure (Fig. 21.11) as does uterine myoma, but confusing the situation at operation by

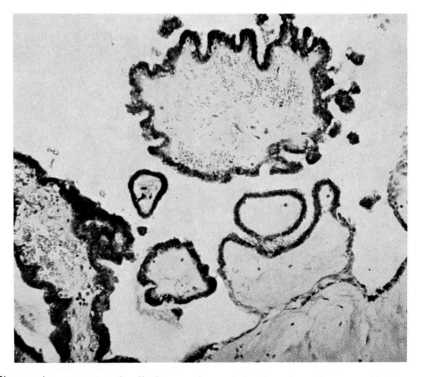

21.9. Microscopic appearance of wall of parovarian cyst showing a low columnar epithelium and often, as in this case, a papillary tendency.

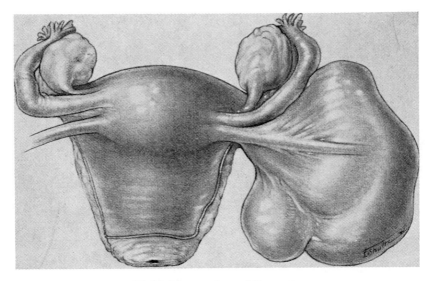

21.10. Myoma of round ligament

grossly distorting and occasionally replacing the round ligament or dissecting under the bladder. Another tumor which is not uncommon is *adenomyoma*, which histologically consists of endometrial tissue islands embedded in a matrix of involuntary muscle. *Sarcoma* is exceedingly rare.

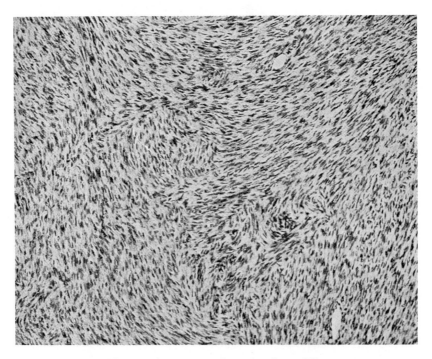

21.11. Microscopic structure of myoma of round ligament

TUMORS OF THE BROAD LIGAMENTS

Although not very common, *myoma* may develop from the involuntary muscle normally included in the structure of the broad ligaments as may sarcoma. *Cysts* may likewise be encountered, arising from the portion of Gartner's duct (vestigial remains of the mesonephric or paramesonephric duct (Bransilver *et al.*) which courses along the lateral margin of the uterus. Imperfect obliteration and cystic distention of portions of this duct give rise to cysts, usually small but sometimes quite large.

Novak, Woodruff, and Novak have pointed out that an identical tumor may be found at any level of the genital tract where *remnants of the mesonephric duct* may be found. In the cervix, vaginal fornices, broad ligaments, or region of the ovary may be found a histologically similar tumor. This may be similar to the ovarian *mesonephroma of Schiller* or the so-called *clear cell adenocarcinoma*, but admixtures are frequent. In the broad ligament region it is of moderate malignancy.

In recent years a paramesonephric origin has been suggested. The recent case report by Czernobilsky would support this thesis. Perhaps there is more than a single means of genesis.

TUMORS OF THE UTEROSACRAL LIGAMENTS

Although *myoma* occurs, the most common tumor of the uterosacral ligaments is *adenomyoma* (Fig. 21.12). In cases of pelvic endometriosis these ligaments are frequently the seat of endometrial "implants" (Fig. 21.13). These often consist of very superficial islands of endometrial tissue but in some cases the ectopic endometrium excites a marked local muscular reaction, producing nodular adenomyomas which must be considered probably neoplastic. These nodules vary in size from a few millimeters to several centimeters in diameter. They are often multiple. Because of the responsiveness of

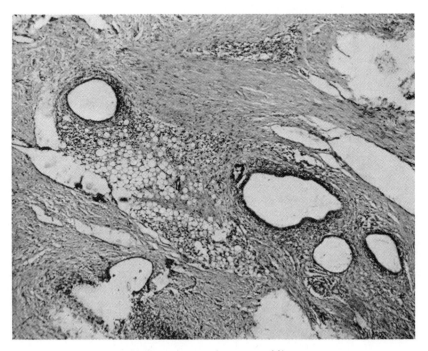

21.12. Adenomyoma of uterosacral ligament

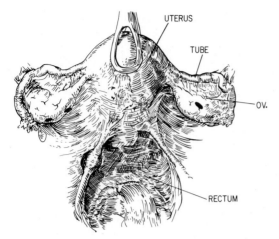

UTERUS

TUBE

OV.

RECTUM

21.13. Adenomyoma of uterosacral ligaments; endometrial implants in ovaries.

the contained endometrium to the ovarian hormones, the growths are usually dark, bluish red. The same menstrual responsiveness gives rise to menstrual pain, which is referred to the rectum or the lower sacral or coccygeal regions. This symptom, coupled with the presence of palpable nodules in the uterosacral regions, justifies a presumptive diagnosis of pelvic endometriosis, although it is often impossible to know if this represents diffuse external endometriosis or an extension of internal (adenomyosis) disease. In any case, both represent examples of misplaced uterine mucosa.

The adenomyomatous growth may involve the adjoining rectal wall and may infiltrate the rectovaginal septum (*adenomyoma of rectovaginal septum*). When such growths are encountered as a part of the picture of extensive pelvic endometriosis, as they so often are, complete removal of ovarian tissue leads to their regression. Adenomyosis or endometriosis of the upper vagina can be distinguished only by biopsy from the unusual case of *posthysterectomy prolapse* of the tube.

REFERENCES

Abrams, J., Kazal, H. L., and Hobbs, R. E.: Primary sarcoma of fallopian tube. Amer. J. Obstet. Gynec., *75:* 180, 1958.
Boronow, R. C.: Chemotherapy for disseminated tubal carcinoma. Obstet. Gynec., *42:* 62, 1973.
Boutselis, J. G., and Thompson, J. N.: Clinical aspects of primary tubal carcinoma. Amer. J. Obstet. Gynec., *111:* 98, 1971.
Bransilver, B. R., Ferenczy, A., and Richart, R. M.: Female genital tract remnants. Arch. Path., *96:* 255, 1973.
Cavallero, G., and Rossi, R.: Contribution to the study of malignant mixed tumors of the Fallopian tube (carcinosarcoma). Pathologica, *51:* 443, 1959.
Cron, R. S., and Claude, J. L.: Primary papillary carcinoma of uterine tube. Obstet. Gynec., *13:* 734, 1959.
Cullen, T. S.: Adenomyoma of round ligament. Bull. Johns Hopkins Hosp., *7:* 112, 1896.
Czernobilsky, B., and Lancet, M.: Broad ligament adenocarcinoma of Müllerian origin. Obstet. Gynec., *40:* 238, 1972.
Dede, J. A., and Janovski, N. A.: Lipoma of the uterine tube—a gynecological rarity. Obstet. Gynec., *22:* 461, 1963.
Dodson, M. G., Ford, J. M., Jr., and Avenette, H. E.: Clinical aspects of fallopian tube carcinoma. Obstet. Gynec., *36:* 935, 1970.
Erez, S., Kaplan, A. L., and Wall, J. A.: Clinical staging of carcinoma of the uterine tube. Obstet. Gynec., *30:* 547, 1967.
Frankel, A. W.: Primary carcinoma of the fallopian tube. Amer. J. Obstet. Gynec., *72:* 31, 1956.
Gardner, G. H., Greene, R. R., and Peckham, B.: Tumors of the broad ligament. Amer. J. Obstet. Gynec., *73:* 563, 1957.
Goldman, J. A., Gans, B., and Eckerling, B.: Hydrops tubae profluens—a symptom of tubal carcinoma. Obstet. Gynec., *18:* 631, 1961.
Green, T. H., Jr., and Scully, R. E.: Tumors of the fallopian tube. Clin. Obstet. Gynec., *5:* 886, 1962.
Grimes, H. G., and Kornmesser, J. G.: Benign cystic tumor of the oviduct. Obstet. Gynec., *16:* 85, 1960.
Hanton, E. M., Malkasian, G. D., Dahlin, D. C., and Pratt, J. H.: Primary carcinoma of the fallopian tube (27 cases). Amer. J. Obstet. Gynec., *94:* 832, 1966.
Hayden, G. E., and Potter, E. L.: Primary carcinoma of the fallopian tube. Amer. J. Obstet. Gynec., *79:* 24, 1960.
Hurlbutt, F. R., and Nelson, H. B.: Primary carcinoma of the uterine tube. Obstet. Gynec., *21:* 730, 1963.
Janovski, N. A., and Paramanandhan, T. L.: *Ovarian Tumors, tumorous and Tumorlike Conditions of the Ovaries, Fallopian Tubes, and Ligaments of the Uterus.* W. B. Saunders Co., Philadelphia, 1973.
Kneale, B. L. G., and Attwood, H. D.: Primary cancer of the fallopian tube. Amer. J. Obstet. Gynec., *94:* 840, 1966.
Larsson, E., and Schooby, J. L.: Positive vaginal cytology in primary carcinoma of the fallopian tube. Amer. J. Obstet. Gynec., *22:* 1369, 1956.
Mazanella, P., Okagi, T., and Richart, R. M.: Uterine tube teratoma. Obstet. Gynec., *39:* 381, 1972.
McQueeney, A. J., Carswell, B. L., and Sheehan, W. J.: Malignant mixed Mullerian tumor primary in uterine tube. Obstet. Gynec., *23:* 338, 1964.
Momtazee, S., and Kempson, R. L.: Primary adenocarcinoma of the fallopian tube. Obstet. Gynec., *32:* 649, 1968.
Novak, E., Woodruff, J. D., and Novak, E. R.: Mesonephric origin of certain female genital tumors. Amer. J. Obstet. Gynec., *68:* 1222, 1954.
Pauerstein, C. J., Woodruff, J. D., and Quinton, S. W.: Developmental patterns in "adenomatoid lesions" of the fallopian tube. Amer. J. Obstet. Gynec., *32:* 649, 1968.
Pauerstein, C. J., and Woodruff, J. D.: Cellular patterns in proliferative and anaplastic disease of the fallopian tube. Amer. J. Obstet. Gynec., *95:* 486, 1966.
Riggs, J. A.: Wainer, A. S., Hahn, G. A., and Farell, D. M.: Extrauterine tubal choriocarcinoma. Amer. J. Obstet. Gynec., *88:* 637 1964.

Roberts, C. L., and Marshall, H. K.: Fibromyoma of the fallopian tube. Amer. J. Obstet. Gynec., *82:* 364, 1961.

Ryan, G. M.: Carcinoma in situ of the fallopian tube. Amer. J. Obstet. Gynec., *84:* 198, 1962.

Schiller, H. M., and Silverberg, S. G.: Staging and prognosis in primary carcinoma of the fallopian tube. Cancer. *28:* 389, 1971.

Sedlis, A.: Primary carcinoma of the fallopian tube. Obstet. Gynec. Survey, *16:* 209, 1961.

Teel, P.: Adenomatoid tumors of the genital tract. Amer. J. Obstet. Gynec., *75:* 1347, 1958.

Thompson, J. D., Dockerty, M. B., Symmonds, R. E., and Hayles, A. B.: Ovarian and paraovarian tumors in infants and children. Amer. J. Obstet. Gynec., *97:* 1059, 1967.

Williams, T. J., and Woodruff, J. D.: Malignant mixed mesenchymal tumor of the uterine tube. Obstet. Gynec., *21:* 618, 1963.

Woodruff, J. D. and Pauerstein, C. J.: *The Fallopian Tube.* The Williams & Wilkins Company, Baltimore, Md., 1969.

Wu, J. P., Tanner, W. S., and Fardal, P. M.: Malignant mixed Müllerian tumor of the tube. Obstet. Gynec., *41:* 707, 1973.

chapter 22

Benign Tumors of the Ovary

In discussing the origin of ovarian tumors, McKay has emphasized the concepts of histological examination, the use of logic, knowledge of ovarian embryology, as well as other data. Also emphasized in our laboratory is a knowledge of ovarian histology in the neonatal and infant years, as described by Curtis. A brief resume of certain practical histological classifications of ovarian tumors follows; clinical classification is noted in the following chapters.

I. BENIGN TUMORS OF THE OVARY

A. *Cystic*
  1. Nonneoplastic
    a. Follicle
    b. Lutein
    c. Stein-Leventhal
    d. Endometrial
    e. Tubo-ovarian inflammatory
    f. Germinal inclusion
  2. Neoplastic
    a. Serous cystadenoma
    b. Mucinous cystadenoma
    c. Dermoid (benign cystic teratoma)

B. *Solid*
  1. Fibroma

  2. Brenner (rarely malignant)
  3. Assorted rare lesions

II. MALIGNANT TUMORS OF THE OVARY

A. *Cystic*
  1. Serous cystadenocarcinoma
  2. Mucinous cystadenocarcinoma
  3. Carcinoma (epidermoid) arising in dermoid

B. *Solid*
  1. (Adeno)carcinoma
  2. Endometrioid carcinoma (often adenoacanthoma)
  3. Mesonephroma

III. OTHER MALIGNANT LESIONS (RARE)

1. Teratoma, entodermal sinus, etc.
2. Choriocarcinoma
3. Sarcoma
4. Lymphoma
5. Melanoma

IV. TUMORS WITH ENDOCRINE POTENTIAL (LITTLE MALIGNANCY)

1. Functioning
  a. Dysgerminoma, generally inert (gonadoblastoma)

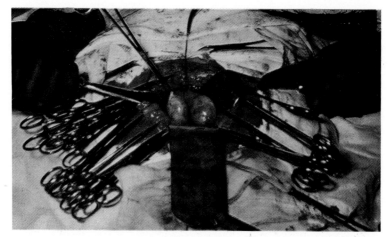

Plate 22.1. Characteristic Stein-Leventhal syndrome; bilaterally enlarged, smooth, oyster-white ovaries with small uterus.

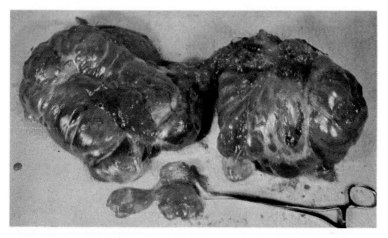

Plate 22.2. Mucinous cyst, which ruptured and produced myxoma peritonei and mucocele of appendix, the latter being seen in the lower part of the picture.

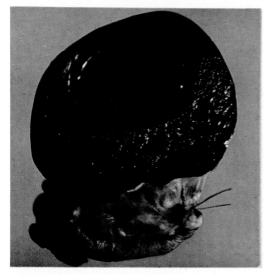

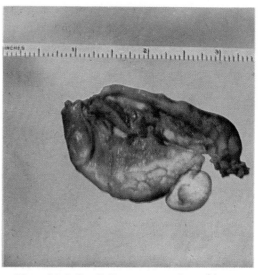

Plate 22.3. Torsion of pedicle of small ovarian cyst showing dark gangrenous picture produced by interference with circulation.

Plate 22.4. Small fibroma on surface of ovary

b. Granulosa theca (with luteinization), generally feminizing ⎫
c. Arrhenoblastoma, generally virilizing ⎭ Gonadal Stromal

2. Adrenal rest tumor, generally virilizing
3. Hilus cell, generally virilizing
4. Tumors with functioning matrix

V. METASTATIC OR BY EXTENSION

Pattern similar to primary lesion
Krukenberg tumor

Another excellent method of classification of ovarian tumors is that proposed by Hertig and Gore which considers ovarian tumors as originating in (1) *germinal epithelium* as serous, mucinous, and endometrioid cystadenomas and cystoadenocarcinoma, and others; (2) *connective tissue* tumors as sarcoma, fibroma, etc.; (3) *germ cell* tumors such as dysgerminoma, teratoma, and choriocarcinoma; (4) *gonadal stromal* tumors as arrhenoblastomas and the granulosa-theca cell neoplasm; (5) *vestigial rest* tumors such as mesonephroma or hilus cell tumor; (6) *metastatic* tumors. Frankly, this classification has considerable merit, and we are in the process of adapting to it.

However, the Cancer Committee of the International Federation of Gynecology and Obstetrics has proposed the following classification for the *epithelial* tumors of the ovary. Although the FIGO scheme refers only to the epithelial tumors of the ovary, it is a first step towards uniformity and presumably is a prelude to a complete scheme of classification.

HISTOLOGICAL CLASSIFICATION OF THE COMMON PRIMARY EPITHELIAL TUMORS OF THE OVARY

I. Serous cystomas
  A. Serous benign cystadenoma
  B. Serous cystadenomas with proliferating activity of the epithelial cells and nuclear abnormalities, but with no infiltrative destructive growth (low potential malignancy)
  C. Serous cystadenocarcinomas

II. Mucinous cystomas
  A. Mucinous benign cystadenomas
  B. Mucinous cystadenomas with proliferating activity of the epithelial cells and nuclear abnormalities, but with no infiltrative destructive growth (low potential malignancy)
  C. Mucinous cystadenocarcinomas

III. Endometrioid tumors (similar to adenocarcinomas in the endometrium)
  A. Endometrioid benign cysts
  B. Endometrioid tumors with proliferating activity of the epithelial cells and nuclear abnormalities, but with no infiltrative destructive growth (low potential malignancy)
  C. Endometrioid adenocarcinomas

IV. Mesonephric tumors
  A. Benign mesonephric tumors
  B. Mesonephric tumors with proliferating activity of the epithelial cells and nuclear abnormalities but with no infiltrative, destructive growth (low potential malignancy)
  C. Mesonephric cystadenocarcinoma (Not included but a logical addition would be Brenner tumors (although there is also a stromal component) as suggested by the recent ultrastructural study by Bransilver *et al.*)
    a. Benign
    b. Proliferative
    c. Malignant

V. Concomitant carcinomas, unclassified carcinomas (tumors which cannot be allotted to one of the previous groups)

BENIGN CYSTS

By far the most frequent of all ovarian tumors are the cysts, most of which are not genuine neoplasms. This applies particularly to the smaller cystic structures which are frequently found in the ovary and which are to be looked upon as functional retention cysts originating in the follicles or corpora lutea. Many cysts, on the other hand, are true neoplasms

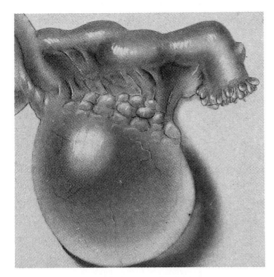

22.1. Follicle cyst of ovary

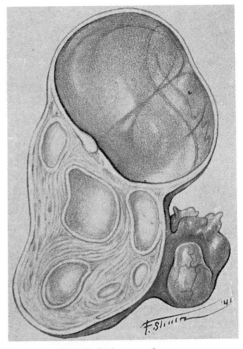

22.3. Follicle cyst of ovary

which may reach enormous size. On the basis of this distinction, therefore, the benign cysts of the ovary may be divided into two groups: (1) the nonneoplastic cysts, and (2) the neoplastic cysts.

Nonneoplastic (Functional) Cysts of the Ovary

Follicle Cysts

These arise from simple cystic overdistention of follicles during the process of atresia (see Chapter 3). Every month a considerable number of follicles are blighted, with death of the ovum, followed soon by degeneration of the follic-

ular epithelium. Frequently the cavity is greatly overdistended with fluid (Figs. 22.1–22.3), producing cysts of clinically important size, although they only rarely exceed the size of a lemon, and are usually much smaller. Hemorrhage into the cyst cavity may take place, producing the so-called follicular hematoma (Fig. 22.4).

Symptoms. The symptoms of follicle cysts are not characteristic, but dis-

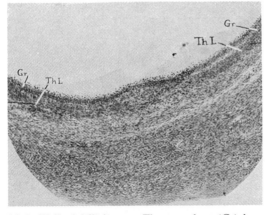

22.2. Wall of follicle cyst. The granulosa (*Gr*) has almost disappeared and beneath it is seen the theca (*ThL*).

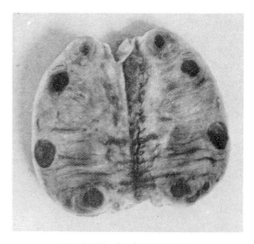

22.4. Follicular hematomas

tinctive effects on menstruation may be produced. When the cyst is sufficiently large, it may cause a sensation of heaviness or a dull aching discomfort in the affected side. As with any other type of ovarian cyst *torsion* of the pedicle may occur (Plate 22.3), and in rare cases, *spontaneous rupture with intraabdominal bleeding* producing a clinical picture simulating ruptured tubal pregnancy. Far more frequently, however, *spontaneous resorption* takes place, just as in the normal process of atresia folliculi.

Diagnosis. The diagnosis can be made only by palpation of the cyst, but it is not possible at one examination to be sure whether the cyst is of the nonneoplastic variety or whether it is a genuine cystic tumor such as cystadenoma. One should, therefore, avoid prompt operation for small ovarian cysts. It is a common observation that cysts are frequently evanescent, and the gynecologist who is absolutely certain at one examination that he feels a cyst as large as a lemon may find on reexamination a few weeks later that the ovary has regressed to normal size. By contrast the neoplastic type of cyst not only persists but gradually increases in size. With younger women, expectant therapy is indicated over the course of eight to ten weeks before deciding on laparotomy; in the middle age group, evaluation should not be so prolonged, and in the postmenopausal patient, any adnexal enlargement warrants prompt laparotomy. (Barber and Graber)

Treatment. When small follicle cysts are found at operation, they are best treated by either simple puncture (needling) or excision, depending upon their size. When the cyst is larger, it can be shelled out, often intact, with conservation of the normal ovarian tissue.

Lutein Cysts (Figs. 22.5, 6)

The term "lutein cyst" is generally used collectively, although it is important clinically to consider the possibility of pregnancy lest removal of the cyst increase the chances of abortion, especially in the first trimester of pregnancy. Lutein cysts may, of course, occur in the absence of pregnancy.

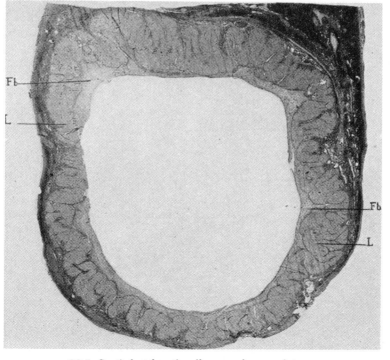

22.5. Cystic but functionally normal corpus luteum

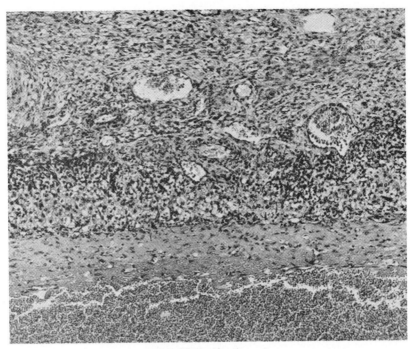

22.6. Wall of lutein cyst

The origin of the true lutein cyst is usually from a corpus luteum hematoma. The latter, in turn, is brought about by an exaggeration of the hemorrhage which normally takes place into the corpus cavity in the so-called stage of vascularization. When the bleeding is excessive, a large *corpus luteum hematoma* is produced, characterized chiefly by a thinned out, bright yellow lutein wall about the blood-filled central cavity. Gradually, however, there is a resorption of the blood elements, leaving a clear or slightly bloody fluid.

Symptoms. The symptoms of lutein cysts cannot always be correlated with their histological appearance. In the most interesting group, the symptoms resemble those of early tubal pregnancy. Menstruation is apt to be slightly delayed, followed by persistent scant bleeding, with often pain in one or the other of the lower quadrants, and with the presence on pelvic examination of a small tender swelling in the corresponding side of the pelvis. This represents the characteristic symptomatology of early tubal pregnancy, and yet not infrequently one may find at operation a lutein cyst instead.

There is some belief that such cases represent very early abortion of a fertilized but as yet unimplanted egg, although there is no direct evidence to substantiate this view. Others look upon the syndrome as identical with that of the so-called *corpus luteum persistens*, in which, for some unknown reason, the normal regression of the corpus is deferred, with persistence of the progestational phase in the endometrium, through a mechanism which may be similar to the pseudopregnancy observed in some of the lower animals.

A rare type of lutein cyst is that found in some cases of hydatidiform mole and choriocarcinoma. In some cases of this sort the wall of the cyst is formed by luteinized granulosal cells, but usually the cyst is composed of paralutein (*thecalutein*) cells of connective tissue rather than epithelial origin (Fig. 22.2). A few such theca-lutein cysts have been reported during the course of a normal pregnancy (Girouard *et al.*). A more recent review by Caspi *et al.* records 29 cases not associated with molar pregnancy. These cystic changes may be produced by administration of HCG.

Diagnosis. The diagnosis of lutein cysts is obviously difficult, and in the majority of cases their presence is not suspected before operation. When of considerable size they can of course be palpated. In a small group of cases the presence of a cyst of this character can be at least suspected when a symptom complex like that of tubal pregnancy is produced. When such a problem arises, pregnancy tests may be of service, for they are often positive in tubal gestation, and negative in the corpus luteum cysts. Culdoscopy or laporoscopy is more conclusive.

Treatment. The treatment of lutein cysts or hematomas consists of observation, for most of them undergo spontaneous disappearance. In the case of hemorrhagic cysts of considerable size, or where there is evidence of intraperitoneal bleeding, excision is the proper treatment, for massive hemoperitoneum may occur. At times the yellowish shimmer of the wall gives a clue to the lutein character of the cyst, and in such cases the surgeon should, before removal of the cyst, consider the possibility of very early gestation. In a large proportion of cases the lutein character of the cyst is not suspected before laboratory examination.

It has been noted that functional cysts are relatively uncommon in women taking birth control pills as a result of suppression of the pituitary. This may be of

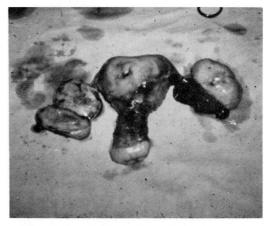

22.8. Recurrent Stein-Leventhal ovaries after earlier successful wedge resection.

assistance clinically—if a cyst persists after two months of pill therapy, it is more likely neoplastic rather than functional.

Stein-Leventhal Ovary

In 1928 Dr. Irving Stein focused gynecological attention on a certain group of patients who were characterized by infertility, oligo-amenorrhea, occasionally interspersed with menorrhagia, and less commonly hirsutism, an enlarged clitoris, and obesity. The clinical details of this so-called Stein-Leventhal syndrome will be dealt with more fully in Chapter 31, but it seems feasible to discuss the pathological aspects of this ovarian enlargement here, although the "S.-L." ovary should probably not be regarded as a true neoplasm.

Stein has always been careful to emphasize that the validity of this syndrome is dependent upon a characteristic pathological appearance of the ovaries, and this is important if successful diagnosis and treatment be achieved. Bilateral enlargement of the ovaries is the rule, although possibly it may not be noted in incipient stages of the disease. In a typical case, however, the examiner will note three equal-size pelvic masses, a small uterus, and bilaterally enlarged ("hen's egg") ovaries (see (Figs. 22.7, 8).

The enlargement of the ovaries is usually bilateral, although one side may predominate. The ovarian surface is

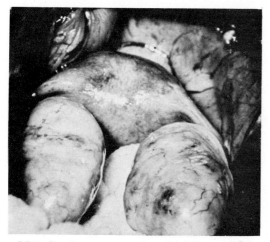

22.7. Small uterus anterior with bilateral Stein-Leventhal ovaries (after HCG stimulation).

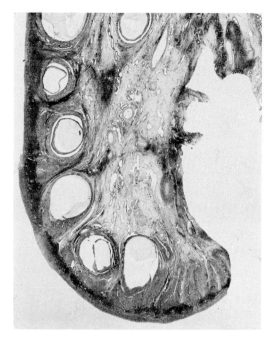

22.9. Cut surface of so-called multiple cystic ovary.

found to be smooth, thickened, and pearly gray or oyster-white in color (Plate 22.1). So fibrotic is the capsule that the operator, on cutting into the ovary, will note a very characteristic "gritty" consistency, and although the ovary is polycystic due to many follicular cysts, there is no evidence of a corpus luteum (Fig. 22.9).

Microscopically there is a characteristic pattern showing a thickened fibrotic and sometimes hyalinized cortical tunica albuginea, below which are many follicles in all stages of maturation and atresia, seemingly incapable of penetrating the thickened cortex (Fig. 22.10). One often sees hyperplasia of the theca interna in the walls of the cystic follicles (Fig. 22.11), and there is some belief that these luteinized theca cells (*hyperthecosis*) may produce an androgenic substance leading to some of the virilizing tendencies seen on occasion (Shippel). Of paramount importance is the absence of corpora lutea;

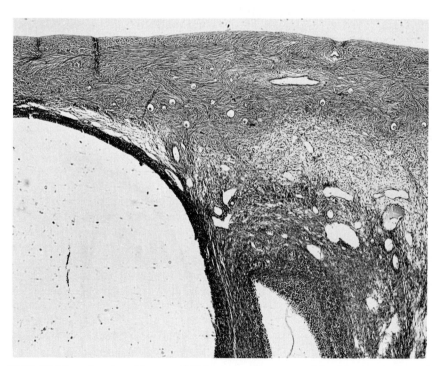

22.10. Thickened cortex with many follicles in varying stages of development and atresia.

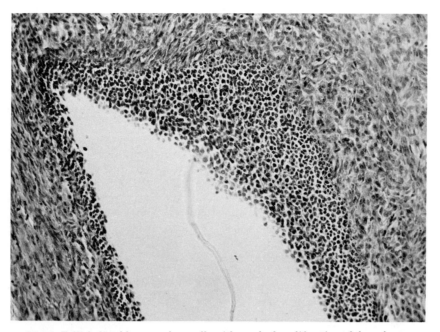

22.11. Follicle lined by granulosa cells with marked proliferation of theca layer

whereas the finding of a single corpus luteum should not completely invalidate the diagnosis, the S.-L. syndrome is characterized by recurrent anovulation with persistent estrogen and an absence of progesterone.

The polycystic ovary is found uniformly with the S.-L. syndrome; however, it is by no means pathognomonic, for essentially the same ovarian pattern may be found in many cases of recurrent anovulation where bleeding is the presenting problem. There are probably many closely related varieties of "polycystic ovarian disease" which may produce a variety of endocrine dysfunctions. It is our laboratory policy to avoid a definite diagnosis and speak of ovarian tissue removed at surgery as being merely "compatible with a Stein-Leventhal syndrome."

Judd *et al.* also indicate an indefinite borderline between polycystic ovarian disease and hyperthecosis, and suggest that they may represent variations of the same basic disease process. Both may have a familial basis. Cooper *et al.* have suggested that transmission of the hereditary potential for the S-L syndrome is consistent with a dominant mode of inheritance, probably autosomal.

Treatment. Stein originally proposed surgical wedge resection of the bilaterally enlarged polycystic ovaries, and removal of approximately one-half to two-thirds of the ovarian tissue is accomplished, the remaining ovarian substance being approximated by lock suture of triple zero catgut. Originally it was believed that resection of the densely thickened cortex might remove a mechanical barrier to ovulation and subsequently permit more ready passage of the ovum out of the ovary. Since, however, following wedge resection the ovarian cortex is re-approximated, this suggestion is difficult to accept, and other students have attempted to explain the successful results of surgery by postulating the law of "follicular constancy"; *i.e.,* removal of a certain amount of ovarian tissue might permit greater stimulation by a given amount of gonadotrophin to the degree that ovulation may be incurred. Our own feeling is that the S.-L. ovary differs from the usually "anovulatory ovary" only in the matter of size, which is in accord with Evans and Riley's belief that the polycystic ovary as seen in the S.-L. gonad represents merely an advanced degree of anovulation. Perhaps reduction of ovarian tissue leads to a decreased estrogen which is followed by a greater gonadotrophic stimulus; many other explanations have been offered.

It also would seem that the beneficial results following wedge resection of the ovary are probably due to sheer reduction of ovarian bulk which may prompt query as to why unilateral oophorectomy might not be just as effective. It probably is, as has been noted by Greenblatt, but is not done as a routine merely because most gynecologists are inclined to be extremely conservative about even unilateral ovariectomy in the young women. In addition, the S.-L. ovary is not infrequently associated with other tumors, generally dermoids, but we are aware of granulosa-theca tumors and arrhenoblastoma among others; it is speculative whether the S.-L. endocrine dysfunction is in any way causative of the tumor.

Surgery is by no means the only type of treatment for the S.-L. syndrome. Goldfarb has reviewed the literature and reported his own results with clomiphene citrate (clomid), and Gemzell has published a similar study on therapy with various gonadotrophins. Currently our own feeling is that surgical wedge resection gives better results with subsequently normal menstruation and pregnancy in over 85% of all cases as noted by Stein, and with little likelihood of multiple pregnancy. Clomiphene is used occasionally as treatment where the menses do not regulate postsurgically. Goldfarb has suggested that operation allows for better response to clomiphene. Gonadotrophin and hypothalamic LRF are used only rarely and seem most helpful where there is a proven pituitary dysfunction. Fuller details in regards treatment will be found in Chapter 31.

Benedict *et al.* feel that biopsy of both ovary and adrenal in cases of hirsutism and virilism will show certain evidence of adrenal hyperplasia, thus suggesting a pluriglandular disorder with the hypothalamic-pituitary axis as the primary culprit. We find it difficult to disagree with this thesis, which conforms closely to the expressions of Taymor, Clark, and Sturgis who feel that no typical clinical picture, ovarian size, or laboratory findings are constant; unlike these authors, however, we would not accept a diagnosis of a Stein-Leventhal ovary if numerous corpora lutea (with presumed ovulation) are present. Nor could we be as precise as Fienberg who attempts to establish specific clinico-pathological groups of thecosis, as suggested earlier by Shippel. It seems difficult to refute the likelihood that some type of hypothalamic-pituitary defect is the basic defect in this problem.

Association with Endometrial Adenocarcinoma

Jackson and Dockerty have reported a 40 per cent incidence of adenocarcinoma, frequently low grade adenocanthoma, in conjunction with "Stein-Leventhal" ovaries, although Stein himself states he has never observed this sequel. Although it is unlikely that endometrial carcinoma is a frequent concomitant of the S.-L. syndrome, we see several cases a year, either of our own or referred for a pathological opinion. Kaufman, Abbott, and Wall have reported a group of women whose endometria were extremely adenomatous and proliferative to the degree that a diagnosis of early adenocarcinoma had to be considered. Up to a certain point, however, wedge resection of the ovaries was followed by regression of the endometrium to normalcy. Just what that "critical point" may be is difficult to state with assurance, but anovulation and unopposed estrogen is the obvious stimulus.

In reviewing a recent case with metastases, Cameron has carried out an extensive review of the literature which would leave little doubt that real endometrial malignancy *does* exist with this particular form of ovarian dysfunction. Stein has been, of course, the leading student of this disease, and probably noted the problem early, before the advent of endometrial adenocarcinoma;

his diligence in performing surgery may have spared certain women the advent of fundal cancer. The recent therapeutic effects of clomiphene and the different gonadotrophins will be discussed in Chapter 31.

Our own feeling is that the microscopic differentiation between the typical Stein-Leventhal ovary and ovarian pathology associated with endometrial hyperplasia is extremely difficult, both being characterized by a myriad of small follicular cysts. Indeed, such excellent pathologists as Roberts and Haines question the validity of a S-L syndrome. Clinically there are all kinds of intermediary ovarian forms between the S-L pattern and various types of functional bleeding. Wedge resection is frequently curative for the former, but only in the classic syndrome as described by Stein and Leventhal. Desultory ovarian surgery ("whittling") is not recommended for the uncertain forms.

Yet it seems that the S-L syndrome should be regarded as a discrete entity, when there is a combination of the characteristic clinical stigmata along with the pathological features as noted, al-though neither one in itself is distinctive. Taw and Jones echo our sentiments in regard to the extreme difficulty in correlating the laboratory and clinical findings. Jeffcoate has stressed the biosynthesis and the bisexual problems present in this syndrome, at the same time indicating that the polycystic ovary may be of only secondary importance. This will be discussed more fully in the section on amenorrhea.

Recurrence of the S-L syndrome may be seen even where initial therapy seemed quite successful. A recent patient had a wedge resection followed by two pregnancies within three years. Ten years later, persistent menorrhagia ultimately led to hysterectomy, and characteristic S-L ovaries were also removed (Fig. 22.8).

Germinal Inclusion Cysts (Fig. 22.12)

These need only brief mention, as they are never of clinical importance. They are produced by invagination of the germinal epithelium of the ovary, so that they are most common in middle-aged and old women, when this invagination tendency

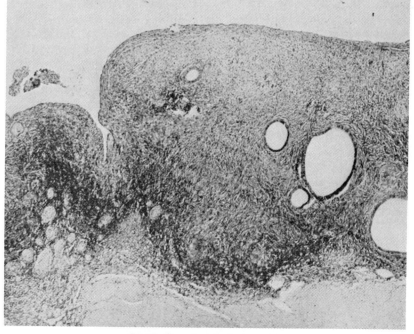

22.12. Germinal inclusion cysts

is most marked. They are always very small and usually of microscopic size, and they produce no symptoms. Metaplasia of these germinal inclusion cysts may occur.

Endometrial and Inflammatory Cysts

These are discussed in appropriate chapters.

Neoplastic or Proliferative Cysts of the Ovary

There are three chief varieties of cystic neoplasms of the ovary, as follows: (1) serous cystadenoma, (2) mucinous cystadenoma, and (3) dermoid cysts. The cystadenomas are far more common than the dermoids, constituting the most frequent of all ovarian tumors, solid or cystic. The mucinous tumors are those rich in the nonprotein substance mucin, whereas the serous growths are rich in the blood proteins, serum albumin, and serum globulin. There is no doubt that serous tumors predominate, at least in our own clinic material.

Serous Cystadenoma (FIGO 1)

Although serous cysts may reach a size of many pounds, they do not as a group attain the enormous proportions of some cases of the mucinous variety.

Grossly the external appearance may be similar to that of the mucinous cysts, but in other cases the surface presents papillomatous outgrowths which may in some instances resemble a cauliflower pattern (Fig. 22.13). In fact, if one notes this papillary external growth, it is reasonably certain that the cyst is of serous type.

The content is generally a thin watery fluid, but may be hemorrhagic or brownish in color. The inner wall of the cyst may be entirely smooth, so that, with the smaller growths, it is difficult to distinguish the cyst from one of simple follicular variety. More characteristically, one finds warty excrescences, sometimes small and discrete, in other cases filling the cyst cavities. Unlike the mucinous cystadenoma, this *papillomatous ten-*

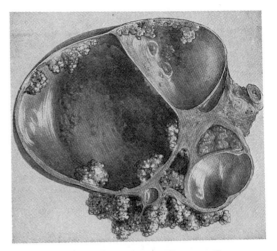

22.13. Papillary serous cystadenoma of ovary.

dency is very characteristic of the serous growths.

Microscopically (Fig. 22.14), the epithelium of serous cysts in quite different from that of the mucinous tumors, and it presents much more variation in the individual case. In general it is of much lower columnar type, with ciliation of many of the cells, so that there is a striking resemblance to tubal epithelium, which likewise is made up of ciliated and nonciliated columnar cells. In other tumors, or in other parts of the same cyst wall, the epithelium may be cuboidal or peg-shaped. The stroma is fibrous, with often hydropic degeneration. Rather characteristic of this variety of cyst is the frequent presence of small calcareous granules, the so-called *psammoma bodies,* an end product of the tumor implants (Fig. 22.15).

Indeed, Aure *et al.* imply that the presence of frequent psammoma bodies is of good prognostic import in that they seemingly represent an effective immunological response to the neoplasm. Since the last edition of this text, considerable work has been done with regard to the antigen-antibody nature of various ovarian tumors, predominantly of the malignant variety, but currently this work seems to be too speculative to draw any sound conclusions. The recent article by

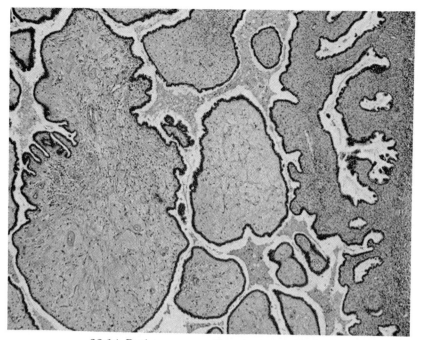

22.14. Benign serous papillomatous cystadenoma

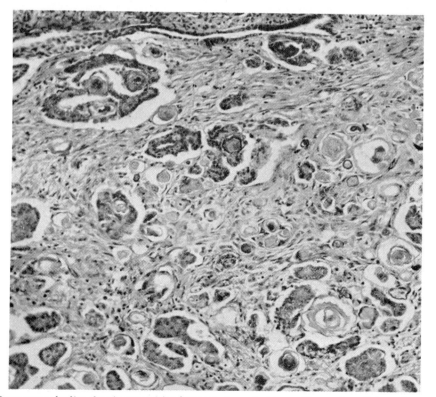

22.15. Psammoma bodies showing transition between recognizable papillae and acellular calcified bodies.

Gall, Walling and Pearl provides a satisfactory review of recent antigen-antibody studies in tumors of the genital tract.

When the epithelium is of the above type, and arranged in a single layer, there is no doubt of the benign nature of the cyst, at least from a histological standpoint. However, departures from this clearly benign pattern are very common, with stratification of the epithelium and evidence of epithelial overactivity so that it is not always easy to determine whether one is dealing with a benign serous cystadenoma or a papillary cystadenocarcinoma (see next chapter).

Histogenesis. Although there may be different origins of mucinous cysts, there is little doubt that the origin of the serous type is from the surface epithelium of the ovary. It is possible to demonstrate microscopically all stages of transition from simple invagination of the germinal epithelium, to invagination plus slight papillary formation, to the typical serous papillomatous cyst (Fig. 22.16).

Fibroadenoma and Cystadenofibroma.

Although the former is not a cystic tumor, and the latter only partly so, they are properly considered here because their histogenesis is so closely allied to that of serous cystadenoma. Like the latter, they arise from the surface epithelium of the ovary, which undergoes invagination, with the formation of long, cleftlike tubules surrounded by hyperplastic fibrous tissue, similar to the ordinary fibroadenoma of the breast. Such lesions are therefore designated as *fibroadenoma of the ovary.* They are usually of small size, and may be found only on microscopic examination (Figs. 22.17 and 22.18).

On the other hand, the invaginations often become cystic and may attain large size, as shown in Figure 22.19. Such tumors, designated as *cystadenofibroma,* are usually partly cystic and partly solid, in varying proportions. When small they form dense whitish, partly cystic nodules near the surface, but when large they may replace all or nearly all the ovarian substance. They are benign, but in rare cases may become malignant.

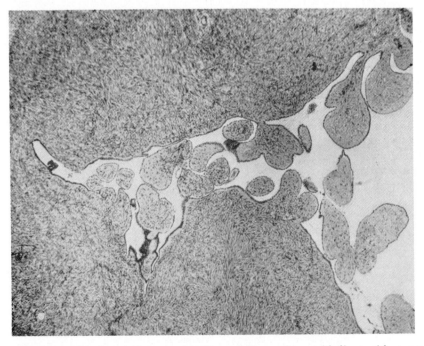

22.16. Photomicrograph showing how invagination of the surface epithelium with a papillomatous tendency brings about the development of what is essentially an early papillary serous cystadenoma.

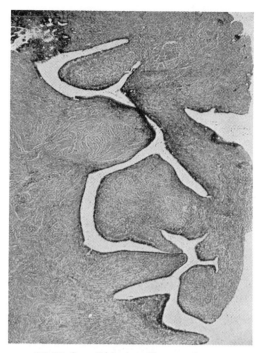

22.17. So-called adenofibroma of ovary

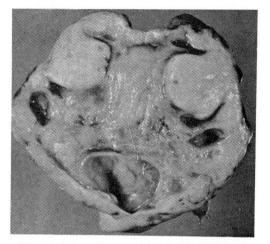

22.19. Gross appearance of rather large cystadenofibroma.

Mucinous Cystadenoma (FIGO II)

This variety may reach huge size, and as a matter of fact, many of the largest human tumors belong to this group. The largest appears to have been that reported by Spohn, 328 pounds, including the weight of frequent preoperative paracenteses, perhaps not a fair appraisal. Symmonds, Spraitz, and Koelshe have recently reported a tumor which, with aspirated fluid, weighed approximately 175 pounds, the largest removed in the last 50 years (Figs. 22.20-21). They have summarized the ten reported largest lesions, including Spohn's case. With four exceptions these occurred before 1900, and the mortality rate is high, although data are incomplete.

Grossly these tumors appear as rounded, ovoid, or irregularly lobulated growths, with a smooth outer surface of whitish or bluish white hue. The wall may in many areas be so thin as to be translucent. Although adhesions to surrounding organs may be present, they usually represent inflammatory adhesions and do not connote malignant extension. The attachment to the broad ligament is by a pedicle which may be quite narrow, but in some cases rather broad, with a markedly increased blood supply.

The *content* of the cyst is generally a clear, viscid fluid, sometimes very thick,

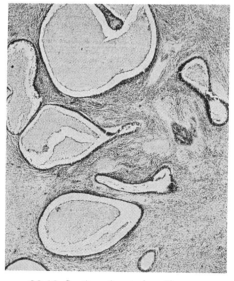

22.18. Section of cystadenofibroma

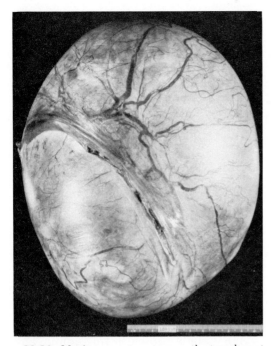

22.20. Mucinous cyst; note smooth, translucent wall.

of tall, pale-staining, secretory epithelium, with nuclei placed at the basal poles of the cells (Fig. 22.23). Goblet cells are often seen. In large cyst cavities the epithelium may be more or less flattened, with patches of immature epithelium lower than the more characteristic picket cells that line most of the cyst. A papillomatous tendency is far less common than with the serous type of cystadenoma. The epithelium has a characteristic adenomatous tendency (Fig. 22.24), producing invaginations which develop into other cysts in the wall of the original cavity (daughter cysts).

Histogenesis. It would appear that a simple metaplasia of the lining germinal epithelium (mesothelium) of the ovary into a mucinous type of cell is the initial step in the evolution of this form of cyst. The multipotency of this germinal (or

at other times thin. Admixture of blood elements may give it a chocolate or brownish hue. The *cut surface* shows the cavity to be divided by septa into a varying number of compartments or locules (Fig. 22.22). These tumors have therefore often been spoken of as *multilocular cysts,* but the designation is not a good one, for two reasons. In the first place, other types of ovarian tumor may be multilocular, and, secondly, one will encounter an occasional mucinous cyst with only a single large cavity produced by the merging of a number of locules into one due to a constant conflict between this merging process and the tendency to multiplication of compartments because of the proliferative tendency of the epithelium. The merging tendency is due to pressure atrophy and absorption of the septa between adjoining locules as they increase in size and distention.

Microscopically, the distinctive feature of mucinous cysts is the characteristic single layer, often of undulating outline,

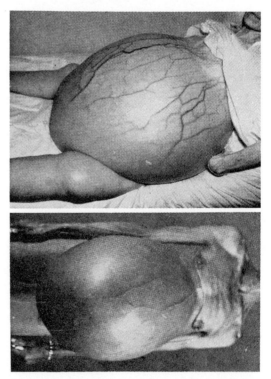

22.21. (*top*) Huge mucinous cyst. (Courtesy of Dr. Richard Symmonds, Rochester, Minnesota, and The Paul Hoeber Company.) (*bottom*) Ovarian cyst weighing 73 pounds. (Case of Dr. Gordon Johnson, New Orleans.)

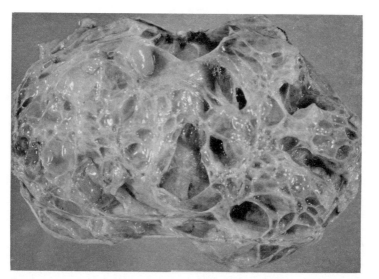

22.22. Mucinous cystadenoma of ovary showing the multilocular appearance on section.

primitive coelomic) epithelium is well known, and it is this invaginated epithelium that normally forms the entire Müllerian or *paramesonephric* ducts of the upper genital tract. Thus it should cause no surprise to note that this lining cell of the ovary may reduplicate tumors seen in the tube, endometrium, or endocervix, for the mucinous ovarian tumor is histologically closely allied to certain

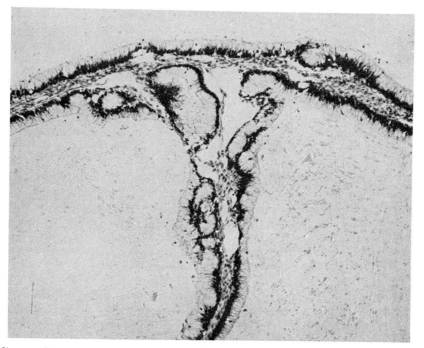

22.23. Microscopic appearance of mucinous cystadenoma. This shows the typical tall epithelium with nuclei at the base.

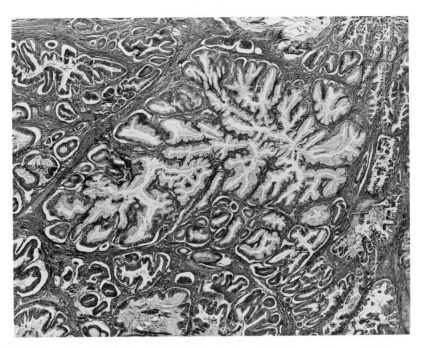

22.24. Very adenomatous but histologically benign pattern in mucinous cystadenoma.

mucinous tumors of the endocervix. Towers has adequately discussed this method of histogenesis.

One must also recognize that some mucinous tumors arise from teratomas in which all other elements have been blotted out by this entodermal tissue. There is considerable evidence for this sequel, such as the frequent occurrence of circumscribed mucinous adenomas in teratomas. The close kinship of the characteristic epithelium of mucinous tumors with the entodermic epithelium of the intestine is suggested by the occurrence of this epithelium in the mucocele of the appendix (Fig. 22.33 and Plate 22.2). Finally, a few mucinous tumors are noted in association with a Brenner tumor; whether there is mucinous metaplasia of the epithelioid cells or an epithelioid change of a primary mucinous pattern is uncertain, but we suspect that either may occur.

In conclusion then, it might appear that the mucinous cystadenoma may have diverse methods of histogenesis.

Various combinations of combined serous, mucinous, clear cell, and endometrioid patterns may be seen in a single tumor. This would offer additional evidence as to the multi-potential differentiating capacity of the mesothelium and reinforce the probability that this is indeed the source of all of these tumors. Indeed, the generic term of *mesothelioma,* further qualified by the predominent cell type, does not seem an illogical method of classification. A tubal-like type of epithelium is also seen not infrequently in any of these epithelial ovarian tumors.

Endometrioid Tumors (FIGO III)

See Chapter 25.

Mesonephric Tumors (FIGO IV)

See Chapter 23.

Dermoid Cysts

The dermoid cyst is the most common germ cell neoplasm and comprises approximately 10% of all ovarian lesions.

These germ cell tumors include a (benign cystic) subdivision of ovarian teratoma and comprise the most common type of ovarian tumor found in the young girl less than 20 years old, as noted by Abell and Holtz. In a study of ovarian neoplasms in the *adolescent* female, they found nongerm cell tumors in 40% of 188 young girls as compared to 60% germ cell neoplasms. Booth has indicated that germ cell tumors represent the most common tumor in association with pregnancy (about one in 600 pregnancies).

The cystic tumors are distinguished from the more serious solid tumors chiefly on the basis of their cystic character, their usually non-malignant malignant nature, and the fact that the foreign elements which they exhibit are dominantly ectodermal, with at times considerable mesodermal admixture, although elements of all three germ layers may occasionally be found. The solid teratomas always show a conglomeration of structures derived from all three fetal layers. The component elements of a dermoid cyst are always of mature differentiated type, in contrast with the malignant teratoma, in which the elements are of immature variety. This undoubtedly explains the benign nature of dermoid and the malignant behavior of teratoma, made up, as it is, of unripe elements with consequently greater malignant potentiality.

Dermoid cysts rarely reach large size, but they are occasionally combined with large mucinous cystadenomas. They show a rather thick, opaque, whitish wall, and on cross section the dermoid nature is at once indicated by the presence of hair and a large amount of offensive, greasy, sebaceous material (Fig. 22.25). At times teeth (Figs. 22.26, 27) and cartilaginous or osseous nodules are to be seen or felt in the cyst wall, and if these are found in preoperative x-ray the diagnosis is likely.

Microscopic examination shows skin-like stratified squamous epithelium lining the wall, but in the larger cysts this is often limited to a comparatively small raised area spoken of as the *mamilla,* from which arises also the hairy growth. Besides the stratified squamous epithelium and the hair follicles, there are sebaceous and sudoriferous glands, and often cartilage, the latter not infrequently in the wall of small ducts lined by ciliated epithelium, and resembling the trachea in structure. Neural tissue is common. Endodermal elements, such as gastrointestinal mucous membrane, may also occasionally be found. A characteristic finding in the vicinity of the wall is the presence of sievelike areas in which are scattered large *giant cells,* often polynuclear (Fig. 22.28). These are of foreign body type, resulting from the penetration of the cyst

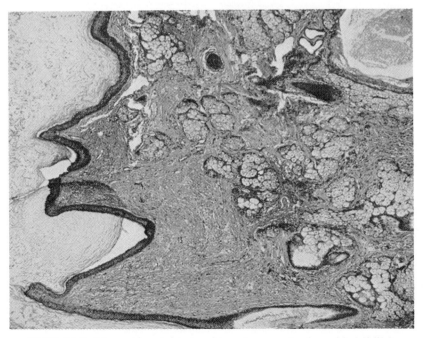

22.25. Wall of dermoid cyst showing skin, sebaceous glands, and hair follicles

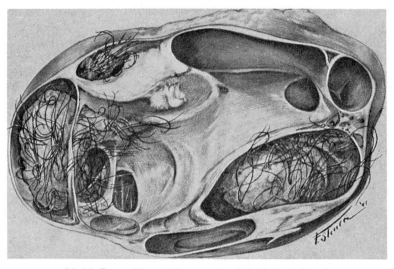

22.26. Dermoid cyst of ovary containing hair and teeth.

wall by lipoid material. The wall of the cyst except at the mamillary area is often devoid of epithelium, and may show numerous endothelial leukocytes (*pseudoxanthoma cells*) as well as foreign body giant cells and cholesterol crystals. Considerable amounts of thyroid tissue (*struma ovarii*) (Fig. 22.29) may occur

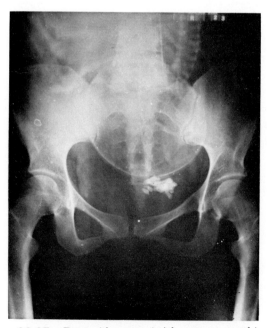

22.27. Dermoid cyst (with many teeth) obstructing labor. (Courtesy of Dr. Albert Brown, Wilmington, N.C.)

which can be thyrotoxic or undergo characteristic thyroid malignant degeneration.

Carcinoid tumors may arise from argentaffine cells of the gastrointestinal tract, and metastasize to the ovary. However, these occur primarily with the dermoid cyst, and sometimes produce characteristic symptoms primarily due to *serotonin.* Cutaneous flushing, diarrhea, and various cardiovascular symptoms may be manifest, and these symptoms in conjunction with a palpable ovarian tumor might suggest a carcinoid syndrome. A rather rare complication associated with dermoid cysts is *hemolytic anemia,* and some 15 cases have been noted in a recent review by Adcock. Abnormal antibodies may be noted, but the anemia is completely reversible following removal of the ovarian tumor. Should *rupture* of a dermoid cyst occur, a profound peritonitis with fistula formation may result.

Malignant degeneration can occur in primarily benign dermoid cysts. This sequence can be assumed when the unquestionably malignant lesion occurs in a definitely localized area of a dermoid which is otherwise entirely benign (Fig. 22.30). Carcinoma of the *epidermoid* type is seen in a small proportion of cases (one to three per cent). In one or two interesting personal observations we have

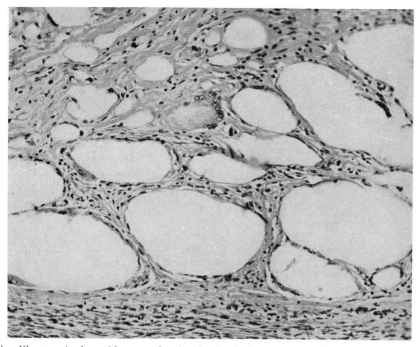

22.28. Sievelike area in dermoid tumor showing foreign-body giant cells. Such areas are produced by the penetration of fatty material through the wall of the dermoid.

even observed areas of typical *carcinoma in situ* (Fig. 22.31). *Sarcoma* and malignant melanoma may also be seen, but are less frequent. A fine point of nomen-clature is sometimes argued as to whether secondary malignant change in a benign dermoid justifies a diagnosis of a malignant teratoma. This seems unwarranted, the designation of malignant teratoma having a different connotation, as will be discussed in a later chapter (Chapter 23). Even when a dermoid is quite benign, recurrent intraperitoneal lesions may occur, presumably because of intermittent leakage and subsequent growth.

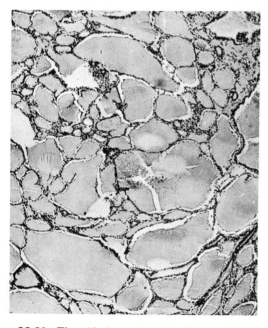

22.29. Thyroid tissue in wall of dermoid cyst (struma ovarii).

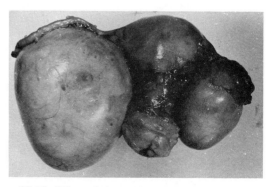

22.30. Bilateral dermoid tumor "overriding" the uterus. An extreme anterior location suggests a dermoid tumor.

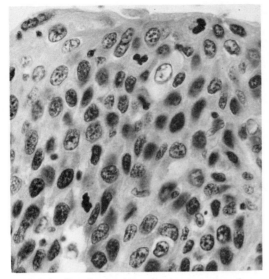

22.31. Carcinoma in situ may arise from epidermal elements. (Courtesy of Dr. B. L. Klionsky, Pittsburgh, Pa.)

An intermediate form should be recognized, *a benign solid teratoma,* as noted by Peterson. This is made up of tissues derived from all the fetal layers, but all very mature. Some of these have been extremely large, and some have occurred in children, so that one might at first suspect such tumors to be the malignant types of teratoma seen chiefly in children and usually fatal. The particular group we are describing, however, have all been benign clinically.

Origin. There are two chief theories as to the origin of dermoids. One ascribes them to the imperfect development in later life of blastomeres which have lain dormant since early stages of embryonic development. The other, which is more popular, is that they arise from spurious parthenogenetic activity of the unfertilized ova which abound in the ovary, as noted in discussion of ovarian teratoma.

Symptomatology of Neoplastic Cysts

There is little of a characteristic nature in the symptomatology of cystadenomas of the ovary. For example, no distinctive influence is exerted on the *menstrual function* although bleeding from a hyper-

plastic endometrium (an estrogenic effect) or virilization (an androgenic result) have been recorded. Plotz is uncertain whether the ovarian steroid stimulus is in the tumor epithelium or the adjacent stroma, but it is generally accepted that the stroma is the source as a result of "irritation" by epithelial cells.

Dysmenorrhea may or not be a symptom, but with the larger growths there is likely to be a sense of *heaviness or pressure.* In a large proportion of cases, the first intimation of trouble comes when the patient herself notices a *mass* in the lower abdomen, often to one side of the midline. On the other hand, it is remarkable what size a tumor may attain before the patient suspects any abnormality.

With serous papillary tumors the presence of the ovarian cyst may be altogether unsuspected until *ascites* has developed, for this variety of cyst, even when histologically benign, can at times produce ascites. This is because papillary tumors may implant themselves on the general peritoneal surface, producing irritation and exudation of serous fluid. Far more frequently, however, ascites is a feature of the malignant ovarian tumors. When ascites is pronounced, it may be impossible to palpate a mass in the lower abdomen until after paracentesis has been performed. Because there are many other possible causes of ascites, it is easy to understand that the problem of differential diagnosis may be difficult.

Complications

Torsion of the Pedicle. The most frequent complication of ovarian cyst is torsion or twisting of the pedicle, and the acute symptoms thus precipitated are occasionally the first indication of the presence of an ovarian tumor. This complication is more common with tumors of small or moderate size than with the very large ones. The twisting of the pedicle is generally in a clockwise fashion, and it may be slight or so extreme that several complete twists of the pedicle are demonstrable (Fig. 22.32). The circulatory disturbance produced by the torsion

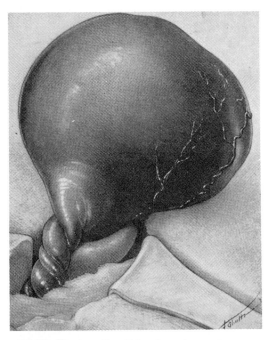

22.32. Torsion of pedicle of ovarian cyst as seen at operation.

usually affects chiefly the veins, with intense venous stasis, so that the cyst becomes dark bluish or even black (Plate 22.3). In extreme cases the arteries are also occluded, with resultant gangrene. The cyst may even, if unrecognized or neglected, twist itself off completely.

The occurrence of torsion of the pedicle is associated with *pain* which may be sharp and persistent, but which in other cases may be only moderately severe and transitory. The latter is true when the twisting of the pedicle corrects itself, as it not infrequently does. A common history in cases of ovarian cyst of moderate size is that from time to time the patient has experienced attacks of sharp pain, with spontaneous disappearance after a short time.

In a considerable proportion of cases, however, the symptoms produced by torsion of the pedicle are much more urgent with sudden excruciating pain. When the cyst is on the right side, the simulation of acute appendicitis may be made all the more perfect by the occurrence of *nausea and vomiting,* and by the

development of tense *rigidity* over the right lower abdomen. The *pulse* is accelerated and the *temperature* elevated, although it rarely rises to more than (perhaps) 101°F. Examination of the blood shows a moderate *leukocytosis.* It is not surprising, therefore, that many patients with this condition are operated upon with the mistaken diagnosis of acute appendicitis. Surgery is often performed by a general surgeon who may with all respect have no concept of the potential lethal nature of certain ovarian lesions so that inadequate operation is common.

Rupture of Cyst. This is relatively infrequent, but may occur either spontaneously or as result of trauma. In either case it is characterized by *pain,* often *nausea and vomiting,* and with varying degrees of *prostration,* where the rupture is attended with marked intraperitoneal bleeding. In such cases the peritoneal cavity may be filled with blood, with the rapid development of *shock,* characterized by rapid, thready pulse, subnormal temperature, air-hunger, and cold clammy skin. Such extreme bleeding, however, is rare, as in the majority of cases the rupture involves only an individual locule of the cyst. The initial pain and other symptoms may therefore subside after a few hours, although there may be tenderness and rigidity over the lower abdomen for a number of days, with moderate fever. There is no doubt that spontaneous disappearance of the symptoms occurs in a considerable proportion of cases.

Rupture of small thin-walled locules may happen without producing any immediate symptoms. It carries with it the risk, however, of dissemination of the cyst contents into the general abdominal cavity, and of possible implantation of the lining epithelium on the peritoneum. With *mucinous* tumors there is thus produced the rather rare *(pseudo)-myxoma peritonei,* in which the abdomen may contain huge amounts of a gelatinous exudate. Evacuation of this exudate is followed by reaccumulation within a comparatively short time, because of the continued secretion of the peritoneal implants, and a fatal termination is noted in almost all cases.

An interesting lesion of the appendix, the so-called *mucocele,* is a frequent but not invariable occurrence with (pseudo)myxoma peritonei (Campbell *et al.*), although the mucocele itself can produce the peritoneal fluid. The appendix may be enormously distended with gelatinous material, and large translucent gobs of the latter may be attached to the outer surface of the organ. The normal appendix epithelium in such cases is largely replaced by tall secretory epithelium identical with that seen in the wall of mucinous cysts. Because mucocele can occur even in the absence of mucinous cysts, it would seem that there must be a close kinship between mucinous and intestinal epithelium, and this further suggests a probable teratomatous origin of some mucinous cysts (Fig. 22.33).

Suppuration of Cyst. Secondary infection and suppuration of a cyst may follow torsion of its pedicle; but quite independently of the latter accident, in-

fection of the cyst may occur through the hematogenous or lymphatic route, although often the mechanism may be obscure. Dermoid cysts appear to be more prone to infection than do the cystadenomas, possibly because of the irritating character of their content and the fact that the weight of such cysts is more apt to bring about predisposing circulatory disturbance. Secondary infection of an ovarian cyst is characterized clinically by symptoms not unlike those of the ordinary type of acute pelvic inflammatory disease.

Malignant Change. Secondary malignant change may occur with any of the benign neoplastic cysts. In some cases this sequence is easily demonstrable, as when a localized malignant area is found in the wall of a benign cyst. This is a not infrequent observation with *mucinous cystadenoma,* in which, moreover, the histological differentiation between the benign and the malignant can be drawn more sharply than with the serous papillary cysts. From five to ten per cent of mucinous cysts become malignant.

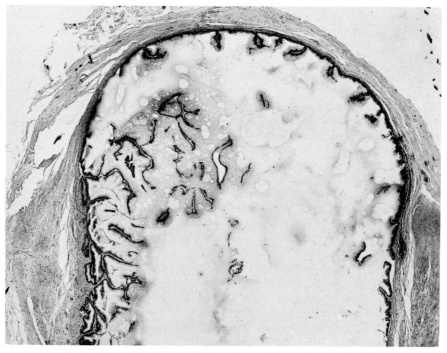

22.33. Mucocele of appendix lined by typical mucinous epithelium

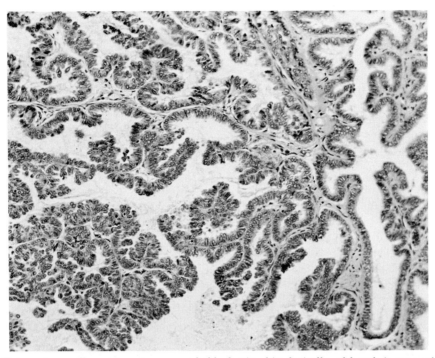

22.34. Extremely papillary serous tumor, probably benign histologically, although it may exhibit malignant clinical trends.

With the *serous papillary cystadenoma* the problem is more complex, particularly because the histological differentiation between the benign and the malignant is much more difficult (see Fig. 22.34), and because even cysts which histologically are benign not infrequently exhibit essentially malignant characteristics such as implantation, infiltration of surrounding organs, recurrence, and ultimately the death of the patient. As a group the serous papillary cystadenomas unquestionably are more lethal than the mucinous group. It is often impossible to be sure whether a malignant papillomatous growth has been so from the beginning or whether it has arisen secondarily in a previously benign serous cyst, although Meyer and others believe that the latter is the more frequent. At any rate, the incidence of malignant change in the serous papillary cyst is much higher than in the mucinous variety, being commonly put at no less than 25%. Abell notes the ratio of serous to mucinous malignancies as 4:1. This approximates our own clinic material.

Woodruff and Novak point out the extreme difficulty in distinguishing between the benign and malignant serous tumors and speak of a "borderline" group, characterized by multiple papillae with early stratification of the lining epithelium and invasion of the stroma (Stage 0). They emphasize the importance of multiple blocks to obtain a true composite picture of the tumor.

Malignant degeneration of *dermoid cysts* is relatively uncommon, 3% or less. It usually assumes the form of epidermoid or squamous cell carcinoma, but sarcoma may occasionally be seen.

Differential Diagnosis

Although the diagnosis of ovarian cyst is often easy, there are numerous cases in which the differentiation from other conditions is extremely difficult or impossible. The recent usage of laparoscopy has been most helpful. Among the more important of these lesions which may simulate ovarian cyst, or *vice versa*, the following may be mentioned.

Pregnancy. Either early or late gestation may be confused with ovarian cyst, or *vice versa,* as palpatory findings in themselves may not always be conclusive. Pregnancy tests, sonar, x-ray for a fetal skeleton, and auscultation for a fetal heart should be decisive.

Ascites. Marked ascites may cause extreme enlargement of the abdomen not unlike that seen with the large cysts, although generally there is much more bulging in the flanks. With the encysted fluid of ovarian cysts, *percussion* shows dullness anteriorly over the growth and tympany in the flanks. The reverse is the case with ascites, in which there is dullness over the flanks, with tympany over the front of the abdomen. *Palpation* of the abdomen in patients who are not too obese will often permit the definite outlining of the tumor mass in cases of ovarian cyst.

Tuberculous Peritonitis. Although not common, this disease can bring about a perfect simulation of an ovarian cyst. This is because the ascites of tuberculous peritonitis is frequently of the encysted variety, giving the exact feel of an ovarian cyst, as well as the same percussion findings. A history of pulmonary tuberculosis may be obtained, and there may be a slight evening elevation of temperature; tuberculin tests may also be of some help. The encysted mass may be well above the pelvic zone, and the pelvic findings may simulate a cyst with an unusually long pedicle. However, tuberculous endometritis may coexist and be revealed by curettage.

Myoma of Uterus. A soft intraligamentary myoma, or a pedunculated uterine growth arising from the side of the uterus, gives palpation findings which may puzzle even the expert examiner. The decision between an ovarian and uterine growth is usually based upon the demonstrable separateness of the former from the uterus, and in the latter on its continuity with the uterine surface. Where there is any doubt, however, exploration or endoscopy is indicated because of the malignant potential of ovarian tumors.

Abdominal Obesity. Certain types of obesity are characterized by huge abdominal deposits of fat which may lead to the suspicion of a large ovarian cyst. Elimination of the latter is usually easily made by percussion and pelvic examination. When the patient's abdominal wall is very thick and tense, palpation under anesthesia may be necessary to eliminate tumor.

Diverticulitis. This may be unassociated with gastrointestinal symptoms and may simulate perfectly a left ovarian tumor, so that it is a wise precaution to obtain barium enema whenever there is a left adnexal mass. An appendiceal abscess may cause confusion on the other side.

Treatment

As a rule it is unwise to advise immediate operation in the young patient for asymptomatic cysts which are no larger than a lemon, because a considerable number of these are of follicular or corpus luteum type, and not infrequently undergo spontaneous shrinkage and disappearance, so that reexamination in even a few weeks may reveal an ovary of normal size. Certainly, however, reexamination should always be insisted upon, and genuinely neoplastic cysts will show persistence and later gradual increase in the size of the tumor. With a 20-year-old patient, it is permissible to defer surgery for two or three months, although procrastination is not advisable in the postmenopausal woman. A general rule— the older the woman, the shorter the period of observation.

When cysts of considerable size or solid tumors are discovered, and whether or not they are producing symptoms, operation is almost always advisable. One may hesitate to give this advice to a patient who has had no symptoms whatsoever, but the reasonable certainty of increasing growth, and the ever present possibility of torsion of the pedicle as well as the more serious risk of malignant change, especially in women over 40, make this plan the proper one. There is no doubt that the malignant potentialities of ovarian growths are considerable. Furthermore, once ovarian cancer has developed, the patient's prospects of cure are slim with any method of treatment. A tactful and reassuring explanation will almost always ensure the patient's cooperation, and it should be emphasized that the exact extent of the surgery cannot always be predicted. This must be left up to the surgeon's best judgment. For obvious reasons, this should ideally be tape recorded or stated before reliable witnesses.

The type of operation must depend upon the type of cyst and also upon the age of the patient and the importance or unimportance of preserving the possibility of pregnancy. It is advisable to open the cyst immediately after removal before closure of the abdomen. If it is thin-walled, and especially if there is no papillomatous or solid ingrowth into the wall, one can be reasonably certain of its benign nature, so that conservative surgery is justified. On the other hand, even an innocuous appearing cystic tumor may reveal, on cut section, a vegetative, granular, or solid internal growth, so that there is a strong probability of malignancy, in which case the proper procedure would be removal of the entire uterus and the adnexa of both sides.

Serious problems of judgment often arise in the presence of unilateral papillomatous cysts in women of the child-bearing age, and in general the risks of conservatism with tumors of this group are definitely greater than with mucinous or dermoid cysts. When such unilateral cysts are thin-walled, without discretely scattered papillomata on the surface or within the cavity, the uterus and the uninvolved adnexa may be left with reasonable safety. In the presence of extensive papillomatous growths, especially with infiltration of the surrounding tissues, complete operation is much the safer plan. With women beyond the menopause, the wiser policy with neoplastic cysts of any variety is hysterectomy, with bilateral salpingo-oophorectomy. *Frozen section* is often the decisive factor, and where there is a unilateral lesion, it is preferable to send the whole tumor to the pathologist for careful rather than random biopsy.

Ovarian Tumors and Pregnancy. When small benign cysts are discovered in early pregnancy, most gynecologists are inclined to postpone their removal, for fear that the corpus luteum may be located in the ovary with the tumor, and that its removal might predispose to abortion, as Fraenkel found to be true in his early experiments on rabbits. Although it has been clearly established that the risk of abortion is far less in humans, it is still considered wise to defer operation until after the first trimester unless some more urgent indication should arise, such as torsion of the pedicle. By the same token, many gynecologists try to minimize the hazard of operations of this type by the substitutional administration of progesterone, although even without this the pregnancy will not usually be disturbed.

Whether or not an ovarian cyst should be removed promptly if discovered late in pregnancy should be decided on the basis of its size, its position, its rate of growth and the stage of gestation. If it is of moderate size, and riding high, its removal can often be deferred until after delivery. If the consistency of the tumor suggests that it may possibly be malignant, its prompt removal is indicated. Only recently we have examined sections of a highly malignant papillary cystadenoma which had been treated expectantly until acute symptoms arose at the sixth month of pregnancy. It is evident, therefore, that each case must be judged on its individual merits, and mistakes can easily occur.

The association of ovarian tumor and pregnancy is quite rare. Beischer *et al.* were able to report only 164 such cases in a 23-year span at the Royal Womens Hospital, and in over one-half of the cases the tumors concerned were either benign dermoid cysts or mucinous cystadenoma; the incidence of malignancy in their series was only 2.5%. Diagnosis of even large tumors was sometimes difficult because of the concomitant enlarged gravid uterus, although acute abdominal pain, because of associated torsion of the pedicle was not uncommon. In an earlier study Jubb has also noticed this sudden method of presentation.

In his study Jubb was able to note only 24 cases of malignancy in the world literature from 1882 to 1963, and in their more recent review Chung and Birnbaum suggest that the number of cases is probably less than 50. They record 6 cases of carcinoma, only 1 of whom is living 5 years following surgery. It is their feeling that laparotomy should be performed during pregnancy when an ovarian tumor is large enough or symptomatic enough "to require laparotomy," irrespective of the stage of the pregnancy. With a low grade epithelial tumor confined to the ovary (FIGO Stage IA) unilateral adnexectomy may be carried out, and surgery is most opportunely car-

ried out in the mid trimester of pregnancy. If a solid or suspicious ovarian tumor is found, laparotomy with frozen section should be carried out and definitive surgery be performed. The clinician should always be cognizant of the possibility of a luteoma of pregnancy (as will be noted in the next chapter). The prevailing concept is that this represents merely a physiological enlargement of the ovary rather than a true neoplasm, and as such requires only confirmatory diagnosis rather than ablation. In his recent report of 37 cases White discussed this association.

A very rare and rapidly fatal case of Burkitt's lymphoma has recently been reported in a gravid 24-year-old Caucasian who had never left the U.S.A. It is speculated that pregnancy may afford a favorable milieu for its growth.

A recent unpublished review of our own

Table 22.1

Epithelial Tumors

| | FIGO | Cases | Five Year Survival | | Dead | % 5 Year Survival |
			A and W	A with Rec.		
Serous	A	13	13	0	0	
	B	10	8	1	1*	
	C	2	0	0	2	
		25	21	1	3	84
Mucinous	A	5	4	0	1**	
	B	2	1	1	0	
	C	1	0	0	1	
		8	5	1	2	63
Endometrioid	A	1	1	0	0	
	B	2	2	0	0	
	C	3	0	0	3	
		6	3	0	3	50
Mesonephric	A	2	2	0	0	
	B	2	1	0	1	
	C	2	1	0	1	
		6	4	0	2	66
Total		45	33	2	10	75

* Death unrelated to tumor (plane crash)
** Pseudomyxoma peritonei

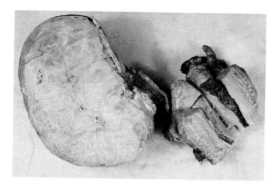

22.35. Fibroma of ovary

from the Emil Novak Ovarian Tumor Registry records 100 cases associated with pregnancy (Tables 22.1, 2). This is a very specialized group of neoplasms, since it is unnecessary to submit the average dermoid which comprise the most common tumor seen during gestation. The high salvage reflects the favorable nature of the pathology encountered.

Benign Solid Tumors of Ovary

Fibroma

This is a not uncommon tumor of the ovary, appearing sometimes as a small nodule on the surface (Plate 22.4) or in the substance of the ovary, while in some cases it may attain huge size, filling most of the abdominal cavity and weighing many pounds. The tumors are generally solid, but in the larger ones cavities may form as a result of cystic degeneration. The cut surface is whitish or yellowish white, and is of either homogeneous or of trabeculated appearance (Fig. 22.35).

Microscopically (Fig. 22.36) the structure is that of fibrous tissue of varying morphology. In some areas the cells are stellate or fusiform, but in other areas, the cells are rather closely packed and spindle-shaped, and may show an admixture of muscle cells (*fibromyoma*). In other tumors, areas of cartilage or bone may be found (*fibrochondroma* or *fibroosteoma*), suggesting a teratomatous origin. Admixtures of *theca* cells are common if routine fat stains are performed.

The small growths produce no *symptoms*. With those of larger size the patient herself notices the tumor sooner or

later, and there is likely to be pain and heaviness in the affected side. There are no characteristic effects on menstruation, but menorrhagia and dysmenorrhea may be noted. Because of the heaviness of the growths, partial twisting or angulation of the pedicle may occur, with venous obstruction and, therefore, ascites.

MEIG'S SYNDROME

Meigs called attention to a peculiar syndrome which may occur with these tumors, characterized by *hydrothorax* as well as *ascites,* and a considerable group of such cases has been described. The mechanism of this syndrome is not completely understood, but various lymphatics through the diaphragm seem the likely route for ascitic fluid into the chest. Contrary to an earlier belief, it is not distinctive of fibromas, as it has been noted with Brenner tumors, granulosal and thecomatous growths, and carcinoma, even in the absence of pleural metastasis. Hodari and Hodgkinson have performed lymphangiography on a single patient with Meig's syndrome and have noted accumulation in only the right thoracic cavity and not intraperitoneally. They propose different mechanisms for the formation of hydrothorax and ascites in

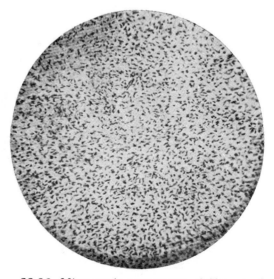

22.36. Microscopic appearance of fibroma of ovary.

Table 22.2

Other Tumors

	Cases	Five Year Survival		Dead	% 5 Year Survival
		A and W	A with Rec.		
Germ Cell:					
Dermoid	10	9	0	1*	
Dysgerminoma	19	13	3	3	
Malignant teratoma	3	1	0	2	
Endodermal sinus	1	0	0	1	
	33	23	3	7	76
Gonadal Stromal:					
Feminizing	11	9	1	1	
Virilizing	3	3	0	0	
	14	12	1	1	85
Sarcoma:	2	1	0	1	50
Metastatic:					
Krukenberg	2	0	0	2	
Other	4	1	0	3	
	6	1	0	5	16

Note. Of the 14 deaths listed in these 100 cases, 7 were postoperative.

this syndrome, but are uncertain as to its nature.

Because ascites is often combined with carcinoma of the ovary, and because the feel of a fibroma on bimanual examination is quite like that of some cancers, the *diagnosis* is not usually possible, although thoracentesis and paracentesis may be helpful. When a sharply defined solid unilateral ovarian tumor is encountered in a younger individual its fibromatous nature can at least be suspected, although it may prove otherwise.

The *treatment* of fibroma is surgical, and this results in complete disappearance of chest and peritoneal fluid where there is a *Meigs syndrome*. As a matter of fact, operation is indicated in any solid tumor of the ovary, although distinction from a pedunculated fibroid is not easy.

Brenner Tumors of the Ovary (FIGO V)

It is only in recent years that this interesting tumor form has been recognized, largely through the investigations of Robert Meyer. Its *gross* (Fig. 22.37) characteristics are not unlike those of fibroma, and the *microscopic* (Fig. 22.38) structure of these tumors is characterized by the presence of *epithelial cell* nests or columns in a *fibromatous matrix*. The distribution of these cell nests throughout the stroma may at first suggest malignancy, but the cells show a remarkable uniformity, with not the

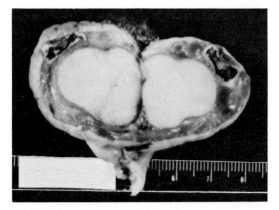

22.37. Brenner tumor arising from medullary or hilar area. Note intact cortex.

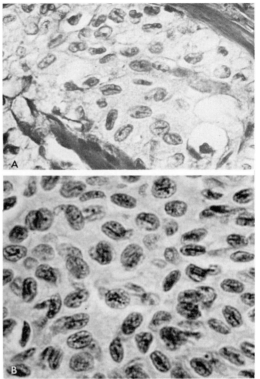

22.39. Characteristic longitudinal grooving to produce "coffee bean" pattern. (Courtesy of Dr. John MacKinlay, Glasgow, Scotland.)

slightest suggestion of anaplastic activity. The epithelioid cells often show a rather characteristic longitudinal "coffee-bean" grooving (Fig. 22.39).

The characteristic cell nests often show a tendency to central cystic degeneration (Fig. 22.40), the cavity often containing a cytoplasmic mass which superficially resembles an ovum within a follicle. This indeed was the original interpretation, which led to the earlier designation of these tumors as "oophoroma folliculare."

Another interesting characteristic of some of these tumors is a tendency for *mucinous transformation* (Fig. 22.41), so the cyst may contain areas resembling mucinous cystadenoma. Large cysts of the latter type may thus arise from Brenner tumors, although this is not the common origin of this type of cystadenoma, as described previously.

Symptoms. Brenner tumors are rather rare, and they occur usually in older women, the majority of patients being beyond 50. They produce no characteristic symptoms, and the smaller ones are usually accidental findings in operations for other indications. The larger ones, however, may weigh up to 20 pounds (Averbach), with symptoms like those of large fibromas. The large size is attained by an enormous fibromatous overgrowth

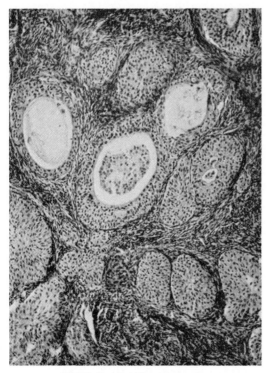

22.38. Typical Brenner tumor

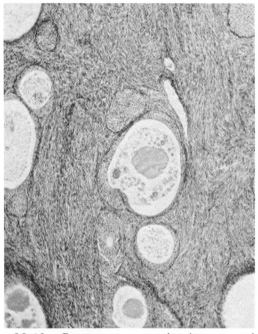

22.40. Brenner tumor showing central degeneration of epithelial nests.

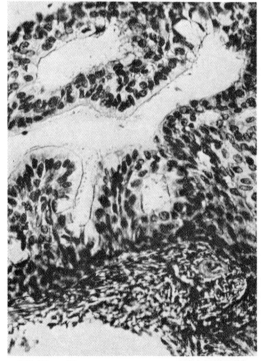

22.41. Brenner tumor with mucinous transformation of epithelium, sometimes giving rise to large cysts.

around the characteristic cell nests, and hence all presumably fibromatous tumors should be carefully studied for these. Bilaterality occurs in less than 10% (Kendall and Bowens).

Although there is some doubt as to the *histogenesis* of Brenner tumors, the explanation originally generally accepted was that suggested by Meyer, who believed that they arise from the so-called Walthard cell islets. These are collections of so-called indifferent cells, appearing as squamous plaques or as small clumps of gland acini, on or just below the surface of the ovary or on the tube or uterine ligaments. However, Greene and his coworkers have presented evidence that Brenner tumors may arise from other sources, including the surface epithelium of the ovary, the rete ovarii, and at times from the ovarian stroma. Arey's recent study by serial section and reconstruction would leave little doubt that certain Brenner tumors can arise from surface epithelium, with subsequent downward cordlike growth. That Brenner tumors may arise from a transitional type of epithelium (uroepithelial) is suggested by the 57 cases reviewed by Ehrlich and Roth.

Woodruff and Acosta believe that Brenner nests should be interpreted merely as a metaplastic phenomenon, and just as we find squamous metaplasia in the endocervix, these epithelioid cells may occur in conjunction with mucinous epithelium in the ovary. McKinlay does not agree that the only genesis is metaplasia, and he has kindly made some direct answers to our questions. "(a) Only the large tumors are associated with mucinous cysts, for the smaller ones show only a small percentage of mucoid cells. (b) Where both cell types are present, the mucoid are central, indicating a more recent formation. (c) Many mucinous cysts occur but very few show Brenner cells; the rare Brenner tumors show a high proportion." For such reasons he is inclined to believe that mucinous degeneration of a Brenner tumor is the rule. Our own ideas are that either may occur, and it might appear that there is more than a single mechanism to explain this particular appearance, as well as diverse methods of histogenesis.

Malignancy. In past years it had always been stressed that Brenner tumors are to be regarded as benign, and this is still the general rule; but in the last decade numerous cases of malignant Brenner tumors (Fig. 22.42) have been reported in the review by Idelson. Today there must be at least 50 such cases. On occasion a mucinous cystadenocarcinoma has seemed to arise from this type of epithelium, which may be found in particular tumors; much more frequent has been malignancy arising in the epithelioid cells with a poor prognosis.

Roth has recently reported a few cases of a so-called *"proliferating"* Brenner tumors. These are characterized by increased degrees of epithelial proliferation, but without frank invasion of the stroma. Morphologically these resemble low grade transitional cell carcinomas of the bladder, and add additional support to a concept of an origin from urinary tract epithelium. His photomicrographs seem extremely convincing and it would certainly seem logical to include a benign Brenner, proliferating, and malignant among the epithelial tumors of the ovary in the recent FIGO classification, although a marked fibromatous hyperplasia seems essential for the diagnosis of this type of tumor.

Hormonal Activity. A recent well studied case by Shay and Janovski reports an endometrial carcinoma in conjunction with a malignant Brenner tumor, the first reported coassociation. Extensive histochemical studies suggest that the Brenner cells are rich in glycogen, but the stroma may contain much lipoid, the latter suggesting an endocrine effect.

Although it had previously been believed that most of these tumors have been inert, it is increasingly apparent that some do appear hormonally active. A number of these neoplasms have been observed to be associated with postmenopausal endometrial hyperplasia, and adenocarcinoma as noted by Eton and Parker, McKinlay, as well as others. A recent review by Farrar and co-workers would appear to afford considerable circumstantial evidence of estrogen effect, for they found this to be present in 7.5%

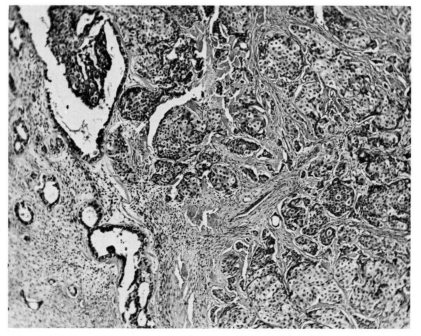

22.42. Malignant Brenner tumor. (Courtesy of Prof. Hans Limburg, Hamburg.)

of over 400 cases studied. Since endometrium was available for study in only a fraction of cases, it would appear that this figure might in reality be considerably higher. Ming and Goldman have performed similar studies of 69 postmenopausal endometria associated with Brenner tumors, and found an atrophic pattern in only 14, with hyperplasia, polyp, and adenocarcinoma accounting for the other 55, nearly 80%. Nissen and Goldsmith add a recent case of a 75-year-old woman with breast engorgment, endometrial hyperplasia and a Brenner tumor, in which the stromal cells seem to have been converted into a thecalutein cell as indicated by differentiated stains and various histochemical techniques. The latter may be utilized to pinpoint oxidative enzyme activity which is an indication of steroidogenesis. On the other hand, a recent three-part study by Ullery and his associates report a Brenner tumor with clinical masculinization, presumably due to testosterone, and their excellent histochemical studies are convincing.

TUMORS WITH A FUNCTIONING MATRIX

(See also Chapter 24.) Morris and Scully, as well as others, have indicated that various ovarian tumors might have an endocrine effect, although not of the typical "functioning" variety morphologically. They suggested that the ovarian stromal cell may under certain conditions be converted to a cell capable of producing various hormones (hyperthecosis or Leydig cell transition). Presumably it is the irritation of malignant cells that converts the stroma into an active agent, and these cells show increased lipoid activity, indicating the likelihood of a steroid content.

Many such tumors have been reported with a "functioning matrix," which has been usually estrogenic, occasionally androgenic, and rarely productive of progesterone. These tumors include not only the Brenner, but Krukenberg tumors, mucinous and serous lesions, and a variety of others. Jakobovitz has reported

nine miscellaneous tumors with an endocrine effect.

The recent histochemical study by Woodruff, Williams, and Goldberg would afford additional support to the fact that the stroma is occasionally endocrinologically active; histochemical studies of a variety of gonadal neoplasms have pointed to the ovarian stroma as a source of endocrine activity. The stroma, derived from the mesenchyme, is of course notorious for its remarkable powers of differentiation potential.

Other benign solid tumors, such as lymphangioma, hemangioma, fibroadenoma, and adenomyoma are very rare, so that their mere mention will suffice. The diagnosis cannot be made before operation, and rarely before pathological examination.

OVARIAN TUMORS IN CHILDREN

Although many young teen-age females are quite mature, it seems expedient to utilize the age of 16 years as the upper limit of childhood. Ovarian tumors represent a rather infrequent neoplasm in the youthful female. If such functional cysts as follicle or lutein are excluded, the most common gonadal neoplasm would appear to be the dermoid cyst (benign cystic teratoma), which represents approximately $\frac{1}{3}$ to $\frac{1}{2}$ of tumors in the young female. In a review of 992 cases reported in the literature (1935–1961) Huffman reports 298 teratoma (benign or malignant) as well as 97 other germ cell tumors; 115 gonadal stromal tumors are noted along with 177 carcinomas of all types. In his own series of 75 cases Ein has indicated that an ovarian tumor in the child has a nearly 85% chance of being benign even if functional cysts are included. Nevertheless Jensen and Norris record 67 patients less than 20 years of age with primary epithelial tumors, of which 8 were malignant or borderline malignant with at least 2 deaths. A considerable proportion ($\frac{1}{3}$) of these tumors occurred in conjunction with pregnancy.

Moore, Schiffrin and Erez, record 127

youthful patients in 35 years with ovarian tumors of which 9 per cent were malignant. Those occurring before the menarche were generally neoplastic; those after were generally functional. Endometriosis is noted in 7 instances; in 3 less than 14 years of age there was a bicornuate uterus and other anomalies. Benign dermoids, functional cysts and polycystic ovaries were the most common findings, but malignant disease occurred in 11 instances. Acosta, Kaplan and Kaufman find approximately the same distribution in their series of ovarian tumors, although they have not included endometrial or Stein-Leventhal ovarian disease.

Symptoms, Diagnosis and Treatment

The symptoms of ovarian tumors in children are quite similar to those in the adult, but many parents may assume that the young female complaining only of vague abdominal discomfort is simply "coming of age," and it is frequently not until there is a protuberant abdominal mass that the girl is presented to the gynecologist, unless a hormone-producing tumor leads to endocrine stigmata. Rupture, hemorrhage, or torsion of the pedicle may produce acute abdominal symptoms similar to appendicitis.

Treatment in young females obviously should be directed toward the conservative approach if circumstances permit. The surgeon must be guided by frozen section and pathological consultation, but his own pathological expertise is important. As a general rule the gonadal stromal and germ cell tumors (barring teratocarcinoma and endodermal sinus tumor) are of low grade malignancy and warrant lesser degrees of surgery as noted in the appropriate chapters of this text. In separate studies Barber and Graber and Smith *et al.* indicate the disproportionate frequency of germ cell tumors which may grow rapidly in the child. Where malignancy has occurred, there have been occasional favorable responses to triple drug therapy.

REFERENCES

Abell, M. R., Johnson, V. J., and Holtz, F.: Ovarian neoplasms in childhood and adolescence. I. Tumors of germ cell origin. Amer. J. Obstet. Gynec., 92: 1059, 1965.

Abell, M. R., and Holtz, F.: Ovarian neoplasms in childhood and adolescence. II. Tumors of nongerm cell origin. Amer. J. Obstet. Gynec., 93: 850, 1965.

Abitbol, M. M., Pomerance, W., and Mackles, A.: Spontaneous intraperitoneal rupture of benign cystic teratomas. Obstet. Gynec., 13: 198, 1959.

Acosta, A., Kaplan, A. L., and Kaufman, R. H.: Gynecologic cancer in children. Amer. J. Obstet. Gynec., 112: 944, 1972.

Adcock, L. L.: Unusual manifestation of benign cystic teratoma. Obstet. Gynec. Survey, 27: 476, 1972.

Arey, L. B.: The origin and form of the Brenner tumor. Amer. J. Obstet. Gynec., 81: 743, 1961.

Aure, J. C., Hoeg, K., and Kolstadt, P.: Psammoma bodies in serous carcinoma of the ovary. Amer. J. Obstet. Gynec., 109: 113, 1971.

Averbach, L. H., Promin, D., and Hanna, G. C., Jr.: Brenner tumor of the ovary; a case of unusually large size. Amer. J. Obstet. Gynec., 74: 207. 1957.

Azoury, R. S., et al.: Dermoid cyst of the ovary containing fetus-like structures. Obstet. Gynec., 73: 887, 1973.

Barber, H. R. K., and Graber, E. A.: The PMPO (postmenopausal palpable ovary) syndrome. Obstet. Gynec., 37: 921, 1971.

Barber, H. R. K., and Graber, E. A.: Gynecological tumors in childhood and infancy. Obstet. Gynec. Surv., 28: 357, 1973.

Beacham, W., et al.: Ovarian/uterine tumors weighing more than 25 pounds. Amer. J. Obstet. Gynec., 109: 1153, 1971.

Beck, R. P., and Latour, J. P. A.: Review of 1019 benign ovarian neoplasms. Obstet. Gynec., 16: 479, 1960.

Beischer, N. A.: Ovarian tumors in pregnancy. Obstet. Gynec. Survey, 27: 429, 1972.

Benedict, P. H., Cohen, R. B., Cope, O., and Scully, R. E.: Ovarian and adrenal morphology in cases of hirsutism on virilism and Stein-Leventhal syndrome. Fertil. Steril., 13: 380, 1962.

Booth, R. T.: Ovarian tumors in pregnancy. Obstet. Gynec., 21: 189, 1963.

Bransilver, B., Fenenczy, A., and Richart, R. M.: Brenner tumors and Walthard cell nests. Arch. Path., 98: 76, 1974.

Brenner, F.: Das Oöphoroma folliculare. Frankfurt Z. Path., 1: 150, 1907.

Cameron, W. J.: Endometrial carcinoma with ovarian metastasis in association with Stein-Leventhal syndrome. Obstet. Gynec., 22: 12, 1963.

Campbell, J. S., et al.: Pseudomyxoma peritonei et ovarii with occult neoplasm of the appendix. Obstet. Gynec., 42: 897, 1973.

Caruso, P. A. et al.: Study of 305 teratomas of the ovary. Cancer, 27: 343, 1971.

Caspi, E., Schreyer, P., and Bukovsky, J.: Ovarian lutein cysts in pregnancy. Obstet. Gynec., 42: 388, 1973.

Chung, A., and Birnbaum, S. J.: Ovarian cancer with pregnancy. Obstet. Gynec., 41: 211, 1973.

Cooper, H. E., et al.: Hereditary factors in the Stein-Leventhal syndrome. Amer. J. Obstet. Gynec., 100: 371, 1968.

Doucette, J. W., and Estes, W. B.: Primary ovarian caretinoid. Obstet. Gynec., 25: 94, 1965.

Ehrlich, C. E., and Roth, L. M.: The Brenner tumor. Cancer, 27: 32, 1971.

Ein, S. H.: Cystic and solid tumors in children. J. Ped. Surg., 5: 148, 1970.

El-Minawi, M. F., and Hori, J. M.: Malignant melanoma in bilateral dermoid cysts. Int. J. Obstet. Gynec., *11:* 218, 1973.

Esposito, J. M.: An unusual theca-lutein cyst. Obstet. Gynec., *30:* 260, 1967.

Eton, B., and Parker, R. A.: Endometrial abnormalities including carcinoma associated with ovarian Brenner tumors. J. Obstet. Gynaec. Brit. Comm., *65:* 95, 1958.

Evans, T. N., and Riley, G. M.: Polycystic ovarian disease; a clinical and experimental study. Amer. J. Obstet. Gynec., *80:* 873, 1960.

Evans, T. N., and Riley, G. M.: Thecoma and polycystic disease of the ovaries. Obstet. Gynec., *18:* 52, 1961.

Fallahzedeh, H., Dockerty, M. B., and Lee, R. A.: Leiomyoma of the ovary. Amer. J. Obstet. Gynec., *113:* 394, 1972.

Farrar, H. K., Jr., Elesh, R., and Libretti, J.: Brenner tumors and estrogen production. Obstet. Gynec. Survey, *15:* 1, 1960.

Farrar, H. K., and Greene, R. R.: Bilateral Brenner tumors of the ovary. Amer. J. Obstet. Gynec., *80:* 1089, 1960.

Fienberg, R.: Thecosis: A study of diffuse stromal thecosis of the ovary and superficial collagenization with follicular cysts (Stein-Leventhal ovary). Obstet. Gynec., *21:* 687, 1963.

Finkle, H. I., and Goldman, R. L.: Burkitt's lymphoma— gynecological considerations. Obstet. Gynec., *43:* 281, 1974.

Finkle, H. I., Goldman, R. L., and Sung, M.: A proliferating Brenner tumor. Obstet. Gynec., *40:* 39, 1973.

Foda, M. S., and Shafeek, M. A.: Malignant Brenner tumor. Obstet. Gynec., *13:* 226, 1959.

Gall, S. A., Walling, J., and Pearl, J.: Tumor associated antigens. Amer. J. Obstet. Gynec., *115:* 387, 1973.

Gemzell, C.: Induction of ovulation with human gonadotropins. Acta Endocr. (Suppl. 67), 49, 1962.

Greenblatt, R. B.: *The Hirsute Female.* Charles C Thomas, Springfield, 1960.

Greene, R. E.: Diverse origin of Brenner tumors. Amer. J. Obstet. Gynec., *64:* 878, 1952.

Groeber, W. R.: Ovarian tumors during infancy and childhood. Amer. J. Obstet. Gynec., *86:* 1027, 1963.

Hodari, A. A., and Hodgkinson, C. P.: Lymphangiogram of Meigs' syndrome. Obstet. Gynec., *32:* 477, 1968.

Huffman, J. W.: *The Gynecology Of Childhood and Adolescence.* W. B. Saunders Co., Philadelphia, 1968.

Hughesdon, P. E.: Thecal and allied reaction in epithelial ovarian tumors. J. Obstet. Gynaec. Brit. Comm., *65:* 710, 1958.

Hull, M. G. R., and Campbell, G. R. Malignant Brenner tumor. Obstet. Gynec., *42:* 527, 1973.

Idelson, M. G.: Malignancy in Brenner tumors of the ovary, with comments on histogenesis and possible estrogen production. Obstet. Gynec. Survey, *18:* 246, 1963.

Jackson, R. L., and Dockerty, M. B.: Stein-Leventhal syndrome and endometrial carcinoma. Amer. J. Obstet. Gynec., *73:* 161, 1957.

Jeffcoate, T. N. A.: The androgenic ovary, with special reference to the Stein-Leventhal syndrome. Amer. J. Obstet. Gynec., *88:* 143, 1964.

Jensen, R. D., and Norris, H. J.: Epithelial tumors of the ovary. Arch. Path., *94:* 29, 1972.

Jorgensen, E. O., *et al.:* Clinicopathological study of 53 Brenner tumors. Amer. J. Obstet. Gynec., *108:* 122, 1970.

Jubb, E. D.: Primary ovarian carcinoma in pregnancy. Amer. J. Obstet. Gynec., *85:* 345, 1963.

Judd, H. L., *et al.:* Familial hyperthecosis. Amer. J. Obstet. Gynec., *117:* 976, 1973.

Kaufman, R. H., Abbott, J. P., and Wall, J. A.: The endometrium before and after wedge resection of the ovaries in the Stein-Leventhal syndrome. Amer. J. Obstet. Gynec., *77:* 1271, 1959.

Klionsky, B. L., Nickers, O. J., and Amontegui, A. J.: Squamous cell carcinoma in situ in adult cystic teratoma. Arch. Path., *93:* 161, 1972.

Kendall, B., and Bowens, P. A.: Bilateral Brenner tumors of the ovary. Amer. J. Obstet. Gynec., *80:* 439, 1960.

Leventhal, M. L.: The Stein-Leventhal syndrome. Amer. J. Obstet. Gynec., *76:* 825, 1958.

Lynch, M. J. G., Kyle, P. R., Raphael, S. S., and Bruce-Lockhart, P.: Unusual ovarian changes (hyperthecosis) in pregnancy. Amer. J. Obstet. Gynec., *77:* 335, 1959.

McKinlay, C. J.: Brenner tumors of the ovary. J. Obstet. Gynaec. Brit. Comm., *63:* 58, 1956.

McKinlay, C. J.: Personal communication.

Malkesian, G. D., Dockerty, M. B., and Symmonds, R. E.: Benign cystic teratoma. Obstet. Gynec., *29:* 719, 1967.

McKay, D. G.: The origin of ovarian tumors. Clin. Obstet. Gynec., *5:* 1181, 1962.

Meigs, J. V.: Meigs' syndrome. Amer. J. Obstet. Gynec., *67:* 962, 1954.

Meyer, R.: Uber verschiedene Erscheinungsformen in der als Typus Brenner bekannten Eierstocksgeschwulst. Arch. Gynaek., *148:* 541, 1932.

Miles, P. A., and Harris, J. J.: Proliferative and malignant Brenner tumors. Cancer, *30:* 174, 1972.

Ming, S., and Goldman, R.: Hormonal activity of Brenner tumors in postmenopausal women. Amer. J. Obstet. Gynec., *98:* 913, 1967.

Moore, J. G., Schifrin, B. S., and Erez, S.: Ovarian tumors in infancy, childhood and adolescence. Amer. J. Obstet. Gynec., *99:* 913, 1967.

Morris, J. M., and Scully, R. E.: *Endocrine Pathology of the Ovary.* C. V. Mosby, Company, Amer. J. Obst. Gynec., *98:* 913, 1967.

Morris, J. M., and Scully, R. E.: *Endocrine Pathology of the Ovary.* C. V. Mosby Company, St. Louis, 1958.

Morrison, C. W., and Woodruff, J. D.: Fibrothecoma and associated ovarian stromal neoplasia. Obstet. Gynec., *23:* 344, 1964.

Nelson, W. W., and Greene, R. R.: Histology of human ovary during pregnancy. Amer. J. Obstet. Gynec., *76:* 66, 1958.

Nissen, E. D., and Goldstein, A. I.: Ovarian tumors with functioning stromal cells (feminizing Brenner). Int. J. Obstet. Gynec., *11:* 213, 1973.

Novak, E., and Novak, E. R.: *Gynecologic and Obstetric Pathology,* Ed. 6. W. B. Saunders Company, Philadelphia, 1967.

Novak, E. R., Lambrou, C., and Woodruff, J. D.: Ovarian tumors in pregnancy. An Ovarian Tumor Registry Report (in press).

Ony, H.: Functional ovarian cysts and oral contraceptives. J.A.M.A., *228:* 68, 1974.

Ottaway, J. P.: Ruptured hemorrhagic ovarian cysts during pregnancy. Obstet. Gynec., *21:* 379, 1963.

Peterson, W. F.: Solid histologically benign teratomas of the ovary. Amer. J. Obstet. Gynec., *72:* 1094, 1956.

Peterson, W. F., Prevost, E. C., Edmunds, F. T., Hundley, J. M., Jr., and Morris, F. K.: Benign cystic teratoma of ovary. Amer. J. Obstet. Gynec., *70:* 368, 1955.

Plate, W. P.: Pathologic anatomy of the Stein-Leventhal syndrome. Fertil. Steril., *9:* 545, 1958.

Roberts, D. W. T., and Haines, M.: Is there a Stein-Leventhal syndrome? Brit. M. J., *1:* 1709, 1960.

Rosenthal, A. H.: Rupture of the corpus luteum, including four cases of massive intraperitoneal hemorrhage. Amer. J. Obstet. Gynec., *79:* 1008, 1960.

Roth, L. H., and Sternberg, W. H.: Proliferating Brenner tumors. Cancer, *27:* 687, 1971.

Sawai, M. M., and Sirsat, M. V.: Ovarian tumors in children and adolescence. Ind. J. Cancer, *10:* 302, 1973.

Shaaban, A. H., Tabdine, F. A., and Youssef, A. F.: Functioning Brenner tumor of the ovary. J. Obstet. Gynaec. Brit. Comm., *67:* 138, 1960.

Shay, M. D., and Janovski, N. A.: Malignant Brenner tumor associated with endometrial adenocarcinoma. Obstet. Gynec., *22:* 246, 1963.

Shinata, T., Tsukui, J., and Matsumoto, S.: Estrogen synthesis by Brenner tumor. Amer. J. Obstet. Gynec., *116:* 408, 1973.

Shippel, S.: The ovarian theca cell. Part IV. The hyperthecosis syndrome. J. Obstet. Gynaec. Brit. Comm., *62:* 321, 1955.

Smith, J. P., Rutledge, F., and Sutow, W.: Malignant gynecological tumors in children. Amer. J. Obstet. Gynec., *116:* 261, 1973.

Spohn, W.: Cited by Lynch, F. W., in *Pelvic Neoplasms,* edited by F. W. Lynch and A. Maxwell. Appleton-Century-Crofts, Inc., New York, 1922.

Stein, I. F.: Ultimate results of bilateral ovarian wedge resection; 25-year follow-up. Internat. J. Fertil., *1:* 333, 1956.

Symmonds, R. E., Spraitz, A. F., and Koelsche, G. A.: Large ovarian tumor. Obstet. Gynec., *22:* 473, 1963.

Taw, R. L., and Jones, E. G.: Polycystic ovaries and menstrual irregularities. Amer. J. Obstet. Gynec., *86:* 626, 1963.

Taym, M. L., Clark, B. J., and Sturgis, S. H.: The polycystic ovary. Amer. J. Obstet. Gynec., *86:* 188, 1963.

Towers, R. P.: A note on the origin of pseudomucinous cystadenoma of the ovary. J. Obstet. Gynaec. Brit. Comm., *63:* 253, 1956.

Ullery, J. C., Hamwi, G. J., Byron, R. C., Besch, P. K., Vorys, N., Teteris, N. J., Barry, R. D., Meiling, R. D., Boutselis, J. G., and George, O. T. (combined contributions in different parts): Testosterone synthesis by a Brenner tumor, Parts I and II. Amer. J. Obstet. Gynec., *86:* 1015, 1963; Parts III. *87:* 463, 1963.

White, K. C.: Ovarian tumors in pregnancy. Amer. J. Obstet. Gynec., *116:* 544, 1973.

Woodruff, J. D., and Acosta, A. A.: Variations in the Brenner tumor. Amer. J. Obstet. Gynec., *83:* 657, 1962.

Woodruff, J. D., and Novak, E. R.: Papillary serous tumors of the ovary. Amer. J. Obstet. Gynec., *67:* 1112, 1954.

Woodruff, J. D., Williams, T. J., and Goldberg, B.: Hormone activity of the common ovarian neoplasm. Amer. J. Obstet. Gynec., *87:* 679, 1963.

chapter *23*

Malignant Tumors of the Ovary

The mortality associated with carcinoma of the ovary approximates uterine malignancy, and it seems to be increasing in frequency, so that it is the leading cause of pelvic cancer fatality in many areas of the world. It may be primary in the ovary or secondary to cancer in other organs.

Malignant ovarian neoplasms may be solid or cystic, and our own laboratory material would suggest that the latter is about twice as common. Due consideration must be given to the cystic degeneration which certain solid tumors undergo as well as the proliferative tendencies of the primarily cystic lesions. In other words, it is not easy to make a sharp distinction between certain cystic and solid ovarian neoplasms.

Malignant tumors often arise in bilateral fashion, but where there is evidence of generalized pelvic disease, it is sometimes impossible to be certain if there have been initial bilateral primary lesions or if a single tumor has spread to the contralateral ovary (and elsewhere) via direct extension or the richly communicating lymphatics. Our estimate would be that bilateral malignancy occurs in 25 per cent of all cystic cancer, and less commonly with solid carcinoma. Certain ovarian tumors as the gonadal stromal, mesonephroma, and Brenner varieties are rarely bilateral (less than 10 per cent).

The specific ratio between benign and malignant neoplasms must also represent an uncertain figure, for certain laboratories will have different criteria as to what constitutes malignancy in a variety of pathological entities, such as papillary serous tumors, various cystic teratomas, and others. There would seem little purpose in even attempting to suggest a ratio between benign tumors and ovarian malignancies because there are simply too many variables. As a rule, cystic tumors are benign, and most solid ones are malignant, but any combination may be encountered with varying degrees of malignancy.

It is manifestly impossible to cite the actual *incidence* of carcinoma of the ovary, because of the diverse interpretations between the benign and malignant. Randall, however, using figures from New York State where cancer is a reportable disease, estimates that at age 40 the *probability* or a woman's developing ovarian cancer is approximately 0.9 per cent, although the actual incidence rises to a peak of 4 per cent at age 70.

CLINICAL CLASSIFICATION

It seems certain that the most important prognostic factor in evaluating ovarian cancer is the extent of the disease, and many schemes of clinical classification have been devised. These have been almost completely replaced by a uniformly accepted one. The Cancer Committee of the International Federation of Gynaecology and Obstetrics (FIGO) has proposed a classification, which is more cumbersome, but does have sufficient groups and subgroups to fit almost any degree of ovarian cancer. As such, it will be of value in comparing results in treated patients in many categories, and this FIGO classification has been endorsed by most organizations.

Definitions of the Different Stages of Primary Carcinoma of the Ovary Based on Findings at Clinical Examinations and Surgical Exploration

Stage I. (Growth limited to the ovaries.)

Stage Ia. Growth limited to one ovary; no ascites. 1) Capsule ruptured. 2) Unruptured.

Stage Ib. Growth limited to both ovaries; no ascites. 1) and 2) As above.

Stage Ic. Growth limited to one or both ovaries, ascites present with malignant cells in the fluid. 1) and 2) As above.

Stage II. (Growth involving one or both ovaries with pelvic extension.)

Stage IIa. Extension and metastasis to the uterus and tubes only.

Stage IIb. Extension to the other pelvic tissues.

Stage III. (Growth involving one or both ovaries with widespread intraepithelial metastasis to the abdomen (the omentum, the small intestine and its mesentery.))

Stage IV. (Growth involving one or both ovaries with distant metastasis outside the peritoneal cavity.)

Special Category. Unexplored cases which are thought to be ovarian carcinoma (surgery, explorative or therapeutic, not having been performed).

Note: The presence of ascites does not influence the staging for Stages II, III, and IV.

PRIMARY CYSTIC CARCINOMA OF OVARY

Although a carcinoma of the ovary may arise as a cystic tumor, it can unquestionably develop in a previously benign cystadenoma of the ovary. There can be no doubt as to the frequent occurrence of secondary carcinomatous changes in cystadenomas. It is not rare, for example, to encounter carcinoma at some portion in the wall of benign cysts which have been known to be present for many years. Again, in many carcinomas large areas of entirely benign cystadenoma may still be observed. In any event, the adenocarcinomas of the ovary are to be looked upon as the malignant prototypes of the benign cystadenoma, arising from the same elements which gave rise to the latter. On the above basis we may distinguish three of four chief varieties of primary cystic ovarian carcinoma.

Serous Cystadenocarcinoma

This represents the malignant form of serous cystadenoma. It is much more common than the mucinous variety, and is almost always characterized by a papillary architecture. The papillary growth is not infrequently present on the surface as well as within the cavity (Fig. 23.1). All grades of transition may be seen between the picture of benign papillary serous cystadenoma and that characterized by almost solid papillary masses. Indeed, Woodruff and Novak have indicated that one must recognize a borderline low grade type of papillary malignancy characterized histologically by a marked papillary growth (Fig. 23.2–4) and a tendency to implant on peritoneal surfaces with the production of ascites (see preceding chapter). They have likewise stressed the importance of repeated pathological sections from many areas of the lesion, for an ovarian tumor can show a highly variegated appearance,

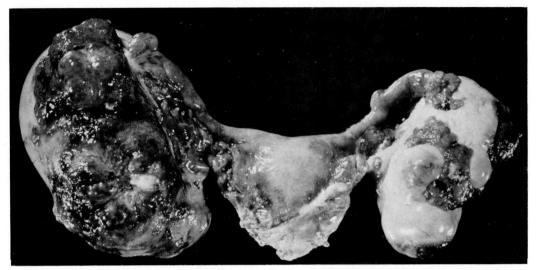

23.1. Bilateral papillary cystadenocarcinomas (note external papillae).

from the extremely benign to the highly malignant.

The *microscopic examination* often presents considerable difficulty, especially in the cases in which the gross appearance is much like that of the benign serous cysts. The epithelial elements present an increased papillary pattern but only moderate and perhaps doubtful anaplastic activity with histologically low-grade lesions, especially where confined to the ovary. Julian and Woodruff indicate a good prognosis. In such cases of papillary tumors, we have found mitosis count of

considerable prognostic importance, and this has led us to utilize these in grading this variety of tumor (Table 23.1). Even in the absence of very clear-cut evidence of histological malignancy, such tumors often exhibit clinical malignancy, especially as regards peritoneal implantation. It is usually safer, therefore, to err on the side of safety, and to consider them in the malignant group, with treatment consisting of removal of both adnexa as well as the uterus.

In the majority of cases, however, the malignant nature of this group of tumors

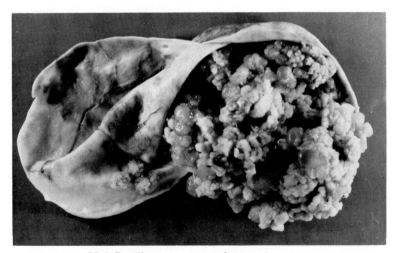

23.2. Papillary serous cystadenocarcinoma

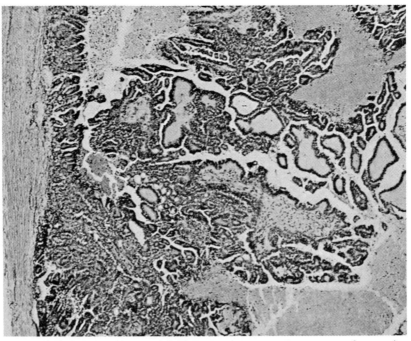

23.3. Histologically malignant papillary vegetations lining interior of serous cystadenocarcinoma although capsule is smooth (six-year-old girl). (Courtesy of Dr. Don. Walcott, San Jose, California.)

is more clearly defined, with many layers of epithelium, showing disparity in size and shape of the cells and especially the nuclei, hyperchromatosis, and marked mitotic activity. Invasion of the stroma by the epithelium is likewise often evident (Fig. 23.5). The structure is definitely papillary, and the epithelial tissue may or

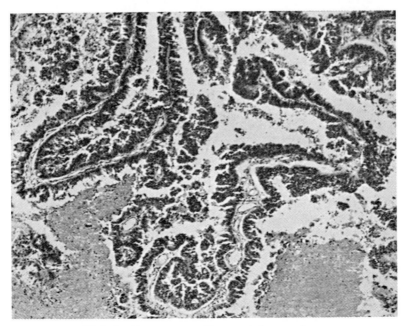

23.4. Another serous papillary cystadenocarcinoma

Table 23.1

	Number of Cases	Living	Dead	5-Year Salvage
				%
Grade 0 (0–1 mitosis)	14	12	2	85
Grade 1 (2–5 mitoses)	21	9	12	41
Grade 2 (6–15 mitoses)	29	3	26	10
Grade 3 (16+ mitoses)	16	0	16	0
	80	24	56	30

may not show a definitely glandular pattern.

Mucinous Cystadenocarcinoma

This is the malignant prototype of mucinous cystadenoma, or arises from the same tissue elements which give rise to the latter. Only about 5 to 10 per cent of these undergo malignant degeneration; this occurrence is much less common than with the serous. The malignant disease may affect only a localized area of the cyst, but in most cases the latter is replaced by solid tumor (Figs. 23.6, 7).

The *microscopic examination* shows the typical picture of adenocarcinoma (Fig. 23.8), but all degrees of differentiation are possible. The cells usually retain their mucoid tendencies to a greater or less extent, and hence one often finds large or small cavities filled with gelatinous material (Fig. 23.9). Stromal invasion occurs along with stratification of the lining epithelium. Unquestionably, borderline malignancies occur with these lesions, as noted by Hart and Norris. Papillary budding in mucinous tumors suggests incipient malignancy (Fig. 23.10) and is associated with aneuploidy (Weiss *et al.*).

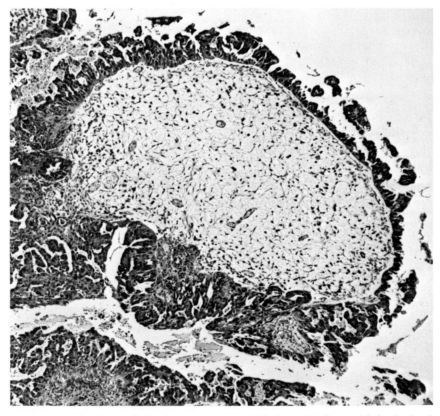

23.5. Increased stratification and adenomatous pattern of lining epithelium with beginning invasion of stroma. All these are indicative of malignant trend.

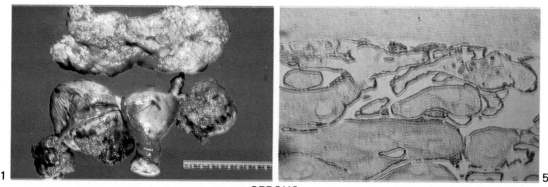

SEROUS

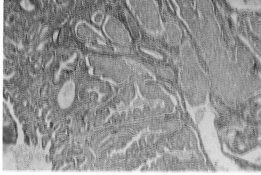

MUCINOUS

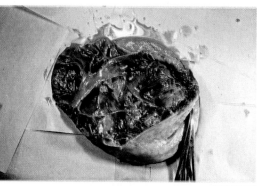

ENDOMETRIOID

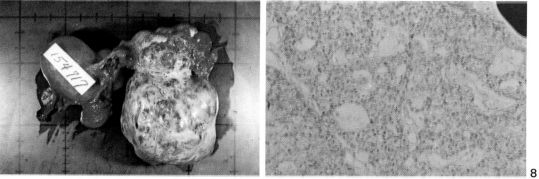

MESONEPHRIC

Plate 23.1

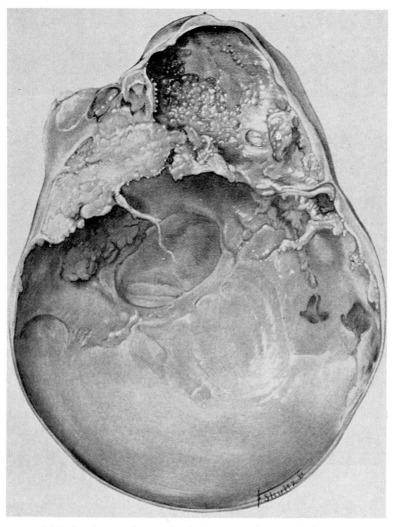

23.6. Carcinoma of ovary developing in mucinous cystadenoma

Secondary Carcinoma in Dermoid Cysts

This is rare, occurring in only one to three per cent of dermoid cysts and usually in the form of epidermoid carcinoma, since it develops from the skinlike elements in such tumors. On several occasions we have seen a genuine intraepithelial pattern.

ENDOMETRIOID CARCINOMA (See Chapter 25)

PRIMARY SOLID CARCINOMA OF OVARY

Types

The classification of solid primary ovarian cancer is also unsatisfactory from a pathological standpoint. We are obliged to have recourse chiefly to general pathological criteria of classification based chiefly on the growth pattern assumed by the tumors, except perhaps for certain germ cell tumors and those arising from the gonadal stroma. Aside from these the following variations of pattern may be noted in primary solid carcinoma.

(1)*Adenocarcinoma* (Fig. 23.11), the most common form, is characterized by its gland architecture, which may present various degrees of differentiation. In one type there is marked resemblance to endometrial adenocarcinoma, so that if both ovary and endometrium are involved, it is

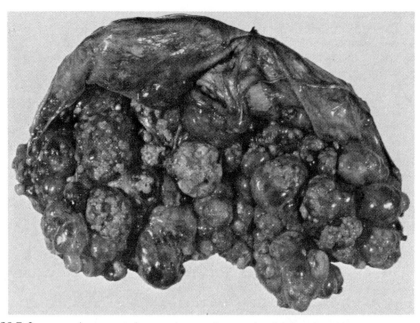

23.7. Large mucinous cystadenocarcinoma of ovary showing interior of large cyst cavity.

impossible to know which is the primary tumor or if there is a multicentric malignant trend of uterine and ectopic endometrium. This will be discussed more fully in the chapter on endometriosis.

(2) *Carcinoma,* also very frequent, is characterized by an absence of an adenomatous pattern. Various descriptive terms may be affixed, for example, papillary (Fig. 23.12), medullary, alveolar, scirrhous, etc. Multiple blocks and microscopic sections are necessary,

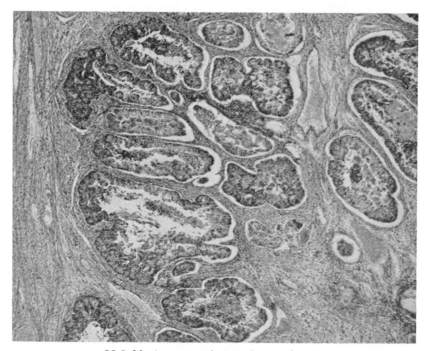

23.8. Mucinous cystadenocarcinoma of ovary

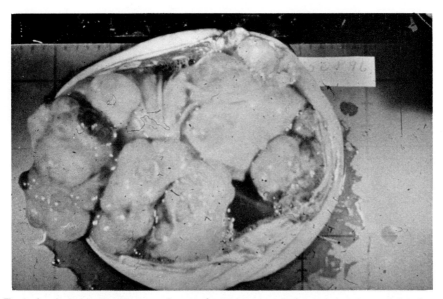

23.9. Typical gelatinous appearance of opened mucinous cystadenocarcinoma, multilocular and nonpapillary.

for a malignant pattern (Fig. 23.13) may coexist with a predominantly benign cystic one (Figs. 23.14–16).

Gross Characteristics

The size of solid ovarian carcinomas is very variable, although most of them give rise to symptoms which call for treatment before they have reached more than a moderate size. They may, however, fill the whole lower abdomen and weigh many pounds. As a rule the external surface is smooth, but it may present many nodular thickenings or excrescences. On cutting into the tumor, the surface may be of grayish granular appearance, but often

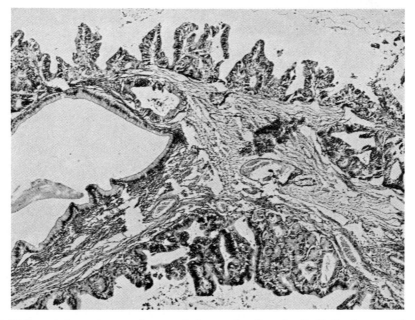

23.10. Malignant change in a mucinous cystadenoma (portion of wall of latter is seen at the *left*).

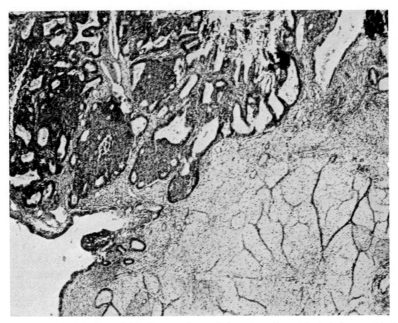

23.11. Adenoacanthoma arising from endometrial cyst; endometriosis below and to left.

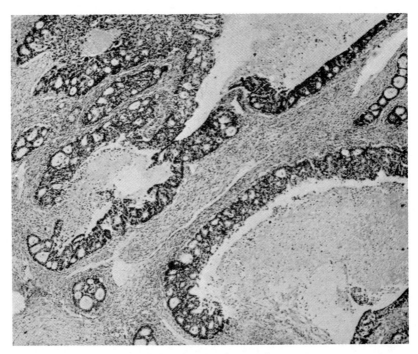

23.12. Papillary carcinoma of ovary

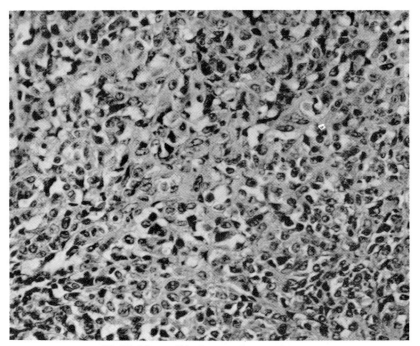

23.13. More solid adenocarcinoma of ovary

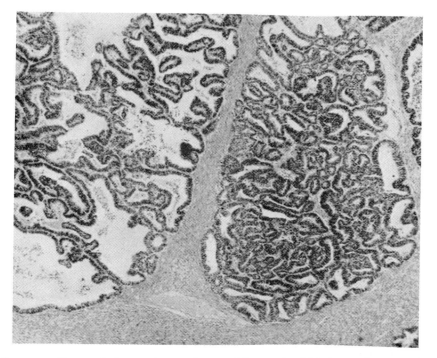

23.14. Serous papillary cystadenocarcinoma of ovary. Other parts of this tumor show a much more solid and anaplastic pattern.

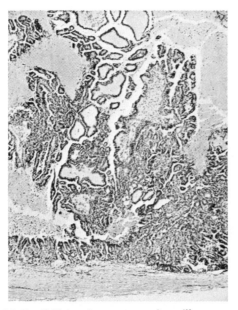

23.15. Still another pattern of papillary serous cystadenocarcinoma.

tissue is brainlike and pultaceous, with frequent ragged looking cavities produced by extensive necrosis. In the smaller group of scirrhous tumors the consistency may be firm and fibrous. In the earlier stages the tumor is commonly unilateral, but there is an increasing tendency to bilaterality as the disease advances.

Mesonephroma of the Ovary (Fig. 23. 17)

In 1939, Schiller published several articles concerning a certain type of ovarian lesion that he believed originated from mesonephric duct remnants. These tumors were tubular, and the lumina were lined by a flat, hobnail, cuboidal epithelium, with occasional intraluminal projections (Fig. 23.18), strongly suggestive of primitive glomeruli. This pattern was considered a specific entity, and was referred to as "Schiller's mesonephroma."

Somewhat later Saphir and Lackner reported a few cases of clear cell adenocarcinoma of the ovary which they believed were identical to renal tumors. These hypernephromas or "hypernephroid" tumors of the ovary were thought to be of mesonephric origin (Fig. 23.19).

Various publications by Novak and Woodruff appear to have established two very important points. (1) Certain tumors may show various admixtures of both the Schiller pattern and the clear cell architecture. (2) Such lesions are found exclusively in areas where there are remnants

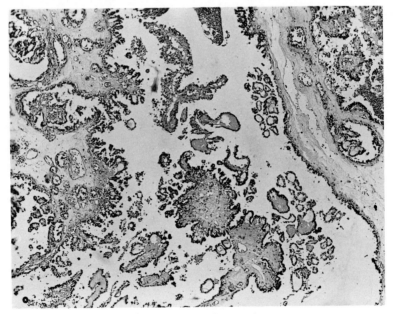

23.16. Medullary carcinoma of ovary

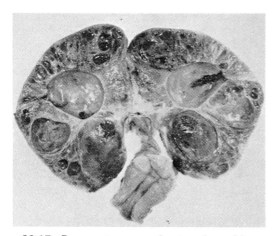

23.17. Gross appearance of cut surface of large mesonephroma (other ovary previously removed.

from extraovarian vestiges of the mesonephric tubules, with subsequent involvement of the gonad.

An early publication by Novak *et al.* noted 13 cases of mesonephromas occurring in the lower genital tract; a more recent article concerns 35 ovarian mesonephromas gathered from the Ovarian Tumor Registry. Mesonephromas represent merely a variety of adenocarcinoma; they are usually partially cystic and solid.

Although histology is similar irrespective of the site at which they occur, ovarian mesonephromas seemed considerably more lethal. Even where the lesion is confined to the ovary, mortality approximates 35 per cent despite any type of surgical and irradiation therapy. Where there is extraovarian extension there is practically no salvage. The high mortality rate, as compared to that of a similar tumor at a lower level, may well be a sequel of the intrapelvic location of the ovarian lesion where its presence is

of the mesonephric apparatus, and the tumors are identical irrespective of the level at which they occur. Such sites as the vagina, vaginal fornices, and broad ligament may be affected. Similarly, the ovary may be the seat of mesonephroma, although the lesion may actually arise

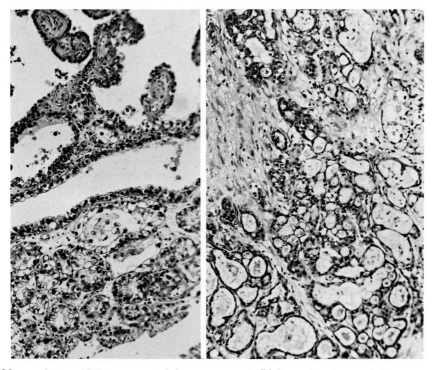

23.18. Mesonephroma (different areas of the same tumor). *Right* portion shows tubular pattern lined by peglike epithelium; *left,* higher power to show clear cells lining tubules.

silent and not so apt to cause bleeding as vaginal and cervical mesonephromas. Wherever the tumor lies, it is endocrinologically inert.

Scully and Barlow's concept stresses the mullerian origin of mesonephroma rather than an origin from mesonephric duct remnants (discussed in Chapter 25). In a more recent study Rogers *et al.* have reviewed 95 cases of mesonephroma from the Ovarian Tumor Registry, and it is their feeling that the data do not support a paramesonephric (or mullerian) source. They believe that the associated patterns suggest an origin from the multipotent mesothelium and that this would explain the occasional concurrent presence of other paramesonephric elements.

Gray and Barnes reported a mesonephric pattern in an endometrial cyst and Villa Santa and Rutledge have separately recorded mesonephric adenocarcinomas of the endometrium. We believe that on occasion focal areas of clear cells found in an endometrioid tumor may be a simple degenerative form of endometrioid adenocarcinoma, just as we find lipoid degeneration occurring in certain areas of an endometrial adenocarcinoma. Silverberg comments on the electronmicroscopic similarity of clear cell tumors of the ovary and the Arias-Stella reaction.

Kurman and Craig report finding clear cell and endometrioid carcinoma in certain cases, and other authors have reported an association of serous, mucinous, clear cell, and endometrioid carcinoma on occasion. This would support a common origin from the surface epithelium of the ovary, so in essence then, any or all of these tumors do appear to have a mesothelial origin. Thus it might be logical to include all of these lesions under the generic term *mesothelioma,* and indeed we are speaking of them as such in our own laboratory. However, these descriptive terms (serous, mucinous, etc.) have been in such long usage that it might be confusing to try to change them. We are not, however, completely willing to discount the origin of certain "mesonephromas" from certain cell rests of mesonephric origin.

The distinction of certain clear cell (Fig. 23.19) or lipoid tumors is difficult. Such terms as hypernephroma or masculinovoblastoma should be dis-

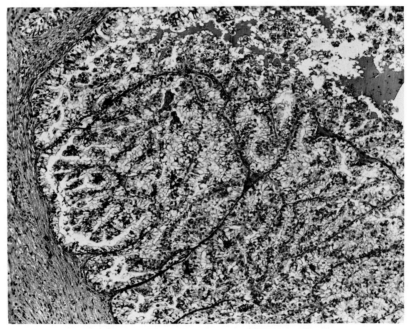

23.19. Clear cell appearance of mesonephroma of ovary

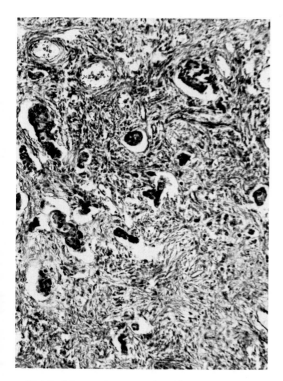

23.20. Metastatic tumor from breast, a common primary source for ovarian lesions.

carded, and the term luteoma retained only for that tumor of pregnancy as noted by Scully and Sternberg.

SECONDARY OR METASTATIC CARCINOMA OF OVARY

Carcinoma of almost any type may occur in the ovary as a result of metastasis from primary sites in other parts of the body, especially in the latter stages of such malignant processes. A not infrequent variety of secondary ovarian cancer is that seen in association with carcinoma of the gastrointestinal tract or breast (Fig. 23.20). This may present the same histological pattern in the ovary as in the primary tumor, this usually being adenocarcinoma.

Krukenberg Tumor

There is one particular variety of secondary ovarian carcinoma, however, which assumes special characteristics, and to which the designation of Krukenberg tumor is applied. This may be an accompaniment of primary carcinoma

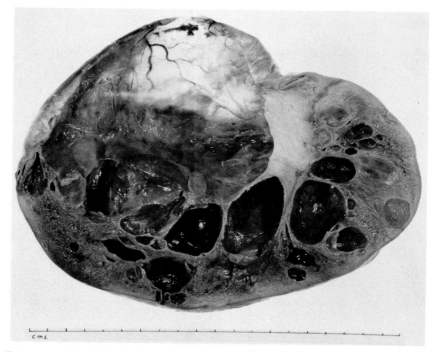

23.21. Primary unilateral Krukenberg tumor of ovary. Gastrointestinal lesion well excluded; classic microscopic Krukenberg features. (Courtesy of Dr. Agnes Scott, Dumfries, Scotland.)

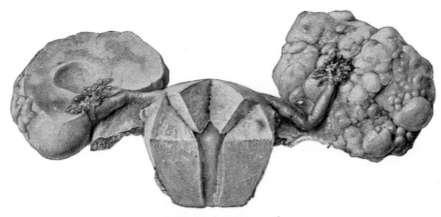

23.22. Krukenberg tumor of ovary

elsewhere, but especially in any portion of the gastrointestinal tract (Fig. 23.21), most frequently the pylorus, but not infrequently the colon, rectum, small intestine, liver, or gall bladder. In 81 cases, Hale noted the stomach to be the primary site in 76 instances. It should be emphasized that the term "Krukenberg tumor" should not be applied to any ovarian tumor secondary to a gastrointestinal lesion. The designation is made purely on a histological basis.

Although it is generally believed that Krukenberg tumors are almost always metastatic, Woodruff and Novak have pointed out that about 20 per cent *seem primary* in nature. An origin from teratoma, mucinous cyst, or mucoid degeneration in a Brenner tumor would seem to furnish the proper ovarian environment for a Krukenberg pattern to evolve. Prolonged salvage without gas-

trointestinal signs or symptoms, or autopsy on women dead from other causes, would leave little doubt as to a not infrequent primary ovarian origin. One or two cases have occurred during pregnancy, as noted by Lawrence *et al.,* and among the Ovarian Tumor Registry material utilized by Woodruff and Novak. The latter have found one 10-year salvage in a patient who had a characteristic uni-

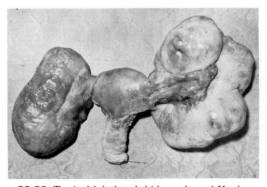

23.23. Typical lobulated, kidney shaped Krukenberg tumors. (Courtesy of Dr. Albert Brown, Wilmington, N. C.)

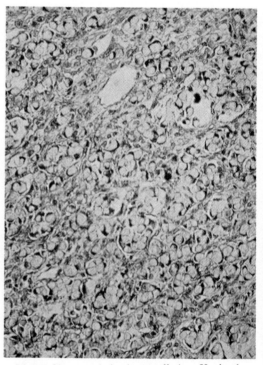

23.24. Characteristic signet cells in a Krukenberg tumor.

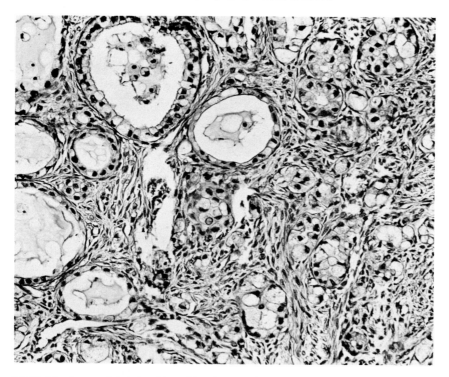

23.25. Mucinous acini, *left,* with melting down to form signet-ring pattern on *lower right.*

lateral primary Krukenberg tumor removed during pregnancy. The case of a Krukenberg tumor associated with a Meigs' syndrome reported by Brenner and Scott also seems to be a primary ovarian Krukenberg tumor, although admittedly there is no prolonged follow up.

There has been considerable discussion as to the route by which carcinoma cells make their way to the ovary from such primary sites as the pylorus. Most students believe that retrograde lymphatic transplantation is the important factor, whereas in some cases the hematogenous route plays the important role.

The tumors are generally bilateral (over 50 per cent). They are solid and they have a tendency to retain the original ovarian contour, so that they are ovoid or kidney-shaped (Figs. 23.22, 23). The surface is smooth, although often nodular, and the cut surface of variegated appearance, with frequently areas of gelatinous consistency.

Microscopically, the pattern of the Krukenberg tumor is quite distinctive, and the diagnosis is dependent only on the histological pattern, not on an associated or prior gastrointestinal lesion. Small nests or acini of epithelial cells are distributed throughout a fibrous or myxomatous stroma, and especially characteristic are the so-called *signet cells* Figs. 23.24, 25), in which the mucoid accumulation in the cytoplasm displaces the flattened nucleus to one side of the cell. A marked stromal hyperplasia mimicking sarcoma may be present, and this stromal (thecal) reaction may lead to bleeding from a hyperplastic endometrium as noted by some authors. Indeed, the striking stromal proliferation led to the original description as *sarcoma ovarii mucocellulare carcinomatodes.*

Endocrine Activity

In our study comprising outside cases submitted to the Ovarian Tumor Registry, there were none associated with any endocrine activity. Many such tumors, however, were sent in from small rural areas where the opportunity for adequate study simply did not exist. That the Krukenberg tumor may be associated with hormone function has been adequately documented, and our own clinic material has afforded several examples of the seemingly functional behavior of this tumor type.

Over 10 years ago, Turenen discussed the *estrogenic* capabilities of Krukenberg tumors with a study of pre- and postoperative urinary estrogens, along with the clinicopathological findings of postmenopausal uterine endometrial hyperplasia and bleeding. The presumed feminizing agent is the ovarian stroma or the stroma of the tumor matrix which is converted into a theca-like type of cell. More recently, an androgenic role has been ascribed to the same cells presumably due to conversion into a cell whose behavior parallels that of the interstitial cell. This is easily comprehensible if one is cognizant of the common ancestry of the potentially active stromal cell as well as the biochemical similarity of the androgens and estrogens which permit ready convertibility. In any event, a number of cases have been collected in which the Krukenberg tumor has been associated with virilism (such as Ober's well studied report), and the even more intriguing study by Spadoni in which pregnancy also concurred, with virilism of the ensuing female infant.

EXTENSION OF OVARIAN CARCINOMA

The other ovary becomes involved in more than one-half of all cases of ovarian carcinoma, whereas the tube and the uterus are not infrequently the seat of metastatic extension, as one might expect from the richness of lymphatic intercommunication of these various organs. Even where the contralateral ovary appears grossly normal, cancer is found in the hilar lymphatics in 25 to 50 per cent of cases. Especially frequent is extension to the peritoneum, as well as the omentum and mesentery, occurring in over 75 per cent of all cases. The lymphatic glands, especially those of the lumbar group, are involved in a very large proportion of the cases, especially in the later stages of the disease. Finally, metastases may occur to such distant organs as the liver, pancreas, lungs, pleura, and long bones.

CLINICAL CHARACTERISTICS OF OVARIAN CARCINOMA

The most important symptoms of ovarian carcinoma are unfortunately rather late ones, as the onset of this disease is almost always very insidious and "silent" in nature. The presence of a *mass* in the lower abdomen is the first indication of the disease in a considerable proportion of cases, and unfortunately by this time other organs are often involved. Moderate *heaviness* or occasional *pain* may be noted, but are more apt to be absent. Irregular or postmenopausal *bleeding* is an infrequent finding. *Thrombophlebitis,* otherwise unexplained, may be due to silent tumor in proximity to the large veins. It has been amply demonstrated that the finding of tumor cells in the blood does not necessarily imply metastases.

Ascites is a relatively common accompaniment of ovarian cancer, especially of the papillary varieties. It is all too frequently indicative of peritoneal extension of the growth, but may be due merely to venous obstruction caused by partial torsion of the tumor, as in any other ovarian neoplasm. The ascites may be so extreme as to make palpation of the tumor impossible, and paracentesis is often needed to palpate the lower abdominal or pelvic masses.

For some reason various ovarian tumors may be associated with *hypercalcemia* even when there is no osteolytic lesion. Ferenczy *et al.* note that this is disproportionately common with mesonephroma. The proposal that the neoplasm produces a parathyroid-like substance is usually supported, but it is very speculative why mesonephroma should be most likely to produce a high calcium level.

Ovarian Carcinoma in Pregnancy (see preceding chapter)

Diagnosis

In a large proportion of cases the malignant nature of the tumors is not suspected before operation, and often not until pathological examination. In many, however, a strongly presumptive diagnosis is possible, chiefly on palpatory findings. Vaginal smear rarely demonstrates exfoliated tumor cells, but Rubin and Frost note a frequent estrogenic effect in the maturation index (see Chaps. 36, 37). Preoperative culdocentesis may be helpful if the removed fluid is studied cytologically. This has been suggested as part of a routine "check-up" of even normal women by Graham. It is estimated that one per cent of asymptomatic patients will be found to show abnormal cells. It is difficult to decide how much should be included as part of a routine examination.

If pelvic examination reveals a mass occupying the position of the ovary, and if the mass is hard, fixed, and firm, ovarian carcinoma should be suspected, especially if the patient is in the cancer age. Benign solid tumors of the ovary, such as fibroma, give somewhat the same feeling but are less common. Benign cystic tumors, on the other hand, give a softer, elastic sensation to the examining hands, and are usually smoother in contour, as compared to the more nodular contour of most cancers. Laparoscopy may be decisive when there is uncertainty if an adnexal mass is uterine or ovarian in origin.

When such a tumor is associated with ascites, there can be little doubt as to its malignant nature. When the ascites is extreme, the tumor may be impalpable, and other causes of ascites, such as hepatic and cardiorenal disease or tuberculous peritonitis, may have to be eliminated. Occasionally paracentesis may be necessary to permit proper palpation of the pelvic organs, and a definite mass may be felt for the first time. Micro-

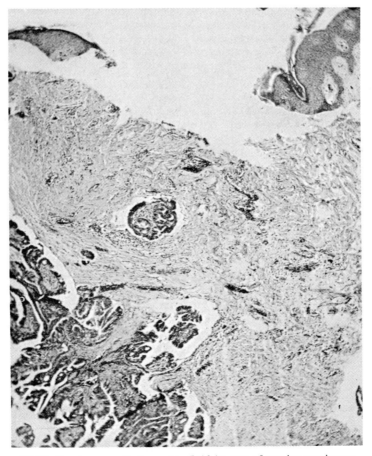

23.26. Carcinoma cells in ascitic fluid in case of ovarian carcinoma.

Table 23.2

Serous Carcinoma

Clinical Stage	Number of Cases Treated	Alive 5 Years	%
1 a	212	116	54.7
1 b, IIa	138	50	36.2
II b	209	52	24.9
III	414	26	6.3
IV	137	4	2.9
Total	1 110	248	22.3

Table 23.4

Endometrioid and Mesonephric Carcinoma

Clinical Stage	Number of Cases Treated	Alive 5 Years	%
I a	102	64	62.7
I b, II a	78	41	52.6
II b	120	58	48.3
III	134	10	7.5
IV	35	0	
Total	469	173	36.9

scopic examination of the centrifuged ascitic fluid may show typically malignant cells (Fig. 23.26).

Peritoneal washing at laparotomy has been suggested by some as being of prognostic value, if performed before operative manipulation and immediately after entry into the abdomen. This should be done, but the surgeon should be mindful of the vagarious nature of ovarian tumors. Sometimes an apparently localized lesion is followed by massive recurrence. In other instances extensive disease seems compatible with longevity.

Even at the time of surgery, the exact nature of an ovarian tumor may be uncertain, and in such instances a *frozen section* may be helpful. It is perhaps preferable to remove the whole adnexal mass, and allow the pathologist to select likely areas for section rather than remove blindly one or two areas for evaluation. Although this may minimize errors, permanent sections will on oc-

casion show malignancy that had not been noted on frozen section, so that the trained gynecologist will also strongly consider the gross appearance of the lesion at surgery.

Prognosis

The outlook for the patient with ovarian carcinoma is very grave, especially if one omits from consideration the gonadal stroma group (granulosa-theca cell tumor, arrhenoblastoma, and dysgerminoma) in which the results are far better. There are few writers who report a five-year survival rate of much more than 30 per cent, and indeed in some areas such as New York, ovarian cancer accounts for more deaths than cervical malignancy due to improved detection of the latter disease.

It should be apparent that the results with ovarian carcinoma depend to a considerable degree as to what histological types of tumor are included. Tables 23.2–6 depict the cumulative results by 23

Table 23.3

Mucinous Carcinoma

Clinical Stage	Number of Cases Treated	Alive 5 Years	%
I a	104	76	73.1
I b, II a	51	22	43.1
II b	50	21	42.0
III	76	12	15.8
IV	24	0	
Total	305	131	43.0

Table 23.5

Unclassified Carcinoma

Clinical Stage	Number of Cases Treated	Alive 5 Years	%
I a	65	37	56.9
I b, II a	28	11	39.3
II b	67	10	14.9
III	200	9	4.5
IV	76	3	3.9
Total	436	70	16.1

Table 23.6

Cases of So-Called Low Potential Malignancy.
All Types

Clinical Stage	Number of Cases Treated	Alive 5 Years	%
I a	188	157	83.5
I b, II a	90	62	68.9
II b	71	46	64.8
III	76	33	43.4
IV	26	5	19.2
Total	451	303	67.2

clinics as reported in the most recent FIGO results, the first time ovarian carcinoma has been included in this report. It is obvious that any report containing a large proportion of mucinous, or endometrioid-mesonephric carcinoma will show a considerably better result than one with a majority of more lethal serous carcinoma, or when the tumor is so anaplastic as to become unclassified. It is likewise apparent that histologically low grade tumors yield a fairly respectable salvage in particular where the disease is not clinically too advanced. Munnell indicates that the salvage of 235 cases studied from 1952 to 1961 has risen to 40 per cent which is attributed to increasingly radical surgery and improved methods of irradiation and chemotherapy.

Treatment

The proper treatment of ovarian carcinoma is *surgical*. Operation should be performed as early as possible, and should ideally comprise hysterectomy and bilateral salpingo-oophorectomy. Even when peritoneal involvement is disclosed (Fig. 23.27), the primary lesions should be removed if this is safely possible, as there is rather general agreement that this retards the progress of the secondary extensions. Some degree of omentectomy decreases recurrent ascites, although it may predispose to intestinal obstruction.

Munnell makes a very strong case for unilateral salpingo-oophorectomy only in the young patient with an encapsulated lesion confined to one ovary, particularly when the pathology reveals a relatively favorable type of neoplasm such as mucinous. Admittedly total "pelvic clean out" may afford a slightly better salvage, but Munnell suggests there is only a negligible improvement. Where conservative procedures are contemplated, bisection of the contralateral ovary is mandatory, for there is a 12–15% chance of involvement of a grossly normal gonad. Peritoneal washing is likewise of value. We are in accord with this rationale in the young female desiring further pregnancy, although there may be a slight calculated risk.

Advanced Disease. Most gynecologists feel that ovarian carcinoma warrants exploration despite suggestive evidence of extrapelvic disease and even pulmonic or pleural spread. Admittedly the prognosis is poor but surgery is worthwhile (1) as a diagnostic measure, (2) in obviating incipient obstruction, and (3) as a palliative procedure by reducing tumor bulk, omental lesions, and ascites. Rarely there is profound regression following removal of the parent lesion, and modern

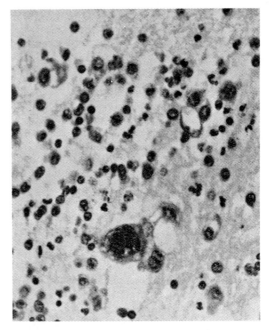

23.27. Metastasis of papillary serous cystadenocarcinoma of ovary to umbilicus (see skin epithelium *above* and to the *right*). The histology is similar to that of primary ovarian growth.

methods of chemotherapy and irradiation often lead to prolonged remission although cure is minimal. The exact role of the "second look" procedure for ovarian malignancy as noted by Smith *et al.* seems uncertain; this should be preceded by laparoscopy and cell washings.

Irradiation

The postoperative employment of *irradiation therapy* has been almost universal, and is of undoubted value in prolonging life in many instances, with little regard as to tumor histology. Burns *et al.* are convinced that total body radiation prolongs longevity; occasionally this M. D. Anderson group combines it with chemotherapy. There is scant evidence, however, of any curative effect.

More recently, *radioactive* colloidal gold or *phosphate* has been placed into the peritoneal cavity and seems of considerable aid in preventing the recurrent ascites which is such a frequent problem in the implanting papillary tumors. Damage to the intestinal tract has been decreased by replacing gold with chromic phosphate P_{32}, which is considerably less penetrative because it emits almost exclusively beta rays. Nevertheless, uneven distribution due to adhesions and localization in the postoperative patient may lead to complications. It is of no assistance where there are large masses and of course is rarely curative, merely palliative in increasing the life span. Details are available in the papers of Decker *et al.* and of Moore and Langley.

Chemotherapy

Chemotherapy should be considered in all cases where the surgeon feels that all of the tumor was not removed or peritoneal washings show tumor cells. It is of less value where there is much bulk tumor but certainly both irradiation and drug therapy deserve consideration where there is residual tumor. Different clinics will have preferences for one or another method; on occasion both will be used simultaneously.

The *chemotherapeutic* agents fall basically into three different groups. The *alkylating agents* include Thiotepa, chlorambucil (Leukoran), Cytoxan (cyclophosphamide), sarcolysine (Alkeran), and others. The *antimetabolites* consist of such folic acid antagonists as methotrexate, or aminopterin, and the pyrimidine and purine analogues such as 5-fluorouracil and 6-mercaptopurine. Lastly are the antibiotics, primarily actinomycin D. In essence all chemotherapeutic drugs included in this category are cellular poisons which affect DNA and/or RNA and therefore cellular reduplication so that as such they all must be considered to be quite toxic.

Toxicity seems related to the dosage, which should depend on body weight (Hreshchyshyn). Toxicity may be profound with extensive bone marrow depression, severe stomatitis, and other profound gastrointestinal effects including nausea, vomiting, diarrhea, along with severe ulceration of the gastrointestinal tract, as well as liver and kidney damage. Alopecia and various types of dermatitis may occur. As has been stated earlier the mode of action is interference with either DNA or RNA synthesis, either through inhibition of protein metabolism or by replacing normal proteins in the synthesis of DNA or RNA with the production of fraudulent nuclear protein.

With most of the epithelial tumors the drug of choice seems to be Chlorambucil, which may be given orally over long periods of time. Patients so treated should be followed initially by weekly hematocrit, white blood count, and platelet count, with the dosage being decreased should there be any significant drop of either the blood elements. Temporary discontinuance should be practiced if the white count should drop below 3,000, the hematocrit below 30, or the platelets below 150,000. Should there be a significant drop in the white count, broad spectrum antibiotic therapy and isolation should be carried out. Therapy should be continued unless there is severe toxicity or if there is no apparent response to the tumor. In such instances another alkylating agent such as cyclophosphamide (Cytoxan) may be considered.

In certain instances of rare tumors such as the endodermal sinus or other germ cell tumors triple chemotherapy may be utilized with Actinomycin D, cyclophosphamide, and 5-fluorouracil as advocated by the M. D. Anderson Hospital. This type of therapy has been relatively favorable for these generally extremely fatal tumors and we have had several similar satisfactory cases. It should be emphasized that in most cases chemotherapy should not be considered necessarily curative, but may provide long remissions.

Frick *et al.* and Burns *et al.* prefer Sarcolysin, and various clinics have different preferences.

Parker and Singleton feel that there is increased longevity in certain treated patients, and this is in accord with Rutledge's findings with Sarcolysin; a 50 per cent objective response was noted in 338 patients.

We regard perfusion as a truly heroic and very dangerous procedure, and have utilized this only when there was absolutely no alternative type of therapy.

It has been established that (ovarian) cancers evoke a specific *immune reaction,* and Bhattachanya and Barlow indicate a common antigen for serous and mucinous cystadenocarcinoma. A so-called carcinoembryonic antigen (CEA) related to endodermal structures has many other chromosomally related systems. Elevation of CEA is apparent in a considerable proportion of women with malignant ovarian tumors, but not with benign lesions. The finding of tumor specific antigens in various neoplasms seems of potential diagnostic and therapeutic value; however, the current status of immunotherapy today is that of chemotherapy 20 years ago. Such studies as that of Order (although in rabbits and mice) seemingly demonstrate increased salvage with advanced transplantable ovarian tumor of mice following injection of rabbit antibodies.

SARCOMA OF OVARY

Sarcoma of the ovary is far less common than carcinoma, its *incidence* as compared with carcinoma being about 1:40. It *may occur at any age.* Most authors emphasize that it is frequent in children, but this is open to doubt, as so many ovarian tumors in children which were formerly diagnosed as sarcoma are now recognized as either gonadal stromal carcinoma, dysgerminoma, or lymphomas.

Various types of sarcoma are found in the ovary, the spindle variety (Fig. 23.28) being more common than the round cell, although mixed forms often occur. The lymphomas, occasionally primary, and angiosarcoma are also described, but it appears that in the latter the perivascular arrangement of the cells is due to the fact that extensive degeneration has occurred except where the cells are near to their blood supply. Endometrial or mixed mesodermal sarcomas seem probable sequelae of endometriosis. Symptoms are identical to those of carcinoma.

Azoury and Woodruff have recently reviewed 43 cases of primary ovarian sarcomas from the Emil Novak Ovarian

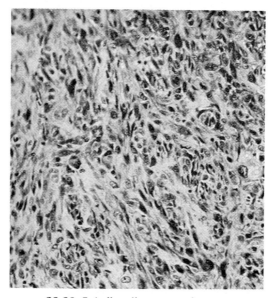

23.28. Spindle cell sarcoma of ovary

Tumor Registry. They felt it was possible to divide these into 3 different categories (excluding lymphomas) as follows: (1) teratoid sarcomas—most common in youthful patients with a very poor prognosis, (2) mesenchymal or stromal—occurring at any age with the malignancy definitely comparable to the degree of histologic malignancy, (3) paramesonephric sarcomas—occurring at any age, not infrequently in association with endometriosis, and with a very poor prognosis.

TERATOMA

Teratoma of the ovary may be *cystic or solid.* The cystic form is represented by the benign dermoid, already described in the chapter on benign ovarian cysts. The *solid teratoma* (Fig. 23.29) differs from the simple dermoid not only in that it is a solid tumor, but also because it is malignant, and that it contains elements derived from all three of the fetal layers. The term *embryonal carcinoma* is utilized for extremely bizarre teratoid lesions, and closely related to this is the *endodermal sinus tumor* (derived from extra-embryonic structures) as described by Teilum (Fig. 23.30); both have a very poor prognosis. The ability of the latter to synthesize alpha fetoprotein noted by Wilkson *et al.* may be of diagnostic and therapeutic import.

The *histogenesis* of teratoma is not clearly known, the two chief theories

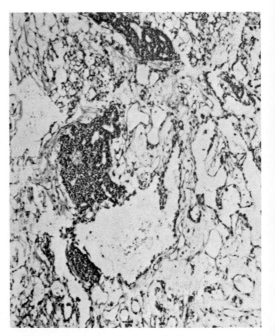

23.30. Typical endodermal sinus tumor with some resemblance to mesonephroma but showing characteristics noted by Teilum

being: (1) an origin from segregated blastomeres, and (2) an origin from unfertilized sex cells. According to the first of these, blastomeres may be segregated in early stages of embryonic development, lying dormant until later life, when for some unknown reason they begin to differentiate into the tissues which they were originally designed to form. The weakness of this concept is that it does not explain why the ovary is such a seat of predilection for such teratomatous growths.

Perhaps somewhat more popular is the second theory. This is based on the fact that the ovary normally contains large numbers of germ cells, capable after certain preparatory changes of producing another human body if fertilized by the male element. Even without the latter, it is thought possible that a species of *parthenogenetic* development may occur because of certain stimulating if unknown factors which may arise, and that abortive and imperfect formation of various fetal tissues may thus occur.

According to this hypothesis, it will be

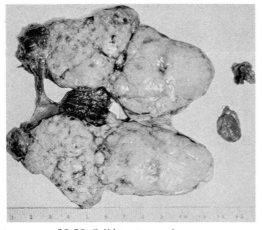

23.29. Solid teratoma of ovary

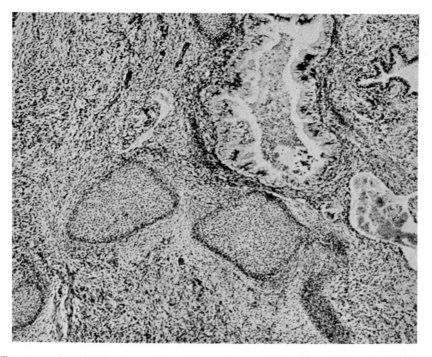

23.31. Teratoma of ovary showing cartilage plates and a cavity lined by entodermic epithelium like that seen in pseudomucinous cystadenoma.

seen that the histogenesis of teratoma is somewhat allied to the phenomenon of twinning. In this connection, it is worth noting that the chromosomal test for sex differentiation has been applied by Hunter, Lennox, and Durk to the study of a group of 21 teratomas, 12 occurring in females and 9 in males. All the teratomas in women were found to be chromatin positive, but of those in males four were male and five female. No important lesson can be drawn from these findings in view of our ignorance as to the histogenesis of teratomas. Aneuploidy is frequent in most ovarian malignancies; Arias-Bernal and Jones, however, indicate diploidy in one teratoma studied cytogenetically.

Teratoma may occur at any age, but is *more common in younger individuals.* The tumors are usually of small or only moderate size. They are firm and solid, with often cartilaginous or bony areas (Fig. 23.31), and not infrequently with small cavities produced by degeneration.

Microscopically almost any of the tissues or organs of the body may be re-

produced in the tumor, although usually imperfectly. Cartilage, bone, teeth, brain tissue, intestine, and many other tissues may be found, although they are not always easy to differentiate, especially as they are often of immature embryonic type. Woodruff suggests that the presence of undifferentiated neural tissue markedly impairs the prognosis. Recently

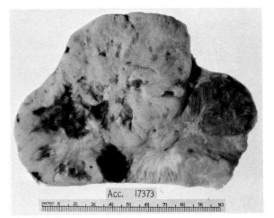

23.32. Struma ovarii with associated thyroid carcinoma.

Albites has noted a case of a benign teratoma with malignant transformation of benign glial implants. *Choriocarcinoma* of the ovarian tumor may occur with lung metastasis as commonly as with the usual trophoblastic lesion of the uterus. A limited experience with this rare lesion indicates that it responds less favorably to drug (MTX) therapy than the trophoblastic growths of the uterus.

A specific subdivision of teratoma is the so-called *struma ovarii*, or thyroid tumor of the ovary (Fig. 23.32). In this variety the thyroid tissue blots out other elements in large areas of the tumor (Fig. 23.33), although usually at least some other teratomatous elements are found.

An interesting clinical feature of some cases of struma ovarii has been that the thyroid tissue is functionally active or even overactive, producing systemic manifestations of hyperthyroidism, with pronounced increase of the basal metabolic rate. Removal of such tumors will cure the hyperthyroidism.

The mere finding of a small amount of mature thyroid tissue does not justify the designation of struma ovarii, as such islands are not rarely seen in simple

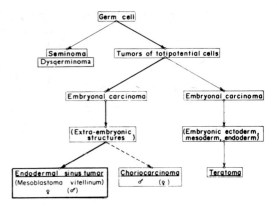

23.34. Teilum's concept of germ cell tumors. (Courtesy of Dr. Gunnar Teilum)

dermoids. The term should be used only when the thyroid tissue forms a dominating fraction of the tumor, although no mathematical rules can be laid down. Another interesting characteristic of teratoma is that in some cases there is a dominance of endodermic epithelium which morphologically resembles that so characteristic of mucinous cystadenoma. As a matter of fact a commonly accepted theory is that the origin of some mucinous cystadenomas is teratomatous, from the endodermic epithelium just described.

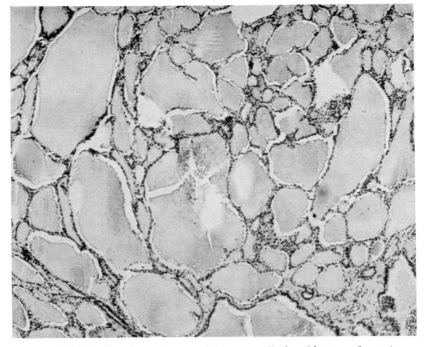

23.33. Microscopic appearance of struma ovarii (thyroid tumor of ovary)

Unquestionably, mucoid metaplasia of the germinal epithelium can occur and be a potential source of genesis for mucinous lesions (see Fig. 23.34).

A small group of carcinoid tumors arising from argentaffine cells has been reported by Nissen to arise in teratomas. They are of low grade malignancy, but may, when extensive, produce a metabolite that may produce vasomotor changes. These have been discussed more extensively in the previous chapter (Fig. 23.35).

The *symptoms* of teratoma are the presence of an *ovarian mass, occasionally slight bleeding* and not infrequently *ascites*. The course is definitely *malignant,* and *metastases* occur not only in various abdominal locations, but also in distant organs even where there is an intact capsule and no gross extension. Nogales and Oliva have discussed rather recently the rare occurrence of peritoneal gliomatosis, teratomas containing immature neural tissue with perforation, peritoneal dissemination, and subsequent maturation of the spilled neural tissue.

The *treatment* is of course surgical, but even so the prognosis is unfavorable in most cases. In the recent series of 97 cases reported by Woodruff *et al.,* only 37 patients were free of recurrence after two years. Breen and Neubecker in their study of 17 patients suggest complete hysterectomy and adnexectomy despite an average age of slightly more than 16 years. Our own preference would be to perform conservative surgery if the tumor capsule is intact, admittedly as a calculated risk. Radiotherapy appears to be of little or no value, but we have experienced some success with the use of triple drug therapy. If, however, we include cases of solid but well differentiated tumors, the prognosis is much improved. Our own preference is to use the term teratoma to indicate a malignant process, but to modify this by the prefix "benign" if there is an orderly arrangement of well differentiated cell patterns.

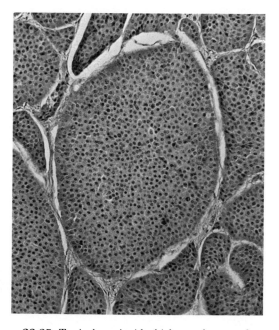

23.35. Typical carcinoid which may be secondary to gastrointestinal lesion, but which occurs primarily in a benign cystic teratoma.

REFERENCES

Abell, N. R., and Holtz, F.: Ovarian neoplasms in childhood and adolescence. I. Tumors of germ cell origin (with Johnson, V. J). Amer. J. Obstet. Gynec., *92:* 1059, 1965. II. Tumors of non-germ cell origin. Amer. J. Obstet. Gynec., *93:* 850, 1965.

Abell, N. R.: Undifferentiated malignant germ cell neoplasm (embryonal carcinoma) of ovary with stromal luteinization and viralism. Amer. J. Obstet. Gynec., *101:* 570, 1968.

Acosta, A., Kaplar, A. L., and Kaufman, R. H.: Gynecological cancer in children. Amer. J. Obst. Gynec., *112:* 944, 1972.

Albites, V.: Solid teratoma of the ovary with malignant gliomatosis peritonei. Int. J. Gynec. Obstet., *12:* 59, 1974.

Anderson, M. C.: Endometrioid tumor of the ovary with serous and mucinous components. Amer. J. Obst. Gynec., *113:* 686, 1972.

Arias-Bernal, L., and Jones, H. W.: Chromosomes of a malignant ovarian tumor. Amer. J. Obstet. Gynec., *100:* 785, 1968.

Aure, J. C., Hoeg, K. and Kolstadt, P.: Mesonephroid tumors of the ovary. Obstet. Gynec., *37:* 860, 1971.

Aure, J. C., Hoeg, K., and Kolstadt, P.: Clinico-histological studies of ovarian carcinoma. Obstet. Gynec., *37:* 1, 1971.

Aure, J. C., Hoeg, K., and Kolstadt, P.: Psammoma bodies in serous carcinoma of the ovary. Amer. J. Obstet. Gynec., *109:* 113, 1971.

Azoury, P. S., and Woodruff, J. D.: Primary ovarian sarcoma. Obstet. Gynec., *37:* 920, 1971.

Bhattachanya, M., and Barlow, J. J.: Immunologic study of carcinoma of the ovary. Amer. J. Obstet. Gynec., *117:* 849, 1973.

Breen, J. L., and Neubecker, R. D.: Malignant teratoma of the ovary. Analysis of 17 cases. Obstet. Gynec., *21:* 669, 1963.

Brenner, W. E., and Scott, R. B.: Meigs-like syndrome secondary to Krukenberg tumor. Obstet. Gynec., *31:* 40, 1968.

Burns, B. C., Jr., Rutledge, F. N., Smith, J. P., and Delclos, L.: Management of ovarian carcinoma. Surgery, irradiation, and chemotherapy. Amer. J. Obstet. Gynec., 98: 374, 1967.

Chon, S. Y., Koffler, D., and Cohen, C. J.: Cell mediated immunity with ovarian carcinoma. Amer. J. Obstet. Gynec., 115: 467, 1973.

Creasman, W. P., and Rutledge, F.: The value of peritoneal cytology. Amer. J. Obstet. Gynec., 110: 773, 1971.

Creasman, W. P., Rutledge, F., and Smith, J. P.: Carcinoma of the ovary associated with pregnancy. Obstet. Gynec., 38: 111, 1971.

Czernobilsky, B., and Corrog, J. L.: Squamous adenoacanthoma. Obstet. Gynec., 37: 555, 1971.

Decker, D. G., Malkasian, G. D., and Johnson, C. E.: Adjuvant therapy for advanced ovarian malignancy. Amer. J. Obstet. Gynec., 97: 171, 1967.

Decker, D. G., Webb, M. J., and Holbrook, M. A.: Radiogold treatment of epithelial cancer of ovary. Amer. J. Obstet. Gynec., 115: 751, 1973.

Drukker, B. H., and Hodgkinson, C. P.: Ovarian carcinoma—preoperative for the 70's. Amer. J. Obstet. Gynec., 109: 825, 1971.

Fenn, M. E., and Abell, M. R.: Carcinosarcoma of the ovary. Amer. J. Obstet. Gynec., 110: 1066, 1971.

Ferenczy, A., Okagaki, T., and Richart, R. M.: Paraendocrine hypercalcemia in ovarian neoplasms. Cancer, 27: 427, 1971.

Frick, H. C., Tretter, P., Tretter, W., and Hyman, G. A.: Disseminated carcinoma of the ovary treated by L-phenylalanine mustard. Cancer, 21: 508, 1968.

Friedman, N. B.: The comparative morphogenesis of extragenital and gonadal teratoid tumors. Cancer, 4: 265, 1951.

Gibbs, E. K.: Suggested prophylaxis for ovarian carcinoma. Amer. J. Obstet. Gynec., 111: 756, 1971.

Graham, R. M., Schueller, E. F., and Graham, J. B.: Detection of ovarian cancer at an early stage—routine culdocentesis. Obstet. Gynec., 26: 151, 1965.

Griffiths, C. T., Grogan, R. H., and Hall, T. C.: Advanced ovarian cancer. Cancer, 29: 1, 1972.

Hale, R. W.: Krukenberg tumors of the ovary. Obstet. Gynec., 68: 221 1968.

Hall, J. E., Caband, P. G., and Sullivan, T.: Squamous carcinoma in previously benign cystic teratoma. Obstet. Gynec., 6: 93, 1955.

Hart, W. R., and Norris, H. J.: Borderline and malignant mucinous tumors of the ovary. Cancer, 31: 1031, 1973.

Hilaris, B. S., and Clark, D. G. C.: Postoperative intraperitoneal radio colloids in early carcinoma ovary. Amer. J. Roentgenol., 112: 749, 1971.

Hasilag, F. B., and Rutledge, F. N.: Metastatic breast cancer in the ovary. Amer. J. Obstet. Gynec., 74: 989, 1957.

Hreshchyshyn, M. M.: Basic considerations of chemotherapy of gynecological cancer. Clin. Obstet. Gynec., 11: 334, 1968.

Hunter, W. F., Lennox, B., and Durh, M. D.: The sex of teratomata. Lancet, 2: 633, 1954.

Huntington, R. W., Jr., and Bullock, W. K.: Yolk sac tumors of the ovary. Cancer, 25: 1357, 1970.

Jakobovitz, A.: Hormone production by miscellaneous ovarian tumors. Amer. J. Obstet. Gynec., 85: 90, 1963.

Johnson, C. E., and Soule, E. H.: Malignant lymphomas as a gynecological problem. Obstet. Gynec., 10: 149, 1957.

Julian, C. G., and Woodruff, J. D.: The role of chemotherapy in the treatment of primary ovarian malignancy. Obstet. Gynec. Surv., 24: 1307, 1969.

Julian, C. G., and Woodruff, J. D.: Biological behavior of low grade papillary cystadenocarcinoma. Obstet. Gynec., 40: 860, 1972.

Keetel, W. C., Fox, M. R., Longnecker, D. S., and Latourette, H. B.: Prophylactive use of radioactive gold in the treatment of primary ovarian cancer. Amer. J. Obstet. Gynec., 94: 766, 1966.

Krukenberg, F.: Über das Fibrosarcoma ovarii mucocellulare carcinomatodes. Arch. Gynaek., 50: 287, 1896.

Kurman, R. R. J., and Craig, J. M.: Endometrioid and clear cell carcinoma of the ovary. Cancer, 29: 653, 1972.

Lathrop, J. C.: Pelvic lymphomas. Obstet. Gynec., 30: 137, 1967.

Lawrence, W. D., Larson, P. N., and Hauge, E. T.: Primary Krukenberg tumor of the ovary in pregnancy. Obstet. Gynec., 10: 54, 1957.

Leo, S., Robat, E., and Parekh, M.: Malignant melanoma in dermoid cyst. Obstet. Gynec., 41: 205, 1973.

Malkasian, G. D., Symmonds, R. E., and Dockerty, M. B.: Malignant ovarian teratoma. Obstet. Gynec., 25: 810, 1965.

Malpas, P.: Pseudomyxoma peritonei. J. Obstet. Gynaec. Brit. Comm., 66: 247, 1959.

McGowan, L., Davis, R. H., and Bunrag, B.: Biochemical diagnosis of ovarian cancer. Amer. J. Obstet. Gynec., 116: 760, 1973.

Meyer, R.: In *Handbuch der spezielle pathologische Anatomie und Histologie,* edited by F. Henke and O. Lubarsch, Vol. 7, Part 3; Vol. 8, p. 396, Julius Springer, Berlin, 1930.

Moore, D. W., and Langley, I. I.: Routine use of radio-gold following operation for ovarian cancer. Amer. J. Obstet. Gynec., 98: 624, 1967.

Morris, J. M., and Scully, R. E.: *Endocrine Pathology of the Ovary.* C. V. Mosby Company, St. Louis, 1958.

Munnell, E. W.: The changing prognosis and treatment in cancer of the ovary. Amer. J. Obstet. Gynec., 100: 790, 1968.

Munnell, E. W.: Conservative therapy in stage 1A cancer of the ovary. Amer. J. Obstet. Gynec., 103: 641, 1969.

Neubecker, R. D., and Breen, J. L.: Embryonal carcinoma of the ovary. Cancer, 15: 546, 1962.

Nissen, E. D.: Consideration of the malignant carcinoid syndrome. Obstet. Gynec. Survey, 14: 459, 1959.

Nogales, F. F., Jr., and Oliva, H. A.: Peritoneal gliomatosis produced by ovarian teratomas. Obstet. Gynec., 43: 915, 1974.

Novak, E., Woodruff, J. D., and Novak, E. R.: Probable mesonephric origin of certain female genital tumors. Amer. J. Obstet. Gynec., 68: 1222, 1954.

Novak, E. R., and Woodruff, J. D.: Mesonephroma of the ovary. Amer. J. Obstet. Gynec., 77: 632, 1959.

Ober, W. B., Pollak, A., Gerstman, K. E., and Kupperman, H. S.: Krukenberg tumor with androgenic and progestational activity. Amer. J. Obstet. Gynec., 84: 739, 1962.

Order, S. E., Donahue, V., and Knapp, R.: Immunotherapy of ovarian carcinoma. Cancer, 32: 573, 1973.

Parker, R. T., and Shingleton, W. W.: Chemotherapy in genital cancer: systemic therapy and regional perfusion. Amer. J. Obstet. Gynec., 83: 981, 1962.

Parker, R. T., Parker, C. H., and Wilbanks, G. N.: Cancer of the ovary. Amer. J. Obstet. Gynec., 108: 878, 1970.

Peterson, W. F.: Solid, histologically benign teratomas of ovary; report of four cases and review of literature. Amer. J. Obstet. Gynec., 72: 1094, 1956.

Piven, M. S.: Management of patients with ovarian carcinoma. Obstet. Gynec., 40: 411, 1972.

Plate, W. P.: Clear-cell adenocarcinoma in an endometrioid ovarian cyst. Obstet. Gynec., 27: 428, 1966.

Plotz, E. J., Wiener, M., and Stein, A. A.: Steroid synthesis in cystadenocarcinoma of the ovaries. Amer. J. Obstet. Gynec., 94: 189, 1966.

Plotz, E. J., Weiner, M., and Stein, A. A.: Enzymatic activities related to steriod synthesis in common ovarian cancer. Amer. J. Obstet. Gynec., 97: 1050, 1967.

Pomerance, W., and Moltz, A.: Ten year survival in carcinoma of the ovary. Obstet. Gynec., 37: 560, 1971.

Rogers, L. W., Julian, C. G., and Woodruff, J. D.: Mesonephroid carcinoma of the ovary. A study of 95 cases from the Emil Novak Ovarian Tumor Registry. Gynec. Oncol., *1:* 76, 1972.

Rubin, D. K., and Frost, J. K.: The cytologic detection of ovarian cancer. Acta Cytologica, *7:* 191, 1963.

Rutledge, F.: Chemotherapy of ovarian cancer with melphalan. Clin. Obstet. Gynec., *11:* 354, 1968.

Sampson, J. A.: Carcinoma of tubes and ovaries secondary to carcinoma to body of uterus. Amer. J. Path., *10:* 1, 1934.

Saphir, O., and Lackner, J. E.: Adenocarcinoma with clear cells (hypernephroid) of ovary. Surg. Gynec. Obstet., *79:* 439, 1944.

Schiller, W.: Mesonephroma ovarii. Amer. J. Cancer, *35:* 1, 1939.

Scully, R. E.: Ovarian tumors of germ cell origin. *Progress in Gynecology,* Vol. V. Sturgis and Taymor, eds., Grune & Stratton, New York, 1970.

Scully, R. E., and Barlow, J. F.: "Mesonephroma" of ovary, Cancer, *20:* 1405, 1967.

Silverberg, S. G.: Clear cell carcinoma ovary. Amer. J. Obstet. Gynec., *115:* 394, 1973.

Silverman, B. B., O'Neill, R. T., and Mikuta, J. J.: Multiple malignant tumors with primary carcinoma ovary. Surg. Gynec. Obstet., *134:* 244, 1972.

Smith, J. P., and Rutledge, F.: Chemotherapy in cancer of the ovary. Amer. J. Obstet. Gynec., *107:* 691, 1970.

Smith, J. P., Rutledge, F., and Sutow, W.: Malignant gynecologic tumors in children. Amer. J. Obstet. Gynec., *116:* 261, 1973.

Smith, J. P., Rutledge, F., and Wharton, J. T.: Chemotherapy in cancer of the ovary. Amer. J. Obstet. Gynec., *116:* 261, 1973.

Spadoni, L. R., Lindberg, N. C., Moffet, N. K., and Herrman, W. L.: Virilization coexisting with Krukenberg tumor during pregnancy. Amer. J. Obstet. Gynec., *92:* 981, 1965.

Sternberg, W. H.: Nonfunctioning ovarian neoplasms. In *The Ovary,* International Academy of Pathology Monograph No. 3, edited by H. G. Grady and D. E. Smith, p. 209. The Williams & Wilkins Company, Baltimore, 1963.

Taylor, H. C.: The diagnosis and treatment of ovarian carcinoma. Clin Obstet. Gynec., *1:* 1078, 1958.

Teilum, G.: Endodermal sinus tumors of the ovary and testis. Cancer, *12:* 1092, 1959.

Thompson, J. D.: Primary ovarian adenoacanthoma. Obstet. Gynec., *9:* 403, 1957.

Thurlbeck, W. M., and Scully, R. E.: Solid teratoma of the ovary. Cancer, *13:* 804, 1960.

Toews, H. A., Katayama, P., and Jones, H. W.: Chromosomes of normal and neoplastic ovarian tissue. Obstet. Gynec., *32:* 465, 1968.

Van Orden, D. E., McAllister, W. B., Zenne, S. R. M., and Morris, J. M.: Ovarian carcinoma (the problems of staging and grading). Amer. J. Obstet. Gynec., *94:* 195, 1966.

Weiss, R. R., Richart, R. M., and Okagaki, T.: DNA content of mucinous tumors of the ovary. Amer. J. Obstet. Gynec., *103:* 409, 1969.

Wilkinson, E. J., Friederich, E. G., and Hasty, T. A.: Alpha fetoprotein and endodermal sinus tumor. Amer. J. Obstet. Gynec., *116:* 711, 1973.

Wolfe, S. A.: Metastatic carcinoid tumors of ovary. Amer. J. Obstet. Gynec., *70:* 563, 1955.

Woodruff, J. D., NoliCastillo, R. D., and Novak, E. R.: Lymphoma of the ovary. Amer. J. Obstet. Gynec., *85:* 912, 1963.

Woodruff, J. D., and Novak, E. R.: Papillary serous tumors of the ovary. Amer. J. Obstet. Gynec., *67:* 1112, 1954.

Woodruff, J. D., and Novak, E. R.: Krukenberg tumors of the ovary. Obstet. Gynec., *15:* 351, 1960.

Woodruff, J. D., Protos, P., and Peterson, W. F.: Ovarian teratomas. Amer. J. Obstet. Gynec., *102:* 702, 1968.

Woodruff, J. D., *et al.*: Metastatic ovarian tumors. Amer. J. Obstet. Gynec., *107:* 202. 1970.

Ziegerman, J. H., Imbriglia, J., Makler, P., and Smith, J. J.: Ovarian lymphosarcoma. Amer. J. Obstet. Gynec., *72:* 1357, 1956.

chapter 24

Functioning (Special) Tumors of the Ovary

Certain rare ovarian tumors, all of low grade (25 to 35 per cent) malignancy may conveniently be discussed together because they had been thought to originate from some innate defect in the gonad, possibly during embryonic life, and because they may on occasion show evidence of functional activity. These tumors include (1) the *dysgerminoma,* which is generally hormonally inert, (2) the frequently estrogenic *granulosa-theca cell tumor,* and (3) the often androgenic *arrhenoblastoma.* Less common virilizing tumors are the *hilus cell* and *adrenal* neoplasms. *Struma* ovarii, a simple teratoma with an excess of thyroid tissue leads to production of the thyroid hormone (Chapt. 23).

Ten years ago the problem of these tumors seemed a simple one. Dysgerminomas of neutral germ cell origin were almost always inert, arrhenoblastoma, presumably derived from the primitive sex cords and tubules as a transitory effect even in the female, were considered potentially virilizing, and granulosa-theca tumors, derived from the early mesenchyme, were invariably thought of as feminizing. Today, however, due to the studies of Teilum, MacKinlay, Shippel, Nokes, and many others, the exact behavior of ovarian cells is subject to considerable disagreement, and this will be fully discussed at the end of this chapter. In any case it seems questionable whether the granulosa-theca cell lesions and arrhenoblastomas should necessarily be regarded as *dysontogenetic* since they may evolve from the mature stromal cell.

DYSGERMINOMA

Dysgerminoma is not usually regarded as an active tumor as far as endocrine effect is concerned. Because it is generally discussed with other functioning tumors which had been presumed to originate from some disorder in embryonic life (*dysontogenetic*), it seems logical to include it in this chapter.

Incidence

Morris and Scully note that dysgerminoma comprises 3 to 5 per cent of all malignant ovarian tumors. Less than 1500 cases have been reported, three-fourths of them occurring in the second or third decade of life. There is a not infrequent association with other types of germ cell neoplasm.

Origin

This interesting tumor type is believed to arise from cells which date back to the early undifferentiated phase of gonadal development. In this stage the *germ cells* have not as yet acquired either male or female characteristics, so that, as might be expected, dysgerminoma has no effect on the sex characteristics of the patient. Such an origin, first suggested by Meyer, is given much support by the fact that an identical tumor occurs in the testis, where it is commonly designated as *seminoma.*

The probable correctness of this theory is further indicated by the fact that in a considerable proportion of the reported cases the tumor has occurred in individuals showing some degree of gonadal dysgenesis, varying from minor degrees to actual pseudohermaphroditism. Barr *et al.* stress the frequency with which these germ cell tumors occur in phenotypic females with an XY sex chromosome complement and "streak" gonads, and McDonough *et al.* record 18 cases of gonadoblastoma occurring in the rudimentary "streak" ovary. Taylor *et al.* likewise indicate the importance of karyotype study. There is general agreement that when a dysgerminoma occurs with "streak ovaries," a high incidence of malignancy (15%) is found in the contralateral ovary if a Y chromosome is present. Various mosaic patterns have been recorded.

Heinz has noted that the majority of 10 cases studied showed a negative (male) sex chromatin pattern, although this discrepancy between the sex of the tumor and host was not present in the case of testicular seminoma. Obviously, in such cases the tumor has no causal relation to the sex abnormality, which persists even when the tumor is removed. This is in contrast with certain gonadal stroma tumors which produce direct changes in sex

characters, with return to normal after removal of the tumors.

Because a small proportion of dysgerminomas show various alien elements, there are some who look upon these tumors as of teratomatous origin, but the prevailing concept is that most cases of dysgerminoma originate as described above. However, the presence of teratoid elements impairs the prognosis. An origin from the mature oocyte, as suggested by Hughesdon, seems implausible.

Pathology

Grossly, these tumors are of solid type, although when large, they often show degeneration and cystic cavities (Fig. 24.1). They may be very small, measuring only a few centimeters in diameter, or they may reach such large size as to fill most of the abdominal cavity. They are, when small, surrounded by a rather dense capsule, which, however, is often broken through as the tumor grows, with later infiltration of surrounding organs. The cut surface of the tumor is grayish pink with areas of hemorrhagic degeneration. The consistency is doughy but at times firm and rubbery. The growth is usually unilateral, although bilateral tumors have been noted in a few cases. (Chauser *et al.* and Williamson).

Microscopically, there are few tumors of the ovary which present such a distinctive picture, so that the diagnosis in most cases is easy, once one is familiar

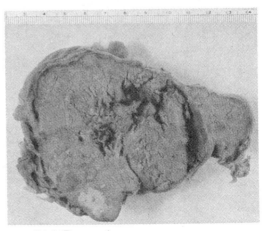

24.1. Dysgerminoma—gross appearance

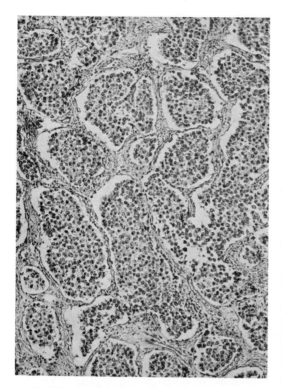

24.2. Dysgerminoma—microscopic appearance

with this picture (Fig. 24.2). The tumor is made up of rather large round or ovoid cells, arranged characteristically in alveoli separated by septa of partially hyalinized connective tissue which shows a characteristic infiltration with lymphocytes (Fig. 24.3). The nuclei of the epithelial cells are large and rather deeply staining, and a varying number of mitoses are to be seen, although usually they are not numerous. Occasionally one finds large symplasmic giant cells, which have at times led to the mistaken diagnosis of associated tuberculosis.

Malignancy

This tumor undoubtedly belongs in the malignant group, but there is much variation in individual cases. Certainly the degree of malignancy is not to be compared to that of the common types of primary ovarian cancer, and cure has in many cases followed simple removal of the adnexa on the involved side. When the tumor is well encapsulated, the prognosis is in general good, but in the infiltrating

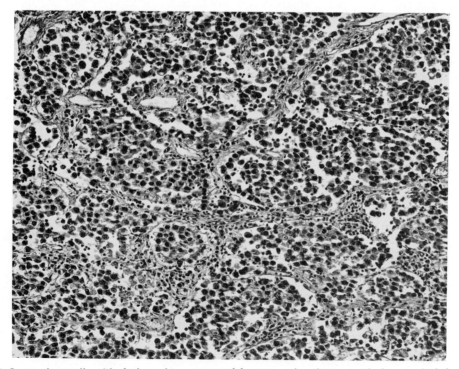

24.3. Large clear cells with dark nucleus separated by connective tissue matrix in a typical dysgerminoma. Characteristic lymphocytic infiltration.

variety, associated as it is with involvement of adjoining viscera and sometimes distant metastases, the outlook is very unfavorable. Estimates as to its degree of malignancy vary widely. At one

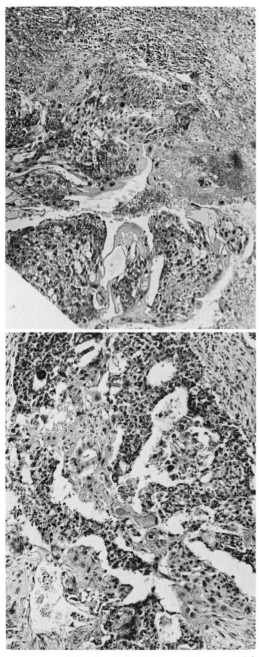

24.4. A, Dysgerminoma in association with typical choriocarcinoma, B. (Courtesy of Dr. L. Stent, Manchester, England.) B, Higher magnification of trophoblast with dysgerminoma.

extreme is the gloomy 27 per cent salvage noted by Pedowitz, but the 68 per cent figure in Ovarian Tumor Registry patients noted by de Lima seems more realistic. The prognosis worsens if (a) there are bilateral tumors, (b) the capsule is not intact, (c) there is spillage at operation, or (d) there are associated teratomatous or trophoblastic elements (Fig. 24.4). Actually where the capsule is intact and the disease is unilateral, de Lima notes an 80 per cent salvage. Malkasian and Symmonds record an 80.9 per cent five-year survival following conservative surgery as compared to 87.5 per cent when treatment was more extensive, and the AFIP figures (Assadourian and Taylor) are even more favorable.

Clinical Characteristics

The incidence of these tumors appears to be about one-third of granulosa cell tumors, which in turn makes up something like 10 per cent of all primary malignant ovarian tumors (Fauvet). Dysgerminoma is characteristically a *tumor of early life* ("carcinoma puellarum"). It occurs not infrequently in very early childhood, and is common in the second and third decades. A certain number of cases have been associated in conjunction with pregnancy, and Smith and Ward report 24 recorded cases. In addition Neigus has commented on a positive A-Z test in the complete, proved absence of pregnancy, and he feels that this type of bioassay represents an ominous prognostic point due to combined trophoblastic elements. With this exception, and the few cases of endocrine activity as noted by Jakobowitz, Scully, and Usizama, dysgerminoma is usually hormonally inert. An exception is the case of precocious puberty with virilism due to a combined germ cell-gonadal stromal tumor which produced both estrogen and androgen (Drobnjak), and Scully has noted certain virilizing trends due to a functioning stroma.

Symptoms

As with so many other types of ovarian tumor, the first evidence of its presence is often the detection of a *mass* in the lower abdomen. There is *no characteristic effect on menstruation,* although it must be remembered that dysgerminoma often occurs in women who have had amenorrhea as a result of gonadal deficiency. Where other marked sex abnormalities such as

Table 24.1

105 Dysgerminomas

Age
  Before age 20, 43.8 per cent
  Before age 30, 86.67 per cent
  Most patients, 15–24 years
  Youngest, 19 months
  Oldest, 67 years
Symptoms
  Nondescript, most
  Menstrual history, normal (90%)
    Amenorrhea (7), metrorrhagia (7)
    One pregnancy test positive
  "Somatic sexual" changes, 15 per cent
  Fertility, normal
Operative Findings
  Ascites, 30.5 per cent
  Bilaterality, 3.8 per cent
  Intact capsule, 90 per cent (12 metastases)
  Rupture capsule, 10 per cent (poor prognosis)
  Tumor free, 60 per cent
  Tumor adherent, 40 per cent
Tumor Spread
  None: limited to one ovary, 78 per cent
  Spread (in order of frequency), 22 per cent
    (1) Peritoneum, adjacent tube, omentum
    (2) Lymph nodes (retroperitoneal), uterus, other ovary (?)
    (3) Bowel, liver, lung, etc.
  Note: tumors <15 cm. localized; >15 cm. extend
Recurrence Most Likely
    (1) Young age group, <20 years
    (2) Spillage or bilateral tumors
    (3) Large tumors, >15 cm.
    (4) Medullary (cellular) or where emboli (L.N. or B.V.)
    (5) Anaplastic or associated with teratoma or chorio
Salvage, 68 per cent
  "Pure," 73 per cent (94 cases)
  Mixed (with teratoma or chorio), 27 per cent (11 cases)
  Unilateral SO recommended (11 pregnant at operation)
  "High incidence, postoperative pregnancy"
  Confirms radio sensitivity.

(Courtesy of F.O.A. de Lima, São Paulo, Brazil, 1966.)

(pseudo-) hermaphroditism are present, the strong possibility of dysgerminoma should be considered when an ovarian tumor is diagnosed. On the other hand, the majority of cases have occurred in ostensibly normal women with often one or more pregnancies before the development of the tumor, and it may concur with pregnancy. *Ascites* has been observed with these tumors, as with other solid ovarian growths. Table 24.1 represents various abstracted statistical data collected from the important contribution of de Lima, which considers 105 authentic, well studied cases from the files of one Ovarian Tumor Registry.

Treatment

Localized Tumors

Although there is no difference of opinion as to the advisability of surgical treatment, there is still some uncertainty as to the extent of the operation in the individual case. Most of these patients are very young, so that there is a natural tendency to avoid radical operations if possible. In the case of young patients with *well encapsulated unilateral tumors,* conservative operation, consisting commonly of unilateral salpingo-oophorectomy, appears fully justified by the good results obtained in many reported cases. Rationalization suggests that if the tumor has exceeded the confines of the ovary, cure is unlikely. If the tumor is confined to the ovary, complete surgery is not necessary, although some 10 per cent of patients will have metastases despite an intact capsule.

There is no question but that hysterectomy and bilateral adnexectomy is the proper procedure where there are no further procreative desires, irrespective of age. Thoeny *et al.* have noted that patients undergoing conservative salpingo-oophorectomy have a higher incidence of recurrence (43 per cent of 14 patients) even with no apparent extension of the disease at the original operation.

The *optimal* treatment seems to be complete operation with additional irradiation if there is any evidence of local or lymphatic extension. *Conservative* surgery, however, should be reserved for the young individual with a slight calculated risk, but we know of many young women treated conservatively who have become pregnant as reported recently by Ayerst and Johnson. It does not seem that women treated conservatively should be subjected to routine radiotherapy (even with the remaining ovary shielded), as suggested by Brody. If this approach seems too conservative it is because of our belief that the tumor is generally of rather low grade malignancy, which frequently involves an extremely youthful patient very anxious for further pregnancy.

The recent study by Asadourian and Taylor indicates an 88.6 per cent 10-year salvage of 71 patients with a unilateral tumor treated only by salpingo-oophorectomy. The authors point out, however, that deaths from other causes than tumor are excluded, and their cases include only "pure" dysgerminomas without teratomatous components. Their figures are comparable to those of de Lima, and Malkasian and Symmonds (as noted previously).

Dysgerminoma may coexist with pregnancy, and indeed germ cell tumors are among the most common neoplasms noted during gestation (see Chapter 22). Prognosis is generally good, although the diagnosis is frequently delayed so that there is time for the lesion to extend. In a recent unpublished review of 100 ovarian tumors with pregnancy (Ovarian Tumor Registry), 19 cases of dysgerminoma were tallied with 18 5-year survivors (3 alive with recurrence) despite frequent conservative surgery.

Infiltrative Tumor

When, on the other hand, the tumor is infiltrative or extensive, complete removal of the pelvic organs is indicated, and this should be followed by various forms of *irradiation therapy*. Today there is general agreement that dysgerminoma is usually quite radiosensitive, and studies by Brody and Thoeny *et al.* seem convincing, but we would not advocate irradiation therapy if only conservative unilateral adnexectomy is done. Not only may it

defeat the purpose of conservatism, but there is a high incidence of mental deficiency if pregnancy should occur.

GONADOBLASTOMA

Morris and Scully originally described the *gonadoblastoma,* a germ cell tumor combined with such mesenchymal elements as granulosa-theca cells, or Leydig cells, along with frequent areas of calcification (Fig. 24.5). This tumor has only recently been accepted as a specific entity. Teter notes various androgenic and estrogenic combinations with these primarily germ cell tumors, but utilizes the term *gonocytoma* and designates several types according to the endocrine effect produced by the elements contained in the cell. As with dysgerminoma, *gonado-*

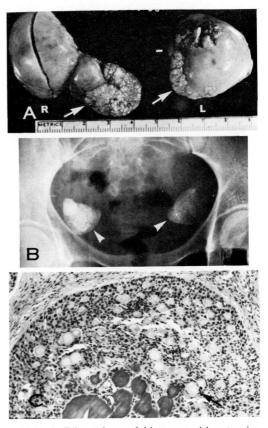

24.5. A. Bilateral gonadoblastoma with extensive calcification. B. Pre-operative flat plate. C. Characteristic microscopic pattern. (Courtesy of Dr. R. S. A. Prentice and *Archives of Pathology.*)

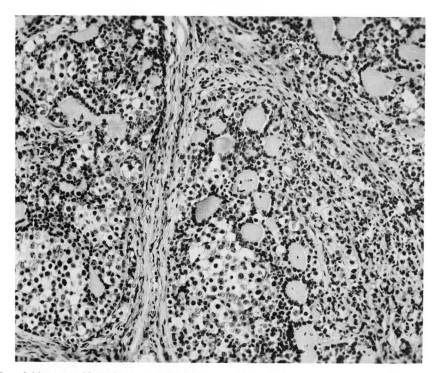

24.6. Gonadoblastoma. Note the germ cells with abundant pale cytoplasm and other cell type often arranged in tubular or rosette-like pattern. None of the frequent areas of calcification visible here. (Courtesy of Dr. John M. Morris, New Haven, Connecticut.)

blastoma often occurs in the dysgenetic gonad or in the hermaphrodite.

The sex chromatin pattern is usually negative, a generally 46-XY with occasional mosaicism, although other patterns may be noted less frequently. As Patel and Prentice indicate it seems there is no one consistent karyotype pattern with these neoplasms. Indeed a calcified ovarian tumor in conjunction with ambiguous sex characteristics might suggest the possibility of gonadoblastoma, irrespective of the karyotype.

Scully has recently reported 74 cases of gonadoblastoma, most of which arose in gonads of "unknown nature." The largest lesion was 8 cm, and the clinical course and histological pattern seemed generally benign (Fig. 24.6), although various other malignant germ cell tumors such as dysgerminoma or teratoma may be superimposed. On occasion all combinations of germ cell and stromal tumors may occur. More recently Talerman has noted combined dysgerminoma and gonadoblastoma in siblings with dysgenetic gonads, and has recorded 2 other similar cases.

GRANULOSA-THECA CELL TUMORS (FEMINIZING GROUP)

These neoplasms are properly discussed together, since it seems probable that they have a common origin and biological effect. They are given their special designations chiefly because of the different morphological patterns which they may assume. Not all authors, however, are convinced of the wisdom of any sharp separation, especially since mixed forms are not infrequent; indeed some admixture is the rule. For convention, however, we shall allude to granulosa and theca cell lesions as if they are discrete tumors. Opinion today is that only the theca cells produce estrogen, and that granulosa cell tumors are feminizing only by virtue of any associated thecal cells.

Histogenesis

The exact histogenesis is far from certain, but the prevailing concept of the origin of granulosa cell tumors has been that they arise from cells of the early ovarian mesenchyme or gonadal stroma. The latter is the mother tissue of both granulosa and theca cells, so that tumors of such mesenchymal origin can assume the morphological characteristics of either granulosa or theca cell with occasional luteinization. In many tumors one finds mixtures of these various elements, and various studies have given substantial support to the concept of their common origin from the mesenchyme. There appears to be no acceptance of the hypothesis of McKay and his co-workers that granulosa cell tumors may have their origin from granulosa cells in atretic follicles and thecomas in cortical stromal hyperplasia. Thompson *et al.* have reported six cases arising in a cystic teratoma; this should not imply that this is the usual method of genesis.

Pathology of Granulosa Cell Tumors

Grossly (Figs. 24.7, 8) these tumors vary in size from only a few millimeters in

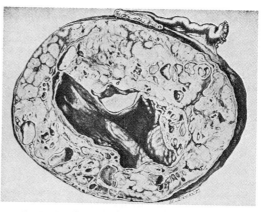

24.8. Another granulosa cell tumor of ovary.

diameter to tumors filling a large part of the abdominal cavity and weighing over 150 pounds (Robertson). The larger tumors often show one or many cystic cavities. The intervening solid tissue is of friable or granular consistency, and of grayish-yellowish hue. In a study of 25 cases, Fathalla finds that many small but functionally active tumors occur in normal-sized ovaries and are often missed. In a recent study of the feminizing tumors in the Ovarian Tumor Registry we have encountered several predominantly cystic papillary lesions (Fig. 24.9).

Microscopically, the diagnosis of granulosa cell tumor is based upon the *granulosal character of the constituent cells* and upon the *growth characteristics* of these cells, which are quite like those of normal granulosa. For example, there is a tendency to the formation of tiny cystic areas of liquefaction, corresponding to the Call-Exner bodies so characteristic of the granulosa which gives rise to the frequent *folliculoid* pattern. The epithelial elements may dominate the picture in *diffuse* varieties of the tumor, with only a small amount of trabeculating connective tissue, often hyalinized. In such cases the epithelial cells have a tendency to arrange themselves in rosette-like or horseshoe-shaped clusters, resembling the primitive follicles. A very common variety is the cylindroid in which the presence of much larger amounts of connective tissue brings about an arrangement of the cells in

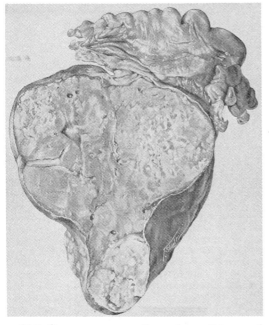

24.7. Gross appearance of granulosa cell tumor of ovary.

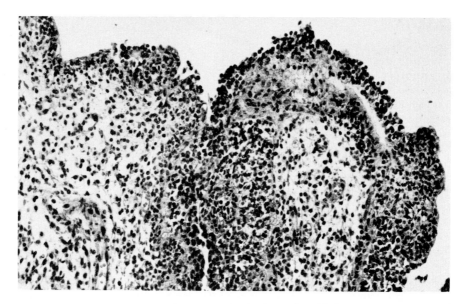

24.9. Papillary and cystic tumor. Outer core of granulosa cells with loose myxomatous matrix.

columns or cylinders (Fig. 24.10) which often anastomose. A relatively uncommon type (Fig. 24.11) is characterized by large round masses of granulosa cells with often central cystic degeneration, simulating very large follicles (formerly called *folliculoma malignum*). If exaggerated, the pattern may be *pseudoadenomatous* (Fig. 24.12), due to cystic liquefaction of the connective tissue. Many different patterns may be found in a single tumor.

Pathology of Thecoma

Gross. In a certain proportion of cases, a fibroma-like character may be given to the histological picture by the presence of

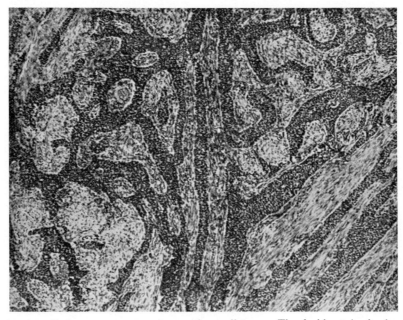

24.10. Strikingly cylindromatous pattern in granulosa cell tumor. The darkly stained columns are made up of granulosa cells.

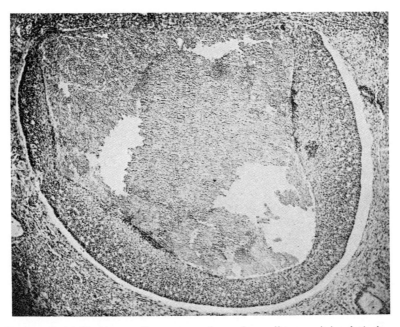

24.11. The so-called folliculoma malignum type of granulosa cell tumor; it is relatively uncommon.

large numbers of connective tissue elements. The term of fibrothecoma seems appropriate, although the general term, thecoma, is most commonly employed. Such tumors are commonly firm and fibrous (Fig. 24.13) in appearance and consistency and are less likely to show a tendency to cystic degeneration. The contralateral ovary may show evidence of profound overgrowth of stromal cells, the so-called *"diffuse thecomatosis,"* and this is a frequent finding with many ovarian

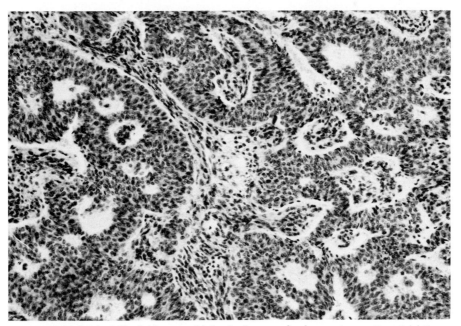

24.12. Multiple *folliculoid* areas with beginning *pseudoadenomatous* pattern (*right*).

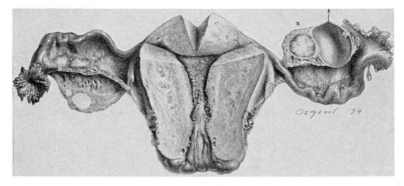

24.13. Small thecoma of ovary (x) in a woman 57 years of age. Regular menstrual bleeding recurred 10 years after the menopause. In the other ovary are two small fibromas.

tumors, especially where there is apparent endocrine activity (Fig. 24.14).

Microscopically they are distinguished especially by the presence of bundles of broad spindle cells distributed in an irregular interlacing manner throughout the tumor (Fig. 24.15), separated by varying sized bands of connective tissue and often hyaline plaques. Stress is laid also upon the presence of doubly refractile fat in large amounts within the cells and to a lesser extent in the surrounding connective tissue. Lipoid staining (Fig. 24.16) shows the presence of fat, practically always intracellular, suggestive but not pathognomonic of steroid activity. In these thecal tumors, however, one often finds areas of what are apparently definite granulosa cells, so that one must question the advisability of too sharp a division

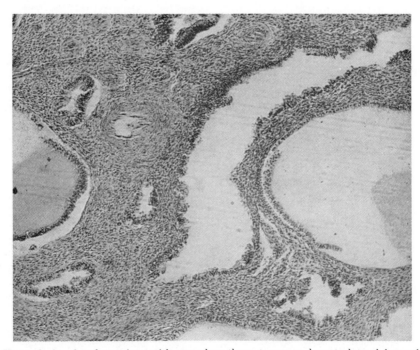

24.14. Hyperplasia of endometrium with granulosa-theca tumor and contralateral hyperthecosis in a woman 62 years of age.

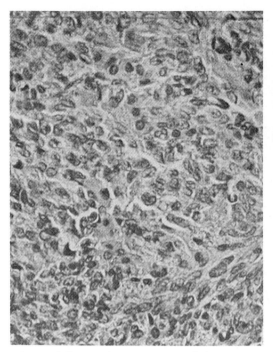

24.15. Microscopic appearance of thecomatous type of tumor shown in Figure 24.13.

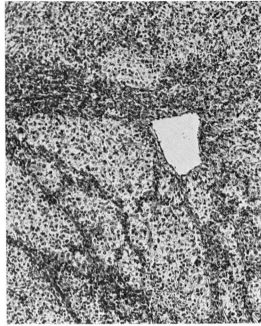

24.17. Granulosa cell tumor type with partial luteinization of the tumor.

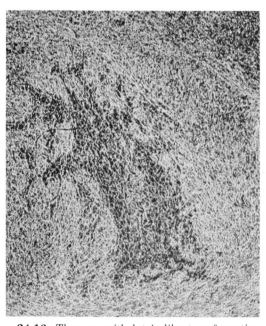

24.16. Thecoma with lutein-like transformation in certain areas.

between the granulosal and thecal tumors, especially in view of their identical endocrine effects.

Luteinization of Granulosa-Theca Cell Tumors (Figs. 24.17, 18)

An interesting histological characteristic of this tumor type is that the constituent granulosa or theca cells may at times undergo transformation into what are typical lutein cells. We have seen a considerable group in which such a transition is in progress, so that parts of the tumor have a lutein appearance, whereas others are still typically granulosal in character. It seems desirable to call these simply *"luteinized granulosa-theca tumors."* Although the term "luteoma" was formerly utilized, we feel it is misleading and reserve it exclusively for the *luteoma of pregnancy.* The term *"folliculoma lipidique"* is often applied to markedly luteinized granulosa cell tumors, often tubular, although Teilum has indicated that the origin is the Sertoli cell (see Fig. 24.19).

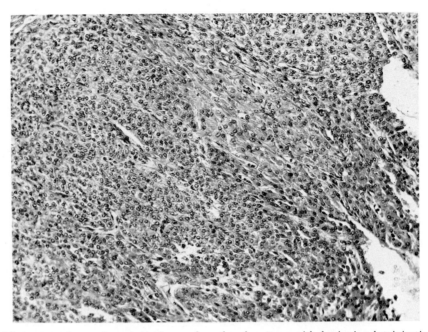

24.18. Most areas show only a typical granulosa-thecal pattern with beginning luteinization in *right central area.*

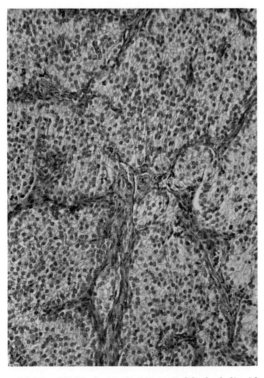

24.19. "Folliculoma lipidique." Marked lipoid changes in a granulosa (or Sertoli) cell tumor.

In at least a small group of reported tumors associated with luteinization, progesterone effects upon the endometrium have been noted in such transformed tumors, differing from the purely estrogenic effects which characterize granulosa cell tumors in general. Occasionally an exaggerated progesterone effect with a frank decidual response may be noted (Fig. 24.20). In other luteinized tumors, it would seem that the cells may be morphologically but not functionally like lutein cells, and they are perhaps better spoken of as pseudolutein rather than lutein cells. In any case a feminizing effect is produced, rather than virilism which is so characteristic of the almost identical tumors of hilus cell origin. However, association of cell type and endocrine effect is inconstant.

Peutz-Jeghers Syndrome

Scully has described certain lipid sex-cord tumors with associated *intestinal polyps* and *melanin spots* on the aural mucosa and skin; the so-called *Peutz-Jeghers syndrome.* Actually this synd-

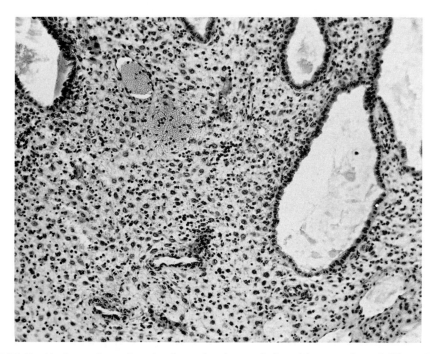

24.20. Decidual transformation of endometrium in association with tumor shown in Figure 24.18.

rome may occur with many varieties of ovarian tumors. However, in discussing the granulosa cell combination of tumor with the syndrome, Christian has suggested that granulosa cells may evolve from certain endodermal sources; in any case it is an extremely rare entity.

Pregnancy Luteoma

Sternberg describes a "pregnancy luteoma" as an ovarian enlargement (up to 12 cm.), which is generally solid, composed of eosinophilic, polyhedral cells, which are not a part of the corpus luteum of pregnancy, and may on occasion be bilateral. It was not certain whether this is a true neoplasm or merely a physiological response to pregnancy, similar to the theca lutein cysts so frequently seen in trophoblastic disease, and occasionally with normal pregnancy. Greene indicates that this particular picture should be regarded as a preexisting thecoma, which merely portrays the hormonal influences of pregnancy. In reporting 15 cases, Norris and Taylor strongly imply that this ovarian pattern is simply a physiological hyperplasia of stromal theca lutein cells,

perhaps due to an abnormal stimulus or an unusual response to FSH.

Recent study by Rice *et al.* would suggest that androgen production (Δ^4-androstene-3,17-dione) is quite characteristic of luteoma irrespective of whether there is clinical virilization, a not uncommon sequel. This virilization is frequently passed on to any female infant.

Most of these cases of ovarian enlargement regress spontaneously despite no other treatment than biopsy, which would further indicate a physiological rather than a neoplastic origin. However, Barclay reports a case where lutein enlargement persisted and necessitated surgery (Fig. 24.21). Whether a true neoplasm followed this physiological advent must be left open for speculation. Focal stromal luteinization is common in the ovary removed during pregnancy, and this would seem a logical beginning to the luteoma of pregnancy (Fig. 24.22).

Although we have seen a limited number of such ovarian enlargements, our own impression would be that it represents merely a profound *exaggerated physiological response* of the ovary to the

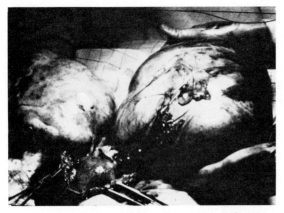

24.21. Massive luteomas of pregnancy. (Courtesy of Dr. D. L. Barclay, New Orleans, La.)

increased endocrine stimulus of gestation. In the cases personally observed, it would be extremely difficult to exclude a hilus cell tumor on a purely morphological basis, although the concomitant pregnancy and absence of Reinke crystalloids is helpful.

Clinical Characteristics of Granulosa-theca Tumors

The granulosa cell neoplasms of the ovary may be considered a fairly common tumor, comprising probably nearly 10 per cent of all solid malignant ovarian neoplasms. The thecoma is much less frequent, although admixture is common. These tumors may occur at any age—before puberty, during the reproductive epoch, or after the menopause. Although the larger tumors, like other ovarian neoplasms, may cause such symptoms as pain or discomfort, the more distinctive symptomatology is dependent upon the capability of the tumor cells to produce the estrogenic hormone. However; perforation of the tumor with intraperitoneal hemorrhage may lead to acute symptoms simulating those associated with a ruptured ectopic pregnancy (French, and Gondos and Monroe). Bilaterality is rare (approximately 5 per cent).

When the tumor occurs *during reproductive life,* as it does in a large proportion of cases, the clinical syndrome is not so striking as when it occurs against the background of the prepubertal or postmenopausal phase, during which there is normally little or no estrogenic hormone in the circulation. The age distribution of over 200 patients with granulosa-theca tumors is noted in Table 24.2. It is apparent that there is *not* the predeliction for the young woman as occurs with dysgerminoma and arrhenoblastoma.

During the reproductive years, on the other hand, the tumor merely adds quantitatively to the cyclical hormonal content of the blood. No change would be expected in the secondary sex characters, for example, because these have long since been developed, whereas the effect upon menstruation would be merely a quantitative one, not unlike that which characterizes the relative hyperestrogenism which is associated with most cases of functional bleeding. Hyperestrogenism may be associated with normal menstruation, with hypermenorrhea, or with long

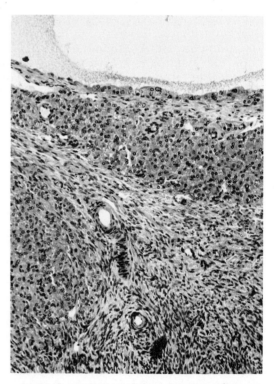

24.22. Luteinization of theca interna and stroma in ovary removed during pregnancy. If exaggerated, it might progress to a full-fledged luteoma.

Table 24.2

Distribution of Tumor by Age Group

Age by Decade	Granulosa	Granulosa-theca	Thecoma	Luteinized	Total in Round Numbers	
					No.	(%)
0–9	1	3		3	7	2
10–19	3	8	4	6	21	7
20–29	9	17	14	10	50	16
30–39	13	21	13	2	49	16
40–49	18	20	14	5	57	19
50–59	8	22	19	5	54	17
60–69	12	14	18	2	46	15
70–79	5	9	5	2	21	7
80–89	2				2	1
Total	71	114	87	35	307	

periods of amenorrhea, as noted in Table 24.3, and these varying effects upon menstruation are noted with granulosa cell carcinoma.

Nevertheless, pregnancy may concur with granulosa-theca cell tumors, and Diddle and O'Connor have noted this association in 37 of nearly 1200 reported cases of this type of lesion. In a recent review of *virilizing* ovarian tumors occurring during pregnancy Verhoeven records 9 arrhenoblastomas as well as many other varieties of ovarian tumors, not microscopically classically virilizing. Indeed their material includes 5 presumably estrogenic granulosa-theca cell tumors. The authors conclude that since an excess of androgen production usually inhibits ovulation the marked androgenic features occurred after the onset of pregnancy. In a number of the female infants in his series there was profound transitory virilization.

When, on the other hand, such tumors occur *in young children,* long before the inauguration of the normal estrogenic function of the ovary, the clinical manifestations of precocious puberty are evoked, *viz.,* precocious menstruation and the premature appearance of secondary sex characters, such as hypertrophy of the

Table 24.3

Predominant Symptoms and Signs (307 Patients)

Symptom or sign	Predominantly granulosa	Granulosa-theca	Predominantly theca	Luteinized	Total
Precocious puberty		5		1	6
Mass		Frequent with all tumor types			
Normal menses	16	6	13	5	40
Oligomenorrhea	10	12	11	5	38
Menometrorrhagia	19	21	11	6	50
Virilism	2	2	1	1	6
PMB	13	21	19	8	61
Prior hysterectomy	5	5	2	0	12
Pregnant	1	3	3	6	13
Ascites	14	19	11	0	44
Incidental finding	6	13	14	2	33

Some patients had various predominant findings.

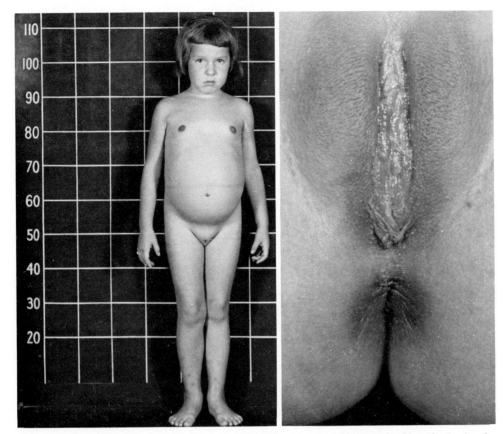

24.23. (*left*) Five-year-old girl with large granulosa-theca tumor (luteinized). Note beginning breast development, prominent labia, and abdominal distention. (*right*) Adult labia in same child.

breasts, the appearance of axillary and pubic hair, pubertal development of the external genitalia (Figs. 24.23, 24), and also hypertrophy of the uterus. With the removal of the tumor, these manifestations promptly regress, constituting a crucial biological demonstration of the direct causal role of the tumor in the production of the symptoms.

Instances are recounted in which, after the removal of a unilateral tumor and disappearance of the abnormal symptoms, a recurrent tumor has developed in the remaining ovary, with again the production of precocious pubertal symptoms followed by disappearance after the removal of the second tumor. It is of interest to note that the precocious menstruation of this syndrome is of the anovulatory type, in which respect it differs from certain other types of precocious puberty and menstruation in which both ovulation and

menstruation occur. In the latter group, insemination may incur pregnancy at abnormally early ages.

In the *postmenopausal* group of cases occurring at a life phase at which little or no estrogenic hormone is found in the blood, the tumors may produce a re-establishment of periodic menstruation-like bleeding, an estrogenic type of cytological specimen, and hypertrophy of the uterus, with cases noted up to 84 years of age. No effect is seen upon secondary sex characters, presumably because of the higher threshold or unreceptivity of these at this phase of life. With the removal of tumors at this age, the abnormal menstruation of course ceases and, interestingly enough, the patient may experience a second menopause from the standpoint of the characteristic vasomotor phenomena.

It is generally accepted that estrogen is

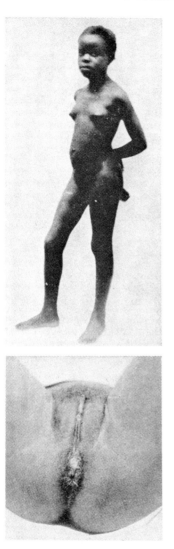

24.24. Precocious puberty due to granulosa cell tumor in 7-year-old child showing pubertal type of external genitalia.

produced by associated theca cells. Our ideas in the past have always been that both granulosa and theca cells are capable of estrogenic production. More recently, however, Falck, utilizing intraocular transplants for study of various cell systems of granulosa and theca cells, has indicated that it is the *theca* interna cells that are actually responsible for the secretion of *estrogen,* but only where there is continuity with granulosa cells.

This impression is based on granulosa and theca cells found in the normal follicle where the granulosa cells seem primarily concerned with progesterone excretion. However, in the follicle the granulosa cell layer is devoid of a blood supply for most of the month. In a hyperemic ovarian tumor endocrine function could be be somewhat different.

Malignancy

In an earlier study Busby and Anderson found a 22% index of malignancy among the granulosa cell tumors encountered in the first 500 cases in the Ovarian Tumor Registry (OTR). More recently we have reviewed this entire group of tumors, including the earlier cases reported by the above authors for a total of 414 such cases among approximately 2300 tumors in the Registry (Table 24.4). Of these it was possible to obtain an adequate follow up in 280 cases with a 5 year salvage of 78%, yet one should recall that there may be occasional late recurrences, after more than 20 years, as has been noted by Simmonds and Sciarra, and Sommers, Gates, and Goodof. Like Flick and Banfield we found that thecoma is considerably less malignant than the predominantly granulosa cell tumors as noted in Table 24.5. Since, however, there is a frequent admixture of epithelioid and connective tissue-like

Table 24.4

Five-Year Followup

Followup	Current Series	Busby and Anderson	Composite Series
	184/307	96/107	280/414
Living and well	136	74	210
Living, recurrence	8	2	10
Living No.	144	76	220
(%)	78.2	79.2	78.5
Died No.	40	20	60
(%)	21.9	20.8	21.5
Total	184	96	280

Table 24.5

Five-Year Followup and Survival of 184 Patients

Followup and Survival	Granulosa		Granulosa-theca		Thecoma		Luteinized	
	No.	(%)	No.	(%)	No.	(%)	No.	(%)
Living and well 5 years or more	27	55	46	67	45	92	18	100
Living with recurrence 5 years or more	3	6	4	6	1	2	—	
Death (tumor)	16	33	15	22	2	5	—	
Death (other)	3	6	3	5	1	3	—	
Total	49		68		49		18	9.8

components, it is difficult to be precise. Norris and Taylor propose a salvage of over 90% in these feminizing tumors due to careful follow up with exclusion of patients known to have died of other causes.

Goldston *et al.* feel that it is possible to separate the granulosa cell tumor from the thecoma, and they too have found that the granulosa cell tumor is considerably more malignant than the thecoma. They likewise note several cases of late recurrences.

Association of Endometrial Carcinoma with Feminizing Tumors

Various investigators have found that from 15 to 25 per cent of postmenopausal women with feminizing tumors of the ovary develop endometrial carcinoma. In our recent review of OTR material, adenocarcinoma was encountered in 23% and hyperplasia in an additional 68% (Fig. 24.25). This association emphasizes the probable predisposing role of postmenopausal stimulation of the endometrium by estrogen in the development of cancer. The study by J. W. Greene, reviews all the previous studies.

A frequent observation is that a predominant thecoma apparently exerts a much stronger carcinogenic effect on the endometrium than where there is a preponderance of granulosa cells. This would seem to support the view that theca rather than granulosa cells are the source of estrogen, as previously noted. In making the diagnosis of endometrial carcinoma with feminizing ovarian tumors, one should bear in mind that benign hyperplasia may appear in a highly proliferative and atypical form which may simulate adenocarcinoma.

Treatment

Little need be said on the subject of treatment, which is, of course, surgical. When the tumors are small and unilateral, as they have been in practically all the prepuberal cases, unilateral salpingo-oophorectomy has frequently resulted in permanent cure. Preferable to random *frozen section* is removal of the total tumor so that the pathologist can select the most suspicious areas for microscopic evaluation; on the basis of this the clinician is in a better position to make a decision as to the extent of the operation, although the degree of differentiation and mitotic activity of these "special" tumors does not always parallel their malignant potential.

In any case, one must realize that conservative operation is attended by some slight risk and periodic postoperative examinations are of obvious importance. In most of the cases occurring in adult women, complete operation would seem wise if the nature of the tumor is recognized at operation. Unfortunately this is usually not the case; therefore the problem not infrequently arises as to whether a unilateral operation should be followed by subsequent complete removal

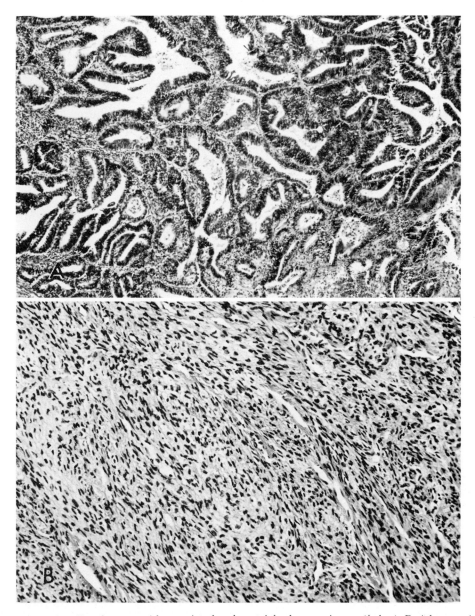

24.25. A. Benign fibrothecoma with associated endometrial adenocarcinoma (*below*). B. Adenocarcinoma of endometrium.

of the pelvic organs. In our experience with *recurrences* following conservative operation for granulosa-theca cell tumors, the retained adnexa has not been involved by recurrent tumor, which is generally of diffuse intra-abdominal nature. Considerable individualization should be practiced, according to age, parity, extent of the tumor, whether encapsulated, etc.

MASCULINIZING OVARIAN TUMORS

In contrast with the feminizing group, the masculinizing tumors are much less common, and we would estimate that they are perhaps one-tenth as frequent, according to the statistics of the Ovarian Tumor Registry. Estimates seem proper because of the extreme difficulty in making a diagnosis in many of these histologically complex tumors. The term "arrhenoblastoma" was originally applied by Meyer to a group of ovarian tumors whose common characteristic seemed an origin from the male gonadogenic structures at one phase or another of development, with differing histological pictures corresponding to the varied degrees of differentiation. Pcdowitz's study (1960) records only 240 such tumors although they represent by far the most common type of virilizing gonadal neoplasm.

ARRHENOBLASTOMA

Histogenesis

As described previously, the early development of the ovary is identical with that of the testis, and, in the later stages of female differentiation, certain elements of male differentiating potency may be left in the medullary portion of the ovary. From these, tumors were thought to develop in later life with the capacity of producing the male hormone, with striking effects upon the sex characters of the woman. This, at any rate, was the view championed by Meyer and was accepted by most investigators, although today there is speculation that the adult stromal cell (of mesenchymal origin) may be converted into an estrogen- or androgen-secreting cell. Scully among others prefers to consider arrhenoblastoma as a Sertoli-Leydig cell tumor; *i.e.,* tumors of male cell type although possibly possessing bisexual endocrine influence, for the Sertoli cells of the testis are capable of estrogen secretion.

Our preference is to avoid such terminology as Sertoli cell for ovarian tumors, for this involves an element foreign to the female gonad. It would appear that the ultimate cell that evolves into most mature structures of functioning tumors in the ovary is the *mesenchyme* or the *gonadal stromal cell.* Although the belief

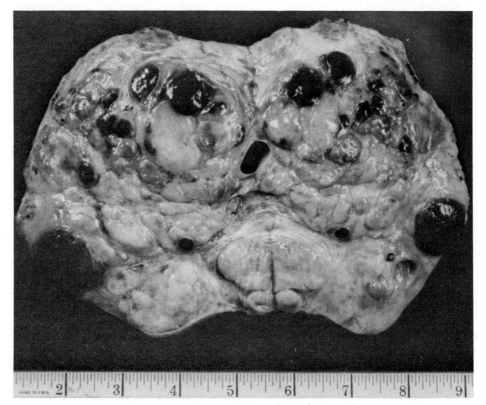

24.26. Frequent areas of cystic and hemorrhagic degeneration are present

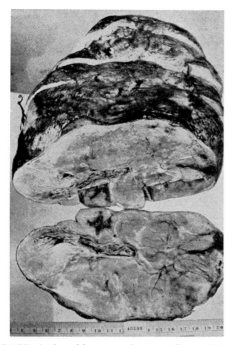

24.27. Arrhenoblastoma of ovary. (Case of Dr. R. K. Hancock).

that persistent cell rests (Cohnheim) may give rise to certain neoplasms is passe, current ideas that various reserve or mature cells may undergo metaplastic changes is still a very real one.

Pathology

Gross. These tumors, as encountered at operation, are usually of moderate size, and may be very small, although in a number of reported instances they have reached large proportions, up to 26 pounds in our recent study. Pedowitz notes a number of tumors greater than 25 cm. in diameter and indicates that they are 96 per cent unilateral. Characteristically, especially when small, they are solid tumors, although they not infrequently exhibit cystic areas, and in the larger tumors the cysts may be of considerable size. The color and consistency are variable, depending upon their widely differing histological structure. They may be grayish, frequently with areas of definitely yellowish hue (Plate 24.1), but in some the cut surface is bluish or reddish blue. The consistency may be quite firm in some cases, but degenerative changes with hemorrhage are common (Figs. 24.26, 27).

Microscopic. A description of the microscopic characteristics of arrhenoblastoma is not easy, because of the extreme variations which may be encountered in certain cases, and in different parts of the same tumor. At one extreme is the highly *differentiated* variety corresponding to the *testicular adenoma* described by Pick in 1905, and characterized by a very definite tubular structure, reproducing more or less perfectly the structure of normal testicular tubules. At the other extreme is the very *undifferentiated* variety which, at first sight, may be considered a typical sarcoma, and in which only very careful study of many blocks may reveal the presence of structures like sex cords (Fig. 24.28), imperfect tubules (Fig. 24.29), or lipoid-containing cells corresponding to *interstitial cells* identical to those of the testis and the presumed source of the androgenic stimulation. Finally, in the group designated by Meyer as the *intermediate,* one usually finds a varying number and distribution of definite tubular structures, interstitial cells, and of cell columns ar-

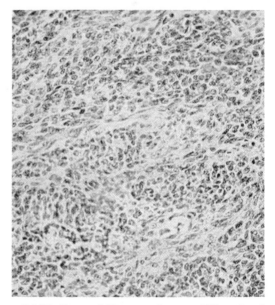

24.28. Sex-cord like areas in an undifferentiated type of arrhenoblastoma.

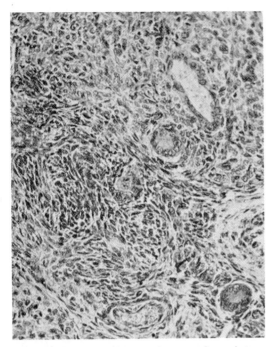

24.29. Microscopic appearance of an intermediate variety of arrhenoblastoma showing imperfect efforts at testicular tubule formation.

ranged in rather zig-zag fashion, quite like the sex cords seen in the early development of the gonads.

It is clear, therefore, that the microscopic recognition of these tumors presupposes some familiarity with the various phases of development of the seminiferous apparatus. It is likely that the impetus to virilism is the *interstitial* or *Leydig cells* (Fig. 24.30), and it is interesting that these are uncommon in the highly differentiated "Pick's adenoma" which is rarely associated with an androgenic trend. Berendsen *et al.* have recently recorded the electron microscopic features of the Leydig cell. The Sertoli cells found in the testis are thought to be potential producers of estrogen although histochemical studies in our laboratory suggest that they are relatively inert insofar as steroid excretion is concerned.

Malignancy

Although arrhenoblastoma is properly classified as a malignant tumor, there is no doubt that its degree of malignancy,

like that of granulosa cell carcinoma, is much less than that of ovarian cancer in general. On the other hand, it must be remembered that many of the reports of this interesting tumor type have been made very soon after treatment so that one cannot always be certain whether or not later recurrence had occurred. Even so, there are already available sufficient reports to indicate that in at least some cases the tumor may exhibit highly malignant characteristics. A recent review of the Ovarian Tumor Registry cases by Novak and Long would suggest a 33 per cent recurrence rate.

Clinical Features

Arrhenoblastoma of the ovary occurs most frequently in relatively young patients, the decade between 20 and 30 showing the largest incidence; we have recently encountered a 30-month-old girl with this type of lesion. In our recent study, 75 per cent of the patients were less than 40 and 66 per cent less than 30, al-

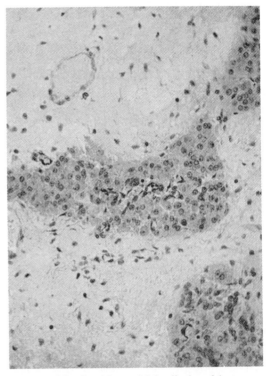

24.30. Islands of interstitial cells found in tumor pictured in Figure 24.29.

though women of 70, 67, and 64 were found to have an arrhenoblastoma (Table 24.6).

The clinical course of these patients is characteristically divisible into two phases. There is first a stage of *defeminization* in which certain typical feminine characteristics are subtracted from the patient, and this is followed, with possible overlapping, by a stage of *masculinization,* in which certain positive masculine stigmata are added. Chief among the defeminization symptoms are amenorrhea, atrophy of the breasts, and loss of the subcutaneous fatty deposits which are responsible for the rounding of the feminine figure. The masculinization signs include hypertrophy of the clitoris, hirsutism, and deepening of the voice.

The first symptom noted by most patients is *amenorrhea,* which may come on abruptly. *Regression of the mammary glands* (Fig. 24.31) soon occurs. *Changes in body contour* may not be conspicuous and are often not noticed by the patient herself, or not at least until *hirsutism* has developed.

A *change in the patient's voice* is often very noticeable, she herself often attributing this to a persistent "cold" or laryngitis. A normally soft, high-pitched feminine voice may be changed to a baritone or even to a basso, with often hoarseness or roughening of the voice. These vocal changes are due to lengthening of the vocal cords, while in marked cases there is overgrowth of the laryngeal cartilages with the development of a prominent "Adam's apple."

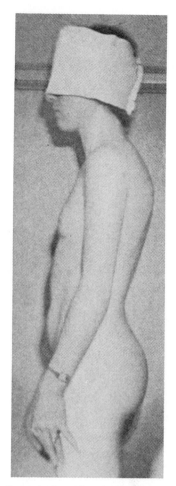

24.31. Lateral view of patient with arrhenoblastoma to show flattening of breasts.

With reference to the *hypertrophy of the clitoris*, here again there are marked individual variations. In some cases it is only slight; in others the clitoris may assume the proportions of a miniature penis. As noted earlier eight cases of concomitant pregnancy with arrhenoblastoma have been recorded. Transient virilism of a female child was noted occasionally.

Hormone Studies. In these days of blood and urine hormone studies, the question arises as to the possible value of such investigations in the diagnosis of such tumors. In the present state of our knowledge it appears that by no means all cases have a definitely elevated level of 17-ketosteroids to the degree found in

Table 24.6

Age Groups of Patients

Ages	Number of patients
Under 20	27
20 to 30	40
30 to 40	18
40 to 50	11
50 to 60	8
60 to 70	7
Total	111

adrenal tumors, although Mahesh has reported such a case. Scully points out that very small amounts of testosterone may be potently virilizing, although incapable of elevating the 17-ketosteroids. Other steroids, not nearly as androgenic, may feature an increased assay with no clinical evidence of masculinization. Nor does adrenocorticotrophic hormone (ACTH) or cortisone cause any appreciable change in the level of the 17-ketosteroids.

Various hormonal assays which have been carried out by Younglai *et al.* on a recent case of arrhenoblastoma seem to prove various points such as (1) certain androgens produced by the arrhenoblastoma lead to virilization, and at the same time suppress normal ovarian function; and (2) both Δ^5 and Δ^4 pathways are responsible for the biosynthesis.

Effects of Tumor Removal on Symptoms. The ultimate clinical test in the substantiation of a diagnosis of arrhenoblastoma is the regression of the abnormal masculinization symptoms after the removal of the tumor. Although this regression may not be complete in every

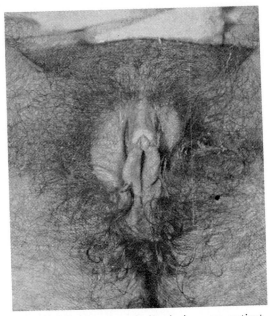

24.33. Hypertrophy of clitoris in same patient (Fig. 24.31).

case, it is usually striking in most cases of arrhenoblastoma. The return of menstruation is the first manifestation of returning femininity, and in general the symptoms disappear in the order of their appearance. The positive manifestations of masculinization, however, disappear much more slowly than those of defeminization, and often incompletely. Some degree of hirsutism and enlarged clitoris has persisted for over 20 years in the patient shown in Figures 24.32–34.

Treatment

The treatment of arrhenoblastoma is surgical, and conservatism appears to be fully justified in the case of young women in whom future pregnancies are important. Our review of the Ovarian Tumor Registry material suggests that the 5-year salvage is in the nature of 65 per cent despite frequent conservative surgery. Where the true nature of these tumors is not recognized until after histological examination, an expectant plan of treatment is advisable, with periodic examination. In the older woman complete operation is preferable; should there be extension, irradiation may be

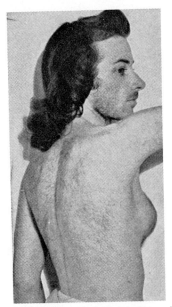

24.32. Appearance of patient with arrhenoblastoma showing extensive hirsutism with moderate flattening of breasts; she had not menstruated for 3 years.

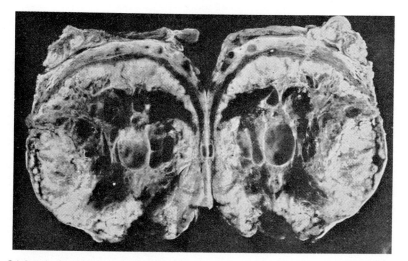

24.34. Arrhenoblastoma of ovary found in patient shown in two preceding figures

considered although the efficacy of radio-therapy and chemotherapy is uncertain in this rare group of tumors.

GYNANDROBLASTOMA

The name gynandroblastoma was applied by Meyer (1930) to a rare type of ovarian tumor which histologically shows components of both granulosa cell carcinoma and arrhenoblastoma. Only a small group of such cases has been described, and the dominant biological effect in most of these has been a masculinizing one, although at times such estrogen effects as endometrial hyperplasia with excessive bleeding have been noted. Although gynandroblastoma is excessively rare, and some cases are to be considered as a misinterpretation of the microscopic appearance, it is difficult to deny such a case as illustrated by Figure 24.35.

We suspect that increasing awareness of the bisexual potential of normal and neoplastic cells, confirmed by histochemical techniques, may reveal that many tumors secrete both androgenic and estrogenic substances. If these be considered gynandroblastomas, the number will certainly increase.

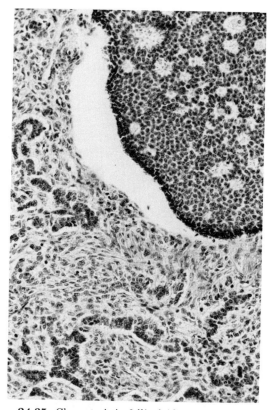

24.35. Characteristic folliculoid pattern of granulosa cells, *upper right;* tubular arrangement with interstitial cells elsewhere. Case showed slight virilization.

ADRENAL TUMORS OF THE OVARY

The chief interest of this group lies in the fact that it gives rise to a clinical syndrome almost identical with that described above for arrhenoblastoma (Fig. 24.36). Only a very small group of cases has been reported, most recently by Sobrinho and Kase. The tumors are small usually, and are made up of tissue similar to that of the adrenal cortex. They are almost uniformly benign.

There has been much confusion in the literature with regard to the differentiation of these "lipoid-cell tumors." Our own preference is to avoid such terms as ovarian hypernephroma, luteoma, and masculinovoblastoma and simply to use the term "adrenal cell tumor." For a further discussion of this subject the reader may be referred to the recent review by Scully.

VIRILIZING HILUS CELL TUMORS

A very scant group of cases, estimated at 50 by Dunniho *et al.*, has been regarded as true hilus cell tumors. Be-

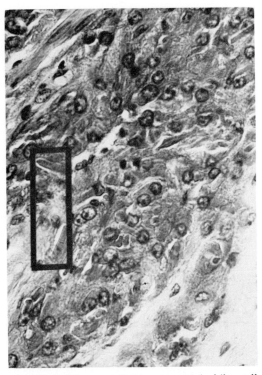

24.37. Reinke crystalloids apparent in hilus cell tumor. Though pathognomonic, they are not mandatory for diagnosis. (Courtesy of W. Peterson, Washington, D.C.)

cause all these tumors have shown masculinization effects, support is given to the prevailing view that the hilus cells are the homologues of the interstitial or Leydig cells of the testis, especially as the tumor cells have been found to show the Reinke albuminoid crystals (Fig. 24.37) so characteristic of the Leydig cells in some but by no means all cases. Dunniho feels that demonstration of these crystaloids should be mandatory, but this view is not uniformly held. The precise nature of these crystalloids is very uncertain, as noted by Janko and Sandberg. An earlier review of 18 cases by Novak and Mattingly has indicated that these tumors were always small (less than 5 cm.), unilateral, benign, and uniformly virilizing (Fig. 24.38). An interesting if inexplicable association has been the presence of endometrial hyperplasia where uterine tissue was obtained; Jeffcoate and Prunty find that both estrogens and androgens were

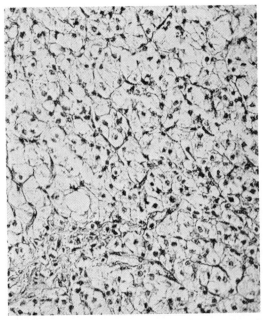

24.36. Microscopic appearance of rare adrenal tumor of ovary characterized by a syndrome identical with that of arrhenoblastoma.

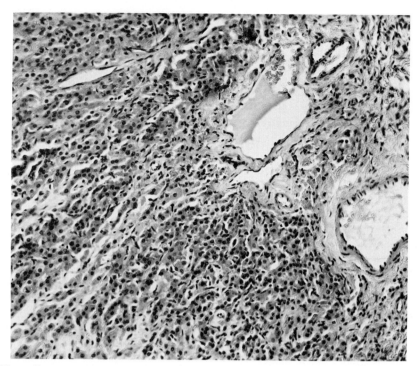

24.38. Hilus cell tumor of ovary producing masculinization symptoms which regressed after removal of tumor.

synthesized by a hilus cell tumor studied biochemically.

Sternberg and Roth have recently reported the occurrence of a virilizing presumed hilus cell tumor (with Reinke crystalloids) well removed from the hilar area. While it might be difficult to distinguish these from certain arrhenoblastomas with interstitial cells, this should not detract from the fact that hilus cells may evolve from the ovarian stromal cell.

Stewart and Woodard have recorded the first malignant hilus cell tumor. Since the authors were kind enough to permit us to study their material, we can unanimously agree with their impressions of this clinically and histologically lethal tumor despite certain disagreement as noted in an addendum to the article by Boivin and Richart. In the material reviewed by us, Reinke crystalloids were plentiful. A second metastatic hilus cell tumor has recently been reported by Echt and Hadd, and massive testosterone excretion (10,000 times normal) was found in this clinically virilized patient. The concurrence of hilus cell hyperplasia and tumors with gonadal dysgenesis and the "streak ovary" has been summarized by Warren, Erkman, and Cheatum.

An addition to the Ovarian Tumor Registry has been a hilus cell tumor (with obvious Reinke crystalloids and a 17 K.S. of 300 mg) associated with pregnancy. The patient was virilized as was the female infant, but clinical information is somewhat sketchy.

Tumors with Functioning Matrix (See also Chapter 23)

It is becoming increasingly apparent to all pathologists that a certain number of ovarian tumors, not morphologically of the endocrinologically productive variety, possess hormonal activity. Indeed, these tumors may be of many types, both benign or malignant, and may produce either estrogenic or androgenic features.

It would appear that the *ovarian stroma* is capable of conversion into a steroid secreting cell similar to a theca (lutein) or Leydig cell, apparently as a result of stimulation or irritation by adjacent tumor. Consequently, a great many supposedly inert tumors such as Brenner, Krukenberg, and various carcinomas have seemed to exert a *feminizing* influence. Fewer androgenic tumors have been reported, but a recent review by Scully notes 11 diverse tumors with virilizing tendencies. In the next chapter Figures 25.24 and 25 portray an endometrioid tumor with a seeming *progestational* effect in a patient who had received *no hormone therapy*. Scully has observed a virilized patient whose endometrium showed a frank decidual reaction in association with a metastatic ovarian tumor secondary to a gastric cancer. A progestational pattern is a rare finding in the endometrium and should always raise the question of exogenous hormones.

From our own clinic Woodruff, Williams, and Goldberg have provided strong histochemical proof that certain tumors not usually recognized as endocrinologically active are capable of a hormonal effect. It would seem likely that increasing knowledge of biosynthetic pathways will suggest that many tumors regarded as inert will show evidence of an endocrine effect even though on occasion any estrogenic trend may be nullified by an equal androgenic effect. This represents a premature impression of various ovarian neoplasms that have been studied by certain histochemical techniques in our own laboratory.

GONADAL STROMAL TUMORS

In previous editions this text has indicated that the criterion for the diagnosis of steroid-producing tumors should be the histological appearance rather than endocrine effect. At that time it was assumed that *arrhenoblastoma* was a tumor arising from vestigial remnants of the sex cords, originating in invaginated coelomic epithelium, and possessing androgenic potentiality due to the evanescent trend toward maleness which is common to all females. The *granulosa-theca cell* tumor was thought to arise from

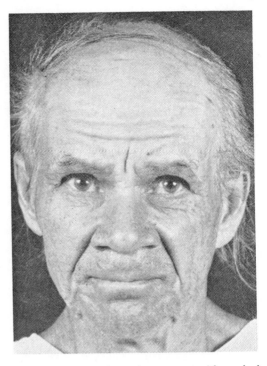

24.39. Patient with mucinous tumor with marked hyperplasia of "stromal cells" showing profound virilism. "Stromal cells" histochemically resembled interstitial cells of the testis.

redundant clumps of granulosa cells unused in the process of follicle formation, the so-called "granulosa ballen" (Meyer). Today it would seem that our earlier concepts are open to a certain amount of doubt in view of the following facts.

(1) It is frankly impossible to distinguish between certain patterns of arrhenoblastoma and granulosa-theca tumors without reference to the endocrine effect. This was quite apparent from our recent study of arrhenoblastoma, and in a review of granulosa-theca tumors by Busby and Anderson and our own study in which hirsutism, reversible postoperative, occurred in some 5%.

(2) Morphologically typical tumors show an endocrine effect exactly opposite to the histological pattern. Shippel has written extensively on thecomas with associated virilism; arrhenoblastomas with feminization have been recorded. Various bisexual effects are also noted

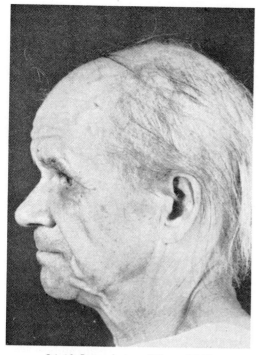

24.40. Lateral view of Figure 24.39

with hilus cell tumors, wherein there is profound general virilism along with endometrial hyperplasia, a presumed estrogen effect.

(3) If sufficient sections are obtained, various transition forms between classic arrhenoblastoma and granulosa-thecoma may be found on occasion. McKinley indicates that there is ready convertibility of granulosa and theca cells, normally estrogenic, into hilus or luteinized cells capable of androgen secretion.

(4) Various tumorigenic agents (Warner) lead to all variants of arrhenoblastoma and granulosa-theca tumors in rodents and poultry. The capability of the ovarian stromal cell in many types of ovarian neoplasms to produce any type of steroid such as estrogen, testosterone, and even progesterone seems to afford additional proof.

Today we subscribe to the thoughts of Sandberg that *endocrine effect* rather than morphology should be the decisive diagnostic factor. We suspect that both granulosa-theca tumors and arrhenoblastoma may arise from the mesenchyme or gonadal stroma, and that the uncertain sex cord arises from the mesenchyme rather than the germinal epithelium.

A great variety of patterns may be found in any single tumor, and it is conceivable that both estrogen and androgen may be produced (Jeffcoate) with the predominant steroid determining the clinical effect. In a histochemical study of normal and abnormal postmenopausal ovaries we observed this bisexual reaction as indicated by enzyme activity suggestive of steroidal biosynthesis. Plotz has confirmed this, using biological techniques, and has indicated that the androgens are precursors to estrogen in the plasma pool, and may be converted to estrogen. It would seem that a bisexual endocrine activity might occur in many functional tumors, and that any type of active tumor may produce any of the biochemically closely related steroids. Indeed we might conjecture that such tumors are in reality forms of *gynandroblastoma* in that many types of steroids are manufactured with the endocrine effect being determined by the most potent steroid. Thus in formulating a diagnosis for these neoplasms it does not seem illogical to utilize the term *gonadal stromal tumor*, qualified by *feminizing, virilizing or inert.*

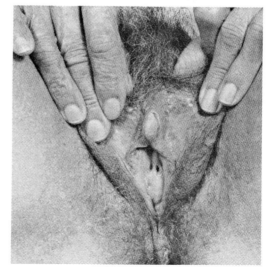

24.41. External genitalia (Figs. 24.39, 40) with marked enlargement of clitoris.

It seems possible that the ovarian stromal cell is capable of many histological variations, culminating in all the diverse forms of granulosa theca tumors and arrhenoblastoma, with all types of steroidal activity, though whether this is a capability of the adult stromal cell or a result of certain "reserve cells" as suggested by Warner *et al.* seems relative academic. Utilizing electron microscopy, Kempson has indicated that stromal tumors contain cells identical to the normal ovarian stroma.

In a recent provocative publication, Fathalla reaffirms the endocrine potential of a number of miscellaneous ovarian tumors with observed thecal change of the ovarian stroma. A similar mechanism is proposed for the hormonal stimulus of granulosa cell tumors and arrhenoblastoma; *i.e.*, the altered ovarian stroma rather than the tumor itself produces the active steroid as a result of stimulation by the epithelial elements in the neoplasm. At the same time the author admits the impossibility of distinction between an altered ovarian stroma, and thecal or interstitial tissue (as the case may be).

As support to such a unique opinion, Fathalla utilizes the following facts, substantiated by numerous case reports (which we have not reviewed individually). Where there is recurrence of a granulosa cell tumor or arrhenoblastoma, a recurrent endocrine effect is the rule, *only if* there is involvement of the ovary, but *not if* there is merely extra-ovarian extension. One might imagine certain instances where all of the ovary and stroma) is obliterated by tumor so that no endocrine effect would be possible, and it is a fact that not all granulosa-theca tumors or arrhenoblastomas are endocrinologically active. It would be a fascinating concept to suggest that such neoplasms are capable of steroid production where there is available alterable stroma, but become inert when this is destroyed. This would be difficult to prove, and is not compatible with the usual history of progressive increasing virilism or feminization seen on occasion when recurrence followed complete operation with presumed removal of all ovarian stroma. However, this concept deserves consideration.

We have already commented on the ability of the normal ovary to secrete both estrogenic and androgenic hormones. Study of many functioning tumors has led to the belief that some produce a mixture of androgens and estrogens, with one or the other predominating and leading to the clinical effect observed. The close chemical kinship of the virilizing and feminizing hormone with the likelihood of a variable equilibrium would seem to make this a very real possibility, irrespective of the histological pattern concerned.

If this basic point is accepted, it may seem desirable at some time to completely delete such uncertain designations as androblastoma, gynandroblastoma, and even granulosa-theca and arrhenoblastoma from the literature. Admittedly Gunner Teilum has performed a real service in portraying homologous ovarian and testicular tumors which contain the same basic stroma, yet considerable confusion has arisen from the terms evolved. It is our sincere belief that the term *gonadal stromal tumor*, whether *virilizing, feminizing,* or *inert* is best suited as a "family" name for these tumors.

Today various biochemical studies are available which permit direct analysis of tumor tissue. Certain incubation techniques and use of radioactive substances have permitted more precise determination of biosynthetic pathways, intermediate metabolites, and quantitative steroid production. For a fuller discussion of the complex methods involved, the excellent studies by Kase and Conrad, and others are recommended. Increasing understanding of the various forms of electronmicroscopy will almost certainly prove valuable.

HISTOCHEMICAL STUDIES

Because of the morphological uncertainties in distinguishing between certain functioning ovarian tumors, it would seem that more recent methods of

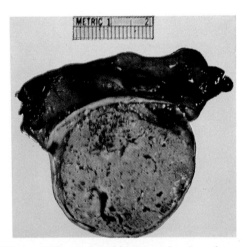

Plate 24.1. Arrhenoblastoma showing characteristic yellowish color with focal hemorrhage and smooth capsule. (From Novak, E. R., and Woodruff, J. D.: *Gynecologic and Obstetric Pathology,* Ed. 5 W. B. Saunders Company, Philadelphia, 1962.)

diagnosis might be utilized. Various histochemical techniques can be applied to cryostat sections of frozen ovarian tissue incubated with various substrates. Any resultant enzymatic activity may be considered highly suggestive (although not conclusive) of certain biosynthetic pathways necessary to steroid formation. For example, with dehydroepiandrosterone (DHA) as substrate, Goldberg, Jones, and Woodruff have indicated intense activity for steroid 3-β-ol dehydrogenase in tissues normally producing progesterone (corpus luteum, placenta, or adrenal), but less appreciable activity in tissues or tumors producing estrogen or testosterone. Since DHA is an intermediate metabolite in the progression to estrogen and testosterone, enzyme activity is highly suggestive of steroid activity in morphologically equivocal tumors. Many substrates are available and useful in indicating precise cellular function, including steroidogenesis.

Other similar studies of enzyme histochemistry of the biosynthetic pathways are currently being utilized. Unquestionably they will add considerably to our knowledge of the behavior of various tumors, although interpretation of the biochemical data is often so complex that it may be beyond the scope of the average clinical gynecologist. Currently, histochemical methods of absolutely distinguishing between estrogen and androgen producing cells by virtue of enzyme response are not perfected.

REFERENCES

Abell, M. R., Johnson, V. J., and Holtz, F.: Dysgerminoma: current opinions on clinical problems. Amer. J. Obstet. Gynec., 86: 693, 1963.

Abell, M. R., Johnson, V. J., and Holtz, F.: I. Ovarian neoplasms in childhood and adolescence. Amer. J. Obstet. Gynec., 92: 1059, 1965: II. Non-germ cell tumors. Amer. J. Obstet. Gynec., 93: 850, 1965.

Asadourian, L. A., and Taylor, H. B.: Dysgerminoma. Obstet. Gynec., 33: 370, 1969.

Barr, M. L., Carr, D. H., Plunkett, E. R., Soltan, H. C., and Wiens, R. G.: Male pseudohermaphroditism and pure gonadal dysgenesis in sisters. Amer. J. Obstet. Gynec., 99: 1074, 1967.

Berendsen, P. B., Smith, E. B., Abell, M. R., and Jaffe, R. B.: Fine structure of Leydig cells from an arrhenoblastoma of the ovary. Amer. J. Obstet. Gynec., 103: 192, 1969.

Berger, L.: La glande sympathicotrope due hile de l'ovaire; ses homologies avec la gland interstitielle du testicule. Les rapports nerveuses des deux glandes. Arch. Anat., 2: 255, 1923.

Biskind, G. R., and Biskind, M. S.: Experimental ovarian tumors in rats. Amer. J. Clin. Path., 19: 510, 1949.

Boivin, Y., and Richart, R. M.: Hilus cell tumors of the ovary. Cancer, 18, 231, 1965.

Brody, S.: Clinical aspects of dysgerminoma of the ovary. Acta Radiol., 56: 209, 1961.

Busby, T., and Anderson, G. W.: Feminizing mesenchymomas of ovary. Amer. J. Obstet. Gynec., 68: 1391, 1954.

Chan, L. K. C., and Prathrop, K.: Virilization in pregnancy with mucinous cystadenoma. Amer. J. Obstet. Gynec., 108: 946, 1970.

Chauser, B. J., Green, J. P., and Klein, H. Z.: Bilateral metachronous dysgerminoma with 15-year interval. Cancer, 27: 939, 1971.

Christian, C. D.: Ovarian tumors and Peutz-Jeghers syndrome. Amer. J. Obstet. Gynec., 111: 529, 1971.

Creasman, W. T., Rutledge, F., and Smith, J. B.: Carcinoma of the ovary and pregnancy. Obstet. Gynec., 38: 111, 1971.

De Lima, F. O. A.: Disgerminoma do ovario, contribuacao para o seu estudo anatomo-clinico. São Paulo, Brazil, 1966.

Dickman, S. H., and Toker, C.: Strumal carcinoid with masculinization. Cancer, 27: 925, 1971.

Diddle, A. W., and Devereux, W. P.: Ovarian mesenchymomas. Obstet. Gynec., 13: 294, 1959.

Diddle, A. W., and O'Connor, K. A.: Feminizing ovarian tumors and pregnancy. Amer. J. Obstet. Gynec., 62: 1071, 1951.

Drobnjak, P., et al.: Precocious puberty with masculinization due to teratochorio-gonadoblastoma. J. Obstet. Gynaec. Brit. Comm., 78: 845, 1971.

Dunniho, D. R., Grieme, D. L., and Wolfe, R. J.: Hilus cell tumors of the ovary. Obstet. Gynec., 27: 703, 1966.

Echt, C. R., and Hadd, H. E.: Androgen excretion patterns in a patient with metastic hilus cell tumor of the ovary. Amer. J. Obstet. Gynec., 100: 1055, 1968.

Emig, O. R., Hertig, A. T., and Rowe, F. J.: Gynandroblastoma of the ovary. Obstet. Gynec., 13: 135, 1959.

Falck, B.: Site of production of estrogen in rat ovary as studied in micro-transplants. Acta Physiol. Scand. (Suppl. 163), 47: 5, 1959.

Farber, M., Palmer, P. G., and Bull, M. J.: Pure gonadal dysgenesis with bilateral gonadoblastoma in first cousins. Obstet. Gynec., 35: 444, 1970.

Fathalla, M. F.: The role of the ovarian stroma in hormone production by ovarian tumors. J. Obstet. Gynaec. Brit. Comm., 75: 32, 1968.

Fathalla, M. F.: The occurrence of granulosa and theca tumors in clinically normal ovaries. J. Obstet. Gynec. Brit. Comm., 71: 279, 1967.

Felmus, L. B., and Pedowitz, P.: Clinical malignancy of endocrine tumors of the ovary and dysgerminoma. Obstet. Gynec., 29: 344, 1967.

Flick, F. H., and Banfield, R. S., Jr.: Theca and granulosa cell tumors. Bull. Sloane Hosp. Wom., 2: 31, 1956.

Francis, H. H.: Granulosa cell tumor of the ovary at the age of 85 years. J. Obstet. Gynaec. Brit. Comm., 64: 274, 1957.

French, W. G.: Clinical behavior of granulosa-cell tumor of ovary. Amer. J. Obstet. Gynec., 62: 75, 1951.

Furth, J., and Butterworth, J. S.: Neoplastic diseases occurring among mice subjected to general irradiation with X-ray. Amer. J. Cancer, 28: 666, 1936.

Gillibrand, P. N.: Granulosa-theca tumors of the ovary associated with pregnancy. Amer. J. Obstet. Gynec., 94: 1108, 1966.

Goldberg, B., Jones, S. E. S., and Woodruff, J. D.: A histochemical study of steroid 3β-ol dehydrogenase activity in some steroid-producing tumors. Amer. J. Obstet. Gynec., 86: 1003, 1963.

Goldstein, D. P., and Lamb, E. J.: Arrhenoblastoma in first cousins. Obstet. Gynec., 35: 444, 1970.

Goldstein, D. P., and Piro, A. J.: Combination chemotherapy in germ cell tumors containing choriocarcinoma. Surg. Gynec. Obstet. 134: 61, 1972.

Goldston, W. R., et al.: Clinicopathological studies in feminizing tumors. Amer. J. Obstet. Gynec., 112: 422, 1972.

Gondos, B., and Monroe, S. A.: Cystic granulosa cell tumor with massive hemoperitoneum. Obstet. Gynec., 38: 683, 1971.

Graber, E. A., O'Rourke, J. J., and Sturman, M.: Arrhenoblastoma of the ovary. Amer. J. Obstet. Gynec., 81: 783, 1961.

Greene, J. W., Jr.: Feminizing mesenchymomas (granulosa and theca-cell tumors) with associated endometrial carcinoma. Amer. J. Obstet. Gynec., 74: 31, 1957.

Greene, R. R., Holzwarth, D., and Roddick, J. W., Jr.: "Luteomas of pregnancy." Amer. J. Obstet. Gynec., 88: 1001, 1964.

Gusberg, S. B., and Karden, P.: Endometrial response to theca-granulosal cell tumors. Amer. J. Obstet. Gynec., 111: 633, 1971.

Heinz, H. A.: Investigations on the determination of the sex of dysgerminoma from the morphology of the cellular nuclei. Geburtsh. Frauenheilk, 21: 144, 1961.

Hughesdon, P. E.: The structure and origin of theca-granulosa tumors. J. Obstet. Gynaec. Brit. Comm., 65: 540, 1958.

Hughesdon, P. E.: Structure, origin and histological relations of dysgerminoma. J. Obstet. Gynaec. Brit. Comm., 67: 566, 1959.

Jakobovits, A.: Hormone production by miscellaneous ovarian tumors. Amer. J. Obstet. Gynec., 85: 90, 1963.

Janko, A. B., and Sandberg, E. C.: The Reinke crystalloid. Obstet. Gynec., 35: 493, 1970.

Jeffcoate, S. L., and Prunty, F. T. G.: Steroid synthesis in vitro by a hilar cell tumor. Amer. J. Obstet. Gynec., 101: 684, 1968.

Jones, G. S., Goldberg, B., and Woodruff, J. D.: Enzyme histochemistry of a masculinizing arrhenoblastoma. Obstet. Gynec., 9: 328, 1967.

Kase, N., and Conrad, S. H.: Steroid synthesis in abnormal ovaries. I. Arrhenoblastoma. II. Granulosa cell tumor. Amer. J. Obstet. Gynec., 90: 1251, 1964.

Kempson, R. L.: Ultrastructure of ovarian stromal cell tumors. Arch. Path., 86: 492, 1968.

Koudstall, J., Bossenbroek, B., and Hardonk, M. J.: Ovarian tumors investigated by histochemical and enzyme histochemical methods. Amer. J. Obstet. Gynec., 102: 1004, 1969.

Krause, D. E., and Stembridge, V. A.: Lutenomas of pregnancy. Amer. J. Obstet. Gynec., 95: 192, 1966.

Lewis, P. D., and Percival, R. C.: Combined thecoma and teratoma. J. Obstet. Gynaec. Brit. Comm., 72: 447, 1965.

Liebert, K. I., and Stent, L.: Dysgerminoma of the ovary with choriocarcinoma. J. Obstet. Gynaec. Brit. Comm., 67: 627, 1960.

Mackinlay, C. J.: Male cells in granulosa cell ovarian tumors. J. Obstet. Gynaec. Brit. Comm., 64: 512, 1957.

Mahesh, V. B., McDonough, P. G., and Deleo, C. A.: Endocrine studies in arrhenoblastoma. Amer. J. Obstet. Gynec., 107: 183, 1970.

Malkasian, G. D., Jr., and Symmonds, R. E.: Treatment of unilateral encapsulated ovarian dysgerminoma. Amer. J. Obstet. Gynec., 90: 379, 1964.

McDonough, P. G., Greenblatt, R. B., Byrd, J. R., and Hastings, E. V.: Gonadoblastoma (Gonocytoma III). Obstet. Gynec., 29: 54, 1967.

McKay, D. G., Hertig, A. T., and Hickey, W. F.: Histogenesis of granulosa and theca cell tumors of human ovary. Obstet. Gynec., 1: 125, 1953.

Meyer, R.: Pathology of some special ovarian tumors and their relation to sex characteristics. Amer. J. Obstet. Gynec., 26: 505, 1933.

Morris, J. M., and Scully, R. E.: Endocrine Pathology of the Ovary. C. V. Mosby Company, St. Louis, 1958.

Meuller, C. W., Topkins, P., and Laff, W. A.: Dysgerminoma of ovary; an analysis of 427 cases. Amer. J. Obstet. Gynec., 60: 153, 1950.

Neigus, I.: Ovarian dysgerminoma with chorionepithelium. Amer. J. Obstet. Gynec., 69: 838, 1955.

Nokes, J. M., Claiborne, H. A., and Reingold, W. N.: Thecoma with associated virilization. Amer. J. Obstet. Gynec., 78: 722, 1958.

Norris, H. J, and Taylor, H. B.: Luteoma of pregnancy, Amer. J. Clin. Path., 47: 557, 1967.

Norris, H. J., and Taylor, H. B.: Prognosis of granulosa-theca tumors of the ovary. Cancer, 21: 255, 1967.

Novak, E. R.: Gyandroblastoma of the ovary (review of eight cases from the Ovarian Tumor Registry). Obstet. Gynec., 30: 709, 1967.

Novak, E. R., and Long, J. H.: Arrhenoblastoma of the ovary. A review of the Ovarian Tumor Registry. Amer. J. Obstet. Gynec., 92: 1082, 1965.

Novak, E. R., and Mattingly, R. F.: Hilus cell tumors of the ovary (with a review of 18 cases). Obstet. Gynec., 15: 425, 1960.

Novak, E. R., Woodruff, J. D., and Linthicum, J. M.: Evaluation of the unclassified tumors of the Ovarian Tumor Registry 1942–1962. Amer. J. Obstet. Gynec., 87: 999, 1963.

Novak, E. R., et al.: Feminizing gonadal stromal tumors. Obstet. Gynec., 38: 701, 1971.

Patel, S. K., and Prentice, R. S. A.: Gonadoblastoma. Arch. Path., 94: 165, 1972.

Pedowitz, P., Felmus, L. B., and Grayzel, D. M.: Dysgerminoma of the ovary; prognosis and treatment. Amer. J. Obstet. Gynec., 70: 1284, 1955.

Pedowitz, P., and O'Brien, F. B.: Arrhenoblastoma of the ovary. Obstet. Gynec., 16: 62, 1960.

Persaud, V., Patterson, A. W., and Pathak, U. N.: Theca cell tumor associated with pregnancy. Int. Surg., 53: 48, 1970.

Pfleideren, A., and Teufely, G.: Incidence and histochemical investigation of enzymatically active cells in stroma of ovarian tumors. Amer. J. Obstet. Gynec., 102: 907, 1968.

Pick, L.: Über Adenome der männlichen und weiblichen Keimdrüse. Klin. Wschr., 42: 502, 1905.

Plate, W. P.: Oestrogenic functie van de Tussencellen in de gonade. Nederl. T. Verlosk., 63: 83, 1963.

Robertson, M. G., and Miller, R. E. C.: Massive cystic granulosa-theca cell tumor. Amer. J. Obstet. Gynec., 109: 407, 1971.

Sandberg, E. C.: The virilizing ovary. Obstet. Gynec. Survey, 17: 165, 1962.

Schellhas, H. F., et al.: Germ cell tumors associated with XY gonadal dysgenesis. Amer. J. Obstet. Gynec., 109: 1197, 1971.

Scott, J. S., Lumsden, C. E., and Levell, M. J.: Ovarian endocrine activity in association with hormonally inactive neoplasia. Amer. J. Obstet. Gynec., 97: 161, 1967.

Scully, R. E.: Androgenic lesions of the ovary. In The Ovary, International Academy of Pathology Monograph No. 3, edited by H. G. Grady and D. E. Smith, p. 143. The Williams & Wilkins Company, Baltimore, 1963.

Scully, R. E.: Gonadoblastoma (74 cases). Cancer, 25, 1340, 1971.

Scully, R. E., and Richardson, G. S.: Luteinization of the stroma of metastatic cancer involving the ovary and its endocrine significance. Cancer, 14: 427, 1961.

Segall, F., et al.: XO-XY gonadal dysgenesis and gonadoblastoma in childhood. Obstet. Gynec., 41: 536, 1973.

Shippel, S.: Ovarian theca cell. J. Obstet. Gynaec. Brit. Comm., *57:* 362, 1950.

Simmons, R. L., and Sciarra, J. J.: Treatment of late recurrent granulosa cell tumors of the ovary. Surg. Gynec. Obstet., *124:* 65, 1967.

Smith, A. H., and Ward, S. V.: Dysgerminoma in pregnancy. Obstet. Gynec., *28:* 502, 1966.

Sobrinho, L. G., and Kase, N. G.: Adrenal rest cell tumor of the ovary. Obstet. Gynec., *36:* 895, 1970.

Sommers, S. C., Gates, O., and Goodof, I. I.: Late recurrence of granulosa cell tumors. Obstet. Gynec., *6:* 395, 1955.

Spadoni, L. R., Lindberg, M. C., Mottet, N. K., and Herrmann, W. L.: Virilization coexisting with Krukenberg Tumor during pregnancy. Amer. J. Obstet. Gynec., *92:* 981, 1965.

Steenstrup, E. K.: Ovarian tumors and Peutz-Jeghers syndrome. Acta Obstet. Gynec. Scand., *51:* 237, 1972.

Sternberg, W. H.: Nonfunctioning ovarian neoplasms. In *The Ovary*, International Academy of Pathologists Monograph No. 3, edited by H. G. Grady and D. E. Smith, p. 209. The Williams & Wilkins Company, Baltimore, 1963.

Sternberg, W. H., and Barclay, D. L. Luteoma of pregnancy. Amer. J. Obstet. Gynec., *95:* 165, 1966.

Sternberg, W. H., and Roth, L. M.: Ovarian stromal tumors containing Leydig cells. Cancer, *32:* 940, 1973.

Stewart, R. S., and Woodard, D. E.: Malignant ovarian hilus cell tumor. Arch. Path., *73:* 91, 1962.

Talerman, A.: Germ cell-sex-cord tumor. Obstet. Gynec. *40:* 473, 1972.

Talerman, A., Huyzinga, J., and Kuipens, T.: Dysgerminoma. Obstet. Gynec., *41:* 137, 1973.

Taylor, H., Barter, R. H., and Jacobson, C. B.: Neoplasms of dysgenetic gonads. Amer. J. Obstet. Gynec., *96:* 816, 1966.

Teilum, G.: *Special Tumors of the Ovary and Testis.* J. P. Lippincott, Philadelphia, 1971.

Teter, J.: A mixed form of feminizing germ cell tumor (gonocytoma II). Amer. J. Obstet. Gynec., *84:* 722, 1962.

Teter, J.: Germ cell tumor in dysgenetic gonads. Amer. J. Obstet. Gynec., *108:* 894, 1970.

Thoeny, R. H., Dockerty, M. B., Hunt, A. B., and Childs, D. S.: Study of ovarian dysgerminoma with emphasis on role of radiation therapy. Surg. Gynec. Obstet., *113:* 692, 1961.

Thomas, E., *et al.*: Bilateral luteomas of pregnancy with virilization. Obstet. Gynec., *39:* 577, 1972.

Thompson, J. P., Dockerty, M. B., and Symmonds, R. E.: Granulosa cell carcinoma arising in a cystic teratoma of the ovary. Obstet. Gynec., *28:* 549, 1966.

Traut, H. F., and Butterworth, J. S.: The theca, granulosa, lutein cell tumors of the human ovary and similar tumors of the mouse's ovary. Amer. J. Obstet. Gynec., *34:* 987, 1937.

Tweeddale, D. N., Dockerty, M. B., Pratt, J. H., and Hranilovich, G. T.: Pregnancy with a recurrent granulosa cell tumor. Amer. J. Obstet. Gynec., *70:* 1039, 1955.

Usizama, H.: Ovarian dysgerminoma associated with masculinization. Cancer, *9:* 736, 1956.

Vande, Wiele, R. L.: Studies of the androgenic function of the ovaries. Bull. Sloane Hosp., *6:* 82, 1960.

Verhoeven, A. T. M., *et al.*: Virilization in pregnancy. Obstet. Gynec. Surv., *28:* 597, 1973.

Warner, N. E., Friedman, N. B., Bomze, E. J., and Masin, F.: Comparative pathology of experimental and spontaneous androblastomas and gynoblastomas of the gonads. Amer. J. Obstet. Gynec., *79:* 971, 1960.

Warren, J. C., Erkman, B., and Cheatum, S.: Hilus-cell adenoma in a dysgenetic gonad with XX/XO mosaicism. Lancet, *1:* 141, 1964.

Waugh, D., Venning, E. H., and McEachern, D.: Sympathicotropic (Leydig) cell tumors of ovary with virilism. J. Clin. Endocr., *9:* 486, 1949.

Williamson, H. O., and Pratt-Thomas, H. R.: Bilateral gonadoblastoma with dysgerminoma. Obstet. Gynec., *39:* 263, 1972.

Wong, T. W., and Warner, N. E.: Ovarian thecal metaplasia in the adrenal gland. Arch. Path., *92:* 319, 1971.

Woodruff, J. D., Williams, T. J., and Goldberg, B.: Hormone activity of the common ovarian neoplasm. Amer. J. Obstet. Gynec., *87:* 679, 1963.

Younglai, E. V., *et al.*: Arrhenoblastoma. Amer. J. Obstet. Gynec., *116:* 401, 1973.

chapter 25

Endometriosis

One of the most interesting lesions encountered in gynecological practice is pelvic endometriosis, a clinical and pathological entity publicized primarily by the classic contributions of Sampson in 1921. It may be defined as the condition in which tissue resembling endometrium is found in various extrauterine locations, but chiefly in the pelvic cavity. Even before Sampson's studies, aberrant uterine mucosa had been described from time to time, and as far back as 1899 Russell had reported such findings in the ovary.

SITES OF ENDOMETRIOSIS

The endometrial islands may be found in many possible locations, of which the following are the most common: (1) ovaries; (2) uterine ligaments (round, broad, uterosacral); (3) rectovaginal septum; (4) pelvic peritoneum covering the uterus, tubes, rectum, sigmoid, or bladder; (5) umbilicus; (6) laparotomy scars; (7) hernial sacs; (8) appendix; (9) vagina; (10) vulva; (11) cervix; (12) tubal stumps; (13) lymph glands. In rare cases, still other locations, such as the arm, thigh, or pleural and pericardial cavity have been reported.

HISTOGENESIS

Since Sampson's original paper in 1921, there has been much discussion as to the origin of the aberrant endometrium in cases of pelvic endometriosis. There are various theories on this point.

(1) Sampson's original concept of *transtubal regurgitation of menstrual blood* and endometrial particles at the time of menstruation, with their subsequent implantation and growth on the ovaries and elsewhere in the pelvis (Fig. 25.1).

(2) The so-called *celomic metaplasia doctrine,* according to which the aberrant endometrium develops as a result of abnormal differentiation changes in the germinal epithelium and various parts of the pelvic peritoneum which are embryologically derived from the celomic epithelium.

(3) The *lymphatic dissemination* theory of Halban, who believed that the aberrant tissue is derived from endometrium entering the uterine lymphatic vessels of the uterus at the time of menstruation, being thus disseminated throughout the pelvis (Fig. 25.2).

(4) *Hematogenous* spread of endometrium, as an explanation for certain rare cases of endometriosis which would be

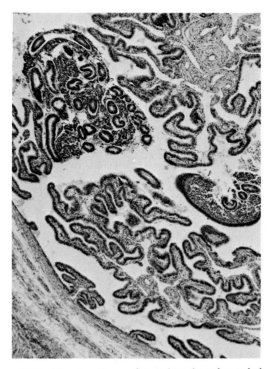

25.1. Menstruating endometrium in tube; tubal wall left lower quadrant.

difficult to explain on any other basis (see Plate 25.3).

Sampson's view, as expressed in his original papers, was that the aberrant endometrium arises from the implantation on the surface of the ovaries, or elsewhere in the pelvis, of bits of uterine mucosa which during menstruation are regurgitated from the uterine cavity through the tubes. In other words, he believed that transtubal regurgitation of menstrual blood into the peritoneal cavity is relatively common, particularly in the presence of retroflexion or some degree of cervical stenosis. Sampson himself later modified his views considerably, agreeing that the tubal regurgitation concept cannot explain all cases of pelvic endometriosis and certainly not such types as umbilical endometriosis. The experimental studies of Scott and Wharton have indicated the probability that in the monkey the desquamated and regurgitated endometrium is capable of peritoneal growth. McCann has suggested that the monkey and the human female may

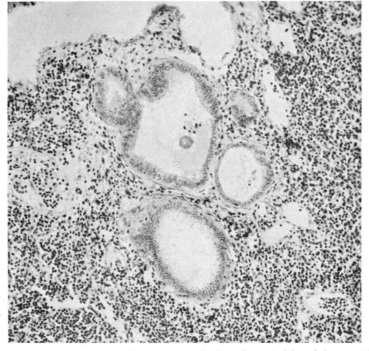

25.2. Endometrium in lymph gland. A fairly common finding (Javert) although it cannot be interpreted to support Halban's lymphogenic theory of etiology of pelvic endometriosis in general.

have a somewhat different menstrual mechanism.

Such cases as the six young women reported by Hanton *et al.,* who found endometriosis associated with such obstructive conditions in the lower genital tract as a nonpatent cervix or absent vagina add additional support to this concept. Moore and Schiffrain in separate studies record various teen-age patients with some type of congenital abnormality, which acted as a barrier to unobstructed menstrual flow. That implantation results in certain such cases seems likely; we cannot be as dogmatic as Ridley who insists there is no other possible method of histogenesis.

Merrill has suggested that perhaps endometrium does not necessarily implant but contains an inductor. He has utilized an endometrium-filled, escape-proof Millipore filter to produce endometriosis in adjacent tissues.

The majority of those who have taken issue with Sampson (Meyer, Novak, etc.) believe that a more rational and more inclusive explanation is one based on a study of the embryology of the genital organs. The mucosa of almost the entire genital canal, as well as the germinal epithelium of the ovary, represents only varying degrees of *modification* of the *celomic epithelium,* the primitive peritoneum. The germinal epithelium represents a segment of this tissue which is relatively undifferentiated, possessing therefore a great deal of unused differentiating potentiality, and it would seem a reasonable speculation that various inflammatory (Meyer) or endocrine (Novak) stimuli might activate this.

It is not surprising, therefore, that at times areas of this epithelium may show differentiation phases beyond that normal in the ovary (prosoplasia), giving rise most frequently to endometrium. At times, on the other hand, the abnormal areas may be identical with that of the tube, this being a well recognized subvariety of endometriosis, designated as *endosalpingiosis.* Gray and Barnes have pointed out a high association of endometrial and endocervical abnormalities

with endometriosis which might imply a general response to some kind of stimulus on a potentially reactive tissue.

There is much evidence for, as well as against, both the above mentioned theories, but it would be a long story to review this. Suffice it to say that the question is still unsettled and that the adherents of both views have seemed to manifest a less rigid policy. For example, Sampson finally accepted the importance of the metaplasia factor in a considerable group of cases, whereas most of his opponents admit that, although implantation is not the important primary factor in most cases of ovarian or extragenital endometriosis, it is difficult to deny its importance in the secondary deposits so commonly found throughout the pelvis and the lower genital tract.

We do not believe that the occasional finding of endometrial tissue in the pelvic lymph glands, as reported by Javert, has more than academic interest at this time; it adds little to Halban's theory as to the *lymphatic etiology* of ordinary pelvic endometriosis. In spite of the finding of endometrium in the pelvic lymph nodes, no one has ever described any clinical entity of pelvic lymph gland endometriosis, although Koss has reported a small adenoacanthoma in a surgically removed lymph node, an incidental finding. That it evolved from endometriosis is strongly suggested by the excellent figures depicting transition forms. Lastly, *hematogenous* spread of endometrium almost has to be invoked to explain a few rare cases of thigh, lung, or pleural endometriosis, although no one feels this to be the common method of origin or spread of the disease. Labay and Femen record a case of malignancy evolving in pleural endometriosis.

Indeed, *most critical gynecologists believe that there is more than one mode of origin for endometriosis, and that no single theory explains all cases.* The implantation doctrine seems a likely one for the majority of cases of endometriosis. Recent experiments, wherein human subjects were given injections of their own exfoliated endometrium months before elective laparotomy, have suggested that this implantation may lead to endometriosis, not only in the monkey but in the human. Plantation of endometrium into the abdominal wall of patients subsequently scheduled for laparotomy by Ridley has suggested growth of the implanted tissue in a few, but by no means a majority of women.

PATHOLOGY

Gross

The gross picture in cases of endometriosis is extremely variable. The surgeon on opening the abdomen and exposing the pelvic organs may find a small adherent mass in one or both sides of the pelvis, usually attached to the posterior surface of the uterus quite low down. On loosening these adhesions to rotate the adnexa into the field of operation, there is a gush of chocolate-colored or dark, rusty-looking fluid, and this should at once make him think of endometriosis. Examination of the ovary may disclose a cyst with a dark

hemorrhagic lining (Fig. 25.3), which has been opened in bringing up the adherent adnexa.

The cyst may be only a centimeter or so in diameter, and is rarely larger than a grapefruit (Fig. 25.4). The tube is usually quite normal, with a patent fimbriated extremity, although it may be surrounded by peritoneal adhesions with a number of rather puckered hemorrhagic areas of dark bluish color, in one or both uterosacral ligaments. Similar areas may be seen on the anterior surface of the sigmoid or rectum, or elsewhere in the pelvis.

This, then, is the typical picure, but it may present all sorts of degrees and variations. In a few mild cases the adnexa may initially seem quite normal, but close inspection of the ovaries may reveal a number of reddish-blue, fibrin-like areas representing tiny endometrial islands or "implants" with occasional bloody ascites (Fig. 25.5).

At the other extreme are cases in which the pelvis may be filled with a "frozen"

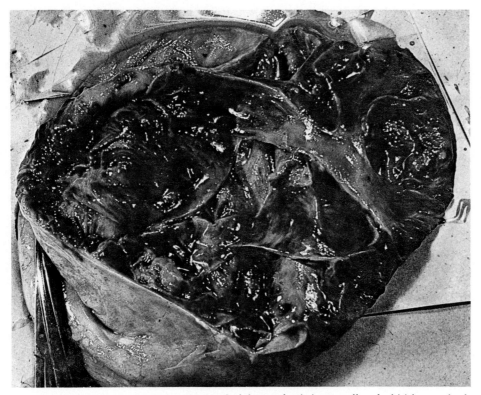

25.3. Cut surface of endometrial cyst showing dark hemorrhagic inner wall and whitish capsular layer.

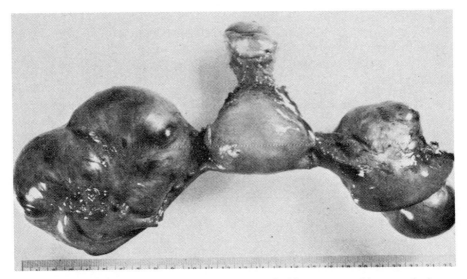

25.4. Large bilateral endometrial cysts removed without rupture (the exception)

mass, consisting of a uterus with adenomyosis, firmly adherent adnexa, bilateral endometrial cysts, and extensive endometrial invasion of the rectal or sigmoidal wall. In fact, the bowel may be so enormously infiltrated as to simulate malignancy, or to produce complete obstruction, and Davis and Truehart have thoroughly discussed surgical management of colonic endometriosis. Oophorectomy rather than difficult bowel surgery seems desirable, except in the occasional young woman. At times the invading endometrium may push far down into the rectovaginal septum. Like Cavanagh, we are inclined to believe that endome-

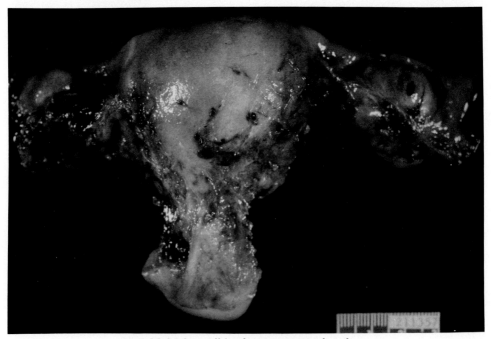

25.5. Multiple small implants over serosal surfaces

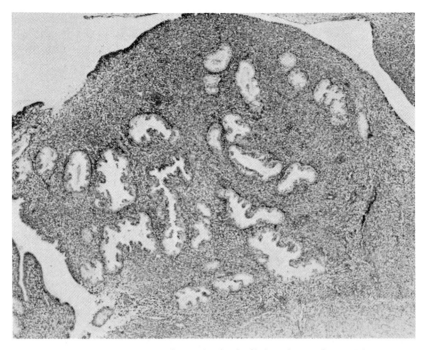

25.6. Marked premenstrual reaction in the lining of an endometrial cyst

triosis may progress rapidly in the youthful (less than 30 years) patient. Endometrial cysts may enlarge enormously within a few months as a result of extensive intracystic hemorrhage.

Microscopic

From a microscopic standpoint, there is considerable variation, the essential criterion being the presence of endometrial tissue in the wall of the cyst, preferably stroma as well as glands. It should be remembered that the aberrant tissue resembles the uterine mucosa not only histologically but also physiologically, so that it may sometimes, but not by any means always, show evidence of response to menstrual and pregnancy stimuli (Fig. 25.6–8). Because of the constant recurrence of menstrual desquamation, with perhaps the pressure of the retained menstrual blood in the cyst cavities, the endometrial lining of the latter may be almost completely absent (Fig. 25.9), and in its place one may see only reactive con-

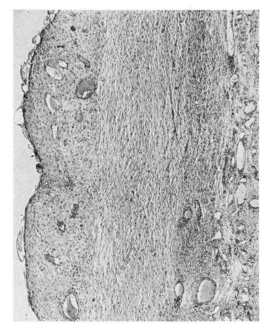

25.7. Decidual changes in wall of endometrial cyst in pregnancy. Pseudodecidual changes may occur in the nonpregnant ovary (Bassis) in the absence of endometriosis.

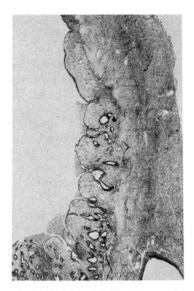

25.8. Endometrial cyst with lining endometrium identical with that of the uterus.

nective tissue elements, with usually a large number of endothelial leukocytes heavily laden with blood pigment (*pseudoxanthoma cells*) (Fig. 25.10). Indeed, in about one-third of all cases of typical, even extensive "clinical" endometriosis as seen at operation, there

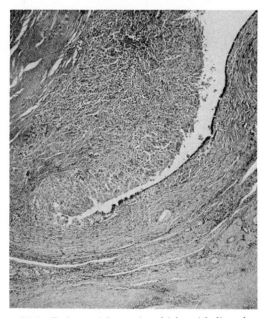

25.9. Endometrial cyst in which epithelium has been lost over considerable areas. No glands or stroma are to be seen.

may be no histological proof of its existence, even if many pathological sections are made. Tissue committees should be aware of this fact.

The term *"chocolate cyst"* of the ovary has come into general vogue as synonymous with "endometrial cyst." The latter term, however, is a much better one, in spite of the expressiveness of the former. There are some surgeons who forget that other types of ovarian cyst may have a chocolate-colored content; *e.g.,* follicle or corpus luteum hematoma, cystadenoma, etc., so that when a cyst discharges such a fluid, it should not categorically be concluded that endometriosis is present.

Malignant degeneration of an ovarian cyst may occur, but so rarely that it does not influence the handling of the patient. The usual lesion is adenoacanthoma, a relatively low grade type of malignancy (Figs. 25.11–13) and acanthosis is a frequent finding with uterine adenocarcinoma.

ENDOMETRIOID CARCINOMA OF THE OVARY

In 1962, the Cancer Committee of the International Federation of Gynecology and Obstetrics (FIGO) heard Professor L. Santesson of Stockholm state that tumors of the ovary similar to endometrial carcinoma accounted for 24.4 per cent of all malignant tumors, less than papillary serous cystadenocarcinoma (39.3 per cent) but more than mucinous tumors (9.4 per cent). The most recent FIGO report would indicate that serous lesions are nearly four times as common as mucinous lesions and more than twice as common as endometrioid malignancies.

The term "endometrioid carcinoma" was accepted as one of the tumors of epithelial origin, and has been popularized in this country by Long and Taylor as a suggested diagnosis for certain ovarian tumors which have a histological similarity to endometrial adenocarcinoma. This would include most adenoacanthomas which are often observed to occur in conjunction with pelvic endometriosis, although it is on occasion impossible to demonstrate a frank transition

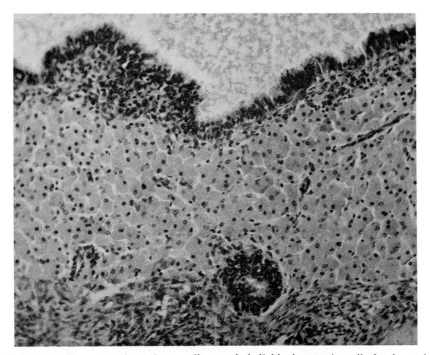

25.10. High power of large pseudoxanthoma cells or endothelial leukocytes in wall of endometrial cyst.

between benign and malignant ovarian endometrium, which Sampson insisted should be mandatory in indicating an endometrial origin. Long and Taylor have listed other criteria, which, aside from acanthosis, are difficult to apply. In addition, histologically similar tumors may arise from either the ovary or endometrium, so that it is impossible for any one to categorically state that this pattern of tumor is of endometrial origin, particularly when there is no other evidence of pelvic endometriosis. Because the term "endometrioid tumor" is FIGO approved, it would seem we must be prepared to accept it.

In their study of 20 women with this type of ovarian tumor, Long and Taylor note a 70 per cent salvage, Kistner and Hertig report 64 per cent salvage, and in a larger group of 56 patients, Malloy and Pratt record an 80 per cent salvage. Schiller and Kirol likewise suggest the prognosis is twice as good as with most ovarian tumors, and this improved survival is in accord with our own impressions.

Scully and Barlow have suggested that *mesonephromas* should be regarded as merely a variant of endometrioid tumor, and their premise is based on the not infrequent co-association of endometriosis and mesonephroma. One must recall, however, that pelvic endometriosis is a common lesion; it would be reasonable to expect that diverse ovarian tumors may arise in an endometriotic ovary without any direct causal relation. Scully's concept would suggest a Müllerian origin for mesonephroma rather than an origin from mesonephric duct remnants.

Gray and Barnes have reported a mesonephric pattern in an endometrial cyst, and Villa Santa and Rutledge have separately recorded mesonephric adenocarcinomas of the endometrium. Perhaps fuller studies of the endometriosis-mesonephroma relationship are warranted, and we suspect that on occasion mesonephroma may be purely a degenerative form of any ovarian or endometrial adenocarcinoma.

Kurman and Craig find that about 15% of ovarian adenocarcinomas are endometrioid in type, and have reaffirmed the previously known increased salvage with

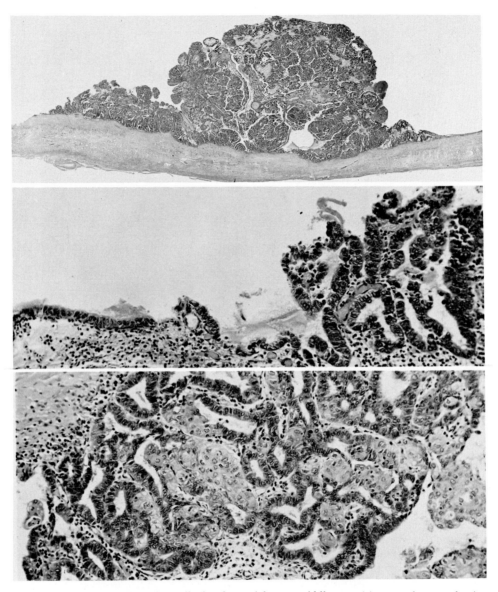

25.11. *Top,* lesion arising from the wall of endometrial cyst; *middle,* transition zone between benign and malignant; *bottom,* full-fledged adenoacanthoma. (Courtesy of Dr. Dan Thompson, Atlanta, Georgia.)

this type of tumor, which in all series amounts to around 60%, considerably better than cancer of the ovary in general. They further indicate that in a considerable proportion of cases (approximately one-third) there may be an admixture of serous or mucinous elements. They have further extended their studies to clear cell carcinomas of the ovary, and again have noted a frequent co-association of this with other types of epithelial carcinoma. This would imply that the germinal epithelium (mesothelium) might be the source of the clear cell type of tumor as with other epithelioid lesions of the ovary. It would not seem illogical to believe that either mesonephric or paramesonephric elements may give rise to the clear cell type of ovarian neoplasm.

Fathalla also comments on the frequency of malignant changes in endome-

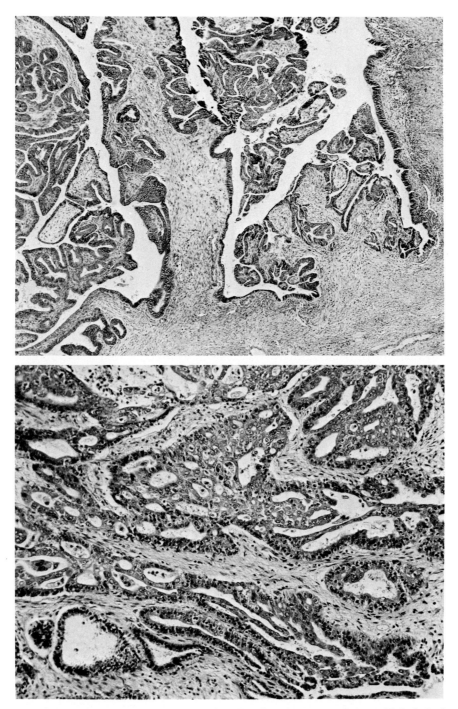

25.12. *Top,* Transition zone endometriosis and early adenocarcinoma. *Bottom,* Full fledged adenoacanthoma in other areas.

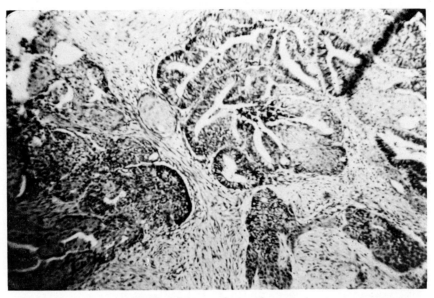

25.13. Adenoacanthoma of ovary

triosis, and he found this accounted for 12 per cent of ovarian tumors studied. Gray and Barnes discuss the increased frequency of malignancy occurring or being recognized in conjunction with endometriosis in the last 10 years. They indicate that in addition to adenoacanthoma many other types of histological pattern may be found due to the multiple differentiation potency of the Müllerian epithelium. Whatever the stimulus is, these authors feel it may affect not only the ovary but also the other structures evolving from the Müllerian tissue (tubes, uterus, and endocervix), because of a high incidence of extra-gonadal lesions. Carcinosarcoma may occur as a sequal to endometriosis on rare occasion (Fenn and Abell).

OTHER SITES OF ENDOMETRIOSIS

Uterosacral Ligaments

This location is very common, and this is one of the arguments by those who favor Sampson's theory, inasmuch as endometrial particles regurgitating through the tube might be expected to gravitate toward the cul-de-sac and implant themselves on the uterosacral ligaments. In this region the endometriosis occurs in the form of bluish, somewhat puckered nodules, which may be minute or the size of a walnut so that they may be easily palpable through the vaginal vault. There is the usual perforative tendency of endometriosis, with peritoneal irritation and the formation of dense adhesions to the rectum or adnexa.

Rectovaginal Septum

As an extension of uterosacral endometriosis, one may find endometrial tissue extending downward along the rectovaginal septum, with sometimes enormous infiltration of the rectum and cyclic rectal bleeding. In other cases such growths may penetrate into the vagina (Figs. 25.14, 15), producing *vaginal endometrial polyps* which may bleed with each menstrual period or following such contact as intercourse or douche.

Round Ligaments

These may be involved in the form of small superficial endometrial "implants," or in the form of nodules of adenomyosis, in which both endometrium and muscle are to be found.

Umbilicus (Figs. 25.16–18)

Many cases of umbilical endometriosis have been reported. This group is of

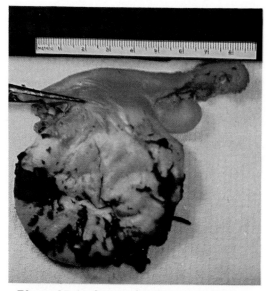

Plate 25.1. Ovary showing superficial endometrial lesion and typical chocolate-colored the other side. Note the puckered appearance produced by the superficial lesions.

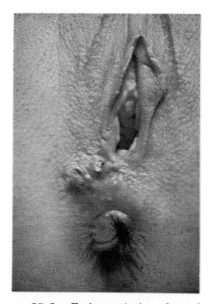

Plate 25.2. Endometriosis of perineum developing in episiotomy scar. The wound had broken down and curettage had been necessary shortly afterward, suggesting probable endometrial implantation. (Courtesy of Dr. G. R. Cheatham, Endicott, New York.)

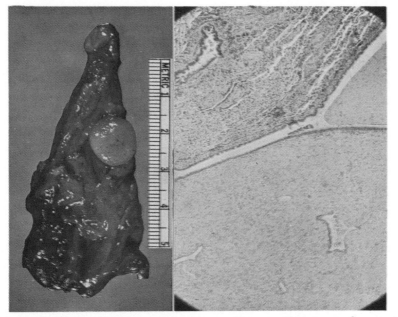

Plate 25.3. Lobectomy during pregnancy because of x-ray diagnosis of lung tumor. Gross and microscopic appearance of decidua in lung. (Courtesy of Dr. R. Lattes.)

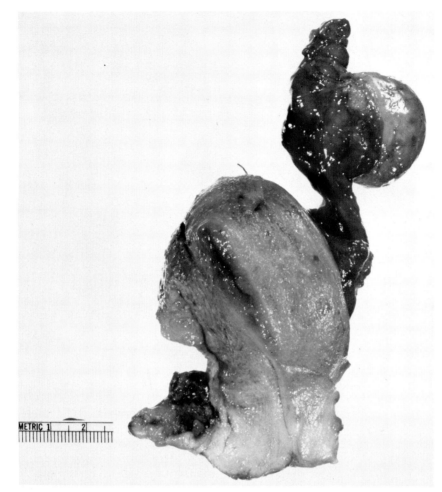

25.14. Typical endometriosis of rectovaginal septum (just above ruler) which had also extended into vagina. Small endometrial cyst of ovary is also present.

interest as it seems impossible to rationalize by Sampson's theory, although explainable by the metaplasia theory, inasmuch as remnants of celomic epithelium are normally found at the umbilicus. More recently, Scott *et al.* have described Cullen's sign occurring with endometriosis due to transplantation of blood and menstrual debris from the peritoneal cavity *via* certain umbilical lymphatics.

Umbilical endometriosis presents in the form of small nodules which may, when they approach the surface be of bluish hue. They increase in size at the menstrual periods, when they become tender, painful, and sometimes break through the skin, with periodic external bleeding.

Laparotomy Scars

This interesting group likewise has evoked much discussion by the proponents of the two principal theories of histogenesis. The postoperative development of endometrial nodules in laparotomy scars, sometimes long after the original operation, may be noted after any type of laparotomy and not, as was originally suggested by some, only in those in which direct implantation of endometrial tissue seemed mechanically possible. As a matter of fact, it is uncommon after cesarean section, although a small group of such cases has been observed. Indeed, endometriosis has been noted in McBurney scars long after appendec-

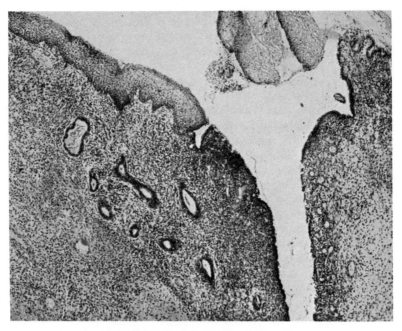

25.15. Endometriosis of vaginal vault

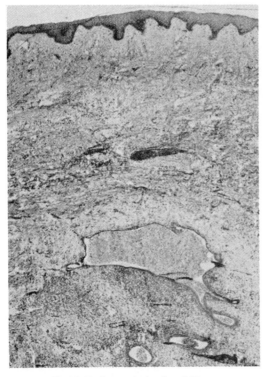

25.16. Endometriosis of umbilicus

tomy in the prepubertal female. The endometrial nodules in laparotomy scars may reach considerable size, and they show the same characteristic cyclic menstrual swelling, pain, tenderness, and sometimes external bleeding described for the umbilical form.

Other Sites

The chief locations have already been enumerated, and it should again be emphasized that any portion of the *pelvic peritoneum* may be involved. In some instances only a single tiny island may be observed, without involvement of the ovaries, and without clinical significance. At the other extreme one may find extensive pelvic dissemination, usually including the ovaries. The appendix, small intestines, rectum, sigmoid, bladder, lymph glands, hernial sacs—any of these may show endometriosis (see Figs. 25.19-22). Complete obstruction at any level of the gastrointestinal tract may occur as described by Williams (in postmenopausal patients). A few cases of

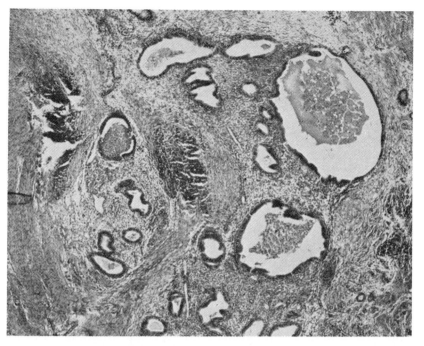

25.17. High power of Figure 25.16

carcinoma of the rectum have been noted with concomitant endometriosis. A case report by Lash and Rubenstone gives due credit to the seven cases reported by Dockerty.

In discussing the urological location of endometriosis Ball and Platt note such complications as intravesical endometrioma, endometriosis of the ureter, etc. with operative damage to the urinary

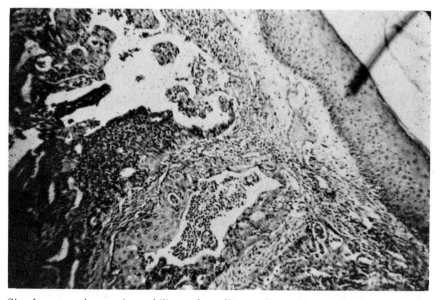

25.18. Simultaneous changes in umbilicus; the solitary other evidence of adenoacanthoma shown in Figure 25.13. Should this be interpreted as a single metastasis or simultaneous acanthosis in two logical sites for endometriosis? We suspect the latter.

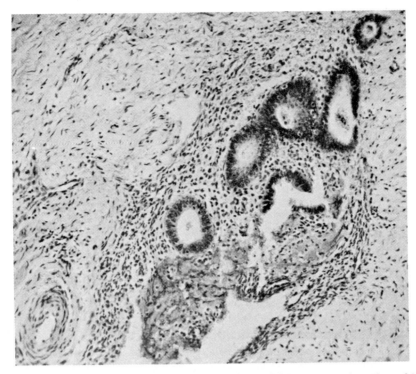

25.19. Endometrioma, measuring $3 \times 3 \times 1$ cm., excised from McBurney scar in patient of 30, whose appendectomy had been done at age of 10, several years before menarche at 13. Such a case would seem to speak against menstrual regurgitation theory and tend to support that of celomic metaplasia. (Courtesy of Dr. Harold Schwarz, Chattanooga, Tennessee.)

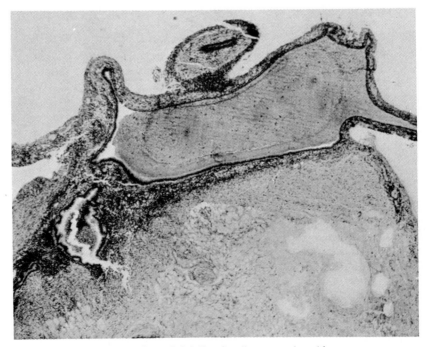

25.20. Superficial "implant" on rectosigmoid

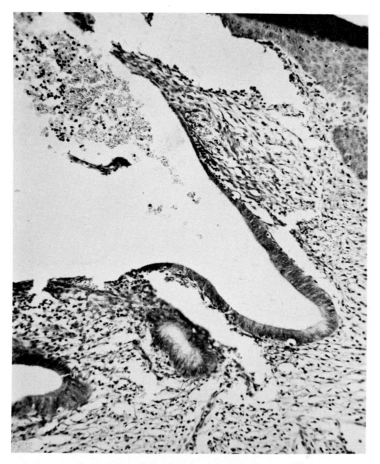

25.21. Endometriosis on surface of pars vaginalis of cervix (see the stratified squamous epithelium above and to the right). Such a picture would justify suspicion of surface implantation although, in many cases of cervical endometriosis that we have seen, the aberrant endometrium has involved deeper tissues and not the surface.

tract in 0.5 per cent of all cases; although minor degrees of the disease are common. Simon *et al.* discuss the possibility of complete ureteral obstruction in their report of 10 cases, including an apparent case of bilateral disease, necessitating reimplantation into the bladder. They urge the utmost discretion in pelvic operations, but seem to advocate major urological surgery rather than castration. Whether this is justified in view of our adequate and diversified means of replacement therapy seems questionable. Endometriosis of the kidney has been observed and would seem to arise from a hematogenous or lymphatic basis (Hajdu and Koss).

The cervix, the vagina, and even the vulva will occasionally harbor endometriosis as may the perineum, especially in the region of episiotomy scars. In reporting 35 cases, Williams and Richardson enlarge on cervical endometriosis, and Novak and Hoge have discussed the occurrence of lower genital tract endometriosis with particular reference to the responsiveness of the surface implants to the progestational hormone. This is in contrast to a frequently refractory endometrial response within the pelvis and may suggest a different etiology.

Finally, there are a number of reported instances of what is apparently unques-

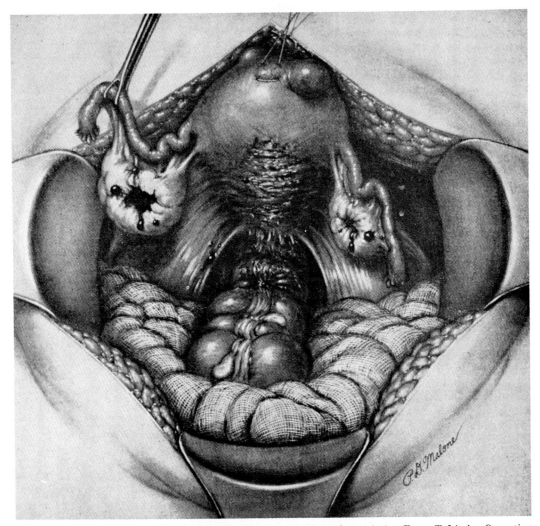

25.22. Uterosacral, rectovaginal, and ovarian involvement in endometriosis. (From TeLinde: *Operative Gynecology,* 3rd ed. J. B. Lippincott Co., Publishers.)

tionable endometriosis of both the upper and lower extremities. One would be inclined to invoke the hematogenous route in the explanation of these bizarre cases except for the difficulty of explaining how the endometrium could get through the pulmonary capillaries if it were transported from the uterus. A mechanism which might possibly be invoked would be the pathway along the vertebral veins or by the lung "shunts" which have apparently been demonstrated between pulmonary arteries and veins, bypassing the capillaries.

Similarly, there have been a few cases in which the pleural cavity or lung was involved. Lattes' patient was pregnant at the time of her thoracotomy, and had a three-year history of intermittent hemoptysis, following previous cesarian section. The removed lung tissue showed classic decidual changes (see Plate 25.3) as well as glands. Park and Hartz have both reported cases in which decidua alone occurred in the lung as a pure embolic phenomenon from the placental site and via the same mechanism as "deportation of villi" (Chapter 27). Williams *et al.* note 11 cases of thoracic endometriosis, but suggest direct extension through a diaphragmatic defect rather than by a hematogenous route.

That endometriosis can be made to develop in the pericardium of dogs has been demonstrated by Sensenig *et al.* After hysterectomy, at which time endometrium was implanted into the pericardium, endometriosis was incurred if the animal was placed on daily stilbestrol for approximately 4 months.

CLINICAL CHARACTERISTICS OF ENDOMETRIOSIS

In most series 75 per cent of the patients with endometriosis are between the ages of 25 and 45. However, Fallon has reported a considerable group below the age of 20, and Schiffrain has also commented on teen-age endometriosis in a more recent publication. There seems no doubt that endometriosis is much more common in the white private patient than in the dispensary clientele. Early or frequent pregnancy with interruption of cyclic menstruation in the clinic patient is suggested as having some kind of guarding effect against the disease, and there is general agreement that pregnancy may incur some regression of endometriosis, although McArthur and Ulfelder have reported 24 cases which do not conform to this thesis.

As to the *incidence,* the condition is not as frequent as was originally suggested by the figures of Sampson, who reported finding 104 instances of endometriosis in a series of 466 patients, the largest group of these representing the ovarian type. In most clinics the incidence is considerably less, and it is obvious that it will vary with the degree of thoroughness of microscopic study.

Although there are no characteristic symptoms, and although in a large proportion of cases none whatsoever are referable to the endometriosis, *disturbances of menstruation* are often present. *Dysmenorrhea* is a frequent symptom, being noted in about one-third of all series studied. It may be moderate or very severe, the latter being the case only when the endometriosis is extensive. When the rectovaginal septum or uterosacral region

is involved, as is so often the case, the dysmenorrhea is often referred to the rectum or to the lower sacral or coccygeal regions. This is due to the premenstrual and menstrual swelling of the endometrium in the uterosacral islands.

In cases of moderate or slight degree, there is ordinarily no *pelvic* or *abdominal pain* or discomfort, but in the more extensive cases these may be present, resembling the symptoms of chronic pelvic inflammatory disease. *Dyspareunia* is often complained of, especially in the cases of uterosacral involvement or vaginal extension (Fig. 25.20). In the same group of cases *constipation* and *pain on defecation* may be noted. However, there is no correlation between the amount of endometriosis and the symptoms. On occasion *minor degrees of the disease lead to severe pain; however, massive amounts of endometriosis are compatible with no symptoms.* Indeed, the clinician is often struck by this disparity which may be difficult to justify to the pathologist.

An endometrial cyst can leak blood, causing considerable pain; perforation may occur and produce a clinical picture much like a ruptured ectopic pregnancy or appendix. Golditch indicates that nearly 10 per cent of cases with endometriosis present with acute symptoms which may require exploration for diagnosis and treatment. Ranney has made similar observations and his contributions on the behavior of endometriosis are recommended for all readers.

Sterility is present in the majority of cases, Sutton giving the proportion as 75 per cent of all cases, and only about 20 per cent of patients have had more than one child. Other authors report an even higher incidence of sterility. The reason for this is not clear, as the tubes are usually patent, although often adherent. Perhaps adhesions around the capsule of the ovary may interfere with the normal mechanics of ovulation. Yet, if pregnancy should occur, the woman may be reassured that, despite her endometriosis, the gestation will not be complicated by the disease, and that, if anything, her symptoms will be improved. Spangler *et al.* have recently reviewed our infertility-endometriosis patients and have indicated the success of conservative surgery.

DIAGNOSIS

It can be seen that no characteristic symptoms are to be expected in endometriosis. This fact, together with the complete absence of symptoms in many cases, and the further fact that endometriosis so often coexists with other lesions which obscure it symptomatically, explains why diagnosis is often difficult or impossible before operation. There are, however, certain helps in diagnosis which may be yielded by history and pelvic examination. The most distinctive of the symptoms, although it is present in only a fraction of the cases, is *menstrual pain referred to the rectum, the lower sacral, or coccygeal regions,* as described above.

In many instances the findings on bimanual examination may be exactly the same as in chronic adnexitis, there being palpable in one or both sides of the pelvis a tender, irregular mass, consisting of the adherent tube and ovary. A successful Rubin's test in equivocal cases will favor the likelihood of endometriosis.

In a certain proportion of cases, however, the internal examining finger reveals *nodular thickening in the uterosacral ligaments,* corresponding to endometrial islands in this location. Sometimes the nodules are small and shotlike, but they may reach the size of a hickory nut and be single or multiple. Such a finding, when noted in a patient who otherwise exhibits the symptoms and signs of chronic pelvic inflammatory disease, should suggest the probability of endometriosis, and usually this suspicion is verified by operation. A fixed retroflexion of the uterus is present in cases of this description, but there are exceptions to this. *It is hazardous to make a diagnosis of endometriosis on the basis of symptoms alone, in the complete absence of palpatory findings.*

TREATMENT

It is our own feeling that symptomatic endometriosis is best treated by surgery.

For *one* thing, the diagnosis of endometriosis by palpation may be difficult, and more than one carcinoma of the ovary has been preceded by conservative management of a presumed endometrial cyst. *Second,* hormone therapy over any long period of time is expensive, often unsatisfactory, sometimes complicated, and never definitive. Indeed, Wharton and Scott have indicated that serious defects occur in the fetal genitalia of monkeys whose mothers were treated by certain hormones during pregnancy. Although this cannot be directly applied to humans, it might suggest caution.

Surgical

In the treatment of endometriosis it is usually accepted that the continued growth and development of the aberrant endometrium is entirely dependent upon the internal secretion of the ovaries, although the Mayo group (Kempers *et al.*) noted significant endometriosis in women up to 79 years. On the other hand, it should be emphasized that only a proportion of all cases of endometriosis justify complete ovarian ablation. More conservative procedures are indicated in many cases, especially in the relatively young women in whom preservation of the childbearing function is of prime importance. Kistner notes that conservative surgery is successful in relieving pain, improving coitus, preventing bleeding, and increasing fertility. The surgeon must, therefore, adapt the treatment to the needs of the individual patient, as indicated in the review by Parsons.

First of all, it should be remembered that *in not a few cases endometriosis is a symptomless condition.* At times, in the course of operations for other indications, the observant surgeon will note tiny patches of endometriosis on the ovary or elsewhere in the pelvis as an incidental finding. When such small areas are noted at operation by the surgeon who has trained himself to detect them, it is probably best, when they are easily accessible, to destroy them with the cautery or to excise them.

When the surgeon encounters a *unilateral endometrial cyst* in a young woman who is very anxious for future pregnancy, it is advisable, as a rule, to remove only the adnexa of the involved side along with a suspension and presacral neurectomy as indicated by symptoms and operative findings. In the majority of cases there is no recurrence of the endometriosis, although there are exceptions to this. Even if there is later recurrence of the trouble, the woman may have had one or more children in the meantime, so that a later more radical procedure will not seem so tragic to her. In numerous patients, however, in whom conservative operations are performed, there has been complete relief, with no recurrence of endometriosis and subsequent pregnancy in 25 to 50 per cent. In others the presence of nodules in the uterosacral regions indicates a persistence of at least mild degrees of endometriosis, although without significant symptoms.

On the other hand, when a unilateral endometrial cyst in encountered in a woman who is approaching the menopausal age, and who has already had all the children she desires, it is probable that most surgeons would be inclined toward hysterectomy, although frequently one ovary may be spared in the young woman without any sequel. Indeed *hysterectomy alone* may often incur prolonged relief of symptoms up to and through the menopause despite conservation of one adnexa. All sorts of individual variations in the problem may arise, and the conservatively inclined surgeon will find that the patient's social and marital status are factors often quite as important in guiding his decision as are the pelvic pathological findings. If a woman has had one conservative procedure, however, any necessary subsequent operation should include castration.

Finally, in the much less common group of *cases in which the endometriosis is very extensive,* with bilateral endometrial cysts, endometrial "implants" at many points in the pelvis, and perhaps adenomyosis of the uterus with firm fixation of the pelvic viscera, nothing short of hysterectomy with bilateral salpingo-oophorectomy may be expected to cure the patient. In such operations the complete removal of ovarian tissue is essential, and if this is accomplished, the patient is reasonably sure to get well even though all endometrial tissue cannot be removed.

Frequently it is impossible to remove all the aberrant endometrium, for it may, for example, infiltrate the bowel wall and perhaps invade the rectovaginal septum. At one time, colostomy was practiced for such cases, but now this is rarely justified, because removal of the ovaries produces regression of the endometrial growth. Occasionally, bowel resection (Fig. ?5.23) is preferable to castration in the young patient, but in this era of oral hormones, such treatment should be rare and generally when the uterus is saved for procreative purposes.

Hormone Therapy Postoperative

Since endometriosis seems dependent on estrogen stimulation, the question often arises as to whether hormone therapy is indicated in the symptomatic post-castrate woman who has had extensive endometriosis. Theoretically it might be expected to stimulate any residual endometrium not removed at surgery. Actually the small dosage of estrogen necessary to suppress vasomotor symptoms would probably not cause en-

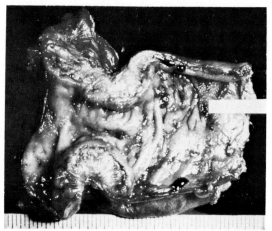

25.23 Bowel resection because of partial obstruction. Intact mucosa with marked extrinsic lesion. (Courtesy of Dr. Edward Ingalls, Minneapolis, Minnesota.)

dometrial activation, although some gynecologists might prefer birth control
(estrogen-progesterone) pills because of
the anti-estrogen effect of progesterone.

Nonsurgical

In a symposium on the treatment of endometriosis, Carter comments on the
protean manifestations of the disease, and
stresses certain considerations before
treating the disease. Above all, the disease
must be proven to be endometriosis, for a
few unfortunate women have had "typical
endometriosis" ultimately proved to be
ovarian carcinoma. The extent of the
disease, childbearing faculties, and
cooperation in regard to long-term follow-
up are likewise important. Like Carter,
we feel that the best treatment for
symptomatic endometriosis (and mandatory if there is an ovarian mass) is
operative intervention. Radiotherapy for
recurrent endometriosis after a diagnosis
has been made seems feasible only in the
bad risk patient, but let us remember that
true neoplasms may occur in any patient,
and the finding of endometriosis at one
operation does not mean that any subsequent ovarian mass is endometrial in
nature.

Hormone therapy has many advocates,
and Kistner's work with the oral progestogens is promising, especially where
there are no adnexal masses and biopsy
proven evidence of cul-de-sac endometriosis. Indeed he finds an 85%
improvement in symptoms where hormones without surgery are utilized. Long
standing amenorrhea, or *"pseudopregnancy,"* with remission of symptoms may
be produced, although the dosage (and
cost) must be continuously increased over
the course of months up to 40 mg. a day
to prevent bleeding (Fig. 25.24). Kistner is
currently using smaller dosages for as long
as a year with a subsequent pregnancy
rate of 40%. However, the recent study by
Andrews and Larsen seems to indicate the
pregnancy rate following conservative surgery is better than that following
progesterone therapy. Small dosage of
testosterone (5 mg. orally) may cause
amelioration of symptoms without

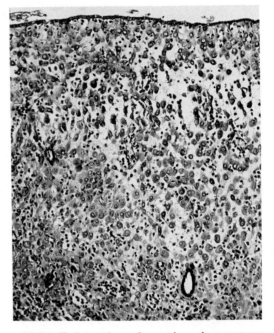

25.24. Endometrium after prolonged progestogen
therapy. Note glandular exhaustion along with decidual reaction and edema.

impairing ovulation and is worth a trial in
the young woman anxious for pregnancy.

It would appear that any hormone
therapy should be temporary and short-
lived. On the basis of experimental work
on monkeys, Scott and Wharton indicate
that the new progestogens are not curative
and should be utilized purely as a tempo-
rizing measure. Our own preference is to
reserve if for those who desire further
pregnancy.

Retroprogesterone is reputedly progestational, although not antiovulatory,
but there has not been wide-spread
usage of this agent in the treatment of endometriosis, although it may be helpful
for dysmenorrhea in the young woman desiring pregnancy. More recently, Danazol,
a derivative of 17-α-ethinyltestosterone,
has been suggested as an inhibitor of
gonadotrophin with resultant anovulation
and amenorrhea. Preliminary studies by
Greenblatt *et al.* and Friedlander suggest
excellent symptomatic results and
improved fertility after a course of
therapy (800 mg daily for 6 months). Side

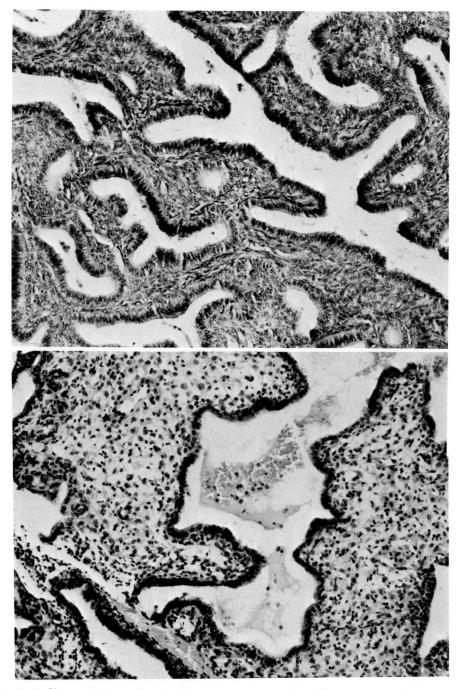

25.25. (*top*) Characteristic endometrioid carcinoma ovary with OTR consensus. (*bottom*) Decidual reaction endometrium incurred by above tumor. Patient had received no hormones. Although estrogen and testosterone effects are observed with various tumors, a progesterone effect is rare in the nonpregnant untreated patient. (Courtesy Dr. Sydney Katz, Trenton, Michigan.)

effects are usually minor, and our limited experience has been favorable.

Lastly, it should be mentioned that endometrioid tumors of the ovary are capable of steriod function even in the postmenopausal era (Fig. 25.25) (see Chapt. 24).

REFERENCES

Acosta, A. A., *et al.*: Proposed classification for endometriosis. Obstet. Gynec., *42:* 19, 1973.

Allen, E., Peterson, L. F., and Campbell, Z. B.: Clinical and experimental endometriosis. Amer. J. Obstet. Gynec., *68:* 356, 1954.

Andrews, W. C., and Larsen, G. C.: Endometriosis; Treatment with hormonal pseudopregnancy and/or operation. Amer. J. Obstet. Gynec., *118:* 643, 1974.

Bachman, E.: Paradoxical metastasis and trans-pulmonary cancer spread. Amer. J. Roentgenol., *72:* 409, 1954.

Ball, T. L., and Platt, M. A.: Urologic complications of endometriosis. Amer. J. Obstet. Gynec., *84:* 1516, 1962.

Barnes, J.: Endometriosis of the pleura and ovaries. J. Obstet. Gynaec. Brit. Comm., *60:* 823, 1953.

Campbell, J. S., Magnen, D., and Fourrier, P.: Adenoacanthomas of ovary and uterus occurring as coexistent on sequential primary neoplasmas. Cancer, *14:* 817, 1961.

Carter, B.: Treatment of endometriosis (as part of a symposium). J. Obstet. Gynaec. Brit. Comm., *69:* 783, 1962.

Cavanagh, W. F.: Endometriosis. Bull. Sloane Hosp., *6:* 115, 1960.

Charles, O.: Endometriosis and hemorrhagic pleural effusion. Obstet. Gynec., *10:* 309, 1967.

Crist, T., Brenner, W. E., and Edwards, J. R.: Adenoacanthoma originating in endometriosis of the ovary. Obstet. Gynec., *37:* 419, 1971.

Czernobilsky, B., and Cornog, J. L.: Squamous predominance in adenoacanthoma. Obstet. Gynec., *37:* 555, 1971.

Davis, C., Jr., and Truehart, R.: Surgical management of endometrioma of the colon. Amer. J. Obstet. Gynec., *89:* 453, 1964.

Dockerty, M. B.: Malignancy complicating endometriosis. Amer. J. Obstet. Gynec., *83:* 175, 1962.

Ecker, J. A., Deere, W. A., and Dickson, Endometriosis of the gastrointestinal tract. Amer. J. Gastroent., *41:* 405, 1964.

Fallon, R.: Endometriosis. Amer. J. Obstet. Gynec., *72:* 557, 1956.

Fathalla, M. F.: Malignant transformation in ovarian endometriosis. J. Obstet. Gynaec. Brit. Comm., *74:* 85, 1967.

Fenn, M. E., and Abell, M. R.: Carcinosarcoma of the ovary. Amer. J. Obstet. Gynec., *110:* 1066, 1971.

Ferreira, H. P., and Clayton, S. G.: Three cases of malignant change in endometriosis, including two cases arising in rectovaginal septum. J. Obstet. Gynaec. Brit. Comm., *64:* 41, 1958.

Fertano, L. R., Hertz, H., and Carter, H.: Malignant endometriosis. Obstet. Gynec., *7:* 32, 1956.

Friedlander, D. L.: The treatment of endometriosis with Danazol. J. Reprod. Med., *10:* 197, 1973.

Gardner, G. H., Greene, R. R., and Ranney, B.: The histogenesis of endometriosis. Amer. J. Obstet. Gynec., *78:* 445, 1958.

Golditch, I. M.: Endometriosis presenting as an acute abdominal emergency. Obstet. Gynec., *26:* 180, 1965.

Gray, L. A.: Endometriosis of the bowel. Southern Med. J., *58:* 815, 1965.

Gray, L. A., and Barnes, M. L.: Relation of endometriosis to carcinoma of the ovary: Report of seven cases. Ann. Surg., *163:* 713, 1966.

Gray, L. A., and Barnes, M. L.: Endometrioid carcinoma of the ovary. Obstet. Gynec., *29:* 694, 1967.

Grayburn, R. W.: Ureteric obstruction due to endometriosis. J. Obstet. Gynaec. Brit. Comm., *67:* 74, 1960.

Greenblatt, R. B., Borenstein, R., and Hernandez, S.: Experiences with danazol in the treatment of infertility. Amer. J. Obstet. Gynec., *118:* 783, 1974.

Greene, J. W., and Enterline, H. T.: Carcinoma arising in endometriosis. Obstet. Gynec., *9:* 417, 1957.

Hajdu, S. I., and Koss, L. G.: Endometriosis of the kidney. Amer. J. Obstet. Gynec., *106:* 314, 1970.

Hanton, E. M., Malkasian, G. D., Jr., Dockerty, M. B., and Pratt, J. H.: Endometriosis in young women. Amer. J. Obstet. Gynec., *98:* 116, 1967.

Hartz, P. H.: Occurrence of decidual-like tissue in the lung. Amer. J. Clin. Path., *26:* 48, 1956.

Hawthorne, H. R., Kimbrough, R. A., and Davis, H. C.: Concomitant endometriosis and carcinoma of the rectosigmoid. Amer. J. Obstet. Gynec., *62:* 681, 1951.

Hughesdon, P. E.: Structure of endometrial cysts of the ovary. J. Obstet. Gynaec. Brit. Comm., *64:* 481, 1957.

Javert, C. T.: Spread of benign and malignant endometrium in the lymphatic system with a note on co-existing vascular involvement. Amer. J. Obstet. Gynec., *64:* 780, 1952.

Kempers, R. D., Dockerty, M. B., Hunt, A. B., and Symmonds, R. E.: Postmenopausal endometriosis. Surg. Gynec. Obstet., *111:* 348, 1960.

Kistner, R. W.: Endometriosis and adenomyosis. Vol. II, Chapter 43, *Gynecology and Obstetrics.* Davis, Hagerstown, Md., 1968.

Kistner, R. W.: Endometriosis. Fert. Steril., *13:* 237, 1962.

Koss, L. G.: Miniature adenoacanthoma arising in an endometriotic cyst in an obturation lymph node. Cancer, *16:* 1369, 1963.

Kottmaier, H. L. (editor): *Annual Report on the Results (1954-63) of Treatment in Carcinoma of the Uterus, Vagina, and Ovary,* Vol. 15, Stockholm, Sweden, 1973.

Kovarik, J. L., and Toll, G. D.: Thoracic endometriosis with recurrent spontaneous pneumothorax. J.A.M.A., *196:* 221, 1966.

Kurman, R. J., and Craig, J. M.: Endometrioid and clear cell carcinoma of the ovary. Cancer, *29:* 1653, 1972.

Labay, G. R., and Femen, F.: Malignant pleural endometriosis. Amer. J. Obstet. Gynec., *109:* 478, 1971.

Lane, R. E.: Endometriosis of the vermiform appendix. Amer. J. Obstet. Gynec., *79:* 372, 1960.

Lash, S. R., and Rubenstone, A. I.: Adenocarcinoma of the rectovaginal septum probably arising from endometriosis. Amer. J. Obstet. Gynec., *78:* 299, 1959.

Lattes, R.: A clinical and pathological study of endometriosis of the lung. Surg. Gynec. Obstet., *103:* 552, 1956.

Long, M. E., and Taylor, H. C.: Endometrioid carcinoma of the ovary. Amer. J. Obstet. Gynec., *90:* 936, 1964.

Malloy, J. J., Dockerty, M. B., Welch, J. S., and Hunt, A. B.: Papillary ovarian tumors. II. Endometrioid cancers and mesonephrome ovary. Amer. J. Obstet. Gynec., *93:* 880, 1965.

McArthur, J. W., and Ulfelder, H.: The effect of pregnancy upon endometriosis. Obstet. Gynec. Survey, *20:* 709, 1965.

McCann, T. O., and Myers, R. E.: Endometriosis in the rhesus monkey. Amer. J. Obstet. Gynec., *106:* 516, 1970.

Meigs, J. V.: An interest in endometriosis and its consequences. Amer. J. Obstet. Gynec., *79:* 625, 1960.

Melody, G. F.: Endometriosis causing obstruction of the ileum. Obstet. Gynec., *8:* 468, 1956.

Merrill, J. A.: Endometrial induction of endometriosis across Milipore filter. Amer. J. Obstet. Gynec., *94:* 780, 1966.

Moore, J. G., Schiffrain, B. S., and Erez, S.: Ovarian tumors in infancy, childhood and adolescence. Amer. J. Obstet. Gynec., *99:* 913, 1967.

Novak, E. R.: Pathology of endometriosis. Clin. Obstet. Gynec., *3:* 413, 1960.

Novak, E. R., and Hoge, A. F.: Endometriosis of the lower genital tract. Obstet. Gynec., *12:* 687, 1958.

Nunn, L. L.: Endometrioma of thigh. Northw. Med., *48:* 474, 1940.

Overton, O. H., Wilson, R. B., and Dockerty, M. B.: Primary endometriosis of the cervix. Amer. J. Obstet. Gynec., *79:* 768, 1960.

Parsons, L.: Conservative surgical management of external endometriosis. Obstet. Gynec., *32:* 576, 1968.

Paul, T., and Tedesch, L. G.: Endometriosis at the site of an episiotomy scar. Obstet. Gynec., *40:* 28, 1972.

Pratt, J. H., and Shamblin, W. R.: Spontaneous rupture of endometrial cysts. Amer. J. Obstet. Gynec., *107:* 76, 1970.

Prince, L. N., and Abrams, J.: Endometriosis of perineum. Amer. J. Obstet. Gynec., *73:* 890, 1957.

Ranney, B.: Endometriosis. I. Conservative operations. Amer. J. Obstet. Gynec., *107:* 743, 1970; II. Emergency operations due to hemoperitoneum. Obstet. Gynec., *36:* 437, 1970; III. Complete operations. Amer. J. Obstet. Gynec., *109:* 1137, 1971; IV. Hereditary tendencies. Obstet. Gynec., *37:* 734, 1971.

Ridley, J. H.: The histogenesis of endometriosis. Obstet. Gynec. Surv., *23:* 1, 1968.

Ridley, J. H.: Primary adenocarcinoma in an implant of endometriosis. Obstet. Gynec., *27:* 261, 1966.

Ridley, J. H.: The validity of Samperson's theory of endometriosis. Amer. J. Obstet. Gynec., *82:* 777, 1961.

Rodman, M. H., and Jones, C. W.: Catamenial hemoptysis due to bronchial endometriosis. New Eng. J. Med., *266:* 805, 1962.

Sampson, J. A.: Perforating haemorrhagic (chocolate) cysts of the ovary. Arch. Surg., *3:* 245, 1921.

Sampson, J. A.: Peritoneal endometriosis due to the menstrual dissemination of endometrial tissue into the peritoneal cavity. Amer. J. Obstet. Gynec., *14:* 422, 1927.

Sampson, J. A.: Pathogenesis of postsalpingectomy endometriosis in laparotomy scars. Amer. J. Obstet. Gynec., *50:* 597, 1962.

Schiffrain, B. S., Erex, S., and Moore, J. G.: Teen-age endometriosis. Amer. J. Obstet. Gynec., *116:* 973, 1973.

Schueller, E. F., and Kirol, P. M.: Prognosis in endometrioid carcinoma of the ovary. Obstet. Gynec., *27:* 850, 1966.

Scott, R. B., and Wharton, L. R., Jr.: Effects of progesterone and norethindrone on experimental endometriosis in monkeys. Amer. J. Obstet. Gynec., *84:* 867, 1962.

Scully, R. E., and Barlow, J. F.: Mesonephroma of the ovary: tumor of Müllerian origin related to the endometrioid carcinoma. Cancer, *20:* 405, 1967.

Sensenig, D. M., Serlin, O., and Hawthorne, H. R.: Pericardial endometriosis: An experimental study in dogs. J.A.M.A., *198:* 645, 1966.

Sheets, J. L., Symmonds, R. E., and Banner, E. A.: Conservative management of endometriosis. Obstet. Gynec., *23:* 625, 1964.

Shmuel, J., Stamler, B., and Suprun, H.: Endometriosis of the appendix with acute symptoms. Int. J. Obstet. Gynec., *8:* 38, 1970.

Simon, H. B., Zimet, R. R., Schneider, E., and Morgenstern, L. L.: Bilateral ureteral obstruction due to endometriosis. J.A.M.A., *183:* 191, 1963.

Spangler, D. B., Jones, G. S., and Jones, H. W.: Infertility due to endometriosis. Amer. J. Obstet. Gynec., *109:* 850, 1971.

Steck, W. D., and Helwig, E. B.: Cutaneous endometriosis. J.A.M.A., *191:* 101, 1965.

Stevenson, C. S. (Editor): Symposium on endometriosis. Clin. Obstet. Gynec., *3:* 411, 1960.

Tate, G. T.: Acute obstruction of the large bowel due to endometriosis. Brit. J. Surg., *50:* 771, 1963.

Te Linde, R. W., and Scott, R. B.: Experimental endometriosis. Amer. J. Obstet. Gynec., *60:* 1147, 1950.

Wharton, L. R., Jr., and Scott, R. B.: Experimental production of genital lesions with norethindrone. Amer. J. Obstet. Gynec., *89:* 701, 1964.

Williams, C., Jr.: Endometriosis of the colon in elderly women. Ann. Surg., *157:* 974, 1963.

Williams, G. A., and Richardson, A. C.: Endometriosis of cervix uteri. Obstet. Gynec., *6:* 309, 1955.

Williams, J. F., Williams, J. B., and Harper, J. W.: Thoracic endometriosis. Amer. J. Obstet. Gynec., *84:* 1512, 1962.

Wynn, T. E.: Endometriosis of the sigmoid. Arch. Path., *92:* 42, 1971.

chapter 26

Ectopic Pregnancy

Definition

The term ectopic pregnancy is applied to pregnancy following implantation of the fertilized egg on any tissue other than the mucous membrane lining the uterine cavity. It is a better and more inclusive term than extrauterine pregnancy, as a pregnancy may be ectopic and yet be situated within the uterus, as in the case of interstitial or cervical pregnancy.

TUBAL PREGNANCY

Much the most common type of ectopic pregnancy is that which occurs in the tube (Fig. 26.1). The latter normally is concerned in the transportation of the fertilized egg to the uterus, but under certain conditions the egg may plant itself on the tube wall. The latter is ill adapted for either satisfactory nidation or later continuance of the gestation, so that with rare exceptions the embryo succumbs at an early stage.

Etiology

The causes ascribed for tubal pregnancy may be placed in two chief groups, *viz.,* (1) factors which delay or prevent the passage of the fertilized egg into the uterine cavity; and (2) factors which

increase the receptiveness of the tubal mucosa to the fertilized egg.

(1) Factors Which Delay or Prevent Passage of Fertilized Egg into Uterine Cavity. This is probably the more important of the two groups of causes. Partial obstruction of the tube by *chronic salpingitis* is most often concerned, not only because of the mechanical factor but also because of the impairment of sperm capacitation, ciliary activity, and muscle peristalsis, all so important in the propagation of the egg. The study by Kleiner and Roberts would support this concept. Follicular salpingitis especially is believed to be a frequent cause, because of the formation of blind gutters into which a fertilized egg may stray.

Articles by Halbrecht and by Nokes *et al.* have pointed out that any pregnancy ensuing after *chemotherapy for pelvic tuberculosis* is likely to be ectopic in nature. Halbrecht reports an astounding 66 per cent incidence of extrauterine pregnancies in patients becoming pregnant after antituberculous treatment, and he feels that a significant cause of ectopic pregnancy in general is spontaneous healing of unrecognized tubal tuberculosis, whereas the scarring and fibrosis may be a factor in

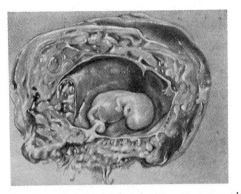

26.1. Cut surface of tubal pregnancy sac at $2\frac{1}{2}$ months showing embryo alive at time of operation.

the production of partial obstruction. This entity must be extremely less common in the United States than in Israel. A few cases of *post-laparoscopy* gestations in the tube have occurred in this area; how common this is will not be known for a few years.

Congenital abnormalities of the tube, especially diverticula and accessory ostia, may likewise be concerned, as may also be *partial occlusion by adhesions or tumors* outside the tube. Persaud records a high incidence of diverticula and believes this to be the most frequent cause of tubal gestation. Finally, the occasional role of *transmigration of the ovum* is indicated by the fact that the gestation may occur in the tube opposite to the ovary containing the corpus luteum of pregnancy.

Implantation does not occur until after the burrowing apparatus, the trophoblast, has developed, and this normally takes place after the egg has reached the uterus. Retardation of its progress is probably an important factor in tubal pregnancy, permitting development of the trophoblast while the egg is still in the tube. Iffy has concluded that pregnancy may antedate the last menstrual period (LMP) and has provided a very persuasive correlation between the last menstrual period, the measurements of the early embryo, and any observations on the dates of coitus. His suggestion that menstruation may dislodge an early implantation with subsequent expulsion through the cornu and secondary tubal pregnancy is difficult to

accept or deny. Because, however, pathological examination of tubes removed during menstrual bleeding only rarely reveals endometrium, it would seem that Iffy's suggestion explains only a minority of cases of tubal gestation.

(2) Factors Increasing Receptiveness of Tubal Mucosa to Fertilized Egg. The second group of causes is less clearly demonstrable, although of undoubted importance in some cases. In some instances areas of *typical endometrium may be found in the tube,* and in such cases it is easy to understand how a fertilized egg may implant itself. Again, in certain cases of tubal pregnancy a greater or less degree of *decidual response* can be demonstrated histologically, indicating a responsiveness at least approaching that of the endometrium.

Incidence

Whereas it has been frequently quoted that one out of 300 pregnancies is ectopic, Fontanilla and Anderson, in an excellent statistical study, indicate that the occurrence is considerably more frequent. In Baltimore, ectopic gestation occurs once in 200 pregnancies among white women, once in 120 among black patients, nearly an 80 per cent difference. The authors feel strongly that inflammatory disease is the responsible factor, and obviously consideration of any reported incidence should include the racial percentages. Breen's New Jersey study records one ectopic to every 87 deliveries in an 85% black group of women.

The recent study by Bobrow and Bell from the Harlem Hospital in New York notes one ectopic pregnancy to every 64 live births, which would indicate the highest ratio ever recorded for any large American series, and approaches the figure of one ectopic in 28 pregnancies reported from Jamaica by Douglas. That repeat ectopic pregnancy may recur in the remaining tube in approximately 10 per cent of cases (Schiffer) has been accepted by most gynecologists, although normal intrauterine gestation is much more common (approximately 25%).

Pathology

Once the fertilized egg has implanted itself on the tubal mucosa, the early nidation changes are much like those seen in uterine pregnancy, except for an absence of the striking decidual reaction in the endometrium. The erosive action of the villous trophoblast causes penetration of the tubal wall, and this may extend through the muscularis. The invasion of blood vessels causes bleeding into the lumen, the tubal wall, or the peritoneal cavity. The environment is therefore a very unfavorable one, and the embryo usually succumbs within a few weeks, although a certain number of *full term, viable tubal pregnancies* are on record, and are diagnosed by hysterogram and sonar.

Bleeding into the lumen of the tube converts the latter into a *hematosalpinx* (Fig. 26.2). Indeed, when hematosalpinx is found at operation or in the laboratory the first thought should always be of tubal pregnancy. When the latter is in the outer portion of the tube, the fimbriated orifice may be distended by an extruding blood clot.

Microscopically, the pathognomonic feature of tubal pregnancy is the *finding of chorionic villi* (Fig. 26.3) in the blood-filled lumen, sometimes penetrating the wall. The villi may be well preserved or they may show marked degeneration and hyalinization, although even then the characteristic outline is sharply preserved. However, care should be taken not to mistake for villi the organized thrombi not infrequently seen. The latter

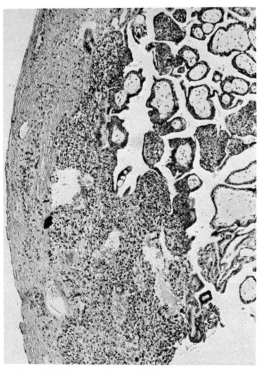

26.3. Tubal pregnancy with numerous young villi and marked trophoblastic invasion of tubal wall which is often mistaken for decidua (*below right*).

show an absence of any cellular stromal structure and of an epithelial covering. Even old villi, on the other hand, are likely to show a flattened degenerated epithelium and some persistence of cellular structure in the stroma.

When the villi are well preserved, they show the characteristic histological features of young villi. Two layers of trophoblastic epithelium are seen on the surface. The inner (layer of Langhans or *cytotrophoblast*) is cuboidal, the outer *syncytium* is represented by a thin ribbon of cytoplasm with nuclei placed at regular intervals although no cell differentiation is seen. As in uterine pregnancy, the Langhans layer often shows a localized heaping up (trophoblastic nodules) and the syncytium shows frequent budding outgrowth, cross sections of which constitute the so-called syncytial or placental giant cells. These contain large, dark staining nuclear masses, often multiple.

There has been much discussion as to

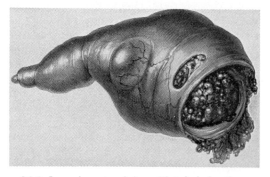

26.2. Large hematosalpinx with tubal abortion

the frequency of a *decidual reaction* (Figs. 26.4, 5) in the tube. That genuine decidual response may occur is certain, and for that matter, even with uterine pregnancy one may, in rare instances, find fields of typical decidual cells in the tube. On the other hand, there is also no doubt that trophoblastic cells invading the tubal wall are often mistaken for decidual cells, especially where only cytotrophoblast is evident, for this is not nearly so distinctive as the mature syncytial cell. Finally, even when a decidual response is demonstrated, as it is in a minority of cases, it is always of patchy and incomplete nature, in contrast to the massive and uniform response seen in the uterus.

Possible Terminations of Tubal Pregnancy

(1) Tubal Rupture. This may occur as a result of the erosive action of the trophoblast, with bleeding into the peritoneal cavity, sometimes slight, sometimes profuse or even fatal. As a result of the

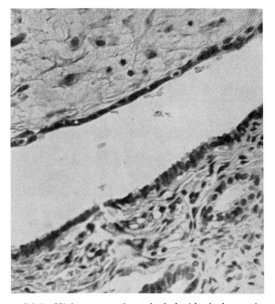

26.5. High power of marked decidual change in tubal fold (*above*) well removed from implantation site.

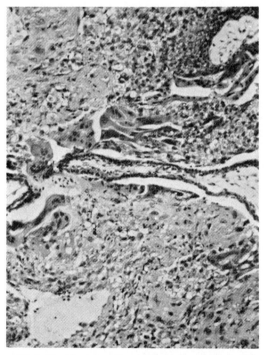

26.4. Decidual reaction in the tube which in this section is distinguishable from trophoblastic invasion.

rupture of the imperfectly formed capsularis, *intratubal hemorrhage* (Fig. 26.6) takes place. In both conditions there may be free bleeding from the fimbriated end of the tube, although tubal perforation generally produces much more massive hemoperitoneum.

(2) Tubal Abortion. This refers to an actual separation of the ovum from the tubal wall, with bleeding from the fimbriated orifice, which may be stuffed with clots. Tubal abortion is frequently unrecognized, with only minor degrees of bleeding that ceases spontaneously (Fig. 26.7).

(3) Secondary Abdominal Pregnancy. The older descriptions of secondary abdominal pregnancy would lead one to believe that when tubal rupture occurs, the product of conception may be expelled into the abdomen, and reimplant itself upon the peritoneal surface of the tube, broad ligament, or small intestine. Such a reimplantation is obviously impossible; instead more and more of the still attached placenta emerges, to grow external to the tube. Finally, the whole placenta is weaned away from the tubal lumen and continues its growth externally

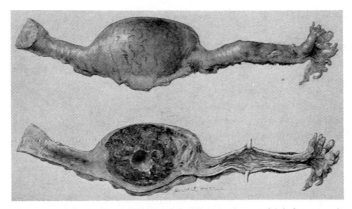

26.6. Unruptured tubal pregnancy but with intratubal hemorrhage which has terminated the life of the egg.

on the peritoneal surface, perhaps even to full term, although this is rare.

(4) Broad Ligament or Intraligamentary Pregnancy. When the tubal perforation is along the line of attachment of the mesosalpinx, the embryo escapes between the folds of the broad ligament, and is gradually followed by the still attached placenta, as described in the pre-

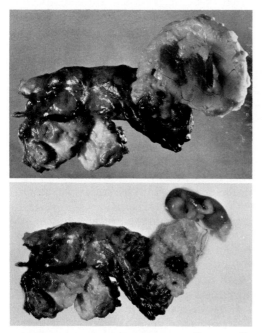

26.7. (*top*). Tubal abortion protruding out fimbria. (*bottom*). Opened specimen.

ceding paragraph. Such pregnancies may advance to late stages, and in a considerable number have progressed to full term.

(5) Spontaneous Regression. A good many tubal pregnancies undoubtedly pass unrecognized, and never reach operation at the time, but come to laparotomy at a later date for various reasons. On occasion there is evidence in the tubes of old hyalinized villi long after a possible pregnancy (Figs. 26.8, 9). Careful retrospective analysis of the histories of such patients often elicits the probability of a tubal gestation, perhaps many years previously. In such cases the embryo has evidently succumbed at a very early phase, with retrogression of the placenta, and with symptoms not severe or acute enough to compel medical attention.

(6) Mummification of the Fetus. This may occur in unrecognized ruptured tubal pregnancies which have advanced to a later stage, whereas in other cases extensive *calcification* may convert it into a so-called *lithopedion*. On occasion fetal bones may be passed vaginally, rectally, or through an abdominal sinus tract.

(7) Term Abdominal Pregnancy. A number of these cases have occurred, and are only occasionally diagnosed as an abdominal pregnancy. A hysterogram may be helpful if one is quite certain the pregnancy is extrauterine; sonar may likewise be informative.

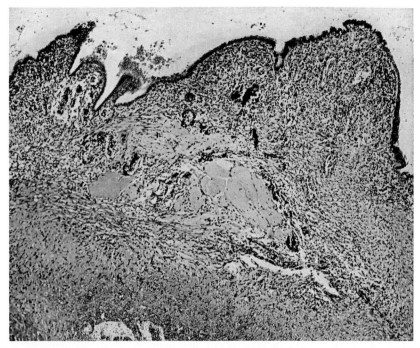

26.8. Old hyalinized villi found in tubal wall of patient operated on for another indication, and representing remains of tubal pregnancy which had occurred long before.

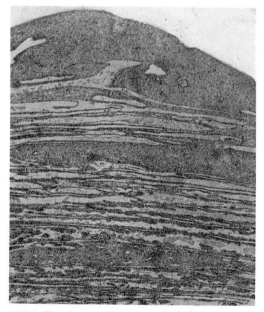

26.9. Decidua vera in a case of tubal pregnancy in which the embryo was living at $2\frac{1}{2}$ months (case pictured in Figure 26.1). Note the superficial compacta with its broad fields of decidual cells, and the spongiosa made up largely of very tortuous glands here shown running parallel with the surface, as is often the case. The basalis is not shown.

Behavior of Uterine Mucosa in Cases of Tubal Pregnancy

No matter where a pregnancy is located, the uterine mucosa responds by a decidual reaction (Fig. 26.10) to the hormonal stimuli set in motion by the implanted egg. As long as the latter is alive, this decidual reaction in the uterus is maintained. With the death of the embryo, however, the uterine decidua is cast off, generally piecemeal and in fragments, but on occasion as a single cast of the uterine cavity. When an entire cast is passed, the patient usually believes she has had a miscarriage, and the same error is frequently made by her physician.

One must remember that a decidual reaction in the endometrium is present in only about one-third of the patients with a tubal pregnancy on whom a curettage is performed, because in many instances fetal death and subsequent passage of the

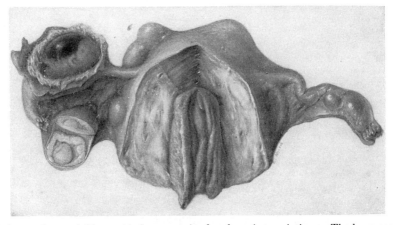

26.10. Tubal gestation sac laid open to show contained embryo in amniotic sac. The large corpus luteum of pregnancy is seen in the ovary of the same side, while the interior of the uterus shows the very thick decidua.

decidua has allowed the re-establishment of ovulation and any type of endometrial pattern. In addition, the finding of a decidual reaction, without villi, is not pathognomonic of a tubal pregnancy. Even in the absence of pregnancy some endometria can overrespond in an exaggerated fashion to contraceptive pills or the usual progestational hormones to produce a decidua-like appearing endometrial pattern.

Arias-Stella Reaction

In 1954 Arias-Stella described certain endometrial glandular changes supposedly pathognomonic of pregnancy whether intra- or extrauterine, or as a result of trophoblastic disease. These changes are characterized by cellular enlargement with significant hyperchromatosis, pleomorphism, and mitotic activity, a tendency for the cellular lining to be almost decapitated so that the nucleus is exfoliated into the gland lumen, and a generalized tendency to appear neoplastic (Figs. 26.11, 12). These changes are usually focal and associated with a stromal decidual change and a hypersecretory glandular pattern, although this is not invariably so. Indeed it has been stressed by many authors that these ASR changes can be very helpful in making a diagnosis of an ectopic pregnancy even though the endometrium shows no other evidence of potential pregnancy and may appear as proliferative, interval, etc.

It should be noted that Sturgis adequately described and depicted these endometrial changes long before Arias-Stella. In a recent publication Sturgis has pointed out without rancor and with amusement that his several publications have long preceded the articles by Arias-Stella, and review of his material leaves little doubt. While it may be difficult to get away from the established term "ASR," one should recognize Sturgis' pioneer work.

The incidence of the ASR in conjunction with an ectopic or other pregnancy varies tremendously in different laboratories from less than 5% to nearly 75%, as noted by numerous authors. It has been observed as early as 22 days after the last missed period. As to how late in pregnancy it may present or how long it may persist after fetal death seems open to considerable question. With the ever increasing frequency of therapeutic abortion and hysterectomy for abortion-sterilization there is ample opportunity to study the gravid endometrium. It is our belief that the ASR is rarely apparent after 14–16 weeks of pregnancy, perhaps due to glandular exhaustion, and that it does not persist longer than 4–6 weeks after fetal death. As has been noted by many authors, it seems just as common after therapeutic as after spontaneous abortion, which would imply that it represents a response to trophoblast rather than a degenerative sequel.

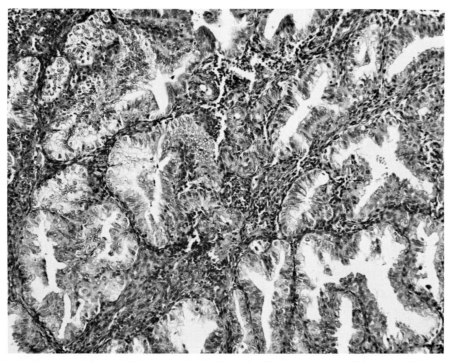

26.11. Adenomatous pattern with intraluminal tufting of tall pale secretory cells; some cellular atypia and mitotic activity present in this *Arias-Stella reaction.*

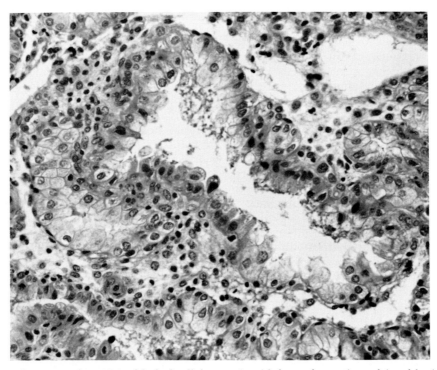

26.12. Higher power than 26.11. Marked cellular atypia with hyperchromatic nuclei and beginning extrusion into gland lumen.

Where there is evidence of an abortion or an intrauterine pregnancy, so that the pathologist is alerted to look for an ASR, it is often impossible to establish that diagnosis. Indeed in many respects we rue the day when Arias-Stella presented his findings. When the tissue reveals a florid and readily apparent pattern, there is no problem. However, one becomes a little irritated at the clinician with no pathological background who palpates an adnexal mass at the time of curettage, and sends his specimen to the laboratory with the accompanying note "rule out pregnancy."

If the clinician had any inkling of what a borderline subjective diagnosis this is (as indicated by the less than 5% to over 75% frequency recorded in various laboratories), perhaps he would not be so optimistic. In only a very small minority of cases is the pathological picture so obvious that it may be possible to specifically state that an ASR is present. In the majority the report must be something like "hypersecretory endometrium with possible ASR." The clinician should remember that this has been noted after contraceptive pills, clomiphene, and occasionally as a physiological response to the hormones elaborated during a normal cycle. While highly suggestive, it is not pathognomonic of pregnancy.

Pildes and Wheeler have described such endometrial patterns as highly suggestive of an adenocarcinoma, and to the novice pathologist this would be an easy mistake. Roach, Guderian, and Brewer also comment on this atypical picture which of course reverts to normal following termination of the pregnancy. Wagner and Richert find that polyploidy is a common finding in the endometrium with the Arias-Stella pattern, unlike the aneuploidy or diploidy often found with adenocarcinoma. Electron microscopy (de Brux and Ancia) suggests the microscopic appearance is due to an excessive secretory action with absence of glycogen.

Expulsion of a decidual cast (Figs. 26.13, 14) in cases of tubal pregnancy signifies the death of the embryo, but a considerable interval, often several days, may elapse before the cast is thrown off.

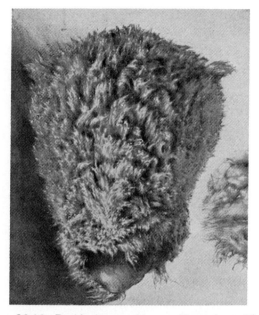

26.13. Decidual case thrown off at about 6th week of extrauterine pregnancy.

Most cases of tubal pregnancy do not come under observation until after the embryo has succumbed, sometimes not until weeks afterward. The endometrium in the meantime has regenerated itself, so that if it is examined at the time of operation for tubal pregnancy, it may show little or no suggestion of decidual change. For this reason, *curettage* and microscopic examination of the endometrium *is of limited value* in the diagnosis of tubal pregnancy; nevertheless, it may be helpful if the clinician is aware of its shortcomings, and it should present the opportunity for examination under anesthesia.

If the embryo is still viable, typical decidua may be obtained on curettage, with no villi. Often the curettage is contraindicated under such circumstances, as there is usually scant external bleeding, and the possibility of early uterine gestation cannot be eliminated. When, on the other hand, curettage is performed in patients who have been bleeding for many days or weeks, the endometrium may be entirely normal (Fig. 26.15) or it may still show a persistence of decidual change, depending on the time which has elapsed since embryonic death.

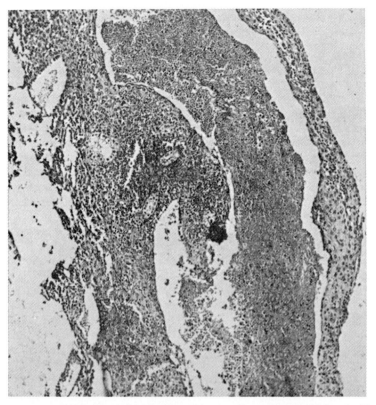

26.14. Structure of a decidual cast. In other cases the cast shows a much thicker decidual layer.

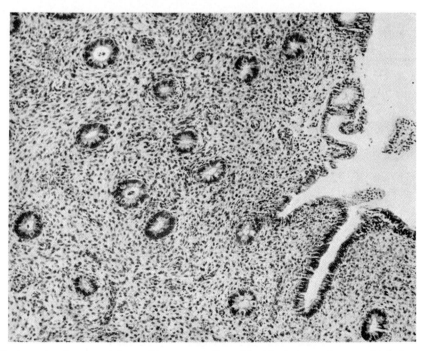

26.15. Postmenstrual endometrium with no suggestion of decidual change in case of tubal pregnancy. In other cases more or less pronounced decidual change may still be present.

As already intimated, the external bleeding so common with tubal pregnancy is generally of uterine origin, but there are exceptions to this, as in the case of interstitial pregnancy (Fig. 26.16). Even with a living embryo in the tube, slight bleeding may at times be noted, probably due to "ovular unrest" at the implantation area. There is rather general acceptance of the view that the persistent slight bleeding characterizing most cases of tubal pregnancy is of endometrial origin, and that it is initiated by separation of the decidua.

Pregnancy Tests in Tubal Gestation

The universal use of the various tests of pregnancy has been of only slight diagnostic value in cases of suspected tubal pregnancy. Not only must one distinguish by other methods between uterine and extrauterine gestation if the test is positive, but one must remember that a negative test by no means excludes the possibility of tubal pregnancy. Where large dosage of progesterone (such as Produosterone) have been utilized as a pregnancy test, the results have been varied, with bleeding only on occasion.

Symptoms and Signs

The first symptom noted by the patient is apt to be a 7- to 14-day *delay in menstruation,* followed by slight bleeding which persists, with perhaps only a scant show of blood almost every day. Although this *spotting type of bleeding* is rather characteristic, not infrequently the bleeding may be somewhat freer, but rarely so profuse as with an incomplete abortion. Again, instead of the menstrual period being delayed, there may be an ap-

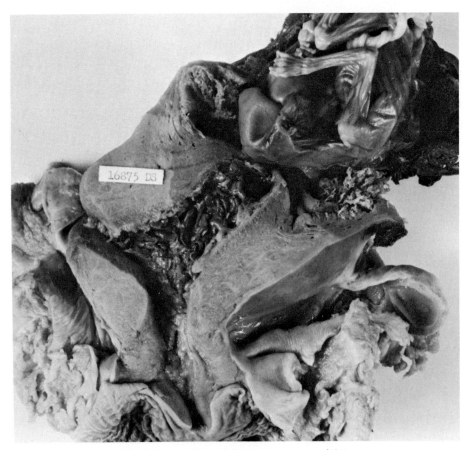

26.16. Interstitial tubal gestation (*upper right*)

parent anticipation of the flow by a few days. In still other cases, where the embryo survives sufficiently long, amenorrhea may continue for two or even three months, or in the rare cases of ectopic pregnancy which continue to term, for the full duration of the pregnancy.

Pain is an early symptom although sometimes very slight. In the beginning there may be only a vague soreness in the affected side of the pelvis, but often the patient complains of sharp colicky pain occurring from time to time. When rupture or tubal abortion takes place, the pain may be very severe, and associated with faintness or actual syncope, and often nausea and vomiting. These symptoms are the result of the peritoneal reaction produced by the escape of blood from the tube. Pain in the right shoulder may be noted, as a result of the diaphragmatic reflex excited by free blood in the peritoneal cavity. *Expulsion of a cast* may or may not be noticed by the patient.

When the hemorrhage is slight, the pain may subside quickly, leaving only *soreness.* With recurrence of bleeding repeated attacks may occur. If the intraperitoneal bleeding is very profuse, *symptoms of shock* occur, *viz.,* a rapid, thready pulse, extreme pallor of the skin and mucous membranes, air-hunger, a cold, clammy skin, and a subnormal temperature. In the occasional case in which prompt treatment is not instituted, death may occur in a short time. In only a small proportion of cases, about 5 per cent, is the intraperitoneal bleeding of such cataclysmic proportions, the hemorrhage being much more often of the moderate and repeated type. Most cases, for that matter, are of the ambulatory type, and Parker and Parker aptly described "*chronic ectopics*" with various types of pelvic hematocele but without acute symptoms.

Subjective signs of pregnancy, such as morning nausea and enlargement of the breasts, are not often seen because of the usually early termination of the gestation, although in later cases they may be noted. *Laboratory findings* are of little value in the cases with moderate internal bleeding, with the possible exception of the pregnancy tests, already discussed. When bleeding is free, the hemogram shows varying degrees of anemia, with a low hematocrit. Under such conditions slight leukocytosis is the rule, rarely exceeding a white cell count of 12,000. When the blood loss is great, however, the degree of leukocytosis is apt to be higher. The temperature with mild bleeding may be normal, but with more abundant hemorrhage it is slightly elevated, although with extreme hemoperitoneum, it is subnormal.

Physical Signs. *Abdominal examination* may be entirely negative or there may be only slight tenderness over the lower abdomen, usually more marked on one side. When the stage of the pregnancy or the intratubal bleeding makes the tubal mass correspondingly large, it may even be felt through the lower abdominal wall, if this is very thin and lax, but this is unusual. *Percussion* comes into valuable play in cases in which free abdominal bleeding is suspected, and it frequently gives evidence, especially by dullness in the flanks, of free fluid in the abdomen.

Even *inspection* may be of value in the occasional case. Where there has been repeated bleeding into the abdomen for a considerable time, a bluish, bruise-like discoloration may be found surrounding the umbilicus (*Cullen's sign*), especially if the latter is very thin or if there is an umbilical hernia. This sign, only rarely observed, is due to deposit of blood pigment absorbed by way of the lymphatics in the umbilical region. *Tympanites* and *abdominal distention* are not infrequently associated with free abdominal bleeding.

Pelvic Examination. Of the greatest importance are the findings on pelvic examination. The cervix may become patulous and softened. The uterus may enlarge slightly (Fig. 26.10), even in early tubal pregnancy, but this is rarely noticeable in the average case. Where the tubal mass is large, the uterus may be pushed somewhat to one side. The distinctive finding is the presence of a *tender mass on one side of the pelvis.* The opposite side of the pelvis may show no demonstrable abnormalities, although not infrequently there may be evidence of chronic adnexitis. Where bleeding into the pelvis has been profuse, *pelvic hematocele* is produced, with a doughy consistency in the cul-de-sac.

Diagnosis

The clinical picture of tubal pregnancy is so typical in many cases that diagnosis is very easy, but many errors are made, and it may well be considered a disease of diagnostic surprises. The physician who has extrauterine pregnancy "on the brain" will rarely fail to diagnose it when it exists. On the other hand, one who is not alert to its possibility will meet with many surprises which greater care could have avoided.

When a woman presents herself with a history of slight spotting beginning a few days after an expected missed period, with pain in one side of the pelvis, and when examination in such a patient reveals a unilateral tender pelvic mass, the first thought should be of tubal pregnancy, and often this will prove to be the case. *Pelvic aspiration or puncture* (culdocentesis) with a large bore needle or *endoscopy* is of frequent value; the former where there is some degree of hemoperitoneum, the latter if the tube is unruptured. Indeed, the physician's familiarity with the culdoscope or laparoscope (Steptoe) will spare many patients needless laparotomy in many of the conditions noted below. *Posterior colpotomy* is likewise helpful, and occasionally definitive treatment can be carried out via this approach, although we do not believe in the usual adnexal surgery per vagina.

The conditions with which tubal pregnancy is most easily confused are: (1) incomplete or threatened abortion of intrauterine pregnancy, (2) pelvic inflammatory disease, (3) ovarian cyst with twisted pedicle, (4) corpus luteum or follicle cyst, and (5) torsion of adnexa. The percentage of error given by all authors is quite large, varying from 15 per cent to as much as 35 per cent.

(1) Uterine Pregnancy with Threatened or Incomplete Abortion. The amenorrhea preceding the beginning of bleeding is almost always of longer duration than with tubal pregnancy, the uterus is likely to be larger and softer, the pain less severe and situated in the midline rather than on one side of the pelvis, and the bleeding generally more profuse in the case of incomplete abortion. Not infrequently there is associated expulsion of portions of obviously placental tissue and no such unilateral enlargement is palpable as is characteristic of tubal gestation. In cases of ectopic pregnancy the degree of anemia is out of all proportion to the external blood loss if free intraperitoneal hemorrhage has occurred, whereas with incomplete abortion the blood picture more or less parallels the blood loss. Nevertheless, errors are not infrequent.

(2) Pelvic Inflammatory Disease. This may simulate tubal pregnancy, and *vice versa.* Perhaps most important in the diagnosis is the fact that salpingitis is commonly bilateral, although the enlargement may be predominantly unilateral. There may be metrorrhagia, but this is far less common than is the spotty bleeding so characteristic of tubal pregnancy. In the more acute cases of salpingitis the fever, the higher leukocytosis, and the increased sedimentation rate are all of value in diagnosis, but these evidences of infection are rarely apparent with an old hydrosalpinx.

(3) Ovarian Cyst with Twisted Pedicle. The sudden onset of pain, with often nausea and vomiting, may resemble the severe pain of tubal rupture or abortion, but there is frequently no menstrual abnormality. Pregnancy tests are of dubious value, and the surgeon will generally operate without waiting for these, because of the urgency of the condition and the fact that surgery is indicated in any event (Fig. 26.17).

(4) Lutein or Follicle Cysts. These may cause delay in menstruation followed by persistent slight bleeding, just as does tubal pregnancy. Moreover, the

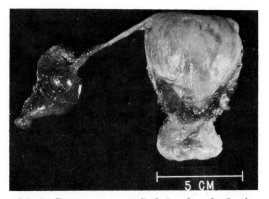

26.17. Pregnancy near fimbriated end of tube. This would be difficult to distinguish from an ovarian cyst.

enlargement of the ovary constitutes a unilateral mass sometimes difficult to distinguish from that of a tubal gestation. Such cases may represent very early abortion of possibly even an unimplanted egg, and the corpus luteum cyst may in reality be a cystic corpus luteum of pregnancy.

Actually, the corpus luteum with a normal intrauterine pregnancy may occasionally bleed into the peritoneal cavity, and massive degrees of hemoperitoneum may occur. The bleeding may be so scant as not to warrant operative intervention, but may well be the cause of the not infrequent pains that the obstetrician may find difficult to explain in the first trimester.

On occasion, hemorrhage may be very profuse and may simulate the shocklike pattern seen in certain forms of ruptured tubal pregnancy. Although such symptoms as external bleeding and pelvic mass are lacking, the natural suspicion in the presence of alarming intraabdominal bleeding is of tubal pregnancy, and this is the diagnosis usually made. In cases of abdominal bleeding of ovarian origin which are of moderate degree, the suspicion of their true nature is often confused by the absence of amenorrhea, external bleeding, or demonstrable pelvic mass, but in most cases laparotomy is indicated.

(5) Torsion of Tube or Adnexa. This is another rare occurrence and not usually associated with menstrual abnormalities. It has been fully discussed in earlier chapters.

Treatment

Once tubal pregnancy has been diagnosed, the indication for surgical treatment is clear. Even in patients who are ambulatory, and whose symptoms are relatively mild, there should be no undue delay in recommending operation, because of the ever present possibility of life-endangering hemorrhage from tubal rupture or abortion. In the comparatively small proportion of cases in which such alarming hemorrhage has occurred, the operation should be performed at once. In such cases, transfusion before or during the operation is of prime importance.

It is generally preferable to spare the ovary and remove just the tube, excising the cornu to avoid subsequent pregnancy in the cornual stump. Because there is little doubt that the woman with one ectopic gestation is more likely to have another, conservation of the ovary where possible seems desirable. When the second tube must be removed for a second tubal pregnancy, hysterectomy is generally preferable in the good risk, sensible woman. Appendectomy is routine, even with a ruptured ectopic gestation, unless contraindicated by the general condition of the patient.

We feel strongly that excision of the pregnancy or salpingostomy with reparative procedures should be a rather unusual treatment for tubal pregnancy. Plastic surgery on the tube, even under ideal circumstances, is attended by a mediocre number of full term pregnancies, although a "repeat ectopic" in the operated tube is not unusual. Indeed, we have seen a woman with three ectopics in two years, the last of which was treated by hysterectomy with complete accord by the patient.

In any case, Grant feels that irrespective of the operative procedure utilized, subsequent fertility will be much impaired because of damage to the unremoved or uninvolved tube. This damage seems a sequel to the irritating blood clot in the tube and the adjacent peritoneum which leads to fibrosis and obstructive adhesions.

However, it would seem that removal of the products of conception with conservation of the tube should be confined to the woman who has had the other tube removed and who is anxious fur further pregnancy, as indicated by the study by Timonen and Niemonen. Let us remember that many women have a tubal pregnancy and subsequently deliver per vagina with no problems.

OTHER TYPES OF ECTOPIC PREGNANCY

Interstitial (Cornual)

In this rare form, the pregnancy is located in that portion of the tube which traverses the uterine wall. Diagnosis is difficult and is most likely mistaken for a soft myoma, with perhaps an early abortion of an intrauterine pregnancy. The symptoms are similar to those of tubal pregnancy, although the pain may not be as severe and the amenorrhea preceding any vaginal bleeding a little prolonged due to a more favorable implantation site. Should rupture occur, intraperitoneal bleeding may be very profuse (Figs. 26.18, 19).

Ovarian Pregnancy

This is extremely rare, and until recent years its occurrence was doubted. There is now, however, a considerable group of well authenticated cases; and these have been reviewed by Tan and Yeo. The generally accepted criteria of diagnosis

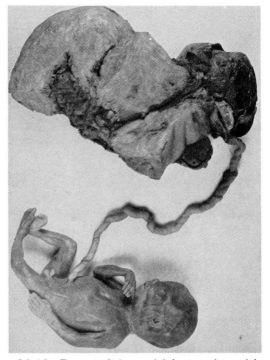

26.19. Ruptured interstitial gestation with embryo.

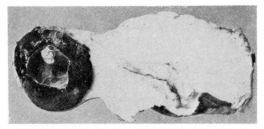

26.18. Cut surface of uterus and cornual pregnancy. Note the thick decidua still in situ although evidences of its impending separation are already present.

are those originally postulated by Spiegelberg. They are: (1) that the tube, including the fimbria ovarica, be intact and the former clearly separate from the ovary, (2) that the gestation sac definitely occupy the normal position of the ovary, (3) that the sac be connected with the uterus by the ovarian ligament, and (4) that unquestionable ovarian tissue be demonstrable in the walls of the sac. (Figs., 26.20–22).

The rarity of ovarian pregnancy, in view of the ready accessibility of the ovary to the spermatozoa and the portals offered by ruptured follicles, is probably due to the fact that the ovum as given off from the ovary has not reached maturation, this being normally completed in its passage through the tube. Several cases of ovarian pregnancy in association with an intrauterine contraceptive device have been noted by Piver *et al.*

The recent study by Lehfeldt *et al.* is concerned with nearly 1,500 accidental pregnancies in 30,000 women in association with the IUD, either in situ or at an

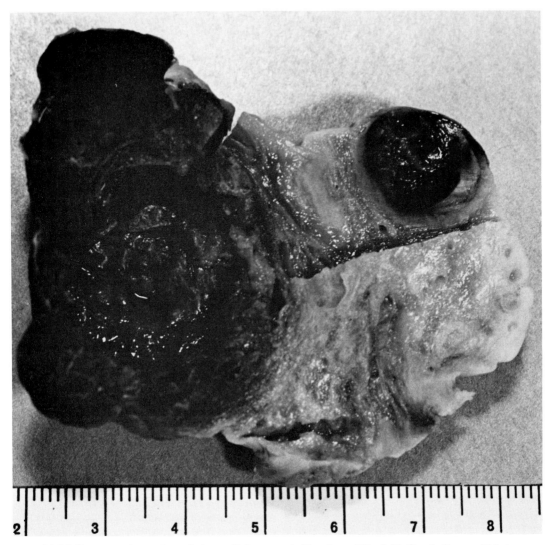

26.20. Pregnancy in ovarian substance. Tube normal. (Courtesy of Dr. J. M. Croak, Oregon, Ohio.)

undetermined location. With the device in situ they found a disproportionately large percentage of ectopic gestation (1 in 23), with 13 women having ovarian pregnancy. This is not meant to imply that the IUD causes ectopic or in particular ovarian pregnancy, but the higher proportion is due to the fact that the IUD prevents uterine more effectively than tubal or ovarian pregnancy. The authors further suggest that the IUD produces some type of antifertility factor which appears to be maximal in the endometrial cavity, weaker in the tube and absent in the ovary. Helde *et al.* suggest that many cases of a presumed ruptured corpus luteum are in reality early ovarian pregnancies, diagnosed if ovarian resection is performed. In reviewing many such cases, this suggestion is not confirmed in our experience.

Primary Abdominal (Peritoneal) Pregnancy

Until recently there had been much skepticism as to the possibility of the fertilized egg implanting itself directly on the pelvic peritoneum, outside the genital

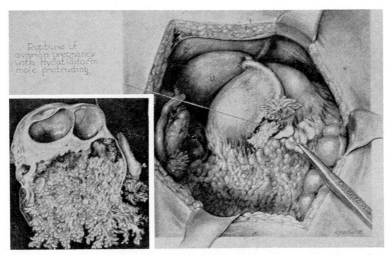

26.21. Ovarian pregnancy associated with hydatidiform mole. (Case of Dr. Henry G. Bennett.)

canal, but the case reported in 1942 by Studdiford seems to establish this possibility beyond question. A few similar cases have been reported, as noted in Cavanagh's recent review. Studdiford suggests the following criteria on which proof of this type of pregnancy must rest: (1)

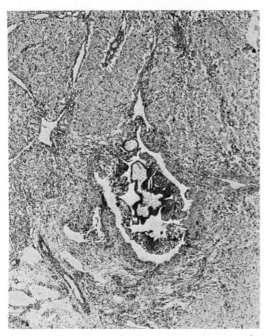

26.22. Chorionic villi in ovarian pregnancy in which the implantation may have been in the corpus luteum which can be seen surrounding the villi in this section.

that both tubes and ovaries are normal with no evidence of recent pregnancy; (2) the absence of any evidence of a uteroperitoneal fistula; and (3) the presence of a pregnancy related exclusively to the peritoneal surface and young enough to eliminate the possibility of secondary implantation following a primary nidation in the tube.

It may be well to mention that the surgeon, in dealing with an abdominal pregnancy, should generally not attempt to remove the placenta, which may be firmly fixed to the mesentery and the abdominal viscera (Fig. 26.23). Profuse hemorrhage can occur on manipulation, and the placenta if left in situ, resorbs without sequelae in most instances, although bowel obstruction may be a late complication. Removal of the fetus with ligation of the cord is usually the wise procedure. Hreshchyshyn *et al.,* Lathrop and Bowles, and others have suggested the use of methotrexate to facilitate devascularization and absorption of any unremoved placenta; this concept is not uniformly accepted.

Cervical Pregnancy

Although exceedingly rare, the possibility of cervical pregnancy does exist. Just as, in placenta praevia, the egg may implant itself in the region of the internal os, so it may, in rare instances, implant

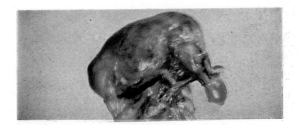

Plate 26.1. Unruptured tubal pregnancy with extensive intratubal hemorrhage.

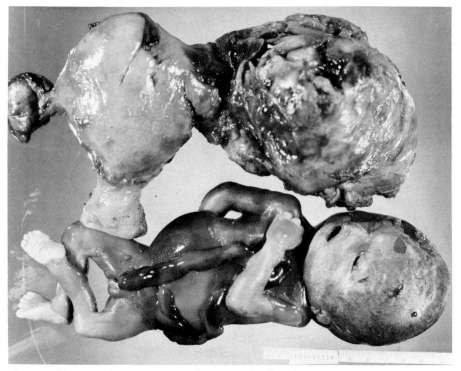

26.23. Presumed intra-uterine pregnancy with attempted saline abortion was ultimately revealed to be an abdominal pregnancy. Placenta (*upper right*) with fetus in peritoneal cavity. A similar case is reported by Walton and Nikrui.

on the cervical mucosa. As would be expected, this bizarre type of pregnancy produces profuse bleeding in the early months of pregnancy and necessitates surgical intervention (hysterectomy), which may be of difficult and serious nature. In reporting a recent case, Resnick notes only some 65 instances of a true cervical pregnancy in his exhaustive review of reported cases. He points out the difficulties in diagnosis and the mortality (20 per cent), primarily due to hemorrhage, understandably due to repeated pelvic examinations in an effort to establish the diagnosis (Fig. 26.24). Roth and Birnbaum, and Jauchlen and Baker likewise emphasize the frequent need for hysterectomy.

Combined Pregnancy (Intra- and Extra-uterine)

There are now several hundred reported cases of combined pregnancy, one embryo being implanted normally

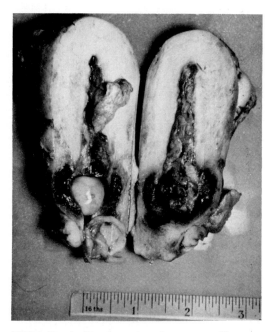

26.24. Cervical implantation of pregnancy (Courtesy of Dr. L. Resnick, South Africa.)

within the uterus, the other ectopically in the tube. Interesting diagnostic problems may arise with such a combination. For example, rupture of the tubal pregnancy may cause serious intraabdominal bleeding, with none from the vagina, since the integrity of the uterine decidua is maintained by the presence of the lining intrauterine pregnancy. For a discussion of the clinical connotations of combined pregnancy, however, the reader must be referred to textbooks of obstetrics. Schaefer feels that the pathogenesis is a double-ovum twin pregnancy in which both ova are fertilized at a single coitus and separates this (combined) form from a compound pregnancy where an intrauterine is superimposed upon a preexisting resolving ectopic gestation. In any case diagnosis is seldom made because the slightly enlarged boggy uterus is felt to represent merely a decidual reaction. In adding an additional case, Brody and Stevens bring up to 506 the cases of combined pregnancy as well as providing an extensive review of the literature.

Simultaneous pregnancy in both tubes may occur and many such cases have been noted as well as simultaneous intrauterine gestation. Less common is *unilateral twin pregnancy.* Only 84 cases have been noted by Loh and Loh, who emphasize that such twins are usually monozygotic. Forbes and Natale have recently reported a *triplet tubal pregnancy* (Fig. 26.25).

Posthysterectomy Ectopic Pregnancy

Although we have seen a few cases of prolapsed fallopian tubes following hysterectomy, where the tubal fimbria protruded through the vaginal vault, it has been our impression that an ectopic pregnancy would be unlikely. The physiology of such a prolapsed tube without an intermediate uterus would seemingly be impaired so that the possibility of pregnancy would seem minimal.

Although tubal pregnancy posthysterectomy is rare, the careful clinician cannot absolutely promise the woman patient that she will not become pregnant following removal of the uterus. Hanes

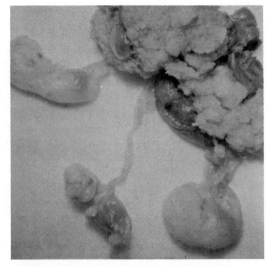

26.25. Placenta and three fetuses from tubal pregnancy. (Courtesy of Dr. Don Forbes, Springfield, Massachusetts.)

has reported 11 cases of pregnancy following abdominal or vaginal hysterectomy. In four instances the pregnancy probably antedated the operative procedure, with conception occurring before and not recognizable at the time of

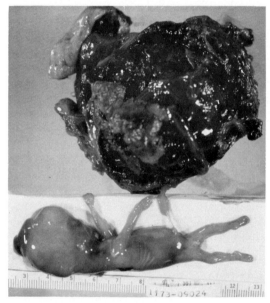

26.26. Tubal pregnancy three months after vaginal hysterectomy ("stormy postoperative course with low HCT—presumed pelvic hematoma").

surgery. Perhaps this occurs much more often than realized, with subsequent anemia and pelvic induration being construed as intraabdominal bleeding incurred by the surgery itself. Often this is self-limited, and does not require operative intervention, but not always (Fig. 26.26).

In other instances years have occurred between the hysterectomy and the ectopic gestation so that we have no recourse but to assume that there is some tract whereby the sperm cell can ascend to fertilize an extruded ovum. Kornblatt, and Bruden and Vigilante have reported additional cases. We might also speculate that passage down the tube by the fertilized egg has been retarded, allowing the trophoblast and villi to undergo sufficient development to permit implantation in the tube or less commonly the abdomen. It might be considered mental cruelty to even mention this remote possibility to the younger posthysterectomy woman.

REFERENCES

Acker, D., Jensen, A. B., and Tenn, G. K.: Abdominal pregnancy with IUD. Obstet. Gynec., 42: 36, 1973.

Arias-Stella, J., and Gutierrez, J.: Frequencia y significando de las atypias endometriales en al embarazo cotopico. Rev. lat-amen. Anat. pat., 1: 81, 1957.

Beacham, M. D., Herrquist, W. C., Beacham, D. W., and Webster, D. H.: Abdominal pregnancy at Charity Hospital in New Orleans. Amer. J. Obstet. Gynec., 84: 1257, 1962.

Bernhard, T. R. N., Bruns, P. D., and Drose, V. E.: Atypical endometrium associated with ectopic pregnancy (the Arias-Stella reaction). Obstet. Gynec., 28: 849, 1966.

Bisca, B. V., and Felder, M. E.: Coexistent interstitial and intrauterine pregnancy following homolateral salpingo-oophorectomy. Amer. J. Obstet. Gynec., 79: 263, 1960.

Bobrow, M. L., and Bell, H. G.: Ectopic pregnancy: a 16-year survey of 905 cases. Obstet. Gynec., 20: 500, 1962.

Breen, J. L.: A 21-year survey of 654 ectopic pregnancies. Amer. J. Obstet. Gynec., 106: 1004, 1970.

Brody, S., and Stevens, F. L.: Combined intra- and extrauterine pregnancy. Obstet. Gynec., 21: 129, 1963.

Bruden, M. L., and Vigilante, M.: Ectopic pregnancy after total hysterectomy. Obstet. Gynec., 41: 891, 1973.

Cavanagh, D.: Primary peritoneal pregnancy. Amer. J. Obstet. Gynec., 76: 523, 1958.

Clark, J. F. J., and Bourne, J.: Advanced ectopic pregnancy. Amer. J. Obstet. Gynec., 78: 340, 1959.

Crawford, J. R., and Ward, J. V.: Advanced abdominal pregnancy. Amer. J. Obstet. Gynec., 10: 549, 1957.

Cullen, T. S.: Bluish discoloration of umbilicus as diagnostic sign when ruptured extrauterine pregnancy exists. In *Contributions to Medical and Biological Research*, edited by W. Osler, Vol. 1, p. 420, 1919.

de Brux, J., and Ancia, M.: Arias-Stella endometrial atypias. Amer. J. Obstet. Gynec., 89: 661, 1964.

Dehner, L. P.: Advanced extrauterine pregnancy and fetal death. Obstet. Gynec., 40: 525, 1972.

Demick, P. E., and Cavanagh, D.: Unilateral tubal and intra-uterine pregnancy. Amer. J. Obstet. Gynec., 76: 533, 1958.

Douglas, C. P.: Tubal ectopic pregnancy. Brit. Med. J., 2: 838, 1963.

Fontanilla, J., and Anderson, G. W.: Further studies on racial incidence and mortality of ectopic pregnancy. Amer. J. Obstet. Gynec., 70: 312, 1955.

Forbes, D. A., and Natale, A.: Unilateral tubal triplet pregnancy. Obstet. Gynec., 31: 360, 1968.

Foster, H. W., and Moore, D. T.: Abdominal pregnancy. Obstet. Gynec., 30: 249, 1967.

Franklin, E. W., Zeiderman, A. N., and Laemmle, P.: Tubal ectopic pregnancy. Amer. J. Obstet. Gynec., 117: 220, 1973.

Goodno, J. A., and Sentry, W.: Coexistent interstitial and intrauterine pregnancy. J.A.M.A., 179: 135, 1962.

Graff, G., Lancet, M., and Czernobilsky, B.: Ovarian pregnancy with IUD. Obstet. Gynec., 40: 535, 1972.

Grant, A.: The effect of ectopic pregnancy on fertility. J. Clin. Obstet. Gynec., 5: 861, 1962.

Grody, M. H., and Otis, R. D.: Ectopic pregnancy after total hysterectomy (report of a case). Obstet. Gynec., 17: 96, 1961.

Halbrecht, I.: Healed genital tuberculosis; new etiologic factor in ectopic pregnancy. Obstet. Gynec., 10: 73, 1957.

Hanes, M. V.: Ectopic pregnancy following total hysterectomy. Obstet. Gynec., 23: 882, 1964.

Harralson, J. R., Von Nagell, J. R., and Roddick, J. W.: Operative management of ruptured tubal pregnancy. Amer. J. Obstet. Gynec., 115: 995, 1973.

Helde, M. D., et al.: Detection of unsuspected ovarian pregnancy by wedge resection. Canad. Med. Ass. J., 106: 237, 1972.

Holmes, E. J., and Lyle, W. H.: How early in pregnancy does the Arias-Stella occur? Arch. Path., 95: 302, 1973.

Hreshchyshyn, M. M., Naples, J. D., Jr., and Randall, C. L.: Amethopterin in abdominal pregnancy. Amer. J. Obstet. Gynec., 93: 286, 1965.

Hubbard, L. T.: Secondary abdominal pregnancy. Amer. J. Obstet. Gynec., 74: 431, 1957.

Iffy, L.: The role of premenstrual postmidcycle conception in the aetiology of ectopic gestation. J. Obstet. Gynaec. Brit. Comm., 70: 996, 1963.

Jauchlen, G. W., and Baker, R. L.: Cervical pregnancy. Obstet. Gynec., 35: 370, 1970.

Kinschnen, R., and Kimball, H. W.: Interstitial pregnancy following unilateral salpingectomy. J.A.M.A., 175: 146, 1962.

Kleinen, G. J., and Roberts, T. W.: Current factors in the causation of tubal pregnancy. Amer. J. Obstet. Gynec., 99: 21, 1967.

Kornblatt, M. B.: Abdominal pregnancy following a total hysterectomy. Obstet. Gynec., 32: 488, 1968.

Laiuppa, M. A., and Cavanagh, D.: The endometrium in ectopic pregnancy. Obstet. Gynec., 21: 155, 1963.

Lathrop, J. C., and Bowles, G. E.: Methotrexate in abdominal pregnancy. Obstet. Gynec., 32: 81, 1968.

Lehfeldt, H., Tietze, C., and Gonstein, F.: Ovarian pregnancy and IUD. Amer. J. Obstet. Gynec., 108: 1005, 1970.

Levin, S., Cospi, E., and Hirsch, H.: Ovarian pregnancy and IUD. Amer. J. Obstet. Gynec., 113: 843, 1972.

Lloyd, H. E. D., and Fienberg, R.: The Arias-Stella reaction: A non-specific involutional phenomenon in intra- and extrauterine pregnancies. Amer. J. Clin. Path., 43: 428, 1965.

Loh, W., and Loh, H. C.: Unilateral tubal twin pregnancy with intraperitoneal rupture. Obstet. Gynec., 19: 267, 1961.

Mackles, A., Wolfe, S. A., and Posner, S. N.: Cellular atypia in endometrial glands (Arias-Stella reaction) as an aid in the diagnosis of ectopic pregnancy. Amer. J. Obstet. Gynec., *81:* 1209, 1961.

Mall, F. P.: *On the Fate of the Human Embryo in Tubal Pregnancy.* Contributions to Embryology Publication No. 221, Carnegie Institute of Washington, Washington, D. C., 1915.

McGowan, L.: Intramural pregnancy. J.A.M.A., *192:* 63, 1965.

Overbeck, L.: Tubal pregnancies concurrent with active tuberculous salpingitis. Gerburtsh. Frauenheilk., *24:* 700, 1964.

Parker, S. L., and Parker, R. T.: "Chronic" ectopic tubal pregnancy. Amer. J. Obstet. Gynec., *74:* 1174, 1957.

Payne, S., Duge, J., and Bradburg, W.: Ectopic pregnancy concomitant with twin uterine pregnancy. Obstet. Gynec., *37:* 905, 1971.

Persaud, V.: Etiology of tubal ectopic pregnancy. Obstet. Gynec., *36:* 257, 1970.

Pildes, R. B., and Wheeler, J. D.: Atypical epithelial changes in ectopic pregnancy. Amer. J. Obstet. Gynec., *73:* 79, 1957.

Piver, M. S., Baer, K. A., and Zachary, T. V.: Ovarian pregnancy intrauterine device. J.A.M.A., *201:* 107, 1967.

Pugh, W. E., Vogt, R. F., and Gibson, R. A.: Ovarian pregnancy and IUD. Obstet. Gynec., *42:* 218, 1973.

Resnick, L.: Cervical pregnancy. South African Med. J., *36:* 73, 1962.

Riggs, J. A., Warner, A. S., Hahn, G. A., and Farrell, D. M.: Extrauterine tubal choriocarcinoma. Amer. J. Obstet. Gynec., *88:* 637, 1964.

Roach, W. R., Guderian, A. M., and Brewer, J. L.: Endometrial gland atypism in presence of trophoblast. Amer. J. Obstet. Gynec., *79:* 680, 1960.

Rosenblum, J. M., Dowling, R. W., and Barnes, A. C.: Treatment of tubal pregnancy. Amer. J. Obstet. Gynec., *80:* 274, 1960.

Ross, P. D., and Gunther, R. E.: Combined pregnancy. Amer. J. Obstet. Gynec., *107:* 1263, 1970.

Roth, D. J., and Birnbaum, S. J.: Cervical pregnancy. Obstet. Gynec., *42:* 675: 1973.

Schaefer, G.: Extrauterine pregnancy with concomitant term uterine pregnancy. Clin. Obstet. Gynec., *5:* 875, 1962.

Schiffer, M. A.: A review of 268 ectopic pregnancies. Amer. J. Obstet. Gynec., *80:* 264, 1963.

Seward, R. N., Israel, R., and Ballard, C. A.: Ectopic pregnancy and IUD. Obstet. Gynec., *40:* 214, 1972.

Sherwin, A. S., and Berg, F. P.: Cervical pregnancy. Amer. J. Obstet. Gynec., *79:* 259, 1960.

Simpson, J. W., Alford, C. D., and Miller, A. C.: Interstitial pregnancy following homolateral salpingectomy. Amer. J. Obstet. Gynec., *82:* 1173, 1961.

Speert, H.: The uterine decidua in ectopic pregnancy. Amer. J. Obstet. Gynec., *76:* 491, 1958.

Spiegelberg, O.: Zur casuistik den ovarial-schwangenschaft. Arch. Gynaek., *13:* 73, 1878.

Steptoe, P. C.: *Laparoscopy in Gynecology.* E. & S. Livingston, London, 1967.

Stromme, W. B.: Conservative surgery for ectopic pregnancy. Obstet. Gynec., *41:* 215, 1973.

Stromme, W. B., McKelvey, J. L., and Adkins, C. D.: Conservative surgery for ectopic pregnancy. Obstet. Gynec., *19:* 294, 1962.

Studdiford, W. E.: Primary peritoneal pregnancy. Amer. J. Obstet. Gynec., *44:* 487, 1942.

Sturgis, S. H.: Arias-Stella phenomenon. Amer. J. Obstet. Gynec., *116:* 589, 1973.

Tan, K., and Yeo, O.: Primary ovarian pregnancy. Amer. J. Obstet. Gynec., *100:* 240, 1968.

Timonen, S., and Niemonem, O.: Tubal pregnancy: choice of operative methods of treatment. Acta Obstet. Gynec. Scand., *46:* 237, 1967.

Wagner, D., and Richart, R. M.: Polyploidy in the human endometrium with the Arias-Stella reaction. Arch. Path., *85:* 475, 1968.

Walton, L. A., and Nikrui, N.: "Salting out" an abdominal pregnancy. New York J. Med., *73:* 2782, 1973.

Webster, H. D., Barclay, D. L., and Fischer, C. K.: Ectopic pregnancy: A 17-year review. Amer. J. Obstet. Gynec., *92:* 23, 1965.

Winer, A. E., Bergman, W. O., and Fields, C.: Combined intra- and extra-uterine pregnancy. Amer. J. Obstet. Gynec., *74:* 170, 1957.

Zlatnick, A. P., Weld, S. L., Schochet, S. S., Jr., and Schochet, S. S.: Combined tubal and intrauterine pregnancy. Amer. J. Obstet. Gynec., *76:* 536, 1958.

chapter 27

Trophoblastic Disease (TRD)

Because they both originate from trophoblast, hydatidiform mole and choriocarcinoma are generally discussed together, although there is considerable variation in the malignant potential as well as a possible difference in the genesis of the two diseases. Although rare in the United States, trophoblastic disease (TRD) represents an unusually provocative and incomprehensible problem.

Any understanding of the extremely abnormal behavior of TRD must be prefaced by a short and perfunctory explanation of trophoblastic activity in the course of normal pregnancy. Without this background, it is totally impossible to have any complete comprehension as to the highly unpredictable nature of these lesions. It must be understood that the placenta with even a normal gestation shows certain features that are usually attributed to malignant disease. For this reason, it is important to know the behavior of *human chorionic gonadotrophin* (HCG) during normal pregnancy, for determination of *HCG* is vital in the diagnosis and malignant potential of certain types of TRD. Although the actual level of HCG may vary in different laboratories, the excretion rate approximates that depicted in Figure 27.1.

PSEUDOMALIGNANT BEHAVIOR OF THE TROPHOBLAST

Of *primary* interest is the ability of the chorionic villi to exhibit rather extensive degrees of invasion into and through the maternal decidua. Trophoblastic buds may often burrow down into the myometrium as discrete small foci of cells (*syncytial myometritis*), although there is often rather abrupt termination of their invasive propensities at the myometrial-decidual junction (*layer of Nitabuch*), presumably due to some type of local inhibition. It is by no means rare, however, to note, following cesarean section-hysterectomy, foci of trophoblast deep in the myometrium. Hertig indicates that villi form during the 14th day of fetal life, and adds that late ovulation incurs a higher frequency of abnormal pregnancies as abortion and mole.

Second is the frequent (50%) possibility of migration of the trophoblast to the

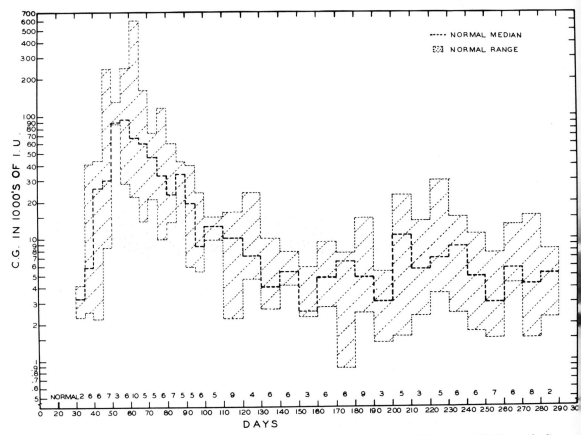

27.1. Serum chorionic gonadotrophin throughout normal pregnancy in 24 women (Delfs method). Gonadotrophin in international units (I.U.) is plotted against duration of pregnancy in days, counting from Day 1 of the last menstrual period. *Heavy black line* shows average gonadotrophin level. *Cross-hatched area* indicates extreme variation for the period with the number of determinations in each. Plotted on semilogarithmic graph scale. (From Jones, G. E. S., Delfs, E., and Stran, H. M.: Chorionic gonadotrophin and pregnanediol values in normal pregnancy. Bull. Johns Hopkins Hosp., *75:* 359, 1944.)

lungs as noted originally by Schmorl in 1893. This so-called "deportation of villi" is an accepted possibility in a not inconsiderable number of normal pregnancies, although probably not as frequently as documented by Schmorl. Yet this form of pulmonary "metastasis" does not behave like a malignant embolus, for there is rarely more than minor transitory difficulty as far as the maternal host is concerned. Attwood and Park, as well as Douglas, have confirmed the frequent finding of blood-borne trophoblast (40%), although formed villi are rare. Again, it is necessary to postulate some defense mechanism that is capable of obliterating pulmonary deposits of trophoblast.

Thus to have any comprehension of the complex behavior of TRD, one must accept some kind of mechanism that operates during a normal gestation to check the pseudomalignant behavior of the trophoblast. Seemingly this immune reaction is impaired in even normal pregnancy, as indicated by Nelson *et al.* Indeed, there is probably a double type of defensive arrangement, one *local* and operating at the uterine level, to limit myometrial invasion of the chorionic villi. The second *systemic* agent appears to limit and suppress the growth of extrauterine trophoblast. Despite the frequency of trophoblast in the blood stream after 18 weeks of pregnancy this tissue only rarely persists and grows.

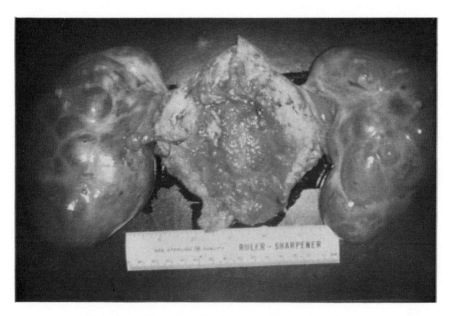

Plate 27.1. Huge theca lutein cysts with choriocarcinoma

Only if we can conceive of a dual guarding effect, local and generalized, is it possible to rationalize the vagarious behavior of certain of these TRD. Although proof of this mechanism is difficult to pinpoint, the clinical pattern exhibited by certain moles and choriocarcinomas seemingly indicates that no other explanation is possible. It seems to operate through some type of immunological channel such as an antigen-antibody effect, but the exact mechanism is still very uncertain to all of us. However, acceptance of some form of *maternal immunizing agent* is vital if there is to be any rational approach to comprehension of trophoblastic abnormalities, which, even in normal pregnancy, show such a striking parallel to malignant disease as local invasion and distant pulmonary metastasis. Bardawil, Hertig, and Tedeschi and Toy have contributed important studies regarding the regression of trophoblast.

Grafts of the husband's skin to the female with choriocarcinoma are not rejected in the usual fashion, as noted by Robinson *et al.* This might reflect some impairment of the expected antigen-antibody reaction in the patient harboring this allograft, and such is the prevailing concept of the immunological defense mechanism in response to trophoblast, although the specific details are still uncertain (Holland and Hreshchyshyn, Billingham, etc.).

Koren *et al.* using a fluorescein technique in certain animals indicates that trophoblastic cells are potentially antigenic, but precisely why these antigenic properties are not expressed is unclear. Douthwaite and Urbach suggest that a sialomucin coating of the trophoblast prevents the expected antigen-antibody reaction. Adcock *et al.* speculate that HCG may represent a trophoblastic cell surface antigen which blocks rejection of the trophoblast by maternal lymphocytes. The recent review by Behrman *et al.* with subsequent discussions touches on many important aspects of the immunological reaction, and points out that trophoblast is specifically antigenic and produces antibodies against pregnancy. This fibrinoid barrier has been presumed to prevent sensitization of the maternal host, but Wynn, utilizing electronic microscopy, implies that fibrinoid acts only in an ancillary role. That antibodies are produced in the maternal host seems certain; why rejection of the foreign trophoblast does not occur is unknown.

Incidence of Trophoblastic Disease

In the United States, hydatidiform mole is generally believed to occur about once in 2500 pregnancies, and choriocarcinoma is less than 5 per cent as common. From the Far East, Acosta Sisson reports a much higher incidence in the Philippine Islands, and in Taiwan, Wei and Ouyang record the startling frequency of one case of TRD to 82 pregnancies. Indeed, in this hemisphere certain Mexican authors find one case of hydatidiform mole per 200 pregnancies. The high incidence of TRD in conjunction with malnutrition, parity, and advancing age has been repeatedly documented. An inadequate diet, notably a protein deficiency rather than an excess of rice, is suggested as the cause for the preponderance of this disease in the Far East. It is the lowest socioeconomic group wherein there is literally almost an absence of dietary protein that is most likely to exhibit this condition.

Fox and Tow note considerable ethnic difference in the incidence of TRD in a multiracial community. There have been case reports of a 12-year-old girl with a hydatidiform mole, yet many postmenopausal women have been noted, and indeed the instance of TRD is increased in the aging procreative female.

Hydatidiform Mole

Hydatidiform mole is a condition in which the chorionic villi become enormously overdistended with fluid, appearing as translucent grapelike vesicles which vary in size from a few millimeters to that of a cherry. Often the whole uterine cavity is filled with vesicular molar tissue, but on other occasions only a small portion of the placenta is involved. Even where the disease is rather massive, however, normal pregnancy has been reported, and of course many instances of routine deliveries will reveal a placenta that shows certain localized areas of hydatid degeneration. Carr points out that it is sometimes very difficult to distinguish between major degrees of hydatid degeneration and a true molar pregnancy. Park stipulates that hydropic villi with trophoblastic hyperplasia should be designated hydatidiform mole; without chorionic proliferation, 'hydropic change' is indicated. Pregnancy in the tube or ovary may be associated with molar disease or choriocarcinoma on rare occasions.

Pathology. There is some uncertainty as to whether the disease is of *neoplastic* or *degenerative* character, but it is agreed that the chief microscopic characteristics are (1) proliferation of the lining trophoblast of the villi, (2) marked edema and enlargement of the villi, and (3) disappearance or extreme scantiness of the villous blood vessels. Of these the first is probably the most important, but it is of variable degree. In portions of the mole within the uterine cavity, or in extruded portions, there may be little or no tropho-

blastic overgrowth (Fig. 27.2), although in the same lesion villi still receiving a good blood supply from the uterine wall may show marked trophoblastic proliferation.

The studies of Hertig strongly imply that mole is often a result of mere accumulation of fluid after complete agenesis or early degeneration of the embryonic cardiovascular system in the third to fifth weeks. The continued presence of a maternal circulation with an absence of a fetal one along with a functioning trophoblast seems essential for the formation of the fluid. Thus it is apparent that moles may be a form of early missed abortion, and certain clinical admixtures may occasionally be found.

Park, however, suggests that the primary cause of molar disease is an abnormal trophoblast with secondary hydrops and fetal death. He has indicated no particular abnormalities in sex chromatin in both benign mole and malignant choriocarcinoma. However Tominaga and Page suggest that most benign trophoblastic tumors have an XX constitution, but true choriocarcinoma arises by

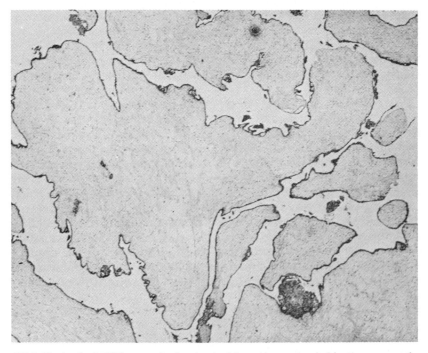

27.2. Benign hydatidiform mole showing in this section no trophoblastic overgrowth

chance. Baggish *et al.* indicate the almost inevitable presence of a chromatin body in trophoblast, but their study embraced primarily benign mole. Carr finds that triploidy is the rule in most moles, although various data from other sources suggest consistent aneuploidy with trophoblastic disease, mole exhibiting 43 chromosomes and choriocarcinoma a count of 86.

The characteristic *macroscopic* appearance of a hydatidiform mole is that of a bunch of grapes (Fig. 27.3), because of the enormous edema of the villi. Ordinarily there is no trace of a fetus, because of the involvement of the entire chorionic surface. However, in a small proportion of cases, *partial hydatidiform mole* or *hydropic degeneration,* only a fraction of the chorion is involved. For that matter, in an occasional instance of this very limited type, the nutritional function of the placenta is not materially impaired, so that pregnancy may continue to term,

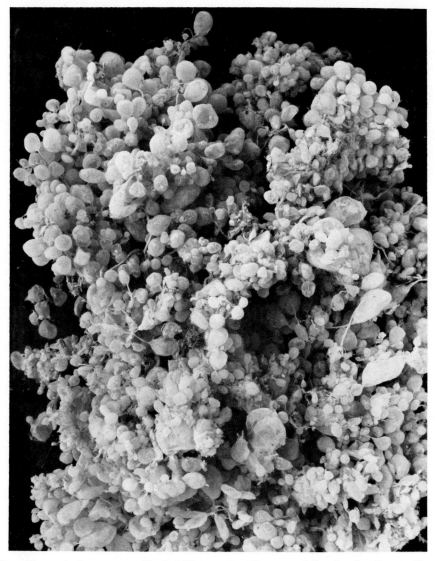

27.3. Grapelike vesicular pattern of hydatidiform mole. (Courtesy of Dr. Jan Smalbraak, Bloemendaal, The Netherlands.)

with delivery of a living child. Obviously this occurrence is not compatible with complete agenesis of the fetal cardiovascular system unless as a twin pregnancy from a single placenta. Baggish *et al.* suggest an origin from the second polar body. Perhaps there is more than one form of origin, both degenerative and neoplastic.

In a recent extensive review Beischer has reported 92 cases of mole associated with a fetus and in the vast majority of cases the fetus was stillborn due to prematurity (see Fig. 27.4). Triploidy has

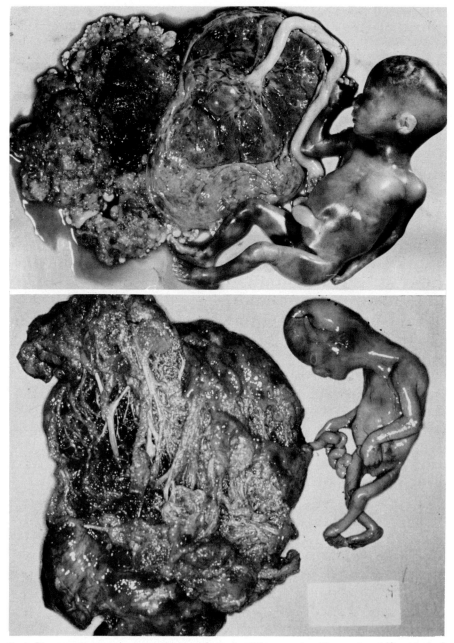

27.4. (*top*) Six month fetus in association with hydatidiform mole. (Courtesty of Dr. N. A. Beischer, Melbourne, Australia.) (*bottom*) Similar fetus. (Courtesy of Drs. C. M. Cabaniss and J. F. Clark, Washington, D.C.)

been observed in certain cases of the mole-fetus "syndrome," and the fetus has been male in 25 per cent of the observed cases. Carr has noted hydatidiform degeneration predominantly in women who have recently discontinued oral contraceptives. The chromosomal pattern (triploidy) is more suggestive of a malformation than a neoplasm, although with the capability of subsequent neoplastic development. Baggish stresses the extreme difficulty in karyotyping TRD but suggests a progression to aneuploidy as malignancy evolves.

Repeated moles in the same patient are uncommon, but do occur as tabulated recently by Hsu *et al.* Only one of their six cases culminated in choriocarcinoma, but Wu reports up to nine recurrent moles in one patient with no progression in malignancy. This would seem to cast some doubt on the statement that TRD is an inevitably continuous spectrum; it may progress, but only rare moles eventuate in choriocarcinoma.

Malignant Mole (Chorioadenoma Destruens). In a small proportion of moles, not always differing histologically from the benign moles previously described, the hydatidiform villi penetrate to undue degree, so that they may perforate the uterine wall and cause alarming or even fatal abdominal hemorrhage (Fig. 27.5). As a rule, there is increased trophoblastic proliferation with a preserved villous pattern. The proliferative villi may invade the parametrium or the vaginal wall, although there is rarely evidence of metastasis. It is this variety of mole which has so often wrongly been diagnosed as choriocarcinoma. It differs very crucially from the latter, not only microscopically, but in that it rarely metastasizes, so that it, unlike choriocarcinoma, has been usually cured by hysterectomy, although the treatment of this era is often nonsurgical.

This benign course is usual but not inevitable with chorioadenoma. Tow notes a very definite mortality (up to 10% in some series), due to hemorrhage, with certain lesions having an intact villous pattern, and feels that in due time a chorioadenoma will proliferate, lose its

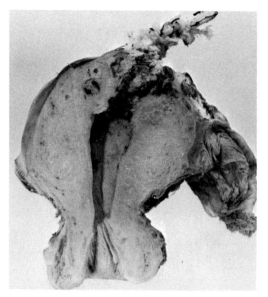

27.5. Invasive mole, perforating dome of fundus. (Courtesy of Dr. M. S. Baggish, Hartford, Conn.)

villi, and become a true choriocarcinoma. For this reason, he would favor utilizing the term "villous choriocarcinoma" for chorioadenoma destruens, as opposed to the "avillous" or classical choriocarcinoma. However, the biological behavior of these lesions does not always conform with their microscopic pattern.

Just why some benign moles secondarily become neoplastic with local invasion is unclear. A few, probably less than 5 per cent, progress to true choriocarcinoma, but a larger number show marked evidence of local infiltration only. Occasionally, this may occur with the most inactive histological type of mole, although frequently there is evidence of trophoblastic overgrowth. Nevertheless, local invasion can be extensive, and the logical explanation is a breakdown of the *locally invasive* defense barrier, although the *generalized systemic* mechanism remains intact and guards against distant extension.

It is this variety of *locally invasive mole* to which Ewing in 1910 gave the ill chosen designation of *chorioadenoma destruens,* which has become rather fixed in the literature. The term is rather vague and confused as to its exact definition, and it is applied not only to the *abnormally*

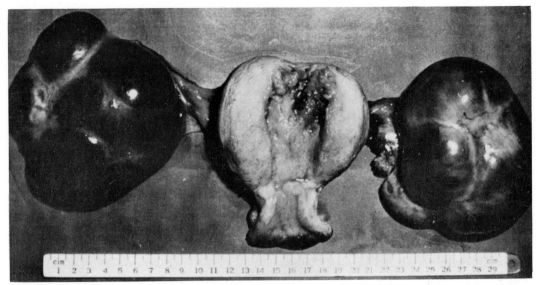

27.6. Invasive mole, with bilateral theca lutein cyst. (Courtesy of Dr. M. S. Baggish, Hartford, Conn.)

penetrative and locally invasive type just described, but also to moles showing abnormally excessive trophoblastic proliferation, although here the factor of individual interpretation comes into play. To summarize, therefore, the designation of malignant mole or chorioadenoma destruens is applied to moles characterized by abnormal penetrativeness and *local invasion* along with *excessive trophoblastic proliferation.* It seems unwise to consider chorioadenoma

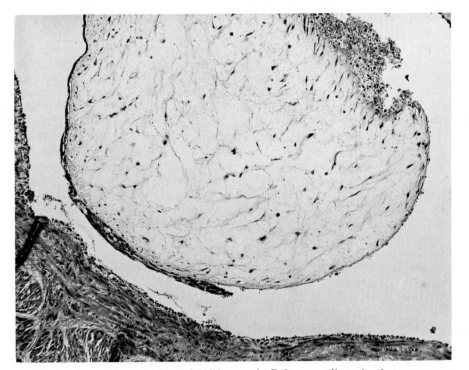

27.7. Villous in blood vessel with hydatidiform mole. Pulmonary dissemination may ensue.

as anything like an "in situ" choriocarcinoma, but as a potentially rather than an inevitably malignant lesion. Ovarian theca lutein cysts may concur (Fig. 27.6 and Plate 27.1) with all forms of TRD.

PULMONARY TROPHOBLAST

Although invasive mole does not usually incur persistently growing or fatal deposits in the lung, there seems little doubt that even benign trophoblast may occasionally be found in the lung, as with deportation of villi (Fig. 27.7). In reporting this sequel, Canlas makes a very real similarity to extrauterine "syncytial endometritis," wherein the residual trophoblast may be a source of sustained HCG, but will ultimately disappear, presumably due to the ill defined, but probably very valid, maternal defense mechanism. More striking is the study by Wilson *et al.*, who found pulmonic trophoblast (often biopsy proven) with invasive moles in 8 of 20 cases, yet invariably the patient continued in good health without any definitive treatment (Fig. 27.8). Obviously, there must be some systemic agent that suppresses continued growth of the pulmonic trophoblast with mole, but is lacking in choriocarcinoma, and permits extensive and often fatal lung

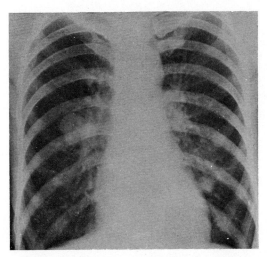

27.8. Pulmonic trophoblast. Spontaneous regression with no definitive treatment. (Courtesy of Dr. M. S. Baggish, Hartford, Conn.)

disease. There is considerable logic in adopting McCrae's suggestion that trophoblastic lesions be divided into only two categories, *localized* and *generalized* choriomas (or localized and metastatic TRD).

LOCAL COMPLICATIONS OF MOLE

Further observations by Thiele and de Alvarez, and Hsu *et al.* indicate a definite morbidity and even mortality, with presumed nonmalignant TRD. On the basis of hemorrhage and sepsis alone, as well as occasional metastasis, the latter suggest hysterectomy for the multiparous woman, and with this tenet we would not disagree. It is well established that older women have a higher incidence of malignant degeneration of TRD, which may approach 25% as the woman passes 35. Although chorioadenoma destruens should be regarded as a benign disease in general, there are exceptions, and fatalities may occur due to uterine hemorrhage or rarely extrauterine disease, even with histological evidence of seemingly only a proliferative mole.

CLASSIFICATION OF MOLES

Douglas has made an attempt to divide moles into six different categories according to cellular anaplasia and proliferation, infolding into the villi, and various other criteria as a prognostic index. Although it is probably true that the more proliferative moles are followed by a higher incidence of complication, a considerable number of invasive or malignant tendencies develop after even the most innocuous appearing mole (see Fig. 27.9). For this reason, it is desirable to reecho the sentiments voiced by Emil Novak as to the impossibility of "pigeon-holing" the bizarre histological patterns of trophoblast. Indeed, Hertig and Sheldon, who originally formulated a similar rigid set of diagnostic criteria, have since modified their division of cases into much more logical *benign, potentially malignant,* and *apparently malignant* groupings. As will be noted subsequently, it would seem that the biological behavior

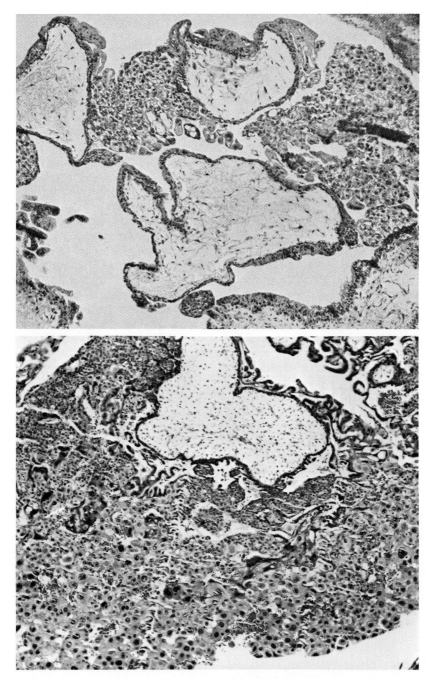

27.9. A. Benign mole with moderate trophoblastic proliferation. B. Invasive mole with excessive tropho-blast.

of trophoblast is even more important than the histological pattern.

Classification. The International Union Against Cancer has proposed the following classification for TRD.

Trophoblastic disease
1. Gestational
2. Non-gestational
Clinical diagnosis
1. Non-metastatic

2. Metastatic
  a. Local (pelvic)
  b. Extra-pelvic
Morphological diagnosis
  1. Hydatidiform mole
    a. Non-invasive
    b. Invasive
  2. Choriocarcinoma
  3. Uncertain

Clinical Characteristics. The chief symptom of hydatidiform mole is *bleeding,* which appears usually in the third and fourth month of pregnancy. Examination shows the *uterus larger than normal for the presumed phase of pregnancy.* There are, however, numerous exceptions to this, as large masses of the molar material have not infrequently been expelled before the patient comes under observation. Despite an enlargement of the uterus above the umbilicus, *no fetal heart sounds* are audible, and *no skeletal shadow* is revealed by the x-ray. The patient is sometimes helpful by extruding small or large masses of the characteristic vesicular tissue. The subjective signs of pregnancy are present, with a high association of first or second trimester toxemia and occasional thyrotoxicosis.

In the *malignant type of mole* the growth may perforate the uterine wall, with sometimes severe or even fatal intra-abdominal bleeding. This destructive variety may likewise invade the vascular channels, and very occasional metastases may appear in the vagina, vulva, or lungs, as in the more frankly malignant choriocarcinoma. Characteristically, however, chorioadenoma destruens is *locally rather than systemically invasive* (Figs. 27.10, 11).

Diagnosis. The occurrence of bleeding and the disproportionately large size of

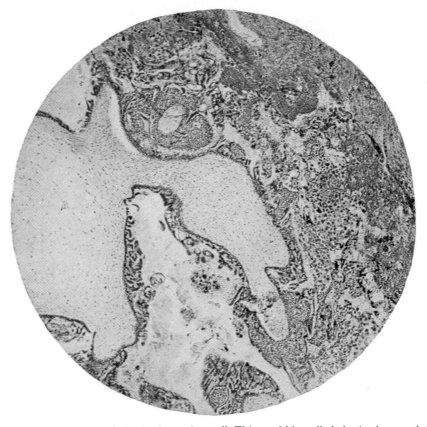

27.10. Highly proliferative mole in situ in uterine wall. This would be called chorioadenoma destruens by most pathologists.

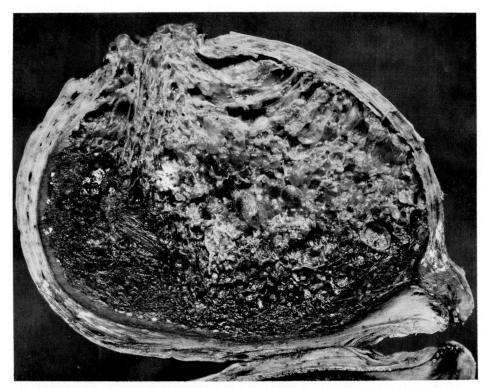

27.11. Gross appearance of mole. (Courtesy of Dr. Jan Smalbraak, Bloemendaal, The Netherlands.)

the uterus should lead to the suspicion of hydatidiform mole and suggest the advisability of obtaining quantitative HCG (see later). Further suspicion is justified when, in the presence of a uterus corresponding to a five or six months' pregnancy, there is an absence of fetal movements, heart sounds, or x-ray evidence of a skeleton. Goldstein and Reed have advocated intrauterine injection of 20 ml. of such a radiopaque substance as *Hyopaque*; subsequent x-ray will reveal a characteristic "motheaten or honeycombed" appearance (Fig. 27.12).

Ultrasound. The use of ultrasound as a method of visualizing internal structures has been well documented, and has been increasingly utilized since the last edition of this text. While various endocrinological tests are available, and an intrauterine dye injection may be of value, ultrasound is among the best available methods in the sometimes difficult diagnosis of hydatidiform mole (Figs. 27.13, 14). In a young woman with a rapidly enlarging uterus the ultrasound picture will produce a very characteristic pattern. Of course the recognition of fetal parts generally excludes the diagnosis of mole except in a rare instance where there is a twin pregnancy (molar and normal). Arteriography is likewise useful (Fig. 27.14).

The most frequent problem is distinction of persistent TRD from a new pregnancy, because both present an enlarged uterus with an elevated HCG. Pregnancy is characterized by a high estriol and pregnandiol level; with TRD, these are low, and this is so valuable a distinction that Beischer (personal communication) feels that attempts at pregnancy are feasible after methotrexate treatment has produced a negative titer (without a year or two of contraception) (see Treatment). Elston and Bagshawe have summarized the difficulties in establishing a diagnosis.

CHORIONIC GONADOTROPHIN (HCG)

During the early months of normal pregnancy there is a markedly elevated level of HCG, although Fox and Tow indicate certain differences in varied ethnic groups. Where the possibility of molar disease is suspected, it is imperative to obtain quantitative determination of the chorionic gonadotrophin (HCG). This index of biological activity is of even greater importance than the pathological picture, for the latter does not invariably indicate the morphology of all the functioning trophoblast. For example, curettage will not be completely informative if there is myometrial invasion, nor will hysterectomy lead to adequate evaluation of extrauterine trophoblast. Nevertheless, any available tissue deserves the closest pathological scrutiny, but the clinician should always remember (1) that this is not always representative of the total trophoblast, (2) biological behavior does not always parallel the usual histological pattern.

Normally, during the 50th and 80th days of the average pregnancy there is a sharp peak of gonadotrophic output, so that the urine may contain amounts of HCG as large as with many hydatidiform moles. Twin or supernumerary pregnancy may lead to an inordinately high titer. A steadily increasing titer is of more significance than a single high assay (over 100, 000 I.U.). All bioassays must be interpreted by the standards of any individual laboratory.

If, after the evacuation or discharge of a hydatidiform mole, the hormone studies once more become positive, or persist after eight weeks, either a new pregnancy or a choriocarcinoma should be suspected. This, however, is not always the case, because in a number of instances in which tests have been even highly positive the subsequent course has shown that nests of trophoblastic tissue have remained in the

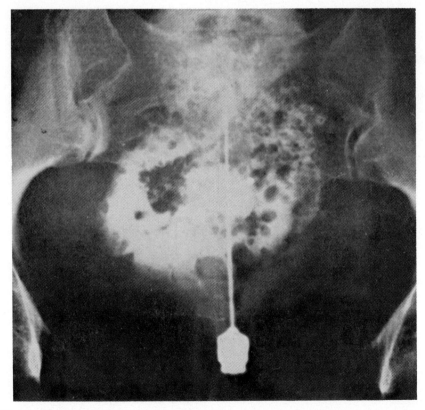

27.12. X-ray of uterine cavity in patient suspected of having a molar pregnancy taken approximately 5 minutes after injection of 20 ml. of radiopaque material (Hyopaque). "Moth-eaten" or "honeycombed" pattern is diagnostic for molar pregnancy. (Courtesy of D. P. Goldstein and D. E. Reid, Clin. Obstet. Gynec., *10:* 313, 1966.)

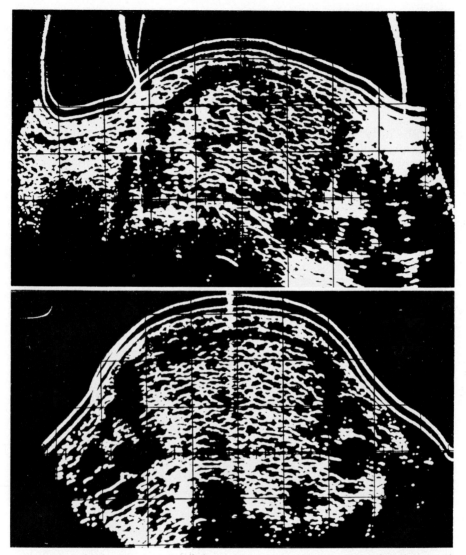

27.13. *A*. Right marker is at pubis; *left,* umbilicus. Note characteristic honeycomb molar mass in center. Each grid 3 cm. *B*. Transverse view. Note absence of fetal sac. Diffuse echoes with "snowstorm effect" (high sensitivity settings).

uterine wall, usually deep in the blood vessel spaces, so that they would be inaccessible to the curette, the so-called *syncytial myometritis.*

Nevertheless, Delfs has pointed out the extreme value of bioassays following evacuation of a mole. In 81 patients studied, 75% showed a normal chorionic gonadotrophin test (HCG) within 60 days, with a few more showing a slower decrease to average range. The residual cases, however, exhibited a high incidence of invasive mole or choriocarcinoma; therefore, a persistently positive HCG after more than two months should be regarded as suggestive. If positive after hysterectomy, the prognosis is poor, for spread to other organs seems likely.

Brewer finds that after evacuation of a mole, HCG is elevated in 40% of patients as late as 60 days; of this 40 per cent, one-half regress more slowly but the others often progress into invasive mole or choriocarcinoma. We might regard *60*

have described a (3) complement fixation method of quantitating the number of International Units (I.U.) of HCG in serum, and their carefully controlled study suggests more accuracy and fewer complications than with bioassays involving animals. Taymor has discussed the comparative values of bioassay and immunoassay of HCG. Although Fox and Tow question the reliability of such latex agglutination tests as described by Wide and Gemzell, their accuracy is attested to by Haskins, although when the level of HCG is low, there seems some error. One must always be mindful of different results from different laboratories and in different ethnic groups. In our own clinic it is unusual for a normal single pregnancy to show a level of HCG exceeding 100,000 I.U. although there are rare exceptions at days 60 to 70.

Recently it has become apparent that both bio- and immunoassays are desirable since they seem to reflect entirely different activities: hormonal action (bioassay) versus the formation of complexes by antigen with only fairly specific antibody (immunoassay). A good bioassay

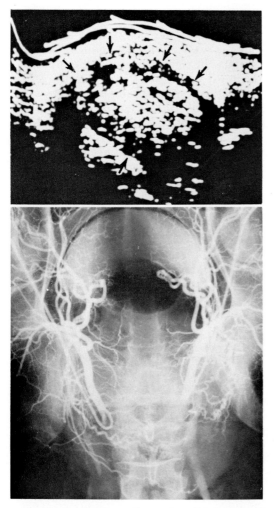

27.14. *A*. Uniform "snowstorm" of internal echoes corresponds to grape-like macrostructure of hydatidiform mole. Ventral line at left indicates umbilicus; arrows outline uterine margins. *B*. Arteriogram of above case. (Courtesy of Dr. J. C. Birnholz, Boston, Mass.)

days as the critical time where some decision must be made as to management of this still biologically active lesion.

Quantitative Determinations of the Chorionic Gonadotrophin

(1) An increased weight of an immature rat or mouse uterus, or (2) a spermatozoa response in male frog or toad, with the use of various dilution factors of serum or urine have been utilized in past years. More recently, however, Lau and Jones

Table 27.1

Current Concepts in Management of Molar Pregnancy

Early Diagnosis
   Clinical suspicion
   Intrauterine dye injection
   Sonar and arteriograms
Method of Delivery
   Intravenous oxytocin → suction-currettage
   Abdominal hysterectomy with mole in situ
   Prophylactic chemotherapy
Follow-up
   Weekly gonadotrophin determinations until normal
   Chest x-rays every two weeks until gonadotrophin excretion is normal
   Repeat gonadotrophin assays at monthly intervals for six months, then bimonthly for six months
   Avoid pregnancy for at least one year

(Courtesy of D. P. Goldstein and D. E. Reid, Clin. Obstet. Gynec., *10:* 313, 1966, with recent additions.)

like the Delfs assay is accurate to levels down to 500 I.U. per liter (0.5 I.U./ml serum); commonly employed immune methods, on the other hand, are accurate to only 1000 I.U./L (1.0 I.U./ml), but specialized radioimmunoassays can get down to the milliunit range. The two different methods used together can indicate certain diagnostic criteria not obtainable by a single method. The results of the two methods generally parallel one another in evaluating HCG and a disparity of results between the different methods of HCG determination might suggest chemotherapy in the untreated patient or a change in therapy in the treated patient. Lau cites the analogy between the lines plotting HCG values by bioassay and immunoassay and the lines plotting temperature and pulse on a patient's chart.

Generally the temperature and pulse lines rise and fall together with the temperature charted below the pulse. When this no longer occurs and the lines cross with temperature rising and pulse falling, the prognosis is impaired. Similarly, the bioassay and immunoassay lines rise and fall together in a normal pregnancy with the bioassay results equal to or just below those of the immunoassay (B/I ratio = 1). When this no longer occurs, and either the plotted lines cross or the values of the two methods diverge, the prognosis for the patient with TRD is impaired.

Further studies on the various subunits of HCG, especially specific types of beta subunits associated with normal pregnancy and different types of TRD, will probably increase our knowledge as to the applicability of these findings, for HCG can be detected specifically (without LH). It should be noted that certain cancers with a primary source outside the genitourinary tract, for example, the breast and gastrointestinal tract, seemingly revert to trophoblast which produces HCG. Perhaps tests for HCG should be a uniform part of the preoperative work-ups for cancer, especially when metastases are suspected. A recent study by Floyd and Cohn adequately reviews the literature.

Associated Ovarian Changes

In at least some cases of hydatidiform mole, as well as of its malignant prototype, choriocarcinoma, the ovaries exhibit an interesting change, in the form of a marked polycystic enlargement, with exaggerated luteinization of predominantly theca rather than granulosa cells. The incidence of these changes in hydatidiform mole would seem to exceed 50% if sonograms are performed, for small cysts may not be palpable. It has also been observed on occasion with normal intrauterine pregnancy. The ovarian enlargement may be only moderate, or it may reach enormous proportions, the masses in some cases being described as of the size of a man's head. The time of appearance of such *theca lutein cysts* seems to be variable, and in some cases they have not appeared until after the evacuation of the mole (Fig. 27.15).

These ovarian changes, including the characteristic *hyperreactio luteinalis,* probably represent an exaggerated response of the ovarian tissue to the abnormally high trophoblastic hormone produced by the molar tissue, although the exact mechanism is not altogether clear. The multiple lutein ovarian cysts thus produced spontaneously disappear within a few months after removal of the mole, and no active treatment is indicated. Shet-

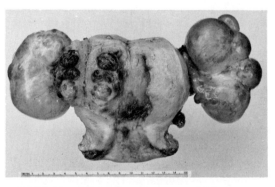

27.15. Note bilateral ovarian cysts which may occur in conjunction with any type of trophoblastic disease. (Courtesy of Dr. Clayton Beecham, Philadelphia, Pennsylvania.)

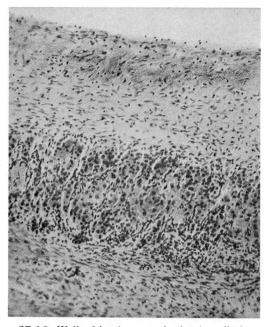

27.16. Wall of lutein cyst, the lutein cells here being obviously of theca cell origin.

tles has recorded recurrent lutein cysts in successive pregnancies. Girouard, Barclay, and Collins have noted 17 cases unassociated with mole or choriocarcinoma where these enlarged cystic ovaries occurred, probably as a response to gonadotrophin stimulation, during a presumably normal pregnancy (Fig. 27.16). Caspi *et al.* have observed similar findings, as noted in Chapter 22.

Treatment. Once hydatidiform mole is diagnosed, the proper treatment is encouragement of evacuation of the uterus preferably by *Pitocin stimulation,* which is usually successful, but otherwise by surgery. This, of course, is followed by careful postoperative supervision with bioassays because of the possibility of later choriocarcinoma. Hysterectomy seems justifiable where the patient has had all desired children and is elderly, for older women seem to show a considerably higher incidence of malignant degeneration (up to 25%), although the usual malignant change is probably less than 5 to 10% Table 27.1.

Vaginal evacuation should be done with much care, to avoid penetration of the thinned-out uterine wall, but at the same time it should be done as thoroughly as possible. Retention of tissue, aside from malignant potentialities, may cause persistence of highly positive pregnancy tests for many weeks or even months, with the later unjustified assumption of choriocarcinoma.

We have been able to utilize suction evacuation in most cases followed sometimes by cautious employment of the curette. An injection of posterior pituitary extract during the procedure will "harden" the uterine wall and lessen the danger of perforation, although bleeding may be free, necessitating a uterine pack, transfusions, etc. If the uterus is enlarged above the umbilicus, however, hysterotomy is less bloody and permits more adequate evacuation of the uterine contents. The use of saline (hypertonic) seems to lead to a high morbidity.

Because diagnosis is rarely made early, *hysterotomy* had been the usual operative approach in this country; Tow (Singapore) on the basis of vast personal experience, impossible for an American, has suggested that hysterotomy is rarely necessary irrespective of the size of the uterus. He states that initial bleeding during curettage may be extreme due to liberation of blood already trapped in the uterine cavity. After initial hemorrhage, however, bleeding becomes much more moderate, especially if pitocin is utilized during operation; blood for transfusion is always available, and today hysterotomy is indicated only rarely with suction-curettage the routine treatment. It is difficult to disagree with so experienced a clinician, and indeed American authors simply do not have the extensive personal experience of various Asian gynecologists in management of trophoblastic lesions.

The *importance of after-supervision* cannot be overemphasized, and bimonthly assays should be continued until the biological tests are repeatedly negative. If the tests are persistently positive, there will be no question as to the presence of actively functioning trophoblastic tissue in the uterus or elsewhere, and this may or may not be due to malignancy. It is usually advisable to obtain periodic x-ray examination of the lungs, which are frequent seats of metastasis in choriocarcinoma.

In the light of present knowledge, no conscientious gynecologist or obstetrician would fail to follow up such cases biologically. Sometimes the tests become negative within two weeks, but often they remain positive for months, indicating definitely the presence of functioning trophoblastic tissue. It is advisable that patients under study practice contraception, as an intercurrent new pregnancy could be very misleading. The currently popular "birth control pill" is acceptable and suppresses the confusing pituitary LH assays, although intermenstrual "break-through" spotting may be disquieting.

If the test continues positive, and especially if the patient has bleeding, and the uterus remains more or less subinvoluted, a second thorough curettage is indicated. This may reveal residual molar tissue or only necrotic portions of decidua. *If the test still remains positive, and especially if the quantitative titer becomes higher,* more definitive therapy must be considered. There is general belief in the efficacy of such drugs as methotrexate as the primary treatment of choriocarcinoma (see "Treatment"), as well as other types of trophoblastic disease of uncertain nature where there is a persistently high or rising titer, and where further pregnancies are desired. An abnormal titer of HCG after evacuation of a mole should merit consideration of some type of specific treatment.

On the other hand, hysterectomy should be considered in the *older parous woman* where there is no evidence of extra-uterine disease, and in many instances it will afford considerable insight into the exact pathological nature of the TRD (as well as obviating the much higher incidence of malignant degeneration or hemorrhage that occur in the older woman). Otherwise there is only evidence of increased HCG which may be due to diverse causes.

In the "premethotrexate days" a persistently rising level of HCG, irrespective of the histological appearance of the curettings, was considered a valid indication for hysterectomy, even in the young patient, with the hope of curing an occasional early choriocarcinoma. At the same time, it was appreciated that most cases would show no more than residual trophoblast in the myometrium where it is inaccessible to the curette. In other words, a number of hysterectomies were performed in the hope of curing an occasional early choriocarcinoma. Management of the *younger* patient with a postmolar elevated HCG is much more sophisticated today.

CHORIOCARCINOMA (CHORIONEPITHELIOMA)

This highly malignant neoplasm (Figs. 27.17, 18), for which both of the above names are used interchangeably, is derived from the chorionic epithelium. It may develop after full term delivery, abortion, or hydatidiform mole although previous pregnancy is not always recognized. Indeed many cases suggest the probability that an initial pregnancy may "go bad" and give rise to choriocarcinoma without a previous mole, abortion, or pregnancy, and Beischer refers to these as

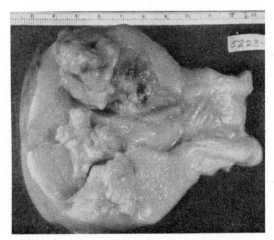

27.17. Choriocarcinoma of uterus of intramural type. (Courtesy of Dr. Laman A. Gray, Louisville, Kentucky.)

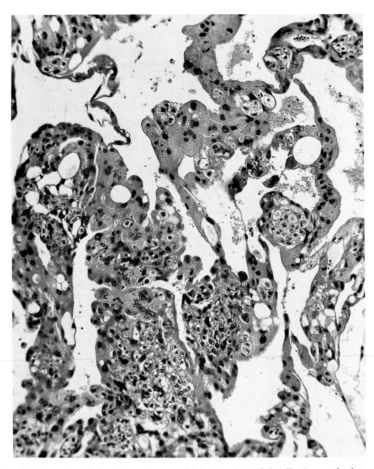

27.18. Curettings from a case of choriocarcinoma which terminated fatally 5 months later with multiple metastases.

"de novo choriocarcinomas." Recently a 17-year-old nulliparous clinic patient was explored because of a suspected ruptured ectopic pregnancy; a definite choriocarcinoma with myometrial perforation and hemoperitoneum was found, and resection of the tumor with conservation of the uterus and subsequent chemotherapy performed. (Incidentally, the titer is negative after 5½ years.) This girl had never experienced pregnancy, and in the three or four years in which she had menstruated could recall nothing to even suggest the possibility of gestation. Yet it is generally believed that previous pregnancy has occurred, possibly in too early a form as to be recognizable except in rare instances.

In proportion to the relative frequency of these three antecedent pregnancy conditions, the incidence after hydatidiform mole is disproportionately high. Fully 50 per cent of all cases of choriocarcinoma are believed to follow vesicular mole, 25 per cent after incomplete abortion, and the rest after preceding or (rarely) concomitant pregnancy. It should be repeated, however, that only in a very small proportion of cases of moles, probably less than 5 to 10 per cent, does malignancy develop, the benign mole being far more common than choriocarcinoma. The latter, indeed, is a very rare disease, and in many rather large clinics only an occasional case has been encountered. Furthermore, because of the frequent difficulty in microscopic diagnosis in this group of cases, it is quite certain that many cases reported as choriocarcinoma have really been highly proliferative but benign hydatidiform moles. It must be remembered that choriocarcinoma is a malignant tumor arising from the fetal trophoblast and not a tumor of the uterus itself. We thus have the curious condition of a tumor of one individual growing in and invading the tissue of another.

Although trophoblastic tumors are not usually found spontaneously in animals, Lindsey and Wharton reported a case in a Rhesus monkey. They have, however, been produced by Shintari *et al.* in certain pregnant rats. After fetectomy, benzanthrocine stimulation was carried out, and this was followed by the development of choriocarcinoma as well as other malignant neoplasms.

Pathology. The tumor appears as a dark, hemorrhagic, grumous mass on the uterine wall, or in other cases in the substance of the latter, beneath the surface (intramural variety (Fig. 27.17). It soon shows extensive ulceration, with increasing spread on the surface or with penetration of the musculature. Uterine perforation and hemorrhage may occur.

Microscopically, it is characterized by a disorderly growth of trophoblastic tissue, both syncytium and cytotrophoblast, into the muscle, with destruction of the latter and extensive coagulation necrosis, as well as hemorrhage. The villous pattern usually is soon blotted out, although traces of it may persist in rare early cases, such as those reported by Brewer and Gerbie. In these unusual cases arising in pregnancy or immediately postpartum, malignancy was manifest clinically despite a villous pattern with considerable trophoblastic overgrowth in an ostensibly normal placenta. MacRae, Driscoll, and McKelvey and others report early choriocarcinoma in routine study of early placentas. Van der Werf *et al.* have recently tabulated 17 cases of metastatic choriocarcinoma with pregnancy.

However, the presence of definite villi strongly militates against a diagnosis of true choriocarcinoma, although it does not guarantee that transitory self-limited

trophoblast may not temporarily involve the lung until it is obliterated by the uncertain defense mechanism. Both layers of trophoblast are involved in the malignant process, but in varying degrees. Certain cases of *syncytial endometritis* or *myometritis,* characterized by abnormal persistence and excess of the syncytial tissue which invades the uterine muscle in the implantation area even in normal pregnancy, are frequently mistaken for choriocarcinoma (Figs. 27.19, 20).

Clinical Characteristics. Although choriocarcinoma may rarely occur late in the course of full term pregnancy, it far more often develops after parturition, and especially after expulsion or evacuation of a hydatidiform mole. In some cases the symptoms appear within a few weeks; in some cases many years (Fig. 27.21). Where the latent period is very long, however, there must always be a suspicion of a more recent and perhaps unsuspected pregnancy. *Bleeding* is the chief early symptom, which becomes increasingly profuse, and may be fatal.

Metastases usually appear comparatively early and involve lung, brain, liver, bone, and even skin. Not infrequently it is these which first call attention to the probability of choriocarcinoma. The vagina and vulva are often the seats of such metastases, which appear as dark hemorrhagic nodules, resembling thrombosed varices. *Cough* or *hemoptysis* should always lead to the suspicion of pulmonary metastasis, and this is often confirmed by x-ray examination. As the disease advances, there is increasing *emaciation* and *weakness,* with profound *anemia* from the frequently profuse hemorrhage.

A case of our own concerned a 26-year-old woman who had passed a mole three years ago, but had then been found to have a subsequent normal titer. Two successive abortions occurred, followed by progressive malaise with pulmonary and skin lesions, both of which showed typical and ultimately fatal choriocarcinoma despite chemotherapy, although curettings showed no uterine tumor. In this case, it seems probable that the malig-

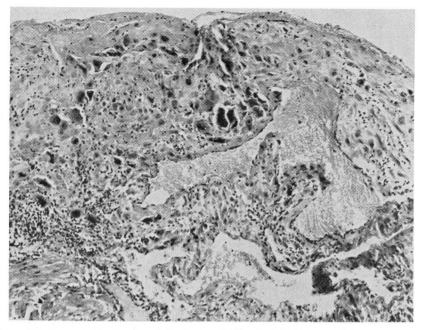

27.19. Syncytial myometritis showing extensive trophoblastic infiltration, chiefly syncytial, of decidual layer. Section from normal pregnancy (Porro operation for myoma). Such a picture is often mistaken for choriocarcinoma.

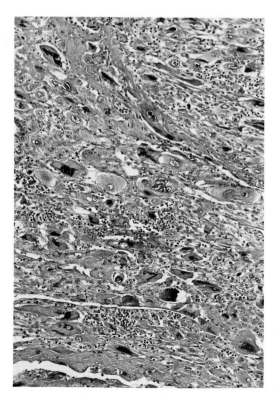

nancy arose not from the earlier mole (which was followed by a normal HCG) but from a later abortion. Cases of reported choriocarcinoma arising from mole with intervening normal pregnancy must be evaluated with caution.

Tedeschi and Toy indicate that it is only malignant trophoblast which has the ability to invade arterial channels. Benign trophoblast may be found in the venous circuit, but is generally arrested in the lung; malignant change with tumor emboli in the pulmonic capillaries encourages bypass of the lung with passage into the arterial system, and the development of cor pulmonale due to right-sided heart failure. *Cerebral accidents* due to intracranial tumor with hemorrhage are a common cause of death in choriocarcinoma. Primary choriocarcinoma of the ovary, as noted by Mar-

27.20. Trophoblastic invasion of myometrium (syncytial myometritis). This type of invasion may be mistaken for choriocarcinoma, but it is common in benign mole and even in normal pregnancy.

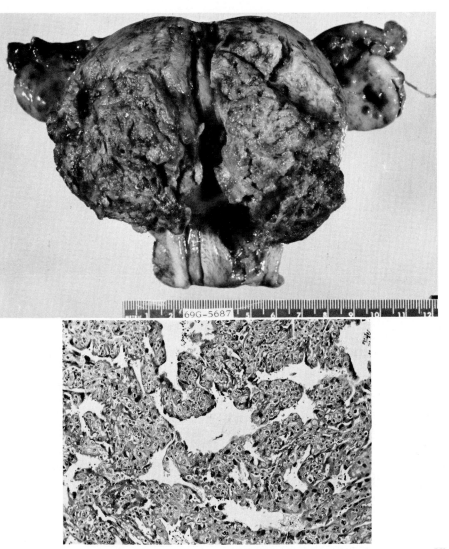

27.21 A. Hydatidiform mole. Six negative currettages for bleeding over a period of seven years. Ultimate choriocarcinoma, as noted. B. Microscopic pattern of above lesion. There is a predominence of cytotrophoblast.

rubini, is perhaps a more logical pattern of teratoma rather than a sequel to the exceedingly rare ovarian pregnancy.

As noted earlier, occasional cases have been reported in conjunction with metastases during pregnancy, and Driscoll and McKelvey in noting very early choriocarcinoma as a chance finding in a normal term pregnancy, suggest that routine study of normal placentas be standard. True choriocarcinoma in both mother and fetus has been reported in a few cases (Buckell and Owen, Mercer *et*

al., and Daamen *et al.*); it is generally fatal. Approximately 60 cases of choriocarcinoma of the tube have been reported by Riggs *et al.*

Although choriocarcinoma is in most cases a highly malignant neoplasm, it is curious that a certain proportion, put by some as almost 5 to 10% (in the prechemotherapy era), seemed to undergo either spontaneous cure or cure after obviously incomplete operations, even in the presence of metastasis. Moreover, it is known that the untreated primary uterine tumor may in rare instances undergo complete regression and disappearance even though the patient dies of metastasis to other organs, and there have been many such cases recorded. We can only speculate as to the explanation of such vagaries, but breakdown of the generalized systemic resistance with a belated resurgence of the local one seems the best explanation.

While choriocarcinoma generally runs a rather rapid and fatal course, if uninfluenced by chemotherapy, certain exceptions may be noted, such as the case of Paranjothy and Samuel. Their patient with presumed choriocarcinoma ("although an occasional villus was found") was treated by hysterectomy without irradiation or chemotherapy, and lived 12 years before returning with characteristic metastatic disease, which lead to rapid demise. (See Fig. 27.22)

The recent study by Elston and Bagshaw points out that the diagnosis of TRD is best made by a combination of clinical, hormonal, histological, and radiological diagnoses, and that curettage alone can make an accurate diagnosis of malignant disease in approximately 20% of the patients.

Diagnosis. Where hemorrhage occurs after any of the pregnancy conditions enumerated above as antecedent to choriocarcinoma, *curettage* (Fig. 27.18) is ordinarily performed, and this may reveal the nature of the disease. It should be pointed out, however, that there are *many pitfalls in diagnosis from curettings*, especially as a certain amount of trophoblastic overgrowth is apt to be found even in normal pregnancy (Fig. 27.20). In addition, the clinician should always be mindful that curettage may yield only the more superficial tissues, which may not be indicative of the activity of trophoblast lying deeper in the myometrium. For this reason, HCG assay might be considered in postpartum or postabortal patients where curettage does not account for or regulate abnormal bleeding.

In a certain proportion of cases, the first suspicion of malignancy comes only after the appearance of *metastases* in the vagina or vulva, or after the occurrence of *hemoptysis* or *cough* leads to x-ray examination of the chest and the demonstration of pulmonary metastasis. Kittredge emphasizes the equivocal nature of the x-ray findings necessitating HCG determination. Finally, it should be emphasized

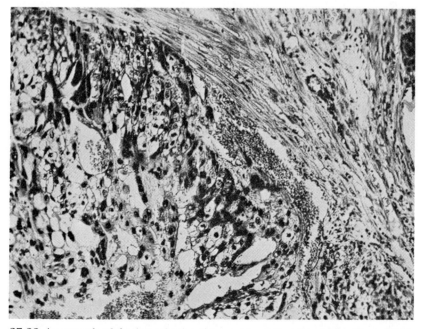

27.22. An example of choriocarcinoma; this must be distinguished from Figure 27.19.

that the *decisive diagnosis of choriocarci-noma should ideally be made both by the microscope and by hormone studies.* A rising titer after evacuation of a mole should make one extremely suspicious of the development of choriocarcinoma, and consideration of an elevated HCG will warrant treatment for choriocarcinoma without specific pathological evidence of even its development.

In study of the material of the Mathieu Choriocarcinoma Registry, it was found that the lesions most often incorrectly diagnosed as choriocarcinoma have been benign hydatidiform mole, chorioadenoma destruens, and syncytial endometritis and myometritis. The latter, pictured in Figure 27.22 (see also Fig. 27.23) is not neoplastic. It is characterized by a scattered infiltration of the endometrium or myometrium, or both, with trophoblastic cells. It is impossible to know how many cases of presumed choriocarcinoma occurring after expulsion of a mole have been subjected to very toxic chemotherapy where the persistently elevated titer was due to only syncytial myometritis.

Hormone Studies with Choriocarcinoma

Much of what has been said as to the application of hormone studies in the management of hydatidiform mole applies to their employment in the diagnosis and prognosis of choriocarcinoma. Unfortunately, these tests offer no absolute means of differentiating between these two conditions; although they suggest excessive trophoblastic activity, the final differentiation is based upon clinical and histological studies. It has been generally accepted that the cytotrophoblast produces HCG which is merely stored in the syncytium. Wynn and Davies, however, in discussing the function of the trophoblast via the electronmicroscope indicate that the syncytium is the productive cell; they have also indicated that the syncytial cells evolve from the more juvenile Langhams cells (cytotrophoblast). Most cases of TRD show hyperplasia of both cell types, though one may predominate—this seemingly does not influence the degree of malignancy on the titer.

Mention has already been made of the

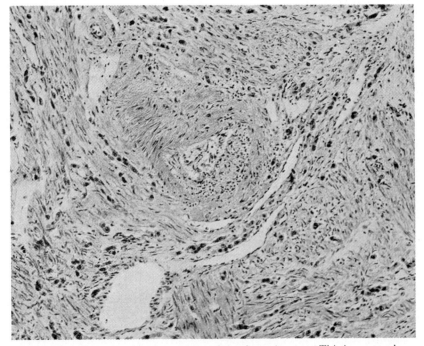

27.23. Trophoblastic invasion of musculature beneath implantation area. This is a normal process, but has at times been wrongly diagnosed as syncytioma or choriocarcinoma.

fact that a persistently high hormone titer after evacuation of a mole is not by any means always indicative of choriocarcinoma, although in some cases the latter does exist; nor does the spinal fluid study differentiate between the two conditions. Finally, it should be remembered that in the occasional case of choriocarcinoma negative phases have been recorded, in which the urinary HCG is negative or only feebly positive. The only explanation which suggests itself to us is that the gonadotrophic hormone, although produced in excess, does not gain access to the maternal circulation because of the extensive necrosis so often produced by the tumor, or that tumor cells are too anaplastic to produce hormone (Browne). In our experience, serum HCG is a much more accurate means of bioassay; with this type of assay we have never studied a choriocarcinoma which was associated with a normal titer prior to treatment.

Vagaries of Benign Moles. Although the previous pages have summarized the usual microscopic and gross pathology of the trophoblastic tumors in relation to their clinical behavior, on occasion one may find a complete disparity between the histological appearance and the course of the disease. For example, we are acquainted with several cases of perfectly benign moles which have metastasized to lung, liver, skeleton, etc., with a fatal outcome. These histologically benign but clinically malignant cases are rare, but do occur (Delfs *et al.*). Perhaps usage of such terms as "non-metastatic and metastatic TRD" may be more informative than such pathological terms as mole or choriocarcinoma, but as a rule the pathological designation seems more precise and specific.

Similarly, we have seen cases in which a benign mole was evacuated, yet later bioassay showed a persistently high level despite repeatedly negative curettings, x-ray of the chest, and even hysterectomy. Sometimes the level would persist for years, before there would appear clinical evidence of a rapidly advancing and fatal choriocarcinoma. How else can one explain such phenomena other than by postulating benign extrauterine trophoblastic elements held temporarily in check by a maternal defense mechanism that finally became attenuated and was overcome? The case report by Kirk, in which a chorioadenoma destruens was treated by hysterectomy, with the appearance of trophoblast in retroperitoneal lymph nodes eleven years after surgery also suggests a defense mechanism that was finally overcome. We can also recall the occurrence of a uterine choriocarcinoma developing in a patient seven years after tubal ligation had been performed following passage of a mole despite negative HCG for over a year postmolar.

TREATMENT

In *past* years the treatment of choriocarcinoma was predominantly *surgical* with hysterectomy and removal of the adnexa the usual operative procedure. Where the level of HCG subsequently became elevated, the outlook was poor, for this usually signified the advent of recurrence, metastasis, and death, although certain cases of metastatic or recurrent tumor were sometimes observed to disappear spontaneously due presumably to an increased host resistance. Where there was a demonstrable recurrent or extrauterine lesion, various other therapy was utilized prior to the past decade.

Irradiation, generally by deep x-ray, seemed to lead to occasional remissions and a few apparent cures of presumed metastatic choriocarcinoma in the lungs. Various *hormones,* both estrogenic and androgenic, were tried, but probably had little clinical effect, although conceivably the level of the HCG might be decreased. *Nitrogen mustard* was given a thorough trial but seemingly with rather meagre results.

Additional surgical procedures such as lobectomy or laminectomy were occasionally utilized for removal of metastatic disease with rather discouraging results, as might be anticipated, because choriocarcinoma spreads diffusely in sarcoma-like fashion via hematogenous channels. Nevertheless, a few presumed remissions were noted, but if one bears in mind the fact that such remissions occasionally have been observed to occur spontaneously, the actual value of such surgery is open to question. Today there must be exceedingly rare indications for this type of extra pelvic surgery, and indeed the role of hysterectomy itself as the primary treatment for choriocarcinoma has been seriously challenged by increasing recognition of the astoundingly beneficial results achieved by chemotherapy with preservation of the uterus and its procreative potentiality. This, of course, is of particular importance in the treatment of a disease that is common in the young female.

MODERN TREATMENT

Approximately 25 years ago, Hertz and his associates at the National Institute of Health began to use various drugs for the treatment of metastatic TRD. Initially *chemotherapy* was utilized merely as adjuvant therapy in patients surgically treated who had continuous or recurrent disease. The drug used was usually methotrexate, and this is still the primary chemotherapeutic agent, although in subsequent years other allied drugs have been developed in the event of drug resistance or as a form of mixed therapy.

The early results with methotrexate (MTX) were most encouraging, in the nature of 60% remission, which was far superior to the results achieved by surgery in all cases of choriocarcinoma. For example, Brewer has recorded 122 patients who had been treated only by surgery. Even without metastases there was a 5-year salvage of only 41%, but where metastatic disease was apparent, there was a marked drop-off to 19%. Actually, Brewer's figures are better than other statistics for choriocarcinoma, which have accrued in earlier years. Indeed, the noted pathologist, James Ewing, stated that, if a patient with choriocarcinoma survived, the diagnosis was incorrect. Today no one will accept this pessimistic statement but there is no question that yesteryear's surgical treatment of choriocarcinoma was quite inadequate.

Chemically MTX is 4-amino-N^{10}-methyl pteroylglutamic acid, a folic acid antagonist which may be given orally or intravenously in dosage according to body weight, but generally 25 mg. a day. Our current *method of therapy* is to give a five-day course, followed by a resting stage of one week during which time repeat quantitative levels of HCG are obtained. If the level continues to decrease, subsequent courses of MTX are administered until the titer becomes negative, and repeated titers are obtained until there is a year of negativity. (Fig. 27.24). Should there be, during therapy, evidence of a rising or sustained HCG, apparent drug toxicity, or other complications, various newer drugs such as actinomycin D or chlorambucil may be administered.

Goldstein believes that actinomycin D is at least as effective as MTX, and is less apt to produce toxicity. He likewise feels that this should be utilized routinely in the treatment of benign hydatidiform mole, but as of this writing most clinicians do not share this belief. Since hydatidiform mole is followed only very infrequently by malignant degeneration, it seems unwarranted to treat all patients with such an extremely toxic agent. With a poorly motivated, unintelligent woman who is unlikely to return for HCG determinations, chemotherapy deserves consideration.

Goldstein finds that mole treated by MTX or low dosage actinomycin D may progress to metastatic disease in about 8% of cases. If, however, large dosage actinomycin is used, there is zero progression. Perhaps improved knowledge of sensitivity tests, as implied by Patillo *et al.*, will lead to more precise therapy.

Toxicity

MTX is an extremely toxic drug, for which reason we do not care to utilize it as a routine prophylactic agent in such a usually benign process as simple hydatidiform mole. Such minor problems as dermatitis, alopecia, and simple nausea and vomiting are frequent. Other more severe possibilities include profound bone marrow depression, renal or hepatic com-

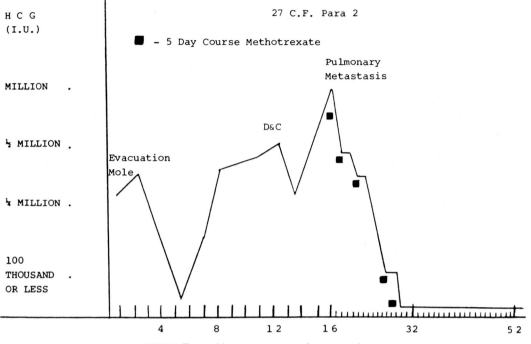

H C G
(I.U.)

27 C.F. Para 2

■ - 5 Day Course Methotrexate

MILLION .

Pulmonary
Metastasis

½ MILLION .

D&C

Evacuation
Mole

¼ MILLION .

100
THOUSAND .
OR LESS

4   8   1 2   1 6   32   5 2

27.24. Favorable response to methotrexate therapy

plications, severe stomatitis and actual ulceration of the gastrointestinal tract. Lewis notes, however, that the deaths from drug toxicity occurred in early patients; with increased familiarity as to the possible toxic sequelae, a protocol for treatment has been developed which has made drug fatality an extremely rare result. Toxicity generally reaches a peak within two to four weeks after inception of therapy.

Considerable care must be taken to avoid too enthusiastic (too much or too rapid) employment of the chemotherapeutic drugs, particularly where there is extensive uterine disease. Severe necrosis and slough of the lesion may ensue with extensive uncontrollable bleeding which may be one of the few indications for hysterectomy. Some of the early fatalities associated with drug therapy occurred in this fashion. (See Fig. 27.25)

Primary Chemotherapy

As a result of the favorable results of metastatic or recurrent choriocarcinoma to chemotherapy, Hertz *et al.* have proceeded to advocate drugs as a *primary* mode of therapy without any surgery, and this concept has truly revolutionized our approach to this disease, particularly in the younger woman. Utilizing a combination of drugs, but with prime reliance on MTX, Hertz *et al.* have treated 111 women with *metastatic TRD*, of whom 75 were presumed to have choriocarcinoma on the basis generally of a high titer following passage of a mole as well as certain x-ray changes, although *histological* evidence of malignancy is not always available. Of the total 111 patients, however, a remission rate of 64% was obtained (Table 27.2); although all remissions were not of 5 years duration, some patients have remained well for over 12 years. In 75 patients with presumed choriocarcinoma, the remission rate was 60%; of 36 additional patients with mole and chorioadenoma destruens it was 75%, although one must question the validity of including patients with such lesions as representing metastatic TRD (Table 27.3). More recently Ross achieved a nearly 75% remission in a smaller series of patients with invasive TRD treated by sequential MTX and actinomycin D (Table 27.4).

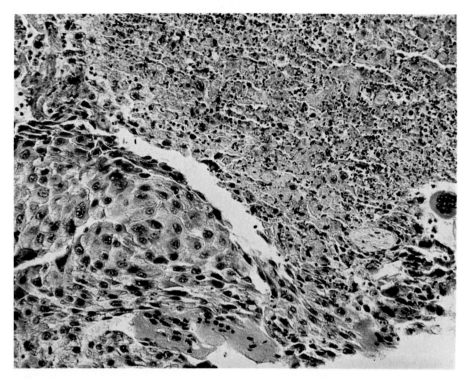

27.25. Uterus removed after two courses of methotrexate because of bleeding. Extreme necrobiotic appearance, *right upper*; viable trophoblast, *left lower*.

There is growing acceptance of the tendency towards dividing TRD into two simple categories, based on the behavior of the disease (*non-metastatic* or *metastatic*) rather than on its histological appearance, and there is considerable logic in it, for what is available for pathological study may be far from representative of the true potential of the tumor.

(1) Nonmetastatic Trophoblastic Disease. A persistently positive titer more than 60 days after evacuation of a mole will suggest residual TRD, and every effort must be made to exclude

Table 27.2

*Results of Chemotherapy in 111 Patients with Metastatic Trophoblastic Disease**

Treatment	Choriocarcinoma		Mole, destruens, and others		Total		
	Cases	Remissions	Cases	Remissions	Cases	Remissions	Per cent
MTX initially	58	29	29	16	87	45	51
Actino after MTX	17	10	6	2	23	12	52
Actino initially	7	3	6	4	13	7	54
MTX after Actino	5	2	2	2	7	4	57
Other†					35	4	9
Total					111	72	64

* 10/1/63.

† Vincaleukoblastine; combination therapy; 6-mercaptopurine; Cytoxan; HN_2; DON. (Courtesy of Dr. R. L. Hertz, Washington, D.C.)

Table 27.3

Complete Remission after Chemotherapy in 111 Cases with Metastases

Histology	Cases	Remissions	Per cent Remissions
Choriocarcinoma	75	45	60
Mole, destruens, and other	36	27	75
Total	111	72	64

(Courtesy of Dr. R. L. Hertz, Washington, D.C.)

metastatic foci by x-ray of the chest, brain and liver scan, and other methods. It is important to obtain quantitative assays of HCG, for the routine pregnancy tests are seemingly insufficiently sensitive to detect HCG at a low level. Should the titer remain high, chemotherapy should be begun according to the routine noted previously. Hertz, Ross, and Lipsett have achieved 93% success in 44 patients with nonmetastatic disease treated only by chemotherapy (98% if two drug failures who have had satisfactory remission following hysterectomy are included).

(2) Metastatic Trophoblastic Disease. Lewis has noted the experience of many clinical attempts at utilizing chemotherapy (primary) in metastatic TRD with remission rates up to 75 per cent. It should not be assumed that all such cases necessarily represent true choriocarcinoma, for histological evidence was not always available, the diagnosis being made purely on the biological behavior of the disease. However, Brewer does report 44 patients (of 85 with TRD) who had specific histological proof of choriocarcinoma, and in these he reports an 80% remission. Once a negative titer has been obtained in a patient treated by MTX, relapse is infrequent, but may occur in 10% of patients so treated (Fig. 27.26.).

Of a group of 50 National Institute of Health patients with metastatic TRD complete remission was obtained in 95% of the women whose HCG was less than 100,000 I.U. per 24 hours and whose therapy was begun within 4 months of the apparent onset of the disease. When the duration was longer than 4 months, and the HCG greater than 100,000 I.U., the remission rate was only 36%. Hammond *et al.* divides patients into good and poor

Table 27.4

Reported Series of Metastatic Trophoblastic Neoplasms Treated with Chemotherapy

Senior author	Year	Drugs	Patients	Complete Remission
				%
Hertz	1961	Methotrexate, vinblastine sulfate	63	48
Hreshchyshyn	1961	Methotrexate	7	57
Li	1961	Methotrexate, 6-diazo-5-oxo-L-norleucine (D.O.N.), chlorambucil, actinomycin D	12	58
Chan	1962	Methotrexate	7	43
Bagshawe	1963	Methotrexate, 6-Mercaptopurine	15	67
Sung	1964	6-Mercaptopurine	58*	44
Brewer	1964	Methotrexate, actinomycin D, Li's "triple therapy"	20	55
Manahan	1964	Methotrexate	28	71
Lamb	1964	Methotrexate	11	36
Ross	1965	Methotrexate, actinomycin D	50	74
Lewis	1966	Methotrexate, actinomycin D	8	75

* Best estimate from inadequate data on patients with choriocarcinoma and metastases. (Courtesy of Dr. J. Lewis, Jr., Obstet. Gynec., *10:* 330, 1966.)

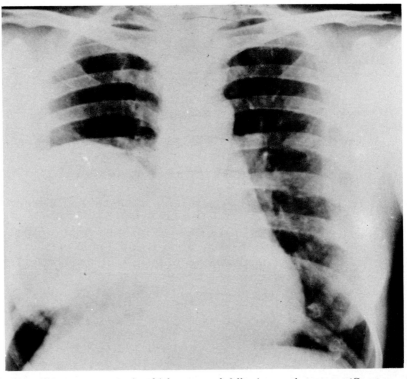

27.26. Massive pulmonary metastasis which regressed following methotrexate. (Courtesy of Dr. M. S. Baggish, Hartford, Conn.)

risk categories on the duration of the disease and the titer, and his results are not dissimilar. However, the poor risk patients seemingly may have a better prognosis if initial treatment consists of combination chemotherapy. There is general agreement that the prognosis is markedly impaired if there are hepatic or cerebral metastasis; in such instances adjuvant irradiation therapy should be utilized.

In a small series of 39 patients, Jones and Lewis report a 100% remission rate of 18 patients with nonmetastatic TRD and an 85% figure with metastatic TRD. Drug resistance was noted in 7.7%. "High risk" patients seemed to respond more favorably to triple drug therapy as has been noted earlier. Lewis has made generalizations about metastatic TRD which are worth repeating verbatim through his kind permission (Table 27.5).

Pregnancy after Drug Therapy

In the younger woman treated for metastatic TRD, chemotherapy permits retention of the uterus with the possibility of subsequent pregnancy, and a considerable number of these cases have been recorded. Van Thiel *et al.* reported a follow up of 50 women who had been treated for both metastatic and nonmetastatic TRD, and subsequently had

Table 27.5

In summary, the generalizations from experience with metastatic gestational TRD are:

1. Patients with metastatic TRD are curable with chemotherapy.
2. Drug toxicity is potentially serious but is predictable.
3. Histological diagnosis is less important once the disease is metastatic.
4. Site of metastases is important prognostically.
5. Duration of disease prior to therapy and the level of HCG excretion are important in predicting response to chemotherapy.
6. Accurate HCG assay is critical for proper diagnosis and management.

(Courtesy of Dr. J. Lewis, Jr., Clin. Obstet. Gynec., *10:* 330, 1966.)

88 pregnancies, with no increase in fetal wastage, congenital abnormalities, or complicated pregnancy, with the possible exception of placenta accreta. Pastorfide and Goldstein indicate that there may be a higher incidence of abortion. Spellacy, Meeker, and McKelvey report a patient with three pregnancies after a genuine choriocarcinoma treated by MTX, and they record 17 pregnancies in 11 patients so treated; additional cases have occurred since.

A negative assay for one full year is considered a prerequisite before pregnancy is allowed, for obviously a new pregnancy with rising HCG would cause considerable confusion as to the status of the patient. Consequently, contraception is recommended for a year. Kistner has indicated that "birth control pills" will in no way influence the HCG and may help to suppress pituitary gonadotrophin, although break-through bleeding may confuse the issue clinically. The offspring of mothers treated by MTX are routinely reported as normal, and in this respect an interesting case is reported by Freedman, which concerns a woman who previously had evacuation of a mole. Because of a rising titer of HCG after the passage of a mole she was treated vigorously with MTX for three months before it was realized that she had a new pregnancy, at which time drug therapy was discontinued. Despite the presumed toxic effects of the MTX the patient subsequently delivered perfectly normal twins.

The Role of Hysterectomy

Hysterectomy seems of decreasing importance in the management of TRD with certain exceptions as noted by Lewis, Ketcham, and Hertz. Where hysterectomy is contemplated it should often be preceded by chemotherapy to minimize the possibility of disseminating tumor emboli. Indications for surgery include the following:

(1) The elderly multiparous patient with a hydatidiform mole;

(2) Such complications as vaginal hemorrhage, uterine perforation, with intraperitoneal bleeding, etc.;

(3) Drug resistance or toxicity;

(4) Certain cases seemingly with the disease confined to the uterus where there seems a good prospect for eradication of the disease without the necessity of prolonged and toxic chemotherapy.

Certainly it is a tremendous boon for the young woman anxious for pregnancy to avoid hysterectomy, retain her uterus, and subsequently become pregnant. Lewis aptly points out that choriocarcinoma starts as a seemingly normal pregnancy which women anticipate eagerly, and then turns out to be a life-threatening, horrible disease that few of them have even heard of. Today these women can be assured that although the treatment may be stringent, cure seems possible with preservation of the uterus and the possibility of normal pregnancy. A trophoblastic lesion of *short duration* and a *low initial titer* seems to afford a much more favorable prognosis.

Admittedly, it is beneficial to the young patient to retain her uterus and still be assured a considerable chance of cure and pregnancy despite what has always been considered as one of the most lethal forms of cancer. From a purely pathological standpoint, however, this form of treatment is somewhat frustrating for in the absence of hysterectomy it may be impossible to know precisely what is being treated except an elevated HCG. Indeed we suspect that not a few cases of presumed metastatic TRD really represent a localized process with a high titer and some nonspecific lung shadow which might have disappeared spontaneously, obviously not Fig. 27.26.

These comments should, however, not be allowed to detract from the truly outstanding work of Hertz and his associates, whose patient efforts have made it seem that chemotherapy can at least partially subjugate or even cure a high percentage of what has always been regarded as a particularly lethal malignancy with an especial propensity for afflicting the younger woman. At the same time, it is often difficult to quote precisely their statistics because they are often utilizing different modalities of drug therapy for diseases where the exact pathological diagnosis must be regarded as uncertain. Indeed, space limitations have compelled us to delete from this edition various references (found in earlier editions) to many cases of malignant choriocarcinoma that were seemingly cured spontaneously or following surgery, irradiation, hormones, nitrogen mustard, and various other agents.

Subsequent editions of this text may stress the important role of immunotherapy in the treatment of TRD. There is considerable preliminary work with regard to improving the immunological response. Increased knowledge of various transplantation techniques will be helpful in that these depend on the absence of various antibodies which are so vital in the treatment of a malignancy. It would seem that a combined immunochemotherapeutic approach is most promising.

REFERENCES

Acosta-Sison, H.: Changing attitudes in management of hydatidiform mole (196 cases). Amer. J. Obstet. Gynec., *88:* 634, 1964.

Adcock, E. W. *et al.*: Human chorionic gonadotropin: its possible role in maternal lymphocyte suppression. Science, *181:* 843, 1973.

Attwood, H. D., and Park, W. W.: Embolism to the lungs by trophoblast. J. Obstet. Gynaec. Brit. Comm., *68:* 611, 1961.

Baggish, M. S., Tow, S. H., and Jones, H. W.: Sex chromatin pattern in hydatidiform mole. Amer. J. Obstet. Gynec., *102:* 362, 1968.

Bagshawe, K. C.: *Choriocarcinoma.* Edward Arnold Ltd., London, 1969.

Bardawil, W. A., Hertig, A. T., and Velardo, J. T.: Regression of trophoblast. Obstet. Gynec., *10:* 614, 1957.

Behrman, S. J., *et al.*: Placental specific antigen. Amer. J. Obstet. Gynec., *118:* 616, 1974.

Beischer, N. A.: Hydatidiform mole with coexistent fetus. J. Obstet. Gynaec. Brit. Comm., *68:* 231, 1961.

Beischer, N. A.: Significance of chromatin pattern in cases of hydatidiform mole with associated fetus. Aust. New Zeal. J. Obstet. Gynec., *6:* 127, 1966.

Bergman, P.: Bilateral multiple lutein cysts of the ovary complicating normal pregnancy. Obstet. Gynec., *21:* 28, 1963.

Billingham, W. D.: Transplantation immunity and the placenta. J. Obstet. Gynaec. Brit. Comm., *74:* 834, 1967.

Birnholz, J. C., and Barnes, A. B.: Early diagnosis of hydatidiform mole by ultrasound imaging. J.A.M.A., *225:* 1359, 1973.

Bobrow, M. L., and Friedman, S.: Hydatidiform mole in 12-year-old girl. Amer. J. Obstet. Gynec., *73:* 448, 1957.

Brandes, J., Grunstein, S., and Peretz, A.: Suction evacuation of the uterine cavity in hydatidiform mole. Obstet. Gynec., *28:* 689, 1966.

Brandes, J., and Peretz, A.: Recurrent hydatidiform mole. Obstet. Gynec., *25:* 398, 1965.

Brewer, J. I., Gerbie, A. B., Skom, I. H., Nagle, R. G., and Torok, E. E.: Chemotherapy in trophoblastic disease. Amer. J. Obstet. Gynec., *90:* 566, 1964.

Brewer, J. I., Rhinehart, J. J., and Dunbar, R. W.: Choriocarcinoma: report of five or more years survival from Albert Mathieu Chorionepithelioma Registry. Amer. J. Obstet. Gynec., *81:* 574, 1961.

Brewer, J. I., and Gerbie, A. B.: Early development of choriocarcinoma. Obstet. Gynec., *94:* 692, 1964.

Brinck-Johnson, T., Sole, J., and Galton, V. A.: Urinary excretion of estrogens with mole and choriocarcinoma. Obstet. Gynec., *36:* 671, 1970.

Brown, E. J., and Effen, S. B.: Induction of labor in hydatidiform mole by intrauterine infusion of hypertonic glucose solution. Amer. J. Obstet. Gynec., *92:* 1160, 1965.

Browne, F. J.: A case of chorionepithelioma of the uterus with pulmonary metastases cured by operation and x-rays. J. Obstet. Gynaec. Brit. Comm., *64:* 852, 1957.

Buckell, E. W. C., and Owen, T. K.: Chorionepithelioma in mother and infant. J. Obstet. Gynaec. Brit. Comm., *61:* 329, 1954.

Canlas, B. D.: Benign lesions of aberrant trophoblast in the lung. Obstet. Gynec., *20:* 602, 1962.

Carr, D. H.: Cytogenetics and the pathology of hydatidiform degeneration. Obstet. Gynec., *33:* 333, 1969.

Chan, D. P. C., and Pang, I. S. C.: Late solitary pulmonary chorionepithelioma following hydatidiform mole. J. Obstet. Gynec. Brit. Comm., *71:* 192, 1964.

Chun, D., Braga, C., Chow, C., and Lok, L.: Clinical observations on some aspects of hydatidiform mole. J. Obstet. Gynec. Brit. Comm., *71:* 180, 1964; Treatment of hydatidiform mole. Ibid., *71:* 185, 1964.

Clark, P. B., Gusdon, J. P. Jr., and Burt, R. L.: Hydatidiform mole. Obstet. Gynec., *35:* 597, 1970.

Coppleson, M.: Hydatidiform mole and its complication. J. Obstet. Gynaec. Brit. Comm., *65:* 238, 1958.

Crisp, W. E.: Choriocarcinoma of the fallopian tube coincident with viable pregnancy. Amer. J. Obstet. Gynec., *71:* 442, 1956.

Daamen, C. B. F., Bloem, G. W. D., and Westerbeek, A. J.: Chorionepithelioma in mother and child. J. Obstet. Gynaec. Brit. Comm., *68:* 144, 1961.

Delfs, E.: Quantitative chorionic gonadotrophin determinations in patients with hydatidiform mole and chorionepithelioma. Ann. N. Y. Acad. Sci., *80:* 125, 1959.

Douglas, G. W., Thomas, L., Carr, M., Cullen, N. M., and Morris, R.: Trophoblast in the circulating blood during pregnancy. Amer. J. Obstet. Gynec., *78:* 960, 1959.

Douthwaite, R. M., and Urbach, G. I.: In vitro antigenicity of trophoblast. Amer. J. Obstet. Gynec., *109:* 1023, 1971.

Driscoll, S. G.: Choriocarcinoma: An "incidental finding" within a term placenta. Obstet. Gynec., *21:* 96, 1962.

Elston, C. W., and Bagshaw, T. K. D.: The diagnosis of trophoblastic tumors from uterine curettings. J. Clin. Path., *25:* 111, 1972.

Floyd, W. S., and Cohn, S. L.: Gonadotropin producing hepatoma. Obstet. Gynec., *41:* 665, 1973.

Fox, F. J., and Tow, W. S. H.: Serial immunological chorionic gonadotrophin assays for diagnosis, treatment evaluation and comparative testing in 16 cases of choriocarcinoma. Amer. J. Obstet. Gynec., *97:* 379, 1967.

Freedman, H. L., Magagnini, A., and Glass, M.: Pregnancies, following chemically treated choriocarcinoma. Amer. J. Obstet. Gynec., *83:* 1637, 1962.

Garancis, J. C., *et al.*: Electronic microscopic and biochemical behavior of trophoblast. Amer. J. Obstet. Gynec., *108:* 1257, 1970.

Girouard, D. P., Barclay, D. L, and Collins, C. G.: Hyperreactio luteinalis. Obstet. Gynec., *23:* 513, 1964.

Goldstein, D. P.: The chemotherapy of gestational tropho-blastic disease. J.A.M.A., *220:* 229, 1972.

Goldstein, D. P., and Reid, D. E.: Recent developments in the management of molar pregnancy. Clin. Obstet. Gynec., *10:* 313, 1967.

Goldstein, D. P., Winig, P., and Shirley, R. L.: Actinomycin D as initial therapy of gestational trophoblastic disease. Obstet., Gynec., *39:* 341, 1972.

Hammond, C. B., Hertz, R., Ross, G. T., Lipsett, M. B., and Odell, W. B.: Diagnostic problems of choriocarcinoma and related trophoblastic neoplasms. Obstet. Gynec., *29:* 224, 1967.

Hammond, C. B., *et al.*: Treatment of metastatic tropho-blastic disease. Amer. J. Obstet. Gynec., *115:* 451, 1973.

Haskins, A. L.: Quantitative assay of human chorionic gonadotropin. Amer. J. Obstet. Gynec., *97:* 777, 1967.

Hershman, J. M., and Higgins, H. P.: Hydatidiform mole: a cause of clinical hyperthyroidism. New Eng. J. Med., *284:* 573, 1971.

Hertig, A. T.: The placenta: some new knowledge about an old organ. Obstet. Gynec., *20:* 859, 1962.

Hertig, A. T., and Sheldon, W. H.: Hydatidiform mole—a pathologic-clinical correlation of 200 cases. Amer. J. Obstet. Gynec., *53:* 1, 1947.

Hertig, A. T.: Human trophoblast: normal and abnormal. A plea for the study of the normal so as to understand the abnormal. Amer .J. Clin. Path., *47:* 249, 1967.

Hertz, R.: Gestational trophoblastic neoplasia. Hospital Practice, *157:* Jan., 1972.

Hertz, R., Ross, G. T., and Lipsett, M. B.: Primary chemotherapy of nonmetastatic trophoblastic disease in women. Amer. J. Obstet. Gynec., *86:* 808, 1963.

Hertz, R., Ross, G. T., and Lipsett, M. B.: Chemotherapy in women with trophoblastic disease: choriocarcinoma, chorioadenoma destruens, and complicated hydatidi-form mole. Ann. N. Y. Acad. Sci., *114:* 881, 1964.

Holland, J. F., and Hreschyshyn, M. M., (Eds.): *Choriocarcinoma.* Springer-Verlag, Berlin, Heidelberg, New York, 1967.

Hreshchyshyn, M. M., Graham, J. B., and Holland, J. F.: Treatment of malignant trophoblastic growth in women with special reference to amethopterin. Amer. J. Obstet. Gynec., *81:* 688, 1961.

Hsu, C., Huang, L., and Chen, T.: Metastases in benign hy-datidiform mole and chorioadenoma destruens. Amer. J. Obstet. Gynec., *84:* 1412, 1962.

Husel, D. H.: Six recurrent hydatidiform moles. Amer. J. Obstet. Gynec., *93:* 287, 1965.

Hutchison, J. R., Peterson, E. P., and Zimmerman, E. A.: Coexisting metastatic choriocarcinoma and normal pregnancy. Obstet. & Gynec., *31:* 331, 1968.

Jackson, R. L.: Pure malignancy of the trophoblast following primary abdominal pregnancy. Amer. J. Obstet. Gynec., *79:* 1085, 1960.

Jacobson, F. J., and Enzer, N.: Hydatidiform mole with "benign" metastasis to lung. Amer. J. Obstet. Gynec., *7:* 868, 1959.

Jones, W. B., and Lewis, J. L.: Treatment of gestational trophoblastic disease. Amer. J. Obstet. Gynec., *120:* 14, 1974.

Kika, K., and Matruda, I.: Primary tubal hydatidiform mole. Obstet. Gynec., *9:* 224, 1957.

Kirk, J. A.: Persistence of abnormal trophoblast. Amer. J. Obstet. Gynec., *92:* 667, 1964.

Kittredge, R. D.: Choriocarcinoma. Aspects of the clinical pathology. Amer. J. Roentgenol., *117:* 637, 1973.

Kohl, G. C.: Hydatidiform mole and 4½-month fetus. Amer. J. Obstet. Gynec., *79:* 1091, 1960.

Koren, Z., Behrman, S. J., and Paine, P. J.: Antigenicity of trophoblastic cells indicated by fluorescein technique. Amer. J. Obstet. Gynec., *104:* 50, 1969.

Lamb, E. J., Morton, D. G., and Byron, R. C.: Methotrexate therapy of choriocarcinoma and allied tumors. Amer. J. Obstet. Gynec., *90:* 317, 1964.

Lau, H. L.: *Tice's Practice of Medicine II,* Chapt. 21: 1, 1970.

Lau, H. L., and Jones, G. S.: Immunoassay of serum HCG by quantitative complement fixation and comparison with the Delfs biassay. Amer. J. Obstet. Gynec., *92:* 483, 1965.

Lewis, J. L., Jr.: Chemotherapy for metastatic gestational trophoblastic neoplasms. Clin. Obstet. Gynec., *10:* 330, 1967.

Lewis, J. L. Jr.: High risk pregnancy: Hydatidiform mole and choriocarcinoma. J. Reprod. Med., *7:* 33, 1971.

Lewis, J. L., Jr., Ketcham, A. S., and Hertz, R.: Surgical in-tervention during chemotherapy of gestational tropho-blastic disease. Cancer, *19:* 1517, 1966.

Lewis, J. L., Jr., Gore, H., Hertig, A. T., and Ross, D. A.: Treatment of trophoblastic disease. Amer. J. Obstet. Gynec., *95:* 710, 1966.

Lindsey, J. R., *et al.*: Intra-uterine choriocarcinoma in a rhesus monkey. Path. Vet., *6:* 378, 1969.

Logan, B. J.: Occurrence of a hydatidiform mole in twin pregnancy. Amer. J. Obstet. Gynec., *73:* 911, 1957.

MacRae, D. J.: Chorionepithelioma occurring during preg-nancy. J. Obstet. Gynaec. Brit. Comm., *58:* 373, 1951.

Manahan, C. P., Manuel-Limson, G., and Abad, R.: Experience with choriocarcinoma in the Philippines. Ann. N. Y. Acad. Sci., *114:* 875, 1964.

Marquez-Monten, H., *et al.* Gestational choriocarcinoma in the General Hospital of Mexico. Cancer, *21:* 1337, 1968.

Marrubinia, G.: Primary chorionepithelioma of the ovary. Acta Obstet. Gynec. Scand., *38:* 251, 1949.

Mercer, R. D., Lammert, A. C., Anderson, R., and Hazard, J. B.: Choriocarcinoma in mother and infant. J.A.M.A., *166:* 482, 1958.

Moore, J. H.: Hydatidiform mole in 53-year-old patient. Amer. J. Obstet. Gynec., *69:* 205, 1955.

Nelson, J. H., Jr.: Effect of trophoblast in immune state. Amer. J. Obstet. Gynec., *117:* 689, 1973.

Novak, E., and Koff, A. H.: Chorionepithelioma, with spe-cial reference to disappearance of primary tumor. Amer. J. Obstet. Gynec., *20:* 481, 1930.

Novak, E., and Seah, C. S.: Choriocarcinoma of uterus. Amer. J. Obstet. Gynec., *67:* 993, 1954.

Novak, E., and Seah, C. S.: Benign lesions in chorionepi-thelioma Registry. Amer. J. Obstet. Gynec., *68:* 376, 1954.

Paranjothy, D. and Samuel, I.: A rare case of choriocarci-noma recurring 12 years after hysterectomy. Amer. J. Obstet. Gynec., *110:* 410, 1971.

Park, W. W.: The occurrence of sex chromatin in chorionepitheliomas and hydatidiform moles. Brit. J. Path. Bact., *74:* 197, 1957.

Park, W. W.: Experimental trophoblastic embolism in the lungs. J. Path. Bact., *25:* 257, 1958.

Park, W. W.: *Choriocarcinoma.* F. A. Davis, Philadelphia, 1971.

Pastorfide, G. B., and Goldstein, D. P.: Pregnancy after hy-datidiform mole. Obstet. Gynec., *42:* 67, 1973.

Pattillo, R. A., *et al.*: Hormone function in trophoblastic tu-mors. Obstet. Gynec., *39:* 632, 1972.

Riggs, J. A., Wainer, A. S., Hahn, G. A., and Farell, D. M.: Extrauterine tubal choriocarcinoma. Amer. J. Obstet. Gynec., *88:* 637, 1964.

Ringertz, N.: Hydatidiform mole, invasive mole and choriocarcinoma in Sweden. Acta Gynec. Scand., *49:* 195, 1970.

Robinson, E., Shulman, J., Ben-Hur, N., Zuckerman, H., and Neuman, Z.: Immunity in chorioepithelioma. Lancet, *1:* 300, 1963.

Ross, G. T., Goldstein, D. P., Hertz, R., Lipsett, M. B., and O'Dell, W. D.: Sequential use of methotrexate and actinomycin D in trophoblastic disease. Amer. J. Obstet. Gynec., *93:* 223, 1965.

Schmorl, G.: Pathologisch-anatomische untersuching uber puerperal eclampsie. Vogel, Leipzig, 1893.

Shintari, S., Glass, L. E., and Page, E. W.: Studies of induced malignant tumors of placental and uterine origin in the rat. II. Induced tumors and their pathogenesis with special reference to choriocarcinoma. Amer. J. Obstet. Gynec., *95:* 550, 1966.

Smalbraak, J.: *Trophoblastic Growths.* Elsevier Publishing Company, Amsterdam, 1957.

Speigel, J. A.: Endarterial choriocarcinoma of the lung. Obstet. Gynec., *24:* 740, 1964.

Spellacy, W. N., Meeker, H. C., and McKelvey, J. L.: Three successful pregnancies in a patient treated for choriocarcinoma with Methotrexate. Obstet. Gynec., *25:* 607, 1965.

Taylor, E. S., Thompson, H. E., Gottesfeld, K. R., and Holmes, J. H.: Clinical use of ultrasound in obstetrics and gynecology. Amer. J. Obstet. Gynec., *99:* 671, 1967.

Taymor, M. L.: Bioassay and immunoassay of human chorionic gonadotropin. Clin. Obstet. Gynec., *10:* 303, 1967.

Tedeschi, L. G., and Toy, B. L.: Experimental transpulmonary migration of trophoblast. Obstet. Gynec., *21:* 55, 1962.

Teow, and Ratnam, S. S.: The malignant sequelae of hydatidiform mole. Int. J. Gynec. Obstet., *11:* 32, 1973.

Thiele, R. A., and de Alvarez, R. R.: Metastasizing benign trophoblastic tumors. Amer. J. Obstet. Gynec., *84:* 1395, 1962.

Tominaga, T., and Page, E. W.: Sex chromatin of trophoblastic tumors. Amer. J. Obstet. Gynec., *96:* 305, 1966.

Tow, S. H.: University of Singapore (Personal communication).

Van der Werf, A. J. M., *et al.*: Metastatic choriocarcinoma as a complication of pregnancy. Obstet. Gynec., *35:* 78, 1970.

Van Thiel, D. H., *et al.*: Partial placenta accreta in pregnancies following chemotherapy for gestational trophoblastic neoplasms. Amer. J. Obst. Gynec., *112:* 54, 1972.

Van Thiel, D. H., Ross, G. T., and Lipsett, M. B.: Pregnancies after chemotherapy of trophoblastic neoplasms. Science, *169:* 132, 1970.

White, T. G. E.: Chorionepithelioma of uterus in a postmenopausal woman. J. Obstet. Gynaec. Brit. Comm., *62:* 372, 1955.

Wilson, R. B., Hunter, J. S., and Dockerty, M. B.: Chorioadenoma destruens. Amer. J. Obstet. Gynec., *81:* 546, 1961.

Wu, F. Y. W.: Recurrent hydatidiform mole. Obstet. Gynec., *41:* 200, 1973.

Wynn, R. M., and Davies, J.: Ultrastructure of transplanted choriocarcinoma and its endocrine implications. Amer. J. Obstet. Gynec., *88:* 618, 1964.

Wynn, R. M., and Harris, J. A.: Ultrastructure of trophoblast and endometrium in invasive hydatidiform mole chorioadenoma destruens. Amer. J. Obstet. Gynec., *99:* 1125, 1967.

chapter *28*

Leukorrhea

Leukorrhea is the term applied to any vaginal discharge other than blood. It is perhaps the most frequently encountered of gynecological symptoms, occurring in at least one-third of all gynecological patients. It is rarely serious, and generally is associated with simple infections of the cervix, vagina, or tube.

Under normal conditions all parts of the genital mucous membrane are kept moistened, either by secretions of their own or by those having their source in a higher segment of the canal. Normally, there is no escape of secretions to the outside, although there are comparatively few women who do not at some time or other in their lives have at least a slight external discharge. The discharge may consist of excess of otherwise normal secretion or may represent abnormal exudates from pathological lesions somewhere in the genital canal.

VULVA

Strictly speaking vulvar secretions should not be considered in the present discussion, as the vulva is an external structure. However, vulvar secretions may contribute to the leukorrhea complained of by the patient, who cannot know the source of the discharge.

In addition to the sebaceous and sudoriferous glands in the vulva, the vulvovaginal gland, Bartholin's gland, is a part of the vulva. This gland plays the most important role in the lubrication of the vaginal introitus and the vulvar mucous membrane. It secretes a thick viscid mucus, which is increased during sexual excitement. Finally, in the periurethral region of the vestibule are situated Skene's ducts and a number of mucous crypts which, likewise, contribute to the lubrication of the vulvar structures.

In infections of Bartholin's gland, there is often a profuse purulent discharge either from the duct or from a ruptured abscess. Such discharge, or those from the periurethral structures, are apt to be interpreted by the patient as of vaginal origin. Although the most frequent cause of inflammation of the Bartholin's, Skene's and periurethral ducts is the gonococcus, other bacterial infections can occur. Persistent or recurrent vulvovaginitis is most often due to a monilial (yeast) vaginitis. Patients with such symptoms and clinical findings should be checked for an associated diabetes.

Treatment of inflammation of the glands of the vulva should be both systemic and local. Systemic treatment is a specific antibiotic selected according to the sensitivity of the organism involved. The local treatment consists of hot sitz baths for 15 minutes 3 or 4 times a day and incision and drainage, if a fluctuant abscess has occurred. Chronically inflamed Bartholin glands frequently need to be surgically removed in a quiescent stage.

VAGINA

Although the vagina is itself devoid of glands, its surface is normally moistened by the secretion of the cervical glands, and to a much less extent by transudation from its own surface. Normally, the secretion found in the vagina is acid in reaction. This acidity is dependent upon the presence of lactic acid produced by the action of vaginal organisms, the chief among these being the large rod shaped bacillus of Döderlein, upon the glycogen content of the vaginal epithelium. The latter undergoes constant desquamation and discharges of vaginal origin are characterized by the presence of many epithelial cells. When actual inflammation and infection of the vagina occurs, an exudate develops which is usually mucopurulent or purulent in character and associated with pruritus.

Although the usual symptomatology is a foul, smelly, irritating discharge, vaginitis can be severe enough to cause a hemorrhagic exudate which can be interpreted as metrorrhagia unless a careful examination is made.

The two most common forms of vaginitis in the mature menstruating woman are those caused by *Candida albicans* and by *trichomonas.* Yeast vaginitis, also called monilial vaginitis associated with the *Candida albicans,* is characterized by a cheesy type of discharge having a sweetish odor. The vaginitis associated with the *trichomonas* infestation is characterized by a bubbly, yellowish, thin discharge sometimes having a foul odor. The diagnosis is made by microscopic examination of a saline wash from the vagina and identification of the organism. The microscopic diagnosis can be confirmed by culture on Sabouraud's media for the *Candida albicans.*

Yeast vaginitis is especially prone to occur during pregnancy, in women taking oral contraception, in the diabetic patient, or after prolonged antibiotic therapy. It can be treated by an antifungicide, nystatin (Mycostatin), 500,000 units 3 times a day given with a 100,000 unit vaginal suppository every night over a 10-day period. Persistent infections can be treated by scrubbing the vagina with Zephiran to remove the colonies and then painting with 2% aqueous Gentian Violet solution. This treatment should be carried out every other day for 3 treatments only, as a chemical vaginitis can be induced due to the Gentian Violet solution if too frequent or prolonged applications are given. If recurrent yeast infections occur, a glucose tolerance test should be done to check the possibility of diabetes. The use of tight slacks or shorts, and prolonged intervals in bathing suits can cause an exacerbation of this vaginitis among women who are predisposed to monilial infections.

Trichomonas vaginitis, which must be regarded as a venereal disease, is treated by metronidazole (Flagyl) 250 mg. 3 times a day for 10 days. It is advisable to prescribe a similar course of treatment for the sexual partner and request that condom protection be used during intercourse. Lang, Fritz, and Menduke have emphasized the frequency of associated trichomoniasis and candida vaginitis. It is, therefore, wise to check for both organisms when the patient returns for her final examination after completion of therapy.

Herpetic lesions of the cervix, vagina and vulva are resistant to most treatments which are currently available. These infections are characterized by painful ulcerations with a recurrent tendency. Development of a vaccine is being attempted.

Rarely one will find a foreign body in the vagina to account for a profuse, malodorous discharge. A forgotten tampon is by far the most common finding, although neglected pessaries are also occasionally found.

The adult vagina is resistant to the gonococcus, but that of the immature child is not, and the most common cause of vulvovaginitis in children, aside from a foreign body infection, is gonorrhea. The diagnosis is made by inspection and lavage to rule out the presence of a foreign body and by a Gram Stain on a direct smear to identify the intracellular diplococci. The treatment is by Stilbestrol vaginal suppository, 0.1 mg. nightly over a period of 2 weeks. This causes maturation of the vaginal epithelium to the adult stage and makes it resistant to the gonococcal organism. It is, of course, necessary to establish the infected contacts and institute treatment both as a public health method and to avoid reinfection of the patient.

At the opposite end of the age scale, senile vaginitis of nonspecific origin, is not uncommon. The decreased ovarian function at the menopause causes the vaginal mucosa to become atrophic and prone to secondary infection. Although usually nonspecific in type, occasionally, as in a child, it is due to the gonococcus. Tiny areas of ulceration can produce not only leukorrhea but also slight vaginal bleeding. Estrogen suppositories (Stilbestrol 0.5 mg.) or creams are usually curative and rarely lead to bleeding even if the uterus is still present.

CERVIX

The mucous glands of the cervix are the chief source of the secretion normally found in the vagina, and it is not strange, therefore, that they are the chief source of leukorrheal discharge. The normal secretion is a clear, viscid, alkaline mucus, which varies in its amount and viscidity at different phases of the menstrual cycle, the greatest amount being at the time of ovulation.

The secretion may be merely increased in amount without alteration in character, as a result of hyperactivity of the glands produced by hyperemic or endocrine factors. However, the histological structure of the cervix, with its numerous gland invaginations, makes it peculiarly prone to persistent infections, characterized by excessive and pathological alterations of the secretion. Cervicitis is etiologically divisible into two major groups; the gonorrheal and the nonspecific. The latter, in which puerperal lacerations often play an important causative role, is the result of infection by various organisms, chiefly of streptococcal and staphylococcal groups. (See Chapter 11 under "Cervicitis.") The diagnosis of gonorrheal cervicitis is made by identification of the organisms from a Gram Stain on a direct cervical smear. It can be suspected when a foul smelling, copious, purulent discharge has developed rapidly in the absence of a pregnancy or a cervical neoplasm. The treatment is as outlined in Chapter 11 under Cervicitis and consists of specific antibiotic therapy and the usual public health measures necessary for such a communicable disease. A serological test for syphilis is indicated.

A syphilitic chancre of the cervix is only a cause of leukorrhea when secondary infection occurs and must be differentiated from a nonspecific ulceration, an herpetic lesion, or a tuberculous granuloma. An examination of a wet smear under dark-field illumination will demonstrate the spirochetes in a syphilitic chancre while a biopsy of the lesion will show giant cells and tuberculous bacilli in a tuberculous granuloma. The treatment for either of these is, of course, specific.

The treatment of nonspecific cervicitis should also be directed towards the systemic treatment of the infection and local eradication of the infected area. Specific antibiotic therapy, both orally and supplied locally, is given in conjunction with hot douches 15 minutes, two or three times a day for two weeks, followed by a cauterization of the lesion if it is on the portio. For more extensive involvement of the cervix, radial cauterization or cryosurgery may be indicated. Such procedure should be followed by cervical dilatation to avoid cervical stenosis.

UTERINE BODY

Although the endometrium contains innumerable glands, these are inactive until the postovulatory phases of the cycle, and even then the secretion adds little to the secretory content of the lower genital canal. However, a certain amount of serous transudation undoubtedly occurs, and this may at times be increased in amount as a result of vascular or endocrine factors, or neoplasia.

Endometritis is of little importance as a cause of leukorrhea. An exception to this is the occasional case of acute septic endometritis, in which a profuse purulent discharge may be present associated with retention of placental tissue. Pyometra with cervical stenosis is also associated with a profuse, foul discharge in the postmenopausal patient.

Finally, uterine polyps, submucous myomas, carcinomas, and other tumors are not infrequently the cause of uterine discharges, particularly when complicated by infection and necrosis. A most unusual cause of copious vaginal discharge is lymphorrhea associated with anomalies and obstruction of the lymphatic ducts. This can only be cured by surgical correction of the defect and has been described by Martorell as chylous metrorrhea.

The treatment of all causes of leukorrhea, originating in the uterine body, is directed towards removal of the etiological factor associated with specific antibiotic therapy.

TUBES

Although rare, leukorrhea of tubal origin may occur, the usual example being that of the so-called profluent salpingitis, in which a hydrosalpinx may periodically expel its content through a partially patent inner orifice into the uterus and thus causes gushes of watery fluid from the vagina. In most cases of hydrosalpinx, however, the uterine end of the tubal lumen is completely closed, so that the above mentioned mechanism must be extremely uncommon.

REFERENCES

Anderson, F. D., Ushijima, R. N., and Larson, C. L.: Recurrent herpes genitalis; treatment with Myobacterium bovis (BCG). Obstet. Gynec., 43: 797, 1974.

Brewer, J. I., Halpern, B., and Thomas, G.: Hemophilus vaginalis vaginitis. Amer. J. Obstet. Gynec., 74: 834, 1957.

Forster, S. A., Raminez, O. G., and Rapaport, A. H.: Metronidazole and trichomonal vaginitis. Amer. J. Obstet. Gynec., 87: 1013, 1963.

Gardner, H. L., Dampeer, T. K., and Dukes, C. D.: The prevalence of vaginitis. Amer. J. Obstet. Gynec., 73: 1080, 1957.

Gray, M. S.: Trichomonas vaginalis in pregnancy: results of metronidazole therapy on mother and child. J. Obstet. Gynaec. Brit. Comm., 68: 723, 1961.

Henricksen, E.: Pyometra associated with benign lesions of the cervix and corpus. Western J. Surg., 60: 305, 1952.

Henricksen, E.: Pyometra associated with malignant lesions of the cervix and uterus. Amer. J. Obstet. Gynec., 72: 884, 1956.

Hesseltine, H. C.: Vulval and vaginal mycosis and trichomoniasis. Amer. J. Obstet. Gynec., 40: 641, 1940.

Johnson, D. G.: Infections of the cervix. Clin. Obstet. Gynec., 2: 476, 1959.

Kauraniemi, T.: Gynecological health screening by means of questionnaire and cytology. Acta Obstet. Gynec. Scand., 48: Supp. 4, 1969.

Lang, W. R.: Genital infections in female children. Clin. Obstet. Gynec., 2: 428, 1959.

Lang, W. R.: Premenarchal vaginitis. Obstet. Gynec., 13: 723, 1959.

Lang, W. R., Fritz, M. A., and Menduke, H.: The bacteriological diagnosis of trichomonal candidal and combined infections. Obstet. Gynec., 20: 788, 1962.

Liston, W. G., and Cruickshank, L. G.: Etiology and pathogenesis of leucorrhea in pregnancy; study of 200 cases. J. Obstet. Gynaec. Brit. Comm., 47: 109, 1940.

Martorell, F.: Chylus metrorrhea. Vascular Diseases, 1: 160, 1964.

McCoogan, L. S.: The treatment of vaginitis. Clin. Obstet. Gynec., 2: 450, 1959.

Reich, W. J., Nechtow, M. J., Zaworsky, B., and Adams, A. P.: Investigation and management of the patient with vaginal discharge. Clin. Obstet. Gynec., 2: 441, 1959.

Watt, L., and Jennison, R. F.: Metronidazole treatment of trichomoniasis in the female. Brit. Med. J., 1: 276, 1962.

chapter 29

Infertility and Abortion

INFERTILITY

Definitions

Sterility is a term which can be correctly applied only to an individual who has some absolute factor preventing procreation. Infertility, however, is the inability to achieve pregnancy within a stipulated period of time, usually stated as one year. This view is adequately based on statistics. For example, Whitelaw found that 56.5% of fertile couples achieve pregnancy within one month and 78.9% within the first six months. Primary infertility is the term used to designate those patients who have never conceived, whereas secondary infertility indicates that the patient has had a pregnancy. This may be further qualified as secondary to term pregnancy, miscarriage, etc.

Occurrence

In the United States, 12% of all marriages are estimated to be involuntarily barren. Thus the problem is one of some magnitude.

Medical Considerations

Medically, infertility is a rather unique condition in that one must consider two individuals. As the husband or wife, or both, may have factors contributing to the condition, both must cooperate in the investigation. Although the woman is usually the most interested and aggressive in her desire for medical help, it is not satisfactory to initiate an infertility investigation without the cooperation of the husband. It is psychologically desirable to begin the evaluation of the husband and wife at the same time as this emphasizes for the couple the dual responsibility which they share in the condition.

Evaluation of the Problem

It has been adequately demonstrated that in formulating a prognosis the age of the wife and the duration of the pregnancy exposure are major factors which must be taken into consideration along with the medical findings. Fertility in women declines after the age of 35 years. Guttmacher has shown that marriages of women between the ages of 16 and 20 years have only a 4.5% infertility rate; the incidence has risen to 31.3% for women married between the ages of 35 and 40 years, and after the age of 40 the infertility rate approaches 70%. This is further substantiated by the relative infrequency of pregnancy after the age of 45 years. This so-called "aging factor" is, however, a difficult one to assess. A routine infertility investigation in older women may fail to reveal any abnormality. In a preliminary study of ovaries removed in the over 50-year-old woman, we have found evidence of recent ovulation in over 20%, despite almost uniform absence of pregnancy beyond the age of 48. Indeed we have found histological proof (corpus luteum) of ovulation in a few women past the age of 55. It may therefore be assumed that the infertility is caused by a defect in the ovum itself, making it unfertilizable. The increased incidence of congenital anomalies and miscarriages in pregnancy among older women might seem to substantiate this theory. The duration of the infertility, which has long been recognized as a reliable yardstick for prognosis, obviously serves as an indication of the seriousness of the condition.

According to statistics from various clinics, 20 to 50% of patients investigated for infertility can be helped. It is estimated that with our present investigative techniques, between 10 and 30% of the patients will be found to have no discernible etiological factors responsible for the infertility.

There is no evidence for fertility differentials of racial origin. Guttmacher estimates the average number of children per couple married before the age of 20 years, without the use of contraception, to be approximately 9.5, and this figure is the same for 5 different nationality groups.

INVESTIGATION

Although it was once thought unjustifiable to initiate an infertility investigation short of three years of barren marriage, it now appears that no couple who seeks medical aid for infertility should be turned away without some consideration of their problem, be it real or fancied. This is scientifically justifiable on the basis of the statistics just cited and psychologically desirable, as often the fears of the overanxious couple can be allayed by a few explanations and suggestions from a sympathetic and well informed physician. Such a discussion may, perhaps, prevent the development of major psychological problems which aggravate or cause infertility.

The Initial Interview

The investigation of the infertile couple begins with a careful history and physical examination which will exclude major medical or gynecological conditions. A proper history must include the age of the patient and her husband, the duration of the marriage, previous marital histories of both parties, and other efforts to obtain medical aid, as well as a medical and social history. Physical examination includes a vaginal smear with maturation index and an examination of the cervical mucus in addition to the usual general examinations of urine for sugar and protein, a hematocrit, and white count. It is generally impossible to make an etiological diagnosis at the first visit. However, it is well to make a tentative diagnosis if there are suggestive factors in the history or physical examination, as these observations are valuable signposts in focusing our attention on important details during the subsequent examinations and tests.

At the first visit it is wise to discuss with the patient and her husband, if possible, the need for a complete investigation, as well as the time and expense involved, the statistical probabilities of help, and the value of the investigation from a prognostic point of view. The couple should be advised that if treatment seems indicated, it is usually necessary to allow at least one year before evaluation of therapy is possible. At this time it is well to set up a subsequent appointment with both the husband and wife to discuss the investigational findings and recommendations.

Fundamental Tests

Pertinent investigations must include tests of the six major factors concerned with fertilization and implantation of an ovum: (1) the occurrence of ovulation, (2) the production of normal sperm, (3) the presence of adequate cervical mucus which can act as a transport medium for sperm and as a sperm repository, (4) the patency of tubes for transport of sperm up and ovum down, (5) the development of the endometrial implantation site which depends upon both ovarian endocrine function and end organ response, and (6) normalcy of the peritoneal factor.

If no abnormalities are found in the above studies, certain ancillary factors must be checked. Some evaluation of thyroid function, a glucose tolerance test, and a 17-ketosteroid assay will detect metabolic disease processes which are associated with infertility problems. However, it is our experience that when there is no evidence of ovarian insufficiency, these diseases are usually not the cause of the infertility. A psychiatric evaluation or a psychological test may be advisable. The blood grouping of husband and wife may also have some significance, as there is statistical evidence to indicate that blood incompatibilities may occasionally be the cause of infertility.

If, at the end of the complete examination, no cause is found for the infertility, and after one year no pregnancy has occurred, a culdoscopic examination shoud be performed. This may reveal unsuspected endometriosis or peritubal or periovarian adhesions. If no cause for infertility is found, no treatment should be given. It is likewise inadvisable to repeat tests after one has satisfactorily established a diagnosis, as such unnecessary procedures or therapy can prove harmful, interfering with the process of fertility rather than improving it.

OVULATION

Of the many methods advocated for the detection of ovulation, four are currently outstanding as clinically proved and applicable: (1) the cornification of the daily vaginal smear pattern or urinary sediment followed by a progestational smear (Fig. 29.1); (2) increased amount and fluidity of the cervical mucus followed by a decreased amount of mucus and absence of the fern formation (Fig.

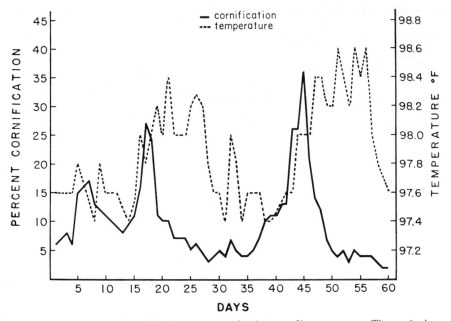

29.1. Ovulation determined by cornification pattern of urinary sediment smears. The vaginal smear pattern parallels that of the urinary cells. Ovulation can be seen to coincide with the cornification peak. (From Vincze, L. O., Taft, P. D., and McArthur, J. W.: J. Clin. Endocr., *19:* 281, 1959.)

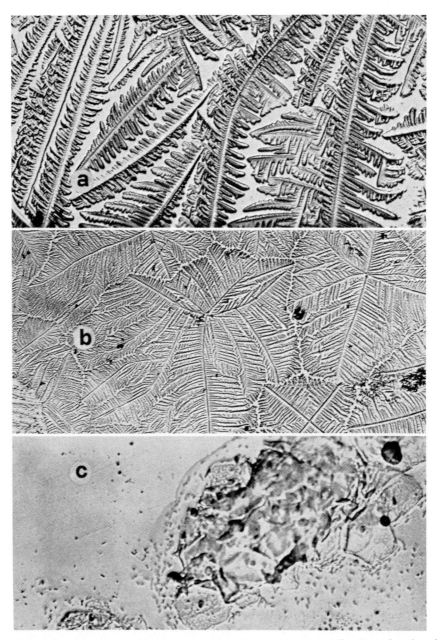

29.2. Ovulation determined by cervical mucus changes. Ovulation occurs at the time when fern formation is strongly positive (*a* and *b*); when progesterone is present the mucus shows a negative reaction or only a slightly positive reaction (*c*).

29.2); (3) the biphasic basal body temperature graph (Fig. 29.3); (4) secretory changes observed in the endometrium (Figs. 29.4 and 29.5).

Of these the first two are most useful in predicting the probable occurrence of ovulation, as the changes take place within the 24-hour period preceding ovulation. However, such findings can be associated with follicular maturation without ovulation and therefore must be interpreted absolutely in the light of knowledge of the entire cycle. The latter two tests are not useful in prediction of

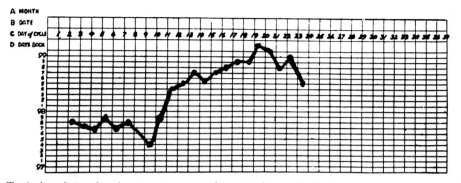

29.3. Typical ovulatory basal temperature record in a 24-day cycle. Ovulation probably occurs at the low point prior to the continuous rise. In this case it would be on Day 10.

ovulation, but are perhaps more reliable in the retrospective evaluation of the cycle, as they are a function of progesterone and therefore imply ovulation by determination of an active corpus luteum.

As far back as 1904, van de Velde reported that the normal basal body temperature throughout the menstrual cycle is biphasic. The temperature is taken orally as soon as the patient awakens each morning, and before she moves about, eats, drinks, or smokes. The low point occurs at or about the time of ovulation, although there is still some uncertainty as to the precise chronological relationships involved.

Methods which depend upon complicated hormone analyses are too expensive and too time-consuming to be clinically applicable; these are the detection of urinary estrogenic peaks which occur about 24 hours before ovulation (Fig. 29.6); measurement of the luteinizing hormone

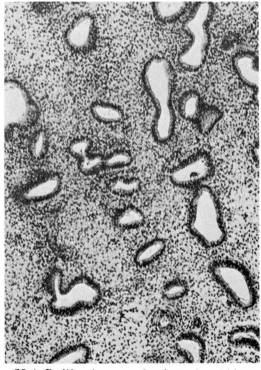

29.4. Proliferative type of endometrium with no suggestion of secretory activity indicating anovulation.

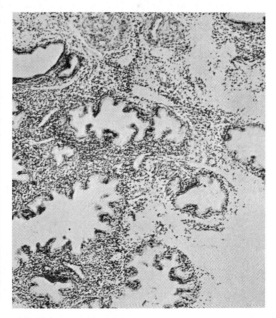

29.5. Normal progestational endometrium removed by suction curette on the 27th day of cycle.

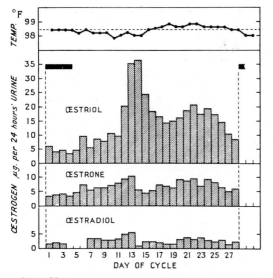

29.6. Urinary estrogen excretion during a normal 28-day cycle correlated with the basal temperature record. The estrogen peak occurs just prior to ovulation. (From Brown, J. B.: *Lancet*, *1:* 320, 1955.)

(LH or ICSH) surge which occurs just prior to ovulation (Fig. 29.7); and urinary pregnanediol excretion (Fig. 29.8), which is a retrospective test for ovulation in that it measures progesterone production by the corpus luteum.

The detection of the preovulatory LH surge in the serum by radioimmunoassay (Fig. 2.17) requires daily blood sampling. Serum estrogen assays, as reported by Baird and Grevera, are of research rather than clinical value at present. The presence of an estrogen midcycle peak in the serum, as in the urine, is presumptive evidence of impending ovulation. Serum progesterone assays, described by Neill *et al.* (Fig. 2.15), although furnishing the best corroborative evidence that corpus luteum function and, therefore, presumptively ovulation has occurred, are likewise of research rather than clinical interest.

For a correlation of some of these

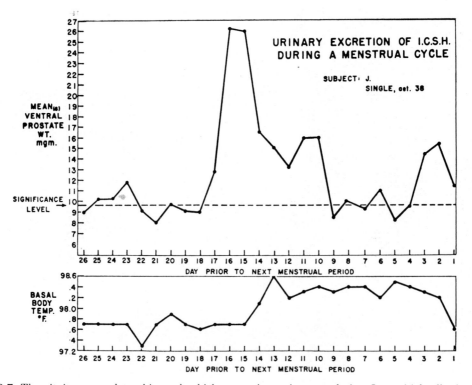

29.7. The pituitary gonadotrophin peak which occurs just prior to ovulation. Interstitial cell-stimulating hormone (*I.C.S.H.*) assay by the McArthur technique. (From Ingersoll, F. M., and McArthur, J. W.: *Amer. J. Obstet. Gynec.*, *77:* 795, 1959.)

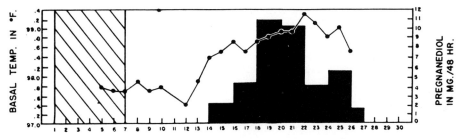

29.8. The basal body temperature charted with the urinary pregnanediol excretion (Astwood gravimetric method). The pregnanediol is plotted in *black blocks,* indicating the amount in milligrams per 48-hour periods. The base line represents the days of the menstrual cycle, counting Day 1 as the first day of menstruation. Pregnanediol excretion begins on the 14th day.

parameters of ovulation with the ovarian histology, the reader is referred to a paper by Taymor.

Ovulation Defects

The etiology of ovulation defects will be discussed in detail in Chapter 30, "Amenorrhea," and will be simply itemized here: (1) central nervous system factors; tumors or scars, functional, drug induced (oral contraceptive or phenothiazine), or heritable defects of the hypothalamus, psychogenic factors, pituitary dysfunctions, tumors, or destructive lesions; (2) intermediate factors; nutrition, chronic illness, metabolic disease (hypo- or hyperthyroidism, diabetes, the adrenogenital syndrome or related disturbances and Cushing's disease; (3) gonadal factors; premature ovarian failure, ovarian tumors, or destructive lesions including autoimmune disease.

The treatment of anovulation depends upon the etiology, and any specific factor found must be specifically treated as indicated, by diet, thyroid, or adrenal hormone. Pituitary insufficiencies or neurogenic disturbances leading to inadequate pituitary excitation and secondarily to inadequate ovarian stimulation should theoretically be best treated by substitution therapy with pituitary hormones. Gemzell and others have demonstrated that this therapy is satisfactory. The use of cyclic steroid hormones, estrogens followed by progestogens, in an effort to stimulate pituitary function, although less expensive and less complicated, is usually unsuccessful. This is probably because there is some disturbance of the normal

feedback control mechanism making the hypothalamus insensitive to the normal steroid signal. Clomiphene is most useful under these circumstances, *e.g.,* in patients with an intact pituitary gland and normal ovaries.

Ovarian tumors must be surgically removed; the Stein-Leventhal ovary must be wedge-resected or treated with clomiphene. Unfortunately, there is no treatment for ovarian failure at this writing, since organ transplant has not been attempted.

SPERM

Evaluation

At least two semen analyses should be performed for proper evaluation of the male factor. If these do not show a satisfactory agreement, samples should be taken until a reasonable assessment of fertility capacity has been reached. Samples should not be collected after a specific abstinence period but in accord with the usual intercourse habits of the couple. A clean, wide-mouthed container should be used for collecting the specimen, which may be procured either by induced ejaculation or by intercourse with withdrawal. A total ejaculate must be obtained, as any loss may seriously influence the sperm count. The sample should be collected and brought to the laboratory within one hour, if possible, marked with the hour of collection and the date of the previous intercourse. Liquefaction of seminal fluid may be expected to occur at room temperature within 20 minutes. Failure of liquefaction indicates a lack of proteolytic enzyme and makes the evaluation of the sample difficult. The quality of the semen is judged by the motility of the sperm, the numbers per milliliter, and the presence of abnormal forms. The total volume is also recorded and is of some importance as the normality of the sample frequently varies inversely, within limits, with the amount of the semen. Thus a large volume is often indicative that the sperm is of poor quality. The total sperm count is not of too great importance. The number of epithelial cells and leukocytes present is obviously significant.

Although absolute criteria of male fertility cannot be obtained with the present rather crude methods of evaluation, the following standards may be considered as representative of the usual fertile male. *Count per milliliter*: normally fertile, above 60,000,000 per ml.; subfertile, between 20,000,000 and 60,000,000 per ml.; infertile, less than 20,000,000 per ml. *Volume:* 2.5 ml. *Motility*: 60% (motility within four hours). *Differential*: less than 25% abnormal forms (Fig. 29.9).

The occurrence of an abnormal differential with an otherwise normal semen analysis is rare. The studies of Leuchtenberger *et al.* have suggested the deoxyribonucleic acid (DNA) content of spermatozoa might be used as a fertility index. These authors' investigations indicate that the DNA value will detect deficiencies in otherwise apparently normal semen. From a theoretical point of view this would be attractive, as the DNA is a measure of chromosomal material and thus would be an accurate measure of genetic abnormalities. Studies by Knudsen in animal husbandry indicate that certain forms of nondisjunction of chromosomes which would give rise to increased or decreased DNA measurements, are incompatible with normal reproductive capacity.

The survival time of sperm in the human female genital tract is at least 96 hours. Investigations by Marshall indicate that 10 days may not be at all improbable. It is also apparent in certain types of experimental animals that sperm require a 24-hour period in the female genital tract in order to acquire fertilizing ability. This property has been called *capacitation* and has been extensively studied in the rabbit by Chang. It probably represents the removal of some substance by enzyme activity which allows the lytic enzyme in the acrosome to be activated. After the reaction, the sperm is able to penetrate not only the cumulus cells and the oocyte, but also the uterine mucosa.

Seminal Insufficiency

Seminal insufficiency can be attributed to constitutional factors such as nutritional problems, acute or chronic illness, general metabolic disease, specific poisonings or occupational hazards, central defects occurring in the pituitary or hypothalamic areas, specific diseases within the genital tract such as infections causing blockage to the vas and scarring of the tubular elements, or congenital defects of testicular development such as the Klinefelter syndrome. A varicocele can also be responsible for a low sperm count or decreased motility, apparently due to the associated increased intratesticular temperature. Diagnosis can be facilitated by a serum testosterone assay, a pituitary FSH assay, and a testicular biopsy. Testicular failure is indicated by a low testosterone and a high FSH assay and confirmed by the microscopic appearance of the testicles. Johnson has proposed a theory to explain oligospermia based on a pathological study of testicular biopsies. Histological fluorescent techniques indicate that some cases of oligospermia may be related to autoimmune disease. Isojima *et al.* described a complement-dependent sperm immobilization test. Nevertheless, in spite of concerted efforts to make an etiological diagnosis, a number of patients with oligospermia must remain in the idiopathic category with spermatogenic arrest of undetermined etiology.

For detailed and specific treatment the reader is referred to urological texts. For the treatment of many constitutional factors general hygiene is important: limitation of smoking and elimination of excessive alcohol, attention to diet and

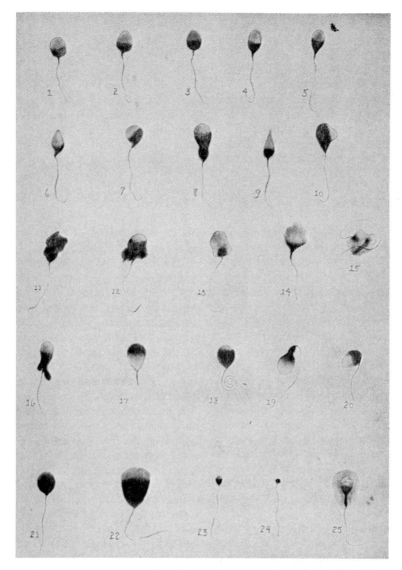

29.9. Drawing of spermatozoa as seen under oil immersion, approximately ×1200. *1-5*, normal variation; *6-10*, common abnormalities of the shape of the head; *11-15* and *25*, immature forms; *16-20*, abnormalities of the size of the head; normal semen contains a maximum of 20 per cent of abnormal forms. (From Israel, S. L.: *Mazer and Israel's Diagnosis and Treatment of Menstrual Disorders and Sterility,* Ed. 4. Paul B. Hoeber, Inc., New York, 1959.)

adequate rest, relief of emotional tension states, treatment of any chronic illness or metabolic disease. Because heat damages testicular tubular function, underwear which holds the testicles in contact with the body are injurious as are excessively hot, prolonged tub baths. Specific hormone therapy has been occasionally successful; this involves the administration of testosterone until the sperm count is reduced to zero, at which time the drug is withdrawn and the pituitary, which has been suppressed, is allowed to resume its function. It is estimated that approximately only 10 per cent of men showing low sperm counts, will show improvement on this form of therapy. Unfortunately, there is no method for detecting which group of patients will respond to the testosterone rebound phenomenon. Human pituitary gonadotrophin therapy has been successful in restoring spermatogenesis and fertility in men with specific hypopituitarism (MacLeod). Clomiphene has been used in men with oligospermia and spermatogenic arrest. It must be given in low dosages and over a prolonged period; 12.5 to 25 mg per day for from 3 months to 1 year. The increased sperm counts recorded are correlated with the increased FSH values. As the process of sperm maturation, from spermatogonia to ejaculation of a mature sperm, takes at least 2 months, an improved count is not expected prior to this time.

For those men having blockage of the vas deferens, surgical therapy may help on occasion. When a varicocele is present, corrective surgery can be offered and is sometimes helpful. For those having destruction of the testis or congenitally defective spermatogenic elements, no therapy is available, and adoption or donor insemination must be considered. In the unusual case in which hypospadias is present so that deposition of spermatozoa on the cervix is inadequate, or in which a neurological cord lesion occurs, semen may be obtained mechanically and artificial insemination attempted.

A more concentrated semen sample can be obtained by collection of a split ejaculate as described by Perez-Pelaez and Cohen. Since the first portion of the ejaculate often contains the majority of sperm this offers a simple method of concentrating specimens of between 20,000,000 and 60,000,000 sperm per ml.; when followed by cervical insemination, some improvement in fertility rate has been reported. Other means of mechanical concentration are centrifugation of the ejaculate and the use of a millipore filter, as described by Perloff. Pooling of multiple samples of frozen semen, and subsequent concentration, is possible where sperm banks are available. However, in normal semen, only 25–50% of the sperm may be motile when unthawed. Unfortunately, sperm from infertile men are more easily damaged by the freezing process and no motile sperm may be recoverable.

Donor Artificial Insemination

The procedure of donor artificial insemination or, as we prefer to call it, semiadoption, is a satisfactory solution for the right couple. The entire subject of artificial insemination in the human is very adequately treated in the book by Schellen.

Any physician who takes it upon himself to perform this service should remember that he accepts a grave responsibility. He is, in effect, placing an adopted child in a home and in so doing must be sure that this home is worthy and capable of contributing happiness and security to the child. It has been our practice to interview couples over a 3- to 6-month period before instituting therapy or to request a psychological evaluation in an effort to estimate the stability of the individuals and their compatibility as a couple. A child, be it natural, adopted, or semiadopted, cannot be regarded as cementing material for a marriage. If there is dissension, the rearing of a baby offers one more matter for disagreement.

In addition to repeated interviews with the couple, there are several rules of thumb which should be followed. (1). The husband must have been aware of his inadequacy for at least a year prior to the first serious consideration of the planning of insemination. (2). The physician must be convinced that the husband is taking the initiative and not being pushed by an overaggressive and overanxious wife. (3). There must be no religious background in either partner which would suggest that either might harbor moral scruples about the procedure. (4). Every possible medical investigation and aid must have been employed to diagnose and treat the cause of the male infertility. (5). A basal temperature chart, Rubin's test, and endometrial biopsy should indicate normal fertility in the female.

In the first interview it is explained to the couple that they must expect at least 3 months, with the possibility of 6 months, of insemination prior to anticipating success. The figures given by Behrman et al. for the occurrence of conception in 50% of the women within 3 months and in 90%

within 6 months are strikingly similar to those quoted for normal fertile couples by Tietze, Guttmacher, and Rubin.

The problem of mixing semen is complicated by the occurrence of sperm agglutination is some specimens. It is therefore practical to request that intercourse be practiced prior to insemination; or, if the couple prefers, the husband's semen is concentrated and used intercervically while the donor's is used in a cervical cap. Intrauterine insemination should probably never be performed. In women with regular menstrual cycles, our figures indicate that a single insemination is as satisfactory as repeated inseminations and this observation is substantiated by Kleegman.

The selection of a donor is of course of utmost importance. He should be physically fit, emotionally stable, intelligent, and free of any history of congenital hereditary defects. In addition, his semen analysis must be in the normally fertile range. Every effort should be made to match his blood group and type with that of the patient to be inseminated.

CERVICAL MUCUS

The examination of the cervical mucus with reference to the amount, quality, and presence or absence of infection should be made at the first office visit. The quality of mucus is judged by the viscosity and *spinbarkeit* (ability to spin a thread) as well as the number of epithelial cells and bacteria and the crystallization patterns. A good estrogenic mucus is watery and clear, has excellent *spinbarkeit* (5 cm. or longer) and few, if any cells. When the mucus is dry, fern patterns may be seen. These are characteristic of the mucus in the preovulatory and ovulatory phase. In the pre- and postmenstrual phase, when estrogen influence is either low or dominated by progesterone, the mucus is scanty, thick, cloudy, and contains numerous cellular elements, and the dried sample does not exhibit ferning. The changes in the mucus throughout the cycle have been described by LaMarr, Shettles, and Delfs (Fig. 29.10) and

elaborated upon by Davajan and Kunitake.

A postcoital examination (the Sims-Huhner test) should be scheduled at approximately ovulation time. The patient is requested to have intercourse within 12 to 24 hours of her visit. It is often well not to make an issue of this as many husbands do not do well with command performances and the patient may be allowed to call for her appointment the day on which she is prepared. In order to make this test as uniform as possible, recordings should be standardized in certain broad aspects. The last menstrual period, the date of the previous intercourse, the hour of the last intercourse, and the hour of the examination must be recorded. Davajan and Kunitake have described a simple method for aspirating and investigating cervical mucus. A No. 14 polyethylene suction catheter, attached to a 10 cc. syringe, is placed in the cervix. The catheter is stabilized and the mucus flow regulated by grasping with an atraumatic cervical tenaculum (Fig. 29.11). When aspiration is completed, the tenaculum is closed, the catheter withdrawn, and any trailing mucus is cut with long curved scissors. The amount of mucus is measured. The quality and presence or absence of infection are recorded, as well as the number of actively progressive sperm per high power field and those with poor or no activity. A successful test is one in which there are five or more actively motile sperm per high power field.

A successful Sims-Huhner test implies (1) satisfactory intercourse techniques, (2) normal mucus for the transport and preservation of sperm, and (3) adequate ovarian estrogenic function, as well as (4) at least the possibility of a normal male fertility. This test, however, does not substitute for a semen analysis but merely complements it. An unsuccessful Sims-Huhner test may result from a variety of causes. Faulty intercourse techniques, oligo- or azoospermia, or poor timing of the test are among the more usual causes since sperm consistently survive and penetrate mucus only in the preovulatory and ovulatory mucus. An inadequate ovarian estrogenic function, cervical in-

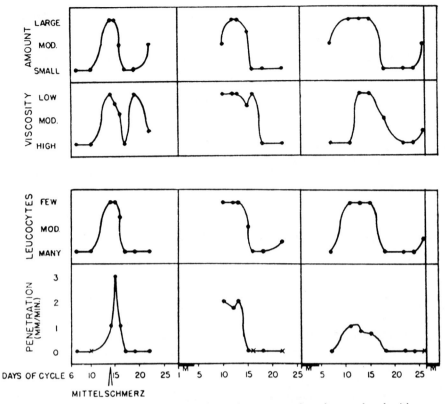

29.10. Characteristics of cervical mucus throughout the menstrual cycle correlated with sperm penetrability. *Curves* are a composite from three cycles of a single individual. (From data reported by LaMarr, J. K., Shettles, L. B., and Delfs, E.: Amer. J. Physiol., *129:* 234, 1940.)

fection, or in rare instances, a specific vaginitis due to *Candida krusei* are other causes. There remains a small residue of cases of unexplained etiology. These are the patients who show no evidence of infection, no evidence of ovarian insufficiency, and whose husbands have a normal semen analysis. Isojima *et al.* have described an immunological factor in cervical mucus, linked with complement, which causes sperm immobilization.

The treatment of the so-called "hostile mucus" depends upon the etiology of the condition. Those patients showing an inadequate estrogenic mucus at the ovulatory time of the cycle can be treated by the daily administration of 0.1 mg. of stilbestrol, or its equivalent, or 0.5 mg. of stilbestrol suppositories every night. If suppositories are used they should be discontinued at the 12th day of a 28-day

cycle or approximately two days prior to the ovulation date. In the majority of patients the dosage of 0.1 mg. of stilbestrol daily is too small to interfere with the menstrual rhythm, and therefore can be administered continuously. If cervical infection is present, this may not always be amenable to cauterization. Chemotherapy should be tried; a broad spectrum antibiotic 4 times a day for 10 days, as advocated by Horne and Rock, has proved successful in the majority of cases. However, as recurrences are frequent it is wise to give medication at the onset of the menstrual period in order to insure a normal mucus at the time of ovulation. If a vaginal infection of *C. krusei* exists, this can usually be eradicated by scrubbing the vagina with surgical soap and painting it with a 2% aqueous solution of gentian violet every other day for 3 times. The use of condom-protected intercourse over a 4-

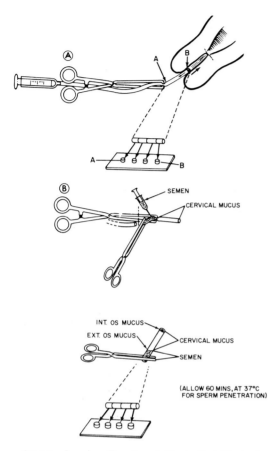

29.11. *In vivo* Fractional Postcoital Test. A. Mucus from external os level; B. Mucus from internal os level. (Davajan, *et al.,* Obstet. Gynec. Survey, *26:* 1970.)

to 6-month period in an effort to allow desensitization of the patient, has been reported to be of some value in the cases of sperm-mucus antibodies. Cortisol therapy has also been advocated but neither is associated with much success. No treatment is known for the normal type of estrogenic-appearing mucus with no evidence of infection which, nevertheless, fails to support sperm activity. Fortunately these cases are extremely rare.

TUBAL FUNCTION

Tubal tests serve not only as diagnostic procedures but also as therapeutic ones in that they tend to overcome minor obstructions. There are three accepted methods for establishing the patency of fallopian tubes. The first is gas insufflation described by Rubin in 1920 and known by his name, Rubin's test. This procedure is the least likely to be associated with any complication and is, therefore, preferable as a first test. The Rubin's test is best performed by using a mercury manometer, and tubal patency is estimated to be normal if gas is heard to pass through the tubes at pressures below 180 mm. of mercury. Partial occlusion is probably present if pressures above 180 and below 200 are obtained, and tubes are completely obstructed for practical purposes if pressures of 200 or over are unsuccessful. By using a mechanical system, Rubin found that tubes requiring 200 mm. of mercury for passage of gas were too small to transport a particle the size of an ovum.

The second method of tubal evaluation is by means of a hysterosalpingogram. This examination is indicated when the Rubin's test in unsuccessful and especially when operative procedures are contemplated. Because of the high amount of radiation to the ovaries which this procedure may entail, it should be limited to carefully selected cases. A water-soluble, opaque medium is preferable to an oil-soluble medium (Fig. 29.12) which carries a greater potential for serious complications such as oil emboli and granulomata. Protagonists of oil-soluble media believe that there is a greater therapeutic value in these media but the facts substantiating these claims are tenuous, and such nebulous evidence does not seem to warrant the additional risks.

The third method of assessing tubal function is by means of culdoscopy or laparoscopy. The Decker culdoscopic procedure (Fig. 29.13), performed simultaneously with the insertion into the cervix of a No. 14 Foley catheter with a 5-cc. bulb (to be inflated to not over 2 ml.), allows the instillation of indigo carmine into the tubes and any blockage may be demonstrated under direct vision. This method is the treatment of choice if there is some question about the accuracy of the Rubin's test or a discrepancy between two tests. It is also useful when extratubal

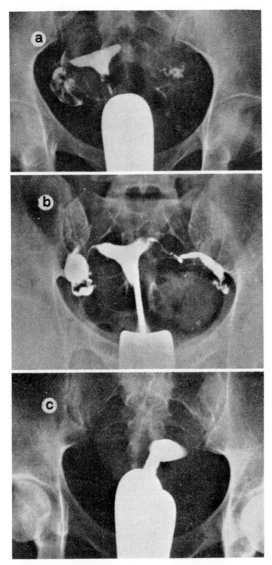

29.12. *a,* normal hysterosalpingogram showing outline of delicate tube and spill into peritoneum on left. The right tube is obscured by massive peritoneal spill on the right. The sweeping, smeared appearance is characteristic when water-soluble media are used. *b,* obstruction at the fimbriated ends of tubes with bilateral hydrosalpinx. There is an arcuate uterus. *c,* bilateral tubal occlusion at the cornu. The uterine cavity has been distorted by overdistention with radiopaque medium.

or periovarian adhesions are suspected. Because of the preponderance of tubal factors responsible for infertility in the female, a culdoscopic examination or laparoscopy should be offered when the infertility investigation has failed to

demonstrate any etiological factor and no pregnancy has resulted within one year after completion of the total investigation.

As a word of warning it must be remembered that neither a Rubin's test nor hysterosalpingogram is infallible. Each can be technically unsatisfactory, giving both false positive and negative results. Therefore, three tests, preferably of different types, must be performed before a diagnosis of tubal occlusion can be made and certainly before considering a tubal plastic procedure. On the other hand, it is not justifiable to perform repeated tubal studies if a normal test has been obtained. As previously stated, if real doubt exists a direct visual examination should be made. No tubal procedures should be repeated before a 3-month interval, as any such intrauterine manipulation produces some tissue damage.

Tubal occlusion may be the result of adhesions from pelvic inflammatory disease due to gonorrhea, tuberculosis, or postabortal or postpartum infections. Adhesions may be due to endometriosis or other more unusual causes of blood in the peritoneal cavity, such as an unrecognized ectopic pregnancy, a ruptured corpus luteum cyst, or a bleeding follicle at ovulation. Extrapelvic inflammatory processes such as an appendiceal abscess may also occasionally cause tubal adhesions with occlusions.

The treatment of tubal occlusion must usually be surgical in the final analysis. However, as indicated, at least three tubal patency tests should be performed in an effort to rupture adhesions. Hydrotubation with solutions of cortisone and an antibiotic is popular in areas other than the United States. A recent survey by Comninos and Manouelides concludes that it is indicated for postabortal or postpartum pelvic adhesions and a pregnancy rate of 17% (16 pregnancies in 94 women) can be expected in this category of tubal disease. As such treatment carries with it the obvious risks of causing pelvic inflammatory disease and peritonitis, it should be used only in the exceptional case.

If the age of the patient warrants the associated delay, medical procedures should be given an adequate trial prior to

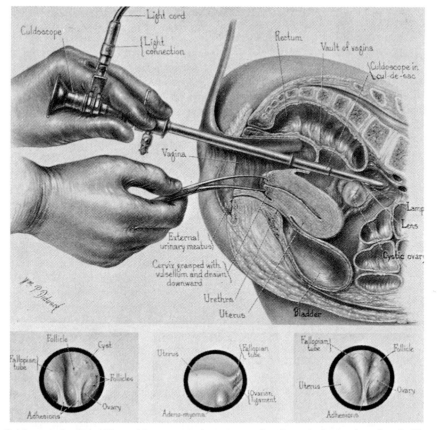

29.13. Culdoscope in place. The culdoscope can be seen passing through the trochar sheath. The trochar is introduced into the cul-de-sac through the posterior vagina, which has been "tented" by pushing the cervix forward and downward. The trochar is then withdrawn and the culdoscope inserted. (From Decker, A.: *Culdoscopy*, W. B. Saunders Company, Philadelphia, 1952.)

consideration of surgery. A tuboplastic procedure in our opinion should be undertaken only if the patient understands the statistical probabilities of success.

Umezaki *et al.* reviewed the tuboplasties performed at The Johns Hopkins Hospital between the years of 1940 and 1972. These authors concluded that the pregnancy rate depended upon the site and cause of the obstruction, which factors also dictated the procedures performed. They found that the duration of the follow-up was important in salpingolysis and fimbrioplasty procedures, as a constant pregnancy rate continued for as long as 5 years postoperatively. Results of resection and anastomosis operations and cornual implantations, on the other hand, could be estimated within 1 year, as all

pregnancies occurred during this interval. These findings suggest that there is no problem with the tubal epithelium in mid-tubal or cornual obstructions. The delay in conception after fimbrioplasty suggests that time is required for the reparative process of the intrinsic tubal damage associated with this form of tubal occlusion. To circumvent the problem of variable follow-up intervals, expectancy of pregnancy was calculated by computer for an indefinite follow-up time (Fig. 29.14). By this algorithm, it was found that 50% of patients could expect pregnancy following tuboplasties of all kinds, 66% after tubolysis, 40% after fimbrioplasty, 50% after anastomosis, 38% after cornual implantation, and 21% after multiple procedures.

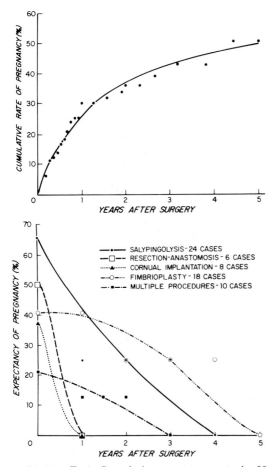

29.14. (*Top*). Cumulative pregnancy rate in 66 cases of salpingoplasty for number of years after surgery. (*Bottom*). Probability of pregnancy for different types of salpingoplasty operation calculated for an indefinite follow-up period. (From figures developed by Umezaki, C., Katayama, K. P., and Jones, H. W., Jr.: Obstet. Gynec. *43:* 418, 1974.)

THE ENDOMETRIUM

A study of the premenstrual endometrium gives information about the implantation site for the fertilized ovum and the ovarian luteal function as well as presumptive evidence concerning ovulation. This, therefore, is an extremely important test.

An endometrial biopsy can be obtained by a Novak curette (Fig. 29.15). The biopsy should be timed according to the basal temperature chart to be approximately two days prior to menstrua-

tion. This time is the most satisfactory for accurate endometrial dating by criteria of Noyes, Hertig, and Rock, and also furnishes an assay of practically the entire luteal function.

Luteal Phase Defect

If the histological dating of the endometrium is two or more days behind the menstrual dating in two or more cycles, the diagnosis of a luteal phase defect can be made. An inadequate endometrium may reflect (1) an inability of the endometrium to respond to hormone stimulation as in endometrial sclerosis, which, in our experience, is unusual, (2) an insufficiency of progesterone production by the ovary or, more unusual, an estrogen-progesterone imbalance.

Luteal deficiency is part and parcel of a broad spectrum of abnormalities of ovulation, comprising failure of follicular development, amenorrhea and anovulation, anovulatory cycles, aluteal cycles and finally luteal phase defects. The etiologic factors responsible for the defect are therefore the same as those discussed under the section on anovulation in Chapter 30. Although the most common clinical symptom of the luteal phase defect is early repeated miscarriages, it can also be a cause of primary infertility.

The treatment of the inadequate luteal phase is dependent upon the etiology.

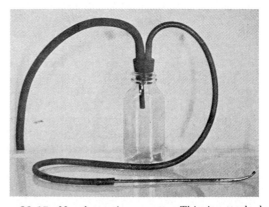

29.15. Novak suction curette. This is attached either to an electric suction apparatus or to a simple water pump although tissue for biopsy may be obtained without either.

However, if the specific factors have been corrected as well as possible or if no specific factors are found, progesterone substitution therapy must be instituted. Fortuitously, if the follicular maturation has been sufficient for ovulation to occur, the ovum is properly prepared for fertilization. Usually the most satisfactory substitution therapy is the administration of 12.5 mg. of progesterone intramuscularly daily, given within 2 days after estimated ovulation and continued until the menstrual period begins. This amount of progesterone is adequate for the repair of the average luteal defect but is not enough to override a normal menstrual period. A repeat biopsy while the patient is on therapy will tell whether or not the defect has been repaired. If this amount of progesterone is inadequate, 25 mg. of progesterone can be given daily until approximately 2 or 3 days before the period is expected, at which time the dosage may be reduced to 12.5 mg. or its equivalent. In this fashion one can prevent a pseudopregnancy reaction.

Synthetic progestogens are not advised since the effect upon the endometrium is often not equivalent to that of progesterone. Additionally, some have been shown to be luteolytic. Although HCG is a potent luteotropic hormone and 2,500 I.U. daily will stimulate the normal corpus luteum to synthesize double the amount of progesterone and prolong luteal function by at least 8 days, the response of an abnormal corpus luteum to HCG is unpredictable (Jones *et al.* 1974). This therapy is therefore to be used only in selected cases. If, in addition to the luteal phase defect, there is an estrogenic deficiency, as judged by an inadequate cervical mucus, 0.1 mg. of stilbestrol daily throughout the menstrual cycle will, as reported by Hughes and Van Ness, sometimes be sufficient to produce a proper endometrial build-up for a progestational response, or initiate more adequate pituitary gonadotrophin stimulation via the hypothalamic steroid feedback mechanism.

If infection is present, proper antibiotic therapy must be instituted. If there is en-dometrial scarring, as in Asherman's disease, repeated gentle curettage may suffice. Tuberculous endometritis as a factor in infertility is discussed in Chapter 20, Genital Tuberculosis.

HABITUAL ABORTION

The usual criterion for the diagnosis of habitual abortion is three or more pregnancies with consecutive losses generally in the third or fourth month. Bishop and Richards have indicated the incidence to be 0.41% of all pregnancies. The clinical symptomatology is not due to a single disease entity, but is characterized by many different etiological factors. For the most successful treatment of the condition, it is important to make a proper etiological differential diagnosis. The etiological factors can be classified under six major headings.

(1) Genetic Factors. Lethal genes which are consistently repetitive are extremely rare even under experimental conditions, and it is estimated that such a cause for repeated abortion in the human would be almost statistically impossible. If, on the other hand, rather than repeated abortions, there is a history of fetal wastage interspersed with normal progeny, a genetic factor can then be suspected. Under these circumstances, the chromosomal karyotype for both husband and wife should be obtained. As there is no known treatment at the present time for such a genetic defect, genetic counseling is all that can be offered to such couples.

(2) Anatomical Uterine and Cervical Defects. The incompetent cervical os, either traumatic or congenital, can be associated with repeated fetal loss. The history is probably the best diagnostic aid. It is characterized by sudden expulsion of a normal sac and fetus between the 18th and 32nd week of pregnancy without prior cramps or bleeding. If a traumatic surgical procedure has been experienced before the first miscarriage or a lesion can be palpated on physical examination, especially at the time of the abortion, the diagnosis is assured. This factor seems to be more prevalent in those areas of the world where abortion is frequent or obstetrical care, at delivery, poor. The traumatic type of cervical incompetence is best treated by an interval trachelorrhaphy as described by Lash. The atraumatic cervical incompetence is probably congenital in origin and is best treated by a cervical suture as described by Shirodkar. This suture must be placed before dilatation of the cervix begins, usually between 12 and 16 weeks, and should be used only when other fetal and maternal endocrine findings are normal.

A double uterus is associated with repeated miscarriage in approximately one-fourth of the cases. This defect is also characterized by delivery of a normal fetus or premature infant usually after the 16th week of pregnancy. It is, however, associated with bleeding and miniature labor. The diagnosis is made by hysterosalpingography and exploration of the uterine cavity. The treatment is surgical, as outlined in Chapter 7.

Submucus fibroids, endometrial polyps, or uterine synechiae which distort the endometrial cavity may also cause repeated abortion. Diagnosis is again made by hysterogram (Fig. 29.16) and the treatment is surgical.

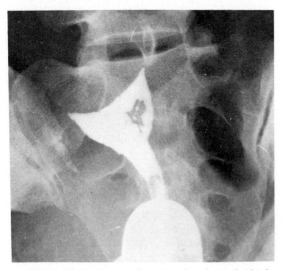

29.16. Hysterogram of uterus of patient who had had repeated early miscarriages following a therapeutic abortion. There is a single area of scarring.

(3) The luteal phase defect. As discussed above, this form of ovarian insufficiency is a relatively frequent cause of repeated miscarriage. It occurred in 34% of the patients studied by Jones and Delfs and was best diagnosed on the basis of the timed endometrial biopsy. If the histological dating of the endometrium is more than two days behind the clinical dating by the onset of the menstrual period in two consecutive cycles, the diagnosis can be established. The etiology of the difficulty can be due to (1) central factors, related to psychogenic, neurogenic, or specific pituitary insufficiency, (2) intermediate disturbances related to nutritional factors, drug toxicity, chronic disease processes, metabolic disease, (3) specific ovarian insufficiency.

Preconceptual therapy should be aimed at correcting the etiological difficulty, if this has been diagnosed, or substitution with progesterone 12.5 mg. in oil daily beginning as soon as it can be established that ovulation has occurred. Oral progestational agents have not been as successful therapeutically and, as they do not reproduce the same histological pattern as progesterone, it is impossible to judge the adequacy of therapy by repeated endometrial biopsy, if these agents are used instead of progesterone in oil. Treatment with progesterone after the first missed period is frequently too late to be effective. By the second trimester, placental steroidogenesis is usually sufficient, and progesterone substitution is no longer necessary.

(4) Infection. Syphilis, brucellosis, listeriosis, toxoplasmosis, cytomegalic inclusion disease and now mycoplasmosis have all been implicated as possible causes of repeated miscarriages. The data, however, in many instances are less than conclusive. In areas where these diseases are endemic, the physician should be aware of the possible relationship.

(5) Blood Incompatibilities. Although Rh incompatibilities are not a cause of repeated miscarriages, certain ABO incompatibilities may be associated with this clinical syndrome. The history under these circumstances is characterized by one normal pregnancy, perhaps with a history of a jaundiced baby, then recurrent abortions at an earlier and earlier duration of pregnancy. This type of abortion is usually indicative of a tissue antibody. Serum antibodies may not be present. At the present time, there is no known treatment for this condition.

(6) Sperm Defects. Although probably a rare cause for repeated miscarriages, when increased numbers of abnormal spermatozoa are found in semen analysis of husbands of patients with repeated miscarriages this factor must be suspected. It occurred in approximately 2% of the series of Jones and Delfs. Joel described semen abnormalities in a select group of men with multiple marriages who had abortions by all wives.

Summary

In summary, the two major etiological factors responsible for repeated miscarriages are anatomical defects involving the cervix and uterine cavity and endocrine defects involving inadequate progesterone production by the corpus luteum. Genetic factors, male factors, and immunological factors, although occasionally involved, are much less frequent. Chronic infections constitute a theoretical but relatively small minority.

The investigation for habitual abortion should include (1) a hysterogram, (2) an endometrial biopsy timed by the basal body temperature chart, for the diagnosis of a luteal phase defect, (3) blood group and type with possible antibody titers for husband and wife to diagnose ABO incompatibilities, (4) a semen analysis with a differential count for the diagnosis of male factors, and (5) a karyotype of the husband and wife, if the history is suggestive of a genetic factor. Ancillary investigations, especially if a luteal phase defect is diagnosed, are a sedimentation rate, white count, and differential, a 17-ketosteroid assay if there is any hirsutism, a three-hour glucose tolerance test if indicated by history or physical findings, a column T-4 or some other equally reliable thyroid test, a nutritional and drug history, an inquiry into psychiatric or emotional instability, and a test for serum antibodies to exclude the possibility of ovarian autoimmune disease. If the patient is seen during an abortion, an examination of the abortus for gross abnormality with karyotype, if possible, is often helpful in giving a prognosis for subsequent pregnancies.

Treatment of repeated miscarriages depends upon the etiology of the condition and may consist of genetic counseling only (Chap. 7). The treatment of a luteal phase defect, to be most effective, consists of progesterone substitution therapy before the first missed period. There is no justification for the empiric use of thyroid therapy in the treatment of pregnancy wastage. If no etiological diagnosis can be made, restricted activity sometimes makes the difference between success and failure, apparently by increasing uterine blood flow, and thereby improving fetal nutrition. At least two serial quantitative serum chorionic gonadotrophin assays should be made early in the pregnancy for assessment of the normalcy of the fetal growth and development. If these values are low, indicating poor trophoblastic development, therapy should be discontinued to avoid the prolongation of an untenable situation. Serum progesterone assays are also valuable in that they furnish an index of maternal luteal function during the first month of pregnancy and will, therefore, indicate when progesterone is necessary and when placental steroidogenesis of progesterone is sufficient to compensate for the maternal defect.

MISSED ABORTION

When embryonic death occurs, the products of conception are generally expelled within a few weeks. In this text we shall concern ourselves only with this complication as it occurs in the first half of pregnancy; at a later date it falls into the fetal death in utero category. When an early perished embryo is not expelled within two months, it is spoken of as a missed abortion (Fig. 29.17).

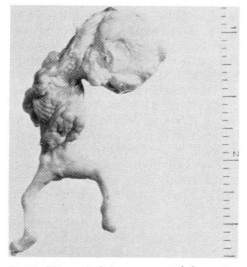

29.17. Mummified fetus evacuated from uterus several months after it had succumbed in a case of missed abortion.

The diagnosis is not easily made but should be suspected when a woman, apparently pregnant, shows no sign of continued uterine growth. Bleeding of some degree, often slight, muddy, and malodorous, may occur, but conversion of a definitely positive to a definitely negative pregnancy test is of course a decisive diagnostic point. The condition is characterized by low spontaneous myometrial activity, low oxytocin sensitivity, and afibrinogenemia. Severe bleeding, after surgical intervention, can occur, due to either uterine atony or coagulation defects.

The cause of the inability of the uterus to expel its contents is uncertain. Bengtsson has suggested that it results when death of the fetus occurs before placental failure. This deprives the uterus of a major estrogen source from the fetal adrenal precursors and causes an estrogen:progesterone imbalance with an excessive progesterone effect. Thus the contractility of the myometrium is depressed and the response to oxytocin inhibited.

Before suction curettage, a fibrinogen determination, prothrombin time, and coagulation studies should be made (Fig. 29.18).

THREATENED ABORTION

Tietze estimates the percentage of abortions in all pregnancies as 10%, although others put the figure as high as 20%. One or more missed periods followed by bleeding and sometimes cramps suggest that a pregnancy is threatened. The persistence of a normal serum chorionic gonadotrophin titer is a good prognostic sign, while low titers are usually a signal of inevitable abortion. The symptoms sometimes subside, and the gestation goes on uneventfully to term. In other instances the bleeding and cramps may increase with ultimate expulsion of the embryo. Although marked bleeding and cramps are rarely compatible with retention of the fetus this may nevertheless occur. If there is no abortion, and the patient goes to term, the expectation of a normal baby is good, although abnormalities of the infant under these circumstances are slightly increased over those seen in the uncomplicated pregnancy.

Where bleeding and cramps are severe, the cervix is often dilated with the products of conception lying just within the os. This is spoken of as *inevitable abortion*. Nothing can be done to salvage this pregnancy.

Actually the fetus has often already been passed and retained placental fragments are the cause of bleeding. Pelvic examination is not helpful except to suggest that some type of intrauterine pregnancy has been in progress; actually large blood clots may make the uterus appear larger than if a pregnancy is still in utero. Where the pregnancy test remains positive after mild bleeding and cramps, it is wise to pursue conservative treatment. Bed rest, sedation, and avoidance of exercise, intercourse, and trauma are indicated. Specific hormonal and uterine therapeutic regimes have not been shown to be effective.

The etiology of abortion is usually uncertain, and fuller discussion will be found under "Habitual Abortion." Suffice it to say here that most authorities agree that minor degrees of trauma or exertion

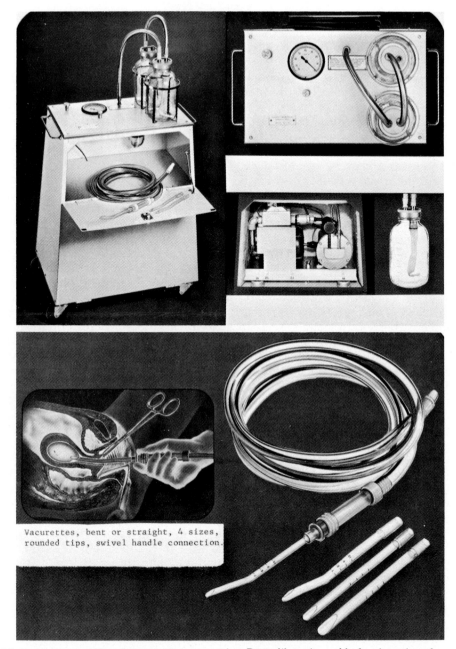

Vacurettes, bent or straight, 4 sizes,
rounded tips, swivel handle connection.

29.18. Apparatus used for uterine suction evacuation. Pratt dilator is used before insertion of vacurette.

can rarely be regarded as instrumental factors. Approximately 25% of spontaneously expelled abortuses have abnormal karyotypes.

INCOMPLETE ABORTION

Where there is continued bleeding, some more concrete form of action is desirable. If the patient has had the foresight to save material passed *per vaginam*, which shows chorionic tissue, the decision to evacuate the uterus is expedited. Meanwhile blood transfusions to combat shock should be under way, for bleeding may be profuse. A pregnancy test is often of little value, as one should understand that in the face of heavy bleeding and cramps there is little likelihood of a sustained pregnancy, even though the fetus has not been expelled; *i.e.,* inevitable abortion.

Sometimes an incomplete abortion can be completed medically by intravenous pitocin, or ergotrate, given every four hours for six doses. More frequently, however, curettage with removal of the retained placental tissue is necessary. Considerable care must be exercised not to perforate the pregnant uterus, which is apt to be soft and mushy. Use of ovum or polyp forceps and a smooth curette is followed by sharp curettage only after intravenous pitocin has been given. The development of the suction curette has obviated most of these problems (Fig. 29.18).

Although Braungardt, Kaufman, and Franklin speak of outpatient management of incomplete abortion, we would hesitate to recommend this as a routine office procedure. It should, of course, never be attempted in the face of sepsis or a uterus larger than twelve weeks of pregnancy.

Where *septic abortion* is present, the plan of therapy is somewhat different, but should be guided primarily by (1) the degree of infection, and (2) the amount of bleeding. There has always been some difference of opinion as to how soon the infected uterus should be evacuated despite severe bleeding. Currently it would seem that majority opinion favors massive antibiotic therapy for 12 to 24 hours, followed by curettage. Such at least is our own policy, although there are some few patients who are too sick for even this simple operative trauma. Sepsis with shock and anuria may occur with localized abscesses and thrombophlebitis.

Occasional clostridium infections occur; massive drainage, often with hysterectomy, plus antibiotic and antiserum therapy are used but the prognosis is poor. Supplementary blood, vasopressors, fluid, cortisone, and other supportive measures are of course necessary, and if there is associated anuria, peritoneal dialysis or an artificial kidney may be considered. *Escherichia coli* with gram-negative septicemia may also be associated with extreme sepsis and shock; a uterine culture with sensitivity tests is always desirable.

Differential Diagnosis between Threatened or Incomplete Abortion and Ectopic Pregnancy

When a patient skips a menstrual period, and then begins to bleed persistently, the first thought is usually of early gestation and threatened abortion. If the bleeding has been rather free and of considerable duration, one is faced with the question of whether or not the embryo has succumbed and been expelled. It should not be forgotten, however, that ectopic gestation characteristically presents a history of menstrual delay, followed by persistent bleeding, usually scanty in amount. One of the commonest errors in the diagnosis of tubal pregnancy is to mistake it for incomplete or threatened early abortion. In the threatened variety, as with tubal pregnancy, the bleeding may be slight, whereas in the incomplete type it may be rather free. Should there be profuse external bleeding, ectopic pregnancy is unlikely.

In early abortion, pain is not a conspicuous symptom, and may be absent. With tubal pregnancy, on the other hand, the bleeding is usually accompanied by attacks of pain in the affected side of the pelvis, sometimes accompanied by nausea, vomiting, or attacks of faintness. Where intraabdominal bleeding is free, pallor, syncope, and rapid pulse are noted. Pregnancy tests are not usually of decisive importance, as they may be positive or negative in both the tubal and the uterine types of pregnancy.

The chief reliance must generally be placed on bimanual examination. In early uterine abortion one can usually make out at least some degree of uterine enlargement, with often softening and patulousness of the cervical canal. Although there is usually no tenderness and no palpable enlargement in either adnexal region, occasionally the corpus luteum of pregnancy may be painful to palpation. Indeed, on occasion it may bleed so that there is no way of distinguishing an ectopic pregnancy except by culdoscopy or laparoscopy.

With tubal pregnancy, on the other hand, the uterus and cervix may show no noteworthy difference from the normal, whereas an adnexal enlargement, sometimes very slight and indefinite, in other cases large and unquestionable, is present in one side of the pelvis. This very unilaterality of the lesion, combined with the menstrual symptoms above mentioned, will usually justify a presumptive diagnosis of tubal pregnancy. Finally, valuable and often decisive help in making the differentiation can be obtained by such diagnostic procedures as culdecentesis, culdoscopy, colpotomy, or laparoscopy.

OTHER PROBLEMS OF PREGNANCY

Diagnostic problems involving the question of pregnancy are constantly obtruding themselves into the practice of the gynecologist. The possibility of gestation must be considered in the differential diagnosis of amenorrhea, as well as uterine enlargement, abdominal tumors, and uterine bleeding.

Diagnosis of Early Pregnancy

In the early weeks of pregnancy there is insufficient enlargement or softening of the uterus to make a positive diagnosis by palpation.

Various quick immunological methods may be utilized for the early detection of human chorionic gonadotrophin in urine or serum.

Where there is no urgency in making the diagnosis, the patient can be instructed to return within a few weeks. At this time, amenorrhea, frequently associated with such subjective symptoms as nausea and vomiting, soreness of the breasts, and bladder irritability, together with softening of the cervix, Hegar's sign, and symmetrical jug-shaped enlargement of the uterus, leave little doubt as to the existence of early pregnancy.

Pregnancy in the Aging Woman

It is not uncommon to find a harassed 45-year-old matron, who comes into the office because she is a week or two overdue for her menses, and is afraid she might be pregnant. Although this is a possibility that must be excluded, the probability statistics are against it. Karen, Zuckerman, and Brzezinski note *no* reported viable births after the age of 49 years in a compilation of reported pregnancies after the age of 46 in contrast to their own experience in Jerusalem where one out of 570 pregnancies occurred in women 46 or older. Both these authors and Stanton describe a high frequency of abortions, congenital anomalies, trophoblastic disease, and other pregnancy complications among women in this older age group. Although a few postmenopausal women have been presumed to become pregnant, it is probable that in most instances there has occurred an episode of functional (often psychogenic) amenorrhea, followed by resumed ovulation and pregnancy; only 1 in 20,000 pregnant women has been in the sixth decade.

Shettles notes that there is diminished ovulation after the age of 35 years, which correlates with the decreased fertility after this age.

Coexistence of Pelvic Lesions and Pregnancy

There are many cases in which a pelvic lesion, such as a large uterine myoma or an ovarian tumor, is known to be present, but in which there is reason to believe that the patient may also be pregnant. As in most such cases, gestation would be an indication for postponement of the operation. Any patient who has a history of amenorrhea or an abnormal menses, particularly if the cervix is softened, deserves a pregnancy test.

Pseudocyesis

This curious condition of imaginary pregnancy occurs in women who are extremely anxious *to* or *not to* become pregnant. It is characterized by amenorrhea, breast enlargement, morning nausea, in some cases imagination of fetal movements. Palpation of a small uterus generally clarifies the problem. During the last 10 years, this interesting psychiatric syndrome has become exceedingly uncommon.

Diagnosis of Pregnancy in Later Stages

In the latter half of pregnancy, diagnosis is usually easily arrived at on the basis of fetal heart sounds, the demonstration of a skeleton by x-ray and fetal movements. In the obese patient with a questionable uterine or ovarian enlargement, the use of ultra-sound has been advocated as a diagnostic technique by MacVicar. As surgery for myomas is rarely an emergency, simple periodic examination with confirmation of a rapidly growing and softening uterus can establish the diagnosis of pregnancy rather than myomas.

Therapeutic Abortion

This procedure has such obvious moral and religious implications that every individual must determine just what his own approach should be. He should first be thoroughly familiar with his own state laws, for different communities vary tremendously, but consultation with two or more confreres is the rule. By far the largest numbers of therapeutic abortions are performed in our present permissive society for socio-economic indications. As stated by Greenhill in a review of the subject as long ago as 1957, ". . . medical therapy has improved so greatly that few illnesses now justify the performance of therapeutic abortion." To this statement, we can now add that technology of birth control has improved to such an extent that this procedure should not often be necessary even for socio-economic indications. Women should be discouraged from using abortion, which carries potential physical and psychological hazards, as a method of family planning. For the true case of rape, abortion also should not be necessary as, under these circumstances, pregnancy can be prevented by giving a high dose of estrogen for a 10-day or 2-week period (Chapter 32) (25 mg. of Stilbestrol daily or its equivalent).

Techniques of abortion depend upon the duration of the pregnancy. Suction curettage can be used up to the 12th week of pregnancy. A saline injection into the amniotic sac can be easily performed as of the 16th week of pregnancy.

If therapeutic abortion is medically indicated, the doctor will also ask if sterilization may not, therefore, be desirable. This obviously does not pertain to the young nullipara or to the patient who is to have an abortion for fetal indications such as German measles. If sterilization is to be done simultaneously, hysterotomy is satisfactory. Caesarean hysterectomy is indicated under certain conditions and is not a difficult procedure, but it does unquestionably carry a greater morbidity than hysterotomy and tubal ligation. Nevertheless, this obviates the return of 10 to 20% of all sterilized women who subsequently have major uterine problems necessitating another laparotomy.

REFERENCES

Adams, C. E., and Chang, M. C.: Capacitation of rabbit spermatozoa in the Fallopian tube and in the uterus. J. Exp. Zool., *151:* 159, 1962.

Aksel, S., and Jones, G. S.: Effect of progesterone and 17-OH progesterone caproate on normal corpus luteum function. Amer. J. Obstet. Gynec., *118:* 466, 1974.

Berhman, S. J., Buettner, J. J., Heglar, R., Gershowitz, H., and Tew, W. L.: ABO (H) blood incompatibility as a cause of infertility; a new concept. Amer. J. Obstet. Gynec., *79:* 847, 1960.

Bengtsson, L. Ph.: Missed abortion, the aetiology, endocrinology, and treatment. Lancet, *1:* 339, 1962.

Brown, J. B.: Urinary excretion of estrogens during the menstrual cycle. Lancet, *1:* 320, 1955.

Campos Da Paz, A.: Crystallization phenomena of cervical mucus in the human being and in animals. Proc. Int. Fertil. Assn., *1:* 595, 1953.

Comninos, A., and Manouelides, N.: Hydrotubation. Int. J. Fertil., *19:* 23, 1974.

Cooper, G., Jr., and Williams, R.: Radiation dosage to female gonads during diagnostic roentgenographic proceedings. J.A.M.A., *170:* 766, 1959.

Corner, G. W., Farris, E. J., and Corner, G. W., Jr.: Dating of ovulation and other ovarian crises by histological examination in comparison with the Farris test. Amer. J. Obstet. Gynec., *59:* 514, 1950.

Davajan, V., and Kunitake, G. M.: Fractional *in vivo* and *in vitro* examination of postcoital cervical mucus in the human. Fertil. Steril., *20:* 197, 1969.

Decker, A.: *Culdoscopy.* W. B. Saunders Company, Philadelphia, 1952.

Gemzell, C. A., Diczfalusy, E., and Tellinger, G.: Clinical effect of human pituitary follicle-stimulating hormone (FSH). J. Clin. Endocr., *18:* 1333, 1958.

Guttmacher, A. F.: Fertility of man. Fertil. Steril., *3:* 281, 1952.

Hansen, K. B., and Hjort, T.: Immunofluorescent studies on human spermatozoa. II. Characterization of spermatozoal antigens and their occurrence in spermatozoa from the male partners of infertile couples. Clin. Exp. Immun., *9:* 21, 1971.

Hanton, E. M., Pratt, J. H., and Banner, E. A.: Tubal plastic surgery at the Mayo Clinic. Amer. J. Obstet. Gynec., *89:* 934, 1964.

Hayes, K.: Prenatal viral infection with particular reference to cytomegaloviruses. Aust. Paediat. J., *10:* 56, 1974.

Heckel, N. J.: Production of oligospermia in man by the use of testosterone propionate. Proc. Soc. Exp. Biol. Med., *40:* 658, 1939.

Heckel, N. J., and MacDonald, J. H.: Rebound phenomena of spermatogenic activity of human testis following administration of testosterone propionate; further observations. Fertil. Steril., *3:* 49, 1952.

Higdon, A. L.: Pregnancy in women over 40. Amer. J. Obstet. Gynec., *80:* 38, 1960.

Horne, H. W., Jr., and Rock, J.: Oral Terramycin therapy for chronic endocervicitis in infertile women. Fertil. Steril., *3:* 321, 1952.

Hotchkiss, R. S., Pinto, A. B., and Kleegman, S.: Artificial insemination with semen recovered from the bladder. Fertil. Steril., *6:* 37, 1955.

Hughes, E. C., and Van Ness, A. W.: In *Progress in Gynecology,* edited by J. V. Meigs and S. H. Sturgis, Vol. 2. Grune & Stratton, Inc., New York, 1950.

Ingersoll, F. M., and McArthur, J. W.: Longitudinal studies of gonadotrophin excretion in the Stein-Leventhal syndrome. Amer. J. Obstet. Gynec., *77:* 795, 1959.

Ismajovich, B., Zemer, D., Revach, M., Serr, D. M., and Sohar, E.: Causes of sterility in familial Mediterranean fever. Fertil. Steril., *24:* 844, 1973.

Isojima, S., Tsuchiya, K., Koyama, K., Tanaka, C., Naka, O., Tedachi, H.: Further studies on sperm-immobilizing antibody found in sera of women with unexplained sterility. Amer. J. Obstet. Gynec., *112:* 199, 1972.

Israel, S. L.: *Mazer and Israel's Diagnosis and Treatment of Menstrual Disorders and Sterility.* Ed. 4. Paul B. Hoeber, Inc., New York, 1959.

Johnson, S. G.: The mechanism involved in testicular degeneration in man. Acta Endocr. (Suppl. 124), *56:* 17, 1967.

Jones, G. E. S., and Pourmand, K.: An evaluation of etiologic factors and therapy in 555 private patients with primary infertility. Fertil. Steril., *13:* 398, 1962.

Jones, G. E. S., Wood, J., Bishop, D., and Donoho, R.: Vaginal fungi and their relation to sperm survival. Amer. J. Obstet. Gynec., *70:* 1271, 1955.

Jones, G. S., Aksel, S., and Wentz, A.: Serum progesterone values in the luteal phase defects; effect of chorionic gonadotropin. Obstet. Gynec., *44:* 26, 1974.

Kleegman, S. J.: Therapeutic donor insemination. Fertil. Steril., *5:* 7, 1954.

Klinefelter, H. J., Jr., Reifenstein, E. C., Jr., and Albright, F.: Syndrome characterized by gynecomastia, aspermatogenesis without A-leydigism and increased excretion of FSH. J. Clin. Endocr., *2:* 615, 1942.

Knudsen, O.: Studies on spermiocytogenesis in the bull. Int. J. Fertil., *5:* 389, 1958.

Kushner, D. H., and Marlow, J.: Therapeutic abortion by aspiration curettage. J. Reprod. Med., *2:* 291, 1969.

LaMarr, J. K., Shettles, L. B., and Delfs, E.: Cyclic penetrability of human cervical mucus to spermatozoa *in vitro.* Amer. J. Physiol., *129:* 234, 1940.

Leuchtenberger, C., Leuchtenberger, R., Schrader, F., and Weir, D. R.: Reduced amounts of desoxyribose nucleic acid in testicular germ cells of infertile men with active spermatogenesis. Lab. Invest., *5:* 422, 1956.

Lorimer, F.: *Culture and Human Fertility.* Columbia University Press, New York, 1954.

Lucas, M., Wallace, I., and Hirschhorn, K.: Recurrent abortions and chromosome abnormalities. J. Obstet. Gynaec. Brit. Comm., *79:* 1119, 1972.

MacLeod, J.: Human semen. Fertil. Steril., *7:* 368, 1956.

MacLeod, J., Artemis, P., and Ray, B. S.: Restoration of human spermatogenesis by menopausal gonadotrophins. Lancet, *1:* 1196, 1964.

MacLeod, J., and Gold, R. Z.: The male factor in fertility and infertility. V. Effect of continence on semen quality. Fertil. Steril., *3:* 297, 1952.

MacVicar, J.: Illustrative examples of ultrasonic echograms. Proc. Soc. Med. Sect. Obstet. Gynaec., *55:* 638, 1962.

Marcus, S. L., and Marcus, C. C.: Cervical mucus and its relation to infertility. Obstet. Gynec. Survey, *18:* 749, 1963.

Mikano, K.: Sex chromosomal anomalies in new-born infants: A 5-year survey of fetal membranes. Obstet. Gynec., *32:* 688, 1968.

Novak, E.: Suction-curet apparatus for endometrial biopsy. J.A.M.A., *104:* 1497, 1935.

Noyes, R. W., Hertig, A. T., and Rock, J.: Dating the endometrial biopsy. Fertil. Steril., *1:* 1, 1950.

Pardanani, D. S., Kothari, M. L., Prudham, S. A., and Mahendraker, M. N.: Surgical restoration of vas continuity after vasectomy; further clinical evidence evaluation of a new operative technique. Fertil. Steril., *25:* 319, 1974.

Perez-Pelaez, M., and Cohen, M. R.: The split ejaculate in homologous insemination. Int. J. Fertil., *10:* 25, 1965.

Pommerenke, W. T.: Cyclic changes in the physical and chemical properties of cervical mucus. Amer. J. Obstet. Gynec., *52:* 1023, 1946.

Quinlivan, W. L. G., and Sullivan, H.: Ratios and separation of X and Y spermatozoa in human semen. Fertil. Steril., *25:* 315, 1974.

Raymon, T. A., Arronet, G. H., and Arrata, W. S. M.: Review of 500 cases of infertility. Int. J. Fertil., *14:* 141, 1969.

Rubin, I.: Non-operative determination of patency of fallopian tubes in sterility; intrauterine inflation with oxygen and production of a subphrenic pneumoperitoneum. J.A.M.A., *74:* 1017, 1920.

Schellen, A.: *Artificial Insemination in the Human.* Elsevier Publishing Company, Amsterdam, 1957.

Sherman, J. K. T., and Char, F.: Stability of Y chromosome fluorescence during freeze-thawing and frozen storage of human spermatozoa. Fertil. Steril., *25:* 311, 1974.

Shirodkar, V. N.: *Contributions to Obstetrics and Gynecology,* p. 65. The Williams and Wilkins Company, Baltimore, 1960.

Siegler, A., and Hellman, L.: Tubal plastic surgery. A retrospective study of 50 cases. Amer. J. Obstet. Gynec., *86:* 448, 1963.

Stenchever, M. A., Jarvis, J. A., and Macintyre, N. M.: Cytogenetics of habitual abortion. Obstet. Gynec., *32:* 548, 1968.

Stone, A., and Ward, M. E.: Factors responsible for pregnancy in 500 infertility cases. Fertil. Steril., *7:* 1, 1956.

Tietz, C.: Statistical contributions to the study of human fertility. Fertil. Steril., *5:* 88, 1956.

Tietze, C., Gutmacher, A. F., and Rubin, S.: Time required for conception in 1727 planned pregnancies. Fertil. Steril., *1:* 338, 1950.

Umezaki, C., Katayama, K. P., and Jones, H. W., Jr.: Pregnancy rates after reconstructive surgery of the fallopian tubes. Obstet. Gynec., *43:* 418, 1974.

Vincze, L. O., Taft, P. D., and McArthur, J. W.: A study of cornification in vaginal, buccal, and urinary sediment smears. J. Clin. Endocr., *19:* 281, 1959.

Zorgnitti, W. A. W., and MacLeod, J.: Studies in temperature, human semen quality, and varicocele. Fertil. Steril., *24:* 854, 1973.

chapter 30

Amenorrhea

GENERAL CONSIDERATIONS

Definitions

Amenorrhea is not a disease but a symptom and may be arbitrarily defined as the absence of menses for three months or longer. *Primary amenorrhea* is defined as the failure of menses to appear initially and should not be diagnosed before the patient has reached the age of 18 years. *Secondary amenorrhea* implies the cessation of menses after an initial menarche. *Physiological amenorrhea* is the normal absence of menses before puberty, during pregnancy and lactation, and after the menopause. *Cryptomenorrhea* signifies that menstruation actually occurs but does not appear externally because of obstruction of the lower genital canal. *Oligomenorrhea* is defined as a reduction in the frequency of menses; the interval must be longer than 38 days but less than three months. This must not be confused with the term *hypomenorrhea,* which is used to designate the reduction in the number of days or the amount of menstrual flow.

Incidence

It is difficult to arrive at a statistical evaluation of the occurrence of amenor-rhea and oligomenorrhea in a general gynecological practice but it probably comprises less than 5% of patients. This figure will, of course, vary with the socioeconomic status of the patients as well as the geographical location. Kaeser finds the incidence of primary amenorrhea among 15,000 gynecological patients, over a 10-year period, to be 0.65%.

Classification

As indicated, amenorrhea and oligomenorrhea are symptoms which may be caused by a variety of etiological factors. A single individual with a constant etiological background may show at various times any or all of the pathological manifestations of menstruation, including dysfunctional uterine bleeding, oligomenorrhea, amenorrhea, infertility, and habitual abortion. It is most satisfactory, therefore, whenever possible, to make the classification of these symptom complexes on the basis of the underlying etiological disturbance. The following outline shows the etiological classification of amenorrhea to be used in the discussion with inclusion of the most common syndromes.

Etiological Classification of Amenorrhea

I. Lesions of central origin
   A. Neurogenic
      1. Organic, destructive lesions, tumors or scars
      2. Idiopathic hypothalamic dysfunction (Stein syndrome)
      3. Inhibition of the prolactin inhibition factor (Chiari-Frommel syndrome)
      4. Iatrogenic
         a. Steroids
         b. Drugs
   B. Pituitary disturbances
      1. Insufficiency
         a. Destructive processes (Sheehan's and Simmonds' disease)
      2. Tumors
         a. Chromophobe adenoma (Ahumada-del Castillo)
         b. Acidophilic adenoma (acromegaly)
         c. Basophilic adenoma (Cushing's disease)
      3. Congenital defects (?)
         a. Hypogonadotrophic eunuchoidism
   C. Psychogenic amenorrhea
      1. Major and minor psychosis
      2. Emotional shock
      3. Pseudocyesis
      4. Anorexia nervosa
II. Lesions of intermediate origin
   A. Chronic illnesses
   B. Metabolic diseases
      1. Thyroid
         a. Hypothyroidism and hyperthyroidism
      2. Pancreas
         a. Diabetes mellitus
      3. Adrenal
         a. Congenital adrenal hyperplasia, adrenogenital syndrome, and related disturbances
         b. Cushing's disease and "stress obesity"
         c. Tumors
   C. Nutritional disturbances
      1. Malnutrition
      2. Exogenous obesity
   D. Excretory and metabolic disease
      1. Liver cirrhosis
      2. Chronic nephritis (?)
III. Lesions of peripheral origin
   A. Ovarian amenorrhea
      1. Insufficiency
         a. Congenital developmental defects — hermaphroditism and related conditions
            (1) Gonadal dysgenesis (Turner's syndrome)
            (2) True hermaphroditism
            (3) Male hermaphroditism
            (4) Testicular feminization syndrome
         b. Premature menopause (autoimmune disease)
         c. Destructive lesions—abscesses, neoplasms, irradiation, and surgical trauma
      2. The insensitive ovary
      3. Tumors
         a. Arrhenoblastoma, hilus cell, adrenal rest
         b. Granulosa cell, thecoma
         c. Nonspecific with steroidogenic stroma
   B. End organ—cryptomenorrhea
      1. Congenital defects
         a. Imperforate hymen
         b. Absence or atresia of vagina
         c. Septum of vagina
         d. Absence of uterus (congenital absence of Müllerian ducts)
      2. Traumatic
         a. Stenosis of vagina
         b. Stenosis of cervix
         c. Sclerosis of uterine cavity (Asherman's disease)
IV. Physiological amenorrhea
   A. Delayed puberty
   B. Pregnancy
   C. Postpartum amenorrhea
   D. Menopause
V. Etiology undetermined

DIAGNOSIS AND TREATMENT

As oligomenorrhea and amenorrhea are symptoms of a great variety of difficulties, from organic brain disease to localized disorders in the pelvis, it is obvious that extensive tests and examinations may be required in order to make a correct etiological diagnosis. Optimal success in the therapy of amenorrhea usually depends upon such a diagnosis. An outline of the clinical methods presently available is shown in Figure 30.1. The most careful observer is occasionally confronted with a patient in whom no etiological factor is demonstrable. It is undoubtedly incorrect to classify all such cases as of psychogenic origin, but such a practice is not uncommon and, until additional evidence is available, no more satisfactory solution can be suggested.

The endometrial findings among a group of amenorrheic and oligomenorrheic patients will show, in the main, atrophic or nonsecretory patterns. However, there will be a moderate number of hyperplastic patterns, a few with endometritis, including tuberculosis and other forms of inflammatory and sclerotic processes, a few with abnormal secretory patterns, and, only rarely, normal secretory patterns.

Investigative Procedures

There is no substitute for a good history. This must include a careful reconstruction of the setting of the amenorrhea, emphasizing such factors as relate to emotional stress; gain or loss of weight; acute or chronic illnesses; accidents or injuries; relationship to pregnancy or possibility of unsuspected pregnancy; symptoms of characteristic metabolic diseases, such as polyuria and polydipsia for diabetes; susceptibility to temperature changes, changes in bowel habits and energy for thyroid disease; and the family history relating to menstrual characteristics, fertility, metabolic disease, or tuberculosis. In the case of primary amenorrhea the early developmental history, as well as a notation of possible birth trauma, is important.

Although a complete investigation for primary amenorrhea need not be undertaken until after the age of 18 years, a history should be obtained and a physical examination, including a pelvic or rectal examination, should be made whenever the patient, or her family, is concerned enough to consult a physician. If this is done, one can detect congenital anomalies at an early age, when the best psychological adjustment of both child and parents is possible.

30.1. Diagnostic methods correlated with anatomical levels at which defects responsible for amenorrhea may occur.

In the investigation of secondary amenorrhea an endometrial biopsy and, if any suspicion of tuberculosis exists, an acid-fast culture should be taken at the initial visit unless the possibility of an intrauterine pregnancy is present. This test is often a diagnostic shortcut and will indicate immediately (1) the ovarian status, (2) the possibility of pregnancy complications, and (3) end organ factors such as tuberculous endometritis and traumatic amenorrhea. A Papanicolaou smear with maturation index and cervical mucus study will also help in the evaluation of ovarian function and should be obtained at the preliminary examination. In all patients with primary amenorrhea a buccal smear for sex chromatin should be taken to exclude problems of intersexuality, including the triplo-X syndrome.

Other examinations will depend upon the specific problems involved and may include special examinations such as neurological and ophthalmological examinations; culdoscopic examination or gynecography; X-ray of the sella turcica and chest; electroencephalogram; hematology with sedimentation rate included; liver and kidney function studies; thyroid function studies; a glucose tolerance test; hormonal analysis, such as 17-ketosteroids, 17-hydroxysteroids, urinary estrogen, and gonadotrophin assays; basal body temperature charts; and steroid withdrawal tests.

General Considerations for Therapy

Each patient must be treated according to the etiological factors involved and such specific therapy will be outlined under the specific headings. Only general considerations will be discussed in the following paragraphs.

Amenorrhea *per se* is not necessarily an indication for therapy. The production of a regular menstrual flow is possible by the administration of steroid hormones whenever there is a functioning end organ with no obstruction of the lower genital passage. Such steroid therapy may be justified as a single course to assess the uterine competence. However, the prolonged use of ovarian hormones to promote monthly menstrual bleeding is rarely, if ever, indicated. Such medication may, in fact, aggravate the condition by causing suppression of the hypothalamic releasing hormones. The appearance of periodic bleeding is also prone to give both the physician and the patient a feeling of false security. The physician must differentiate in his own mind this type of induced menstruation from the induction of ovulation which is quite a different matter. Careful analysis must be made of each individual patient to determine if her symptoms warrant treatment for the induction of ovulation. In patients with oligomenorrhea, there is often no necessity for any treatment other than reassurance and general measures since fertility is usually not appreciably impaired. This advice obviously does not apply to those patients who present clear evidence of endocrinopathy of one sort or another, nor does it mean that such general measures as rest and proper food should not be advised whenever necessary regardless of the patient's age.

There are certain patients in whom efforts at treatment are indicated. These include the following groups.

(1) Young women, married or unmarried, in whom the possibility of future pregnancies is of the greatest importance. As a matter of fact, it is the commonly associated sterility rather than the amenorrhea which prompts the married woman to seek medical advice.

(2) Women who, in spite of the physician's reassurance, are depressed and upset because of absence of menstruation.

(3) Patients who have some associated medical problem.

There are several general methods advocated for the production of ovulation when the amenorrhea is due to factors located in the nervous system, *e.g.*, psychosomatic, neurogenic, or hypothalamic: (1) steroid therapy designed to trigger pituitary function. Although the normal hypothalamic pituitary unit will respond to this type of "feed-back" control, the amenorrheic patient is not normal. This form of therapy is therefore usually unsuccessful and will not be discussed; (2) gonadotrophic therapy designed to replace pituitary function; (3) clomiphene therapy which apparently stimulates pituitary activity via the hypothalamus. As clomiphene is an antiestrogenic drug, it acts on the hypothalamus blocking the estrogen inhibitory effect; and (4) hypothalamic hormone (LRH) stimulation which may directly stimulate synthesis and release of pituitary gonadotrophins. This therapy is still in the research area.

Gonadotrophin Therapy

For the proper use, rather than abuse, of human pituitary gonadotrophin, it is necessary (1) to make an etiological diagnosis in order to select the proper patients for therapy, (2) to arrive at a proper dose schedule, and (3) to be familiar with possible complications which may arise.

Any lesion of central origin (see "Etiological Classification of Amenorrhea," (p. 651)) will respond to gonadotrophic therapy. However, the classic indication is hypogonadotrophic eunuchoidism. It is obvious that pituitary or brain tumors should be carefully excluded and, in consideration of the treatment of patients with psychogenic amenorrhea or Sheehan's disease, factors other than gynecological should play a major role in the selection of suitable patients. Although clomiphene is the treatment of choice in hypothalamic amenorrhea, one may elect to use gonadotrophins in those patients who are clomiphene resistant. It is important that the urinary gonadotrophin assays be consistently in the lowest range. If the patient has a normal pituitary function, this will invalidate the dosage calculation and complications due to overdosage, which are multiple cysts and multiple pregnancies, will arise. The Stein-Leventhal syndrome is specifically excluded as the polycystic ovary is peculiarly sensitive to gonadotrophin stimulation.

A highly purified preparation of gonadotrophins (HMG), has been prepared from the urine of menopausal women. This contains a 1 to 1 ratio of FSH and LH and can be used as a follicle stimulator, FSH, prior to induction of ovulation by HCG, which acts as pituitary LH. Human pituitary extracts are not commercially available.

The dosage schedule which has usually been found satisfactory is 1500 to 2500 IU equivalents of FSH, standardized against the second European standard menopausal urine preparation (IRP-HMG-2). This is given in two injections daily of 75 IU or 75 and 150 IU, for approximately 7 to 10 days. Although patients will respond to less frequent injections, it has been found that daily administration is more efficient. Brown et al. report that it is necessary to induce a urinary estrogen level of approximately 50 μg. per 24 hours to insure proper maturation of the follicle for induction of ovulation. Crooke et al. believe that estrogen values of 150 μg./24 hr. or above, indicate overstimulation and that, under these circumstances, the ovulatory stimulus of HCG should not be given. McGarrigle et al. have reported serum estrogen values for monitoring ovulation induction. The lowest level compatible with ovulation was found to be 150 pg./ml., and 700 pg./ml. the highest level compatible with safety. The clinical evaluation suggested by Igarashi and Matsumoto can satisfactorily be used to judge when the serum or urine estrogen assay should be done but cannot substitute for it. A daily vaginal smear for a maturation index, and observation for the occurrence of cervical dilatation and estrogenic mucus, will indicate when a full estrogenic response has been obtained. This usually occurs between 10 and 14 days after beginning therapy, and, if no response has been obtained by 14 days, treatment should be discontinued. At the full estrogen response, following a 1-day rest period, 5000 IU of HCG is given. In our experience this has usually been an adequate dose schedule to induce ovulation in the hypogonadotrophic, amenorrheic patient, but each patient must be individualized and occasionally a total dose of 3000 IU of HMG will be necessary. Black et al. have found that clomiphene, 100 mg. a day for 14 days, given prior to the

HMG, will potentiate the HMG presumably by inducing endogenous gonadotrophins, thereby reducing the dosage requirement. One must have given a similar Clomid test course prior to adding HMG to determine the patient's response or lack of response to Clomid. FSH and LH serum assays should be done at the end of the Clomid stimulation.

The major complications of gonadotrophin therapy are superovulations with multiple cyst formation and subsequent multiple pregnancies. These complications have led to death through rupture of the cysts, or rupture of the uterus during pregnancy. Therefore, it cannot by emphasized too strongly that, prior to treatment, an etiologic diagnosis must be established and a proper selection of patients must be made to insure that they do not have a significant endogenous gonadotrophic function. A proper exogenous dosage must be employed and frequent pelvic examinations made. Rapid urinary or serum estrogen assays should be available and, if there is evidence of hyperstimulation, e.g., 150 μg. per 24 hours or above, the chorionic gonadotrophin should not be given.

It has been shown, using very pure preparations of FSH with little LH contamination, in patients with severely suppressed endogenous pituitary function, that the exogenous FSH stimulation is initially responsible for the hyperstimulation syndrome. However, the symptoms are not manifested unless ovulation is precipitated by exogenous HCG or endogenous LH. It is the high and unpredictable endogenous LH in patients with the Stein-Leventhal syndrome which makes treatment with pituitary gonadotrophin so hazardous.

Although low dosage irradiation of the ovaries for the correction of menstrual abnormalities has been repeatedly demonstrated to be therapeutically effective, the radiation biologist and geneticist have been so emphatic in their caution against the use of therapeutic X-rays that most gynecologists have abandoned this form of treatment. The viewpoint is summarized by Glass in his review on radiation hazards.

Indirect Methods of Pituitary Stimulation

Clomiphene

A number of years ago, a weak synthetic estrogen, tri-para-anisyl-chloroethylene (Tace) was developed as an antiestrogenic, and possibly an antifertility, drug. Clomiphene citrate (Fig. 30.2), a derivative of this compound, is an effective ovulatory drug in the human. It acts as a competitive inhibitor of estrogen, apparently blocking estrogen at the hypothalamic level, thus removing the inhibition to pituitary gonadotrophin production and allowing a gonadotrophic flood. The increased gonadotrophic secretion causes excessive ovarian stimulation with excretion of urinary estrogen, ovulation and normal corpus luteum function.

The success rate, as with any drug, depends upon the care and skill used in making an etiologic diagnosis when selecting patients suitable for therapy. The classic indication for clomiphene treatment is hypothalamic hypogonadotrophism. The inclusion of the Stein-Leventhal syndrome as a hypothalamic disease can be justified on the basis of experimental evidence and analogy with other endocrine metabolic disease states (p. 659).

Kistner gives the following criteria for selection of patients for clomiphene therapy. First, there should be some evidence of pituitary function, e.g., the total urinary gonadotrophins should be within the low normal range, and clinical evidence of estrogen activity should be present, giving additional evidence that

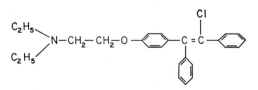

30.2. Clomiphene, 2[p-(2-chloro-1,2-diphenylvinyl)phenoxy]triethyl-amine.

the pituitary FSH and LH function is intact. The thyroid and adrenal function should be normal as should the nutritional status. X-ray of the sella turcica or examination of visual fields should be negative for evidence of intracranial tumors. Those patients who have destruction of the pituitary by either tumors or Sheehan's disease and panhypopituitarism or primary ovarian failure, *e.g.,* premature menopause, pure gonadal agenesis, or Turner's syndrome, should be specifically excluded from therapy.

The most serious complications reported are the occurrence of multiple ovarian cysts with rupture, and multiple pregnancies. As the pathological picture is similar to that seen with pituitary gonadotrophin administration, it seems clear that these effects are the results of pituitary overstimulation. Transitory blurring of vision and hot flushes are infrequent symptoms. If care is taken in using an initial low dosage over a short period and the patient is observed for evidence of ovarian stimulation and not retreated until the initial reaction has subsided, this complication can usually be avoided. Liver function studies should be made if there is a history of any liver disease, because clomiphene is excreted by way of the bile ducts.

Prior to initiation of therapy, the patient should be on a basal body temperature chart, and an injection of 50 mg. of progesterone should be given intramuscularly to induce withdrawal bleeding. This not only ensures the integrity of the endometrium but precludes a pregnancy. Although many dosage schedules have been reported, it would seem that 50 mg. daily for 5 to 10 days, repeated after 30 days if necessary, is a good standard procedure to start with. The lowest dosage should be used in patients with the Stein-Leventhal syndrome. If no effect is observed, the dosage can be increased to 100 mg. daily for 5 days. It is recommended that the total dosage not exceed 600 mg. in one month.

According to Kistner, 77% or 935 of 1731 patients, responded with ovulation to the first course of clomiphene therapy, whereas only 191 ovulated after repeated trials. Although most patients who respond to therapy continue to do so in a surprisingly regular manner, there is an occasional patient who responds erratically. In addition, some patients who do ovulate have evidence of luteal phase defects by endometrial biopsy and basal body temperature records. Grant reports the occurrence of a short luteal phase following clomiphene therapy.

It may be justifiable to assume that patients with a luteal phase defect, or patients who show an estrogenic mucus following clomiphene but no evidence of ovulation, are, in fact, deficient in pituitary LH response. Kistner has suggested that the addition of an LH factor (human chorionic gonadotrophin) will at times be associated with induction of ovulation and more nearly normal corpus luteum function. He adds 4000 units of HCG daily for 4 days following the clomiphene stimulation. Ruehsen and Jones have used a single stimulation of 10,000 units of HCG 3 to 7 days after completion of clomiphene therapy, or when the estrogen flood is detected.

Patients who respond erratically to treatment should be checked periodically with serum FSH assays to rule out the possibility of a premature menopause.

Although no adverse effects on the fetus have been reported in humans treated during early pregnancy, clomiphene has produced fetal anomalies in experimental animals. It is therefore recommended that treatment be avoided during pregnancy.

Luteinizing Release Hormone

Synthetic luteinizing release hormone has been used by a number of investigators in an effort to induce ovulation. Although preliminary results indicate that this hormone can be used for this indication, it seems obvious that the optimum mode of administration has not been attained. Keller was able to induce ovulation with an apparently normal luteal function using 25 μg. of synthetic LRH intramuscularly twice a day for 11 days, followed by 200 μg. given in two doses, as the ovulation inducer (Fig. 30.3).

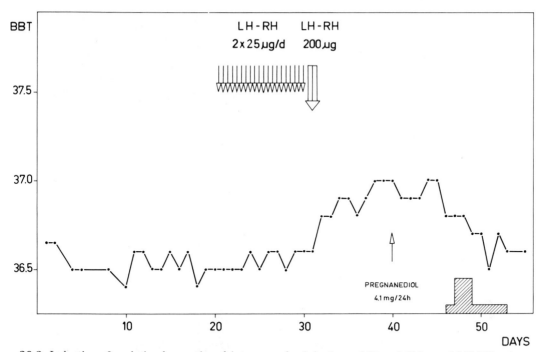

30.3. Induction of ovulation by continued intramuscular injections of 25 and 100 μg. of LH-RH twice a day over a period of 11 days in a woman with secondary amenorrhea (Case 10). (Keller, P. J.: Amer. J. Obstet. Gynec., *116:* 698, 1973.)

Zanartu *et al.* also found that repeated administration over a prolonged period was more effective than a single daily dose schedule. These authors used either 2.1 to 2.6 mg. infused over a 5-hour period, or 0.05 0.1 mg. intramuscularly given every 6 to 8 hours. A polymer-coupled LRH analog has been described which has a slow release and should improve the therapeutic effectiveness (Amoss *et al.*). Although a number of pregnancies have been reported, there has been no report of hyperstimulation or multiple pregnancies. However, it is still too early to know whether this hypothalamic hormone will circumvent the problems which are apparently inherent in the use of pituitary gonadotrophins.

Thyroid

Thyroid has long been advocated as of therapeutic value in the correction of menstrual disorders; however, its empiric and indiscriminate use should be discouraged. It will prove useful only when there is evidence of a low thyroid function as reflected in some reliable thyroid assay. Currently the Murphy Pattee test is used and a TSH, pituitary thyrotrophin, as confirmatory evidence. When such evidence exists adequate thyroid dosage must be used and overdosage avoided; 0.2 to 0.3 mg. of sodium levothyroxine daily is usually sufficient and three months is the shortest possible therapeutic trial period. Repeat thyroid studies should show some improvement at this time. If there is none, however, this is not necessarily an indication for increased dosage, and reevaluation is advisable. There is no evidence that triiodothyronine is more efficient in hypothyroidism than are thyroid hormones; however, a therapeutic effect can be obtained more rapidly. If this drug is used it must be remembered that one cannot rely upon the protein-bound iodine as a standard for judging adequate replacement. The protein-bound iodine will be suppressed as a result of depression of pituitary production of thyrotrophic hormones and resultant thyroid inactivity.

Nutrition

A good nutritional status is mandatory for the ultimate success of any treatment and must not be overlooked in our zeal for less mundane therapy.

LESIONS OF CENTRAL ORIGIN

Lesions of central origin can be subdivided into three major groups: (1) neurogenic, (2) psychogenic, and (3) pituitary. Neurogenic amenorrhea may be further subdivided into organic brain disease and idiopathic or iatrogenic hypothalamic failure; psychosomatic amenorrhea into major and minor psychosis, emotional shock, anorexia nervosa, and pseudocyesis; and pituitary amenorrhea into pituitary insufficiency, tumors and congenital deficiency of gonadotrophic hormone production.

Neurogenic Lesions and Organic Brain Disease

Organic

The diagnosis of organic brain disease is made with the help of the physical examination and history of encephalitis (Fig. 30.4) or related infections, accidents, injuries, or exposure to toxic substances such as lead or carbon monoxide. Laboratory findings are characterized by a low, or low normal, urinary gonadotrophin excretion, lowered urinary estrogen excretion and a moderately atrophic vaginal smear. Depending upon the severity, or the position, of the neurological lesion, there may be associated abnormalities of laboratory findings related to thyroid, adrenal, or pancreatic functions. The neurologic examination and electroenecephalogram are valuable diagnostic aids.

Kinnunen and Kauppinen, in a survey of 78 patients who had amenorrhea following brain injury, indicate that the duration of unconsciousness is a fairly good index of the possibility of amenorrhea. The prognosis in patients with neurogenic amenorrhea is poor except for those following acute trauma. Under these circumstances recovery may occur.

Adequate pituitary hormone therapy

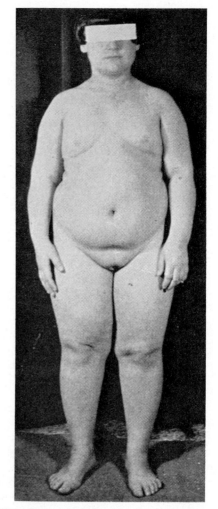

30.4. Postencephalic obesity and absence of sexual development. (From Sevringhaus, E. L.: *Endocrine Therapy in General Practice.* Year Book Publishers, Inc., Chicago, 1938.)

should be successful in bypassing the neurological lesions.

Idiopathic Hypothalamic Insufficiency

In hypothalamic failure it can be postulated that the hypothalamic cells are defective in their secretory ability or excessively sensitive to inhibitory stimulation. In either case there is a lack of stimulation to the pituitary gonadotrophic cells.

The cardinal symptom of idiopathic hypothalamic failure is infrequent, but usually ovulatory, menstruations; the menstrual irregularity dates from the menarche and is often associated with a family history of menstrual irregularities. On physical examination there are no detectable neurogenic or psychogenic factors, and, despite a normal encephalogram, the laboratory findings are similar to those in patients with organic brain disease.

There is usually no indication for therapy among this group of patients, as pregnancy frequently occurs without difficulty. However, if infertility is a problem, regular menstruation with a reasonable expectation of ensuing pregnancy can usually be initiated with clomiphene.

The Stein-Leventhal Syndrome. The Stein-Leventhal syndrome is characterized by bilateral polycystic ovaries in association with infertility and anovulatory menstrual irregularities. These are manifest as either amenorrhea, oligomenorrhea, or dysfunctional uterine bleeding. A mild or marked degree of hirsutism is usually present (Fig. 30.5). The one single criterion which must always be present to substantiate the diagnosis is bilaterally enlarged ovaries. Therefore, the diagnosis cannot be made without some form of visualization of the ovaries. Stein has for many years advocated gynecography; however, culdoscopy or laparoscopy can be used.

The differential diagnosis must often be made between the Stein syndrome and mild adrenal hyperplasia. A prolonged cortisone suppression test is sometimes helpful in this regard. A sufficient amount

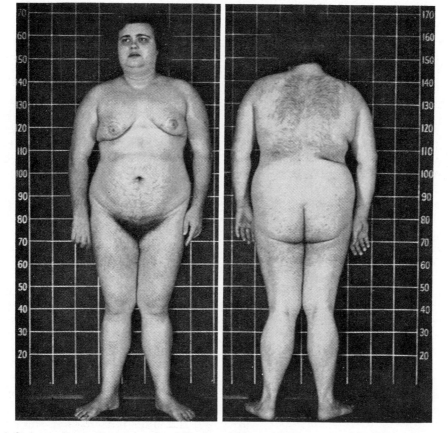

30.5. A Stein syndrome illustrating the difficulty which may be encountered in differentiating the condition from Cushing's syndrome by the physical appearance of the patient.

of adrenal hormone is given to maintain a suppression of 17-ketosteroid secretion to 6 mg. per 24 hours, or below, over a 3-month period; 25 to 50 mg. of cortisone acetate or its equivalent daily is usually satisfactory. The classic response in a patient with the Stein-Leventhal syndrome is a single ovulation usually within the first six weeks of treatment followed thereafter by a reversion to her previous state of anovulation. If continued ovulatory menses do not ensue or suppression cannot be sustained, a Stein syndrome is suspect. An adrenal tumor, however, may also be associated with these laboratory findings, and if the ketosteroid excretion is remarkably elevated, especially if there is also a high dehydroepiandrosterone excretion, this is most likely.

As described in Chapter 22, the ovaries of a patient with the Stein-Leventhal syndrome should be one and one-half to two times enlarged. They are often the size of the uterus which is frequently small, allowing one to feel three structures of equal size in the pelvis. Macroscopically, the ovaries are pearly white in appearance with multiple cysts beneath the capsule. Microscopically, they are characterized by a capsule formed by hyalinization of the interstitial tissue of the cortex directly beneath the germinal epithelium. This hyalinization may engulf the primordial follicles. There are numerous follicular cysts which characteristically have a thin granulosal lining and a marked luteinization of the theca interna. There are no corpora lutea present, although there may be evidence of old corpora albicantia (occasionally, however, even in a typical Stein-Leventhal syndrome a sporadic ovulation can occur). As all of these elements are present at times in the normal ovary and the findings represent simply an exaggeration of the normal, there is no diagnostic pathological picture. Comparison of the "Stein-Leventhal ovary" and the ovary removed with hysterectomy performed for recurrent anovulatory bleeding would suggest that histological differentiation is impossible except for the marked bilateral enlargement of the "S.L." ovary.

Therefore, the diagnosis cannot be made as a pathological entity and one can only report the ovarian findings as "compatible with" those seen with the Stein-Leventhal syndrome. Contrariwise, however, although a positive finding is not diagnostic, a negative correlation, e.g., "not compatible with," is good evidence that one is *not* dealing with a Stein-Leventhal syndrome.

The excessive follicle maturation and hyperluteinization are indications of excessive gonadotrophic stimulation and excessive steroid production. Laboratory investigations indicate that this is indeed the case. As long ago as 1959, Ingersoll and McArthur demonstrated that total urinary gonadotrophins are elevated, and, if a fractionation study is carried out, it is the LH which is responsible for the elevation. These findings have been confirmed by serum radioimmunoassay techniques. In patients who show endometrial hyperplasia and hyperestrogenism (25% of all cases), the urinary estrogen excretion is above normal whereas in patients who show hirsutism, the 17-ketosteroid excretion is usually slightly elevated or in the high normal range indicating excessive androgen secretion. The ovarian vein blood at operation has been found to contain excessive amounts of testosterone and androstenedione. Sandor and Lanthier showed that slices from ovaries of patients with the androgenic form of the Stein-Leventhal syndrome transform Δ_4-androstene-3, 17-dione (ADD) into testosterone at a more rapid rate than those of normal women.

Other laboratory tests such as the vaginal maturation index, and the endometrial biopsy vary depending upon whether or not the ovary is producing excessive androgen or excessive estrogen. When excessive androgen is produced, the maturation index shows a complete shift to the left or a midzone shift with atrophic endometrium. When estrogen is the major steroid produced, the maturation index may be completely shifted to the right and the endometrium may show marked adenomatous hyperplasia (see Chapter 15). These patients are in a high risk category for the development of endometrial cancer.

Stein recognized many years ago that it was impossible to treat the syndrome with suppressive doses of steroids. Keettel, Bradbury, and Stoddard reported apparent hypersensitivity of the Stein-Leventhal ovary to pituitary gonadotrophins and described a remarkable ovarian enlargement which occurred following the use of these substances. A similar hypersensitivity to clomiphene stimulation occurs.

In resumé, the clinical picture represents a patient with the paradoxical finding of *excessive gonadotrophin production* and LH predominance over FSH, in association with *excessive ovarian steroid formation* either androgen or estrogen. Additional *estrogens do not suppress* the *excessive gonadotrophin* production and stimulation with pituitary *gonadotrophins causes a hyperresponse* with multiple cyst formation.

Although the exact pathogenesis of the Stein-Leventhal syndrome is still not completely documented, the existing evidence establishes it as a disease of the neuroendocrine homeostatic control mechanism and places it in the same category as Cushing's syndrome and perhaps some forms of Graves' disease, hyperthyroidism. These diseases are characterized by excessive pituitary activity in the paradoxical presence of excessive target organ hormone formation, hyperresponsiveness to pituitary hormones and lack of response to pituitary suppression in the absence of a pituitary tumor. A possible explanation for these aberrations of physiology is a block in the hypothalamic centers which control the pituitary secretion and release of trophic hormones.

The exact nature of the agents which block the hypothalamic centers in the case of the Stein-Leventhal syndrome is unknown but it would seem, from a review of case histories, that this may be of varied origin. Experiments in the rat by Barraclough indicate that the anterior hypothalamic cyclic-LH center can be blocked by androgen given within three days of birth. That some stimulation early in life may often be responsible for the condition in the human, is indicated by the fact that many patients exhibit symptoms from the onset of the menstrual function. In addition to the possible effect of steroids as blocking agents for the hypothalamic nuclei, one would have to consider emotional stress and other factors in the external environment such as drugs and illnesses. These stimuli, through their effect upon the hypothalamus, alter the secretion and release of the pituitary gonadotrophins, changing the ratio of FSH:LH. It is probably the changing ratio which determines the enzymic mechanism of the ovarian theca cells and sets the equilibrium in favor of either estrogen or androgen production. The high LH in relation to FSH also inhibits ovulation and corpus luteum formation. When additional FSH is given, as in our experiments and those of Crooke *et al.*, ovulation does occur in Stein-ovaries, further substantiating the theory.

Although the pathogenesis is uncertain, the treatment is well documented. A bilateral wedge resection operation will cure the menstrual irregularities in 85% of the patients and pregnancy can be expected in 75% of the married women. The rate of recurrence is low if patients are carefully selected. The explanation for the success of the wedge resection is problematic. Patients with the Stein-Leventhal syndrome also respond remarkably to clomiphene; 305, or 78%, of 391 patients treated ovulated according to the investigator's report in Physicians Drug Monograph on Clomid. As discussed by Cohen, however, there is still some question as to the advisability of this treatment. Clomiphene is not definitive therapy and repeated courses must be given; it also carries a risk of cysts and multiple pregnancies. A number of patients have had associated ovarian neoplasms which would have been, at least temporarily, missed if clomiphene had been the treatment of choice. Cohen concludes that before ovarian resection, a trial course of clomiphene should be given. This is probably a conservative approach.

One would have to surmise that with both methods of therapy, surgical and clomiphene, the gonadotrophic ratio is shifted in favor of FSH against LH. It is easy to explain this syndrome if one accepts the hypothesis that there is an LH inhibitory center in the hypothalamus (Chapter 2) which synthesizes an LH-IH (inhibitory hormone). If this center is blocked, accumulation of LH in the pituitary is prevented, therefore no LH flood can occur to induce ovulation. The tonic center, which is constantly stimulating LH synthesis and release, predominates and a constant high LH prevails with relatively normal FSH values. The ability of the anterior hypothalamic cyclic-LH center to aromatize ADD to estrogen probably establishes a vicious circle perpetuating the syndrome. Tonic LH stimulates more ovarian ADD which in turn continues to block the cyclic center. The efficacy of Clomid in releasing the block confirms the theory that it is caused by estrogen. Therapy by some neurohumoral mechanism unblocks the LH inhibitory center allowing a reaccumulation of LH in the pituitary cells and the mid-cycle signal, presumably estrogen, received by the cyclic LH inhibitory center is once more capable of inducing inhibition of LH-IH and an LH flood occurs as the cell membrane becomes permeable.

The indications for treatment in the Stein-Leventhal syndrome are infertility, and dysfunctional uterine bleeding. Dysfunctional uterine bleeding is an important indication for therapy; as mentioned in Chapter 15, there is evidence that this condition may precede endometrial carcinoma. Medical treatment for the control of the irregular and possibly prolonged bleeding should, of course, be used. This would be either cyclic clomiphene therapy or, perhaps, if reproduction is not desirable, simply some form of cyclic progestational therapy, norethindrone (Norlutin) 5 mg. × 5 days every 28 days, or if the severity of the endometrial pattern warrants it,

megestrol acetate (Megace) 20 mg. twice daily during 3-month intervals (see Chapter 31). In the absence of bleeding or marked hirsutism, it is wise to postpone surgical treatment until such time when fertility is of importance.

Inhibition of the Prolactin Inhibiting Factor (PIF)

The interesting, although rare, syndrome of inappropriate lactation amenorrhea is characterized by atrophy of the vaginal and uterine mucosa with sustained breast development and persistent lactation in association with low pituitary gonadotrophin assays. When observed after a pregnancy, it is designated as the Chiari-Frommel syndrome and theoretically represents a prolonged physiological lactation amenorrhea due to an inhibition of the prolactin inhibiting factor (PIF) of the hypothalamus. When unassociated with a pregnancy and in the absence of demonstrable pituitary tumor, the symptoms are designated as an Ahumada-del Castillo syndrome. The most common causes at present are oral contraceptive drugs or the chronic ingestion of phenothiazine derivatives. Estrogen in the oral contraceptive stimulates the pituitary lactotrophes to secrete prolactin and when the oral contraceptive is withdrawn the breast responds with lactation. Phenothiazine blocks the neurotransmitter, theoretically dopamine, which stimulates the release of PIF and thereby allows the pituitary to produce excessive prolactin. Elevated prolactin levels are almost always associated with depressed LH and FSH values. One is always concerned about the possibility of a microtumor of the pituitary and various function studies have been devised, none of which are completely diagnostic. However, if prolactin does not respond to TRH stimulation briskly or if growth hormone stimulation is blunted, a tumor can be suspected. If, on the other hand, the LRH stimulation shows a brisk response, a tumor is probably not present.

Rakoff *et al.* report a relatively high spontaneous cure rate for the Chairi-Frommel syndrome. However, they also find a high frequency of recurrence following subsequent pregnancies. As will be discussed below, one is always concerned about the possibility of a microtumor of the pituitary when an Ahumada-del-Castillo syndrome is diagnosed. The treatment, until the development of ergocryptine, has been unsatisfactory. Ergocryptine will cause a depression of the elevated prolactin and an almost immediate return to normal of the suppressed gonadotrophin values. Subsequent ovulation and menses can be expected within 4 to 6 weeks after initiation of therapy, and the pregnancy expectation is good. If amenorrhea and an elevation of prolactin recurs after cessation of therapy, the possibility of a microadenoma must be suspected.

Iatrogenic. Drugs, Steroids

Phenothiazine derivatives and oral contraceptive drugs have been referred to above as iatrogenic causes of the inappropriate lactation syndrome. The oral contraceptive drugs are also the most common iatrogenic cause of amenorrhea. These steroids act by inhibiting the hypothalamic gonadotrophic release factors and, in exceptionally sensitive individuals, a prolonged effect can result. Attention has been called to this syndrome by Shearman, who indicates that, although not absolutely related to a history of menstrual irregularities or prolonged administration of the drugs, both of these factors do seem to play a role in post-oral contraceptive amenorrhea. The occurrence is sufficiently rare that other causes for the amenorrhea must always be suspected and investigated. The two most serious problems to exclude in the differential diagnosis are a pituitary tumor and a premature menopause.

The possibility of prolonged hypothalamic suppression should be considered when prescribing contraception for an individual with unproved fertility. If, in addition, irregularity of cycles is characteristic of the past menstrual history, such patients should at least be informed of the possibility prior to prescribing this type of contraception.

It is also wise to interrupt oral contraception over a period of 2 months or so every 2 years to be sure that no unusual hypothalamic suppression has occurred. During such an interruption period, some other type of contraception must be substituted.

The prognosis in this form of amenorrhea is good and no treatment is usually necessary if the patient can be persuaded that menses will recur if enough time is allowed. However, in a patient who is anxious, for one reason or another, to resume menses and ovulation immediately, or if 1 or 2 years have passed, clomiphene therapy should be tried, for it is usually effective. Exogenous pituitary gonadotrophins are indicated when all else fails.

Pituitary Amenorrhea

Pituitary Insufficiency (Sheehan's Disease)

The most common cause of pituitary insufficiency is necrosis of the anterior lobe due to a traumatic labor or delivery, as classically described by Sheehan. Nassar has inferred from experimental work that the use of ergot may predispose to pituitary thrombosis. However, the pituitary is normally enlarged during pregnancy and may, on occasion, thrombose spontaneously. Depending upon the severity of the thrombosis, there is postpartum collapse and hyperpyrexia. After an immediate recovery there is an absence of lactation and amenorrhea. The initial physical signs are uterine and vaginal atrophy with a slight, or occasionally marked, gain in weight (Fig. 30.6). Signs characteristic of the late stages are loss of axillary and pubic hair, lowered blood pressure, and loss of weight as initially described by Simmonds for pituitary cachexia (Fig. 30.7). Such patients are susceptible to infections and other forms of stress and thus live in a precarious state. Sheehan describes acquisition of pigment due to intermedin, and, although theoretically this is possible since the intermediate and posterior lobe of the pituitary are supposedly unaffected

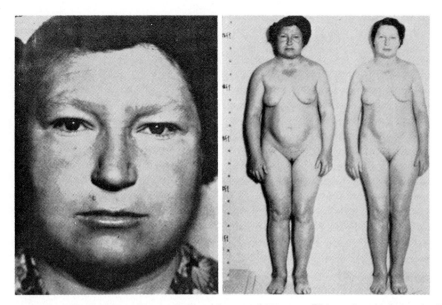

30.6. Late stage of Sheehan's syndrome. *Left,* at the age of 35 years. This patient had amenorrhea of 16-years duration. Her last pregnancy, at 19 years of age, was associated with severe postpartum hemorrhage. *Center,* before treatment. Notice mild obesity, puffiness of face (myxedema), and loss of pubic hair. *Right,* after 8 months of treatment with 2 grains of thyroid daily.

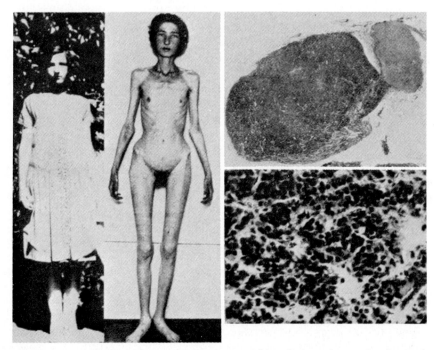

30.7. Cachectic state, resembling Simmonds' disease, caused by pituitary destruction due to chromophobe adenoma. *Left,* at 11 years of age, just prior to onset of illness. *Center,* at the age of 17 years. This patient had amenorrhea of 6 year's duration and a 65-pound weight loss. Notice extreme emaciation and lack of breast development; but pubic hair is still present. *Right,* low and higher power photomicrographs of the pituitary chromophobe adenoma. (From Lisser, H., and Escamilla, R. F.: *Atlas of Clinical Endocrinology.* C. V. Mosby Company, St. Louis 1957.)

by the venous thrombosis, in our experience this finding is unusual.

It is reported that some patients, over a period of years, tend to have an amelioration of the disease probably due to a compensatory hypertrophy of the few remaining pituitary cells. If satisfactory temporary replacement therapy can be obtained, patients have been reported to have become pregnant, and Murdoch and Govan say this is the best treatment of the condition as, under the pregnancy stimulation, the pituitary gland hypertrophies. On the other hand, Israel and Constan warn that this can be dangerous since, as a result of the stress of labor and delivery, collapse and death may occur.

The laboratory findings are characteristic of panhypopituitarism: a lowered or absent gonadotrophin excretion, a low 17-ketosteroid and 11-corticosteroid excretion, a low protein-bound iodine and basal metabolic rate, a flat glucose tolerance test, and anemia.

The treatment is replacement therapy, with 25 mg. of cortisone acetate, or its equivalent, daily. On occasion it may be necessary to use in addition 96 mg. of desiccated thyroid a day to give these patients a general feeling of well-being. Although replacement estrogen therapy will induce menstruation, it is certainly not indicated except for psychological reasons. When sterility is a problem, pituitary gonatotrophin therapy is the treatment of choice if one has the temerity to care for the pregnancy which may ensue under such precarious conditions.

Pituitary Tumors

Although pituitary tumors are uncommon in any series of amenorrhea patients, the reverse is not true, in that amenorrhea is an extremely common symptom among women with pituitary tumors. In a series of 15 young women who had pituitary tumors, all had amenorrhea as one of the presenting symptoms (Jagiello). Thus it is most important to keep this etiological factor in mind and to make the diagnosis when it does occur.

A history of headache and visual disturbances with amenorrhea is suggestive of an intracranial difficulty. However, these may be late symptoms and a slow-growing lesion can exist for years before their onset. The specific laboratory diagnostic aids are (1) an X-ray of the sella turcica, and (2) a color visual field examination, as the first diagnostic sign may be the encroachment of the tumor on the optic tracts with an ensuing defect in red perception.

Any type of pituitary tumor can produce amenorrhea. The most common type, the *chromophobe adenoma,* usually has no specific endocrine symptoms and produces amenorrhea through gross destruction of pituitary tissue. Prolactin-producing chromophobe adenomas are associated with the *Forbes-Albright syndrome.* This is characterized by persistent lactation in the absence of a previous pregnancy, extreme atrophy of the uterus and vaginal mucosa, small ovaries, and a copious milky secretion from the breasts bilaterally. Breast secretion may, on occasion, be enough to cause the patient annoyance and embarrassment, whereas in other instances it may be noticed only by the physician during the breast examination. When an associated defect in the sella turcica is present, the diagnosis is assured. However, in our experience, only about a quarter of the patients show this defect. A case has been reported by Bricaire *et al.* with complete laboratory data including a prolactin assay which was reported as high, 20 pigeon units per 100 ml. of serum.

However, microsurgery promises to be a valuable therapeutic tool, for pituitary function can be preserved. If the pituitary has been destroyed, amenorrhea, of course, persists following operative therapy, and the only curative treatment would be substitution gonadotrophic therapy.

The *basophilic adenoma* is associated with *Cushing's syndrome* which will be discussed in the section on adrenal, under "Lesions of Intermediate Origin." The *acidophilic adenoma* is associated with the signs and symptoms of *acromegaly,* and 85% of young women with acromegaly are said to have menstrual disturbances. The physical appearance of the patient with this condition is usually the best diagnostic aid. There is excessive growth of hands and feet and an increase in coarseness of all of the features. This is associated with an increase in the size of the nose and prognathous of the lower jaw. There may be unusual muscular weakness, polyuria, and polydipsia in the later stages. The laboratory findings are characterized by an increase in serum growth hormone, and decreased gonadotrophins, a diabetic type of glucose tolerance curve, and an increased metabolic rate or protein-bound iodine. It is important to recognize these tumors before the occurrence of severe visual field defects as pressure on the optic nerves may cause blindness. These adenomas are ordinarily radiosensitive, and some form of radiation therapy is usually preferable to surgery. When the condition is arrested, amenorrhea is usually corrected. However, if pressure necrosis of the pituitary has occurred, the amenorrhea may be permanent.

Congenital Deficiency of Gonadotrophic Hormones (Hypogonadotrophic Eunuchoidism)

This condition is extremely rare. It is theoretically due to a specific failure of the pituitary to produce normal biologically active FSH and LH. However, there is no pathological report available on the pituitaries of any of these individuals to date, and LRH stimulation studies indicate that some patients may have hypothalamic defects.

The diagnosis is made when primary amenorrhea occurs with a eunuchoid stature and serum FSH or LH values below normal. A familial occurrence is reported. The pathology of the ovary shows follicles up to the antrum stage, but no evidence of ovulation or corpus luteum formation. The treatment of choice is substitution gonadotrophin therapy. Because of the familial occurrence a protein defect might be suspected. Assay for specific α- and β-subunits of FSH and LH against specific bioassays should help to diagnose

an abnormal, biologically inactive hormone.

Psychogenic Amenorrhea

Psychogenic amenorrhea can be further subdivided into (1) major and minor psychosis, (2) emotional shock, (3) pseudocyesis, and (4) anorexia nervosa.

Major and Minor Psychosis

The diagnosis is made on the basis of the patient's history of psychiatric symptoms. The endocrine assays have been reviewed by Ray, Nicholson-Vailey, and Grappl and are found to show low normal values within the range seen in patients having neurogenic disturbances. This would indicate, as one might expect, that the final common pathway for the production of the amenorrhea is through a depressed pituitary function. The major psychosis most frequently associated with amenorrhea is a depressive state. However, according to Kroger and Freed, amenorrhea may also occur in the less profound psychiatric disturbances and may be a manifestation of emotional immaturity, overtly expressing the patient's subconscious attitude of a distaste for intercourse or a fear of pregnancy.

Some of these conditions are relatively easy to diagnose, as the amenorrhea immediately follows an unfortunate emotional experience. In other patients, the diagnosis is made on an exclusion basis in that no other etiological factor can be found and the patient is emotionally unstable.

The treatment consists of psychiatric care, and, with the present psychiatric approach, the prognosis is poor. Clomiphene therapy is sometimes successful and gonadotrophic therapy is usually successful. However, it is questionable whether such patients should be treated in this substitution fashion until psychiatric care has been administered.

Emotional Shock

Any traumatic experience may be followed by amenorrhea and the history is the most valuable diagnostic criterion. Amenorrhea is usually temporary, and menses may be expected to resume within six months. The laboratory investigation, according to Faierman, indicates lowered pituitary function. Bass reported that amenorrhea occurred in 50% of women interned in concentration camps during World War II; the onset was within 4 weeks of internment and spontaneous remission occurred in 94% of the women in spite of deteriorating food supplies. A nutritional basis would therefore seem to be excluded. A number of such reports have been reviewed by Randall and McElin.

The experience with shock treatments for various psychiatric disturbances has been interesting in this regard; Liepelt reports that 84.7% of 300 patients receiving such therapy have some period of amenorrhea, ranging from 6 weeks to 13 months. The treatment of amenorrhea secondary to emotional shock or trauma is largely reassurance followed by gonadotrophin substitution therapy if necessary.

Pseudocyesis

This condition is characterized by (1) an obsession of pregnancy, (2) weight gain, (3) normal secondary sexual characteristics and pelvic organs, (4) lactation, and (5) an impaired ovulatory mechanism. Since secondary sexual characteristics and pelvic organs are normal, it may be assumed that the estrogenic function is maintained at least to some degree. The lesion would therefore seem to be localized to a disturbance of the FSH:LH ratio. A corpus luteum cyst or ectopic pregnancy may be associated with similar symptoms and these diagnoses, as well as the possibility of a missed abortion, must be excluded.

The laboratory findings are characterized by a low normal gonadotrophin excretion, estrogens within the normal range and a midzone shift in the vaginal smear pattern. A negative serum chorionic gonadotrophin assay will also assist in the differential diagnosis. Endometrial biopsy or curettage should be considered only if an intrauterine pregnancy can be excluded.

Because the basis of this disturbance is often the patient's desire to become pregnant and inability to do so, the problem can frequently be handled by a gynecologist without psychiatric help. A discussion and explanation of her problems, together with the initiation of an infertility investigation, will often suffice.

Anorexia Nervosa

Anorexia nervosa is a disease of adolescence, characterized by severe malnutrition but without an associated lethargy. This presistent feeling of well-being, in spite of profound weight loss, distinguishes the condition from the pituitary cachexia seen with Simmonds' disease. The other characteristic of the syndrome is that the patient is unable to give an accurate account of her food intake and, either willfully or compulsively, falsifies the record. This preoccupation with weight and the inability to eat is the overt manifestation of a severe psychological disturbance. The associated loss of weight is secondarily responsible for the amenorrhea. The physical examination is characterized by emaciation, a fine lanugo type of hirsutism, normal axillary and pubic hair, and atrophy of internal and external genitalia (Fig. 30.8).

The laboratory findings in our experience are compatible with a lowered total pituitary function, apparently related to a depressed hypothalamic function. This is in accordance with Emanuel's findings, although Bliss and Migeon report only a lowered gonadotrophic function. The differential diagnosis between anorexia nervosa and panhypopituitarism of Simmonds' disease is made on the observed activity of the patient in conjunction with the history.

As the etiology is psychogenic, the treatment is psychiatric rather than endocrine. However, because the condition is induced by an obsessive compulsive family, it is frequently difficult to persuade them that psychiatric care is necessary, or desirable. If the patient accepts advice and weight gain is accomplished, menses recur within three months after a minimal ideal weight is regained. Dally and Sargeant have ad-

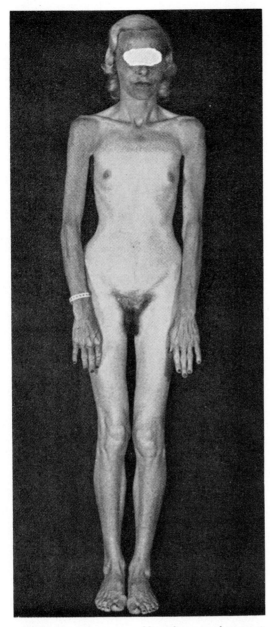

30.8. Anorexia nervosa. Note the normal amount of pubic hair.

vocated a hospital regimen of combined chlorpromazine and insulin. Chlorpromazine is given in massive dosage increasing from 150 mg. a day to as much as 1000 mg. a day. Insulin is started with 5 units and progressively increased to drowsiness, the average morning dose in the reported series being 60 units. The courses are interrupted for three large meals a day. This regimen serves to restore the patient's nutritional status to such an extent that she is able to accept treatment for her psychological problems. The condition is not to be taken lightly, as 10 to 20% of patients with anorexia nervosa develop irreversible, fatal malnutrition.

LESIONS OF INTERMEDIATE ORIGIN

Intermediate problems concerned with the production of amenorrhea are those factors which exert their effect somewhere between the central stimulatory and pituitary gonadotrophic functions and the ovarian or end organ levels. These may be divided into chronic illness, metabolic disease, nutritional factors, and disease of organs concerned with the excretion and metabolism of the steroid hormones.

Chronic Disease

Any chronic disease process associated with inanition can be associated with amenorrhea, an example being tuberculosis. Tuberculosis may exert its influence through constitutional factors or specifically by destruction of the ovary or endometrium. These latter causes have been discussed under the organs involved. Diagnosis of a chronic disease process is suggested by the finding of an increased sedimentation rate. Normal menses reappear when the disease process is arrested or cured.

Metabolic Disease

Disturbances of the pituitary and ovarian function are discussed under these specific headings and metabolic disease is herein divided into three categories: disturbances of the thyroid, the pancreas, and the adrenal.

Thyroid

Both *hypo-* and *hyperthyroid* states may be associated with menstrual irregularities and amenorrhea. These diagnoses must be made by some specific test for thyroid function, the Murphy Pattee being preferred. If the TSH assay is elevated, this measurement is a good index of therapy in hyperthyroidism. The interrelationships between TSH, and LH and TRH and prolactin may explain some of the clinical pathology (Chapter 3). It must be remembered that the diagnosis of hypothyroidism cannot be made in the presence of malnutrition, as lowered thyroid function invariably exists under these conditions. Some clinical signs and symptoms of hypo- or hyperthyroidism should also be present. The classic signs of hypothyroidism are sensitivity to cold, a tendency to constipation, dryness of the skin and hair, and slow reaction time. Hyperthyroidism is characterized by an elevation of the pulse rate, a fine tremor, some loss of weight, excessive perspiration, a lid lag, and occasionally exophthalmos.

The treatment of hypothyroidism is the administration of synthetic thyroxin (Synthroid®). The usual dosage is between 0.15 and 0.2 mg. daily. Therapy must be continued for at least three months and as long thereafter as necessary to maintain the thyroid studies at normal levels. Therapy should be interrupted periodically and patients checked for remissions. There is usually no indication for the use of triiodothyronine in patients with simple hypothyroidism. Either severe hypothyroidism to the point of myxedema or hyperthyroidism warrant medical consultation. In the treatment of hyperthyroidism antithyroid drug therapy is usually the treatment of choice. Propylthiouracil, administered over long periods of time, will usually result in a euthyroid state. Unless there is a suspicion of malignancy, or unless there is resistance to antithyroid drug therapy, thyroidectomy is usually not advisable. Radioactive iodine treatment carries the theoretical possibility of late carcinogenic effects and in addition may produce permanent amenorrhea, perhaps through its effect upon the ovary. Therefore, especially in women of the childbearing age, this type of therapy is not recommended.

When a euthyroid state is achieved in Graves' disease, the menstrual adnormalities are usually promptly corrected and fertility is restored. Among our own patients, however, two women who were treated with radioactive iodine have remained amenorrheic despite apparently adequate thyroid replacement.

Pancreas

Although *diabetes mellitus* is more apt to be associated with dysfunctional bleeding, amenorrhea is occasionally present. There are at least three theoretical causes for the menstrual disturbance. First, the difficulty may be due to the diabetes *per se,* resulting from the insulin deficiency; second, it can be caused by associated nutritional deficiencies; or third, it can be caused by the emotional disturbances which occur so frequently with this disease, especially if the diabetic control is poor.

The classic signs and symptoms are obesity followed by weight loss, polyuria, polydipsia, and nocturia. Often it is the monilial vulvovaginitis, commonly associated with diabetes, which brings the patient to the doctor; therefore the gynecologist may be the first who has the opportunity of making the diagnosis. It should be unnecessary to state that in the presence of these symptoms a determination for urinary sugar must be obtained.

The important laboratory finding is an elevated fasting blood sugar. It has been our experience that when the diabetes is satisfactorily controlled, the menstrual periods become regulated.

An interesting experimental approach to the problem led Foglia *et al.* to conclude that the pancreatectomized rat exhibits alterations of the estrous cycle and disturbances of fertility prior to the development of frank diabetes. As there is some evidence that anatomical changes can be detected in the prediabetic human, these findings are of additional importance.

Adrenal

The two outstanding adrenal syndromes associated with menstrual abnormalities are the *adrenogenital syndrome* and *Cushing's disease.* Adrenal tumors are also usually associated with menstrual abnormalities. Addison's disease is occasionally associated with amenorrhea in its late stages and under these circumstances it is impossible to say that the cachexia is not the major factor rather than the adrenal insufficiency.

Congenital Adrenal Hyperplasia. Probably the most dramatic form of the adrenogenital syndrome has been classically described by Glynn as female pseudohermaphroditism, and the laboratory aspects have been elaborated upon by Wilkins. The characteristic features are the deformity of the external genitalia, precocious virilism, short stature, deep skin pigmentation, and an absence of menses. There are all transitions between severe congenital adrenal hyperplasia diagnosed at birth and the muted form manifested as postpubertal virilization.

The disease is a heritable one, caused by a specific enzyme deficiency which prevents the adrenal from synthesizing cortisol (Chapter 8). Depending upon the peculiar enzyme deficiency which the patient has inherited certain specific urinary metabolites will be increased. In the classic form the urinary ketosteroid excretion is markedly elevated in the adult, usually being in the range of 50 mg. per 24 hours. An elevated pregnanetriol excretion indicates an insufficiency of the 21-hydroxylase enzyme and blockage of adrenal production of cortisol at the 17-hydroxyprogesterone step. The hypertensive form of congenital adrenal hyperplasia has an increased urinary excretion of pregnan-3α, 17α, 21-triol-20-one (THS) indicating defective 11-β-hydroxylation. This form of the disease may be unassociated with an increased 17-ketosteroid excretion (Fig. 30.9), and menses may occur.

Another unusual enzyme deficiency was described by Biglieri. It is a deficiency of 17α-hydroxylase and is also associated with hypertension. The specific metabolite is pregnanediol, the excretion product of progesterone. Elevated pituitary gonadotrophins, FSH and LH, are also present. This occurs because of the inability to make either estrogen or androgen when hydroxylation at the C17 position is impossible (Chapter 3). The syndrome must be differentiated from pure gonadal dysgenesis.

The adrenal pathology is characterized by hyperplasia of the zona reticularis and either anatomical absence of, or failure of steroid accumulation in, the zona fasciculata.

In the severe forms of congenital hyperplasia the deficiency of cortisone causes excessive pituitary adrenocorticotrophin (ACTH) production, which in turn produces the abnormally stimulated adrenal. The steroids which are secreted by the adrenal, in lieu of cortisone, suppress the pituitary gonadotrophins, and ovarian insufficiency and amenorrhea ensue.

There is reason to believe that certain patients with postpubertal virilization also have the same, or a related, problem but to a milder degree. This is evidenced by the course of the disease and the clinical and laboratory findings, and substantiated by the adrenal histology. There are, however, a majority of hirsute patients with many similar clinical findings who apparently do not have a true enzymic insufficiency, as in the congenital form of adrenal hyperplasia, but rather are suffering from a physiological insufficiency induced by stress. There is some evidence that in a predominantly Mediterranean population, where hirsutism is relatively common, the rate of adrenal *androgen* to *cortisol* production is increased. Blackman, in a morphological study of the adrenal of hirsute women, noted an increase in the size of the *zona reticularis* regardless of the cause of the hirsutism. Both observations substantiate the belief that in women with a hirsute tendency there is a "variation" of normal adrenal function.

Dorfman *et al.* have demonstrated that Δ_4-androstenedione inhibits 11β-hydroxylase activity in the adrenal. If a patient has a tendency to synthesize adrenal androgens excessively, under *stress* the increased rate of synthesis of androstenedione might be sufficient to start a vicious circle.

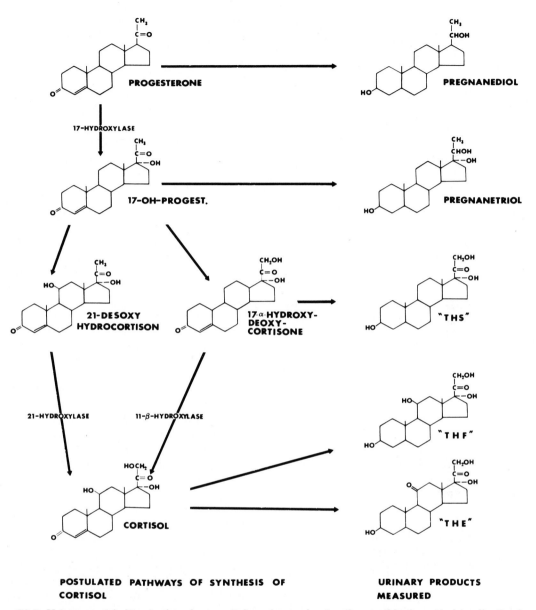

POSTULATED PATHWAYS OF SYNTHESIS OF
CORTISOL

URINARY PRODUCTS
MEASURED

30.9. Urinary metabolites in the adrenogenital syndrome showing the possible theoretical implication in relation to precursor steroids. *THS,* pregnan-3α, 17α-21-triol-20-one; *THF,* pregnan-3α, 11α, 17β, 21-tetrol-20-one; *THE,* pregnan-3α,17α,21-triol-11-20-dione.

Bush and Mahesh have published a fascinating case report of twins, one of whom developed hirsutism under particularly stressful circumstances. Both twins exhibited a high androgen:cortisol ratio following ACTH stimulation. The authors postulate that chronic stress constituted a prolonged ACTH test for the one twin who thereby produced enough androgen to initiate the hirsutism. There may be many such women in the general population who have either a very slight congenitally defective adrenal cortex or simply represent the extreme of the normal variation in the rate of adrenal androgen production. If the adrenal secretion rate is accelerated by stress, symptoms such as hirsutism, acne, oligomenorrhea and infertility appear.

The treatment for congenital adrenal hyperplasia, postpubertal virilization and related disturbances is cortisone substitution therapy; 50 mg. of cortisone acetate or its equivalent, daily by mouth, is usually adequate to maintain ketosteroid excretion suppression to about 5 mg. per 24 hours, which is the desirable level. It is unwise to use such drugs as dexamethasone for therapeutic purposes. The activity of these synthetic compounds is so great that the margin of safety between the effective therapeutic dose and the clinically toxic dose is too small. If it is impossible to maintain an adequate suppression, one must suspect a tumor of the adrenal or ovarian pathology as discussed in this chapter under "The Stein-Leventhal Syndrome."

In the relatively mild forms, it is often possible to maintain a suppression with as little as 25 mg. of cortisone acetate daily (or its equivalent) after the initial suppression has been well established. In the congenital form, which is due to a genetic deficiency of a specific adrenal enzyme, therapy will need to be continued throughout life. However, in the form induced by stress, once the vicious circle has been interrupted, steroid therapy can be discontinued until the next stressful situation develops.

Cushing's Syndrome. In contrast to congenital adrenal hyperplasia, Cushing's disease represents a hyperfunction of the entire adrenal cortex including the cortisone-secreting zona fasciculata. The pituitary-adrenal homeostatic mechanisms are out of control as there is excessive ACTH production in the presence of excessive cortisol. Cushing in his initial publication believed that the syndrome was always the result of a pituitary tumor or pituitary basophilism. Since the initial report, however, it has become clear that bilateral adrenal hyperplasia may occur without a demonstrable pituitary lesion and adrenal tumors are not infrequently responsible for the condition. In addition to these possibilities,

Heinbecker has implicated the hypothalamus as the primary disease site. Thus, when Cushing's disease exists, the differential diagnosis must be made among a pituitary tumor, bilateral hyperplasia of the adrenals due to hypothalamic stimulation and pituitary "basophilism," or adrenal tumor.

In addition to the three principal primary sites of origin for the syndrome, there is a fourth unusual one. Two reports have appeared in the literature of Cushing's disease resulting from an adrenal rest tumor in the ovary (Kepler *et al.* and Rottino and McGrath). In this era of corticosteroid therapy for many diseases, the physician should also be alerted to the possibility of an iatrogenic factor in the production of a Cushing-like picture.

The subject of etiology has been extensively reviewed by Plotz, and according to autopsy findings in 97 cases, carcinoma of the adrenal occurred 16 times, adenoma 11 times, and benign hyperplasia 58 times. A pituitary adenoma was associated with adenomatous hyperplasia 40 times and with carcinoma and benign adrenal adenoma once. There were changes in the paraventricular nucleus in 8 instances, and these 8 instances were distributed evenly among the adrenal carcinomas, hyperplasias, and pituitary adenomas.

Cushing's syndrome is characterized by obesity, amenorrhea, moon face, hirsutism, hypertension, purple striae, erythemic acne, and easy bruisability. The pelvic organs are usually normal and there is no enlargement of the clitoris or marked vaginal atrophy. When the full-blown picture exists, the syndrome is so striking that the diagnosis is blatant; however, in the early stages it may be extremely difficult (Fig. 30.10). The laboratory findings are characterized by an elevation of the urinary and blood corticoids. The urinary 17-ketosteroid assay is usually normal or only moderately elevated; if an adrenal tumor is present it may be markedly elevated. There is polycythemia, diabetic glucose tolerance curve, and X-ray evidence of osteoporosis. The typical response to ACTH

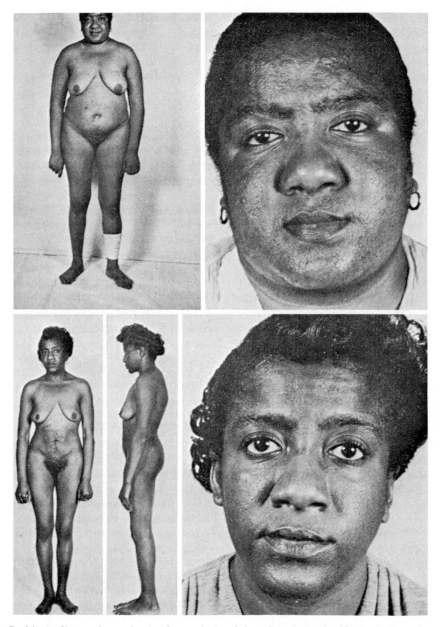

30.10. Cushing's disease due to benign hyperplasia of the adrenal glands. *Upper,* before adrenalectomy the characteristic obesity, moon face, and hirsutism can be seen. Although the purple abdominal striae are not apparent, the acniform rash can be seen on the chest. *Lower,* after operation the patient has regained her normal appearance. Some hirsutism persists. (From Jones, H. W., Jr., and Scott, W. W.: *Hermaphroditism, Genital Anomalies and Related Endocrine Disorders,* 2nd ed. The Williams & Wilkins Company, 1971.)

stimulation is an over-reaction with at least a three-fold increase of the urinary and blood corticoids. It is usually impossible to suppress the urinary corticoids below 10 mg./24 hours by cortisone. When an adrenal tumor is present there is usually no response to ACTH stimulation or cortisol suppression. Unfortunately, however, not all tumors are autonomous and some do show a response.

The treatment of the disease depends upon its etiology. Sosman recommends irradiation of the pituitary for those patients without adrenal tumors. Certainly this is the method of choice if a pituitary tumor can be demonstrated. However, most authorities have recommended adrenal extirpation for bilateral adrenal hyperplasia. The decision between pituitary irradiation and adrenalectomy is further complicated by the difficulty in excluding the possibility of an adrenal tumor. This may be attempted by perirenal carbon dioxide insufflation, by laminography, by simple intravenous pyelograms with attention to the adrenal shadow, or by adrenal angiogram. In our experience none of these is completely satisfactory.

It is often possible to decide at operation, by the appearance of one adrenal, whether or not there is a tumor in the other. If at operation the exposed gland is atrophied, it should be left in situ with a presumptive diagnosis of a contralateral tumor. If, however, the exposed adrenal is hypertrophied it is removed with all or 90% of the opposite gland. When the partial operation is performed there is always a possibility that a second operation will be necessary; however, this seems to be a worthwhile risk to take in an effort to prevent lifelong invalidism with dependence upon prolonged, expensive replacement therapy.

Stress Obesity. A borderline clinical picture with moderately elevated urinary corticoids occurs more frequently than true Cushing's disease. It is thought that this picture represents the response of certain individuals to the *"stress of obesity."* Experimental evidence indicates that Dilantin will inhibit the hypothalamic ACTH-RF and might therefore be of therapeutic value.

Adrenal Tumors. Tumors of the adrenal are usually characterized by marked hirsutism with some associated virilization, *e.g.,* enlargement of the clitoris, fat pad wasting, breast changes and loss of scalp hair. Voice changes are not frequently present. Amenorrhea is often an early symptom but occasionally patients menstruate fairly regularly and have even been known to ovulate and become pregnant. The laboratory diagnosis is made on the basis of an elevated 17-ketosteroid assay which does not suppress with dexamethasone. An elevation of dehydroisoandrosterone is the metabolic fingerprint of adrenal tumors and this assay should always be requested when a neoplasm is suspected. An intravenous pyelogram may show a depression of the renal outline and a suprarenal mass.

As adrenal tumors can be slow growing benign adenomas, the symptoms can be present for many years. As with all tumors, the symptoms are also variable. Depending upon the tumor site, one may have symptoms of an adrenogenital syndrome, Cushing's disease or simply amenorrhea with minor hirsutism.

The treatment is operative removal and the prognosis is guarded.

Nutritional Amenorrhea

The diet is one of the basic influences which determines how any endocrine gland, or indeed any substitution therapy, may act. Richter has ably demonstrated this clinical factor in a laboratory animal, by using self-selective diets in rats. Adrenalectomized, parathyroidectomized, and pancreatectomized animals can all adjust to their deficiencies if allowed a sufficient choice of diet.

In the human, the importance of malnutrition in reproductive function has been demonstrated. Disturbances of reproductive functions can be caused in animal experimentation by specific caloric deficiencies, protein deficiencies, or vitamin deficiencies with special reference to vitamins A, B, and C. Whether one or all of these factors operate in nutritional amenorrhea of the human is undetermined. There is a relatively large literature by European authors on the occurrence of nutritional amenorrhea during World Wars I and II but it is generally difficult for the authors to separate nutritional from psychogenic factors. Heynemann was of the opinion that nutrition played an important part in war amenorrhea, as he observed an increase in the incidence in Germany after 1944 when the deterioration of food supplies occurred. Plotz believed that the protein deficiency aspects were most important and reported that 17 of 19 women with nutritional amenorrhea of over one year's duration responded to an amino acid preparation. The first vaginal bleeding occurred after an average of 31 days of therapy and permanent success was achieved in almost every case.

It is the general opinion, quoted by Seitz, that nutritional amenorrhea is usually reversible; 80% of the patients reviewed recovered with improved nutrition. However, the prognosis is graver when the nutritional damage occurs at or just before puberty. This is in keeping with the experience in animal experimentation, reviewed by Asdell, which indicates that the younger the animal when nutritional damage occurs the more difficult it is to repair. There is also some evidence that residual damage may result; Klebarow reports a 75% incidence of infertility among concentration camp victims of World War II who suffered severe malnutrition, in contrast to a 25% incidence of infertility in the general population. He further states that this may be attributable to damage of the germinal cells, as impaired spermatogenesis, under similar circumstances, was found among males. Stafko, in an examination of ovaries of 120 women who died of starvation, found an absence of primordial follicles and replacement of the cortical layer with scar tissue indicating that the amenorrhea might be primarily due to ovarian damage. The occurrence of amenorrhea in patients with exogenous obesity is somewhat more difficult to explain. The most obvious explanation is that it is secondary to the psychic stress which is the initial cause of the obesity. An alternative explanation is that a relative dietary imbalance has occurred associated with the abnormal caloric intake.

The treatment of both malnutrition and obesity is directed toward general dietary habits—either weight gain or weight reduction, with a well balanced high protein diet (Fig. 30.11).

Disturbances of Steroid Excretion and Metabolism

Chronic Nephritis

As both ovarian steroids and pituitary protein hormones are at least partially excreted through the urinary tract, it is not surprising that patients with chronic nephritis frequently show abnormalities of the menstrual cycle usually characterized by amenorrhea. Goodwin et al. in 1968 studied the effects of uremia and chronic hemodialysis on the menstrual cycle. These investigators found that the menstrual irregularities correlated well with the degree of renal failure and that the irregularities began when the uremic symptoms were first detectable, e.g., when the endogenous creatinine clearance fell to between 10 and 15 ml. per minute. When this level reached 4 or below, amenorrhea ensued. The findings suggest that the amenorrhea may in fact be due to a central disturbance rather than one of steroid clearance.

Liver Cirrhosis

The conjugation and metabolism of estrogens and progesterone take place in the liver; the excretion is accomplished to a large extent through the bile and hepatic portal system to the bowel. In cirrhosis of the liver, impairment of conjugation of estrogen leads to excess circulating active estrogens. This may result in dysfunctional bleeding interspersed with periods of amenorrhea. Although this is certainly the most common menstrual cycle aberration associated with cirrhosis, Green and Rubin report 18 patients having amenorrhea as the menstrual symptom. The diagnosis is made on the basis of the physical findings and liver function tests.

The treatment is medical and the prognosis is poor.

LESIONS OF PERIPHERAL ORIGIN

Ovarian

Ovarian causes for amenorrhea can be classified as follows.

(1) *Ovarian insufficiency*: (a) conge-

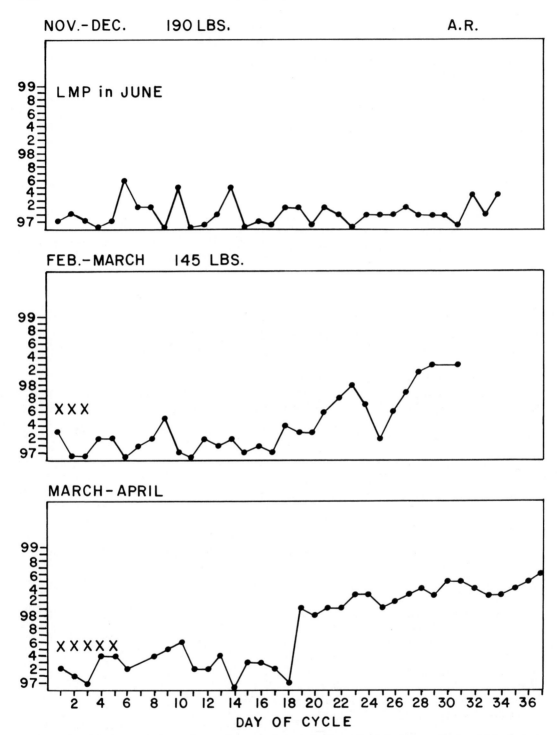

30.11. Basal body temperature charts of amenorrheic, infertile, patient during months in which she lost from 190 to 145 lbs. At this weight she had a recurrence of menses, and ovulated (Feb.-Mar.). She became pregnant in the following cycle (Mar.-Apr.) as indicated by the continuous temperature elevation.

nital defects, gonadal dysgenesis, and related conditions; (b) the premature menopause, congenital and acquired; (c) the insensitive ovary syndrome.

(2) *Ovarian tumors*: (a) arrhenoblastoma, hilus cell tumor, and adrenal rest tumor; (b) theca granulosa cell tumors; (c) dysgerminoma; (d) nonspecific tumors with steroidogenic stromas.

All types of ovarian insufficiency are characterized by elevated pituitary gonadotrophins.

Congenitally Defective Gonads

Gonadal Agenesis (Turner's Syndrome). In 1938 Turner described a syndrome of "infantilism," congenital webbed neck, and cubitus valgus. Albright, Smith, and Fraser, in 1942, demonstrated the association of this syndrome with an elevated urinary gonadotrophin titer, and Wilkins and Fleischmann in 1944 described the pathological condition, which was characterized by absence of gonads and the presence of normally developed but immature Müllerian ducts. The gonads are represented grossly by a primitive streak, white or yellow, and microscopically by stroma only or by stroma and Leydig cells. In 1954, a number of investigators independently reported that a majority of these patients had a negative or male type chromatin pattern, and in 1959 Ford and Jones reported that at least some of these patients with negative chromatin patterns represented not an XY but an XO configuration of sex chromosomes. These contributions provided the building stones for a satisfactory explanation of the syndrome. Those patients who show a 45, X chromosomal configuration can be explained on the basis of nondisjunction of the sex chromosomes. Patients who have a normal XX chromosome pattern, pure gonadal dysgenesis, are usually of normal height and may represent the result of embryonic gonadal damage prior to the eighth week of development.

Every stage of developmental anomaly can be seen in patients with an XY pattern or a Y fragment or translocation—from gonads with a few Leydig cells associated with female genitalia and

hypertrophy of the clitoris only (first described by Pich in 1937), to almost normal testicular development and male external genitalia except for hypospadias. For a complete summary of this abnormal development, see the text by Jones and Scott.

The clinical features of a typical Turner's syndrome are so characteristic that one can recognize such a patient as she walks into the consultation room. There is shortness of stature, webbing of the neck, deformity of the carrying angle, a shield type chest with nipples placed far laterally, no breast development, and scanty or absent axillary and pubic hair. Two other associated congenital defects have been described which are serious health hazards and should therefore always be checked—coarctation of the aorta and absence of one kidney. From the typical picture of Turner's syndrome and dwarf stature there are all gradations through the normal stature with eunuchoid proportions (Fig. 30.12).

The laboratory findings are characteristic in that there must be elevated gonadotrophin assays, and most of the patients exhibit an abnormal chromatin pattern; the buccal smear, therefore, is often the most rapid and least expensive way to make a diagnosis. Thyroid studies are normal. The urinary 17-ketosteroid excretion is normal or low.

Until such a time when transplantation of ovaries is feasible, the treatment of this condition will remain as substitution therapy only. Estrogen is given in interrupted dosage, depending upon the amount of drug necessary to induce vaginal bleeding: 0.5 to 2 mg. of stilbestrol, or its equivalent, daily through the 25th day of each month with a progestational drug associated during the last week for its antimitotic action. Therapy is then discontinued and resumed the first day of the following month. An endometrial biopsy should be obtained periodically to ensure that there is a normal growth pattern, for endometrial cancer has been reported after long-term estrogen therapy. Operation is only advised when the karyotype shows a

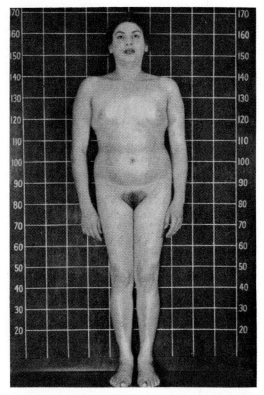

30.12. Gonadal dysgenesis with normal height. Notice typical shield chest with nipples placed far laterally. Buccal smear showed a negative chromatin pattern and the gonadotrophin hormone (FSH) level was elevated.

Y chromosome. Under these conditions removal of the gonads is indicated to prevent tumor formation according to the findings of Teter and Boczkowski.

In cases of dwarfism, if the patient is pubertal and epiphyseal fusion has not occurred, smaller dosages of estrogen over longer periods of time should be tried in an effort to induce a maximal growth spurt prior to epiphyseal closure which will occur with estrogen stimulation. Whitelaw *et al.* report a growth of 9.5 cm. in a year in a patient treated with an anabolic steroid and suggest that this form of therapy should be given until epiphysial closure or failed response occurs. They advise liver function tests and observation for androgenicity.

Therapy may be expected to induce normal breast development, vaginal cornification, and menstruation. The induction of menstruation is usually desirable for psychological reasons. Pregnancy, of course, cannot be expected to occur, and axillary and pubic hair will usually remain scanty or absent unless an androgenic stimulus is supplied. If coarctation of the aorta is present, surgical correction wherever possible should be advised, and if webbing of the neck is deforming, plastic surgery can offer excellent cosmetic results. It is well to have a psychological evaluation, and therapeutic consultations if necessary, to insure that the patient is adjusted to her limitations and will thus be able to live a completely normal life except for ability to bear children.

True Hermaphroditism. True hermaphroditism is extremely rare. A summary of the 82 cases reported in the literature up to 1971 can be found in the textbook on this subject by Jones and Scott. Most true hermaphrodites are raised as men and this was the case in 52 of the 70 patients followed. This indicates, of course, that in a majority of instances the external genitalia are masculine rather than feminine in appearance. The condition should be suspected in patients who show some ambiguity of the external genitalia, associated with breast development. Minimal hirsutism may occur but has been absent in the majority of the reported cases.

These cases are interesting from the point of view of experimental embryology, as they indicate that the male gonad exerts a strong influence on the development of external genitalia. Thus, even in the 16 patients in the literature who showed an ovary on one side and an ovotestis on the other, only eight had been raised as females. The Müllerian duct must be more positively influenced by the ovarian organizer, because a normal uterus was present in about half of the patients. Almost all of these individuals menstruated; thus, in contrast to gonadal dysgenesis, the ovarian tissue present in true hermaphrodites is functioning.

The diagnosis can be suspected by the physical findings, and the laboratory data are of very little assistance. The chromatin pattern can be positive or negative and the 17-ketosteroid and gonadotrophin assays are within normal range. The diagnosis therefore is made by the pathologist at the time of operation, and the treatment is surgical correction.

Male Hermaphroditism. Male hermaphrodites show ambiguous external genitalia, no breast development, minimal hirsutism, and a negative chromatin pattern. This condition has been discussed in Chapter 8 in detail.

Testicular Feminization: Androgen Insensitivity. This interesting form of hermaphroditism is characterized by a normal female appearance with excellent breast development and completely normal female external genitalia. However, in about a third of the cases there is either no axillary or pubic hair, or the axillary and pubic hair is extremely scanty. There is a short or absent vagina and no cervix. The differential diagnosis must be made between this condition and that of congenital absence of the Müllerian ducts. At laparotomy relatively normal testes are present and no uterus. A negative chromatin pattern is confirmatory of a diagnosis of testicular feminization and the karyotype is a normal 46,XY male pattern.

The laboratory findings are bizarre and can vary widely. Some patients show elevated urinary gonadotrophins. Others show urinary gonadotrophins in the normal range. Most patients have a 17-ketosteroid excretion compatible with a normal male, and estrogen excretion compatible with a normal female. Morris has reported a comprehensive survey of his experience with this condition. The findings in the testis have been described in detail in Chapter 8. The assumption is that this is a heritable developmental defect of the testosterone target organs which lack the protein androgen receptor, causing insensitivity to androgen stimulation.

The treatment is operative removal of the testes after the age of puberty because of the predilection to tumor formation, and vaginal plastic procedure if indicated.

Estrogen substitution therapy is usually advisable.

Premature Menopause

Premature menopause is caused by disappearance of oocytes from the ovary, depriving the organ of the stimulus for follicle formation. The etiology can be congenital or acquired. Any germ cell toxin can produce this end result. The insult to germ plasm can occur at any age from the earliest embryo through adulthood. Some factors which interfere with oogenesis or cause damage are known. Anomalies of the X chromosomes make the meiotic division of the germ cell impossible. These defects cause disappearance of germ cells at about the fourth month of life, and are discussed under Gonadal Dysgenesis or Turner's Syndrome in Chapter 8. Cytotoxins such as Busulfan and methotrexate, and irradiation specifically damage germ cells. Nonspecific destruction of ovarian tissue may occur with abscess formation by the tuberculosis bacillus and certain rare tropical diseases, surgical removal of ovarian tissue, or destruction by interruption of the normal blood supply, and, finally, the unusual occurrence of autoimmune disease as described by Irvine *et al.* may all be causes of the premature menopause.

The diagnosis can be suspected when the patient gives a history of hot flushes. As there is a heritable tendency for this anomaly in certain families, a good history of the menopausal ages of all members is important. The laboratory findings of elevated gonadotrophins is the absolute diagnostic criterion. There is no cure for premature menopause and therapy must be substitional only. This is discussed in Chapter 32.

The Insensitive Ovary Syndrome

This very unusual condition is characterized by primary amenorrhea, well developed breasts, axillary and pubic hair, but atrophic vaginal and endometrial mucosa. The serum and urinary gonadotrophins, FSH and LH, are elevated and the estrogens are low. The

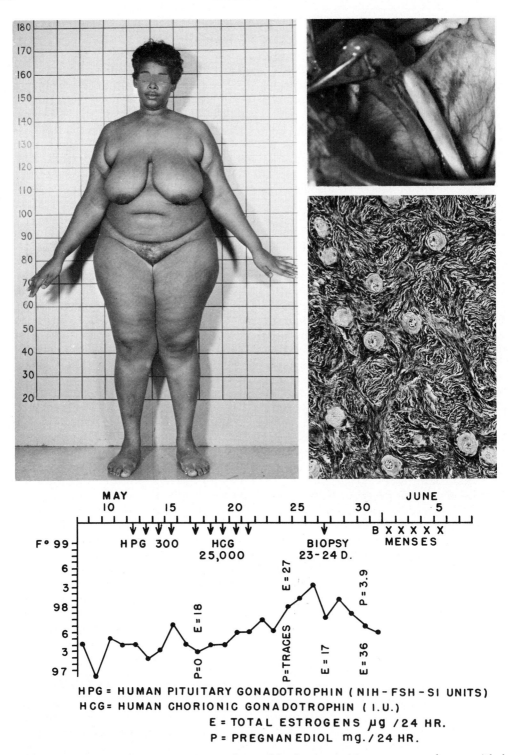

30.13. The clinical appearance of a patient with the insensitive ovary syndrome with hypergonadotrophinuria. Note well developed sexual characteristics and slightly eunuchoid stature. The gross appearance of the ovary, in the upper right, is abnormal and resembles a structure between a prepubertal

ovary grossly resembles a prepubertal organ and microscopically shows numerous primordial follicles but none developed past the antrum stage (Fig. 30.13). Ovulation can occasionally be induced by excessive amounts of exogenous gonadotrophins (3 to 10 times the dosage used for hypophysectomized patients). It is assumed that this syndrome may be due to lack of FSH receptor sites in the ovary.

Ovarian Tumors

Amenorrhea related to ovarian tumors has been discussed in Chapter 24.

End Organ: Uterine and Vaginal Cryptomenorrhea

The conditions embraced under this heading are: traumatic occlusion of the vagina; the imperforate hymen; congenital absence or atresia of the vagina; vaginal septa; congenital absence of the Müllerian ducts; traumatic occlusion of the cervix; and destruction of the endometrium.

Occlusion of the Vagina and Cervix

The term *gynatresia* is applied to occlusion of any part of the genital canal. It may be of congenital or acquired origin.

Causes. The congenital causes embrace any of the forms of congenital occlusion which have been discussed in Chapter 8, "Congenital Anomalies and Hermaphroditism." The most important is imperforate hymen, although occasionally the congenital block involves the cervical or vaginal segment of the canal.

Symptoms. When atresia of the cervix or any part of the vagina is present, or when the hymen is imperforate, the menstrual discharge, if it occurs, is retained behind the obstruction. Of these causes, imperforate hymen is much the most common. The retained blood distends the vagina (*hematocolpos*) whereas with succeeding periods there is distention

of the cervix (*hematotrachelos*), uterine cavity (*hematometra*), and finally even of the tubes (*hematosalpinx*).

With each succeeding period there is increasing pain and discomfort. When the uterine distention becomes marked, a bulging enlargement of the lower abdomen develops, and the patient's discomfort may be extreme, especially at the time of the periods. Difficulty in voiding is a common symptom.

Diagnosis. The diagnosis in such cases is usually easy, especially in the case of imperforate hymen. The distended hymen actually bulges forward from the pressure of the retained blood (see Plates 7.1 and 7.2), and fluctuation can be felt both through the hymen and on rectal examination. In the less frequent cases in which the obstruction is higher up, the diagnosis is not always so obvious, but a history of regularly recurring menstrual molimina, with increasing menstrual discomfort without external menstrual flow, together with the finding of a fluctuating mass on bimanual abdominorectal palpation, will leave little doubt as to the nature of the condition.

Treatment. The treatment in the case of imperforate hymen is simple, consisting simply in slow evacuation of the blood through a cruciate incision in the hymen. Strict asepsis must of course be observed, and most writers, whether justifiably or not, warn of the especial proneness of such patients to infection. After evacuation of the blood, the hymen may be excised, or, as some prefer, gently but widely divulsed, to avoid agglutination and secondary closure.

In the case of obstruction higher up, the problem is not so simple. If the lower vagina is involved, and the septum thin, somewhat the same plan may be followed as with imperforate hymen. But if the obstruction is higher and the intervening mass of tissue thick, much care is necessary in evacuating the blood, and the

ovary and a well developed gonadal streak. The microscopic appearance of the ovary is characterized by numerous primordial follicles, but none beyond the antrum stage. The ovulatory response to exogenous gonadotrophins, as evidenced by biphasic temperature and secretory endometrium, is obtained only when 10 times the usual dosage is given.

later treatment may involve some form of plastic operation for what is essentially absence of the vagina.

Acquired Gynatresia

Gynatresia is by no means always due to congenital factors, and as a matter of fact the acquired variety is more frequent. The portions of the genital canal which by their occlusion may cause retention of the genital discharge are the cervix and the vagina. Especially frequent is the cervix, the canal of which is normally much the narrowest portion of the uterovaginal tract.

Causes. The most important causes of acquired gynatresia are the following.

Senile Contraction. Although atrophy of the genital canal, including its mucosa, occurs normally after the menopause, it may in some women be so extreme as to cause blockage of the cervix and occasionally of the vagina. This is especially true because of the susceptibility of the thin, senile mucous membrane to secondary infection and ulceration. As a result of complete occlusion of the cervical canal in the woman who is no longer menstruating, the retained discharge consists of pus rather than blood, although there may be a bloody admixture because of the presence of granulation tissue in the wall of the retention cavity. Such retention of pus in the uterine cavity is called *pyometra.* It is very gradual in development, with often no symptoms for many months. Attention is called to the condition in many cases by the seepage of slight amounts of blood from the granulation tissue in the cervical canal, whereas in other cases there may be pelvic discomfort or even the development of a mass.

Malignant Disease. One of the most common of all causes of gynatresia is malignant disease, usually of the cervix. Either epidermoid or adenocarcinoma may be responsible, and in most cases there has been an antecedent history of bleeding from the cancer. A not uncommon occurrence, especially in older women, is to encounter the pyometra in the course of diagnostic curettage performed because of postmenopausal bleeding. In other cases, the pyometra develops in the late stages of carcinoma whose existence has long been known.

Radiotherapy and Cauterization. As a result of the radiotherapy universally employed for carcinoma of the cervix, stricture or complete atresia of the cervical canal may occur, with pyometra as the result. Such postradiation strictures might not develop until a long time, even several years, after the application of radium. The widely prevalent and sometimes injudicious or improper use of the cautery in the treatment of cervicitis has left in its wake a definite incidence of strictures of the cervix and even complete atresia of the canal. The same result may follow the use of chemical caustics, such as strong solutions of nitrate of silver, within the cervix.

Surgical Operations. An occasional result of operations upon the cervix is the occurrence of stricture or atresia. This may follow even simple dilatation when associated with laceration of the tissue, but is more likely to occur after cervical cauterization, conization, or such plastic operations as the Sturmdorf tracheloplasty or cervical amputation.

Symptoms. When a previously normal woman ceases to menstruate, but suffers severe colicky pain at the time of the expected period, the possibility of gynatresia should be suspected, especially if there is a history of one of the causative factors enumerated above. The pain recurs at each menstrual date, and pelvic examination will usually, within a month or two, reveal evidence of distention of the uterus if, as is most common, the obstruction is in the cervix. The latter becomes large and broad, and develops a peculiar elastic feel, with sometimes distinct fluctuation. Later the body of the uterus likewise becomes large and fluctuant.

When the gynatresia occurs in postmenopausal women, its development is much more insidious and its recognition more difficult, because the retained genital secretion is far less in amount than the normal menstrual flow. In a large proportion of cases pyometra is found accidentally, as already mentioned. The retained secretion commonly undergoes secondary infection, and there may be fever or chills, in addition to increasing pelvic discomfort and slight bleeding.

Diagnosis. When such symptoms as have been described lead to the suspicion of cervical occlusion, the diagnosis can be made reasonably certain by direct exploration of the cervical canal by the uterine sound, always under strict aseptic precautions. When the occlusion is light, the probe itself may be followed by a telltale trickle of blood or pus. When the blockage is tight even a very fine probe will fail to enter the uterus. In such cases, the diagnosis can be made by passing a large caliber aspirating needle through the cervical wall into the distended cavity.

Treatment. The treatment of the common forms of acquired gynatresia consists of dilatation followed by drainage. The dilatation may be a comparatively simple office procedure, although it must be repeated from time to time, as most strictures of the cervix have a tendency to contract down. Small olive-pointed metal dilators are ordinarily most useful.

Congenital Absence of the Müllerian Ducts

This condition is characterized by a normal development and normal endocrine findings, with absence of the uterus and upper two thirds of the vagina. As mentioned previously, it must be differentiated from testicular feminization and this can be done by the buccal smear, which shows a female percentage of cells with positive Barr bodies. Once the diagnosis is made it must be determined as accurately as possible whether there is absence of the uterus as well as a congenital absence of the upper two thirds of the vagina. In rare instances, there is simply a vaginal constriction band and a normal uterus is present above. In this case, of course, a surgical procedure will assure normal reproductive function, whereas, if the uterus is absent, the only procedure required is either a vaginal plastic operation or the use of a Frank tube to produce a vagina by pressure, as described in 1928.

Destruction of the Endometrium and Traumatic Strictures of the Cervix

This condition has been classically described by Asherman. Although usually associated with secondary amenorrhea, the condition can, very occasionally, be the cause of primary amenorrhea, as when pelvic tuberculosis has involved the endometrium extensively prepubertally. Aside from tuberculosis, cervical stenosis and endometrial sclerosis are almost always secondary to a dilatation and curettage or some other intracervical or intrauterine procedure which has been unduly traumatic or associated with an inflammatory process. A postpartum or postabortion curettage classically predisposes to this type of scarring.

Diagnosis of amenorrhea associated with destructive or congenital lesions of the end organs is made on the basis of an examination and curettage which demonstrate a vaginal or cervical obstruction or scarring of the endometrium. The basal temperature chart indicates ovulation in the absence of menstruation, and after the administration of adequate amounts of estrogen withdrawal fails to induce menstruation. Although frequently advocated as a diagnostic aid in this condition, the hysterogram is usually unsatisfactory.

The treatment of the condition is repeated dilatation of the cervix and curettage. Although this seems paradoxical, the therapeutic effect is probably due to the "freshening up" of the scar tissue, allowing the remains of the basalis layer of the endometrium to regrow. Various operative procedures, originating with that of Strassman, have been advocated for the correction of the condition. These differ mainly only in the use of different materials to substitute for the endometrial lining. Comninos and Zourlas have described the use of a Foley catheter placed in the uterine cavity and gradually inflated with 20 ml of sterile saline. The success obtained with any of these procedures can probably be attributed to the regenerative powers of the endometrium when the cervix is patent.

PHYSIOLOGICAL AMENORRHEA

Physiological types of amenorrhea need only be mentioned briefly as associated with puberty, pregnancy, lactation and the menopause.

Delayed Puberty

The diagnosis of delayed puberty might be best included under lesions of the nervous system, as it is now our concept that puberty is initiated by maturation of the hypothalamus rather than of the pituitary.

Statistically speaking, the diagnosis cannot be made until after the age of 17 years, although any delay of menstruation after 14 years is considered delayed over the average age. The diagnosis is made when the history, physical findings, and laboratory data are all within normal limits, and it is facilitated if there is a family history of delayed menarche. An LRH stimulation characteristically shows a greater FSH than LH response. If in addition one is able to demonstrate an increase in serum LH with sleep, the diagnosis is further substantiated. The causes are numerous, the most important being poor general health, nutrition, or hygiene.

A careful follow-up examination should be made yearly until one is sure that the correct diagnosis has been established. There were three patients among our group with this diagnosis and all three are menstruating regularly at the present time.

Pregnancy and Postpartum Amenorrhea

Any patient presenting with amenorrhea is presumed to be pregnant until proved otherwise. If the physical examination is equivocal, a pregnancy test can be performed to exclude the diagnosis. Postpartum amenorrhea is usual, especially if the patient nurses her baby. The normal duration of this amenorrhea is between six weeks and three months if the patient does not lactate. If the patient has nursed, menses usually return within six months of delivery, or six weeks after cessation of lactation; any period of amenorrhea longer than this can be considered as prolonged, lactation amenorrhea. A differential diagnosis must be made between this physiological condition and true Sheehan's disease, pituitary necrosis caused by the destruction of the gland at the time of the traumatic delivery. If there is a history of a postpartum dilatation and curettage, the possibility of endometrial sclerosis must also be entertained. The diagnosis of postpartum amenorrhea is made on the basis of a history of an uncomplicated delivery and normal laboratory findings. However, this differential diagnosis is not to be made didactically for, if destruction of the pituitary (Sheehan's disease) has not been complete, the findings may be identical with those of postpartum lactation amenorrhea. The Chiari-Frommel syndrome is another variant which is associated with elevated prolactin values.

Time will usually suffice to cure the condition, but cyclic steroid therapy will often suppress the pituitary prolactin and predispose to a more rapid resumption of regular menses. The use of clomiphene citrate in resistant cases is indicated. Ergocryptine has been found to interrupt the production or release of prolactin and thereby facilitate the return of normal FSH and LH values, ovulation and menses.

SUMMARY

In summary, amenorrhea and oligomenorrhea must always be regarded as symptoms, not diseases. The decision as to whether or not these symptoms require investigation or treatment must be made on the basis of the individual case. Investigation is usually indicated if infertility is a complaint, if the patient is anxious or disturbed about the absence of menstruation, or if there are associated signs and symptoms suggestive of a serious physical problem. When primary amenorrhea exists it is always important to determine if an anatomical abnormality of the genitalia exists. No intelligent approach can be made to treatment until a proper etiological diagnosis has been attained. With the addition of human pituitary gonadotrophins and clomiphene to our therapeutic armamentaria, the results of therapy are more encouraging. Although LRH has not yet been developed as a therapeutic tool, it shows great promise. The other therapeutic advances are ergocryptine for the treatment of the galactorrhea-amenorrhea syndrome with elevated prolactin, and the development of microsurgery for pituitary tumors.

REFERENCES

Ahumada, J. C., and Del Castillo, E. B.: Amenorrea y galactorrea. Bol. Soc. Obstit. Ginec., *11:* 64, 1932.

Albright, F., Smith, P. H., and Fraser, R.: A syndrome characterized by primary ovarian insufficiency and decreased stature; report of 11 cases with digression on hormonal control of axillary and pubic hair. Amer. J. Med. Sci., *204:* 625, 1942.

Allen, W. M., and Woolf, R. B.: Medullary resection of the ovaries in the Stein-Leventhal syndrome. Amer. J. Obstet. Gynec., *77:* 826, 1959.

Amoss, M. S., Monahan, M. W., and Verlander, M. S.: A long-acting polymer-coupled LRF analog. J. Clin. Endocr. Metabl., *39:* 203, 1974.

Asdell, S. A.: Reproduction. Ann. Rev. Physiol., *12:* 537, 1950.

Asherman, J. G.: Traumatic intra-uterine adhesions. J. Obstet. Gynaec. Brit. Comm., *57:* 892, 1950.

Barraclough, C. A.: Production of anovulatory, sterile rats by single injections of testosterone proprionate. Endocrinology, *68:* 62, 1961.

Bass, F.: L'amenorrhée au camp de concentration de Terezin (Theresienstadt). Gynaecologia (Basel), *123:* 211, 1947.

Bergman, P.: Clinical treatment of anovulation. Int. J. Fertil., *3:* 27, 1958.

Biglieri, E. G., Herron, A. M., and Brust, N.: 17-Hydroxylation deficiency in man. J. Clin. Invest., *45:* 1946, 1966.

Black, T., Cox, R. I., and Cox, L. W.: Ovulation induction for the treatment of infertility. Aust. New Zeal. J. Obstet. Gynec., *9:* 209, 1969.

Blackman, S.: Concerning the function and origin of a reticular zone of the adrenal cortex; hyperplasia in the adrenogenital syndrome. Bull. Hopkins Hosp., *78:* 180, 1946.

Bliss, E. L., and Migeon, C. J.: Endocrinology of anorexia nervosa. J. Clin. Endocr., *17:* 766, 1957.

Bricaire, H., Moreau, L., Elissade, B., and Bouvier, J. M.: Amenorrhoea and galactorrhoea syndrome in connection with a non-malignant chromophilic tumor of the hypophysis. Ann. Endocr. (Paris), *19:* 719, 1958.

Brown, J. B., Evans, J. H., Adey, F. D., Taft, H. P., and Townsend, L.: Factors involved in the induction of fertile ovulation in the human gonadotrophins. J. Obstet. Gynaec. Brit. Comm., *76:* 289, 1969.

Bush, I. E., and Mahesh, V. B.: Adrenocortical hyperfunction with sudden onset of hirsuitism. J. Endocr., *18:* 1, 1959.

Comninos, A., and Zourlas, P.: Treatment of uterine adhesions (Asherman's syndrome). Am. J. Obstet. Gynec., *105:* 862, 1969.

Crooke, A. C., Butt, W. R., Palmer, R., Morris, R., Edwards, R. L., Gaylor, G. W., and Short, R. B.: The effect of human pituitary follicle-stimulating hormone

and chorionic gonadotrophin in Stein-Leventhal syndrome. Brit. Med. J., *1:* 1119, 1963.

Cushing, H.: The basophil adenomas of the pituitary body and their clinical manifestations (pituitary basophilism). Bull Hopkins Hosp., *50:* 137, 1932.

Dally, P. I., and Sargent, W.: A new treatment for anorexia nervosa. Brit. Med. J., *1:* 1770, 1960.

Decourt, J., and Michard, J.: Les amenorrhees psychogenes. Sem. Hôp. Paris, *25:* 3352, 1949.

Drill, V. A., and Pfeiffer, C. A.: Effect of vitamin B-complex deficiency, controlled inanition and methionine on inactivation of estrogen by the liver. Endocrinology, *38:* 300, 1946.

Emanuel, R. W.: Endocrine findings in anorexia nervosa. J. Clin. Endocr., *16:* 801, 1956.

Everson, C., Williams, E., Wheeler, E., Swenson, P., Spivey, M., and Eppright, M.: The occurrence of five B-vitamins in the tissues of pregnant rats fed rations satisfactory and unsatisfactory for reproduction. J. Nutr., *36:* 463, 1948.

Forbes, A. P., Henneman, P. H., Griswold, G. C., and Albright, F.: Syndrome characterized by galactorrhea, amenorrhea and low urinary FSH; comparison with acromegaly and normal lactation. J. Clin. Endocr., *14:* 265, 1954.

Ford, C. E., and Jones, K. W.: Sex chromosome anomaly in a case of gonadal dysgenesis (Turner's syndrome). Lancet, *1:* 711, 1959.

Furuhjelm, M., and Carlstrom, K.: Amenorrhea following oral contraceptives. Acta Obstet. Gynec. Scand., *52:* 373, 1973.

Gitlow, S., and Kurschner, D. M.: Estrogen, diabetes and menopause. Arch. Intern. Med. (Chicago), *72:* 250, 1943.

Glass, B.: Hazards of atomic radiation to man; British and American report. J. Hered., *47:* 260, 1956.

Goodwin, N. J., Valenti, C., Hall, J. E., and Friedman, E. A.: Effects of uremia and chronic hemodialysis on the reproductive cycle. Am. J. Obstet. Gynec., *100:* 528, 1968.

Green, P., and Rubin, L.: Amenorrhea as a manifestation of chronic liver disease. Amer. J. Obstet. Gynec., *78:* 141, 1959.

Greene, O., Migeon, C., and Wilkins, L.: Urinary steroids in the hypertensive form of congenital adrenal hyperplasia. J. Clin. Endocr., *20:* 929, 1960.

Guinet, P., and Mornex, R.: L'eunuchisme hypogonadotrophique chez la femme. Rev. Lyon. Med., *6:* 39, 1957.

Halmi, K., Brodland, G., and Loney, J.: Prognosis in anorexia nervosa. Ann. Int. Med., *78:* 907, 1973.

Heinbecker, P.: Pathogenesis of Cushing's syndrome. Medicine, *23:* 225, 1944.

Heynemann, T.: Die Nachkriegsamenorrhoe. Klin. Wschr., *26:* 129, 1948.

Igarashi, M., and Matsumoto, S.: Induction of human ovulation by individualized gonadotrophin therapy. Amer. J. Obstet. Gynec., *73:* 1294, 1957.

Ingersoll, F. M., and McArthur, J. W.: Longitudinal studies of gonadotrophin excretion in Stein-Leventhal syndrome. Amer. J. Obstet. Gynec., *77:* 801, 1959.

Irvine, W. J., Chan, M. M. W., Scarth, L., Kolb, F. O., Hartog, M., Bayliss, R. I. S., and Dury, M. I.: Immunological aspects of premature ovarian failure associated with idiopathic Addison's disease. Lancet, *2:* 883, 1968.

Israel, S. L.: Empiric usage of low-dosage irradiation in amenorrhea. Amer. J. Obstet. Gynec., *64:* 971, 1952.

Israel, S. L., and Constan, A. S.: Unrecognized pituitary necrosis (Sheehan's syndrome); a cause of sudden death. J. A. M. A., *148:* 189, 1952.

Jones, G. S., and Ruehsen, M. de M.: A new syndrome of amenorrhea in association with hypergonadotropism and apparently normal ovarian follicular apparatus. Amer. J. Obst. Gynec., *104:* 597, 1969.

Jones, H. W., Jr., and Jones, G. E. S.: Gynecological aspects of adrenal hyperplasia and allied disorders. Amer. J. Obstet. Gynec., *68:* 1330, 1954.

Jones, H. W., Jr., and Scott, W. W.: *Hermaphroditism, Genital Anomalies and Related Endocrine Disorders,* 2nd ed. The Williams & Wilkins Company, Baltimore, 1971.

Jost, A.: Hormonal factors in the development of the fetus. Cold Spring Harbor Symposia Quant. Biol., *19:* 167, 1954.

Jungck, E. C., and Brown, W. E.: Human pituitary gonadotrophin for clinical use; preparation and lack of antihormone formation. Fertil. Steril., *3:* 224, 1952.

Kaeser, O.: Zur Aetiologie der primaren Amenorrhoe, Gynaecologia, *127:* 220, 1949.

Keettel, W. C., Bradbury, J. T., and Stoddard, F. J.: Observations on the polycystic ovary syndrome. Amer. J. Obstet. Gynec., *73:* 954, 1957.

Keller, P.: Treatment of anovulation with synthetic luteinizing hormone releasing hormone. Amer. J. Obstet. Gynec., *116:* 698, 1973.

Kepler, E. J., Dockerty, M. V., and Priestley, J. T.: Adrenal-like ovarian tumor associated with Cushing's syndrome (so-called masculinovoblastoma, luteoma, hypernephroma, adrenal cortical carcinoma of the ovary). Amer. J. Obstet. Gynec., *47:* 43, 1944.

Kinnunen, O., and Kaupinen, M.: The effect of brain injury on the menstrual cycle. Acta Endocr. (Kobenhavn), *6:* 183, 1951.

Klebarow, D.: Fertilitatsstorungen als spatfolge chronischen hungers und schwerer seelischer Traumen. Geburtsh. Frauenheilk., *9:* 420, 1949.

Kroger, W. S., and Freed, S. C.: Psychosomatic aspects of sterility. Amer. J. Obstet. Gynec., *59:* 867, 1950.

Liepelt, A.: Die Auswirkungen der Elektroshockbehandlung auf den Menstrationszyklus bei psychiatrischen Erkrenkungen. Z. Geburtsh. Gynaek., *132:* 65, 1950.

Loeser, A. A.: Effect of emotional shock on hormone release and endometrial development. Lancet, *1:* 518, 1943.

Mattingly, D., Mills, I. H., and Prunty, F. T. G.: Postpubertal adrenal virilism with biochemical disturbances of the congenital type of adrenal hyperplasia. Brit. Med. J., *1:* 1294, 1960.

McGarrigle, H. H. G., Radwanska, E., Little, V., and Swyer, G. I. M.: Plasma estradiol and progesterone estimations in the monitoring of the induction of ovulation by HMG and HCG. Proc. Soc. Endocr. (XXXI), J. Endocr., *63:* 1974.

Morris, J. M., and Mahesh, V. B.: Further observations on the syndrome "testicular feminization." Amer. J. Obstet. Gynec., *87:* 731, 1963.

Murdoch, R., and Govan, A. D. T.: Therapeutic effect of subsequent pregnancy in Simmonds' disease. J. Obstet. Gynaec. Brit. Comm., *58:* 18, 1951.

Mussey, R. D., and Haines, S. F.: Amenorrhea and oligomenorrhea associated with low basal metabolic rates. Amer. J. Obstet. Gynec., *27:* 404, 1934.

Nassar, G., Greenwood, M., Djanian, A., and Shanklin, W.: The etiological significance of ergot in the incidence of postpartum necrosis of the anterior pituitary; a preliminary report. Amer. J. Obstet. Gynec., *60:* 140, 1950.

Novak, E., and Hurd, G. B.: Use of anterior pituitary luteinizing substance in treatment of functional uterine bleeding. Amer. J. Obstet. Gynec., *22:* 501, 1931.

Parlow, A. F., and Shome, B.: Specific, homologous radioimmunoassay (RIA) of hight purified subunits of human pituitary follicle stimulating hormone (h FSH). J. Clin. Endocr. Metab., *39:* 195, 1974.

Pich, G.: Über den angeborenen Eierstockmangel. Beitr. Path. Anat., *98:* 218, 1937.

Plotz, C., Knowlton, A., and Ragan, C.: Natural history of Cushing's syndrome. Amer. J. Med., *13:* 597, 1952.

Plotz, J.: Die Bedeutung der Aminosauren fur die Ebstehung und Behandlung der Nechkriegsamenorrhoe. Z. Geburtsh. Gynaek., *132:* 13, 1950.

del Pozo, E., Varga, L., Wyss, H., Folis, G., Friesen, H., Wenner, R., Vetter, L., and Uelfwiler, A.: Clinical and hormonal response to bromoscriptin (CB-154) in the galactorrhea syndromes. J. Clin. Endocr. Metab., *39:* 18, 1974.

Randall, L. M., and McElin, T. W.: *Amenorrhea.* Charles C Thomas, Springfield, Ill., 1951.

Rankin, J. S., Goldfarb, A. F., and Rakoff, A. E.: Galactorrhea-amenorrhea syndromes: postpartum galactorrhea-amenorrhea in the absence of intracranial neoplasm. Obstet. Gynec., *33:* 1, 1969.

Ray, J. H., Nicholson-Vailey, U., and Grappl, A.: Endocrine activity in psychiatric patients with menstrual disorder. Brit. Med. J., *2:* 843, 1957.

Reiss, H. E.: Primary amenorrhoea as a manifestation of tuberculosis. J. Obstet. Gynaec. Brit. Comm., *65:* 735, 1958.

Robertson, J. D.: Glinski and aetiology of Simmond's disease (hypopituitarism). Brit. Med. J., *1:* 921, 1951.

Seitz, L.: Die sequndare Amenorrhoe in ihrer Abhangigkeit von Stoffwechsel und Psyche. Geburtsh. Frauenheilk., *10:* 165, 1950.

Sheehan, H. L.: Post-partum necrosis of anterior pituitary. J. Path. Bact., *45:* 189, 1937.

Sherman, H. C., Campbell, H. L., and Ragan, M. S.: Analytical and experimental study of the effects of increased protein with liberal calcium and riboflavin intakes; complete life cycles. J. Nutr., *37:* 317, 1949.

Simmonds, M.: Über embolische prozesse in der Hypophysis. Arch. Path. Anat., *217:* 226, 1914.

Solomon, D. H., Beck, J. C., Vander Laan, W. P., and Astwood, E. B.: Prognosis of hyperthyroidism treated by anti-thyroid drugs. J.A.M.A., *152:* 201, 1953.

Sosman, M. C.: Cushing's disease—pituitary basophilism; Caldwell Lecture. Amer. J. Roentgen., *62:* 1, 1949.

Starup, J., and Sele, V.: Premature ovarian failure. Acta Obstet. Gynec. Scand., *52:* 259, 1973.

Stein, J. F.: Diagnosis and treatment of bilateral polycystic ovaries in the Stein-Leventhal syndrome. Int. J. Fertil., *3:* 20, 1958.

Stein, J. F., and Leventhal, M. L.: Amenorrhea associated with bilateral polycystic ovaries. Amer. J. Obstet. Gynec., *29:* 181, 1935.

Strassman, E. O.: Surgical reconstruction of a functional uterine cavity in 6 patients having complete atresia. Southern Med. J., *49:* 458, 1956.

Teter, J., and Boczkowski, K.: Occurrence of tumors in dysgenetic gonads. Cancer, *20:* 1301, 1967.

Tompkins, P.: Treatment of imperforate hymen with hematocolpos; a review of 113 cases in the literature and a report of 5 additional cases. J.A.M.A., *113:* 913, 1933.

Turner, H. H.: A syndrome of infantilism, congenital webbed neck, and cubitus valgus. Endocrinology, *23:* 566, 1938.

Whitacre, F. E., and Barrera, B.: War amenorrhea. J.A.M.A., *124:* 399, 1944.

Whitelaw, M. J., Thomas, S. F., Graham, W., Foster, T. M., and Brock, C.: Growth response in gonadal dysgenesis to the anabolic steroid Norethandrolone. Amer. J. Obstet. Gynec., *84:* 501, 1962.

Wilkins, L.: *The Diagnosis and Treatment of Endocrine Disorders in Childhood and Adolescence.* Charles C Thomas, Springfield, Ill., 1950.

Wilkins, L., and Fleischmann, W.: Ovarian agenesis; pathology, associated clinical symptoms and bearing on theories of sex differentiation. J. Clin. Endocr., *4:* 257, 1944.

Wilson, J. G., and Warkany, J.: Malformations in the genito-urinary tract induced by maternal vitamin A deficiency in the rat. Amer. J. Anat., *83:* 357, 1948.

Zanartu, J., Dabacens, A., Rodriguez-Bravo, R., and Schally, A. V.: Induction of ovulation with synthetic gonadotrophin-releasing hormone in women with comitant anovulation induced by contraceptive steroids. Brit. Med. J., *1:* 605, 1974.

Zondek, B.: Hypophysenvorderhappen. Arch. Gynaek., *144:* 133, 1930.

chapter 31

Abnormal Uterine Bleeding

Abnormal uterine bleeding can be classified under two major etiological headings, (1) anatomical and (2) functional. Bleeding is *anatomical* in origin if it is caused by a lesion in some part of the genital tract. The characteristic history is menometrorrhagia. Although bleeding episodes may appear at irregular and unpredictable times, the patient is often able to identify regular menstrual intervals in addition to the abnormal bleeding phases. This is because there is no interference with the ovarian ovulatory phenomena.

Dysfunctional uterine bleeding (or functional) is abnormal bleeding unassociated with tumor, inflammation, or pregnancy. As the condition is usually associated with an ovarian dysfunction and anovulation, the characteristic history is one of complete irregularity of the menstrual interval, prolonged menses frequently alternating with episodes of amenorrhea.

ANATOMICAL FACTORS

This group embraces lesions of the uterus, tubes, or ovaries (Fig. 31.1).

Among the more important anatomical causes of abnormal uterine bleeding are the following.

Cervical Polyps

The bleeding with cervical polyps is characteristically slight and intermenstrual, being provoked by muscular exertion, such as defecation, and especially by coitus (*contact bleeding*). Many polyps cause no bleeding at all, being discovered only accidentally. The slight intermenstrual or postcoital bleeding which often occurs is like that seen in the early stages of cervical carcinoma, and the gynecologist breathes a sigh of relief when, in a patient with such suspicious symptoms, he finds instead of carcinoma one or more cervical polyps protruding from the canal.

Cervical Erosions or Ectropion

With either erosion or ectropion the cervical mucosa may be reddish, granular, and vascular, producing slight bleeding of the type described for cervical polyp. When the tissues are very vascular,

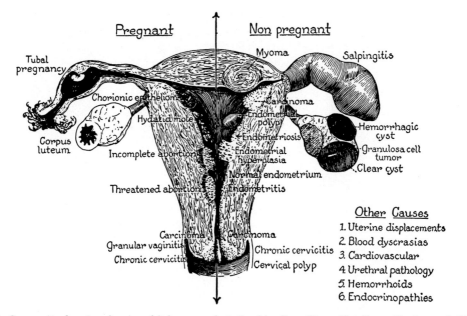

31.1. Composite drawing showing chief causes of uterine bleeding. (From Henriksen, E.: Amer. J. Obstet. Gynec., *41:* 179, 1941.)

bleeding on slight touch, there should always be a suspicion of carcinoma, and biopsy is indicated.

Carcinoma of Cervix

By far the *most important cause of uterine bleeding,* from the standpoint of its life-and-death significance to the patient, has been uterine cancer, especially of the cervix. Characteristically this, in the early stages, is of the spotting, intermenstrual type, and is frequently noted especially after coitus. Such bleeding is always suspicious of a cervical lesion, such as cancer or polyp, and always demands careful examination of the cervix. Such an examination, moreover, must always include a speculum examination under the best possible light, a Papanicolaou smear, and where a suspicious lesion is found, biopsy must be taken to determine whether or not cancer is present. The bleeding in cancer is the result of the surface ulceration seen even in the early stages of malignancy.

Endometrial Polyps

These are much less likely to cause bleeding than cervical polyps, because of their protected position within the uterine cavity. As a matter of fact, the smaller endometrial polyps ordinarily cause no symptoms at all, being found accidentally on curettage or hysterectomy for other indications. In the larger polyps, and especially those which develop pedicles sufficiently long to allow obtrusion of the polyp into the cervical or even the vaginal canal, bleeding is a common symptom. It is the result of ulcerative changes in the dependent portion of the polyp, and at times of necrosis due to interference with the blood supply.

Retention of Gestation Products

This is *one of the most common of all causes of uterine bleeding,* chiefly because of the frequency of abortion, both spontaneous and induced, although placental tissue is not infrequently retained after full term delivery as well. The bleeding may be slight or it may be exceedingly profuse. The continuance of bleeding after abortion usually indicates retention of gestational products (Fig. 31.2). In some cases considerable masses of placenta may be retained for long periods of time with little or no bleeding, whereas in

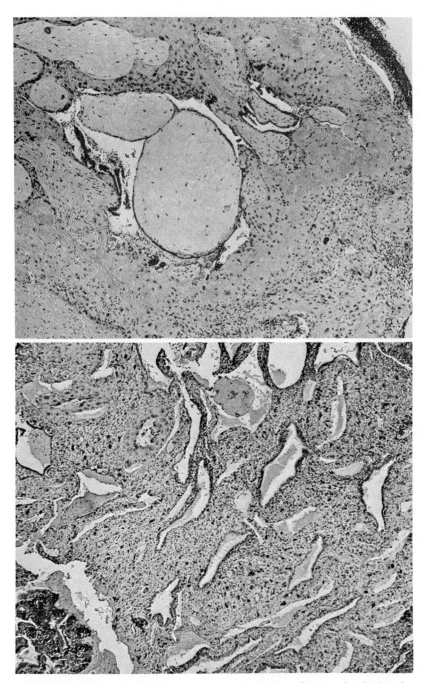

31.2. *Top,* old degenerated "shadow" villi in postabortal curetting. *Bottom,* decidual and trophoblastic cells in curettings following recent abortion.

others only small particles may be associated with prolonged and profuse bleeding. Occasionally, such retained tissue becomes firmly incorporated with the uterine wall, and may form large or small *placental polyps* (Fig. 31.3). The bleeding is sometimes due to failure or inability of the uterine muscle to contract, but in other cases is due to the opening up of large venous sinuses when the uterus

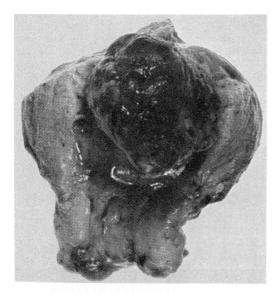

31.3. Large placental polyp of uterus

tries to expel portions of placental tissue still attached to the uterine wall.

Chronic Endometritis

Endometritis is not a common cause of uterine bleeding and, when the association occurs, it is probable that the factor responsible for the bleeding is the chronic metritis which, as Schwarz has shown, is not infrequently associated with the endometritis, and which interferes with uterine contractility.

Subinvolution of the Uterus

This condition is seen most frequently in association with marked retroflexion and retroversion of the acquired type. The incompleteness of the normal involution of the puerperal uterus leaves it large, boggy, and congested, and menstrual excess is not uncommon as a result of the uterine hyperemia.

Carcinoma of the Corpus Uteri

Adenocarcinoma of the uterine body is a common cause of uterine bleeding, especially of the postmenopausal type. In about one-fourth of the cases this disease develops during reproductive life, when the abnormal bleeding may be both menstrual and inter-menstrual, the latter being the more significant. In early stages it is only slight and occasional, appearing often as a blood-tinged watery discharge. In those patients who develop adenocarcinoma after the menopause, the early bleeding is of the same slight degree, but later it becomes increasingly persistent and more profuse.

Sarcoma of the Uterus

Sarcoma of either the cervix or corpus uteri is far less common than carcinoma, and it produces bleeding of the same type as the latter.

Myoma of Uterus

This exceedingly common cause of uterine bleeding is most likely to occur when the tumors are of the submucous or interstitial variety, the subperitoneal growths having no tendency to cause hemorrhage. Even when a myoma is present, the *bleeding is often due to associated ovarian dysfunction.* Furthermore, it should be remembered that the finding of myomas in a patient who is bleeding does not justify the conclusion that the tumors cause the bleeding, which may be due to some very different intrauterine condition, such as cancer or retained placental tissue.

Hydatidiform Mole and Chorionepithelioma

These lesions are occasionally encountered by the gynecologist, although the latter is exceedingly rare. The bleeding of hydatidiform mole appears in the early months of pregnancy, usually the third to the fifth, and is often associated with a disproportionately large uterus as compared with the duration of the pregnancy. *Quantitative serum chorionic gonadotrophin assays* are often of value in arriving at a diagnosis. Chorionepithelioma manifests itself by persistence of bleeding after the evacuation of a hydatidiform mole, or after miscarriage or full term delivery. Here again quantitative chorionic gonadotrophin tests may be helpful, although the diagnosis is often not made until later stages, and sometimes not until metastases have appeared (Chapter 27).

Ectopic Pregnancy

In few other conditions is the menstrual history as suggestive as with ectopic pregnancy. Menstruation is usually delayed for a few days or several weeks, followed by uterine bleeding which is typically of a spotting character, accompanied by pain in one side of the pelvis. Such a history, together with the finding of a unilateral adnexal mass, should always lead to the suspicion of tubal gestation. Although a definite anatomical lesion is present in such cases, the mechanism of the bleeding is at least partly due to hormonal factors, as discussed in Chapter 26, "Ectopic Pregnancy."

Tuberculosis of the Genital Tract

The usual primary seat of genital tuberculosis is in the tubes, but the endometrium is secondarily involved in the majority of cases. Bleeding is frequent but not invariable, and amenorrhea or hypomenorrhea may be noted in some cases, especially in late stages.

Adnexitis

Inflammatory disease of the tubes and ovary may cause not only uterine bleeding, but also disturbances of menstrual rhythm, especially in the form of shortened intervals (polymenorrhea). In many cases, the probable immediate factor is ovarian dysfunction rather than pelvic hyperemia.

Tumors of the Ovary

Although any type of ovarian neoplasm may at times cause uterine bleeding, the proportionate incidence of this symptom is greater with those tumors characterized by the production of estrogen. This group includes especially granulosa cell carcinoma and thecoma, although other tumors not of the "endocrine variety" may likewise exert a hormonal influence, in most instances by virtue of hyperactive stromal cells. Even large growths of other types, malignant or benign, are most frequently accompanied by no external bleeding.

Tumors of the Tube

These are extremely rare, but the most important of them, carcinoma, is not infrequently associated with bleeding. The blood undoubtedly finds its way into the uterus from the ulcerating intratubal neoplasm giving a serosanguinous discharge referred to as hydrosalpinx perfluens.

Treatment

The treatment of uterine bleeding due to any of the anatomical causes enumerated above must obviously be directed toward removal or correction of these various etiological factors. Each is discussed under the appropriate chapter heads.

DYSFUNCTIONAL UTERINE BLEEDING

Definition

Dysfunctional uterine bleeding may be defined as abnormal bleeding from the uterus unassociated with tumor, inflammation, or pregnancy. Although apt to occur at the extremes of the menstrual life, such bleeding may occur at any age and is one of the most common gynecological complaints.

Pathology

Schröder, in 1915, by a correlated histological study of the uterus and ovaries, concluded that the bleeding disorder to which he gave the name of metropathia hemorrhagica, is produced by abnormal persistence of unruptured follicles, with consequent absence of functioning corpora lutea and with the production of hyperplasia of the endometrium as a result of the abnormally persistent and unopposed or excessive estrogenic stimulation. This is still the accepted explanation for perhaps the largest number of cases of dysfunctional bleeding. However, it leaves us the fundamental pathology, the disruption of the central feed-back control, unexplained.

Pathological studies have shown that although such uterine bleeding can be associated with any type of endometrial pathology, the most common finding is a nonsecretory pattern. In a survey of 158 patients with this diagnosis, 85 were found to have endometrial hyperplasia, 38 a nonsecretory pattern including atrophic endometrium, and 35 a secretory pattern. The division of patients into those with nonsecretory and secretory patterns is important as it distinguishes *anovulatory* from *ovulatory* types of bleeding. The classification is of clinical significance, as these two types of dysfunctional uterine bleeding have different etiological backgrounds and respond to different forms of therapy.

Bleeding associated with a secretory pattern must be regarded as anatomical until proved otherwise. If all anatomical factors can be excluded, the functional disturbance is considered to be of a poorly understood neuromuscular, vasomotor, or hematological origin, not endocrinological, whereas anovulatory bleeding can usually be considered of endocrine origin.

Diagnosis

The diagnosis of dysfunctional bleeding can be made with certainty only after a careful bimanual examination and curettage and it is only under exceptional circumstances that this procedure should be waived. An example might be the case of a pubertal child who has had only one or two episodes of bleeding which were not too severe.

Ovulatory Bleeding

In order to make the diagnosis of *ovulatory bleeding* it is obviously important to obtain curettings in the postovulatory or secretory phase of the cycle. When there is no recognizable cycle, this may be difficult. A basal temperature chart is a valuable diagnostic tool under these circumstances if bleeding is not severe enough to require an immediate curettage as a therapeutic measure (Fig. 31.4). Once the diagnosis of ovulatory bleeding is established it is imperative to exclude the possibility of some obscure anatomical cause for the bleeding. In addition to a thorough dilatation and curettage, exploration of the uterine cavity with a polyp forceps is always indicated and occasionally a hysterogram will demonstrate a polyp when other methods have failed (Fig. 31.5). Hysteroscopy may also be used under these circumstances. Sequential serum progesterone assays, especially if correlated with the LH surge, are also diagnostic but hardly useful as routine clinical methods.

Having established that the patient is bleeding from a secretory type of endometrium, it is important to make an etiological diagnosis. If there is an associated ovarian cyst, *Halban's disease* or persistent corpus luteum must be suspected. This syndrome must be differentiated from an ectopic pregnancy, as the history and pelvic findings are often similar.

The diagnosis of *irregular shedding* must be made by proper timing of the curettage which, according to McLennan, should be on the fourth day of bleeding. At this time both secretory and nonsecretory endometrium must be present. The clinical symptomatology is characterized by a prolongation of the menstrual flow, theoretically due to the prolonged desquamation phase. The condition is rather unusual; Marin and Botella discount the pathological finding as responsible for the bleeding, since they found this form of irregular shedding in 17% of a series of 220 normally menstruating women.

If there is severe hypertension the possibility of so-called *apoplexy uteri* must be entertained. A hematological investigation will eliminate the possibility of *blood dyscrasias*: anemias, thrombocytopenic purpura, or disturbances of the bleeding or clotting time. Because lupus erythematosus can occasionally give rise to menorrhagia, a lupus cell preparation should be requested, if indicated by history or physical findings.

Anovulatory Bleeding

If the curetting has established the diagnosis of anovulatory dysfunctional uterine bleeding it is essential to make an etiological diagnosis. The cause of the disturbed ovarian function can be (1)

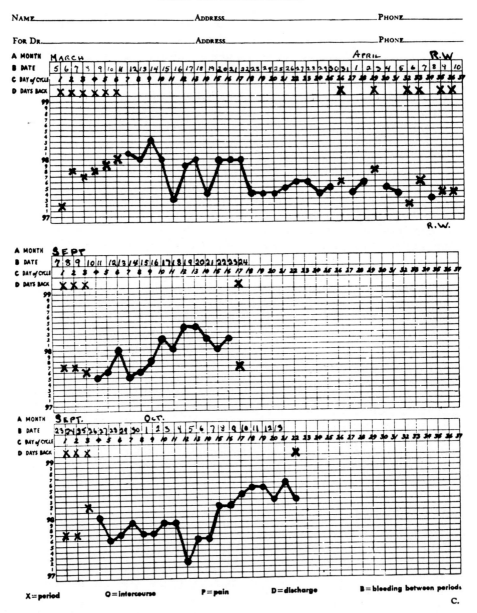

31.4. *Upper,* basal temperature chart of a patient with irregular, sporadic type of bleeding. The temperature graph is monophasic, indicating an anovulatory pattern. *Middle* and *lower,* basal temperature charts of a patient with profuse vaginal bleeding at irregular intervals, from 17 to 27 days. The charts are biphasic, indicating ovulatory bleeding with an occasional excessively short menstrual interval. At curettage a submucous myoma was diagnosed.

central, secondary to psychogenic, neurogenic (including a hypothalamic imbalance and the Stein-Leventhal syndrome) or pituitary factors; or (2) *peripheral,* due to ovarian factors *per se* or to disturbances of steroid metabolism and excretion as in hepatic cirrhosis and chronic nephritis. Ovarian factors can be categorized as functional ovarian tumors or ovarian dysfunction of undetermined type. The third major group of factors responsible for anovulatory functional bleeding are (3) *constitutional factors*; *i.e.,* nutritional deficiencies, metabolic disease, and acute or chronic illness. In a study of 50 patients with cystic glandular hyperplasia, Benjamin found that 84% had some abnormality of the glucose tolerance test (GTT); 22% of these had a true diabetic type curve.

It is helpful to consider the possible etiologic diagnosis of this disease in relation to age, as etiologic factors do tend to cluster according to the three major age groups; perimenarcheal, menstrual and perimenopausal. It is, however, obvious that, in every age group, ovarian tumors must be considered and the diagnosis eliminated. Constitutional factors also tend to cluster in the menstrual age group, probably because this makes up the largest category of women.

The perimenarcheal period is associated with dysfunctional bleeding due to delayed, asynchronous or abnormal hypothalamic maturation and is cate-

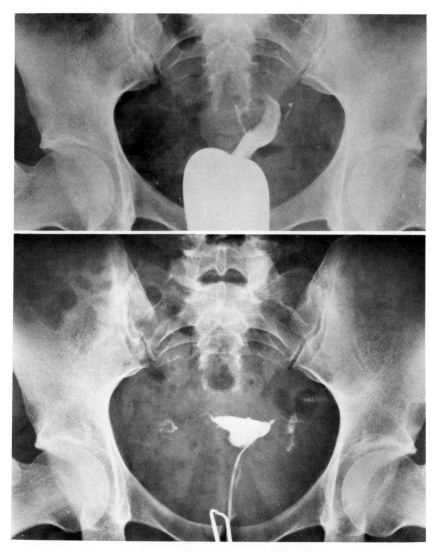

31.5. *Top,* hysterogram demonstrating a submucous myoma. The patient was having prolonged irregular menses. The uterus was normal is size by pelvic examination and two curettages have been performed. At second curettage the submucous myoma was mistaken for a uterine septum. *Lower,* appearance of the uterus postoperatively.

gorized by low FSH, absence of the LH surge, or a low tonic LH. The most frequent type of bleeding is related to a shortened menstrual interval, but no real prolongation, or increase in flow. Such cycles, if studied intensively, are frequently found to be oligo- or aluteal and, therefore, not truly anovulatory. They are readily amenable to treatment during the short interval prior to full hypothalamic maturation. True anovulatory cycles, which fortuitously occur less frequently, are characterized by grossly irregular intervals with prolonged and profuse bleeding phases. These patients may also be showing a transient manifestation of a normal physiologic variant. If so, lowered serum gonadotrophin assays are to be expected and establishment of a normal ovulatory cycle is to be anticipated within 2 years. When the pattern persists, especially if characterized by elevations of serum LH above the levels found in normal cycles during the follicular phase, a Stein-Leventhal syndrome is suspected. The diagnosis is important to make, as both the older study of Southam, and a more recent one by Fraser *et al.,* indicate that the reproductive capacity of such patients is jeopardized, and they are in a high risk cancer category. These young patients respond, as do older ones, to clomiphene and, when indicated, wedge resection operation. More rarely in this age group, the ovary is the primary site of pathology. A buccal smear and/or karyotype may be diagnostic if a mosaic pattern is found indicating a chromosomal abnormality associated with decreased numbers of oocytes and follicles. Transient or persistent elevations of FSH confirm the diagnosis. Visualization of the ovaries is also sometimes helpful. Ovarian biopsy is a definitive diagnostic method but, as these patients have a compromised ovarian function, the advisability of this technique is questionable. Clomiphene has sometimes proved successful in inducing ovulation and even an occasional pregnancy in the young patient with these findings. Among the constitutional factors responsible for dysfunctional bleeding in the perimenarcheal group, nutritional deficiencies are the most frequent.

In the mature woman, the most common cause of dysfunctional uterine bleeding is the Stein-Leventhal syndrome. The characteristic gonadotrophin pattern is a persistent, pulsatile elevation of LH above the expected normal range for the follicular phase of the cycle, a high, but within normal, FSH assay and absence of an LH surge. The pathogenesis of this syndrome is discussed in Chapter 22. It is apparently a hypothalamic disease caused by many different etiologic factors. Among these are heritable defects of the nervous system, scars, psychogenic factors or iatrogenic drugs, such as oral contraceptions, estrogens or androgens. The diagnosis can be made by palpation of bilateral ovarian enlargement confirmed by some technique for ovarian visualization and a persistent elevation of LH assays. An active response to an LRH infusion is further confirmation of the diagnosis. As stated above, these patients are in a high risk category for the development of adenocarcinoma of the fundus and, therefore, the endometrial pathology should be checked periodically. The response to clomiphene or wedge resection (Chapter 22) is usually good. Although ovarian factors are unusual in this age group, constitutional factors occur frequently. These would be metabolic disease and acute and chronic illness, including kidney and liver disease. Nutritional deficiencies are less common than in the younger age group, although obesity is not an infrequent finding.

Obviously, in the perimenopausal group, the etiology is usually related to a failing ovarian function. It is interesting that the FSH values in such patients may be elevated, while the serum LH assays remain normal (Fig. 31.6). Serum estrogen assays may be either normal, relatively low, or markedly elevated. After episodes of elevation, gonadotrophic values may return to normal, and cycles be reinstituted (Fig. 31.7). This pattern seems to represent the ability of the ovary and pituitary to reestablish normal function, probably by way of hy-

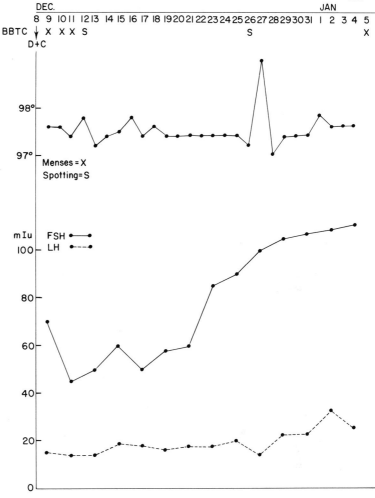

31.6. Anovulatory basal body temperature chart (BBTC) of a 49-year-old woman with dyfunctional bleeding. Dilatation and curettage showed cystic hyperplasia. LH values are within normal range but FSH values are markedly elevated and continue to rise. This patient had the menopause and no further bleeding. (From Aksel, S., and Jones, G. S.: Obstet. Gynec., *44:* 1, 1974.

pothalamic modulation and probably at different levels in relation to a failing ovarian function. The preferential and primary elevation of FSH indicates that the ovarian follicle and/or oocyte does indeed exert some type of feedback at the hypothalamic or pituitary level.

Because of the varied etiology of the condition, the diagnostic procedures involved may be extensive and the physician must be guided by the symptoms of the patient. We found, in a study of 135 patients with dysfunctional uterine bleeding, 47 of central origin, 13 psychogenic and 22 with a Stein syndrome (hypothalamic imbalance). There were no cases due to specific hypophysial lesions.

The diagnosis of neurogenic etiology is made on the basis of neurological findings and the electroencephalographic changes, as well as a history of brain damage, epilepsy, or neurological diseases. Aberrations of normal physiology, *e.g.,* abnormal bleeding at puberty or after pregnancy should also be included in this category. The diagnosis of psychogenic dysfunctional bleeding is usually made on the basis of a history of acute psychic trauma. An elevated pituitary gonadotrophin is indicative of ovarian failure, but may also be seen in the Stein-Leventhal syndrome. The diagnosis of this condition has been discussed in Chapter 30. Thirty-one patients had dysfunctional bleeding of

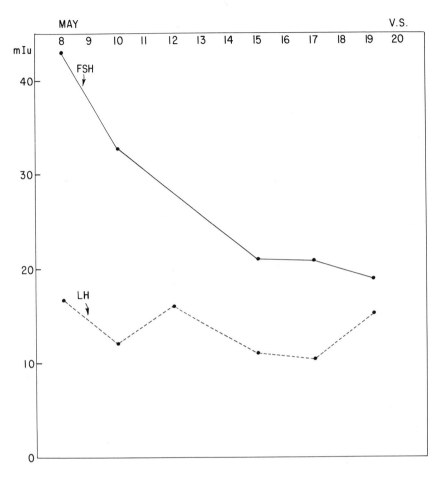

31.7. FSH and LH values in a 54-year-old woman with dysfunctional uterine bleeding. The LH values are within the normal range while the FSH values are initially elevated, but return to normal level within this 2-week interval. This patient resumed fairly regular menses during the following year and then ceased menstruating at age 56.

ovarian origin due to menopausal changes either at the expected time or prematurely. Ovarian tumors had been screened in this series.

The remaining 57 patients were diagnosed as having constitutional factors, nutritional deficiencies, metabolic diseases, and acute or chronic illnesses responsible for the dysfunctional bleeding. Twenty-three women had nutritional insufficiencies, diagnosed by the weight and nutritional history. In 26 the bleeding was associated with metabolic diseases. Of these, 13 had hypothyroidism and three had hyperthyroidism diagnosed by the protein-bound iodine; six had diabetes diagnosed by a glucose tolerance test; and four had Cushing's disease, the diagnosis of which is discussed in Chapter 30. In eight the bleeding was associated

with a chronic disease process. This diagnosis is facilitated by the sedimentation rate, differential and white count, in addition to the medical examination.

There were no patients in the group with dysfunctional bleeding from cirrhosis of the liver or nephritis resulting in increased amounts of circulating active estrogens. These diagnoses would, of course, be made on the basis of the liver function and kidney function tests. An interesting aspect of this problem is the hypermenorrhea which occurs in young women after hemodialysis. Goodlin believes that the bleeding is anovulatory, but Rice suggests it may be associated with the anti-coagulant used to prevent cannula clotting. It would seem that the severe anemia present in many of these patients might also be a contributory factor.

Treatment

As has been previously emphasized, the symptom of abnormal uterine bleeding must always be considered a serious one until proved otherwise, and as anatomical until proved functional. Treatment should be initiated by a thorough curettage which will both establish a diagnosis and serve as definitive therapy. It has been found by Jones and Te Linde that 42% of patients will require no further procedures. If bleeding recurs after curettage, treatment depends upon the severity of symptoms and the age of the patient. After the child bearing years a hysterectomy may be expedient. Intracavitary irradiation, although quick and convenient, has the disadvantage of occasionally causing cervical stenosis with its ensuing complications as well as carrying the risk of subsequent development of endometrial carcinoma.

Ovulatory Dysfunctional Bleeding

Although applicable to both the ovulatory and anovulatory type of dysfunctional bleeding, the curettage is probably most effective in the sporadic forms of ovulatory dysfunctional bleeding caused by a persistent corpus luteum cyst (Halban's disease) or irregular endometrial shedding. Dysfunctional uterine bleeding associated with a secretory endometrial pattern will rarely if ever respond to hormonal therapy and must be controlled by general medical regimen such as diet, iron, and Ergotrate, the latter being given during the first few days of the menstrual flow (1/320 grain every 4 hours until 8 tablets have been given).

It has been our experience that blood dyscrasias and anemia can cause abnormal uterine bleeding, and this fact is well substantiated in the literature as reviewed by Radman. Seaman and Benson report 6 women in a series of 43 with functional uterine bleeding who showed a hemorrhagic diathesis characterized by prolonged bleeding time. Mitch *et al.* report severe menorrhagia in 3 of 4 patients studied with thrombocytopenic purpura.

Experience has demonstrated that ovulatory bleeding cannot be controlled by short cyclic progesterone withdrawal therapy. This finding is substantiated by the knowledge that, in the estrogen-primed castrate, withdrawal bleeding can be induced by amounts of progesterone which are far below the level required for a response in the histological pattern. Therefore, if the patient is producing a suffient amount of progesterone to show a secretory (even though apparently inadequate) endometrium, additional progesterone cannot be expected to affect the bleeding. There is some evidence that the synthetic progestational-like compounds, 19-*nor*-testosterone derivatives, given 24 days throughout the cycle, will suppress abnormal bleeding from secretory types of endometrium. If one has excluded the possibility of anatomical lesions to the best of one's ability by a careful examination under anesthesia and a dilatation and curettage, it is permissible to try this. The success of such therapy apparently depends upon complete suppression of the patient's cycle. Under these circumstances, the endometrial response to exogenous stimulation is theoretically not as great as to the endogenous stimulation. A progestational agent without estrogenic activity is to be preferred; 2.5 mg. of norethindrone given daily for 24 days and repeated beginning five days after the onset of withdrawal bleeding, will often control menorrhagia of hematological or vascular origin. If after several cycles, bleeding fails to occur, small amounts of stilbestrol, 0.1 mg. to 0.2 mg., can be added. Ross has reported the successful treatment of 4 young girls with menorrhagia from serious blood dyscrasias by complete suppression of menstrual bleeding using 10 mg. daily of norethindrone continuously for a 2-year period. Any of the long-acting progestational drugs such as Depo-Provera or Delalutin can be used in a similar way. Under such circumstances this can be a life saving therapy.

Anovulatory Dysfunctional Bleeding

The disturbance of physiology in anovulatory dysfunctional bleeding is the same regardless of the underlying etiology. Therefore all patients can be treated symptomatically to control the bleeding while the primary cause is being investigated. In the younger age group the problem of maintaining reproductive function is important and it is among these patients that endocrine therapy is the treatment of choice. The Stein syndrome responds to a specific form of treatment, wedge resection operation, or clomiphene therapy, and, therefore, this diagnosis must always be suspected and confirmed or disproved by a culdoscopic examination or some other form of ovarian visualization.

Progesterone. It has been shown that the endometrial pattern among the *anovulatory* dysfunctional bleeding group is hyperplastic or nonsecretory in 98% of the cases and atrophic in 2%, indicating that almost all patients have either normal or excessive estrogen stimulation and deficient progesterone. Substitution therapy of progesterone, therefore, in a cyclic manner will establish regular menses in 98% of the patients. It is necessary to give additional estrogens only in the 2% who exhibit a deficiency as manifest by an atrophic endometrial pattern.

An inexpensive and convenient regimen is the administration of 25 mg. of progesterone in oil intramuscularly once every 28 days for 3 months, as advocated by Holmstrom. If the patient is bleeding at the initiation of treatment, however, it is usually necessary to administer additional oral progestogens for the following 3 days—30 mg. daily of ethisterone or its equivalent. Three courses of therapy are usually sufficient and, following this, the treatment should be interrupted in an effort to determine whether or not the patient will establish her own cycle. A basal temperature chart is of value in identifying a therapeutic "breakthrough" (Fig. 31.8). Sixty per cent of the patients will need further treatment within a year.

Forty per cent will resume regular menstrual cycles.

It must be remembered that progesterone is not a hemostatic drug and that it exerts its action only on withdrawal, thus producing a type of chemical curettage. Therefore, if the patient is bleeding at the time therapy is instituted, bleeding will not be controlled until six or eight days after cessation of therapy. If the patient is not bleeding when treatment is begun, her menstrual period usually begins within 2 to 4 days after cessation of therapy. In the 2% of patients who require adjunctive estrogen, 1 mg. of stilbestrol, or its equivalent, may be given immediately with the progesterone and for 17 consecutive days preceding the next cycle of progesterone therapy.

Progestational Drugs. When progestational-like compounds are used to control dysfunctional bleeding these are given either cyclically as progestogens in small doses (5.0 mg. daily for 5 days) or continuously in large doses (10 to 30 mg. daily for 2 to 3 weeks) as pituitary suppressants. The larger dose is said to have the advantage of suppressing bleeding within 24 to 48 hours. Suppression is ideally maintained throughout the course of therapy. Unfortunately, these theoretical ideals are often not obtained. Bleeding may not be immediately controlled and "breakthrough" bleeding, during the course of therapy, is not uncommon.

A number of steroids have been synthesized which have some progestational activity orally or intramuscularly. The majority of these, however, also have certain androgenic properties and some even show inherent estrogenic characteristics. It is therefore extremely important that one should not think of such drugs as interchangeable with "progesterone." It is necessary to know the specific effect of the specific type of steroid one is using. These drugs are primarily useful as oral contraceptive agents but, because of the progestational effect, have also been useful in the control of anovulatory dysfunctional uterine bleeding.

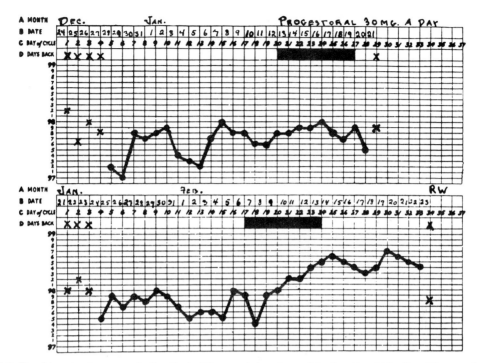

31.8. Basal temperature record of patient with anovulatory type of dysfunctional bleeding. The *top chart* is monophasic. The *black area* indicates the time during which 30 mg. of oral ethisterone were given daily. This dosage is insufficient to produce any thermogenic effect. Withdrawal bleeding occurred 2 days after cessation of therapy. The *lower chart* is ovulatory. Bleeding does not occur until 10 days after cessation of therapy, indicating a "breakthrough" or escape.

A list of the more frequently used progestogens with the trade names and dosages used for the treatment of anovulatory dysfunctional bleeding is given in Table 31.1.

Chorionic Gonadotrophin. Although the use of chorionic gonadotrophin seemed theoretically promising and initially practical, most subsequent reports have been disappointing. Bergman, however, reports a series of 361 patients with excellent clinical results using 4500 IU of chorionic gonadotrophin, given in 3 doses of 1500 IU each, on 3 consecutive days each month. With this regimen ovulation was apparently induced. This is largely of historic interest.

Estrogens. The use of high dosages of oral estrogens (25 mg. or more of stilbestrol daily), or of intravenous estrogen as a hemostatic agent, is undesirable, because a vicious circle is established. Although intravenous estrogens have been

reported as having hemostatic properties, Kudish and Rapaport were unable to demonstrate that they affected the plasma clotting time in humans. Kelly has reviewed the evidence for the rationale of the use of intravenous estrogen and concludes that "there is no concrete experimental evidence to justify the endorsement of estrogen given by the intravenous route for any therapeutic indication."

The great individual variation in response to estrogens makes it extremely difficult to establish a satisfactory routine dosage and withdrawal schedule. The rationale of estrogen therapy in dysfunctional bleeding was initially based on the theory that the abnormal bleeding resulted from a drop in the estrogen level. Estrogen was therefore given in an effort to maintain a uniform estrogen milieu. The metabolic studies of Brown *et al.* have failed to substantiate this theory.

Table 31.1

Progestational Therapy for Anovulatory Dysfunctional Bleeding

Mode of Administration	Generic Name	Trade Name	Dosage
Intramuscular	Progesterone in oil		50 mg. stat. and q. 28 da. × 3 mo.
	17α-Hydroxyprogesterone caproate	Delalutin	125 mg. stat. & q. 28 da. × 3 mo.
Oral	Ethindrone	Progestoral	30 mg. q.d. × 5 da. q. 28 da. × 3 mo.
	Norethindrone	Norlutin	5 mg. q.d. × 3–5 d. q. 28 da. × 3 mo.
	Megestrol acetate	Megace	40 mg. q.d. × 3 mo.

The later rationale of giving estrogen to mimic the normal cycle and induce the characteristic feed-back effect, the LH surge, and ovulation is untenable because these patients are unable to evoke the "normal" feed-back response.

Estrogen as a single agent in the treatment of dysfunctional uterine bleeding is not to be recommended, because the instance of unpleasant side effects is high and the results are uncertain and unreproducible. Likewise, the use of sequential steroid therapy, *e.g.*, estrogen followed by a progestational agent (Chapter 34) is not to be recommended.

Testosterone. Treatment with testosterone is certainly not justifiable now that so many other types of drugs are available. This is particularly true, because the dosage which is necessary to cause consistent cessation of bleeding is in the androgenic area, that is, over 250 mg. per month; therefore, some degree of virilism is a possibility. Likewise, the addition of testosterone to other regimens of therapy is unnecessary and increases the complexity of the treatment and the cost to the patient.

Clomiphene. In 1964 Charles *et al.*, and subsequently many others, reported the use of clomiphene for the induction of ovulation in a series of patients with anovulatory dysfunctional bleeding.

These authors gave 100 mg. daily for 21 days each month and were successful in inducing normal ovulatory cycles which persisted after three courses of therapy. Although most subsequent investigators have used somewhat lower and shorter dose schedules (Chap. 30), this drug has proved to be of great value in this condition. Because clomiphene is the most successful drug for the induction of ovulation, it is the treatment of choice in those patients who are primarily concerned about infertility.

Specific Therapy. Cyclic progesterone therapy should be considered as a substitution therapy to be used to control bleeding while the underlying etiological factors are being investigated, as described under diagnostic methods. Specific therapy should then be directed toward these factors: supportive therapy with extra calories and vitamins when malnutrition occurs; thyroid in adequate dosage, sodium levothyroxine (Synthyroid) 0.2 mg. daily, and over a prolonged interval when hypothyroidism can be demonstrated; diabetic regulation when diabetes is associated with dysfunctional uterine bleeding; and reassurance and mild sedatives or psychiatric care when emotional disturbances are responsible for the condition.

It should be stressed that the Stein syndrome can be associated with dysfunctional uterine bleeding and, when no other factors can be found to account for the condition, a culdoscopic examination should be performed. Southam has emphasized the importance of this finding, especially among the younger patients who have exhibited symptoms almost since menarche. Although the definitive therapy is still operative ovarian wedge resection, it does respond to clomiphene therapy as reported by Kistner in 1960.

SUMMARY

In summary, after a Papanicolaou smear, a thorough curettage is preliminary to any treatment for abnormal uterine bleeding, as this at once establishes the diagnosis and initiates the most universally effective therapy. When dysfunctional bleeding exists, it is of paramount importance to differentiate ovulatory from anovulatory types, and once this pathological diagnosis is made an etiological diagnosis must be attempted. When ovulatory bleeding occurs one must be sure that anatomical lesions have been satisfactorily excluded; a hysterogram must be performed when necessary. A complete hematological investigation is also indicated. Anovulatory dysfunctional bleeding is most apt to be caused by nutritional insufficiency, metabolic disease, or emotional disturbances and these etiological factors should be carefully checked. Severe, persistent anovulatory bleeding in young women may be caused by polycystic ovaries, and a culdoscopic examination is indicated under these conditions.

In the older woman who has completed her childbearing career, hysterectomy may be the treatment of choice. In the younger woman in whom the reproductive function is important, cyclic progestational therapy should be used while efforts are being made to discover the etiology of the condition and to institute specific therapy. When no etiological factor can be found, an anti-estrogenic agent, clomiphene, may prove effective in restoring ovulation and fertility. When steroid therapy is used for the control of symptoms let the clinician then not delude himself that this type of hormone therapy will cure the condition. He should realize that he is merely providing some form of hormonal hemostasis and substitution therapy. It should be stressed that such treatment should never be continued in an uninterrupted fashion, unless for the treatment of life-threatening blood dyscrasias. After a three- or four-month period hormone therapy should be discontinued and the patient observed. Fortunately, there is a high spontaneous cure rate in this disease and only by such sporadic cessation of any hormone regimen can this sequel be observed.

PRECOCIOUS PUBERTY

Definition

Precocious puberty can be said to occur if sexual development and menstrual bleeding begin before the age of 10 years. Such development can occur at any time after birth.

Classification

The condition can be divided into two major categories: (1) *complete precocity, true precocious puberty,* indicative of total ovarian function with ovulation, and (2) *incomplete precocity, pseudo-precocious puberty,* of secondary sex characteristics only, with no evidence of ovulation, indicative of estrogen stimulation. The major clinical significance of the classification is that children with complete precocity are able to conceive and suitable precautions must be taken to prevent this serious sequel. A working classification is as follows.

Complete Precocity: True Precocious Puberty
  Neurogenic lesions
    Pineal tumors
    Hamartomas and lesions of the hypothalamus and connecting tracts
    Neurologic lesions
    Albright's syndrome—polyostotic fibrous dysplasia
  Hypothyroidism
  Idiopathic

Incomplete Precocity: Pseduo-precocious Puberty

Ovarian tumors

    Feminizing mesenchymomas, chorionepithelioma, teratoma

Adrenal tumors or hyperplasia producing masculinization

Iatrogenic

The sex distribution among the various subdivisions reported by Wilkins is interesting in that only one of 22 pineal tumors and 10 of 35 hypothalamic lesions occurred in girls whereas neurogenic lesions involving other areas of the central nervous system were evenly distributed between boys and girls. In contrast to the preponderance of males in the first 2 categories, Albright's syndrome occurred 28 of 29 times among girls. This syndrome is

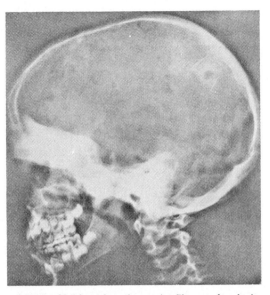

31.10. Child with polyostotic fibrous dysplasia (Albright's syndrome). The characteristic bony sclerosis at the base of the skull is marked.

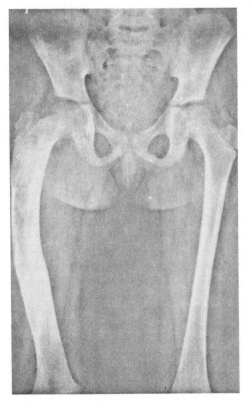

31.9 Femurs of child with typical polyostotic fibrous dysplasia (Albright's syndrome). The sclerotic cortex is seen in both femurs and the cystic characteristics are noted in the head of the right femur.

characterized by areas of increased skin pigmentation, disseminated areas of osseous rarefaction (Fig. 31.9), and a sclerotic overgrowth of the base of the skull (Fig. 31.10). The cause of precocity is unexplained. Precocious puberty of the idiopathic type also occurs more frequently in the female, being 3 to 4 times more common among girls.

As Novak has estimated that 90% of the cases fall into the idiopathic category it follows that precocious puberty in general is more frequently seen in females. Among the patients who are judged to have idiopathic precocious puberty, a constant concern is that a small neoplastic lesion of the hypothalamus or scar in the connecting tracts may be the real etiological factor. Such a case has been reported by Wolman and Balmforth. As indicated under Chapter 2, the current concept is that hypothalamic gonadotrophic centers are inhibited, before puberty, by higher centers, perhaps coordinated in the amygdala and connecting to the hypothalamus by way of the stria terminalis. Therefore scars which interrupt the inhibitory tracts would allow the hypothalamic centers to function. The alternative theorey is that, because of the plasticity of the adrenergic nervous system, injury causes excessive sprouting of nerve endings. This causes increased deposition of catecholamines in the hypothalamus and thereby premature function.

Hypothyroidism associated with precocious puberty and lactation is rare. Only 24 cases have been reported since 1905. The etiology of this syndrome depends upon the cross-reactivity of LH with TSH and the response of prolactin to the stimulation of TRH (Chap. 2). These children have severe hypothyroidism, no negative feedback from T_3 and T_4 at the pituitary level and, therefore, a marked elevation of pituitary TSH and eventually hypothalamic TRH. The excessive TSH gives an LH-like biologic effect stimulating ovarian estrogen secretion. The estrogen, however, is unable to turn off TSH; therefore precocious puberty ensues and occasionally dysfunctional anovulatory uterine bleeding. The TRH stimulates excessive prolactin production and galactorrhea. The treatment of this condition is obviously thyroid replacement.

Ovarian tumors comprise a major group of patients with incomplete precocity. Of 78 cases collected from the literature, Wilkins reports 33 were caused by granulosa cell tumors, 30 by an unidentified type of ovarian tumor, four by chorionepitheliomas, six by teratomas, and five by luteomas. Although usually unnecessary, endocrine assays can be used to differentiate idiopathic precocious puberty from that caused by steroid producing tumors. Patients with tumors have some elevation of the serum estrogen levels and low or undectable serum FSH and LH values. With the sensitive radioimmunoassay, it is now possible to demonstrate increased FSH and LH levels compatible with the stage of sexual development, not chronological age, in children with precocious puberty of idiopathic origin. Winter and Faiman have evidence that those patients with precocious thelarche may have an elevation of LH only. The ability to demonstrate this, because of the pulsatile type of LH discharge, apparently depends upon the frequency of the sampling. However, perhaps the most clinically applicable hormone assay in precocious puberty is the pregnancy test. This should be obtained in every case as it is such a simple assay. If positive, the diagnosis of tumor, probably chorionepithelium or teratoma, is assured.

Iatrogenic stimulation is a final etiology which must always be suspected in an unexplained case of incomplete precocious puberty. Vitamin preparations and skin creams should be considered and investigated, because occasionally an infant is given a geriatric preparation with hormones added.

If a proper diagnostic survey is made it is seldom necessary to resort to an exploratory laparotomy. Such a survey should include an examination of the vagina with a small cystoscope to exclude a foreign body, especially when vaginal bleeding is the sole manifestation of precocity and an examination under anesthesia to eliminate the possibility of an ovarian tumor (however, by the time the precocity is recognized the tumors are usually of sufficient size to be palpated abdominally). An enlargement of one ovary is not unusual in the idiopathic type of precocious puberty and may represent only a follicle cyst; therefore, no operative procedure is indicated if regular ovulatory bleeding occurs even in the presence of such an ovarian enlargement. Documentation of ovulation can be made by a basal body temperature chart kept by the mother and serial vaginal or urinary sediment smears. If an incomplete precocity exists and a tumor is diagnosed, a pregnancy test should be done to diagnose a chorionepithelioma. A skull film should be taken to diagnose Albright's syndrome and a careful neurological and ophthalmalogical examination are important, when the syndrome is considered to be of central origin, to eliminate, if possible, the presence of an intracranial lesion. A pneumoencephalogram, however, is usually not indicated as a rapidly growing intracranial tumor will usually cause death within five to seven months, or by the time precocity is established, whereas a hamartoma may be impossible to diagnose even with this diagnostic aid. Finally, a thyroid study is indicated if any signs of hypothyroidism are present.

Treatment of precocious puberty has as its objective two major purposes: (1) suppression of menstruation, ovulation, and fertility, and (2) prevention of excessively short stature. Treatment with progestational agents, preferably those without androgen or estrogen activity, will successfully accomplish the first objective. Provera, 10 mg. daily, is probably as successful as any current therapy available. Long acting derivatives of this compound, medroxyprogesterone acetate (MPA), 100 to 200 mg. every 2 weeks has also been used. This excessive hypothalamic suppression, however, does not seem to be justified, because there is little evidence that such therapy will prevent early epiphyseal closure leading to excessively short stature. Richman et al. concluded that it did not prevent skeletal maturation and that the clinical and laboratory toxicity precluded its further use. The major complication which these authors reported was mild blood pressure elevation. Chlorpromazine in 20-mg. daily doses has also been advocated on the basis of its general depressive effect on the hypothalamus. Too few cases have as yet been sufficiently followed to know if it will effectively combat the skeletal disturbances, and it also seems like a very drastic suppressive therapy. Two experimental drugs are currently being used in research centers. Danazol, an anti-gonadotrophic steroid, has been used with some success, and Bossi et al. have reported a small series of 5 children treated with cyproterone acetate, an anti-androgen. Although their data indicated that both sexual development and skeletal maturation were inhibited by this steroid, Werder et al. concluded that the drug did not affect growth. Tumors of whatever site must be treated surgically or by some form of radiation therapy; whereas precocious puberty associated with hypothyroidism will respond to appropriate replacement therapy.

REFERENCES

Aksel, S., and Jones, G. S.: Etiology and treatment of dysfunctional uterine bleeding. Obstet. Gynec., 44: 1, 1974.

Benjamin, F.: Glucose tolerance in dysfunctional uterine bleeding and in carcinoma of endometrium. Brit. Med. J., 5181: 1243, 1960.

Bergman, P.: The clinical treatment of anovulation. Int. J. Fertil., 3: 27, 1958.

Bishop, P. M. F., and Cabral de Almeida, J. C.: Treatment of functional menstrual disorders with norethisterone. Brit. Med. J., 5179: 1103, 1960.

Bossi, E., Zurbrugg, R. P., and Joss, E. E.: Improvement of adult height prognosis in precocious puberty by cyproterone acetate. Acta Paediat. Scand., 62: 405, 1973.

Brewer, J. I., and Miller, W. H.: Post-menopausal uterine bleeding. Amer. J. Obstet. Gynec., 67: 988, 1954.

Brown, J. B., Kellar, R., and Matthew, G. D.: Preliminary observations on urinary oestrogen excretion in certain gynaecological disorders. J. Obstet. Gynaec. Brit. Comm., 66: 177, 1959.

Charles, D., Barr, W., and McEwan, H. P.: The use of clomiphene in dysfunctional bleeding due to endometrial hyperplasia. J. Obstet. Gynaec. Brit. Comm., 89: 66, 1964.

Collipp, P. J., Kaplan, S. A., Boyd, D. C., Plachte, F., and Kogut, M. D.: Constitutional isosexual precocious puberty: Effects of medroxy progesterone acetate therapy. Amer. J. Dis. Child., 108: 399, 1964.

Corscaden, J. A., Fertig, J. W., and Gusberg, S. B.: Carcinoma subsequent to radiotherapeutic menopause. Amer. J. Obstet. Gynec., 51: 1, 1946.

Costin, G., Kershnar, A. K., Kogert, M. D., and Turkington, R. W.: Prolactin activity in juvenile hypothyroidism and precocious puberty. Pediatrics, 50: 881, 1972.

Faulkner, F. L.: An injection study of the blood vessels of the bleeding uterus. Amer. J. Obstet. Gynec., 61: 766, 1951.

Firat, D., and Stutzman, L. S.: Thrombocyte levels after administration of equine estrogens. Proc. Soc. Exp. Biol. Med., 103: 474, 1960.

Fraser, I. S., Michie, E. A., Wide, L., and Baird, D. T.: Pituitary gonadotropins and ovarian function in adolescent dysfunctional uterine bleeding. J. Clin. Endocr. Metab., 37: 407, 1973.

Gribb, J. J.: Hysteroscopy, an aid in gynecologic diagnosis. Obstet. Gynec., 15: 593, 1960.

Holmstrom, E. G.: Progesterone treatment of anovulatory bleeding. Amer. J. Obstet. Gynec., 68: 1321, 1954.

Jones, G. E. S., and Te Linde, R. W.: An evaluation of progesterone therapy in treatment of endometrial hyperplasia. Bull. Hosp., 71: 282, 1942.

Jones, G. E. S., and Te Linde, R. W.: Survey of functional uterine bleeding with special reference to progesterone therapy. Amer. J. Obstet. Gynec., 57: 854, 1949.

Jones, H. W.: Functional bleeding with special reference to that associated with secretory endometrium. Amer. J. Obstet. Gynec., 35: 64, 1938.

Kelly, J. V.: Intravenous estrogen therapy: an assessment. Obstet. Gynec., 17: 199, 1961.

Kendle, F. W.: Case of precocious puberty in a female cretin. Brit. Med. J., 1: 246, 1905.

Kudish, H. G., and Rapaport, S. I.: The failure of intravenous estrogens (Premarin) to affect plasma clotting factors in humans. J. Urol., 83: 730, 1960.

Lathrop, C. A., and Carlisl, W. T.: Oral toluidine blue in the treatment of hypermenorrhea. Amer. J. Obstet. Gynec., 64: 1376, 1952.

Marin Bonachera, E., and Botella, Llusia, J.:La duración del desprendimiento menstrual en relación con la así llamada descamación irregular del endometrio. Rev. Mex. Cir. Ginec. Cancer, 26: 109, 1958.

Markee, J. E.: Morphological basis for menstrual bleeding. Anat. Rec., *94:* 481, 1946.

Mazer, C., and Mazer, M.: Treatment of dysfunctional uterine bleeding with testosterone propionate. Endocrinology, *24:* 599, 1939.

McLennan, C. E.: Irregular sheeding. Amer. J. Obstet. Gynec., *64:* 988, 1952.

Mitch, W. E., Spivak, J. L., Spangler, D. B., and Bell, W. R.: Thrombotic thrombocytopenic purpura presenting with gynecological manifestations. Lancet, *1:* 849, 1973.

Novak, E.: Hyperplasia of endometrium. Amer. J. Obstet. Gynec., *75:* 996, 1917.

Novak, E., and Hurd, G. B.: Use of anterior pituitary luteinizing substance in treatment of functional uterine bleeding. Amer. J. Obstet. Gynec., *22:* 501, 1931.

Novak, E., and Martzloff, K. H.: Hyperplasia of endometrium; a clinical and pathological study. Amer. J. Obstet. Gynec., *8:* 385, 1924.

Radman, H. M.: Blood dyscrasia as a causative factor in abnormal uterine bleeding. Amer. J. Obstet. Gynec., *79:* 1, 1960.

Rice, G.: Hypermenorrhoea in the young hemodialysis patient. Amer. J. Obstet. Gynec., *116:* 539, 1973.

Ross, R. A.: Blood coagulation defects in obstetrics and gynecology. Amer. J. Obstet. Gynec., *86:* 77, 1963.

Schröder, R.: Anatomische Studien zur normalen und pathologischen physiologie des Menstruationszyklus. Arch. Gynaec., *104:* 27, 1915.

Seaman, A. J., and Benson, R. C.: Coagulation studies of patients with abnormal uterine bleeding. Amer. J. Obstet. Gynec., *79:* 5, 1960.

Sherman, B. M. T., and Koreman, S. G.: Hormonal features of the menstrual cycle in perimenopausal women; evidence for independent ovarian regulation of FSH. Endocrinology, *94:* (Abst. 276, Suppl.) A-193, 1974.

Sluder, H. H., and Lock, F. R.: Incidence and management of uterine bleeding in nonmalignant lesions. Southern Med. J., *44:* 820, 1951.

Southam, A. L.: A comparative study of the effect of the progestational agents in human menstrual abnormalities. Ann. N. Y. Acad. Sci., *71:* 666, 1958.

Southam, A. L.: The natural history of menstrual disorders. Ann. N. Y. Acad. Sci., *75:* 840, 1959.

Te Linde, R. W.: Causes of postmenopausal bleeding. Amer. J. Surg., *48:* 289, 1940.

Werder, E. A., Mürset, G., Zachmann, M., Brook, G. G. D., and Prader, A.: Treatment of precocious puberty with cyproterone acetate. Pediat. Res., *8:* 248, 1974.

Wilkins, L.: *The Diagnosis and Treatment of Endocrine Disorders in Childhood and Adolescence.* Charles C Thomas, Publisher, Springfield, Illinois, 1957.

Winter, J. S. D., and Faiman, C.: Development of cyclic pituitary-gonadal function in adolescent females. J. Clin. Endocr. Metab., *37:* 714, 1973.

Zuckerman, S.: Inhibition of menstruation and ovulation by means of testosterone propionate. Lancet, *2:* 676, 1937.

chapter 32

The Management of the Menopause

For a discussion of the endocrine and anatomical changes during the menopause the reader is referred to earlier chapters. In the present chapter we are concerned with the management of the woman who is passing through this epoch.

PHYSIOLOGY

It has been estimated that there are approximately 500,000 available oocytes at the menarche, and with every menstrual cycle a certain number of these are used up, and ultimately there is a complete loss of the follicles, resulting in gradual withdrawal of estrogen. Prior to this, however, there is complete loss of progesterone, since, in the aging ovary, anovulation is usual, resulting in unopposed estrogen stimulation, with endometrial hyperplasia and frequent irregular bleeding. Although the postmenopausal ovary may be completely lacking in follicles, which normally secrete the steroidal hormones, it should be remembered that many women are not totally devoid of estrogen, since the ovarian stroma may be converted into theca-like cells, with the capacity for steroidogenesis. This so-called "hyperthecosis" may be present in some degree in as many as one-third of all aging women, even though there has been a cessation of bleeding. As will be noted subsequently, the actual steroid produced by the postmenopausal ovary may well be an androgen, which is converted to estrogen at other areas of the body.

By definition, the term menopause means the final cessation of menses, whereas the climacteric implies a transitional period in the life of an individual during which the reproductive function is diminished and lost.

In past years it was estimated that among the women of the United States the average age for the menopause was approximately 48 years, whereas the span of the climacteric was in the nature of 4 years, between the ages of 46 and 50. Today, however, many gynecologists are impressed with the frequency with which apparently regular menstruation may persist into the mid-50s, and it would seem the most important factor in this respect is improved nutrition, although unquestionably certain genetic considerations must play a part.

It is interesting to note that the human female is the only animal incapable of reproduction until death. Since the average life span of the American woman today is almost 75 years, it follows that there is a rather long period of time during which she must get along without any appreciable ovarian function. The importance of this prolonged lack of steroidogenesis has created certain different feelings among various gynecologists, some of whom advocate no treatment, others temporary treatment, whereas a certain minority advocate prolonged replacement therapy for life. We disagree rather strenuously with the last approach, as will be noted subsequently (Treatment), and even more with the suggestion of certain gynecologists that cyclic therapy with sustained menstruation be maintained until the grave.

Until a short while ago, a discussion of the menopause involved only a brief review of the physiological changes occurring at the time, an evaluation of the symptomatology, and a list of the various types of hormonal therapy to be used if necessary, supplemented by a discussion of the place of psychotherapy and symptomatic treatment. In the past few years, there has been a radical change in viewpoint and there is a minority who would regard the menopause as a possible pathological state rather than a physiological one and discuss therapeutic prevention rather than the amelioration of symptoms. This changing viewpoint has been brought about largely through the experimental work which is being done on what, if any, role estrogens play in coronary artery disease and arteriosclerosis. These concepts and their relation to therapy will be discussed below.

SYMPTOMATOLOGY

Before discussing the symptomatology of the menopause, it is necessary to realize that only 25% of all women have any symptoms which are severe enough to take them to the physician. The other 75% simply stop menstruating and life continues as before with health and happiness unimpaired.

The two classic symptoms of the menopause are *vasomotor instability*, characterized by the hot flush, and irregularities or cessation of menses. A veritable host of other problems may be enumerated, many of which are almost certainly of psychogenic origin.

PATHOGENESIS

The menopause (cessation of menses) is undoubtedly due to failing ovarian function, and although it is not known what specific factors initiate the hot flush, it is certainly well substantiated that estrogen withdrawal is paramount.

Many individuals have felt that it is not the low estrogen per se but the resultant high FSH that is responsible for the vasomotor instability. Greenblatt, however, suggests that these are due to a drastically altered hypothalamus, as a result of withdrawal of estrogen. In any case, although the cessation of menses used to be considered synonymous with complete absence of function, it is now recognized that this is not usually the case. Some steroidal activity is maintained in the majority of women over at least a 10-year period.

In certain instances the source of this hormone seems to be the ovary, as indicated by the histochemical studies of E. R. Novak *et al.* (Chapter 15). As noted subsequently, however, the actual steroid produced may be an androgen, which is converted into estrogen in certain poorly defined sites.

According to the studies of Masukawa, *severe atrophy* of the menopausal vaginal smear is found in only 25% of the patients *within* a 10-year postmenopausal period and in only 37% of patients *after* 10 years. Twenty per cent of menopausal women continue to show estrogenic smears for approximately 10 years postmenopausally, and urinary estrogen excretion is maintained at levels compatible with those found in the early follicular phase of the cycle, 5 to 15 µg./24 hours. The source of this residual estrogen has been disputed. Grodin *et al.* calculate that all estrone in menopausal women is derived from peripheral conversion of androstenedione (ADD), which in turn is of adrenal origin. Bullbrook *et al.* have shown that oophorectomy after the menopause lowers the estrogen excretion from a level of 5 to 15 μg. to between 2 and 5 μg./24 hours. These authors also described cyclic excretion of estrogen for a short while, at least in a postmenopausal woman.

Poliak *et al.* report a marked increase in urinary estrogens following the administration of 50,000 I.U. of chorionic gonadotrophin to women at least 15 years postmenopausal. Ovulation with apparently normal corpus luteum steroidogenesis was induced in one woman of 54 years whose last menstrual period had occurred four years previous to stimulation. The menopausal ovary is therefore capable of substantial steroidogenesis. The most likely steroid is ADD, for this is the preferential steroid synthesized by the ovarian stroma.

Thus it would seem that although menopausal women do have an estrogen milieu which is lower than that during the menstrual years, it is not negligible or absent. The menopause can perhaps be regarded as a physiological phenomenon which is protective in nature—protective from undesirable reproduction and the associated growth stimuli.

As estrogen decreases, pituitary gonadotrophin secretion rises in an effort to whip the flagging ovarian function. The increase in the urinary gonadotorphin is seen in Tables 32.1 and 32.2; the mean value between the ages of 36 and 49 years being 21.4 m.u./24 hours while the mean value after the age of 50 years rises to 210 m.u./24 hours. As indicated in Chapter 31, FSH apparently rises prior to LH, substantiating the theory of a modulator of FSH function in the developing follicles. Once elevated, the gonadotrophin level is sustained throughout the remainder of the patient's life.

The vasomotor instability which causes

Table 32.1

The Excretion of Gonadotrophins in Mouse Units per 24 Hours in 64 Postmenopausal Women Aged 51 to 87 Years[*]

50–64 Years		65–74 Years		75–87 Years	
Age	Gonadotrophin	Age	Gonadotrophin	Age	Gonadotrophin
51	320	65	57	75	165
51	450	65	255	75	135
52	290	65	110	77	115
52	270	66	135	77	140
52	80	66	265	77	130
53	66	68	185	77	90
53	320	69	80	77	185
53	205	69	145	77	145
54	70	69	140	77	150
54	250	69	150	77	92
54	425	70	72	79	145
56	145	70	115	79	118
56	140	72	205	79	120
56	230	73	68	79	220
57	200	73	63	79	140
57	215	73	125	80	160
58	78	74	135	81	151
58	64	74	120	84	125
58	280	74	115	86	195
59	120	74	295	87	185
59	240				
61	66				
61	150				
61	265				
Mean 210.0		Mean 141.8		Mean 143.5	
Min. 64		Min. 57		Min. 90	
Max. 450		Max. 295		Max. 220	

[*] From Johnsen, S. G.: Acta Endocr. (Kobenhavn), *41:* 209, 1959.

the hot flush is undoubtedly due to a disturbance or imbalance of the autonomic nervous system, and Reynolds believes that the estrogen exerts a protective action on the subcutaneous blood vessels. When this cushion is removed the response to any stimulus such as heat, emotion, embarrassment, or exercise causes a rapid reaction bringing about the blush. The specific inciting factor, however, is as yet unknown, although it has been fairly well established that it is not serotonin.

Table 32.2

The Excretion of Gonadotrophins in Mouse Units per 24 Hours in 38 Normal Women of Menstrual Age*

18–34 Years		35–49 Years	
Age	Gonado-trophin	Age	Gonado-trophin
18	32	36	66
20	20	36	13
21	13	37	36
22	16	37	12
23	35	37	8
25	35	38	17
26	7	39	8
26	31	39	7
26	15	40	16
27	26	40	28
27	8	41	34
27	9	42	<3 (2?)
27	21	42	10
28	14	42	14
29	11	44	78
30	3	46	20
31	34	46	8
34	13	49	8
34	23		
34	9		

Mean 18.8	Mean 21.4
Min. 3	Min. <3 (2?)
Max. 34	Max. 78

* From Johnsen, S. G.: Acta Endocr. (Kobenhavn.), *31:* 209, 1959.

DIAGNOSIS

Although the clinical symptoms of vasomotor instability in conjunction with irregularities or cessation of menses are pathognomonic, the laboratory finding which confirms the diagnosis of the menopause is an elevated serum pituitary gonadotrophin assay for FSH and LH. Values for FSH by radioimmunoassay are usually 1000 ng/ml or above while LH values are above 400 ng/ml. These laboratory assays must be used *only* in conjunction with the clinical findings and both FSH and LH values obtained as the level of LH can be equally high in the ovulatory phase of the cycle.

Premature Menopause

Diagnosis of the premature menopause, especially in very young girls, is sometimes difficult and it must be remembered that this condition can occur at any age. The youngest reported case of which we are aware was 18 years of age.

If the pituitary FSH values are elevated and the patient complains of hot flushes, the diagnosis is fairly well substantiated. However, if there are no hot flushes, in the presence of an elevated gonadotrophin assay, it may be wise in the very young patient to use a gonadotrophin stimulation test to differentiate between a premature menopause with ovarian failure, the Stein-Leventhal syndrome and various psychogenic forms of amenorrhea. The routine for this test is the same as outlined in Chapter 31 under "Treatment of Hypogonadotrophic Forms of Amenorrhea." Occasionally, it is necessary to perform a laparotomy and actually biopsy the ovaries to make the diagnosis of the insensitive ovary syndrome (Chapter 30).

TREATMENT

General Considerations

The treatment of the menopause is complicated at the present time by the uncertain medical concept that estrogenic hormones may protect against arteriosclerotic cardiovascular disease. These data have been interpreted by some to indicate that all menopausal women should have replacement therapy and that treatment should be continued indefinitely. The increasing life span of women makes such considerations extremely important, for were these tenets accepted a large portion of our population would receive regular daily hormonal therapy. Although estrogens do reduce the abnormal *cholesterol to phospholipid ratio,* the exact relation of abnormal lipid ratio to arteriosclerosis has not been satisfactorily demonstrated. In addition, there are specific medications available for accomplishing these lipid changes. Until a more precise rationale for estrogen therapy has been demonstrated, it would seem wiser to treat *only* those menopausal women who have symptoms or those who have signs of estrogen deficiency and medical findings which warrant therapy or prophylactic estrogen. To embark upon the wholesale administration of ovarian hormones to our aging population is currently unjustifiable, a position by no means unchallenged in other sectors.

However, just as it seems unreasonable and unphysiological to give estrogens to women in the normal menopausal age group, it does seem reasonable and physiological to administer hormones to those patients who are symptomatic or have a premature menopause, be it artificial or spontaneous. This is especially important in view of the predilection for osteoporosis which such patients exhibit.

The therapy for acute menopausal symptoms must be individualized, and although some form of estrogen therapy is specific, reassurance with minimal sedation or tranquilizing agents may be adequate if the symptoms are mild. For those patients in whom estrogens are contraindicated, such as patients who have been treated for estrogen dependent carcinoma of the female genital tract or for breast tumors, sedation, supplemented by vitamin E and B-complex, are used.

Testosterone is a poor substitute for estrogens and usually must be given in androgenic amounts if an effect is to be secured. The masculinizing symptoms can be as distressing to the patient as flushes or sweats. On occasion, however, it may be useful in the patient who develops mastodynia following estrogen alone, or in the frigid woman in an effort to improve libido and general well-being. Androgens may be utilized alone, or more frequently in conjunction with estrogen therapy.

As indicated above there is a broad spectrum of symptoms and reaction to symptoms. Patients requiring therapy are those having (1) flushes severe enough to cause discomfort or embarrassment; (2) sweats and resultant insomnia with or without flushes; (3) dyspareunia, a late symptom usually due to senile vaginitis

and constriction; and (4) osteoporosis, the latest manifestation of all, which is usually managed in conjunction with an internist or an orthopedist and the response to therapy is most gratifying.

Hormone Therapy

The aim of proper hormonal therapy for acute symptoms is to control these as rapidly as possible with as little medication as possible and to discontinue treatment as soon as possible. If one is able to institute therapy at the onset of symptoms, all of these criteria can usually be met. However, if a patient has been suffering from flushes for many years, she will probably require prolonged therapy. In some instances, it may be impossible to discontinue medication under these circumstances, although every effort should be made to achieve this.

Regimens of treatment can be divided into four types: (1) those used for a menopause occurring at the expected time; (2) those used for the premature menopause; (3) those used when symptoms of senile vaginitis or urethritis predominate; and (4) regimens used for the late symptoms of osteoporosis.

Treatment for the Menopause at the Expected Time. A dosage of 1 mg. of stilbestrol or its equivalent daily is usually sufficient to render the patient almost asymptomatic within a two-week period. As the flush is the most common as well as the most objective symptom of the menopause, patients are asked to record on a large calendar page the number of flushes per day and return to the office within two weeks. If this record indicates a sharp reduction of symptoms the dosage can be reduced by half at this time. If symptoms recur, the reduction has been too rapid and a higher dosage must be resumed at once and continued for another week or until reduction can be accomplished without recurrence of symptoms. As there is a great individual variation in response to estrogen therapy, no scheme can be regarded as infallible but must be used only as a norm from which to deviate. Individualization of therapy is highly desirable.

The vaginal smear with maturation index (Chapter 36) has, on occasion, proved to be a valuable adjunct in controlling the estrogen dosage. However, if a record of flushes is kept, this serves the same purpose even though symptomatology and cytopathology do not always parallel one another. The psychosomatic aspects of menopausal symptoms must always be borne in mind.

If too high an estrogen dosage is used over too long a period, vaginal bleeding is apt to occur. Stilbestrol and estradiol are especially prone to produce this untoward complication. When bleeding does occur, a curettage is mandatory despite the presumptive diagnosis of bleeding from exogenous steroid therapy. Headaches, nausea, and breast tenderness or swelling may also be sequelae of estrogenic medication.

Testosterone used in conjunction with estrogens has been advocated for the management of menopausal symptoms, but it does not seem superior to the use of unopposed estrogens. In our experience it does not tend to reduce the problems of bleeding occasionally associated with estrogenic therapy. For those who advocate the use of estrogens to prevent or improve an abnormal serum lipid pattern, testosterone is contraindicated as it nullifies the effect of the estrogen according to Marmorston *et al.*

Some have advocated *progesterone* along with estrogen as treatment for the menopause, with the thought that any hyperplastic or neoplastic effects of estrogen would be minimized by the concomitant progesterone. This seems expensive and needless, for if estrogen is administered in interrupted fashion, there is little likelihood of any serious sequelae. In addition, certain of the progestins are androgenic and may negate the desired effect of the estrogen. Many gynecologists prefer to administer estrogens 3 out of 4 weeks, gradually decrease the dosage over the course of time, and stop it entirely when it no longer seems to be needed by the patient. Hormone therapy may be necessary for a relatively short period of time, although in some individuals a number of years are required before hormonal equilibrium is obtained after which exogenous therapy is unnecessary.

Premature Menopause. When the uterus is present, the type of replacement therapy depends upon whether or not it is psychologically advantageous to produce regular menses. Usually, if sufficient time has been taken to educate the patient this is not necessary. However, when the production of regular menses seems desirable, as in younger girls living in close contact with others in boarding school, the minimal estrogenic dosage which will induce bleeding should be used. This varies in our experience from between 0.2 to 1 mg. of stilbestrol or its equivalent given for the first 25 days of each month. Progesterone or one of the synthetic substitutes must be given during the last three days of estrogen therapy, on the 23rd, 24th, and 25th day of each month; 30 mg. of ethisterone or its equivalent are sufficient for this purpose. There should then be an interruption of 5 or 6 days and pills should be resumed again on the first day of the following month. This rest period allows the endometrium to shed and thus usually prevents the occurrence of irregular or profuse bleeding.

When it is unnecessary to induce a menstrual flow, the amount of estrogen required to produce bleeding is determined and the dosage just under this amount is used in the identical manner as described above: 25 days each month with a 5-day rest period. After regulation is accomplished, patients are checked every 6 months the first year and then at yearly intervals unless bleeding or breast symptoms warrant additional examinations. An endometrial biopsy should be obtained perhaps yearly to ensure that an abnormal growth pattern is not being induced.

For the woman under 40 who needs castration, it is sometimes desirable to insert one or two 25-mg. estradiol pellets into the incision, and, at the 6-week postoperative examination, to prescribe estrogen suppositories (stilbestrol, 0.5 mg.) during the first 3 to 7 days each month, depending upon symptoms and vaginal cytology. Such a regimen usually prevents flushes from developing and maintains vaginal pliability and lubrication (Hunter *et al.*).

Therapy in all cases should be maintained until the age of 45 or 50 years and then should be discontinued slowly over a year's time. Again, no rule of thumb will prove successful for all women and each must be individualized according to her needs.

Considerable care must be utilized in treating these women with estrogens over the course of many years, even though it is given in interrupted fashion. Cutler *et al.* as well as others have reported cases of gonadal dysgenesis with treatment by estrogens where the patients developed adenocarcinoma despite cyclic administration of the drug. This has been discussed more fully in Chapter 15.

Senile Vaginitis and Urethritis. The predominating symptoms of senile vaginitis are discharge, itching, burning, and dyspareunia. The symptoms of senile urethritis are urinary frequency and nocturia unassociated with infection. The most effective therapy for these local symptoms is by the vaginal route.

If constriction of the vaginal lumen has occurred, this is an additional factor causing dyspareunia and some form of manual dilatation will also be necessary to reestablish normal function and painless intercourse. Plastic test tubes or wax candles in graduated sizes make the most satisfactory dilators. The response of senile urethritis to estrogen suppositories is frequently dramatic.

Osteoporosis. Osteoporosis is characterized by the X-ray evidence of decalcification of bone, decrease in stature, kyphosis, and eventually severe joint pain and debility associated with multiple fractures. The role played by steroid hormones in maintenance of calcium in bone has not been completely elucidated by the biochemists, but is clearly demonstrated clinically in the occurrence of epiphyseal closure at puberty and osteoporosis associated with conditions causing gonadal hypoplasia, for example, Cushing's disease and acromegaly.

The incidence of menopausal osteoporosis among the general population is difficult to estimate, as is the frequency of its occurrence after a premature menopause, but it is certainly not an uncommon X-ray finding 10 years or more after cessation of ovarian function. Clinical osteoporosis, "backache and pain associated with objective evidence of fractures or loss of skeletal mineral," is a much more uncommon finding.

The mode of action of estrogen primarily in the rapid relief of symptoms is not determined. Its effect on activation of growth hormone with the associated metabolic improvement is one possibility. A hitherto undetermined effect upon thyrocalcitonin has also been suggested.

An instructive report by Caldwell on the experimental production and treatment of osteoporosis in the rat, indicates that after removal of gonads and adrenal glands all animals developed osteoporosis within 100 days (perhaps the equivalent of 20 years in the human life span). Recovery was most rapid and complete with estradiol treatment alone. Lesser degrees of recovery occurred with combinations of estradiol and testosterone and virtually no improvement was obtained with testosterone only.

The experimental results are in accord with the clinical findings, for although testosterone, cortisone, and the snythetic anabolic steriods have been advocated in the treatment of this condition, it is our experience that none, either alone or in combination with estrogens, has proved more effective than estrogens alone. The most satisfactory, and least expensive, schedule used for the treatment of menopausal osteoporosis is 1 mg. of stilbestrol daily for 25 days each month, ending with a single monthly injection of 50 mg. of progesterone or a 3-day course of an oral progestogen, 30 mg. of ethisterone or its equivalent daily. This schedule will usually produce monthly bleeding which, although troublesome, is warranted by the remarkable relief from painful bone symptoms which ensues. Relief from pain can be expected within the first month and it is not unusual to have a return of function concomitantly.

Initial investigators were surprised and disappointed not to see evidence of X-ray changes associated with the dramatic clinical improvement. It is now thought that the production of such X-ray evidence takes a protracted period of time probably amounting to 10 years or so. Albright suggested using the height as a standard of improvement, because all patients show a progressive loss of height with the passage of time. As improvement occurs and osteoporosis is arrested, the height becomes stationary. Hernberg has demonstrated the value of this criterion and the arrest of height loss by the prophylactic use of estrogens (Fig. 32.1).

Davis, in conjunction with various radiologists, has developed a radiologic technique for evaluating bone density, and they feel that postmenopausal osteoporosis is relatively common. How important a role the lack of estrogen plays in the production of this disease is not completely certain since males do develop osteoporosis, although less commonly than women. Nevertheless, such gynecologists as Krokowski feel that there is no relation between estrogen and osteoporosis, and he feels that the term "postmenopausal osteoporosis" should be abandoned.

Although it is a clinically undisputed fact that estrogen is therapeutically effective for relief of pain in symptomatic osteoporosis, there is some question about the use of estrogen for the prevention of asymptomatic osteoporosis. Data of Aitken et al. seem to substantiate the fact that it is easier to prevent changes than to repair them. It has been shown that density decreases with age and at a steady rate not apparently related to any one event in the female. These data suggest that perhaps the most important factor in maintaining bone density is exercise. Prolonged immobilization from any cause is followed by osteoporosis and no amount of calcium or steroid avail. Only the demands of use will increase the bony matrix. Perhaps a game of tennis or jogging once around the block, if other more productive physical activities are not at hand, is a more effective way of maintaining bony density in aging women than steroid therapy.

More recently it has been suggested that fluoride therapy may be beneficial, since it tends to increase bone density, though in large doses it may cause certain toxic side effects (Rasmussen and Bordier).

Hypertensive Cardiovascular Disease

The clinical observation that vascular disease is less common among young women than among men in a similar age group is complicated by a multiplicity of factors and it cannot be assumed that estrogen is the most important one. To cite only two major causes which are also undoubtedly involved, *stress* from the strenuous competitive activities of man concerned with making a place of social and economic security for himself and family is far greater than the *stress* to which the average woman is exposed. *Excessive smoking,* which has also been

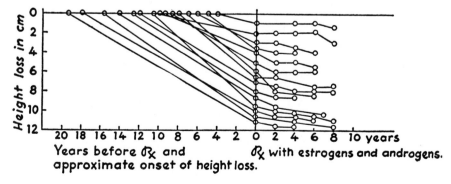

32.1. Treatment of patient with postmenopausal osteoporosis. In most cases there was a cessation of height loss within 2 years after institution of therapy. (From Hernberg, C. A.: Acta Endocr. (Kobenhavn.), *34:* 51, 1960.)

seriously implicated by Hammond and Horn in the production of arteriosclerosis, has, until quite recently, been practiced largely by men.

The two major pieces of evidence which link estrogens with cardiovascular disease are first the statistical studies on the presumed differential occurrence of the disease in normal young men and women, and in menopausal and castrate women with and without estrogen replacement therapy, and second the effect of estrogens on the serum cholesterol to phospholipid ratio. Of still controversial nature is the relationship between these blood changes and arteriosclerosis. Experimental work has demonstrated in the rat that a high cholesterol to phospholipid ratio predisposes to cardiac arteriosclerosis and hypertension. In the rabbit, serum lipids do not change with estrogen administration and estrogens have no effect upon the occurrence of arteriosclerosis in this species.

Findings in the human are interestingly similar to those in the rat in that Wuest, Dry, and Edwards found increased coronary atherosclerosis and hypertensive disease in women who had oophorectomies 10 years or more before death, when compared to normal women of similar ages. Novak and Williams, in a paralled study, investigating atherosclerosis of the coronary arteries and the aorta, found no difference in the amount of atheromatous disease between castrate and normal women in comparable age groups. Davis demonstrated increased electrocardiogram changes and hypertension in postcastrate patients as well as high serum cholesterol to phospholipid ratio. These changes could be reversed by the administration of estrogens. Marmorston et al. in a similar study of the effect of estrogens on serum lipids showed that the addition of testosterone negated the estrogen effect.

Indeed more recent evidence suggests that, far from being beneficial as a prophylaxis against arteriosclerotic vascular disease, estrogen might be an inducing factor. Although the potential dangers of the contraceptive pills are not completely clear at this writing, there is some evidence that they may lead to thrombosis and other cardiovascular complications by virtue of the estrogenic component. It has also been indicated that male patients treated with estrogens because of carcinoma of the prostate develop 3 times as high an incidence of arteriosclerotic heart disease than untreated patients. Berkson has likewise pointed out that in certain non-American communities, such as Bantu Africa, Japan, and Italy, there is an equal incidence of cardiovascular disease in both male and female and not the low incidence in the menstruating female as noted in the American literature. Are we to conclude that the non-American brand of estrogen is less effective in guarding against the advent of cardiovascular disease, or is there some other factor in the American way of life that plays a contributing role? We suspect the latter.

Randall collected statistics from New York State and concluded that, although cardiovascular and hypertensive disease was probably less among a group of estrogen-treated castrate women, the incidence of tumors of all sites was probably increased. Statistics of Mustacchi and Gordan concerning the incidence of neoplastic disease are not as convincing as Randall's figures, because both of these studies are composed of much smaller groups of patients even though they have been followed for a long period.

Most of the clinical experience and investigative work indicate that the average menopausal woman is not truly estrogen deficient. Estrogen levels necessary for adequate maintenance of supporting tissues are much lower than those necessary for physiology of reproduction. Estrogen protection in experimental animals is species specific and can be demonstrated only under specific dietary conditions emphasizing the broad nutritional and metabolic aspects involved. In addition, the great importance of genetic aspects involved has been well substantiated.

One should hesitate to treat menopausal women prophylactically for cardiovascular diseases after a screening process consisting of a vaginal smear and an evaluation of the serum cholesterol to phospholipid ratio. If the vaginal smear is atrophic, indicating a true estrogen deficiency or an elevated serum cholesterol to phospholipid ratio, it may be justifiable to institute prolonged but interrupted estrogen therapy with close observation for any clinical effect. Marmorston *et al.* have demonstrated that small dosages of estrogen are as efficient as large doses in lowering the serum cholesterol to phospholipid ratio. For the comfort, and perhaps the safety of the patient, one should maintain hormonal administration at the lowest therapeutic level. The addition of either testosterone or a progestogen to this therapy destroys its efficacy.

Climacteric Arthritis or Arthralgia

This is an affection concerning which there is no unanimity of opinion. Holmes limits the term to arthritis developing five or six years preceding or following the menopause. Many internists agree that a small proportion of menopausal women develop a rather characteristic mild form of arthritis which affects especially the knees, and which is characterized by pain and moderate swelling of these joints. A frequent feature is tenderness above the condyles. We have observed quite a number of cases which seem to fall into this category. Whatever the exact etiology may be, our experience has been that estrogenic therapy appears to be a valuable adjuvant to other forms of treatment, the condition usually clearing within a few months.

Possible Carcinogenic Hazard of Estrogenic Therapy

A question which has caused some concern is whether or not prolonged estrogen therapy can predispose to, or incite, the development of cancer. This concern is based on the demonstrated chemical interrelation of certain estrogenic and carcinogenic substances, and upon the experimental production of neo-plastic-like and even metastasizing neoplastic lesions by excessive and prolonged estrogen administration. Meissner induced endometrial carcinomas (Chapter 15) which progressed to metastasize and kill the host even after cessation of the exogenous hormone. Thus, there is good reason to accept the correctness of the statement made by Loeb as far back as 1918, that estrogens can be of importance in the development of cancer in those organs and tissues which are normally estrogen dependent, *e.g.,* the genital tract and breasts.

Although the endometrium is the tissue above all others which is responsive to estrogen, it had not, until recently, been possible to produce experimental carcinoma of the endometrium by means of prolonged estrogen therapy. Nevertheless, a number of endometrial cancers in women have been reported following estrogen therapy, and Gusberg has noted this sequel in 23 patients within 20 years. However, such case reports are of little statistical value, since the *post hoc, ergo propter hoc* dictum cannot be ignored. In all experimental studies, it has been emphasized that the uninterrupted prolonged administration of moderate dosage is far more likely to be carcinogenic than is even a huge dosage for a short time. In a few of the reported human cases this feature of prolonged estrogen therapy has been suggestively conspicuous, as in the case reported in 1951 by Novak, in which the patient had been taking 1 mg. of stilbestrol orally for 10 years. We may also refer again to the paper by Randall, Britch, and Harkins discussed under estrogen therapy for the prevention of arteriosclerosis. These authors suggest, from statistical data, that tumors of all sites may be increased in women who are receiving prolonged replacement estrogenic therapy after the menopause.

Any gynecologist who spends time in the pathology laboratory can be impressed by the large number of postmenopausal endometria in which extreme degrees of hyperplasia and even endometrial adenocarcinoma are observed in women who have a history of prolonged estrogen therapy. The recent study by Migaki *et al.* suggests a very high incidence of endometrial carcinoma in cows slaughtered from 1963 to 1969, during which period there was a wide spread practice of adding diethylstilbestrol to cattle feed, although admittedly there is no known incidence of specific bovine cancer in untreated animals. In any case most gynecologists feel much freer to use estrogen therapy in the woman who has had a hysterectomy, and who is suffering from genuine bona fide vasomotor symptoms.

Although it seems clear that estrogen is not carcinogenic in the same sense that methylcholanthrene is, it is undeniably a substance which promotes growth. Evidence of a worrisome nature is beginning to accrue that, at least in certain individuals, it may predispose to cancer. Two male transsexuals, treated for long periods with estrogen, have developed carcinoma of the breast, a very rare occurrence among men. Stamler has reported the occurrence of bilateral breast cancer in one of some 500 men receiving estrogen for prophylactic treatment of cardiovascular disease. Bilateral breast malignancy has never been reported to occur spontaneously in a male.

Supportive Therapy

Often the best supportive therapy for the menopausal woman is a sympathetic listener and a doctor who will take the time to explain the normal physiology underlying the menopause. A word of advice, encouragement, or comfort concerning environmental factors which may be aggravating her physiological readjustment may be more valuble than pills. Phenobarbital, 32 mg., once or twice a day or only when the patient is under stress is an old standby but one which is hard to improve upon. Tranquilizers in moderation will also often carry a patient through a particularly difficult phase; however, it is certainly unwise to prescribe these drugs in lieu of an office visit or a little time spent with the patient.

Psychosomatic Measures

The only treatment necessary for a large proportion of menopausal patients is reassurance and education by the physician. It is surprising how many women, including a good many who are otherwise intelligent, and perhaps well educated, have wrong ideas as to the nature and significance of the menopause. Some believe that it means the end of sexual life and of their physical attractiveness to their husbands. On this point they can be reassured, as the function of the ovary in the human, unlike that in the lower animals, appears to have little to do with libido, in which the psyche and adrenal play far more important roles. Indeed, in many women sexual response may be more highly developed after the menopause than before, especially in women who had been constantly apprehensive about impregnation in spite of contraception. The fear of conception has thus inhibited full enjoyment of coitus, and with the removal of this factor, sex enjoyment is increased.

Other women associate the menopause in a vague way with cancer, and they can of course be told that there is no such association. Again, many women are afraid they will become obese after the menopause; although most women do put on some weight at this time, the gain is usually moderate and easily controllable. To the thin, angular type of female, the menopause may actually be a physical blessing in that the figure becomes more rounded and attractive.

Finally, there are still not a few women who fear that the menopause carries with it a hazard of insanity. Psychoses not infrequently develop in middle life in either men or women, most often of the degenerative or involutional types, but it is age and not the menopause *per se* which is responsible. The slight depressions which a certain proportion of menopausal women exhibit, especially those with severe vasomotor symptoms and those burdened with domestic cares and worries, are not to be mistaken for the actual involutional psychoses. A new intellectual interest—especially if associated with monetary or emotional reward—is the best cure for this type of depression. Many women should be advised, now that families are raised, to refurbish their education and seek employment outside of the home.

SUMMARY

In spite of a healthier attitude among women in general as to the significance of the menopause, there is still a considerable substratum of misconceptions on this point, and the physician must take cognizance of this in the management of climacteric women. The majority of women at this phase need no treatment at all, many require only reassurance and education, and in only a comparatively small proportion is endocrine tharapy necessary.

Although there is perhaps no gynecological disorder in which the indication for organotherapy is more rational than in the treatment of typical climacteric symptoms, especially the vasomotor group, it must be remembered that many symptoms frequently observed in menopausal women are not directly due to the endocrine readjustments of this period, but are more logically explained as due to environmental and psychogenic factors. The physician who depends upon endocrine therapy alone will fall short of the requirements in many cases, and indiscriminate estrogenic therapy should certainly be frowned upon.

The question of the possible hazard of inciting malignancy in cancer-susceptible individuals cannot be decided arbitrarily in the present state of our knowledge, but it is fair to state that no impressive evidence of such a danger has as yet been adduced, after many years of use of the method. Certainly it would at the present time be carrying conservatism and caution to an extreme to deprive the menopausal woman of estrogen therapy when this is otherwise indicated, merely on the basis of this slight theoretical possibility.

REFERENCES

Albright, F., Bloomberg, E., and Smith, P. H.: Postmenopausal osteoporosis. Trans. Ass. Amer. Physicians, 55: 298, 1940.

Aitken, J. M., Hart, D. M., and Lindsay, R.: Oestrogen replacement therapy for prevention of osteoporosis after oophorectomy. Brit. Med. J., 3: 515, 1973.

Berkson, B. M., Stamler, J., and Cohen, D. B.: Ovarian function and coronary atherosclerosis. Clin. Obstet. Gynec., 7: 451, 1964.

Buckholz, R.: Researches on the influence of sex hormones on gonadotrophin excretion in humans. Geburtsh. Frauenheilk., 10: 851, 1959.

Bullbrook, R. D., and Greenwood, F. C.: Persistence of urinary oestrogen excretion after oophorectomy and adrenalectomy. Brit. Med. J., 5020: 662, 1957.

Caldwell, R. A.: The effect of sex hormones in experimental osteoporosis in rats. Brit. J. Exp. Path., 43: 103, 1962.

Cutler, D. S., et al.: Endometrial carcinoma after stilbestrol therapy in gonadal dysgenesis. New Eng. J. Med., 287: 628, 1972.

Davis, M. E.: Estrogen and the aging process. J.A.M.A., 196: 129, 1966.

Davis, M. E., Jones, R. J., and Jarolim, C.: Long-term estrogen substitution and atherosclerosis. Amer. J. Obstet. Gynec., 82: 1003, 1961.

Gardner, W. U.: Tumors in experimental animals receiving steroid hormones. Surgery, 16: 8, 1944.

Greenblatt, R. B.: Estrogen therapy for postmenopausal females. New Eng. J. Med., 272: 305, 1963.

Greenblatt, R. B.: Postmenopausal syndrome. Clinician, Medical Gynecology (Searle Laboratories), 1972.

Grodin, J. M., Siiteri, P. K., and MacDonald, P. C.: Source of estrogen production in postmenopausal women. J. Clin. Endocr. Metab., 36: 207, 1973.

Gusberg, S. B.: Precursors of corpus carcinoma, estrogens and adenomatous hyperplasia. Amer. J. Obstet. Gynec., 54: 905, 1947.

Gusberg, S. B., Jones, H. C., and Tovell, H. M. M.: Selection of treatment for corpus cancer. Amer. J. Obstet. Gynec., 80: 374, 1960.

Hammond, E. C., and Horn, D.: Smoking and death rates; report on forty-four months of follow-up of 187,783 men. I. Total mortality. J.A.M.A., 166: 1159, 1958.

Haymovits, A., and Rosen, J. F.: Human thyrocalcitonin. Endocrinology, 81: 995, 1967.

Hernberg, C. A.: Treatment of postmenopausal osteoporosis with oestrogens and androgens. Acta Endocr. (Kobenhavn), 34: 51, 1960.

Hunter, D. J. S., Akande, E. O., Carr, P., and Stalworthy, J.: The clinical and endocrinological effects of estradiol implants at the time of hysterectomy and bilateral salpingo-oophorectomy. J. Obstet. Gynaec. Brit. Comm., 80: 827, 1973.

Johnsen, S. G.: A clinical routine method for the quantitative determination of gonadotrophins in 24 hour urine samples. II. Normal values for men and women following age groups from prepuberty to senescence. Acta. Endocr. (Kobenhavn), 31: 209, 1959.

Kistner, R. W.: The menopause. Clin. Obstet. Gynec., 16: 106, 1973.

Krokowski, E.: Critical observations on the concept of postmenopausal osteoporosis. Geburtsh. Frauenheilk., 20: 968, 1966.

Lacassagne, A.: Sur la pathogenie de l'adenocarcinome mammaire de la souris. C. R. Soc. Biol. (Paris), 115: 937, 1934.

Lutwak, L.: Symposium on osteoporosis. J. Amer. Geriat. Soc., xvii: 115, 1969.

Margolis, S., and Baker, B. M.: Control of coronary heart

disease: Treatment of hyperlipidemia. Johns Hopkins
Med. J., *124:* 224, 1969.

Marmorston, J., Magidson, O., Lewis, J. J., Mehl, J.,
Moore, F. J., and Bernstein, J.: Effect of small doses of
estrogens on serum lipids in female patients with
myocardial infarction. New Eng. J. Med., *258:* 583,
1958.

Masukawa, T.: Vaginal smears in women past 40 years of
age with emphasis on their remaining hormonal
activity. Obstet. Gynec., *16:* 407, 1960.

Migaki, G., *et al.*: Pathology of bovine uterine adenocarcinoma. J. Amer. Vet. Med. Ass., *157:* 1577, 1970.

Mustacchi, P., and Gordon, G. S.: Frequency of cancer in
estrogen-treated osteoporotic women. In *Breast Cancer*
(*The Second Biennial Louisiana Cancer Conference,
New Orleans, January 22-23, 1958*), edited by A. Se-
galoff, St. Louis, The C. V. Mosby Company, 1958, p.
163.

Nordin, B. E. C., MacGregor, J., and Smith, D. A.: The incidence of osteoporosis in normal women: Its relation to
age and the menopause. Quart. J. Med., *xxxv:* 25, 1966.

Novak, E. R.: Replacement therapy of the menopause.
Johns Hopkins Med. J., *120:* 408, 1967.

Novak, E. R.: Uterine adenocarcinoma in a patient
receiving estrogens. Amer. J. Obstet. Gynec., *62:* 688,
1951.

Novak, E. R., and Williams, T. J.: Autopsy comparison of
cardiovascular changes in the castrate and normal
woman. Amer. J. Obstet. Gynec., *80:* 863, 1960.

Oliver, M. F., and Boyd, G. S.: Influence of reduction of
serum lipids on prognosis of coronary heart disease: a
five year study using oestrogen. Lancet, *2:* 499, 1961.

Poliak, A., Jones, G. E. S., Goldberg, B., Solomon, D., and
Woodruff, D.: Effect of human chorionic gonadotrophin
in postmenopausal women. Amer. J. Obstet. Gynec.,
101: 731, 1968.

Randall, C. L., Paloncek, F. P., Graham, J. B., and
Graham, S.: Causes of death in preclimacteric menorrhagia. Amer. J. Obstet. Gynec., *88:* 880, 1964.

Rasmussen, H., and Bordier, P.: *The Physiological and
Cellular Basis of Metabolic Bone Disease.* The
Williams & Wilkins Co., Baltimore, 1974.

Riley, G. M.: Endocrinology of the climacteric. Clin. Obstet.
Gynec., *7:* 432, 1964.

Robinson, R. W., Higano, N., and Cohen, W. D.: Effects of
estrogen on serum lipids in women. Arch. Intern. Med.
(Chicago), *100:* 739, 1957.

Stamler, J., Best, M. M., and Turner, J. D.: The status of
hormonal therapy for the primary and secondary prevention of atherosclerotic coronary heart disease. Progr.
Cardiov. Dis., *6:* 220, 1963.

Wilson, R. A.: The roles of estrogen and progesterone in
breast and genital cancer. J.A.M.A., *182:* 327, 1962.

Wuest, J., Dry, T. J., and Edwards, J. E.: The degree of
coronary sclerosis in bilaterally oophorectomized
women. Circulation, *7:* 801, 1953.

chapter 33

Dysmenorrhea, Premenstrual Tension and Related Disorders

DYSMENORRHEA

Dysmenorrhea, or menstrual pain, is probably the most common of all symptoms of gynecological disorders, and is the greatest cause of lost work hours among women. In spite of its frequency, and despite the fact that it has been the subject of extensive discussion and study for more than a hundred years, it remained one of the unsolved problems of gynecology.

Definition

Primary dysmenorrhea is menstrual pain observed in the absence of any noteworthy pelvic lesion and due to factors intrinsic in the uterus itself. Characteristically, the pain begins with the onset of menstruation and lasts over a few hours, although in some cases it may continue throughout several days. Although it is most frequently of a colicky, labor-like nature, the pain is sometimes described as of an aching character. It may be severe enough to require bed rest of one to several days each month, and may be accompanied by diarrhea, nausea, and vomiting. In the so-called *secondary variety,* demonstrable pelvic disease, notably endometriosis or intrauterine myomas or polyps, is present and is the apparent cause of the menstrual pain. Although dysmenorrhea may appear with the very first period, in a surprisingly large proportion of patients menstrual pain is not complained of until many months or even several years after the menarche. One explanation for this is that the inaugural cycles of many girls are of the anovulatory or oligoluteal type, and these are painless. When ovulation and normal corpus luteum function begins, primary dysmenorrhea may develop.

Causative Factors and Their Management

Many theories have been advanced to explain the etiology of primary dysmenorrhea. Although it seems clear that a number of factors may be concerned, it is also apparent that the exact pathophysiology is not understood. Some of the more plausible causes are enumerated below, with a discussion of the management of these various factors.

Psychogenic. Although many women suffer no discomfort whatsoever during menstruation, a moderate amount of pelvic heaviness and an occasional cramp may be considered as within normal limits. Indeed, the line between this normal discomfort and real dysmenorrhea is a very shadowy one, and the distinction is commonly made subjectively by the patient herself, on the basis of the incapacity produced. It is this subjective nature of the disorder which has made its study so difficult. It needs no more than a knowledge of human nature to justify the statement that the same degree of peripheral stimulus which in a phlegmatic individual will be expressed as a moderate discomfort will manifest itself in the high-strung, supersensitive girl by severe and perhaps incapacitating pain.

The psychogenic element, therefore, is one which can never be overlooked in the management of cases of dysmenorrhea, and a comprehensive study includes a consideration of factors which may accentuate the subjective element in the particular case. Among these are a congenitally unstable and high-strung nervous system, psychic trauma, especially when related to the menstrual periods, and lack of knowledge as to the significance and normality of the menstrual function. Many times a young girl, at the beginning of her menstrual life, is coddled by an overly anxious mother into the belief that menstruation is a time when she should really consider herself "unwell." To such a girl, especially if reared in a household where one or more members of the female contingent suffer from dysmenorrhea, the transition to menstrual invalidism is an easy one.

So important are these factors that there are some authorities who assert that the cause of primary dysmenorrhea is invariably psychogenic, a view which we do not share. On the other hand, we are convinced of the prime role of the psychogenic factor in many cases. To disclose such etiological factors, it is not necessary to submit the patient to a psychoanalytical examination, but it is important that the physician possess common sense and understanding. He must take the trouble to review the history of the disorder, especially in its inceptional phases, and to set before the patient the fact that menstruation should not normally interfere with work or activities. The physician can soon learn the probable importance or unimportance of the psychogenic factor in the individual case, and thus determine the importance or the futility of intensifying the psychotherapeutic approach. In at least a small proportion of cases, we believe it possible literally to talk a girl out of her dysmenorrhea through a policy of sympathetic understanding, reassurance, and education.

Constitutional. Closely and often indistinguishably linked with the purely subjective group of causes is the factor of constitutional debility of one sort or another, as observed in patients who because of anemia, tuberculosis, diabetes, overwork or many other possible causes, suffer a lowering of the threshold of pain, primarily because of physical factors, but often with a strong admixture of nervous and psychic factors as well. Certainly a part of the treatment of every case of dysmenorrhea should be to outline a regimen calculated to raise the patient's general health level in every possible way, and these measures alone will in some cases cause disappearance or marked amelioration of the dysmenorrhea.

Obstructive and Anatomical. One of the first theories for the explanation of dysmenorrhea was that it was due to obstructive cervical lesions, acute anteflexion of the uterus, or cervical stenosis. Although it is probably true that mechanical obstruction plays a part in the etiology of a small proportion of cases, no one now believes it to play the essential role in dysmenorrhea which was formerly attributed to it. In many dysmenorrheic women the uterus shows no flexion and the cervix is not stenosed, whereas in women who experience no pain whatsoever there may be a sharp anteflexion or retroflexion and the canal may be of pinpoint variety. Pedunculated submucous fibroids or endometrial polyps can also cause dysmenorrhea, because the musculature contracts in an effort to expel the space-occupying lesions. This same mechanism is probably responsible for the dysmenorrhea associated with an intrauterine contraceptive device.

Endocrine Factors. This brings us to the last category of etiological factors, represented by endocrine aberrations of one sort or another. On clinical rather than scientifically demonstrable grounds, the frequently crampy character of primary dysmenorrhea has been rather generally, although not unanimously, accepted as due to *exaggerated uterine*

contractility, and we have learned a good deal as to the endocrine factors which govern the contractility of the uterine musculature. Novak and Reynolds reported studies upon the rabbit uterus which seemed to indicate very clearly that the *normal stimulant of uterine contractility is the estrogenic hormone,* whereas, *progesterone is the normal inhibitor* of this contractility. Csapo's work in vitro substantiates these views.

If the estrogenic hormone is responsible for the heightened uterine contractility which appears to characterize primary dysmenorrhea, there are two clinical observations which seem perplexing and paradoxical. The first of these is the fact that in cases of dysfunctional bleeding, associated usually with a relative excess of estrogen and a deficiency or complete absence of progesterone, menstrual pain is characteristically absent. The second is

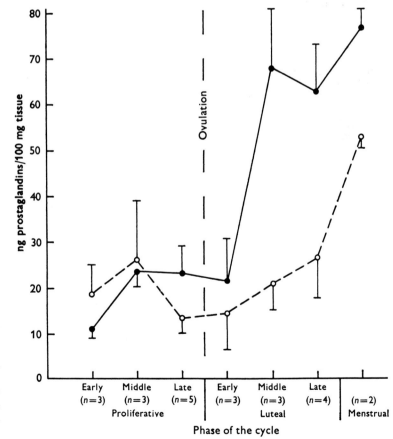

33.1. Levels of prostaglandin $F_{2\alpha}$ (PGF$_{2\alpha}$) (●——●) and prostaglandin E_2 (PGE$_2$) (○——○) in the human endometrium during the menstrual cycle (n = number of separate determinations in each group). (From Downie, Poyser and Wunderlich, J. Physiol., *236:* 465, 1974.)

the fact that primary dysmenorrhea so often does not date from the inauguration of menstruation at puberty, but makes its appearance at a later period, varying from a few months to perhaps two years after puberty.

An explanation was first suggested by the work of Clitheroe and Pickles on prostaglandin production of the endometrium. Under the influence of progesterone, the secretory endometrium synthesizes prostaglandin $F_2\alpha$, a neurohormone which causes contraction of smooth muscles. This is released when the endometrium breaks down at menstruation and the action on uterine muscle and vasculature causes contraction and associated pain. If an excessive amount is released into the circulation, the systemic effects characteristically associated with dysmenorrhea, *e.g.,* diarrhea, nausea, flushing and syncope, occur. The inability to demonstrate differences in $FGF_2\alpha$ serum levels in women with and without dysmenorrhea is understandable when we realize that $PGF_2\alpha$ is rapidly metabolized in the lungs and its action is at the local intracellular level where it is synthesized. The similarity to their dysmenorrhea of the symptoms induced in normal women by a $PGF_2\alpha$ infusion, as well as relief of dysmenorrhea by a $PGF_2\alpha$ antagonist, further substantiate this theory of etiology.

Treatment

Endocrine Therapy. There are several endocrine approaches to the therapy of dysmenorrhea and these may be briefly summarized.

Estrogens. From the studies of Sturgis and Albright, to which reference has already been made, it seems possible to convert an ovulatory cycle into an anovulatory one by administering estrogens in adequate dosage in the early part of the cycle; and often such inhibition of ovulation brings about relief from pain with the next flow. Stilbestrol, 1 mg. or its estrogenic equivalent, given for 20 days beginning shortly after the onset of the period, usually on the first or second day, will abolish ovulation effectively, al-

though much larger doses, 5 mg. daily, are probably necessary to accomplish usually this effect repeatedly in subsequent cycles. Unfortunately, the use of this dosage is associated with nausea and prolonged use is often complicated by excessive bleeding. Because of these disadvantages, synthetic progestogens have replaced estrogens as ovulatory inhibitors.

Although effective in the treatment cycle, the benefits do not usually extend beyond the month of therapy. Even a temporary relief, however, is a boon to the patient who has come to dread the advent of menstruation because of the incapacitation it entails. The effectiveness of this treatment depends upon the inhibition of ovulation; therefore one would not wish to resort to it with any persistence in the case of women anxious for pregnancy.

Progestogens. The widespread use of steroid contraception has decreased the incidence of dysmenorrhea because the efficacy of most methods depends upon inhibition of ovulation. However, some progestational drugs, without estrogen added, can be used to control dysmenorrhea. Unlike estrogens, progestogens can be used in the same dosage month after month with a similar suppression of ovulation and beneficial effects. As little as 2.5 mg. of 19-norethisterone (Norlutin), given daily during the first 25 days of each cycle, is a sufficient dose to suppress ovulation. Side effects are minimal with this small dosage. By avoiding the estrogen which is incorporated into most of the oral contraception regimes, many of the complications and clinical symptoms associated with these drugs (Chapter 34) can be obviated. Dydrogesterone (Duphaston, Gynorest) does not inhibit ovulation, but nevertheless interferes sufficiently with ovarian steroidogenesis to prevent dysmenorrhea.

The same theoretical considerations, of course, apply to the use of progestational agents in the suppression of ovulation as to the use of estrogens, and again the treatment is effective only in the cycle of therapy and no permanent relief is attained. However, as everyone's experience demonstrates that dysmenorrhea is invariably aggravated by general psychic tension, sometimes a course of three to six months of treatment will carry a patient through an unusually difficult time and it will then be possible to control her symptoms with more general measures for several months, after which treatment can be reinitiated if necessary.

Testosterone. Testosterone is of value in the treatment of dysmenorrhea only when endometriosis is the etiological factor. Methyltestosterone, 5 mg. daily over a 6-month period, is usually adequate to control symptoms. This dosage is not associated with any evidence of virilization and will not interfere with ovulation and normal menstruation. An occasional patient who has an acne tendency, however, may find that the acne is exaggerated. It would be important, therefore, to use progestogens if this skin condition exists.

Presacral Neurectomy. The operation of presacral neurectomy or sympathectomy is a rational and frequently effective procedure in an occasional patient with unusually severe dysmenorrhea which has proved intractable to more conservative procedures. It gives complete or almost complete relief from pain in perhaps 60 to 70% of the cases. Although only occasionally indicated in primary dysmenorrhea *per se,* a more frequent application, at least in our hands, has been as a supplementary procedure in conservative operations performed for such conditions as endometriosis when associated with severe dysmenorrhea.

Treatment during Dysmenorrhea Attack. Very little new information can be added to a discussion of the treatment of the dysmenorrhea attack. Once the pain has been initiated, it is apt to run its course. The local use of heat and analgesics such as acetylsalicylic acid and sodium amytal to induce sleep will suffice for all except the occasional case. When nausea is an associated finding, rectal suppositories must be employed. Too much stress cannot be laid on the risk of resorting to the two drugs which will al-

ways relieve the pain, morphine or Demerol and alcohol. It should be unnecessary to emphasize that no habit-producing drug should ever be used, as the condition must be regarded as a chronic illness and under these circumstances the possibility of addiction is too great a hazard. Every attempt should be made to prevent the condition, as it is easier to stop the pain before its inception than after it is well established. This can frequently be done by the use of analgesics, and these in combination with other types of drugs such as psychic energizers and tranquilizers. Two of the most effective ones are Equagesic (150 mg. meprobamate, 75 mg. ethoheptazine citrate, 250 mg. aspirin) and Zactirin Compound-100 (67 mg. ethoheptazine citrate, 227 mg. aspirin, 162 mg. phenacetin, 32.4 mg. caffeine). Medication should be given at the first sign of menstruation and repeated every three hours through the first or second day if necessary. Some patients respond better to an anticholinergic drug such as Trasentine. A smooth muscle relaxant, isoxsuprine hydrochloride (Vasodilan), 10 to 20 mg. 3 or 4 times a day is more effective for others. We have been most encouraged by the results obtained with Indocin, an inhibitor of $PGF_2\alpha$ synthesis. It is most effective if given 24 hours prior to the onset of menses. However, if this is impossible, substantial relief of symptoms is obtained when medication, 25 mg. every 4 hours if necessary, is begun with bleeding.

Summary of Management. No therapy of such a subjective pain disorder as primary dysmenorrhea can be based purely on endocrine considerations, for cognizance must also be taken of constitutional and psychogenic factors as a basis for the management of these patients. Although endocrine factors alone may be responsible in some cases and the same is true of constitutional or psychogenic factors, in most cases more than one of these three chief etiological factors may exist. As a part of the treatment of primary dysmenorrhea, endocrine therapy or surgery may properly be employed, but the physician who depends upon these entirely and who takes no notice of other possible factors is sure to meet with failure in a large proportion of cases. In addition to the general and constitutional measures, psychotherapy and reassurance with advice to try to remain up and about rather than going to bed during the pain of the attack seem preferable to the complications and inconvenience of endocrine therapy. A few doses of aspirin or some antispasmodic will usually suffice. When the dysmenorrhea is more protracted and severe, however, endocrine therapy should be tried before resorting to more radical measures such as presacral neurectomy. The evidence now clearly indicates what has long been suspected, that primary dysmenorrhea is a disorder of ovulating women and that it is probably relievable by preventing ovulation. This can apparently be done for any one particular cycle by progestogen therapy from the 5th through the 25th day of the cycle. The specific etiologic agent responsible for the dysmenorrhea now seems to be $PGF_2\alpha$ synthesized by the endometrial cells under the influence of progesterone. Therefore, specific treatment, *e.g.,* inhibition of $PGF_2\alpha$, should be effective and this does indeed seem to be the case.

PREMENSTRUAL TENSION AND EDEMA

Premenstrual tension in minor degrees is relatively common; extreme degrees are rare and may be very distressing. The milder forms of the condition are characterized by nervousness, depression, or restlessness, whereas the severe types closely approach a psychotic state with striking personality changes and emotional outbursts which make the patient difficult for family and physician alike. On the other hand, the most characteristic complaint may be incapacitating headaches which on occasion are associated with sensory or motor symptoms of cerebral vascular spasms. The symptoms appear to be closely related to premenstrual edema and the two frequently coexist.

Premenstrual edema was described by Thomas in 1933 and a number of reports have since appeared. It must be remembered that many normal women show a slight gain of weight during the premenstrual period. Sweeney, for example, found that 30% of a group of normal women studied by him showed a gain of 3 or more pounds. This agrees with our observations. In the occasional patient, however, the weight gain may be far greater and is obviously due to retention of fluid. There is often a marked edema with puffiness of the face and eyes, swelling of the feet and ankles. In one such patient there was a weight gain of as much as 15 pounds during the cycle; the eyes were almost closed by the edematous eyelids, and there was swelling and pitting of the feet and ankles. The edema usually begins a few days before the onset of menstruation, but may also appear at ovulation time. Toward the beginning of menstruation, or sometime immediately after its cessation, marked polyuria occurs with rapid disappearances of edema. The condition may be noted at any age during the menstrual era, but in our experience it is most common during the fourth decade.

The earliest studies on the problem were made by Frank, who related the symptoms to estrogen retention produced by a high renal threshold of excretion. Although increased blood estrogen levels have yet to be demonstrated early metabolic studies by Thorn, in the human, and Krohn and Zuckerman, in the baboon, confirmed the role of estrogen in fluid retention. However, although some patients do show both preovulatory and premenstrual edema paralleling the ovarian estrogen secretion pattern, as with dysmenorrhea, premenstrual tension usually occurs in the ovulatory cycle, linking it at least circumstantially to progesterone secretion. As with dysmenorrhea also, no abnormality of the ovarian hormone production or metabolism has been demonstrated and the normal hormonal balance is attested by the ability of most patients to retain a normal reproductive function. Because of the associated edema, it has been suggested that the condition may also represent a disturbance of adrenal aldosterone function and Reich has demonstrated an increased aldosterone secretion in normally menstruating women premenstrually. If any hormonal imbalance exists, it must certainly be superimposed on a very specific type of sympathetic nervous system and is influenced by external environmental factors, everyday stress and strain, and dietary indiscretions such as inadequate or infrequent meals, excessive coffee, alcohol, or nicotine. A recent study by Copper has produced some substantiation for this conclusion. His results indicate that there is a definite association of premenstrual tension with a psychotic personality type whereas there is no such correlation with dysmenorrhea.

Thus, it seems that we may consider the condition of premenstrual tension and edema as due to secondary aldosteronism with three major components which contribute to the pathogenesis. First, and certainly fundamental, is the type of nervous system; second, the environmental stress; and third, the shifting ovarian physiology which is, so to speak, the "straw that breaks the camel's back," in producing the secondary aldosteronism. For a better understanding of the physiology a paragraph on aldosteronism seems appropriate.

Aldosteronism. Aldosteronism due to a tumor or hyperplasia of the adrenal *zona glomerulosa* was first described by Krohn and is characterized by hypertension, muscular weakness, polyuria, polydypsia, and high sodium and low serum potassium, but no edema. The absence of edema is explained by Bartter in the following manner. The aldosterone or sodium-retaining factor causes increased sodium resorption by the renal tubules; the expansion of volume of extracellular fluids causes increased cellular filtration rate and thereby an increased sodium secretion. Thus, there is relatively little sodium retention and therefore no edema.

In contrast, secondary aldosteronism described as hypersecretion due to factors outside of the adrenal glomerulosa zone, is usually associated with the state of edema. Some factors known to produce secondary aldosteronism are: corticotrophin, potassium, progesterone, and changes in body fluid volume. In addition to these, surgical trauma and anxiety states have been implicated. It seems apparent that the edema is dependent upon the increased aldosterone secretion, because, under experimental conditions in animals, adrenalectomy will usually eliminate the edema.

Pathogenesis. We are able then to picture a harassed housewife, endowed with a reactive nervous system, who by her fourth decade is burdened with more anxiety than she is able to handle. Having ovulated, she is now producing progesterone and increased amounts of estrogen which lead to mild fluid retention. These two factors, the hormones and the fluid retention, stimulate increased aldosterone production, which then causes more fluid retention, thus creating the vicious circle which produces symptoms of headache, irritability, depression, and swelling (Frank). The intercellular edema itself then causes increased tension, headache, and anxiety. The anxiety further stimulates aldosterone production, and thus the syndrome grows in proportion. It is often difficult to know where the chain begins and how to interrupt it.

It is interesting that the older patients reported by Reich showed more pronounced increases of aldosterone in the premenstrual phase and this may be related to the increased frequency of the condition during the late 30's and early 40's. We have been inclined to attribute this to the additional stress which most patients undergo in association with the greater responsibilities of age.

Treatment. The clinical management of the *premenstrual tension* syndrome is a reminder that medicine is still an art and not an exact science. This statement indicates that the therapy is by no means a standardized one.

In the milder cases and in the younger group of patients, especially when edema is the predominating symptom, ammonium chloride, 0.6 gm. 3 times daily during the last two weeks of the menstrual cycle, associated with a low-salt diet and three regular high protein meals a day, may suffice, if the initial point of attack has been made simultaneously on adjusting the stress and strain of everyday living. For more severe edema problems Diuril, 500 mg. can be given once or twice a day for 2 or 3 days during the onset of swelling. Prolonged, continuous therapy is inadvisable, as marked edema will occur on withdrawal of medication.

When severe emotional disturbances exist these should be treated only in conjunction with a psychiatrist. If recurrent depression is a prominent feature, the use of continuous lithium has proved beneficial. Given as lithium carbonate, 300 mg. 2 or 3 times a day, and monitored with blood lithium values, it controls the depressive symptoms remarkably well but is not effective for the swelling or headache. As lithium can induce hypothyroidism, thyroid function should be checked periodically. It is also teratogenic for experimental animals and is therefore not to be given during pregnancy.

When headache is the major symptom, it has been our experience that 25 mg. of methyltestosterone daily for 2 or 3 days premenstrually and, if necessary, at the time of ovulation, will often prove a great help. When the symptoms are seen in women approaching middle life, especially if headaches are severe and associated with vascular spasms causing unilateral parasthesias, irradiation induction of the menopause may be indicated. Although this specifically does not apply to patients with edema or tension, when done after careful study and consideration with the full understanding and desire of the patient, it has been our experience that this method of treatment is highly satisfactory for the relief of premenstrual headaches. Contrary to the fears of most physicians concerned in handling such patients, they do not have excessive hot flushes or other adverse symptoms of the menopause.

In recapitulation, one can alleviate the symptoms of premenstrual tension and edema by salt restriction and diuretics, by inducing anovulatory cycles, or by giving 25 mg. of methyltestosterone daily for not over a 10-day period each month. When recurrent depression is a predominant symptom, lithium carbonate has proved very beneficial. Little of permanent value can be expected from any therapeutic regimen without concomitant psychotherapy. Let us not resort to operative procedures as a desperate therapeutic attempt. It has been our experience that, especially in those patients with edema, the symptoms will remain even following a bilateral oophorectomy and hysterectomy. A psychiatrist is a much better recourse.

VICARIOUS MENSTRUATION

This is of historical interest mainly and is the designation applied to certain rare cases in which extragenital hemorrhages of one source or another take place at periodic intervals corresponding to the menstrual cycle. The most frequent site of the bleeding is from the nasal mucous membrane in the form of epistaxis. This variety, according to Roth, makes up about 30% of all cases. It has long been known that a biological relation exists between the nasal mucous membrane and the female generative organs. Investigations by Mortimer *et al.* have demonstrated the responsiveness of certain areas in the nasal mucous membrane to estrogen stimulation. The local hyperemia and other vascular changes produced by the ovarian hormones would seem to offer a satisfactory explanation.

Vicarious menstruation has been described as occurring from a great variety of other sources: the stomach, intestines, lungs, mammary glands, skin, and various skin lesions such as ulcers or nevi, kidneys, abdominal fistulas, umbilicus, external auditory meatus, eyes, and eyelids. Many of the cases in the older literature, for example those of umbilical origin, are no doubt explained by the existence of endometriosis or fistulas communicating with the uterus or tubal lumen.

Treatment. The treatment of the condition depends upon the exact diagnosis as well as the source of the bleeding. In the nasal type of vicarious menstruation, cauterization of the nasal spur responsible for the bleeding is usually recommended. When bleeding occurs elsewhere, an investigation for endometriosis should be made and, if confirmed, excision of the area when possible is most expedient. Either methyltestosterone, 5 mg. daily, can be used as described for the treatment of endometriosis or a synthetic progestogen in combination with estrogens, as in the commercial oral contraceptive preparations.

INTERMENSTRUAL PAIN (*MITTEL-SCHMERZ*) AND BLEEDING

These two conditions may be discussed together, in spite of the fact that the pain often occurs without the bleeding, and *vice versa.* They are apparently both linked in some manner with the phenomenon of ovulation, although little is known as to the exact mechanism.

Intermenstrual pain, occurring usually at approximately the midinterval period, with many individual variations as to the exact day of the cycle, was described by Priestley as far back as 1872. Such pain may be slight, or it may be as severe as the more intense forms of dysmenorrhea. The duration may be only a few hours, but in some cases two or three days. There may or may not be associated *bleeding,* sometimes so slight as to cause only a brownish discharge, in other cases sufficiently free and prolonged as to mimic a menstrual flow. To such scanty flows, regularly interpolated between the periods, the Germans have applied the term *kleine Regel* (little period). In the occasional case, this interval type of bleeding is so free that the patient states that she menstruates twice a month. Even when there is no macroscopic bleeding with *Mittelschmerz,* blood corpuscles may often be found in microscopic examination of the vaginal discharge.

Etiology. The chronological relation between intermenstrual pain and bleeding on the one hand, and ovulation on the other, has led to general agreement that there is some sort of causal relation between them. The bleeding would seem logically explainable by the *temporary drop in estrogen* immediately following ovulation, but there is greater difficulty in explaining the pain. As Reynolds states, "one can only speculate upon whether the occurrence of *Mittelschmerz* betokens impending ovulation." Only a few studies of actual *operative findings* in such cases have been reported, the most complete being that of Wharton and Henriksen. In nine of their 21 patients some evidence of bleeding from the ovary was found; in others the findings were negative. Some have suggested that the pain may be most logically explained on the basis of slight intraabdominal hemorrhage.

Treatment. When intermenstrual bleeding is very slight, and has been known to occur with such periodicity that there is little reason to doubt its functional nature, no treatment is necessary except reassurance and perhaps simple analgesics. Where there is doubt on this point, diagnostic curettage may be necessary to eliminate other factors, such as intrauterine lesions. The *curettage* in itself may suffice.

MENSTRUAL EPILEPSY

The occurrence of convulsive seizures in relation to the menstrual period has been repeatedly documented since its description in 1881. Ansell, Clarke, and Laidlow in 1956 again confirmed the findings that epileptic seizures occur more frequently at the time of the menstrual period and less frequently during the luteal phase. These workers have refuted the long accepted theory that the seizures were due to cerebral edema, as their studies indicated no differences between the water balance studies of the epileptic patients and those of normal individuals. All epileptics had a normal total body water volume, and this was the same for those with and those without a menstrual aggravation of seizures. The authors decided that the midluteal reduction in the number of epileptic seizures might be related to an anticonvulsant action of progesterone with an exaggeration of fits when its beneficial effect is withdrawn.

Treatment. The therapy for menstrual epilepsy is similar to that for epilepsy in general. For the occasional patient who suffers severe cyclic seizures which are well documented and who is either in the older age group or who has completed her family, X-ray castration may be advised. Under these circumstances major seizures may be greatly reduced or cease entirely, although petit mal is apt to continue. Endocrine therapy for the suppression of ovulation under these conditions is usually not successful, but there is not yet enough experience with the newer progestational compounds. It may well be that these drugs can be used for the relief of menstrual epilepsy as well as for the relief of dysmenorrhea.

REFERENCES

Ansell, B., Clarke, E., and Laidlow, J.: Epilepsy and menstruation; the role of water retention. Lancet, 2: 1232, 1956.

Browne, O.: Survey of 113 cases of primary dysmenorrhea treated by neurectomy. Amer. J. Obstet. Gynec., 57: 1053, 1949.

Campbell, R. E., and Hisaw, F. L.: Use of corpus luteum in treatment of dysmenorrhea. Amer. J. Obstet. Gynec., 31: 508, 1936.

Clitheroe, H. J., and Pickles, V. R.: The separation of the smooth muscle stimulants in menstrual fluid. J. Physiol. (Lond.), 156: 225, 1961.

Clitheroe, H. J.: The etiology of primary dysmenorrhea. A review. Obstet. Gynec. Survey, 19: 649, 1964.

Copper, A., and Kessel, N.: Menstruation and personality. Brit. J. Psychiat., 109: 711, 1963.

Csapo, A.: Mechanism of effect of the ovarian hormones. Recent Progr. Hormone Res., 12: 405, 1956.

Doyle, J. B.: Paracervical uterine denervation by transection of cervical plexus for relief of dysmenorrhea. Amer. J. Obstet. Gynec., 70: 1, 1955.

Frank, R. T.: Hormonal causes of premenstrual tension. Arch. Neurol. Psychiat., 26: 1053, 1931.

Greenhill, J. P., and Freed, S. C.: Mechanism and treatment of premenstrual distress with ammonium chloride. Endocrinology, 26: 529, 1940.

Henriksen, E., and Horn, P.:Causes of treatment of secondary dyspareunia. Amer. J. Obstet. Gynec., 43: 671, 1942.

Hulme, H. B., and Holmstrom, E. G.: Stilbestrol treatment of dysmenorrhea. Obstet. Gynec., 1: 579, 1953.

Jessen, D. A., Lane, R. E., and Greene, R. R.: Intrauterine foreign body. Amer. J. Obstet. Gynec., 85: 1023, 1963.

Jones, G. S., and Wentz, A.: Transient luteolytic effect of prostaglandin $F_{2\alpha}$ in the human. Obstet. Gynec., 42: 172, 1973.

Keene, F. E.: Treatment of dysmenorrhea by presacral sympathectomy. Amer. J. Obstet. Gynec., 30: 534, 1935.

Kotz, J., and Parker, E.: Endometrial patterns in dysmenorrhea. Amer. J. Obstet. Gynec., 37: 116, 1939.

Krohn, P. L.: Intermenstrual pain (Mittelschmerz) and the time of ovulation. Brit. Med. J., 1: 803, 1949.

Krohn, P. L., and Zuckerman, S.: Water metabolism in relation to the menstrual cycle. J. Physiol. (London), 88: 369, 1937.

McGavack, T. H., Spoor, H. J., Stone, M. L., and Pearson, S.: The treatment of premenstrual pain with a combination of an antihistaminic and a theophylline derivative. Amer. J. Obstet. Gynec., 74: 416, 1946.

Mortimer, H., Wright, R. P., Bachanan, C., and Collip, J. B.: Effect of estrogenic hormone upon nasal mucous membrane of the monkey (Macaca mulatta). Proc. Soc. Exp. Biol. Med., 67: 247, 1948.

Morton, J. H.: Premenstrual tension. Amer. J. Obstet. Gynec., 60: 343, 1950.

Nakano, R., and Takemura, H.: Treatment of dysmenorrhea; a double-blind study. Acta Obstet. Gynaec. Japan, 18: 41, 1971.

Novak, E., and Reynolds, S. R. M.: The cause of primary dysmenorrhoea with special reference to hormonal factors. J.A.M.A., 99: 1466, 1932.

Ogino, K.: Über den Konseptionstermin des Weibes und seine Anwendung in der Praxes. Zbl. Gynaek., 56: 721, 1932.

Roth, A.: Über vikariierende Menstruation. Mschr. Geburtsh. Gynäk., 51: 41, 1920.

Schon, M., Goldfield, M. D., Weinstein, M. R., and Villeneuve, A.: Lithium and pregnancy; report from the register of lithium babies. Brit. Med. J., 2: 135, 1973.

Singer, I., and Rotenberg, D.: Mechanisms of lithium action. New Eng. J. Med., 289: 254, 1973.

Sletten, I. W., and Gershon, S.: The premenstrual syndrome; a discussion of its pathophysiology and treatment with lithium ion. Comp. Psychiatry, 7: 197, 1966.

Sturgis, S., and Albright, F.: Mechanism of estrogen therapy in release of dysmenorrhea. Endocrinology, 26: 68, 1940.

Thomas, W. A.: Generalized edema occurring only at menstrual period. J.A.M.A., 101: 1126, 1933.

Thorn, G. W., Nelson, K. R., and Thorn, D. W.: Study of mechanism of edema associated with menstruation. Endocrinology, 22: 155, 1938.

Waxenberg, S. E., Drellich, M. G., and Sutherland, A. M.: Role of hormones in human behavior. I. Changes in female sexuality after adrenalectomy. J. Clin. Endocr., 19: 193, 1959.

Wharton, L. R., and Henriksen, E.: Studies in ovulation; operative observations in periods of intermenstrual pain. J.A.M.A., 107: 1425, 1936.

Widholm, O., and Kantero, R. L.: A statistical analysis of the menstrual patterns of 8000 Finnish girls and their mothers. Acta Obstet. Gynec. Scand., Suppl. 14, 1971.

Wilson, L., and Kurzrok, R.: Uterine contractility in function dysmenorrhea. Endocrinology, 27: 23, 1940.

chapter 34

Family Planning

INTRODUCTION

Although the scope of this text will not permit a comprehensive discussion of demographic problems and population control, the topic is of too great importance to omit completely. Family planning is population control reduced to the individual rather than to the national or global level. For a proper perspective in either, it seems necessary to have some concept of the problems in both areas.

Few, if any, informed persons fail to recognize the urgency of the need for control of reproduction at all levels, family, national, and world. Demographers relate that the low reproduction rate and the inordinately high death rate of the human allowed for a fairly stable world population from the beginning of time until about 1850 when the first billion population was reached. From this time, the world population trend has taken an incredibly sharp rise upward. By 1930, in slightly less than 100 years, the population had doubled to 2,000,000,000 largely due to the falling death rate and lowered infant mortality. By 1960, less than half the previous time, another billion had been added, and it is esti-

mated that by 2200, the uncomfortable, if not the impossible, number of 500,000,000,000 people will be reached. This is, of course, barring some unforeseen catastrophe or successful planned population control. The problem must not be viewed in light of nutrition only. Such a population density would give the surface of all continents a number of people per square mile equal to that found in Washington, D. C. according to Mayer. We need only to think of this in terms of educational and recreational facilities to realize the seriousness and complexities of such over population.

GENERAL CONSIDERATIONS

There are two major considerations in approaching the subject of either family planning for an individual or population control for a society: (1) motivation which determines who will participate; and (2) methodology which determines how. Studies on motivation indicate that this is influenced first by education, *e.g.,* factual knowledge and understanding; second by cultural backgrounds, *e.g.,* religion and traditional ways of life; and third by specific individual needs dependent, perhaps, upon highly personalized situational factors. It has been demonstrated that the physician who is sincerely interested and adequately trained in contraceptive therapy and practice plays an effective role in motivation. The physician's role in methodology, the imparting of technical knowledge or utilizing of trained skills in this area, is paramount in making voluntary control of reproduction possible.

Demographers agree that the responsible parent today should plan a family of two or not more than three children in an effort to replace, but not increase, the world population. Those individuals emotionally and financially capable of raising larger families should plan to do so by adoption. It is the physician's responsibility to set the example as well as to disseminate knowledge of the seriousness of the world problem.

Because education is a slow process and motivation apparently depends to a large extent upon education, many observers feel that those methods which require the least motivation offer the most promise for rapid results in population control. Although the ideal method has probably not as yet been developed, those currently available are satisfactory, efficient, and offer such a variety of techniques that any individual couple should be able to achieve satisfactory family planning. It is probable that no method, however ideal, will be universally applicable to all couples.

CONTRACEPTIVE METHODS

General Considerations

As stated, there are presently many approaches to family planning, and these can be suited to the needs and capabilities of the individuals involved. Basically, one must consider if a couple is interested in spacing or limiting children, *e.g.,* have they reached the ideal of two or more children, or are they contemplating additional pregnancies. Next, one must assess the motivation, intelligence, cultural background, financial status, and general health as well as the individual's personal preferences, acceptances, and prejudices. The older methods, diaphragm, condom, tablets, and foams replaced still older methods of abstinence, late marriage, coitus interruptus, abortion, and rhythm. The mechanical methods have in turn been supplemented by various forms of oral steroid contraception, long-acting injectable steroids, local vaginal steroids, and the recrudescence of the intrauterine device. Finally, sterilization of either partner has become an accepted means of absolute contraception when the family size is completed, either for socioeconomic or maternal health indications.

Although it has been stressed that each individual should use the method of her choice and, indeed, this must be so if any success is anticipated, nevertheless, there are frequently medical and socioeconomic indications which dictate the preference of one method over another. A skillful and knowledgeable physician can present the evidence in such a way as to insure that the patient makes the proper selection.

Although instruction in family planning was traditionally given in the premarital consultation, our present social climate has for all practical purposes eliminated this custom. Information regarding contraceptive techniques is acquired in sex education courses in high school or from pamphlets disseminated by the college or university student health programs. The high school course is often superficial, given by an inexperienced teacher, and the pamphlet type of self-education, although usually factually correct, does not substitute for the advice and possibility of discussion afforded by a visit with an interested gynecologist. Also, unfortunately, in eliminating the consultation, many are also eliminating the premarital pelvic examination and thus running the risk of overlooking pathology which should be corrected prior to first intercourse. If educational facilities have not been available to the patient before her first pregnancy, the subject should be introduced during the prenatal visits. Initial definitive discussions conducted in the immediate postpartum period have proved ideal as the patient is most receptive to contraception advice at this time.

Coitus Interruptus

Coitus interruptus commonly referred to as "withdrawal" is said to be probably the earliest naturally invented method of contraception and is thought to have been the method of effecting population control during the 19th century in Switzerland and France. It is still probably the most frequently used contraception in Europe. As it simply involves withdrawal of the penis from the vagina when ejaculation is imminent, with completion of ejaculation outside of the vagina, there is no expense involved, nor is technical advice necessary. For successful use of this method, however, it is obvious that the man must have good self control, be highly motivated with a strong sense of responsibility to protect his sexual partner.

It is completely unsatisfactory for men with premature or early ejaculation. It is estimated that the method would be inapplicable to about 50% of all males due to inability to control ejaculation. Although it has often been said to be associated with psychological side effects or the production of chronic prostatitis, neither of these effects can be substantiated. The use failure rate is quoted as between 6 and 16 per 100 women years. Because coitus interruptus is a method which is always available at no cost, it should be learned for those situations in which no other method is possible.

Condom Contraception

Condom contraception or the use of a rubber sheath worn over the penis during coitus is probably the most widely used mechanical contraceptive in the world. The only precautions necessary are to leave a dead space in the condom from which the air has been expelled to receive the ejaculate, to use proper lubrication if necessary, to effect withdrawal of the penis before cessation of the erection, and to grasp the ring of the sheath at the time of withdrawal to prevent it from slipping off. It has the advantage of protecting both against pregnancy and venereal disease and is, therefore, probably the most useful type of contraception in casual intercourse. Its other advantages are relative inexpensiveness, almost universal availability, and ease of usage. An additional advantage of the condom is found for men who have a tendency to premature ejaculation. The condom may blunt the sensation sufficiently to prolong the intercourse time. The delegation of the responsibility for family planning or for pregnancy prevention may increase his feeling of responsibility and family importance.

The disadvantages of the method are that it sometimes interferes with coital sensations both for male and female. It may interrupt the mood as application of the condom requires an erect penis. It is not satisfactory for hot climates because of the deterioration of rubber.

The failure rate is usually given as between 6 and 13 per 100 women years, but some studies show much higher failure rates, the highest being 36 per 100 women years. The failure is largely due to rupture of the condom with the deposition of the entire ejaculate into the vagina. If this type of accident is reported immediately to the physician, a pregnancy can be circumvented by use of a high estrogen dosage recommended by Morris and referred to as the "pill for the morning after" or pregnancy interception.

Vaginal Diaphragm and Spermicidal Jelly

This mechanical method for the female partner is, perhaps, the most sophisticated type of contraception and, therefore, is suitable for the better educated patient. The diaphragm is a mechanical rubber device which must fit snugly behind the pubic bone and over the cervix into the posterior fornix. Too large a diaphragm causes pelvic discomfort, whereas too small a diaphragm can be displaced during intercourse. The diaphragm itself is used to prevent the sperm from being deposited directly onto the cervical mucus, allowing the spermicidal jelly, which is used in the diaphragm and deposited with an applicator in the posterior fornix, time to exert its spermicidal action. The diaphragm should not be removed until eight hours after the last intercourse. The most satisfactory method for using a diaphragm is to insert it each night with jelly before retiring and to remove it, cleanse it, and reinsert it with jelly the following evening. Thus the diaphragm is always in place and its use is, therefore, divorced from the act of intercourse, thus improving the esthetic relationship.

Diaphragm contraception has the advantage of being locally effective and, therefore, unassociated with systemic side effects. It places the responsibility for pregnancy prevention and family planning entirely on the woman's shoulders and, therefore, perhaps affords her more sense of security. It does not interfere with coital sensations. If properly fitted, it should be completely comfortable and neither partner should be aware of its presence. It has the disadvantage of having to be fitted by a competent gynecologist, and it cannot be used in some patients who have vaginal relaxations, uterine descensus, or occasionally marked retroposition of the uterus. As it should be removed and reinserted each evening, it requires constant motivation.

The diaphragm remains medically the most acceptable form of contraception from the point of view of absence of complications. The use failure rate is between 2 and 3 per 100 women years among a private practice group and 33.6 per 100 women years in a Puerto Rican clinic study.

Vaginal Foam

Vaginal contraceptive foams are available as aerosol vials, jells, creams, or tablets. The spermicidal ingredient used is usually p-triisopropylphenolpolyethoxyethanol. The active agents in vaginal foam tablets are tartaric acid and sodium bicarbonate. The aerosol and jells are effective immediately, whereas the tablets require some 5 to 10 minutes to dissolve before effectiveness. The advantages of these methods are that they are inexpensive, easy to use and require no instruction. Because of these characteristics, the method has been found acceptable in the lower socioeconomic levels. The disadvantage is that the failure rate is somewhat higher than among the previously discussed methods, being between 38 and 42 per 100 women years. It is, therefore, a method which could be recommended for patients who are child spacing or to be used in a combination with some other form of contraception such as rhythm or coitus interruptus.

Intrauterine Device (IUD)

A half century ago, Graafenberg devised a metal ring to fit inside the uterus as a contraceptive device. This has been modified, using various plastic materials to form spirals, rings, shields, and loops which can be retained indefinitely in the uterine cavity. The great advantage of this method is the lack of necessity for high motivation. Once the device is in situ, no further action on the part of the patient is necessary. It is, therefore, most suitable for the couple with the lowest income, education, and motivation.

The device should be placed in the uterine cavity by an experienced gynecologist at the time of the menstrual period. This not only allows for ease of insertion when the cervix is relatively dilated, but also assures the patient is not pregnant at the time of the insertion. Although postpartum insertion is at times theoretically desirable, this type of insertion is associated with a greater number of complications, perforation being the most serious, as well as a higher expulsion rate. However, once the device is retained in the pospartum period, it obtains the lowest expulsion rate of all. The disadvantages of this method are the menstrual complications which occur—excessive, profuse periods, irregular bleeding between periods, and abdominal cramps. A cumulative expulsion rate of the device at the present time is said to be approximately 20% in the first 24 months. In addition to the expulsion rate, there is also a failure rate of approximately 2.6%

with the device in situ and failure to protect against ectopic pregnancy.

The method is unfortunately not suitable for some grand multipara with large uteri as well as patients who have myomata with irregularities of the uterine cavity, because the expulsion rate is high.

In spite of the publicity (1974) regarding the dangers of IUDs, more specifically shield devices, a review of the facts indicate that there is no significant difference in complication rates among the commercially available devices. Actually, the complication rate is markedly below that for steroid contraception. Those devices which depend upon copper for effectiveness seem to have two disadvantages; first, the introduction into the system of copper, a potentially toxic metal; second, the necessity for removal and re-insertion every 2 years.

Oral Contraception

Historical. The groundwork for the development of an oral contraceptive was laid in 1940 when Sturgis and Albright described the inhibition of ovulation in the human by estrogen. With the development of potent oral progestational agents, the possibility of consistently inhibiting ovulation, while producing an artificially stimulated menstrual period, became a reality. Rock, Pinkus, and Celso-Garcia described the first successful field trials in humans in 1956, and it was apparent from the outset that the method was remarkably effective and reproducible. Although the side effects were disagreeable enough to cause a 20 to 40% drop-out rate, these were of no medical significance, the most serious being irregular or profuse bleeding and nausea. The first hint of any possible serious complication was given in 1960 when a case of fatal thrombophlebitis, apparently associated with drug administration, was reported.

General Considerations. Oral contraceptives can currently be divided into three major categories. (1) *Combined steroid therapy* consisting of a pill with an estrogen and a progestogen usually taken for 20 days during each month, beginning on the 5th day after the onset of menses. (2) *Sequential steroid therapy* consisting of an estrogen taken for 15 days beginning on the 5th cycle day followed by a progestational agent combined with estrogen for 5 days and, finally, (3) *Microprogestational therapy* which is a low dosage of a progestational drug given continuously. There are 3 general types of progestational agents. Those related to the *androgens* or the *19-carbon compounds,* those more closely ralated to *progesterone,* the *21-carbon compounds* and those with some inherent estrogen activity. The estrogens most commonly used are mestranol and ethinyl estradiol.

The side effects of these oral steroid contraceptives are relative to the specific steroids given and the dosage thereof. There is, however, such an individual patient sensitivity to these synthetic steroids that generalizations are not too accurate or helpful. Kistner has devoted a book to this topic and, for what it may be worth, the generalizations of Dicky and Dorr are reproduced in Table 34.1 with a list of currently available proprietary preparations arranged in order of the relative estimated hormonal dominance.

Method. There are so many oral contraceptive preparations available that it is currently difficult to list them all, but Table 34.1 gives the trade name, manufacturer, and the chemical composition of some of the more frequently used preparations. It is no longer justifiable to use the high-dosage estrogens, over 0.08 mg. daily, and it is to be expected that the microprogestin dosage may be least associated with side effects. This is, of course, the simplest to administer as it is given continuously; however, it is also the least effective. As indicated above, the combination steroids are given beginning on the fifth cycle day and continuing through the 24th, starting again on the 5th day after the onset of bleeding, or on the fifth day after cessation of therapy, if bleeding does not begin. It is extremely important for patients to understand this because, unless they reinstitute their suppressive therapy, the hypothalamic escape will allow a pituitary stimulation

Table 34.1

*Side Effects of Oral Contraceptive Drugs in Relation to Estrogens and Progestins**

Fluid Retention Estrogen Potency in Decreasing Order	Estrogens	Progestogen	Menstrual Problems Progestational Potency in Decreasing Order
Trade Name (Mfg.)			Trade Name (Mfg.)
Oracon (Mead Johnson) Sequential	Ethinyl estradiol 0.1 mg. (21 days)	Dimethisterone 25 mg. (5 days)	Norlestrin 2.5 (Parke Davis)
Ortho-Novum SQ (Or- tho) Sequential	Mestranol 0.08 (20 days)	Norethindrone 2 mg. (6 days)	Norinyl 2 (Syntex) Ortho-Novum 2 (Or-
Norquen (Syntex) Se- quential	Mestranol 0.08 (20 days)	Norethindrone 2 mg. (6 days)	tho) Ovulen (Searle)
Norlestrin 2.5 (Parke Davis)	Ethinyl estradiol 0.05 mg.	Norethindrone acetate 2.5 mg.	Enovid E (Searle) Norlestrin 1 (Parke
Enovid E (Searle)	Mestranol 0.1 mg.	Norethynodrel 2.5 mg.	Davis)
Norlestrin 1 (Parke Davis)	Ethinyl estradiol 0.05 mg.	Norethindrone acetate 1 mg.	Ortho-Novum 1 (Or- tho)
Ovulen (Searle)	Mestranol 0.1 mg.	Ethynodiol diacetate 1 mg.	Norinyl 1 (Syntex) Ortho-Novum SQ (Or-
Norinyl 2 (Syntex)	Mestranol 0.1 mg.	Norethindrone 2 mg.	tho)
Ortho-Novum 2 (Ortho)	Mestranol 0.1 mg.	Norethindrone 2 mg.	Norquen (Syntex)
Ortho-Novum 1 (Ortho)	Mestranol 0.05 mg.	Norethindrone 1 mg.	Oracon (Mead John-
Norinyl 1 (Syntex)	Mestranol 0.05 mg.	Norethindrone 1 mg.	son)

* Taken from Dickey and Dorr: Obstet. Gynec. *33:* 273, 1969.

and ovulation to occur. Sequential therapy is given in this same fashion except the progestational agent is added on the last five days of therapy. Because sequential therapy is associated with a higher complication rate and also a higher pregnancy rate, there seems little indication for the use of this form of contraception. Some preparations are packaged with placebo tablets to take during the five days when steroids are discontinued. This is an especially advantageous package for the poorly motivated, poorly educated patient.

Mode of Action. It has been well documented by a number of investigators that the oral steroids exert their action by inhibition of the hypothalamic-releasing factors, thus blocking pituitary gonadotrophin activity and causing secondary ovarian atrophy. The progestational agents preferentially inhibit the preovulatory LH surge with a lesser effect upon the FSH function. The suppression is directly related to the amount and duration of the dosage. The estrogenic component, on the other hand,

preferentially inhibits the FSH and is also dose-dependent. The longer the period of administration, the more severe the pituitary suppression and ovarian atrophy, with subsequent decreased endogenous estrogen milieu. It is this lowered ovarian estrogen effect which is responsible for the shortened scanty menstrual flow which most women experience after taking oral contraceptives for a number of years.

Advantages. Oral contraception has two great advantages over all other methods of contraception; its remarkable effectiveness and its rather general acceptability. The combined steroid therapy has the theoretical failure rate of zero, and, even if four days of medication are missed, the failure rate is only 2 per 100 women years, which is still lower than any other method. The sequential therapy is not quite as accurate, having a failure rate of 1.4 per 100 women years if taken consistently. The margin of safety with sequential therapy is also less and the failure rate rises to 4 per 100 women years, if even one pill is missed. The microdosage is the least effective, having a failure rate of 3.7 per 100 women years. It also has very little margin of safety, and the failure rate apparently rises rapidly if as few as one or two pills are missed. The high acceptability of the oral contraception method is probably related to the fact that it is completely divorced from the sex act. As it eliminates self handling, it is also especially attractive for those women who find this distasteful.

Disadvantages. The greatest disadvantage of the method is that it involves the administration of potent drugs, which have many diversified systemic effects, to completely well women. The second disadvantage is the time and cost of proper patient supervision. A careful history and complete physical and gynecological examination as well as blood pressure and urine analysis should be made before administration of oral contraception. A gynecological check examination should ideally be made every six months or a year while the individual is on medication. The risk of complications and side effects must be weighed against the possible advantages which will accrue, as well as the advisability and acceptability of some other form of contraception.

Complications. Probably the most serious complication, which has been reported in association with oral contraception, is thromboembolic disease. Three statistical studies from the United Kingdom seem to have conclusively demonstrated that these steroid agents are implicated in a predisposition to thrombophlebitis. The annual death rate from embolism attributed to oral contraception was estimated to be about 3 per 100,000 users. The second possible serious complication, which has been described, is the occurrence of essential hypertension. It has been suggested that the estrogen component causes an increase in renin substrate and this, in turn, may cause an increase in angiotensin. The third medical problem is the associated disturbance of carbohydrate metabolism. The evidence indicates that women who have a diabetic tendency may show a diabetic type of glu-

cose tolerance test when on oral contraception. This seems to be because of the effect of estrogen on growth hormone, which causes hyperglycemia demanding a higher insulin level. Patients who are unable to adjust to this changing blood glucose level, because of an inherent pancreatic insufficiency, will develop diabetes. Finally, Wynn has described certain changes in the blood lipids which resemble those found in early arteriosclerotic vascular disease. The suggestion has been made that, in women who have a predisposition to arteriosclerosis, oral contraception may speed the process. This is as yet a theoretical consideration.

Side Effects. There are certain specific side effects which occur in approximately 40% of the women receiving any form of oral steroid contraception. These are menstrual irregularities, fluid retention, gastric disturbances, increased varicosities, irritability or depression, changes of libido, either plus or minus, melasma, headache, and migraine. None of these side effects is of serious nature, but of sufficient concern to the patient that an estimated 40% of oral contraceptive users discontinue before the end of two years. In Washington, D. C., it is estimated that 50% of welfare patients discontinued within a year.

From a medical point of view, one of the disadvantages of oral contraception is that it interferes with a number of laboratory diagnostic procedures. Among these are the sedimentation rate, tests for protein-bound iodine or thyroxine, blood corticotrophins, and, on occasion, even a Papanicolaou smear; an endometrial biopsy, or cervical biopsy can also present diagnostic difficulties.

Office or Clinic Visits. Probably one of the greatest disadvantages or deterrents for the use of oral contraception is the necessity for a gynecological consultation before administration of medication, and the return for refill of prescription.

In the ideal situation, oral contraception should not be advised without a complete history and gynecological examination including several laboratory investigations. Possible contraindications for oral contraception are found in the family history; if there is a diabetic family history, a history of essential hypertension, or a history of breast or endometrial cancer. Factors in the patient's past history which may contraindicate oral contraception are a history of menstrual irregularities, especially long periods of amenorrhea, breast or endometrial cancer, thromboembolic disease, or liver disease, the history of cardiac or renal disease, depressive reactions or migraine headaches. The physical examination should exclude thyroid and breast nodules, cardiac or renal disease, cervical polyps, and uterine myomas. Every patient should have a blood pressure, urine analysis for albumin and sugar, and a Papanicolaou smear before beginning oral contraception. Only a history of thromboembolic phenomenon or cancer of the breast is an absolute contraindication to therapy, but abnormalities in any of the areas mentioned require special consideration and attention. Each patient should return in two months at which time the blood pressure and urinary sugar test should be repeated and any factors which signal special attention at the first visit should be rechecked. It is then recommended that ideally each patient should be seen every 6 months and contraception should be discontinued over a month or six-week period after approximately 2½ years to be sure that the patient will function normally. If this is done, it must be remembered that some other form of contraception must be provided during the rest period.

Vaginitis. Both yeast vaginitis and trichomonas vaginitis have been reported as frequent complications of oral contraception. Yeast vaginitis might be related to the atrophy of the vagina which occurs due to the low estrogen milieu and also associated with the carbohydrate changes which can take place. This type of vaginitis can, on occasion, be intractable and, although usually it will respond to the recommended therapy, gentian violet and/or nystatin, occasionally oral contraception must be discontinued before the condition can be controlled. Trichomonas vaginitis may be related to a promiscuous way of life rather than to the actual steroid effects on the vagina.

Amenorrhea. After discontinuing oral contraception, the majority of patients resume ovulatory cycles within four to six weeks. However, it is not unusual for a patient to have one or two months of amenorrhea before her first menstrual period. In the 5-year Puerto Rican study, it was estimated that 5% of all women had some period of amenorrhea. More prolonged periods up to 2 years and longer have been reported but are unusual.

Oral Contraception for the Postpregnancy Exposure. Morris has described the use of estrogen as a postintercourse protective drug. This method is useful when there has been a single exposure as in rape or method failure in a single episode. The method has been referred to as "the pill for the morning after." It involves the administration of relatively high amounts of estrogen, 25 mg. of stilbestrol or its equivalent daily. Morris advocates a 4-day administration period but, over the years, we have used a 2-week interval. This insures the production of an abnormal endometrium which will not sustain a normal implantation and, when the pill is withdrawn, a withdrawal bleeding phase ensues. If given immediately after exposure and during the following 2 weeks, it offers absolute protection. It has obvious limited applicability and is especially valuable in cases of rape. It can be associated with gastrointestinal complications, nausea and vomiting, and, occasionally, with excessive bleeding.

Long Acting Injectable Steroids. Medroxyprogesterone acetate (Depo-Provera), 150 mg. intramuscularly every 3 months will inhibit ovulation and menstrual function. Erratic spotty bleeding occurs during the first three months of treatment and sometimes longer. The advantage of this method is the delegation of responsibility for contraception to the physician or the paramedical personnel requiring a house visit by the Public Health officer or an office or clinic visit by the patient only once every 3 months. The disadvantage of the method is the absence of regular menstrual periods and the presence of irregular bleeding which may be prolonged and inconvenient. In addition, the hypothalamic suppression is so efficient that prolonged anovulation and amenorrhea may occur following cessation of injections. Because of these properties, this form of contraception is best suited to those patients who are absolute "limiters," and who, for one reason or another, are unable to take personal responsibility for their birth control. It has been especially useful in patients with serious blood dyscrasias, because complete amenorrhea can be established, and it also has a place in the management of patients who have myomata uteri and, therefore, should receive as little estrogen stimulation as possible.

Vaginal Steroid Therapy. Mishell has reported the successful use of a silastic ring pessary which has been impregnated with a progestational agent. Sufficient absorption can be obtained from the vaginal mucosa in this manner to obtain inhibition of ovulation. The pessary can be inserted by the patient after each menstrual period and removed at the end of a 25-day interval. This form of contraception, of course, requires monthly insertion of the pessary, and, if this is done by a physician, necessitates a monthly visit. It requires less motivation and offers less opportunity for patient failure than daily pill contraception. This technique has not been subjected to a sufficient clinical trial as yet to give any estimate of its effectiveness, but theoretically it seems to offer some advantages in specific circumstances.

Rhythm Contraception; Periodic Continence. The so-called rhythm method of family planning, as proposed by Ogino and Knaus, is based on three fundamental theoretical concepts, and perhaps the efficacy of this method can best be evaluated by examining the validity of these concepts. These are (1) the fertilizable life span of an oocyte is not over 24 hours after ovulation; (2)

sperm survival in the female genital tract is not over 4 days; and (3) ovulation which determines the rhythm of a cycle occurs 14 days before the menstrual flow, and every woman will have cycles which vary within a predictable range. Using these assumptions, Ogino and Knaus calculated the so-called safe period by obtaining cycle records of a woman over a six-month or, preferably, one-year period. Fourteen days were subtracted from the longest cycle to get the latest ovulation date, one day added for ovum survival and one more for good measure, and this date was regarded as the end of the fertile period. Fourteen days were then subtracted from the shortest cycle to calculate the earliest ovulation date and four days subtracted for sperm survival, one additional day was subtracted for good measure, and this date determined the beginning of the fertile period.

Reexamination of the principles upon which the method is based in the light of current knowledge indicates that some of the premises are false. From knowledge based on assumptions derived from animal experimentation, it is probably correct that the life span of the unfertilized oocyte in the female tract is not over 24 hours. However, the second assumption, that human sperm survive with normal fertilizing capacity no longer than 96 hours, seems unjustifiable. Information obtained from donor insemination in the human indicates that four days is not unusual and recent data collected by Marshall, during a study on rhythm contraception, indicated that 10 days is the probable "cut-off" period. The third premise, e.g., all ovulation occurs at 14 days premenstrually, is also probably incorrect, as recent studies by Cargill, Ross, and Yoshimi indicate that at least in young women ovulation may occur much closer to the menses. Thus, it would seem that, instead of a 14-day period, one would, perhaps, need to use a figure of 10 days. The variation of the menstrual cycle is another factor which must be responsible for many rhythm failures. Tietze, in his estimate of the efficacy of rhythm contraception, advises that it can be used for child spacing satisfactorily, but not for child limitation, as within a 2-year period, each woman can be expected to have one cycle which is markedly inconsistent from those characteristic of that individual. This variation is usually caused by factors which disturb the preovulatory cyclic surge of pituitary LH, and are psychogenic stress, acute illnesses, fever, medication, and travel. Women using this method must be alert to these possible interferences and abstain in cycles exposed to such influences.

The other method for circumventing such problems is by the use of the basal body temperature chart. The findings indicate that there is really no "safe period" before ovulation. When basal body temperature graphs are used to pinpoint ovulation and intercourse is confined to the areas *after the thermal shift,* in a small highly motivated group of patients, the method's success rate, according to Sobrero, approximates 100%. According to Marshall, when used in conjunction with the basal body temperature chart in this fashion, the failure rate is 6.6 per 100 women years, whereas, if even as much as a day is added in the preovulatory phase, the failure rate rises to 19 per 100 women years. In summary, to make the method acceptable in regard to its effectiveness, one must pinpoint ovulation with the basal body temperature chart and confine intercourse to the immediate postovulatory area. This limits exposure to approximately 10 days per cycle and is, therefore, impractical for younger couples. The method obviously requires the highest degree of motivation but rates among the least expensive. One of the interesting advantages, which has been reported for the method, is that it leads to some increase in libido due to the long periods of continence. On the other side of the coin, one might say it leads to psychological problems due to frustrations.

Several studies have been made using clomiphene to regularize cycles and thus allow greater predictability of ovulation. The method is not successful enough to permit omission of the basal body temperature chart but can be used to shorten the long cycles. When used in conjunction with the basal body temperature chart, it may have some advantages for patients with grossly irregular, prolonged cycles. The risk of multiple pregnancies in method failures sharply limits its applicability.

Methods for Absolute Limitation

Sterilization: Female. Surgical methods for sterilization of the female are discussed in any gynecological surgical text and range from electrocoagulation and division or mechanical occlusion of tubes at laparoscopy to a more thorough and reliable form of tubal ligation at laparotomy, to hysterectomy. The average gynecologist will employ hysterectomy for the purpose of sterilization only when there are other more generalized indications for removal of the uterus. With reliable types of tubal ligation procedures, not performed in the immediate postpartum period, the failure rate is theoretically low. The disadvantages are that it is frequently an irreversible procedure. There are occasional technical failures. It is an operative procedure with a minimal mortality and morbidity rate. It has become medically acceptable to *consider* sterilization of any patient who requests it. However, the physician must consider it in the light of its possible irreversibility and be sure that the patient understands this aspect of the procedure. Except for maternal health problems or eugenic considerations, it is probably wise to avoid such a final method in relatively young women.

Sterilization: Male. The same considerations apply to male sterilization as have been discussed in female sterilization. However, the method of sterilization in the male is simpler. It is unassociated with the morbidity and mortality accompanying female sterilization. In addition to these advantages, it also has the advantage of being a permanent procedure and the disadvantage of being an irreversible procedure. The theoretical failure rate is low, although occasionally the duct will recanalize. Pregnancy exposure must be avoided over the 3- to 4-month period following operation when the collecting tubules are being emptied of sperm. It is wise to ask the patient to use precautions until a urologist has declared his ejaculate free of sperm. As in the female, it is probably unwise to sterilize a relatively young male, and likewise a husband should not be sterilized because of medical indications in the wife. The fear of serious medical complications associated with autoimmune disease due to the sperm granulomata has not been substantiated.

Abortion

Induced abortion has been a recognized method for family and population control throughout the world. Japan has utilized this technique as the major method of population control and has successfully maintained the lowered stable birth rate necessary for her existence. Hungary is also reported to have a successful abortion program for population control. The success of such a program probably rests upon the availability of broad spectrum antibiotics and the development of the suction curet (see Chapter 29). The first has reduced the morbidity and mortality from infection, while the last has decreased blood loss. The only advantage of the method seems to be its efficacy. The wastefulness of time and expense in terms of physician and hospital utilization, as well as the moral and ethical aspects, allow abortion to be regarded only as a backup procedure for method failures, not as a contraceptive method.

REFERENCES

Baird, D.: Sterilization and Therapeutic abortion in Aberdeen. Brit. J. Psychiat., *113:* 701, 1967.

Barglow, P., and Eisner, M.: An evaluation of tubal ligation in Switzerland. Amer. J. Obstet. Gynec., *95:* 1083, 1966.

Bartzen, P. J.: Cycle Regulation with clomiphene citrate: A double blind study. Amer. J. Obstet. Gynec., *101:* 1032, 1968.

Basavarajappa, K. G., and Belvalgidad, M. I.: Changes in age at marriage of females and their effect on the birth rate in India. Eugen. Quart., *14:* 14, March 1967.

Beckerhoff, R., Luetscher, J. A., Wilkinson, R., Gonzales, C., and Nokes, G. W.: Plasma renin concentration activity, and substrate in hypertension induced by oral contraceptives. J. Clin. Endocr. Metab., *34:* 1067, 1972.

Brakman, P., and Astrup, T.: Effects of female hormones, used as oral contraceptives, on the fibrinolytic system in blood. Lancet, *July 4:* 10, 1964.

Catterall, R. D.: Candida albicans and the contraceptive pill. Lancet, *October 15:* 830, 1966.

Daniel, D. G., Bloom, A. L., Giddings, J. C., Campbell, H., and Turnbull, A. C.: Increased factor IX levels in puerperium during administration of diethylstilboestrol. Brit. Med. J., *March 30:* 801, 1968.

Emerson, L., Gordon, R., Roman, S., Jr., Koike, M., and Speidel, J. J.: Acceptance of family planning among a cohort of recently delivered mothers. Amer. J. Public Health, *58:* 1738, 1968.

Erickson, L. R., and Peterka, E. S.: Sunlight sensitivity from oral contraceptives. J.A.M.A., *203:* 980, 1968.

Garcia, R., Pincus, G., and Rock, J.: Effects of three 19-*nor*-steroids on human ovulation and menstruation. Amer. J. Obstet. Gynec., *75:* 82, 1958.

Haynes, R. L., and Dunn, J. M.: Oral contraceptives, thrombosis, and sickle cell hemoglobinopathies. J.A.M.A., *200:* 186, 1967.

Hollander, C. S., Garcia, A. M., Sturgis, S. H., and Selenkow, H. A.: Effect of an ovulatory suppressant on the serum protein-bound iodine and the red-cell uptake of radioactive triiodothyronine, New Eng. J. Med., *269:* 501, 1963.

Inman, W. H. W., and Vessey, M. P.: Investigation of deaths from pulmonary, coronary, and cerebral thrombosis and embolism in women of child-bearing age. Brit. Med. J., *2:* 193, 1968.

Jordan, W. M.: Pulmonary Embolism. Lancet, *2:* 1146, 1961.

Kissebah, A. H., Harrigan, P., and Wynn, V.: Mechanism of hypertriglyceridaemia associated with contraceptive steroids. Horm. Metab. Res., *5:* 184, 1973.

Kunin, C. M., and McCormack, R. C.: Oral contraceptives and blood pressure. Arch. Intern. Med., *123:* 363, 1969.

Marshall, J.: Congenital defects and age of spermatozoa. Internat. J. Fertil., *13:* 110, 1968.

Marshall, J.: A field trial of the basal body temperature method of regulating births. Lancet, *2:* 8, 1968.

Mayer, J.: Food and population: A different view. Nutrition Rev., *22:* 353, 1964.

Marx, J. L.: Birth control; current technology, future prospects. Science, *179:* 1222, 1973.

McLeroy, V. J., and Schendel, H. E.: Influence of oral contraceptives on ascorbic acid concentrations in healthy, sexually mature women. Amer. J. Clin. Nutr., *26:* 191, 1973.

Mishell, Daniel R., Jr., and Lumkin, Mary E.: Contraceptive effect of varying dosages of progestogens in silastic vaginal rings. Fertil. Steril., *21:* No. 2, February, 1970.

Morris, G. McL., and Van Wagenen, G.: Compounds interfering with ovum implantation and development. Amer. J. Obstet. Gynec., *96:* 804, 1966.

Neumann, H. H., and Frick, H. C., II: Occlusion of the fallopian tubes with tantalum clips. Amer. J. Obstet. Gynec., *81:* 803, 1961.

Orellana-Alcalde, J. M., and Dominguez, J. P.: Jaundice and oral contraceptive drugs. Lancet, *December 10:* 1278, 1966.

Østergaard, E.: Oral anticonception side effects and risks. Acta Obstet. Gynec. Scand., *XLVIII,* Supplement 1: 57, 1969.

Paniagua, M. E., Piedras, R., Vaillant, H. W., and Gamble, C. J.: Field trial of a contraceptive foam in Puerto Rico. J.A.M.A., *177:* 125, 1961.

Poller, L., Thomson, J. M., and Thomas, P. W.: Effects of progestogen oral contraceptives with norethisterone on blood clotting and platelets. Brit. Med. J., *4:* 391, 1972.

Resnik, S.: Melasma induced by oral contraceptive drugs. J.A.M.A., *199:* 95, 1967.

Richart, R. M., Neuwirth, R. S., Iorangkun, C., and Sukhit, P.: Female sterilization by electrocoagulation of tubal ostia using hysteroscopy. Amer. J. Obstet. Gynec., *117:* 801, 1973.

Rutensköld, M.: Pregnancies during oral contraceptive treatment. Acta Obstet. Gynec. Scand., *50:* 203, 1971.

Schaffner, F.: The effect of oral contraceptives on the liver. J.A.M.A., *198:* 155, 1966.

Spellacy, W. N., Carlson, K. L., Birk, S. A., and Schade, S. L.: Glucose and insulin alterations after one year of combination-type oral contraceptive treatment. Metabolism, *17:* 496, 1968.

Spadoni, L. R., Lein, J. N., and Herrman, W. L.: Planned ovulation: Clomiphene citrate to regulate cycles in patients using the rhythm method. Obstet. Gynec., *29:* 18, 1967.

Strieff, R. R.: Folate deficiency and oral contraceptives. J.A.M.A., *214:* 105, 1970.

Sturgis, S. H., and Albright, F.: Mechanism of estrin therapy in relief of dysmenorrhea. Endocrinology, *26:* 102, 1940.

Swartz, D. P., Bullard, T. H., and Felton, H. T.: The introduction of contraception in an urban public hospital. Amer. J. Obstet. Gynec., *97:* 189, 1967.

Tietze, C., Poliakoff, S. R., and Rock, J.: Clinical effectiveness of rhythm method of contraception. Fertil. Steril., *2:* 441, 1951.

Tietze, C., and Potter, R. G., Jr.: Statistical evaluation of the rhythm method. Amer. J. Obstet. Gynec., *84:* 692, 1962.

Tietze, C.: Induced abortion and sterilization as methods of fertility control. J. Chronic Dis., *18:* 1161, 1965.

Vessey, M. P., and Doll, R.: Investigation of relation between use of oral contraceptives and thromboembolic disease. Brit. Med. J., *2:* 199, 1968.

Wynn, Y., Doar, J. W. H., Mill, G. L., and Stokes, T.: Fasting serum triglyceride, cholesterol and lipoprotein levels during oral contraceptive therapy. Lancet, *2:* 756, 1969.

Wynn, V., and Doar, J. W. H.: Some effects of oral contraceptives on carbohydrate metabolism. Lancet, *2:* 761, 1969.

chapter 35

Sex Education

The subject of sex education has been difficult and controversial, perhaps because it concerns divergent disciplines which, for this topic, are so intimately related that experience indicates they cannot be separated. The statement of my British friend is very apropos. When asked if he thought sex education should be taught in the public schools, he replied "I suppose so, but where would you teach it, in Biology or Poetry?" *Sex instruction* is strictly scientific and factual and concerns the anatomy and biology of reproduction, including, of course, family formation and contraceptive methods. *Education in sexuality,* on the other hand, involves ethics, morals, physiology, political science, economics, and all those things which concern the training of the individual to understand himself as a sexual being and to develop successful relationships with other sexual individuals.

Therefore, to a large extent, this topic is of the social sciences. It is regrettable that the factual data which should ideally serve as the content of a course in education for sexuality is virtually nonexistent and what little information is available is so subjective in nature that its reliability is suspect.

An additional difficulty is found in defining the aims of sex education and, therefore, in assessing the success of any program. Most educators, however, agree that the aim should be to develop a well adjusted adult who has lost the egotistical attitude of adolescence and is, thereby, able to use his sexuality (*total personality*) in a responsible manner, thus bringing happiness to himself and others (society). In this area, heretofore, adjustment in the society in which we live in Western civilization has been synonymous with a happy monogamous marriage or a happy unmarried individual without children. As strictly secondary objectives in the total picture, but, perhaps of major importance in some population groups, are the ancillary benefits which would hopefully accrue from such a program; these are a decrease in illegitimacy, venereal disease, and in marital problems supposedly related to sexual difficulties.

The findings in the two countries which have had most experience with sex education programs in the school have indicated that these aims have been difficult to achieve. In Russia the program instituted in 1917 was discontinued in 1948 because, quoting from the Soviet Education Bulletin, "People have incorrectly understood the freedom described in the program and decided sex life can be carried on with a disorderly succession of husbands and wives. . . . Such practices lead to a laxity of orderly relationships unworthy of man, cause difficulties with personality problems, unhappiness and disruption of the family, making orphans of the children." Illegitimacy and venereal disease are increasing in Sweden in spite of a program which has been operating for 15 years and Sjövall says that, "in spite of 40 years of matter of fact instruction in sex education and open-minded discussions, marital sexual difficulties have not decreased, presumably because they are psychologically determined, not biologically." Thus, education for sexuality is at fault, not sex instruction.

The experience of these two nations epitomizes the problem with the programs in general. Education for sexuality, *e.g.,* social responsibility for sexual activity, as defined in Western culture, is apparently difficult, if not impossible, to teach in a school situation, and one can only expect to re-enforce what is learned by example and training in the home situation. Without a stable home background and matrix of education of sexuality, sex instruction must be given very skillfully if the students are not to derive the impression of adult permissiveness. The experience in Russia and elsewhere has been that sex instruction, without education for sexuality, makes for promiscuous sexual behavior, thus thwarting the aims of the well planned program.

The field of sex education and education for sexuality—aside from Masters and Johnson who qualify as experts on techniques, not sexuality—has been largely abandoned by the gynecologist to the psychologist and psychiatrist. This has often led to a theoretical rather than factual approach.

The following sections are written from (1) a review of facts in the literature, (2) experience during 30 years of gynecologic practice among two social extremes, the jet set and the Baltimore ghetto population, and (3) experience as a successful wife and mother of three successful children.

SEX INSTRUCTION

Ottesen-Jensen has outlined a program for sex education, by different age levels, in "Handbook on Sex Instruction" which has been compulsory in the Swedish schools since 1955. It is stated that the purpose of sex instruction in Sweden is to give biological information in such a manner that it will help mold ideals and build character. Thus, it must have an ethical basis and conform with society's demands. Therefore, although this is called a "Handbook on Sex Instruction," education for sexuality is interwoven. The handbook is striving to teach the poetry with the biology, and I would suspect that, in any course of sex instruction, this is a very important warp and woof to weave successfully together.

The following paragraphs, on the content of a course in sex instruction, are based largely, but not entirely, on the considerable experience represented by the Ottesen-Jensen Handbook.

Seven- to Ten-Year Level

During this age level, facts about reproduction in general are learned. Starting with the content, seeds, and seed germination and the development of pure and hybrid strains progress to eggs and fertilization of eggs, hatching of chicks, to the birth of kittens and puppies, and finally to the single cell egg in the human and its union with the sperm. This brings about a realization of the importance of a mother and a father, the differences between the sexes, how the baby develops in the mother and how the child is born and the importance of the family relationship in that the child needs protective care after birth. At this age, it is important to realize that one does not need to go into anatomical details. Instruction is carried out without visual aids. Instruction in anatomy of sexual organs does not need to be given in great detail. The child at this age is usually greatly interested in biological studies and a good teacher can evoke a lively exchange of questions. Such a discussion should complement the factual material reviewed and amplify any details which have been slighted or omitted.

Ages 11 through 13 Years

The major item for discussion during these ages is the development of the internal sexual organs in relation to the development of the secondary sexual characteristics. This involves the description of the relationship of ovarian and testicular function to the maturation of the central nervous system, hypothalamus, and pituitary which gives the individual some comprehension and respect for his total anatomical and physiological integration. The structure and the function of the sexual organs can be discussed in more detail at this age level, allowing for the discussion of menstruation and wet dreams. More detailed discussion of conception and the embryology of the developing fetus, as well as labor and delivery, can be introduced.

In the Jensen handbook, it is advised to discuss certain abnormalities of the sex drive such as homosexuality, exhibitionism, and child molesters. However, it is our belief that such topics are better left for explanation in discussions, if questions regarding them arise. The normal rather than the abnormal is important at this age so that fears are not unnecessarily raised. Every child should, of course, be taught not to go with a stranger under any circumstances, but this can go under the general head of prevention of kidnapping, and sex aberrations do not need to be discussed. Such pathological conditions are fortunately unusual and can be individually explained to the child who has such an experience. Unfortunately, forewarning does not protect the child against such experiences, and a detailed discussion may color his attitude towards normal sexuality. The topic of masturbation, however, is one which might be

casually introduced as a normal adolescent habit pattern which disappears as the individual reaches adulthood.

At this age level, visual aids may be used and blackboard drawings, rather than slides, have been found to be more effective, as it is more personalized and can be better integrated into the individual's own lecture. Moving pictures may also be used, but all of this material should be ancillary, as there is no substitute for a personal explanation by an individual who is respected and trusted by the student. All classes in sex instruction should be followed by an adequate time for questions and answers. The students should also be allowed to write questions, as some will prefer this type of anonymity.

Ages 14 through 16

At this age, discussion of sexual intercourse among adolescents, premarital intercourse, the definition of promiscuity, illegitimate children, and venereal disease is introduced. This is the age, in other words, where the social aspects of sex come into focus. It is, therefore, desirable at this point to introduce the concept of sexuality and education for sexuality. Sex instruction has been completed. The concept of the importance of responsibility in the act of intercourse must be developed—responsibility not only for the new life of a child which may result, but also for the individuals involved. Intercourse as an act of love and sharing must again be stressed. Discussions of the home and family as the basis of our Western society form a nidus for the discussion of adolescent intercourse where family formation is precluded because of financial and educational responsibilities. The problem of sexual continence can be discussed in the light of other physical needs. Everyone recognizes the desirability and necessity of controlling appetite for both food and drink and regulation of sleep and work habits. One has the opportunity here to discuss the difficulties which excesses of alcohol or drugs pose in the responsible management of sexual behavior. One can also develop the concept that a happy monogamous marriage perhaps depends upon the development of this type of continence. There is certainly good evidence to indicate that child rearing is most successful in homes with a happy monogamous marriage.

At this age, discussions should stress the importance of limiting families to two or three children as a social responsibility in our already crowded world. They should develop the theme that sexual intercourse implies the readiness to accept responsibility for our actions, for our own welfare and, more especially, for the welfare of the individuals with whom we are associated. These sessions should also stress that sexual intercourse is a way of life which implies willingness to accept responsibility for the beginning of another life and that this requires emotional maturity, physical work, and financial responsibility. Current reliable contraceptive methods should be enumerated with the statement that every pregnancy should be a planned pregnancy and every baby a wanted baby. No specific discussion of details of contraceptive techniques is called for at this time, but the lecture should conclude with the statement that, before the individual is ready to be married or begin intercourse, he or she should consult a physician for a premarital consultation, at which time a decision can be made about which contraceptive technique would be most suitable for that individual. If the teacher has been successful in securing interest and rapport, those individuals who need further instruction in contraception, because of already established intercourse habits, will find a way to discuss this with the teacher individually.

Techniques and detailed description of intercourse should be reserved for specific courses on sexual anatomy and physiology, either with a prerequisite for routine sex education courses or at the college level.

Because of the difficulty of integrating instruction in sex with education for sexuality which many educators, as well as individuals, feel is best done in the home with a responsible family situation, a series of television programs have been developed for family participation which can be viewed in the home one evening and then discussed in a school general meeting with parents and children the following day. Such a program has a great deal of merit. It has also been suggested that, in the absence of such a television program, sex instruction and education for sexuality can be taught on a voluntary basis outside of school hours with the participation of families and students. The concern of individuals and educators is that this type of so-called sex education may serve only as sex exposure. Richards, in an article on The Role of the Physician in Sex Education, points out that, after the flurry of interest in this subject in 1940, there was a reaction and suggestion that sex education was a cause of promiscuity. As previously stated, one would have to say that this was not sex education but sex miseducation, but there is some evidence that, when this type of material is mishandled, such an adverse result may ensue.

Hoffmeyer gives a concrete example of such a situation. In a boarding school for physically handicapped children in Sweden, it was found that two or three pregnancies occurred each year. It was decided to introduce a course on sex information, including information on contraception, when and how to obtain these devices, and the emotional and ethical aspects of premarital relationships, and the responsibilities involved. A great deal of interest was generated in the course and open-minded discussion ensued. In the year following the introduction of this course, there were 10 rather than 3 girls pregnant. The authors concluded that the open-minded approach had signaled to the children adult permissiveness in this type of relationship. It is interesting and, perhaps, informative that the directive given by the Soviet Education Academy, published in 1948, signaled a change from their former sex education in schools from 1917 through 1948. It is stated that sex education, *e.g.,* explanation of sex and reproductive functions, is not to be taught in the schools but in the home. The parents were instructed that examples of genuine love, mutual respect, and aid between the mother and father is the most important aspect for sexual education. They stressed that talks should be held between father, son, mother, and daughter. This Russian about-face meant that they thought that their permissive education made for promiscuous sexual behavior.

Dr. John Rock, before the American Infertility Society, in a lecture which has never been published, concluded his talk for adolescents with a discussion of primate anthropology. If one studies monkeys, chimpanzees, gorillas, and humans, one finds that polygamy and promiscuity disappear to be replaced by monogamy and constancy. The persistence of this pattern through millennia seems to indicate that it has merit, from the point of view of the individual and society. Dr. Rock was wont to conclude this lecture by the statement "boys, be a man, don't make a monkey out of yourself." This is an extremely good ending for the topic, but today we must broaden the scope by including girls.

PREMARITAL CONTRACEPTIVE ADVICE

Although it has been stated in the "ideal situation," contraceptive advice for a specific couple is best discussed and decided upon in the premarital consultation, it must be recognized that there are many other situations which do not fit this ideal. In cultural areas, where it is recognized that unwed girls are exposed to pregnancy, it is of course mandatory that such information be furnished. In certain socioeconomic areas, it can be expected that young girls may be exposed to pregnancy, with or without consent, at or slightly after their first ovulation. It has been found that one of the best approaches to this problem is a house to house canvass by a visiting nurse from the State Health Department who can discuss the situation with the mother or the individual involved. Both are usually well aware of the problem and anxious to cooperate to prevent such unwanted pregnancies.

The most satisfactory method, at the present time, seems to be oral contraception administered by the mother. If there is no responsible mother or mother-substitute in the house, injectable steroids can be considered. A small intrauterine device may be the contraceptive of choice, as it is difficult and slightly hazardous to maintain young girls on oral contraception over the appropriate number of years. However, it goes without saying, that the health hazard involved is nevertheless minute in comparison to that entailed by a pregnancy and the responsibility of child rearing at such an early age.

The unmarried girl of the upper socioeconomic status who requests contraceptive advice poses a different problem and probably requires a different approach, depending upon her experience. If she has not engaged in intercourse, she deserves the benefit of advice as to the desirability and possible consequence of her contemplated relationship. If she has already been having intercourse, the experience is that she will continue to do so. She needs the same type of advice. From a theoretical point of view, the best type of contraception for this casual intercourse relationship is condom contraception by the male as, in addition to protecting against pregnancy, it also protects from venereal disease. The Swedish experts have suggested that all girls be advised to carry condoms with them and insist that their partners wear them. Such advice is probably valuable, not only because of its soundness, but also because it underlines for the patient the hazards of this way of life. It places it in its realistic perspective, removing the glamour, and pinpoints for her exactly how much responsibility her partner is willing to take. This in turn is a fair index of his concern for her as an individual. If he is unsympathetic and resistant to this form of contraception, the true value of the relationship can be assessed.

Frequently the patient is actually requesting oral contraception but is also anxious not to have parents or guardians informed of her decision. The hazards of this position should be appreciated by the physician and he, in turn, should inform the patient. Because of the possibility, even though remote, of thromboembolic disease, oral contraception is dangerous under these circumstances. Because parents are responsible for the health and welfare of minors, they are entitled to know of medications which can produce serious, even fatal, consequences. If the patient is not a minor, the casual relationship of extramarital intercourse does not provide for the presence of a responsible individual other than the patient who is aware of the possible dangers of thromboembolic disease and is in a position to recognize and report signs or symptoms promptly. For these reasons, and especially when dealing with minors, it is preferable to use an intrauterine device or fit a diaphragm and insist that the patient accept the responsibility for wearing it consistently as described in Chapter 34.

INSTRUCTION FOR SEXUALITY

Sexuality may be defined as the character of maleness or femaleness. Development of our sexuality involves the development of our characters as mature, responsible, adult individuals, therefore happy adult men or women. This further implies a successful relationship with other individuals and society. It is an integral part of each individual and determines the way he talks, walks, sits, dresses, in short all of his actions and activities. It is determined by and, in turn, determines (1) the way he thinks about himself, *his gender role* and (2) the way society regards him, *the social gender*. In short, sexuality involves the development of the character and characteristics of the individual and, therefore, is intimately concerned with his individuality and his place as a member of the society in which he lives. The development of this sexuality or character, if you will, implies

development of standards for self evaluation, and acceptance of such standards implies acceptance of responsibility for personal action. Because sexuality involves the total individual, it must recognize the anatomical aspects of each individual, which are specifically designed for functioning in the sex act, intercourse. As intercourse, which is an expression of sexuality, is an activity which involves another individual, education in sexuality becomes education in interpersonal relationships between individuals and society. An aim of adequate education for sexuality, as stated above, is, therefore, to develop an individual who will accept full responsibility for his actions, not only to himself but to others.

In an International Conference of Sex Education and Family Planning in 1962, the concensus was that the aim of education in sexuality was the development of a well adjusted, happy adult with a responsible nonegotistical attitude toward self and others, which is society. It was thought that, if this aim could be accomplished, the individual would have an appreciation of the positive satisfaction associated with responsible sexual relationships which have, as a foundation, love and consideration for other individuals, rather than the simple relief of sex tensions. Under these circumstances, family stability and an atmosphere of love and respect, so necessary for proper rearing of children, are accomplished.

This brings us very naturally through the full circle to the question of how best to teach children the development of sexuality which involves *ethics,* as it is concerned with the happiness of the individual, *inter-personal relationships* or *morals,* as it intimately involves at least one other individual, and two, if a child is conceived, *sociology,* as it concerns family formation and reaction to society in general and finally, *biology* and *physiology,* as reproduction is an ultimate consequence of this development.

All experts agree that education for sexuality begins at birth. The most and, perhaps, the only effective education is received from the parents or parent-substitutes, within the first two years of life. This education is by action and example, not by verbalization. Thus, the way the parents treat the individual determines, to a large degree, the gender role of that individual. Investigations of Money, and Money and Hamstead, with children who have ambiguous external genitalia and have been raised in a sex contrary to the chromosomal and gonadal sex, indicate that these "social factors" are the major contributions to the development of the gender role. This role has usually been set by the age of two years, and efforts to change the sex of rearing after this age are apt to be unsuccessful. The relation of transvestism to pathological parental attitudes is also suggested by certain case histories. This, however, may merely modify or re-enforce specific embryonic imprinting of the central nervous system through male or female types of steroid hormones.

Not only behavioristic elements of sexuality are influenced by such early parental treatment, but also the basis for interpersonal relationships is established. The observation of a loving, considerate relationship between parents and siblings is, perhaps, the most effective teaching method. It is a well established fact that children from happy homes are prone to make happy marriages, whereas those from broken homes are more apt themselves to have unsuccessful marriages.

A successful educational program can only be developed, if one can define the aims and then evaluate the project in terms of success by accomplishment of these aims. This has become unusually difficult for education in sexuality recently because of the changing concepts of social behavior. In Western culture, education in sexuality had as its proper aim the development of a mature, responsible adult who was, therefore, prepared to enter into a happy, monogamous marriage and become a responsible parent. There may be some question about this structuring of our society in the future. Extramarital relationships were generally frowned upon, although tacitly accepted for men, because the experience was that the habit of multiple sexual relationships did not predispose to the most success in a later monogamous marriage. Promiscuity patterns are notoriously habit-forming for men or women. The use of prostitutes has been generally condemned as degrading to a man's sexuality, because it fosters acceptance of the sex act for relief of sexual tension without proper regard for the other individual involved. Thus, the action degrades the prostitute in relegating her to the status of a possession or convenience. With the dawn of female suffrage and equality, the professional prostitute has begun to disappear, but the non-professional prostitute has appeared. The double standard is also disappearing, because women have tended to accept the casual sexual relationships which were common among a certain element of the male population. Thus, we cannot quote the disappearance of the professional prostitute or the double standard as being completely due to a more mature responsible and adult attitude for the use of sexuality, if by this we mean consideration for the rights and happiness of the other person involved. Although, with current widespread knowledge and technology of birth control, it is possible for women to engage in extramarital intercourse and promiscuous relationships without fear of pregnancy, this, nevertheless, does not insure that the individual has discharged his or her full responsibility in the relationship. Many women assume that, if they are not taking responsibility for beginning another life, they are acting in a responsible manner. This, however, fails to consider the other individual as well as their own sexuality which is involved. Experience has taught us that, in the breaking of such an intimate, warm, and, supposedly, tender, considerate relationship, someone is invariably hurt in the process and, in hurting others, we damage ourselves by blunting our sensitivities. From a woman's point of view, we need only read the autobiographies of famous men's mistresses to know some of the heartaches and bitternesses involved. The divorce courts are also filled with similar accounts involving multiple marriages and divorces, *e.g.,* legal prostitution. When children are the result of these episodes, the damage is compounded, and the courts and psychiatrists' offices are filled with individuals whose problems are apparently the result of such broken homes.

Perhaps the monogamous marriage system was developed throughout the eons as the best protection for proper rearing of children, and, perhaps, we are no longer going to find this the best social system. However, in advising our youth or our patients on the question of extramarital intercourse, it is well to remind them of the simple facts. The first of these, perhaps, is that experience teaches that extramarital promiscuity does not make for a happy, monogamous marriage, that this is a habit pattern which is easily established and broken only with great difficulty. Such an extramarital relationship is obviously entered into with the tacit understanding between the two parties of the possibility of failure. Experience with marriage, contracted with the possibility of divorce in mind, has shown such marriages have less chance of succeeding. It also indicates to both partners that the other member is not completely sure of his or her feelings toward him. In the *ideal* loving situation such reserves cannot exist, therefore the union is immediately labeled as not *ideal,* therefore not the most desirable or the most *ethical.* The thought that such extramarital relationships teach sexual behavior has been shown to be erroneous, especially for the female who frequently achieves the complete response to intercourse only after protracted experience with a thoughtful, loving partner under ideal conditions of comfort and privacy. The usual extramarital relationship does not reproduce such conditions either physically or psychologically. A loving relationship is one in which the other individual is considered, and his or her happiness is the first concern. Although Kirkendall described extramarital relations as "moral," if they develop self-respect, mutual trust, integrity, and self-fulfillment and improved interpersonal relationships or, in other words, as the students say, "if nobody gets hurt" as already stated, unless this is a completely casual relationship between two casual individuals, someone is bound to be hurt. Kirkendall's own research study of college students leads to the conclusion that 82 per cent of the student premarital intercourse was exploitative in nature.

Finally, for the individual whose ultimate aim is a successful, monogamous marriage with family formation, it is probably wise to continue to hold the tenets of the society in which we presently live. Rules governing the way people live together have evolved for very good reasons, and those who do not adhere to these rules must be prepared to take the consequences. It must also be remembered that he or she has involved at least one other individual by his actions. This type of relationship is not an individual's private affair but concerns society in general. This means that, not only he or she who engages in this conduct may be hurt, but that the families may also be legally and financially involved. Sexuality involves other individuals and society, and, therefore, it must have as a basis honesty. We cannot live together as individuals and as families or as communities by practicing or speaking falsehoods.

The advantage of premarital continence is the advantage of anticipation. This is one of the greatest pleasures in life. Giving a child a beautiful and complicated toy before he is ready for it, or even before he has had the opportunity to long for it, destroys some of his pleasure in it, sometimes permanently. It certainly destroys the value which he attributes to it, and the same can be said for sexual activity. The individual who enters into this relationship at too early an age fails to bring to the act the maturity which raises it from a physical reaction to a sacrament between two people, the ultimate mature act of complete sharing and complete consideration for another individual. The emphasis must be on responsibility. As with everything in life, if it is too easy, it is not appreciated. If we do not accept physical and financial responsibility as the price for our sexual pleasure, we have devalued its worth.

CONCLUSIONS

The most effective education for sexuality is by example from the parents or parent substitutes in the home. This can best be re-enforced in the schools by teaching *honesty* and consideration in our daily actions with ourselves and others, the importance of *responsibility* and the difference between freedom and license, the advantages of *self-control,* self-discipline, and anticipation. As physicians, when called upon to counsel individuals in these matters, we must be able to differentiate the perennial, egotistical adolescent who is already fixed in his or her sexual habit patterns, and the individual who is capable of the mature, adult, loving relationship. Marriage and family formation should probably only be entered into by the latter group. If we could develop a society on this basis, we would then have the best theoretical situation for ideal sexual education— happy, loving parents creating a thoughtful, loving home.

THE PREMARITAL CONSULTATION

The purpose of the premarital consultation is often three-fold. Primarily, it provides an opportunity for the novice to acquire knowledge from a competent advisor without embarrassment. Some otherwise well educated women feel insecure about their knowledge of marital relationships and hygiene, and books are no substitute for a personal interview. Secondarily, a premarital pelvic examination reveals a pathological condition in approximately 10 per cent of women. The detection and correction of such conditions as a rigid hymen, congenital malformations of the mid- and upper vagina, endometriosis, and pelvic tumors go far in the prevention of so-called "sexual frigidity" and dyspareunia. In this field an

ounce of prevention is easily worth the proverbial pound of cure. The final purpose of the premarital consultation is to provide advice on family planning. This topic was completely discussed in Chapter 34.

In this day of educational courses on everything, including marital relations, it is often pointless for the doctor to discuss the anatomy and physiology of menstruation and reproduction, which may be well known to the patient. However, she should be afforded the opportunity of asking for information she may have missed in her educational program. It is well to have some diagrams or models of male and female anatomy on hand as office visual aids. The more usual positions for intercourse may be discussed, but she should be told that there is no right or wrong technique and any comfortable posture is satisfactory. However, for the inexperienced couple the usual position, with the wife on her back and the husband above, is certainly the most satisfactory for learning. The reverse position, with the wife above, is often a better position for the wife as she has more control of the situation under these circumstances.

The frequency of intercourse should depend primarily upon the male sex drive, for the male physiology involved requires active physical stress. Few if any women have suffered strokes during intercourse while such are not uncommon in older men. There is a wide divergence of normal—varying from two to three times in 24 hours, for the newly married couple, to once or twice a week. Too frequent intercourse will often cause some local irritation to the female urethra and introitus; and, if this happens, intercourse should be discontinued for 24 or 48 hours and hot Sitz baths should be taken. If a habit pattern of two or more times a day persists, there is some reason to be concerned that fertility may be reduced. Therefore, under these circumstances, the husband should be encouraged to develop an athletic skill or another interest which will help to dissipate his sexual tension. Intercourse less frequently than once a week in a newly married couple may simply reflect a lethargic personality.

The female should be advised to allow her male partner's sex drive to set their pace and she should attempt to gear hers satisfactorily to his. This statement is predicated on the necessity for more active physical participation in the act by the male and the knowledge that there is a certain latency period in the ability of the male to achieve an orgasm. Thus it is easier for the female, physiologically, to control her desires than for the male to increase his activities. Lack of consideration for the male partner's inherent physical drive is a common cause of impotence and reflects an immature attitude of the female who is using her partner for self-gratification. If she finds after several months or years that this is not possible, she is advised to consult her physician as soon as she realizes there is a real problem. In assuming this role of "follow the leader," however, she is cautioned not to make her sexual relations passive. Active participation in the sex act is necessary for full fruition.

The subject of douches is frequently of interest to the patient and she may be told that this is a matter of individual preference but that douching after intercourse is not a necessity for hygienic or esthetic reasons. A tub bath or shower is quite adequate.

The patient should be encouraged to discuss her attitude towards intercourse in order that the physician may evaluate her maturity and knowledge. The importance of the act to her husband in both physical and emotional aspects should be stressed and she should be warned that it may take three to six months and sometimes longer for the inexperienced woman to develop a complete orgasm. The development of satisfactory intercourse techniques depends upon mature love and respect for one another, real interest and desire to learn, and the ability to relax. Sometimes this last factor depends upon such trivial matters as drawn blinds and quiet bedsprings. Complete privacy is, of course, a most important consideration.

All of these factors or any one of them may be concerned in the production of frigidity or dyspareunia and, as indicated above, it is easier to prevent these conditions than to cure them.

Sexual Frigidity and Dyspareunia

Sexual frigidity, by which is meant the inability to respond sexually, is not frequent in the female, although there seems to be little doubt that libido, which is well developed among normal males, appears to be somewhat less highly developed among females. Some believe that sexual unresponsiveness is always indicative of such abnormalities as lack of love for the husband, poor techniques, etc. However, it is often encountered in otherwise entirely normal women who love their husbands devotedly and in whom all the other usually described factors can be eliminated. *Dyspareunia,* or painful coitus, may be due to the presence of an actual lesion or it may be of psychic origin. The latter variety is not infrequently a defense mechanism built up by the woman who for one reason or another finds coitus distasteful.

Etiology. The patient herself, when complaining of either frigidity or dyspareunia, frequently believes, or has been told by her associates or husband, that she must have some anatomical abnormality or endocrine deficiency to account for this symptom. She therefore presents for a diagnosis of her anatomical defect or her physiological insufficiency, and for corrective treatment. She is unprepared for and unreceptive to the statement that these symptoms are usually psychogenic in origin.

The sexual response is a complex phenomenon theoretically divisible into at least three components: *psychogenic, anatomical,* and *hormonal.* The importance of the first factor in the female is undisputed. The importance of the last two factors has been difficult to evaluate. Certainly the majority of cases of dyspareunia or frigidity, or both, undoubtedly fall into the psychogenic category. However, especially in the newly married couple, an inexperienced husband with poor intercourse techniques may be at fault. The function of the clitoris as an erotic sex organ has been commonly accepted, and proper stimulation of both the clitoris and nipples will help to stimulate the hitherto unresponsive partner. Communication is nevertheless important, because some women are very concerned about breast stimulation and a possible relation to breast cancer. Under these circumstances, such sex play is contraindicated until she has overcome her fears.

Certain observations make it clear that endocrine aspects are important in orgasmic response. Thus, the patient who is receiving a high dosage of testosterone for relief of symptoms of recurrent carcinoma of the breast almost invariably has an increase in libido. In fact, in elderly patients this is sometimes a very unpleasant and worrisome complication of the therapy. Less frequently, patients who are receiving much smaller doses of testosterone for either endometriosis or premenstrual tension will volunteer the information that sexual activity is either more satisfying or more desirable during therapy. It was observations such as these that led Greenblatt, Mortara, and Torpin to suggest the use of testosterone for frigidity. Waxenberg, Drellich, and Sutherland by gland extirpation for carcinoma metastasis found that androgens play a role in female sexual responsiveness and that the adrenal gland is an important source for these androgens.

Many cases of sexual frigidity or dyspareunia or both, date from painful honeymoon experiences. Still others are due to poor coital techniques. In the female, a satisfactory sex response with orgasm is usually dependent on a sufficiently long preliminary period of excitation, the so-called amatory prelude, the coitus itself being the final act. There are many husbands who are ignorant of this fact or who disregard it, and the development of sexual passivity or frigidity in the wife is a natural consequence. Other male sex deficiencies, such as impotency or premature ejaculation, are often causes for unsatisfactory sex life

for the woman. Unfortunate psychological experiences as a child and emotional immaturity may also cause aversion to the sex act, making a woman unresponsive or giving her psychological dyspareunia.

In addition to these psychic factors, pelvic lesions may be responsible for dyspareunia. These most frequently affect the lower genital canal, one of the most common causes being a persistent, rigid hymen. Inflammatory conditions of the vulva, Bartholin's glands, or vagina, as well as painful scar tissue from a perineorrhaphy, may also be responsible. These factors are associated with so-called entrance dyspareunia, whereas intrapelvic pathology, chronic pelvic inflammatory disease, endometriosis, parametritis, or neoplasms are not infrequently responsible factors for dyspareunia on deep penetration.

Therapy. From what has been said, it is apparent that the problem is not always an easy one—that many possible factors are to be considered and success in treatment will not always be achieved. If the condition has gone on for months or years, the prognosis is frequently poor unless some obvious anatomical factor is found. Advice to the husband is as important as to the wife, especially when the factor of technique seems to play a part in sexual passivity. In short, the treatment for frigidity must usually stress the educational and psychotherapeutic aspects rather than the patient's pelvic or endocrine status. This is not to say that the latter can be altogether neglected. Jones and Park have reported a relatively simple technique, applicable to an office routine, for systematic desensitization of patients with sexual dysfunction of psychogenic origins.

Conditions in the pelvis which make coitus difficult or painful obviously call for correction. Certainly there is no justification for the superficial habit of those physicians who, without making a thorough survey of the individual woman's problem, merely give her a pat on the back or recommend dilatation of the vagina. Such treatment is quite sure to be unsuccessful. If the physician succeeds in winning the patient's confidence, he may obtain information as to her early background, her sex life, her attitude toward her husband and pregnancy. Such information may point the way toward rational management. In the patients in whom emotional immaturity seems to be an important factor, the physician can sometimes inculcate a healthier attitude toward sex life by discussing the importance of adopting an adult, mature attitude toward life in general, as this problem is usually a manifestation of a much broader and deeper psychological disturbance. When such advice is not acceptable to the patient, psychiatric care should be advised.

Endocrine Treatment. Testosterone has been used to increase female libido under many circumstances. As indicated, the majority of cases are unfortunately due to psychosomatic factors and under these conditions cannot be relieved by any amount of hormone therapy. It is, however, sometimes used successfully in overcoming a habit pattern of acquired dyspareunia from a painful perineorrhaphy or other local pelvic cause. This is particularly true in a patient who has had orgasm, but because of some incidental factor has become unable to respond. It may also be of value in furnishing the last bit of impetus for orgasm to the patient who has almost but not quite reached a climax. Unfortunately, it cannot be used as a panacea. The most effective dose is 25 mg. of methyltestosterone daily for 4 or 5 days in the pre- and post-menstrual phase. It must not be used later than this in the postmenstrual phase, as ovulation may be inhibited. It can, of course, be used only during short periods of time and the androgenic level, 250 mg. of methyltestosterone or its equivalent in a month's time, should not be approached.

Psychogenic Therapy. The treatment of the case in which only a psychic factor is concerned may be simple, or it may be extremely difficult. When there is actual aversion to the coital act as in some sexually frigid women, particularly those who have ceased to love their husbands, the dyspareunia, as already mentioned, is utilized as a means of escaping intercourse. The problem, therefore, is apt to involve psychiatric as well as social angles; this makes the solution difficult and at times impossible. In the specific cases, such as those seen in women with a dread of possible pain based on real pain of the first few experiences, simple reassurance of the patient and re-education with self-insertion of vaginal dilators is satisfactory. Simultaneous instruction to the husband as to the need for consideration and gentleness on his part is often necessary to complete the cure. More resistant cases may require the techniques described by Jones and Park.

Anatomical Treatment. In the group of cases in which dyspareunia is indeed due to anatomical factors, active treatment of the causative lesion is indicated and will ordinarily relieve the dyspareunia. When the cause of the coital difficulty and pain is a rigid, persistent hymen the best treatment is a gentle but complete divulsion of the introitus under light anesthesia with pressure to control the bleeding should any occur. Suture for control of bleeding points is usually unnecessary and excision of the hymen is contraindicated, as both are apt to result in a persistent, painful annular scar. The procedure is best performed, of course, a few weeks before the patient is married, if she has presented herself for a premarital consultation.

REFERENCES

Gebhard, P. H.: Situational factors affecting human sexual behavior. In *Sex and Behavior,* Edited by F. A. Beach. John Wiley & Sons, Inc., New York, 1965.

Hoffmeyer, H.: The role of the family and school-sex education of the child. In Excerpta Medica, International Congress Series #71, p. 152. Excerpta Medica Foundation, Amsterdam, 1962.

Jones, W. J., and Park, P. M.: Treatment of single-partner sexual dysfunction by systematic desensitization. Obstet. Gynec., *39:* 411, 1972.

Kirkendall, L. A.: *Premarital Intercourse and Interpersonal Relationships,* pp. 19 and 254. Julian Press, Inc., New York, 1961.

Kostyashkin, E.: Sex morality and sex education in the Soviet Union. Impact of Science on Society, XVIII, 249, 1969.

Lennart, J.: Factors influencing the spread of gonorrhea. I. Educational and Social Behavior. Acta Dermato-Venereal, *48:* 75, 1968.

Linnér, B.: *Sex and Society in Sweden.* Random House, New York, 1967.

Linnér, B.: The sexual revolution in Sweden. Impact of Science on Society, XVIII, 229, 1969.

Masters, W. H., and Johnson, V. E.: *Human Sexual Response.* Little Brown Co., Boston, 1966.

Masters, W. H., and Johnson, V. E.: *Human Sexual Inadequacy.* Little Brown Co., Boston, 1970.

Ottesen-Jensen, E.: The role of the family and school in sex education of the child. In Excerpta Medica, International Congress Series #71, p. 141. Excerpta Medica Foundation, Amsterdam, 1962.

Richards, F. M. F.: Sex education in the schools: The doctor's role. Canad. Med. Assn. J., *95:* 924, 1966.

Sjövall, T.: Psychological difficulties in sexual relations, Excerpta Medica, International Congress Series #71, p. 183. Excerpta Medica Foundation, Amsterdam, 1962.

Turpeinen, K.: Preparation for Marriage. Excerpta Medica, International Congress Series #71, p. 159. Excerpta Medica Foundation, Amsterdam, 1962.

U. S. News and World Report: Russia Takes a New Line on Sex. (Translated from Soviet Education) v. 27-4, p. 25, 1949.

chapter 36

Cytologic Evaluation of Endocrine Status and Somatic Sex

By John K. Frost, M.D.

The endocrine milieu of an individual is accuately reflected in the response of many of her tissues. The vaginal epithelium is one of the most delicate and dependable responders to a broad spectrum of hormones and endocrinologic conditions. It was this evaluation which was the first practical usage to which vaginal cytology was put.

In the early twentieth century Papanicolaou and others established it as a dependable tool for determining the estrous cycle in rodents and other experimental animals. He later extended his work to man, demonstrating its definite value in characterizing the human menstrual cycle (Plate 36.1) and in recognizing the time of ovulation. The great potential value of clinical cytopathology in the detection, diagnosis, and control of cancer (Chap. 37) then took over the major developmental efforts in the United States while mainly in other countries, especially Latin America and Europe,

workers carried on further development of cytology's potentialities for endocrine evaluation and exploited its use.

Great strides have been made in most areas of the world in defining the parameters of clinical usefulness of cytohormonal evaluation, and in determining strengths and weaknesses therein. With good understanding of the latter, valid experience in the use of this potent tool, and close liaison in each case between the interpreting physician and the clinician, cytohormonal evaluation can be of valuable help in the interpretation of normalcy and disease and in clinical management of endocrinologic states.

Additional clinical assistance in the complex endocrine-intersex problem has been added by Barr's discovery of sex chromatin in mid-century (Fig. 36.1). Mushrooming exploitation of this phenomenon and its close correlation with the rapidly expanding discoveries of

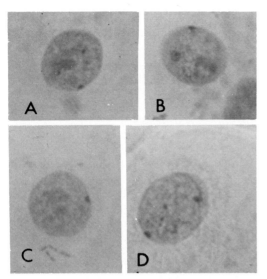

36.1. Normal female sex chromatin, or Barr body, in "chromatin-positive" intermediate cells. The sex chromatin measures around 1.0 μ in diameter, fuses with the nuclear chromatinic rim. It is found at any point around the rim of a well preserved intermitotic (metabolic) nucleus. *A, B,* and *C* are from buccal smears; *D,* is from a Fast smear (single slide, vaginopancervical) ($\times 2000$).

cytogenetics has significantly increased our understanding of these problem cases.

Great clinical insight is gained into the basic causes and efficacious therapy of both simple and complex endocrine-intersex conditions, thorough correlation of *clinical history* and *physical findings* with *cytohormonal evaluation* and *somatic sex determination.*

SEX DETERMINATION AND CYTOGENETICS

Not too long ago it would have seemed that the determination of a patient's sex as female would have to be a prerequisite before consideration in gynecological and obstetrical cytopathology. This paradox has arisen from mounting evidence in the field of cytogenetics which is shedding much light on many clinical problems but, as with any new knowledge, is raising a host of others.

Basis for Determination

Metaphase plate study on air dried or "squash" preparations of the mitotic cell in properly incubated blood, bone marrow, and other cell cultures allows morphological definition of individual chromosomes. In this fashion identification and enumeration of all 44 autosomes and 2 sex chromosomes is possible for detailed cytogenetic study.

In the metabolic (resting) nucleus, chromosomes are threadlike and not individually identifiable. In this state, however, the XX chromosome pair can be determined by the presence of a female sex chromatin or Barr body. Following the work of Barr, many investigators have confirmed the fact that a high percentage of the epidermal cells of human females contain a peripheral clump of chromatin on the nuclear chromatinic rim, which is absent in the male. This sex chromatin (Fig. 36.1) is present in exfoliated cell nuclei in the easily obtainable clinical specimens of both vaginal and buccal smears, preceding the results of complex and time-consuming cytogenetic studies, and at times obviating their necessity.

In the neutrophilic polymorphonuclear leukocyte, this sex difference manifests itself by a small lobe or nuclear "drumstick" appendage in a female's nucleus, which is absent in a male's nucleus. The two methods are in essential agreement but, because of its greater clinical ease of preparation and its more objectively reproducible results, only the sex chromatin of the *exfoliated squamous epithelial cell* will be detailed here.

The Clinical Method

The buccal mucus membrane is scraped above the white dentate line, or linea alba (see Fig. 37.20). The milky cellular fluid so obtained is spread on a glass microscopic slide and *immediately* fixed (*e.g.,* dropped in 95% ethyl alcohol). A good hematoxylin nuclear chromatin stain can be used, such as the routine Papanicolaou or hematoxylin and eosin (H & E) stains. More satisfactory, however, are certain stains which preferentially demonstrate deoxyribonucleic acid (DNA) while deemphasizing the bacteria and granular artifacts. The latter, with hematoxylin, can obscure a clear cut finding. These include aceto-orcein fast green, cresyl violet, Biebrich scarlet, thionine, and Feulgen. Of this group, the former has proved so reliable and valuable that a permanent aceto-orcein fast green mount has been developed and is recommended for routine use of all buccal smear preparations, with a Papanicoloau stain on a duplicate slide if one is available:

Aceto-Orcein Fast Green (Permanent Stain)

Procedure. *Allow cell spread to fix in 95% ethyl alcohol (EOH) 15 minutes or longer. Hydrate slide through 50% EOH and water. Refilter aceto-orcein stain (see below) immediately before each use. Stain in aceto-orcein for 5 minutes. Wash for 10 seconds in gentle stream of distilled water (wash bottle) and dehydrate rapidly through 50% EOH, 70% EOH, 80% EOH, and 95% EOH. Stain in fast green stain (see below) for one minute and rapidly pass through 95% EOH, 100% EOH, and 100% EOH-xylol (equal parts). Clear in xylol for 5 minutes and mount.*

Stain Preparations: *Aceto-orcein Stain. To 45 ml. glacial acetic acid (80° to 85° C.) add 1.0 gm. of orcein with rapid agitation. Gradually add this solution to 55 ml. of distilled water (room temperature), stirring constantly. Cool in running water bath and filter (No. 1 paper). Store in brown screw cap jar. The stain improves with age. It must be refiltered just before each use.*

Fast Green Stain. To 100 ml. of 95% ethyl alcohol add 0.03 gm. of fast green, with agitation to dissolve. Store in screw cap jar.

Identification and Reporting

"Chromatin-positive" is a useful clinical term for individuals with recognizable Barr bodies. To be so identified, these must be chromatin accumulations on the nuclear chromatinic rim of approximately 1μ diameter and which *blend in* with the chromatinic rim. Those individuals whose nuclei do not have Barr bodies in *well prepared* specimens are termed as "chromatin-negative." The use of these terms, rather than "female" or "male," reduces the possibility of psychological trauma of emotionally undesirable information reaching the patient.

Normal childbearing *females* with two X-sex chromosomes are chromatin-*positive*. Normal *males* with one X-sex chromosome and one Y-sex chromosome are chromatin-*negative*.

At birth, a few female infants do not show good Barr bodies. Thus chromatin-negative intersex infants should be repeatedly examined for the first two or three months before definitive male somatic sex is decided upon.

Care must be taken in calling bland nuclei chromatin-negative. Poor fixation, momentary drying before fixation, or poor staining "wash out" the Barr body and can cause a false chromatin-negative diagnosis.

Conversely, poor preservation and interpreting degenerated nuclei can cause chromatin clumps of degeneration to be indistinguishable from Barr bodies with resultant false chromatin positive diagnoses. Good technique and satisfactory preparations are essential.

An extremely small number of cells with sex chromatin (*i.e.,* 1–10%), if one counts *only* the well-preserved nuclei, should make one consider a mosaic situation. Repeat the buccal smear with strict attention to scraping *above* the dentate line (no linea alba contamination) and *immediate* fixation. If the low count persists, cytogenetic evaluation will determine mosaicism.

A consistently extremely small Barr body or extremely large one should be noted and reported in order to detect those rare individuals with abnormally small or abnormally large X-sex chromosomes.

Study of "squash" preparations of metaphase cells reveals 46 chromosomes. Formally thought to total 48, the human chromosomal endowment has been shown, by the more sensitive modern cytogenetic methods, to be 46. These consist of 22 pairs of autosomes (non-sex chromosomes) and one pair of sex chromosomes. In the normal female, the latter are XX; in the male, they are XY. On present evidence, it appears that any cell requires one X-sex chromosome to be in the metabolic phase. Thus, a second X-sex chromosome may be found in the clumped, presumably non-metabolic phase resulting in sex chromatin on the nuclear chromatinic rim of chromatin-positive individuals (Fig. 36.1). The number of Barr bodies per nucleus *plus* one gives the minimum number of X-sex chromosomes present in that nucleus.

Nondisjunction

Many chromosomal aberrations are being discovered. A high percentage are shown clinically to be linked to certain sexual and somatic developmental abnormalities.

In the development of the ovum or sperm, failure of a pair of chromosomes to separate during miotic division is referred to as nondisjunction. When this occurs, both (or neither) chromosomes enter the gamete, while the complement (neither or both) is lost to heredity as a polar body.

In lower forms of life, nondisjunction occurs with increased frequency in older individuals. This aging tendency likewise applies to man in some states, such as mongolism and Klinefelter's syndrome. Mental status, physical makeup, and endocrine balance are frequently affected in the clinical entities produced from nondisjunction.

Sex Chromosomal Nondisjunction. Most individuals with *Turner's syndrome,* or gonadal-agenesis, have an endowment of only 45 chromosomes. The 22 autosomal pairs seem to be intact, but only one X-sex chromosome is present (XO). Although these patients are physically female, they are sex chromatin-*negative.* In addition they do not show estrogenic effect in either their vaginal or buccal smears when untreated. Approximately 25% of individuals who clinically fit Turner's syndrome have 46 chromosomes, including apparently intact X-sex chromosomes on cytogenetic study.

Persons with *Klinefelter's syndrome* or testicular dysgenesis are chromatin-*positive* even though of male habitus. Their total chromosomal count is usually 47. Again the 22 autosomal pairs appear to be intact but there are 3 sex chro-

mosomes, 2 X and 1 Y (XXY). Rarely Klinefelter individuals have 4 sex chromosomes, 3 X and 1 Y giving *double* chromocenters; others are XXYY, etc. The common factor appears to be 2 or more X-sex chromosomes plus at least 1 Y-sex chromosome.

Trisomy for the X-sex chromosome (XXX) has been well known to the geneticists in lower forms of life and referred to there as "superfemales." In man, these individuals possess 22 apparently intact autosomal pairs. In addition, as with the usual Klinefelter's syndrome, they have 3 sex chromosomes, but differ from it in that all are alike (XXX). They are not only chromatin-*positive,* but have *two* sex-chromocenters widely separated on the nuclear chromatinic rim (Fig. 36.2). Such doubled sex chromatins in XXX are to be distinguished from paired or forked sex chromatin which can be found in any Barr body (Fig. 36.2, *right*).

Abnormally small X-sex chromosomes produce small X-sex chromocenters. Although this is a very rare finding, *consistently extremely* small Barr bodies should be reported to determine if cytogenetic studies are indicated.

Other extremely rare variants occur (*e.g.,* XXXYY Klinefelter's with two Barr bodies, XXXXY with three Barr bodies), usually in complicated mosaicism. No individuals have been described without at least one X-sex chromosome (*i.e.,* OY). It is probable that, as with lower species, these produce "lethal variants," with death of the fetuses in utero.

Autosomal Nondisjunction. LeJeune found that mongolian idiocy is associated with an extra chromosome in one of the smallest of the autosome sets (21-trisomy), with an abnormal total of 47 chromosomes resulting. At times, the extra chromosome attaches to another one, which results in a normal total of 46, but with one abnormally large.

Trisomy in other non-sex (somatic) chromosomes occurs usually associated with severe somatic malformations, but with no evident change in the metabolic (resting) nuclear pattern. Thus, in females with somatic trisomy, there is the single sex chromocenter (Barr body).

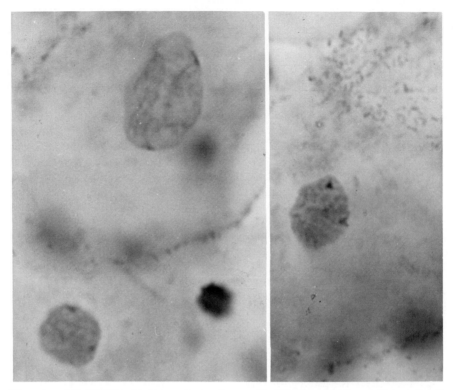

36.2. "Superfemale" (XXX) with 2 sex chromatins, or Barr bodies, in intermediate cells of a buccal smear. *Left,* 2 cells, each having 2 diagnostic sex chromatins widely separated on the nuclear chromatinic rim. *Right,* the same patient with 2 sex chromatin bodies. One, being on the nuclear chromatinic rim in profile, is diagnostic; however, the other one, being on a superior or inferior portion of the nucleus, is not diagnostic as it does not blend in with the chromatinic rim in profile. The diagnostic one is forked; at times it appeared paired in this individual (aceto-orcein fast green, permanent stain, ×2000).

Developments in cytogenetics have been very rapid in recent years and many fundamental concepts are being basically altered; not only concepts of genetics, but also of approaches to many clinical problems. Physiological and biochemical genetics is playing an ever increasing role in recognition, appreciation, and handling of these clinical entities.

Summary

Normal females (XX) have positive nuclear sex chromatin (♀), whereas normal males (XY) have negative sex chromatin (♂) or lack of the Barr body. Male pseudo-hermaphrodites (XY with female external genitalia) have negative chromatin (♂), whereas female pseudohermaphrodites (XX with male external genitalia) have positive chromatin (♀).

Most Turner's syndrome patients (XO with female habitus) have negative sex chromatin (♂). Klinefelter's syndrome patients (XXY with male habitus) have positive sex chromatin (♀). "Superfemales" (XXX with female habitus) and some Klinefelter's (XXXY with male habitus) have "double positive" sex chromatin. Many of the patients reported with nondisjunction of the sex chromosomes are mentally deficient and/or sterile.

ENDROCRINE STATUS EVALUATION BY CYTOHORMONAL STUDIES

Endocrinopathies detected for therapy in today's medical practice are rarely overt. Most are subtle and obscured by structural and functional changes seeming to have other, nonendocrine bases. In ad-

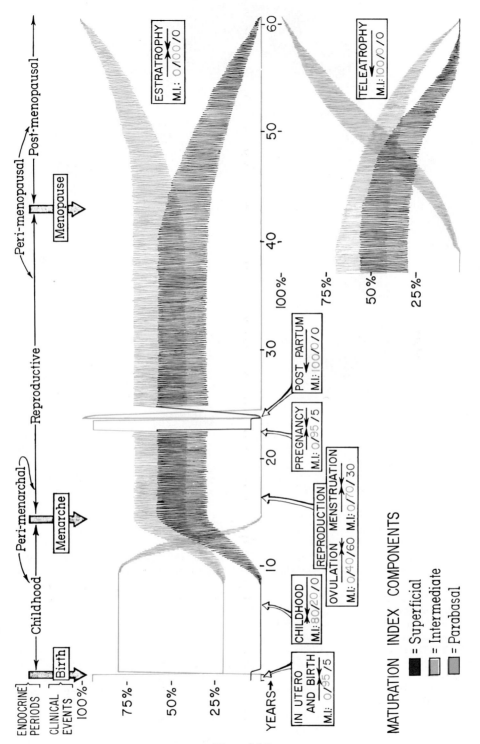

Plate 36.1

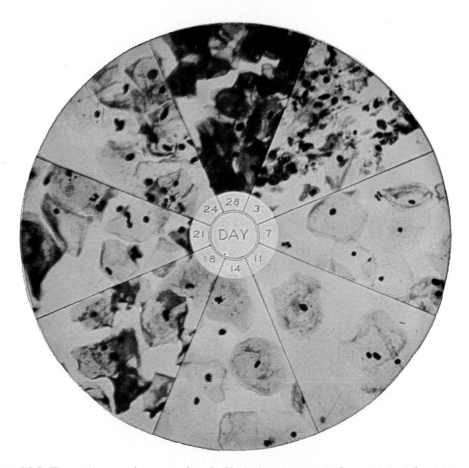

Plate 36.2. *The cytohormonal menstrual cycle.* Vaginal smears were taken at 3- to 4-day intervals of a normal 28-day cycle; menstruation commenced on the 1st and 29th days; age 21. At ovulation (Day 14) the maturation index (M.I.) was $\overline{0/40/60}$, the cells lay singly and flat, and the background was "clean." Immediately before menstruation (Day 28) the M.I. had become $\overrightarrow{0/\overleftarrow{70}/30}$, cells clumped and curled and the background was "dirty." Note endometrial cells on Day 3 ($\times 70$).

Plate 36.1. Maturation indices (M.I.) of a woman's lifetime. The endocrine periods of the female and the corresponding maturation indices (M.I.)—a composite based upon cytohormonal determinations of individual patients. This schematically represents the fluctuations of the 3 levels of maturation of the epithelial surface cell (parabasal, intermediate, superficial) which occur under the influence, mainly, of various hormones.

Estrogen produces superficial cell maturation (M.I. to right, toward $\overrightarrow{0/0/100}$). A moderate degree of this effect is noted at ovulation (M.I., *c.* $\overrightarrow{0/40/\overleftarrow{60}}$ (Plate 36.1).

Progesterone and cortisone cause intermediate cell maturation (M.I. to midzone, toward $\overrightarrow{0/\overleftarrow{100}/0}$). A moderate degree of this effect is noted at menstruation (M.I., *c.* $\overrightarrow{0/\overleftarrow{70}/30}$ (Plate 36.1) and extreme effect at birth (Fig. 36.4) or pregnancy (M.I., $\overrightarrow{0/\overleftarrow{95}/5}$) (Fig. 36.6) and estratrophy or intermediate cell atrophy (M.I., $\overrightarrow{0/\overleftarrow{100}/0}$) (Fig. 36.9). Lack of all maturing factors, or repression of their effect, causes no maturation beyond parabasal cells at exfoliation (M.I. to left, toward $\overleftarrow{100/0/0}$). A moderate degree of this effect is noted during childhood (M.I., *c,* $\overleftarrow{80/\overrightarrow{20}/0}$), and extreme effect at postpartum (Fig. 36.8) and teleatrophy or parabasal cell atrophy (M.I., $\overleftarrow{100/0/0}$) (Fig. 36.10).

The period of childhood, is relatively constant and predictable. The reproductive period is constant from cycle to cycle. Atrophy in the post-menopausal period is fairly constant and of 2 main types: intermediate cell atrophy (M.I., $\overrightarrow{0/\overleftarrow{100}/0}$) (Fig. 36.9), and parabasal cell atrophy (M.I., $\overleftarrow{100/0/0}$) (Fig. 36.10).

Conversely, the patterns of the perimenarchal and the perimenopausal periods are extremely difficult to predict before cytologic evaluation because of the wide range of normal possibilities serving as an unpredictable base line.

In all cytohormonal evaluations it is thus essential to know everything pertinent to the patient endocrinologically, such as: age, date of last menstrual period (LMP), date of previous menstrual period (PMP), characteristics and irregularity of periods, drug therapy, radiotherapy, surgery.

dition, a wide variety of diseases is associated with endocrine abnormalities or produce them as by-products. Prompt determination of the patient's hormonal status, with accurate recognition of its variance from normal, is a key to detection of the underlying cause and to its proper management.

Cytohormonal determination is a readily available tool which has been made easily accessible to the clinician by rapid and simple methods for obtaining specimens. With proper interpretation it can offer valuable assistance which is either detective and directive to more elaborate procedures, or is definitive and diagnostic.

The Cytological Basis for Hormonal Evaluation

Determination of endocrine status is made from an *aliquot,* with extrapolation to the *whole.* Because of this, aliquot samples must be picked with care and full knowledge of limitations, and interpreted wisely. To be complete, knowledge of endocrine status should be gained from all possible sources, including accurate clinical observations, biochemical assay of blood and urine, and cytohormonal evaluation.

Cytohormonal evaluation, as with clinical observation, must recognize the complex *endocrine interplay* which is mirrored in the cellular spread. One is not dealing with a single compound evaluation, as with biochemical determination. Thus the indiscriminate and connotative use of "estrogen evaluation," to cover all cytohormonal evaluation, is out of order and should be replaced by the use of proper and specific, denotative terms.

Individual sensitivity to compounds vary. Further, the presence of undetermined substances may be overlooked by focusing one's attention solely upon the few for which objective determinations can be made by biochemical assay. Cytologically adjudging patient endocrine response is a physiological test of the actual reaction in that individual patient to the hormonal milieu.

Specifically, cytohormonal evaluation is based upon the reactions of certain cells (while *in situ*) to the complex endocrine milieu. It is dependent upon four major factors: the *types* of hormonally active compounds present at that time, their degree of *physiological activity,* their *dose level,* and the ability of the patient's *tissue to respond.* All four are capable of great variations. The latter, for instance, is dependant upon other endocrine-enzymatic systems active at that time, *e.g.,* thyroid status, previous injury to the tissue (*i.e.,* graft, radiation), and differences in response inherited by the tissues of the end organ. In certain clinical situations, cytopathological endocrine determinations yield detective, diagnostic, or therapeutic information unobtainable by other methods.

Virtually all living tissues respond to their endocrine-enzymatic milieu, each in its own way and degree. Some, however, recognizably change their morphological and physiological states with great sensitivity, to reflect accurately the delicate hormonal balance present throughout the body at that time. Such a systemic mirror for the interplay of certain clinically important substances is the vaginal epithelium. Extremely sensitive to the sexually active compounds (estrogens, progestogens, androgens), it is also sensitive in varying degrees to others (corticoids, thyroxines, vitamins, cyclic antibiotics, digitoxins, etc.). The buccal mucous membrane, the urinary tract epithelium, and the external skin show similar responses which are weaker and less dependable.

The epithelium of the middle vagina is the most sensitive indicator of steroidal hormonal status in quality, quantity, and rapidity of response. Regardless of the controversy over its embryological origin, vaginal epithelium faithfully mirrors the status of the Müllerian and associated tissues.

The Specimen

While the total thickness of the vaginal epithelium is affected by its endocrine milieu, cytohormonal evaluation depends upon the state of the epithelial cells lying upon the surface of the epithelium. *Natural* exfoliation therefrom or *gentle* scraping, therefore, yield a reproducibility which cannot be achieved when specimen depth artificially varies due to variations in scraping technique.

Lateral Vaginal Wall Scraping. This specimen obtains material directly from the organ of response (*i.e.,* vaginal epithelium). Thus it does not have to accumulate in the vaginal pool reservoir and is most free of contaminating material from the cervix and endometrium. *Light, uniform* scrapings from the mid-portion of the lateral vaginal wall is the most accurate and preferred specimen for cytohormonal evaluation.

Vaginal Pool Specimen. This is very satisfactory material for accurate cytohormonal evaluation *provided* that one evaluates *only* the *vaginal* wall portions of the pool, recognizing and entirely disregarding those portions coming from the cervix. When this is not possible (*i.e.,* inexperience; severe cervicitis) lateral vaginal wall scraping should be utilized.

Vaginal pool material should be, and usually is, a part of a routine cancer detection specimen, either as a separate slide or a part of a combined single-slide specimen (*i.e.,* Fast vaginopancervical) (p. 806–8). A cervical scraping by itself does *not* suffice for cancer detection, and is *un*reliable for hormonal evaluation.

In this way, therefore, accurate cytohormonal evaluation is available to all patients with routine cancer detection cellular examination if it includes vaginal pool material. A cytohormonal evaluation should be made on all such cancer detection material, and reported upon if abnormal.

Cervical Specimen. This material is *not* reliable for cytohormonal evaluation. Cervical epithelium is frequently the site of abnormalities (*i.e.,* inflammation, regeneration, metaplasia, dysplasia), is less sensitive to endocrine changes and can *unpredictably* be entirely *misleading* in cytologic interpretation. It should *not* be used for cytohormonal evaluation.

Serial Specimen. When serial evalua-

tion is important (*i.e.,* cycle, ovulation, drug response), *daily serial* smears are invaluable. The patient herself can easily take daily vaginal pool smears which are completely comparable, reproducible, and reliable or daily vaginal irrigation smears (p. 809).

Staining by the classical Papanicolaou method is preferred for an accurate evaluation and permanent record, or the more rapid Shorr stain can be used. For an immediate clinical impression, it can be stained fresh by a rapid method (*i.e.,* Rakoff's stain (Paschkiss *et al.*)) and microscopically examined directly. While the latter is a temporary preparation, it allows for immediate recognition of overt abnormalities for prompt institution of therapy but does not allow for cancer screening or for future endocrine reference. The permanent preparation allows a complete evaluation of subtle endocrine changes and comparison with previous and subsequent preparations. A combination of the rapid, temporary office procedure *and* the permanent one is most valuable.

In *children* and the *aged,* great care must be exercised to obtain the specimen only from the vaginal vault. It must not be contaminated by touching either the labia, the vestibule, or the ungloved examiner's fingers. A nonabsorbent cotton swab, moistened with saline and introduced through a nasal speculum or drinking straw, gives an adequate vaginal smear for cytohormonal evaluation of a child (see p. 779).

General Pattern Response

The vaginal epithelium is capable of producing carbohydrates, proteins, and crystalloids in varying aqueous concentrations. Additional quantities come from higher up the tract in the endocervix, endometrium, endosalpinx, and peritoneum. Many of these are under endocrine influence, but other factors also effect them. Nervous and psychic stimuli alter their production. Irritation, inflammation, and bleeding change or obscure them. A few neutrophiles appear and disappear under hormonal influences, but their significance is obscured and invalidated by slight infections.

As the significance of these elements is unpredictable, they are usually of dubious assistance, but occasionally they will clarify an obscure problem.

Cellular Morphology Response

The most dependably valuable information is obtained from cellular morphology. Both the relationships of one cell to another *and* their individual state of cellular maturation are evaluated. The former includes their sticky behavior with clumping *versus* a tendency to remain separate as individual cells, and a tendency to lie flat *versus* a crinkling and retraction of the outer margins of the cytoplasm with a characteristic folding upon itself in a navicular fashion (Plate 36.1).

The state of maturation which the cells of the vaginal epithelium attain at the time of their exfoliation yields by far the *most* objective and reliable information. Thus, natural exfoliation is of basic importance to hormonal evaluation; vigorous scraping can produce artifacts. The endocrine-enzymatic milieu in which the squamous cells are bathed has the greatest influence upon the length of time they remain attached as part of the epithelium and upon the state of maturation they develop. Compounds reach the cells with effectiveness either from the vessels below the basement membrane or from the vaginal lumen above the epithelial surface, with both systemic and suppository therapy producing the characteristic effects.

Cytohormonal pattern parallels the pattern of tissues taken simultaneously at biopsy. The most objective, reproducible, and generally valuable methods for determining endocrine status cytologically are based upon assessing the state of maturation attained by the cells of the squamous epithelium at their time of exfoliation. Numerous indices and values have arisen to more easily and accurately express this maturation.

Numerous indices have been used to describe only the squamous cells, or squames. The percentage of squamous cells with nuclear pyknosis is referred to as the karyopyknotic index (K.I.). The percentage of squamous cells showing cytoplasmic acidophilia is termed the cornification index (C.I.), eosinophilic index (E.I.), or acidophilic index (A.I.).

The maturation index (M.I.) expresses most of the above information *plus* information regarding maturation only to the level of parabasal cell exfoliation as found in atrophy. The maturation value (M.V.) expresses most of the information of the latter index in one figure.

Maturation Index (M.I.)

The maturation index is a concise and objective method for gaining insight regarding the endocrine milieu. This expresses conveniently the level of cellular maturation attained at the time of exfoliation as a delicately changing ratio. A differential of the three major types of cells shed from the stratified squamous epithelium of the lateral vaginal wall, is expressed as percentages present of the parabasal, the intermediate, and the superficial cells *in that order* (Fig. 36.3). The nomenclature used for these three major types of cells shed from squamous epithelium, is the International Nomenclature which was informally agreed upon in 1958. Nomenclature used previously differs from this.

The M.I. of a patient exfoliating no parabasal cells, 55% intermediate cells, and 45% superficial cells is written 0/55/45 and accurately reflects their ratio on the surface of her vaginal epithelium. This order (parabasal/intermediate/superficial) of the M.I. is important to obviate confusion and mistake. It is analogous to the Arneth index in which the level of maturation of the neutrophiles exfoliated from marrow into circulating blood is represented with the least mature cell on the left (*i.e.,* band or stab cell) and the most mature cell on the right (*i.e.,* segmented PMN). Likewise, a shift to the left denotes less mature cells being released (exfoliated), whereas a shift to the right indicates more mature cells. Arrows written over the M.I. may be used to more clearly indicate the direction and degree of the maturation shift (*i.e.,* $\overline{0/55/45}$).

These three normal cells shed from the noncornified, stratified, squamous vaginal epithelium are usually easily told apart:

First, one determines the cytoplasmic thickness (Fig. 36.3). If it is *thick,* the cell is a *parabasal* regardless of the nuclear pattern or cytoplasmic color, size, clear pattern or cytoplasmic color, size, or shape. If the cytoplasm is "wafer-thin" the cell is a squame of either intermediate or superficial type.

Second, if it is a squame, one then determines the nuclear size and chromatin pattern. If the nucleus of this squame is plump and vesicular with an intact chro-

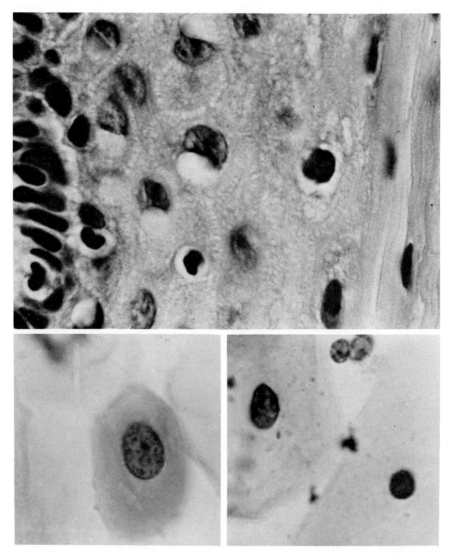

36.3. Noncornified, stratified, squamous epithelium of the vaginal vault and its exfoliated cells. *Upper section from left to right:* basement membrane, true basal cells, parabasal cells, intermediate cells, superficial cells (×1100). *Lower left,* parabasal cell (exfoliated, in vaginal smear); cytoplasm is *thick* from nucleus to cell border (×1500). *Lower right,* intermediate cell (*left*) and superficial cell (exfoliated, in vaginal smear); cytoplasm of both is uniformly "wafer-thin" from nucleus to cell border. The intermediate cell nucleus is vesicular and retains chromatin pattern. The nucleus of the superficial cell is pyknotic, measuring less than 6μ, hyperchromatic, and has lost chromatin pattern. For size reference, a neutrophil is in upper midfield. (×1500).

matin pattern, the cell is termed an *intermediate* (Fig. 36.3); if it is pyknotic, shrunken below 6μ, hyperchromatic, and lacks chromatin pattern, the cell is a *superficial,* regardless of cytoplasmic color.

A sharp distinction is usually obvious with a good nuclear stain, such as the Papanicolaou stain, on properly fixed material. In poor nuclear stains and in dried or poorly fixed cell preparations, a sharp differentiation may be difficult. Under phase contrast microscopy, pyknosis usually is accompanied by a very characteristic red sheen to the nucleus.

Cytoplasmic color is not of assistance in separating a parabasal from a squame. Between an intermediate and a superficial cell, however, there is some rough correlation. With a Papanicolaou stain, Shorr stain, and Rakoff stain, intermediate cells tend to have green, blue, or gray cytoplasm, whereas superficial cells usually are acidophilic with an affinity for yellow, orange, or red. This is *not* an absolute correlation, however, and cytoplasmic color is more unpredictable and affected by artifacts (*i.e.,* inflammation, drying, poor fixation, pH change, stain variations) than is nuclear pyknosis. Cytoplasmic color can give a rapid *albeit* rough impression.

Strict cellular morphology, *i.e.,* cytoplasmic maturation (thick *versus* thin) and nuclear maturation (vesicular *versus* pyknotic), gives the most consistently reproducible endocrine evaluation for clinical purposes. These two are the only factors utilized for determining the M.I.

One must be very careful not to include *dyskaryotic* cells (Fig. 37.9) in the M.I. Such contaminating cells from cervical or vaginal atypias or from dermatological conditions must be recognized as *not* belonging in the *normal* squamous series and therefore must *not* be counted in the M.I. The cells of the dyskaryotic series have larger than normal nuclei. Frequently, the nucleus is hyperchromatic, the nuclear membrane is wavy, and the chromatin is granular and uniformly dispersed (see Fig. 37.9). In severe dysplasia, the cytoplasm of the dyskar-

yotic cell may be scanty and thick, so that the cell would seem to be a parabasal cell to the unwary who did not recognize the enlarged nucleus. This is the greatest cause for incorrectly identifying three cell types as being present in the vaginal smear at the same time, which is very rare. Dyskaryotic cells must *not* be included in the M.I.

Under certain conditions superficial cells can become more mature (hypermature) and lose their nuclei (see Fig. 36.13). As normal vaginal epithelium is nonkeratinizing squamous, these cells are not present in normal vaginal smears. These anucleate superficial cells are usually shed from keratotic epithelium of irritation, reaction, neoplasia, or dermatosis which frequently appears clinically as a leukoplakia. At times, anucleate superficial cells appear with extremely high levels of estrogen or tissue sensitivity to the drug (*i.e.,* excessive therapy, tumors, testicular feminization). It is a normal occurrence in rhesus monkeys at menarche, but not in humans with a normal established cycle.

Under certain conditions parabasal cells can produce orangophilic cytoplasm which may, on rare occasions, be truly keratinized. In addition, some parabasal cell nuclei may occasionally become pyknotic. The true identity of both of these cells as being parabasal is evident from the thickness of their cytoplasm, with failure to show the thin squamification of intermediate and superficial cells. Such abnormal parabasal cells can be found in severe atrophy, inflammation, and an androgen "spread" pattern.

It is obvious from the foregoing that the karyopyknotic index (K.I.), which expresses the percentage of squamous epithelial cells having pyknotic nuclei, and the acidophilic indices (A.I., C.I., E.I.), which express the percentage of cells having yellow, orange, or red cytoplasm usually will approximate closely the right hand figure of the maturation index. The K.I. is exactly the right hand figure, if there are no parabasal cells present (it is rare to have three cell types at the same time). The acidophilic indices, on the other hand, may differ significantly from the right hand cell of the M.I., due, in great part, to the artifacts of drying or inflammation and the variations of staining.

Maturation Value

A useful maturation value (M.V.) is obtained by giving a value of 0 to parabasal cells, 0.5 to intermediate cells, and 1.0 to superficial cells. Thus, an M.I. of 10/90/0 would have an M.V. of 45. Intermediate values can be given to more subtle cell variations.

Other Cytohormonal Expressions

More complicated methods of expression are in use by some, but they appear to offer no more clinical assistance than these mentioned. Recently the terms maturation count and feminity index were introduced briefly, which expressed the *same* cell-types in *reverse* order to the maturation index. This has offered nothing in addition but confusion to the clinician, and it is best to drop the terms.

Cytohormonal Patterns

The *normal patterns* and their *variations* must be thoroughly understood before attempting to interpret abnormalities. For greatest clinical meaning, all of the above facets of the vaginal smear yielding endocrine information must be utilized in evaluating its cytohormonal pattern.

For better comprehension and clinical correlation it is valuable to consider the normal female life span in *five* periods (Plate 36.2). Three of these are clinically well defined—*childhood, reproductive, postmenopausal*—separated by the objective occurrences: *birth, menarche, menopause,* and *death.*

Because of the endocrine turbulence occurring at menarche and menopause, even though clinically they might appear to be fairly sharply defined in most individuals, there is great value in considering the *perimenarchal and perimenopausal* periods in great detail. These, of course, overlap the three major periods.

From the endocrine point of view,

therefore, the normal female life span is conveniently considered in five periods: *childhood, perimenarchal, reproductive, perimenopausal, and postmenopausal.* To understand the endocrine cellular patterns, one should first consider the basic modes in which the vaginal epithelium and its exfoliated cells have to react to individual hormones.

Normal Cytohormonal Patterns of the Basic Stimulating Agent

Estrogens. All layers of the epithelium become thickened and proliferated. This is marked in the squames, where intermediate and superficial cells become most numerous on the surface. A great many of these mature to superficial cells with a resultant shift to the right of the M.I.

Thus, when a patient with a completely atrophic pattern of $\overleftarrow{100/0/0}$ is given increasing doses of estrogens, either systemically or by suppository, there will be a progressive shift of the M.I. to the right, with the degree of shift proportional to the amount of estrogens administered. A moderate dose will produce an M.I. of $\overrightarrow{0/50/50}$, a large dose will approach $\overrightarrow{0/0/100}$. Cellular degeneration and inflammation are strikingly reduced, the smear appears "clean," the cells lie flat, and tend to be distributed singly.

Progestogens. Proliferation of the squames is also a major feature of progesterone, but maturation progresses only through the intermediate cell stage when exfoliation occurs. The M.I. shifts toward the midzone, to $\overleftrightarrow{0/100/0}$ if dosage is sufficient. Superficial cells are not produced on pure progesterone, estrogen being needed to mature the cells to superficial type.

In tissue, the intermediate cells have plump and delicate cytoplasm, which completely collapses on cell spread to a characteristically thin wafer. The edges of the cytoplasm curls and cells appear to be sticky and clump together in masses. The background of the cell spread is "messy" with mucus, neutrophiles, and cellular debris. Mucus is abundant, if the systemic hormonal pattern background is proper; if the epithelium has been "primed" with estrogens, cytolysis may occur.

Androgens. Androgens do not perfectly oppose estrogen proliferation. In fact, proliferation is also the rule under androgens; but the cells on the surface can mature to any or all of the three cell types, depending upon the prior hormonal state of the patient. Thus, one can find parabasal cells lying on the surface alongside superficial and intermediate cells, with an M.I. "spread pattern" approaching $\overleftrightarrow{33/34/33}$, but tending to shift more to the left. In this peculiar androgen pattern, parabasal cells can have orangophilic, thick cytoplasm with karyopyknosis, whereas some superficial cells can have extremely small, wafer-thin cytoplasm.

In other patients receiving androgens, more intermediate cells or parabasal cells are present, approaching in some $\overleftrightarrow{0/100/0}$ and in others $\overleftarrow{100/0/0}$; however, the trend remains for the index to "spread," as androgens do not typically produce 100% of one cell type.

A clue that one may be dealing with androgens may be gained from a "spread" pattern with abnormally small superficial cells (*wafer-thin polygonal* cytoplasm) and small parabasal cells having *thick* orangophilic cytoplasm with nuclear pyknosis. Mucus may be present.

Inflammation also causes "spreading" of the M.I. Thus, as an androgen pattern may appear inflammatory and obscuring, these two conditions can be easily confused. Androgen, therefore, does not produce as diagnostic a pattern as do the estrogens, progestogens, or cortisones. At times, however, it is very suggestive.

Clomiphene. This "anti-estrogen" is actually an extremely weak synthetic estrogen. It has virtually no direct effect upon the vaginal epithelium but apparently blocks estrogenic hypothalamic inhibition to pituitary production of gonadotrophin. This allows increased gonadotrophin secretion (gonadotrophic flood) which stimulates the ovary to follicle growth, estrogen secretion, ovulation, and corpus luteum formation. The level of physiologically active estrogen continues to be mirrored in the response of the vaginal epithelium in spite of clomiphene administration but to a lower degree.

Anovulatory patients, with good cytologically detectable estrogenic effect before clomiphene therapy, seem to have a better chance for ovulation from the drug than those whose pretherapy estrogenic effect is poor.

Cortisone. Drugs having the cortisone effect produce proliferation with many features similar to progesterone. The surface cells mature to intermediate cell type as does progesterone, and the M.I. approaches $\overleftrightarrow{0/100/0}$ according to the dosage.

In contradistinction to progesterone, however, the cells do not tend to curl or stick but they lie flat and separate. Mucus is usually scanty or lacking, and the smear may appear strikingly "clean."

One must bear in mind that the adrenal cortex also produces estrogenic, progestogenic, and androgenic compounds which affect the vaginal epithelium characteristically if in sufficient dosage.

Miscellaneous Substances. Various other compounds may affect the hormonal pattern of the vaginal epithelium. Digitalis produces an intermediate cell maturation, with a midzone shift in the M.I. With prolonged digitalis administration, however, there may be some superficial cell maturation.

Some of the cyclic broad spectrum antibiotics also cause an M.I. shift to the midzone. Absence or severe reduction of some compounds will change the cellular response. Avitaminosis A causes an M.I. shift to the right, whereas *extreme* hypothyroidism or athyroid cretinism causes an M.I. shift to the left.

Compounding Effect. It is important to realize that effects of substances acting in succession or simultaneously may be simply additive, or may qualitatively change each other's response. The effect of progesterone upon an unstimulated atrophic vaginal epithelium, for instance, differs markedly from one "primed" with estrogens.

Birth Control Pills. The cytohormonal effects from antifertility medications

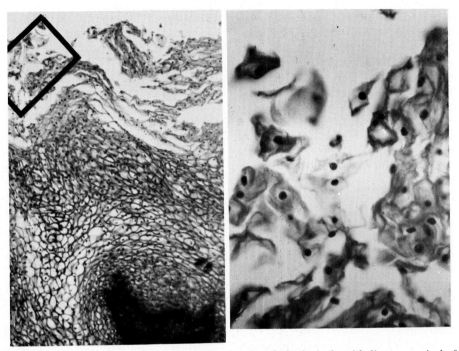

36.4. Vaginal epithelium, female fetus, 6 months gestation. *Left,* the lush epithelium so typical of both a female fetus *en utero* and a pregnant woman (H & E stain, ×40). *Right,* intermediate cells exfoliating from the surface of the same epithelium. Maturation index, 0/95/5 (see Fig. 36.6) (H & E, ×160).

reflect the components making up the drug. Some are simple estrogens, giving the typical estrogenic response. Others are compounds (*i.e.,* estrogen/progestogen) giving the compounding effect, depending upon the levels of activity, sequence, and dosage of each component.

Inflammatory Effect. In addition to bringing forth leukocytes and other inflammatory elements, inflammation alters the level of maturation attained by the surface cells and makes cytohormonal evaluation unsatisfactory. The general effect is to increase the cell types in the minority, at the expense of the cell types in the majority. This "spread" of the M.I. (*e.g.,* $\overleftrightarrow{0/30/70}$, $\overrightarrow{70/30/0}$, and $\overleftarrow{0/95/5}$ all tending to become $\overleftrightarrow{33/34/33}$) is roughly proportional to the severity of the inflammation, and is dependent upon its etiology.

Severe inflammation may result in hypermaturity of the superficial cell sufficient to cause it to lose its nucleus, forming areas of leukoplakia which exfoliate this abnormal, anucleate superficial cell. When severity is restricted to an extremely small area of the epithelium (such as in chronic irritation from a pessary or in a localized dermatosis), such extreme cellular artifacts exfoliated from this area into otherwise healthy vaginal secretions may appear paradoxical. In addition to this alteration of cellular maturation, severe inflammation can be so obscuring and so destructive of cells that the preparation is useless.

Clearing inflammation in any effective way (*i.e.,* triple sulfa, bland douches, Flagyl) which does not employ agents altering the epithelial maturation (do not use, for example, tetracyclines), allows a true hormonal pattern to be evaluated.

Normal Cytohormonal Patterns of the Endocrine Periods

Childhood Period. This period produces one of the most dependable and constant patterns, except for the very beginning and end of the period (Plate 36.2).

At birth the vaginal epithelium of the female infant is thick and lush in response to circulating maternal hormones, including massive progesterones, estrogens, and adrenocortical compounds (Fig. 36.4). The surface cells are mainly of intermediate type, so that the M.I. of the cell spread is characteristic of pregnancy, $\overline{0/95/5}$ (Fig. 36.6). Desquamation rapidly takes place and within a few weeks it becomes the thin atrophic epithelium so characteristic of *childhood,* with the M.I. markedly shifted to the left (*c.* $\overleftarrow{100/0/0}$ or $\overrightarrow{70}/30/0$). The surface cell matures to the parabasal level at exfoliation, with only a few intermediates and with *no* superficials.

Thus, in the absence of inflammation or irritation and with the certainty that the vaginal smear has not been contaminated with introitus cells, the superficial cell is normally absent until the onset of the perimenarchal period. An appearance of this cell in the childhood period is significant (*i.e.,* hormone-producing tumors, adrenogential syndrome).

Perimenarchal Period. Around the age of 8 years, but with great individual variation, there begins a gradual increase of noticeable sex steroid activity until the reproductive level is reached at menarche, about the age of 14 (Plate 36.2). This gradual increase is evidenced in the vaginal epithelium by thickening and proliferation, with increasing numbers of surface cells maturing to the intermediate and superficial types as sex hormone production increases. The vaginal smear mirrors this, with an increasing shift of the M.I. to the right, until the appearance of menses and the full-blown cellular endocrine pattern of the reproductive age.

Therefore, as this perimenarchal period is a continuing transition from childhood atrophy (M.I., *c.* $\overleftarrow{100/0/0}$ to $\overrightarrow{70}/30/0$) to the lush epithelium of the reproductive period, (M.I., *c.* $\overline{0/70/30}$ to $\overline{0/40/60}$), great variation can be encountered. Age is the major factor in evaluating endocrine status of this period.

When the menarche appears, there is still adjustment for many. Some have not yet reached a full reproductive M.I.,

whereas others for a period of time exceed normalcy and have an M.I. with an extreme shift to the right.

Reproductive Period. During the childbearing age, from perimenarche to perimenopause, the endocrine milieu shows great cyclic fluctuation. Following the initial period of endocrine adjustment in the establishment of menses and extending into the disruption of endocrine interplay of the perimenopausal period, the pattern is a series of menstrual cycles (Fig. 36.5). Although the hormonal patterns vary widely between individuals, they are usually mirrored in repetition for a given individual. Their constancy is broken normally only by childbearing, so that the cellular patterns of the *menstrual cycle,* or *pregnancy,* and of the *postpartum period,* are characteristic.

Throughout the *menstrual cycle* with a normal ovulatory pattern (Plate 36.1), superficial cells and intermediate cells vary in exfoliation from 30 to 60% (M.I. from *c.* $\overline{0/40/60}$ around ovulation to *c.* $\overrightarrow{0/70/30}$ around menstruation) in response to estrogen and progestogen levels. At the time of ovulation, high and unopposed estrogen is present (Fig. 36.5) with a moderate shift of M.I. to the right (*c.* $\overline{0/40/60}$) (Plate 36.1). With ovulation, circulating estrogen drops rapidly. Shortly thereafter estrogen rises again with the development of the corpus luteum during the secretory phase, but at this time it is accompanied by progestogens (Fig. 36.5). Just before menstruation the progestogen opposition is at its highest and produces a moderate M.I. shift to the midzone (M.I., *c.* $\overrightarrow{0/70}/30$). During menstruation both estrogen and progestogen sharply drop. Soon, from the developing new follicle, estrogen again rises alone during the proliferative phase, shifting the M.I. to the right until the ovulatory pattern (M.I., *c.* $\overline{0/40/60}$) is once more reached, two weeks before menses.

Except postpartum, the parabasal type cell does not exfoliate normally until the later years of the reproductive period or in the perimenopausal period. In some patients, the parabasal cell may not exfoliate at any time during the reproduc-

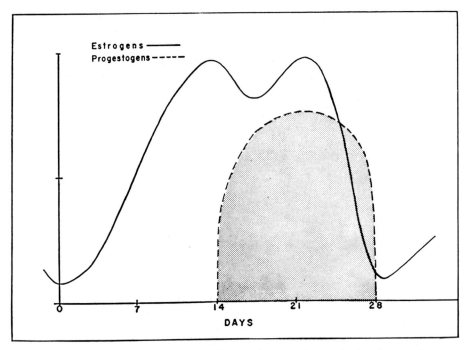

36.5. Menstrual cycle. A diagrammatic composite of the interplay in levels of systemic estrogens and progestogens which occurs during the menstrual cycle of a woman in her reproductive period of life.

tive and postmenopausal periods if at the latter time they go into intermediate cell atrophy ($\overleftrightarrow{0/100/0}$) rather than parabasal cell atrophy ($\overline{100/0/0}$) (Plate 36.2).

As with a single basal body temperature determination, a *single* vaginal smear evaluation gives only limited endocrine information. This is not only because of the great endocrine variations encountered during the menstrual cycle, but also because of the fact that many combinations of dynamic factors can produce similar static cytohormonal patterns. *Daily* vaginal pool aspiration smears obtained and prepared by the patient along with her basal body temperature, are invaluable in detecting ovulation, anovulation, time in cycle, endocrinopathies, etc. Almost as valuable and easier to obtain, are the twice-a-week series taken every 3–4 days (Plate 36.1). Such complete cytohormonal evaluation yields valuable dynamic endocrine information.

In *pregnancy,* the cytohoromonal pattern is characteristic and is "locked in" by massive levels of hormones. With conception the normal luteal phase M.I. shift toward the midzone, proceeds just as in the nonpregnant menstrual cycle; however, when the pattern reaches the menstrual M.I. (*c.* $\overline{0/70/30}$), it does not recede, but continues its midzone climb. Within a few weeks it has reached the pattern so characteristic of pregnancy (Fig. 36.6), with the extreme M.I. midzone shift ($\overleftrightarrow{0/95/5}$) maintained throughout gestation. The levels of estrogens, progestogens, and cortical steroids are so massive in the normal pregnancy (Fig. 36.7) that this M.I. is not altered by usual doses of hormones. This forms the basis for Wied's test for menopausal amenorrhea *versus* pregnancy (see p. 773). Direct effect of infection upon the vaginal epithelium, however, will artificially alter even the hormonal pattern of pregnancy, with a characteristic inflammatory "spread" of the M.I. (*e.g.,* from $\overrightarrow{0/95/5}$ toward *c.* $\overleftrightarrow{33/34/33}$).

In the absence of inflammation, therefore, it is significant when the usual pregnancy M.I. of $\overline{0/95/5}$ varies markedly either to the right or to the left. Hormonal change must be great indeed, to effect such

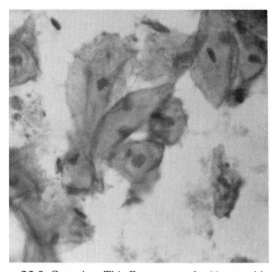

36.6. Gestation. This Fast smear of a 23-year-old woman in her 7th month of gestation shows the "midzone" shift in the maturation index, $\overrightarrow{0/9\overset{\times}{5}/5}$, so typical of pregnancy. It is also found during fetal life and at birth (see Fig. 36.4). The intermediate cells curl at their edges, folding into "navicular" forms. They seem sticky and tend to adhere together. The perinuclear cytoplasm was golden brown. ($\times$160.)

an alteration in a pattern normally held to by massive levels of hormones. Abortions having an endocrine basis are heralded by a bizarre M.I. either to the right or to the left. If this threatened or impending abortion then leads to fetal death, it is signaled by a drastic shift of the M.I. to the left, similar to the postpartum pattern.

The *postpartum* pattern is striking (Fig. 36.8). Around the time of delivery another mammoth hormonal change takes place. The M.I., heavily shifted to the midzone throughout pregnancy, briefly shifts to the right in some patients and then, after delivery, shifts to the left (from $\overline{0/9\overset{\times}{5}/5}$ to $\overline{100/0/0}$) (Plate 36.2). This teleatrophic postpartum or lactational pattern (Fig. 36.8) is striking in a young woman. It can be altered by hormones administered for suppression of lactation. After varying lengths of time it gradually returns to the normal menstrual cyclic pattern.

Of continuing interest is Pundel's report of a significant change in cytohormonal pattern a few days *before* normal termi-

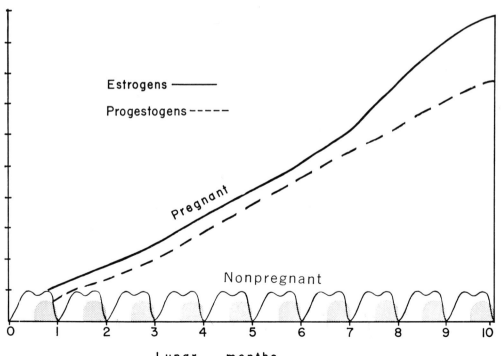

36.7. Gestation. A diagrammatic composite of the systemic estrogens and progestogens of a pregnant patient, superimposed upon those expected if she were not pregnant.

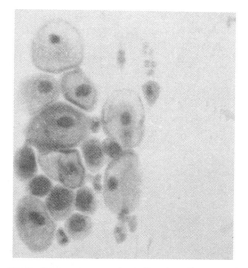

36.8. Postpartum or lactational pattern; maturation index, $\overleftarrow{100/0/0}$. This peculiarly teleatrophic pattern contains only parabasal cells. It occurs abruptly at the end of gestation and is a marked change from the lush intermediate cell exfoliation of pregnancy (see Fig. 36.6) ($\times$160).

nation of pregnancy, with a slight shift to the right and then the significant shift to the left of the M.I. He has used this to indicate extreme postmaturity in a few cases, with successful saving of some of the infants. Others have been unable to confirm entirely the findings in much smaller series.

Determination of fetal sex from alterations of maternal cytohormonal pattern, by fetal endocrine production, has proved fruitless in spite of earlier encouraging reports. The maternal hormonal level which establishes the normal pregnancy pattern is massive, relative to the minute alteration which any fetal production might play.

Perimenopausal Period. For years, both before and after the actual cessation of menses, there are gradually progressive alterations and diminutions in the orderly cyclic endocrine patterns of the reproductive period. These are mirrored in the vaginal epithelium and its cytohormonal pattern (Plate 36.2). This process of alteration begins in the latter part of the reproductive period and continues through the menopause and for years thereafter, with the cyclic hormonal variations decreasing in intensity and

varying in frequency. The onset of this perimenopausal period is gradual and varies greatly among individuals. If cessation of cycles does occur before death, it is insidious and without clinical fanfare.

Cytohormonally, perimenopausal patients appear to fall into two well defined categories, those developing intermediate cell atrophy (towards M.I., $\overleftarrow{0/100/0}$) with apparent lack of any estrogen effect, or *estratrophy* (Fig. 36.9), and those developing parabasal cell atrophy or *teleatrophy* (towards M.I., $\overleftarrow{100/0/0}$) with total absence of evidence of any effect of vaginal maturation (Fig. 36.10). The reasons for the differences are not clear. Adrenal cortical function may well play a larger role than generally ap-

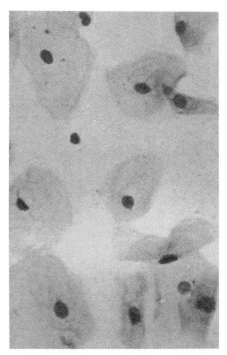

36.9. Intermediate cell atrophy pattern, or estratrophy; maturation index, $\overleftarrow{0/100/0}$. This Fast smear from a 55-year-old woman, 5 years postmenopausal, contains only cells of intermediate type (wafer-thin cytoplasm with vesicular nuclei). Although there is no evidence of estrogenic stimulation (no superficial cells) and this is thus a true estratrophic pattern, there is sufficient stimulation from other substances to mature cells to the intermediate state before exfoliation. This is in contradistinction to the thin, atrophic epithelium of teleatrophy ($\times$160).

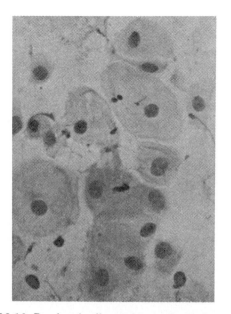

36.10. Parabasal cell atrophy or teleatrophy pattern; maturation index, $\overline{100/0/0}$. This Fast smear from a 66-year-old woman, 12 years postmenopausal, contains only parabasal cells (thick cytoplasm). The thin, atrophic epithelium from which these cells are shed shows no effect of maturing hormones but is usually very sensitive to them. Present in childhood and postmenopause, it is easily infected producing, in the latter, senile vaginitis ($\times$160).

preciated, and probably accounts for the M.I. "midzone" shift of intermediate cell atrophy, even though small levels of estrogens have also been implicated. Why all do not follow this pattern is not clear. Variations in hypophysial response to feedback may underlie these patterns, and at times adrenal androgens are suspected of playing a role.

In the development of intermediate cell atrophy throughout the perimenopausal period, there is an increasing number of intermediate cells exfoliated at the expense of superficials, without significant production of parabasals. This shift toward the midzone of the M.I. may be gradual, with $0/100/0$ being reached years after actual cessation of menses. This is not an atrophic vaginal epithelium, clinically, but is lush and resistant to infection; however, of great importance is the virtual absence of superficial cells (less than 10%). This total lack of ap-

parent estrogen stimulation may reflect relatively high or unopposed cortisone levels.

In the development of the other frequent pattern, that of *teleatrophy* (Fig. 36.10), there is a gradual increase in exfoliation of parabasal cells at the expense of superficial cells, and later of the intermediate cells. Finally complete atrophy, or teleatrophy, appears with total shift of the M.I. to the left $\overline{(100/0/0)}$. Clinically, vaginal atrophy is present and the epithelial resistance to infection is low. Senile vaginitis is frequent in this group.

There is no "normal" or typical pattern of a woman at the time of her last menses, the range of normalcy being extremely wide. Some pass through the menopause with a "young" pattern, whereas others are more atrophic. The established pattern is more one of default than of strong endocrine levels, and is thus labile and sensitive to small doses of hormones or inflammation. Wied (1957) has taken advantage of this in differentiating between a menopausal missed period and pregnancy. The strong endocrine level of the latter is not affected by small doses of *systemically* administered estrogens, whereas the former patient developing postmenopausal intermediate cell atrophy with essentially the same cytohormonal pattern (M.I., c. $\overline{0/95/5}$), will show a marked shift to the right following the same therapy.

With the length of the perimenopausal period so great and variable, and with the uncertainty of the exact pattern to be taken by a given patient, one has a very broad "normal limit" to consider when evaluating patients of this period for endocrine abnormalities. One pattern is clearly abnormal, however—that of extreme estrogen stimulation or marked shift to the right of the M.I. in the absence of inflammation. This is frequently associated with certain "functionally active" ovarian tumors (see Chaps. 24 and 37).

Postmenopausal Period. Either of the two major patterns are assumed as the stormy perimenopausal phase passes into this relatively quiescent postmenopausal period (Plate 36.2), that of intermediate cell atrophy (M.I., $\overline{0/100/0}$) (Fig. 36.9) or of parabasal cell atrophy (M.I., $\overline{100/0/0}$) (Fig. 36.10) with variations in between. Cyclic fluctuations become less intense and frequent. Intermediate cell atrophy, in which the epithelial surface is completely covered with intermediate cells, is usually asymptomatic. This pattern predominates when inflammatory patterns are removed from consideration.

Teleatrophy, or parabasal cell atrophy, frequently becomes inflamed and infected, producing senile vaginitis. At times bizarre parabasal cell changes come about from irritation which, in morphology, can *approach* dysplasia or even closely resemble neoplasia. These problems are dissipated with small amounts of oral or vaginal estrogens, to which the epithelium is very sensitive, and reevaluating cytologically bi-weekly thereafter.

Without extrinsic estrogens and in the absence of inflammation, the presence of significant numbers of superficial cells is abnormal in this postmenopausal period. They rise in infection, chronic irritation (procidentia, etc.), leukoplakia, vaginal dermatoses, and estrogen administration. In the absence of those, however, a significant rise in superficial cells may indicate the presence of certain neoplasms (endometrial, ovarian, mammary, etc.), and hormonal abnormalities. Contamination of the vaginal specimen with vulvar cells must be ruled out.

Abnormal Cytohormonal Patterns

Neoplasms Producing Hormones. Endocrine-producing tumors cause a shift of the M.I. which is characteristic for the hormone or hormones secreted. Although the cytohormonal pattern is of the quality characteristic of the particular hormone produced, its quality or degree of shift of the M.I. depends both upon the clinical effectiveness of the particular compound being produced and its amount.

Estrogens from ovarian granulosa cell tumors are usually potent, shifting the M.I. clearly to the right (toward $\overrightarrow{0/0/100}$) with the squames lying flat and singly in a clear background, if there is no infection present. Estrogens from the adrenal cortex, on the other hand, may be weaker clinically and less physiological in their activity, but produce estrogenic effects proportional to the quality and quantity of the compound. Luteinizing tumors of the ovary producing *progestogens* bring about a midzone shift of the M.I. (toward $\overline{0/100/0}$) and the other features of the cytohormonal pattern of progesterone. *Androgens* are produced by some virilizing ovarian tumors (*i.e.,* arrhenoblastoma, hilus cell tumor, etc.)

Many of the ovarian mesenchymal tumors, however, produce *mixtures* of hormones, such as progestogens and estrogens. In addition, many adrenal cortical tumors also produce androgens, estrogens, progestogens, and corticoids.

Pituitary tumors produce hormones which act upon their specific end organs. If the latter produces hormones, they act upon the vaginal epithelium in characteristic fashion. Under these conditions, the cytohormonal pattern of the vaginal smear, when evaluated with the patient's age and other influential factors, reflects the compounding effects of these multiple agents, each with its characteristic effect.

Neoplasms without Obvious Hormonal Production. Patients with cystic and solid tumors of the ovary (*i.e.,* adenocarcinoma, cystadenoma, serous cystadenocarcinoma) and endometrial adenocarcinoma and hyperplasia are frequently *not* found to have cytohormonal teleatrophy, regardless of age. In spite of the lack of known hormonal secretion of these tumors, the M.I. of the host is frequently shifted toward the right. Frequently, this shift is out of the range of normal (Fig. 36.11), so that greater than 10% superficial cells in a vaginal smear may be the only clue to the presence of disease. This appears to be a reflection of tumor cell influence on the ovarian stroma to produce estrogens (Chap. 25). Whether this represents such an abnormal endocrine level or whether it reflects abnormal tissue sensitivity, it at times will be the only presenting evidence of disease leading to detection of an asymptomatic lesion.

Obviously, this is not an absolute diagnostic finding, as a certain number of patients exhibit this abnormal response

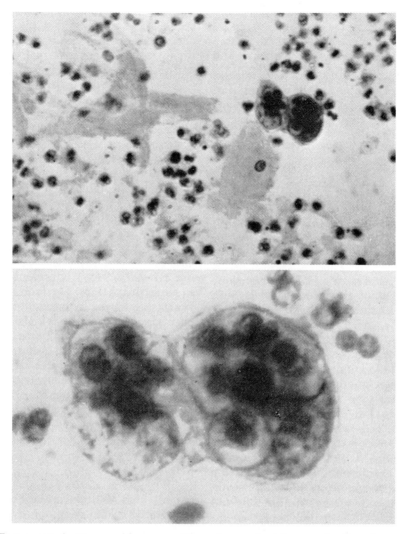

36.11. A Fast smear of a 71-year-old woman with an abnormal cytohormonal pattern for a woman of this age. In spite of the inflammation, the maturation index does not show a spread, but is shifted to the right $(\overline{0/72/28})$. The 2 cancer cells were shed from a serous cystadenocarcinoma of the ovary and traveled down the tubes and uterus into the vaginal pool. They have hyper-distended secretory vacuoles which are filled with phagocytizing, well preserved neurtophils (*top,* ×480; *bottom,* ×2000).

and are in apparent good health on close follow-up. In time, some of these patients with an unexplained abnormal M.I. shift to the right *will* reveal lesions of the breast (fibroadenoma, adenocarcinoma), endometrium (hyperplasia, adenocarcinoma), salpinx (adenocarcinoma), ovary (cysts, benign tumors, primary and secondary cancers), and adrenal cortex (hyperplasia, adenoma, adenocarcinoma). The M.I. shift to the right from estrogen-producing tumors (*i.e.,* granulosa cell tumor) tends to be great (*e.g.,* up to 90% superficial cells). Conversely, that associated with those neoplasms without obvious hormonal production tends to be modest (*e.g.,* 10 to 35% superficial cells). Some of these latter patients bear a history of these lesions in the *past.* About one-quarter of the patients with this modest abnormal M.I. shift to the right appear to harbor *no* disease.

Anovulation. Absence of the biphasic cytohormonal cycle signifies anovulation.

It is demonstrated clearly by an absence of the monthly cyclic change between the superficial cells and intermediate cells, and lack of progestational changes (*i.e.,* cell folding, sticking), which are so characteristic of the normal menstrual cycle (Plate 36.1).

This is best detected by evaluating daily vaginal smears. Clinically, this is a simple procedure (see p. 807), which can greatly augment information obtained from basal body temperature concerning the nature of the basic cause involved.

Ovulation is characterized by the monthly cyclic change of the M.I. from proliferative to secretory pattern and back again (*c.* $\overline{0/40/60} \rightleftarrows \overline{0/70/30}$) (Plates 36.1, .2). This is lacking with anovulation, where the M.I. continues at a *constant* value, in some cases in the high estrogen (*c.* $\overline{0/20/80}$) range, in other cases in a low estrogen (*c.* $\overline{0/80/20}$) range, and others without any estrogen effect (estratrophy, *i.e.,* Turner's, Sheehan's). As the significant finding is not the absolute value of the M.I. but is rather its change around ovulation (from *c.* $\overline{0/40/60}$ to *c.* $\overline{0/70/30}$), a random smear will *not* suffice in this determination.

The earliest sign that ovulation has occurred, before a significant M.I. cycle shift, is the *appearance* of a *progesterone* effect. Curling and sticking of intermediate cells with mucus production and cytolysis (Plate 36.1) usually appears immediately around ovulation. Although a single smear determination during the luteal phase may suggest that ovulation has occurred, some situations can obsure it (*i.e.,* infection) or even mimic the pattern (*i.e.,* pregnancy, tumors, endocrine imbalances) unless the preovulatory smear is present for comparison.

Therefore, at times one can gather information by only two single evaluations, one just before estimated ovulation and the second two weeks later, if there is a definite M.I. shift to indicate ovulation and a sufficient change in pattern to indicate progesterone effect. However, if no alteration is detected, this does *not* indicate anovulation, as the possibility still exists that ovulation occurred at a time different than estimated.

From daily to semi-weekly smears thus are best as they obviate this difficulty by clearly indicating anovulation, and will further provide information for detecting endocrinopathies. Persisting follicular cysts are found in a high estrogenic pattern with an M.I. shift to the right, at times extremely shifted.

The Stein-Leventhal syndrome may be accompanied by either a moderate shift to the right, or a midzone spread. Characteristically, however, the cytohormonal pattern is constant, without the cyclic ovulatory shift in the M.I. Thus the pattern is not of help, but the lack of ovulatory shift is.

Primary Amenorrhea (see Chap. 30). Women of the reproductive age who have never menstruated can be considered to fall within one of a few clinical categories based upon characteristics of three major parameters: the chromosomal sex, the cytohormonal pattern, and the presence or absence of ovulation.

Normal hormonal pattern with *"positive chromatin"* (♀) is found in XX anatomical variants with normal ovaries (*e.g.,* congenital atresias; absence of portions of the generative system, except ovaries; endometrial sclerosis before puberty, as with tuberculosis), or endocrinopathies whose abnormalities are not sufficient to make the hormonal pattern fall outside of the wide range which is within "normal" limits for the childbearing age. In the former, the cyclic ovulatory shift in the cytohormonal pattern (*i.e.,* M.I.; progesterone curling) is usually present; in the latter, it is usually absent or abnormal.

Abnormal hormonal pattern with "positive chromatin" (♀) is present in endocrinopathies. Dysfunctions of the ovary (agenesis, hypofunction, tumor), pituitary (dwarfism, infantilism, Simmonds' disease), thyroid (*marked* hypothyroidism, cretinism), adrenal (hyperplasia, tumor), and chromosomes (XXX, mongolism, miscellaneous trisomy) and systemic illness (*i.e.,* tuberculosis) play major roles in this regard. Ovulation is usually absent, but may provide key evidence as to the site of abnormality. The presence of estratrophy (M.I.,

$\overrightarrow{0/1\overleftarrow{0}0/0}$) indicates lack of ovarian or pituitary function (*i.e.,* Sheehan's) whereas an approach towards teleatrophy (M.I., $\overleftarrow{100/0/0}$) is found in pituitary or adrenal dysfunction, or *extreme* hypothyroidism.

Normal hormonal pattern with *"negative chromatin"* (♂) may be present in testicular feminization (XY) or a Turner's syndrome (XO) who has received estrogen therapy. With adequate estrogen production or therapy, the cytohormonal pattern may well be within normal limits (Fig. 36.12). At times in the former the estrogenic effect is so extreme that the M.I. shifts past the right of normal, with exfoliation of anucleate superficial cells (Fig. 36.13).

Abnormal hormonal pattern with *"negative chromatin"* (♂) is found in untreated Turner's syndrome (XO) and in male pseudohermaphrodites (XY). In younger patients of the childbearing age with Turner's syndrome, estratrophy

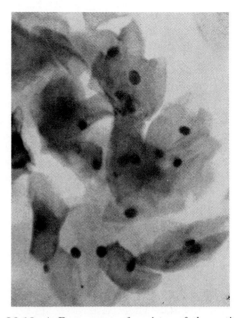

36.13. A Fast smear of a sister of the patient shown in Fig. 36.12. This 17-year-old girl also has testicular feminization, demonstrated at subsequent operation, with negative sex chromatin; however, her cytohormonal pattern shows a more extreme estrogen response, with numerous anucleate superficial cells produced (*upper left*). The maturation index is $\overrightarrow{0/3\overleftarrow{2}/68}$, with 18 of the 68 superficials being anucleate (×160).

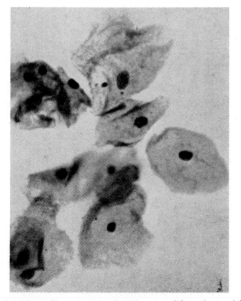

36.12. A Fast smear of a 20-year-old patient with testicular feminization demonstrated at subsequent operation. A normal appearing girl with good breast development and normal external genitalia, she had never menstruated. The nuclei contain no Barr bodies ("chromatin-negative"), and the cytohormonal pattern shows good estrogen production with a normal maturation index of $\overrightarrow{0/6\overleftarrow{2}/38}$ (×160).

$\overline{(0/1\overleftarrow{0}0/0)}$ rather than teleatrophy ($\overleftarrow{100/0/0}$) is usually present in the vaginal smear cytohormonal pattern. Male pseudohermaphrodites may have evidence of androgen in their cytohormonal pattern, but may approach estratrophy or teleatrophy according to their age.

Secondary Amenorrhea or Oligomenorrhea (see Chap. 30). In evaluating unexplained secondary amenorrhea or oligomenorrhea, one should consider the cytohormonal status, the cytogenetic status (*i.e.,* XXX) and the possibility of anovulation. In determining the presence or absence of ovulation in these patients, it is best to obtain daily smears at the time basal body temperatures are taken. Obtaining these specimens should be extended past the usual 30 days in order to detect the extremely long periods encountered with many irregular menses.

The cytohormonal levels of Stein-

Leventhal syndrome patients remain virtually constant and do *not* reveal the cyclic ovulatory shift. Patients with persistent follicular cysts also show anovulation, but their constant daily pattern approximates that found normally at the time of ovulation, *e.g.,* estrogen without progesterone. Only occasional patients with Sheehan's syndrome may retain sufficient partial pituitary function to have a cytohormonal pattern which falls within a low normal range, but they do *not* have the cyclic ovulatory shift.

Mild or moderate hypothyroidism produces cytohormonal patterns within normal range, but without ovulation if the disorder is severe enough. In extreme hypothyroidism and athyroidism, the M.I. is shifted to the left toward teleatrophy. Cytohormonal patterns falling within normal range are also found in systemic illnesses, emotional disturbances, endocrinopathies of borderline severity, simple physical blockage, or endometrial sclerosis (Asherman's disease). The latter two have normal ovulatory patterns in daily vaginal smear cytohormonal evaluation, whereas the former usually have either anovulation or disturbed ovulatory patterns.

Secondary amenorrhea or oligomenorrhea with *abnormal cytohormonal pattern* bespeaks severe systemic illness, endocrinopathy, or emotional disturbances. Four major cytohormonal patterns should be sought, either in pure form or combinations: a shift in the M.I. to the right, the midzone, the left, or the spread of androgens.

The extreme M.I. *shift to the right* (approaching $\overline{0/0/100}$) is that of high estrogen effect. This is found in persisting follicle cysts and in certain ovarian and adrenal tumors. A less marked shift to the right is found in other tumors, some endometrial hyperplasias and adenocarcinomas. In rare instances various miscellaneous hormonally associated states are found with this pattern, such as endometriosis, myomas, and mammary disease (adenofibromas, chronic cystic mastitis, carcinoma); these are not, however, found in any consistent pattern. One must always be alert for exogenous estrogens in its many and frequently overt forms of administration.

The extreme M.I. *shift to the midzone* (approaching estratrophy $\overline{0/100/0}$) bespeaks lack of estrogen effect in the presence of nonestrogenic maturing stimulation. The most frequent situation is ovarian failure with adequate adrenal cortical function remaining. Oophorectomy, either from surgery or adequate irradiation, removes production, leaving adrenal cortical function. During the reproductive age the latter normally is overwhelmingly of cortisone type compounds, which produce exfoliation at the intermediate cell level of maturation $\overline{(0/100/0)}$. The small amounts of estrogen and progestogen compounds produced by the adrenal cortex are normally insufficient to alter this cytohormonal pattern in the face of overwhelming cortisone effect.

Hypopituitary function from tumors, Simmonds' disease, anorexia nervosa, and radiation ablation may be partial with a spread M.I. pattern simulating inflammation. The usual mild or moderate Sheehan's syndrome results from a selective lack of gonadotrophins from partial pituitary apoplexy, and produces a cytohormonal shift to the midzone (M.I., $\overline{0/100/0}$) typical of ovarian ablation with continuing adrenal corticoid production. When pituitary injury has been more marked and widespread in its trophic effects, a severe Sheehan's syndrome will also produce an M.I. shift toward the left and even, in very severe ablation, complete teleatrophy.

Other menstrual disturbances associated with an M.I. midzone shift include functioning ovarian mesenchymal tumors producing progestogens, functional adrenal tumors, and certain drug administrations.

The most frequent cause for secondary amenorrhea with an approximate estratrophy pattern $\overline{(0/95/5)}$ is, of course, pregnancy. This is due not to lack of estrogens, as in true estratrophy $\overline{(0/100/0)}$, but to its overwhelming opposition by progestogens and adrenal corticoids.

The extreme *M.I. shift to the left* (approaching teleatrophy, $\overline{100/0/0}$) is found with secondary amenorrhea or oligomenorrhea when there has been no maturation of the vaginal epithelium past the immature parabasal cell. At times the vaginal epithelium is at fault, but usually the maturing stimuli are absent. In the first instance the vaginal epithelium is incapable of reacting to maturing substances in normal fashion owing to inherent inadequacies following injury (*e.g.*, extensive irradiation for cervical carcinoma) or from lack of elements basic to fundamental cellular metabolism (*e.g.* thyroid deprivation in cretins or extreme hypothyroidism). The second instance is more frequent. A normal vaginal epithelium capable of full maturation may be deprived of sufficient amounts of specific maturing substances such as estrogens, progestogens, corticoids, etc. This is responsible for the teleatrophy of extreme panhypopituitary function found in severe Sheehan's syndrome, anorexia nervosa, Simmonds' disease, and ablation. One must remain aware of the peculiar lactational teleatrophy and amenorrhea which may normally be present postpartum, and which may persist for varying lengths of time (Plate 36.2 and Fig. 36.8).

Mammary Lesions. Some lesions of the breast are associated with bizarre cytohormonal patterns. They are neither consistent nor diagnostic; but, by arousing proper suspicion, they may lead to an earlier clinical diagnosis. Adenofibromas are the most frequent mammary lesions of youth associated with an M.I. shift to the right, at times beyond the wide normal limits of the menstrual cycle. Chronic cystic mastitis, usually with a normal pattern, can also be associated with an M.I. shift to the right, or a spread pattern. Adenocarcinoma is associated with virtually any pattern, either extremely abnormal for the age and history (M.I. to the right, left, or spread), or normal.

Therapy of a patient with *advanced* or metastatic adenocarcinoma of the breast who is within the perimenopausal period can be greatly assisted at times by cytohormonally evaluating her actual endocrine status and monitoring its changes under therapy. The five-year postmenopausal clinical rule-of-thumb for endocrine supplemental or ablative therapy is only rough. It can be made more exact by close correlation with proper cytohormonal evaluation. In the absence of inflammation, this can qualitate and roughly quantitate remaining endocrine activity to evaluate estrogenic stimulation, androgenic effect, or teleatrophy and may thus assist the clinician in choosing the proper therapy to drastically alter the patient's hormonal milieu. In following such patients cytohormonally after therapy, an unexplained change in pattern often heralds, by a few months, a clinical relapse.

Compounding States. It is no rarity for multiple lesions in the above categories to present together. It is well documented that there is an increased frequency of the association and either simultaneous or subsequent occurrence of ovarian tumors, endometrial hyperplasias or carcinomas, myomas, endometriosis, and mammary lesions. Some bizarre cytohormonal patterns persist for years after the removal of a lesion, such as an extreme M.I. shift to the right in an 80-year-old patient, living and well without evident recurrence or related disease, 16 years after hysterectomy for endometrial adenocarcinoma.

Artificial Vagina. Vaginal grafts from the thigh may show varying degrees of endocrine response after becoming well established. This coincides with their secretory ability, as demonstrated by Masters. Their cytohormonal pattern is not entirely normal, however, as they retain some true cornification with an extreme M.I. shift to the right and exfoliation of numbers of anucleate superficial cells.

Childhood Abnormal Cytohormonal Patterns

The cytohormonal pattern of childhood is so constantly predictable, at or near teleatrophy with *no* superficial cells (Plate 36.2), that abnormalities are usually obvious. An adrenogenital syndrome with adrenocortical hyperplasia, is associated with an abnormal cytohormonal pattern varying according to the amounts of estrogens, progestogens, and androgens being produced. As the effect of the latter usually predominates, the corresponding androgenic M.I. spread pattern is the most frequent cytohormonal finding.

An M.I. shift to the right during childhood, especially before perimenarche, is distinctly abnormal and bespeaks estrogens. Ovarian granulosa-theca cell tumors produce significant M.I. shifts to the right. Luteinizing and feminizing produce cytohormonal patterns typical of the hormones secreted by the neoplasm, with varying degrees of progestational effect including those identical with pregnancy.

Exogenous hormones must always be suspected in children, and their presence thoroughly investigated. They vary widely from iatrogenic therapy (*i.e.*, estrogens for childhood vaginitis) to ingestion of *geriatric* vitamins containing steroids intended for a grandparent.

REFERENCES

Barr, M. L.: The sex chromosomes of man. Amer. J. Obstet. Gynec., *93:* 608, 1965.

Barr, M. L., and Bertram, E. G.: A morphological distinction between neurons of the male and female, and the behavior of the nucleolar satelite during accelerated nucleoprotein synthesis. Nature (London), *163:* 676, 1949.

Batrinos, M. L., and Eustratiades, M. G.: Vaginal cytology in primary amenorrhea. Acta Cytol., *16:* 376, 1972.

Benson, R. C., and Traut, H. F.: The vaginal smear as a diagnostic and prognostic aid in abortion. J. Clin. Endocr., *10:* 675, 1950.

Briggs, D. K., and Kupperman, H. S.: Further experience with sex determination from leukocytes. Trans. I.S.C.C., *5:* 79, 1957.

Chu, E. H.: The chromosome complements of human somatic cells. Amer. J. Hum. Genet., *12:* 97, 1960.

Dokumov, S. I., and Spasov, S. A.: Sex chromatin pattern and menstrual cycle. Acta Cytol., *12:* 131, 1968.

Ferguson-Smith, M. A., Johnston, A. W., and Handmaker, S. D.: Primary amentia and micro-orchidism associated with an XXXY sex-chromosome constitution. Lancet (London), *2:* 184, 1960.

Frost, J. K.: Gynecologic and obstetric cytopathology, Chapter 35 in *Novak's Gynecologic and Obstetric Pathology,* Novak, E. R., and Woodruff, J. D. (Editors). W. B. Saunders Company, Philadelphia, 7th ed., 1974.

Frost, J. K.: *The Cell in Health and Disease.* S. Karger, Basel; Williams & Wilkins, Baltimore, 1969.

Frost, J. K., Wood, D. A., and Kearney, J. V.: Vaginal smear hormonal patterns in adenocarcinoma of the breast. Trans. I.S.C.C., *3:* 93, 1955.

Geist, S. H., and Salmon, U. J.: The evaluation of the human vaginal smear in relationship to the histology of the vaginal mucosa. Amer. J. Obstet. Gynec., *38:* 392, 1939.

Gupta, P. K.: Cytohormonal studies in arrhenoblastoma. Acta Cytol., *16:* 1, 1972.

Hsu, T. C.: Numerical variation of chromosomes in higher animals, Chapter 3 in *Developmental Cytology,* Rudnick, D. (Editor). The Ronald Press Company, New York, 1959.

Jacobs, P. A., Baikie, A. G., Brown, W. M., MacGregor, T. N., MacLean, N., and Harnden, D. G.: Evidence for existence of the "super female." Lancet (London), *2:* 423, 1959.

Kahn, R. H.: Vaginal keratinization *in vitro.* Ann. N.Y. Acad. Sci., *83:* 347, 1959.

LeJeune, J., Gautier, M., and Turpin, R.: Etude des chromosomes somatiques de neuf enfants mongoliens. C. R. Acad. Sci. (Paris), *248:* 1721, 1959.

Lencioni, L. J.: Comparative and statistical study of vaginal and urinary sediment smears. J. Clin. Endocr., *13:* 263, 1953.

Lencioni, L. J., Martínez Amezaga, L. A., and Lo Bíanco, V. S.: Urocytogram and pregnancy. I. Methods and normal values. Acta Cytol., *13:* 279, 1969.

Lencioni, L. J., Martinez Amézaga, L. A., Alonso, C., and Camargo, L. A. H.: Urocytogram and pregnancy. II: Correlation with fetal condition at birth in high risk pregnancies. Acta Cytol., *17:* 125, 1973.

Liu, W.: Vaginal cornification in women with uterine cancer. Cancer, *8:* 779, 1955.

Mack, H. C.: A new and rapid method of staining vaginal smears based upon a specific color reaction for glycogen. Harper Hosp. Bull., *1:* 54, 1942.

Masters, W. H.: The sexual response cycle of the human female: vaginal lubrication. Ann. N.Y. Acad. Sci., *83:* 301, 1959.

Masukawa, T.: Vaginal smears in women past 40 years of age, with emphasis on their remaining hormonal activity. Obstet. Gynec., *16:* 407, 1960.

Masukawa, T., Masukawa, N. K., Frost, J. K., Lewison, E. F., Trimble, F. H., and Grow, J. L.: Vaginal cytology of women with advanced breast carcinoma treated by endocrine alteration, p. 43 in *The Proceedings of the First International Congress of Exfoliative Cytology.* J. B. Lippincott Company, Philadelphia, 1962.

Meisels, A.: The maturation value. Acta Cytol., *11:* 249, 1967.

Miles, C. P.: Sex chromatin in cultured normal and cancerous human tissues. Cancer, *12:* 299, 1959.

Mittwoch, U.: *Sex Chromosomes,* Academic Press, New York, 1967.

Moore, K. L., and Barr, M. L.: Nuclear morphology, according to sex, in human tissues. Acta Anat. (Basel), *21:* 197, 1954.

Moore, K. L., and Barr, M. L.: Smears from the oral mucosa in the detection of chromosomal sex. Lancet (London), *269:* 57, 1955.

Moore, K. L., Ohno, S., Miller, O. J., and Uchida, I. A.: Symposium: Sex chromatin, chromosomal errors, and human development. Acta Cytol., *7:* 146, 1963.

Moorhead, P. S., Nowell, P. C., Mellman, W. J., Battips, D. M., and Hungerford, D. A.: Chromosome preparations of leukocytes cultured from peripheral blood. Exp. Cell Res., *20:* 613, 1960.

Moracci, E., and Berlingieri, D.: Hormonal evaluation of vaginal smears from artificial vagina. Acta Cytol., *17:* 131, 1973.

Moraes-Ruehsen, M. D., and Masukawa, T.: The irrigation smear: use in hormonal colpocytology. Acta Cytol., *9:* 307, 1965.

Ng, A. B. P., Reagan, J. W., and Cechner, R. L.: The precursors of endometrial cancer: a study of their cellular manifestations. Acta Cytol., *17:* 439, 1973.

Papanicolaou, G. N.: 159. The existence of a "postmenopause" sexual rhythm in women, as indicated by the study of vaginal smear. Anat. Rec. (Suppl.), *55:* 71, 1932–33.

Papanicolaou, G. N.: The sexual cycle in the human female as revealed by vaginal smears. Amer. J. Anat., *52:* 519, 1933.

Papanicolaou, G. N.: *Atlas of Exfoliative Cytology.* Published for The Commonwealth Fund by Harvard University Press, Cambridge, 1954, with supplements.

Papanicolaou, G. N., and Shorr, E.: Action of ovarian follicle hormone in ovarian insufficiency in women as indicated by vaginal smears. Proc. Soc. Exp. Biol. Med., *32:* 585, 1934–35.

Papanicolaou, G. N., and Shorr, E.: The action of ovarian follicular hormone in the menopause, as indicated by vaginal smears. Amer. J. Obstet. Gynec., *31:* 806, 1936.

Papanicolaou, G. N., and Traut, H. F.: *Diagnosis of Uterine Cancer by the Vaginal Smear.* The Commonwealth Fund, New York, 1943.

Papanicolaou, G. N., Traut, H. F., and Marchetti, A. A.: *The Epithelia of Woman's Reproductive Organs. A Correlative Study of Cyclic Changes.* The Commonwealth Fund, New York, 1948.

Paschkis, K. E., Rakoff, A. E., Cantarow, A., and Rupp, J. J.: *Clinical Endocrinology.* Hoeber Medical Division, Harper and Row, New York, 3rd ed., 1967.

Plunkett, E. R., and Barr, M. L.: Testicular dysgenesis affecting the seminiferous tubules principally, with chromatin-positive nuclei. Lancet (London), *271:* 853, 1956.

Pundel, J. P.: The practical value of the vaginal smear at the end of pregnancy. Trans. I.S.C.C., *7:* 9, 1959.

Riley, G. M., Dontas, E., and Gill, B.: Use of serial vaginal smears in detecting time of ovulation. Fertil. Steril., *6:* 86, 1955.

Rubin, D. K., and Frost, J. K.: The cytologic detection of ovarian cancer. Acta Cytol., *7:* 191, 1963.

Schmitz, H. E., Isaacs, J. H., and Fetherston, W. C.: The value of routine cytologic smears in pregnancy. Amer. J. Obstet. Gynec., *79:* 910, 1960.

Shorr, E.: A new technic for staining vaginal smears: II. Science, *91:* 579, 1940.

Steward, J. S., and Sanderson, A. R.: Fertility and oligophrenia in apparent triple-X female. Lancet (London), *2:* 21, 1960.

Stockard, C. R., and Papanicolaou, G. N.: The existence of atypical oestrous cylce in the guinea pig, with a study of its histological and physiological changes. Amer. J. Anat., *22:* 225, 1917.

Torres, E. F.: Feminization in tumors of Sertoli-Leydig cells. Acta Cytol., *18:* 187, 1974.

Traut, H. F., Bloch, P. W., and Kuder, A.: Cyclical changes in the human vaginal mucosa. Surg. Gynec. Obstet., *63:* 7, 1936.

Wachtel, E.: A simple cytological test for cancer cure. Brit. Med. J., *5061:* 20, 1958.

Wachtel, E., and Plester, J. A.: Hormonal assessment by vaginal cytology. J. Obstet. Gynaec. Brit. Comm., *61:* 155, 1954.

Wells, L. J.: Embryology and anatomy of the vagina. Ann. N.Y. Acad. Sci., *83:* 80, 1959.

Wied, G. L.: The cytologic changes of the vaginal epithelial cells and the leukorrhea following estrogenic therapy. Amer. J. Obstet. Gynec., *70:* 51, 1955.

Wied, G. L.: Climacteric amenorrhea; a cytohormonal test for differential diagnosis. Obstet. Gynec., *9:* 646, 1957.

Wied, G. L.: An international agreement on histological terminology for lesions of the uterine cervix. Acta Cytol., *6:* 235, 1962.

Wied, G. L., Boschann, H.-W., Ferin, J., Frost, J. K., Luksch, F., Meisels, A., Montalvo-Ruiz, L., Terzano, G., Teter, J., and Wachtel, E.: Symposium on hormonal cytology. Acta Cytol., *12:* 87, 1968.

Wied, G. L., and Davis, M. E.: Synergism and antagonism of sex steroids as determined on the vaginal epithelial cells. Ann. N.Y. Acad. Sci., *83:* 207, 1959.

Wilkins, L., Grumbach, M. M., and Van Wyk, J. J.: Chromosomal sex in ovarian agenesis. J. Clin. Endocr., *14:* 1270, 1954.

Woodruff, J. D., Williams, T. J., and Goldberg, B.: Hormone activity of the common ovarian neoplasm. Amer. J. Obstet. Gynec., *87:* 679, 1963.

chapter 37

Gynecologic Clinical Cytopathology

By John K. Frost, M.D.

Health and disease are accurately reflected in cellular patterns. Cellular samples are *micro*biopsies by which the cytopathologist, like the histopathologist using tissue samples, studies the multiple processes of health and disease to arrive at interpretations or diagnoses of conditions present. As extremely small as these specimens might be, they at times hold more information than larger tissue samples removed by surgery.

Although usually coming from the surface of organs, these samples reflect the deeper processes accurately. They cover a wider surface area for examination than biopsies usually can, do not remove viable tissue, and virtually do not bring forth inflammatory or reparative processes. They afford unequaled opportunity not only to detect and diagnose disease but also to study the biologic behavior of disease processes *unaltered* by surgical intervention or surgical removal.

CLINICAL APPLICATION

Papanicolaou and Traut initially introduced this technique into clinical medicine in 1943. It has been accepted into our armamentarium after extensive use and proof of reliability.

In the United States, great clinical emphasis has been placed upon its unequaled ability to detect *early cancer*. This has speeded its development and acceptance, but has overshadowed its cytohormonal and cytogenetic potentials (Chap. 36). Additionally, it has proved very useful in furthering our understanding of the whole problem of *host response* to infections, neoplasias, radiation, and therapy.

Accurate cytopathological evaluation and diagnosis is difficult and complex, requiring extensive proper education and experience. However, the *simplicity* and *rapidity* with which the clinical specimen is obtainable has placed its consultation at the fingertips of *every* practicing physician regardless of specialty, training, or experience.

Physicians' *techniques* for the clinical preparation of these cytopathology specimens are depicted at the end of this chapter.

Both the clinician and the consulting

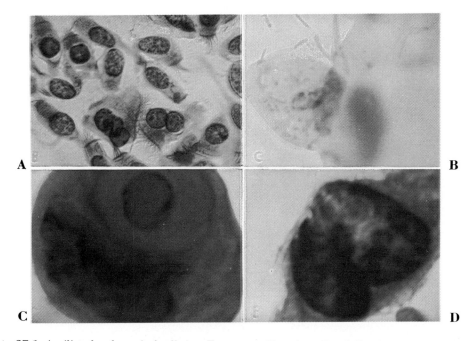

Plate 37.1. *A*, ciliated endocervical cells in a Fast smear. Note the eosinophilic cilia whose rootlets extend into the green cytoplasm as the eosinophilic terminal plate. See Fig. 37.3. (×520). *B, Trichomonas vaginalis, left,* lying on the edge of the cytoplasm of an acidophilic superficial cell. Döderlein bacilli above. Note the pale, but definite, nucleus of the Trichomonas and green cytoplasm containing red granules (Fast smear, ×1378). *C*, malignant "pearl" exfoliated from invasive squamous cell carcinoma of the cervix. These two cells have extremely hyalinized and keratinized cytoplasm. An unusual hypermaturation for cervical carcinomas. The lower nucleus has many malignant criteria (Fast smear, ×1378). *D*, undifferentiated cell from invasive carcinoma (Fast smear, ×1378). Papanicolaou stain.

pathologist must have a clear, accurate picture of each other's problems and perspective in order for cytopathology not to mislead but to guide securely. Together these physicians must strive for a complete understanding of the total patient as a whole.

INFLAMMATION

General Inflammation

A nonspecific inflammatory host response is brought forth by many agents and conditions. This includes trauma, chemicals, radiation, infections, and tumors.

This heavy leukocytic, hemorrhagic, or necrotic exudate often obscures diagnostic elements. The maturation index is "spread," so that cytohormonal evaluation becomes invalid. Neoplastic elements are rendered unrecognizable from obscure degenerative cells; conversely, at times non-neoplastic cells are sufficiently altered morphologically for the unwary to falsely diagnose cancer.

CHRONIC TRAUMA

Irritation, such as from a long-standing pessary, prolapse, or foreign body, produces an M.I. shift to the right (see p. 763) in addition to the general inflammatory exudate. Anucleate superficial cells are exfoliated from leukoplakic areas. Although multinucleated giant cell histiocytes are most frequently associated with trichomonas infection, some foreign bodies (*e.g.,* iodinized solutions to determine tubal patency, embedded sutures) may bring them forth.

INFECTIONS

Viral Infections

The cellular response of the host to infection by virus, changes markedly with the stage of infection. The initial stage of many viral infections is a basic stimulation of the epithelium. As it progresses, the usual background pattern in viral infection is a great leukocytic outpouring with cellular destruction, especially of epithelial cells.

Some viruses produce a fairly characteristic pattern of stimulation and degeneration with inclusion bodies in either the nucleus, the cytoplasm, or both, the former yielding the most diagnostic information. Intranuclear inclusion bodies usually are smudged and have cleared "halo" areas about them (Figs. 37.1, 2) in contradistinction to giant nucleoli or chromocenters (Fig. 37.11). As nuclei with viral inclusions are degenerating, their chromatin is smudged and is both plastered onto the outer edge of the inclusion as well as margined onto the inner surface of the nuclear membrane, leaving a clearing between which forms the "halo." Cytoplasmic inclusion bodies are much less helpful diagnostically as they are difficult to distinguish from debris of phagocytosis or degeneration, as well as from cellular organelles or inclusions of metabolism.

Many different viruses have been identified in the urogenital tract but these undoubtedly represent merely a small fraction of those present either locally or

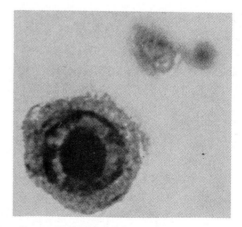

37.1. Congenital salivary gland virus disease of childhood, cytomegalic inclusion disease; renal epithelial cell in urine. The large, dark intranuclear inclusion body with smudged chromatin on its surface, has a cleared parachromatin "halo" about it. This is surrounded by the rest of the degenerated chromatin which has marginated onto the nuclear membrane leaving radially arranged strands behind bridging the cleared gap, or "halo." There are no recognizable cytoplasmic inclusions present in this cell, but the cytoplasm is dark and heavily textured. A leukocyte is in the *upper corner* of the field (Papanicolaou stain, ×1200).

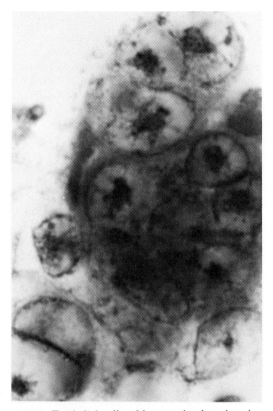

37.2. Epithelial cells of herpes simplex virus infection in a Fast smear. The nuclear inclusions are very irregular and stellate, but have blurring of degeneration. Note the trans-halo chromatin bridges transversing the cleared peri-inclusion halo, and the blurred degenerated chomatin matted against the ballooned nuclear membrane. The right nucleus of the binucleated cell in the lower left corner has some of the peculiar "clay" or "gelatinous" appearance to its degenerated chromatin which is associated with some infected nuclei which have not formed inclusion bodies (Papanicolaou stain, ×1600).

as part of a systemic involvement. Salivary gland viral infection during pregnancy can produce congenital infection in the infant with resultant cytomegalic inclusion disease of the newborn. Although this is a generalized infection of the infant and the mother, it produces characteristic cells in the renal tubular epithelium which exfoliate into the urine (Fig. 37.1) to yield a clinical diagnosis.

Other viral or possible viral-associated diseases have been associated with inclusions in the vaginal smear. Herpes simplex genitalis infection produces charac-

teristic cellular changes whose recognition during pregnancy can be of great clinical assistance to the newborn's well being. The nuclear inclusions are stellate with trans-halo bridges spanning the peri-inclusion halo. Packed multinucleation is prominent, superficially resembling degenerated syncytiotrophoblast from which they are to be differentiated in the child-bearing age. The cytoplasm is scanty and strongly basophilic (Fig. 37.2).

Bizarre cellular changes have been associated with condyloma acuminata with rounded nuclear inclusions and poorly defined cytoplasm. Ciliocytophthoria, as found in sputum with respiratory viral infection (*e.g.,* parainfluenza virus), is at times present in gynecological smears (Fig. 37.3) with varying degrees of inflammation.

Bacterial Infections

The pattern of most acute infections, such as from neisseria, streptococcus, staphylococcus, haemophilus, and pleuropneumonia, is that of exudation of neutrophiles and serum.

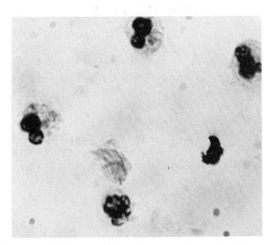

37.3. Ciliocytophthoria in a Fast smear. A ciliary tuft lies just below the middle portion of the figure. It is derived from a ciliated, columnar endocervical cell (Plate 37.1A) and consists of a small bit of cytoplasm from the luminal end of the cell with intact cilia attached, whose rootlets appear as a dotted terminal plate. The cell has pinched off this tuft, leaving behind the nucleus and balance of the cytoplasm. Note the neutrophils for size. (Papanicolaou stain, ×1200.)

Blood is not infrequent in acute infections. There is a marked cellular destruction and obscuring of both cytohormonal pattern and any previously existing evidence of cancer. These acute infections are usually vaginal, whereas the subacute and chronic infections reside in the paraurethral glands, the vulvovaginal glands, and, especially, the endocervical canal and associated glands.

Chronic infections involving the endocervix, including tuberculosis, are usually associated with various stages of epithelial metaplasia and varying degrees of atypia. The latter sheds cells of the dyskaryotic series (Fig. 37.9) corresponding to the degree of atypia or dysplasia present in the epithelium.

The finding of intracellular, biscuit-shaped diplococci within the cytoplasm of neutrophiles, should lead to culture for gonococcus identification. Likewise, multiple small bacteria crowded on the surface of a squame, the "clew cell", should alert one for hemophilus vaginalis.

Doederlein's bacillus, usually a lactobacillus, is associated with health rather than disease. It metabolizes glycogen, resulting in an acid pH which inhibits the growth of most of the vaginal pathogens. When the vaginal epithelial cells are rich in glycogen, as in progesterone opposed by estrogen during the luteal phase or pregnancy, these organisms cause cytolysis with resultant bare nuclei. This "hormonal cytolysis" is thus far different than the "inflammatory cytolysis" from heavy inflammation and necrosis.

Although bacteria can be roughly morphologically classified in a Papanicolaou stained cellular spread, the proper method for accurate identification is culture and Gram's stain in a laboratory of diagnostic microbiology.

Mycotic Infection

Candida albicans is the usual etiological agent of mycotic vulvovaginitis. Its most rapid diagnosis in the hands of a clinician is afforded by a 1.0% NaOH crush preparation of a "cotton patch" between a microscopic slide and a cover glass.

Its discovery in routine vaginal smears prepared for cancer detection is often fortuitous or is laborious and unpredictable. When found it is tentatively identifiable if it consists of both forms: "long" and "round" bodies. The former are septate pseudohyphae (Fig. 37.4), whereas the latter are round, elongate or budding yeast forms. Frequently, only one form is present.

Although acridine orange has proven disappointingly unreliable for cancer detection and diagnosis, it provides an excellent method for rapid detection of fungi, bacteria, and protozoa. When viewed with proper filters in low visible or high ultraviolet light, a few scattered bodies stand out brilliantly under low power (Fig. 37.4). It is usually not associated with the more serious infections (*i.e.*, gonococcus, herpes) or epithelial lesions (*i.e.*, dysplasia, cancer) as are trichomonas or leptothrix.

Other fungi of both the superficial mycoses (dermatophytes) and deep systemic mycoses (actinomycoses, coccidioides, aspergillus, blastomyces) rarely occur in the routine smear. When they are present, however, they usually can be tentatively classified morphologically.

Positive identification of all fungi

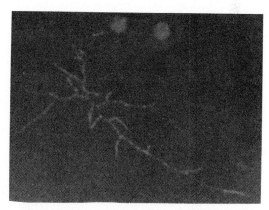

37.4. *Candida albicans.* The red fluorescing long pseudohyphae and yeast buds show brilliantly against the black background, giving a rapid identification under low power. Note the larger nuclei of the patient's two cells (at top), which fluoresce yellow-green. Acridine orange stain with ultraviolet light (×480).

should be made by cultural characteristics. Many contaminating pollens and plant cells closely mimic mycotic morphology. During pregnancy, mycotic infection frequently becomes more severe.

Protozoal Infections

Trichomonas vaginalis can produce a true infection involving the tissues and host response of some women, whereas in others it appears to be merely a superficial symbiote without apparent inflammation.

It is transmitted by sexual contact and has been actively pursued for years as a venereal disease in many areas of the world (*i.e.,* Eastern Europe, Western USSR). It bears a close association with cervical cancer and severe atypias.

The *pathogenicity* varies from strain to strain of the organism. It varies between different hosts (patients), and it varies in a given individual according to her specific state of reaction or of resistance. Its pathogenicity can be more severe when the patient is pregnant or during her late secretory and menstrual phase. The organism has a very narrow pH tolerance and is more florid in the vagina when the vaginal pH is around six. It can be found in virtually any *vaginal* pH, however, for when the pH of the vagina changes or other factors become hostile to the organism, it retreats to the endocervix, the urethra, and the glands. Host factors undoubtedly play a great part in varying degrees of tissue involvement and damage encountered, but the pathogenicity of the organism itself differs greatly among strains.

Its *clinical manifestations* are found in two major phases. The *florid* phase is primarily and symptomatically a vaginitis, whereas the *latent* phase is principally an asymptomatic endocervicitis or urethritis.

During the *florid* vaginitis the patient is troubled and symptomatic. In both the hanging drop and routine vaginal smear, the organisms can usually be identified readily (Fig. 37.5). Routine vaginal smears reveal an acute, obscuring infection with cellular degeneration, debris and, often, old and new blood. The multinucleated giant cell histiocyte is frequent. The trichomonads are numerous and of a fairly large size but, paradoxically, they may be extremely difficult to find and to identify positively in this fixed preparation because of degeneration.

During the *latent* phase of infection with *Trichomonas vaginalis,* in marked contrast, the patient is usually asymptomatic. Mild dysuria may accompany urethral involvement, or a slight discharge may result from a chronic endocervicitis;

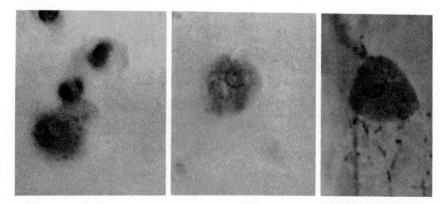

37.5. *Trichomonas vaginalis* on a routine gynecologic smear. Positive diagnostic identification is to be made *only* on well preserved organisms with all of the following critical criteria: There is a small, pale but definite nucleus which is usually eccentric; their rounded bodies take a cytoplasmic stain (neither a bare nucleus or mucus) (see Plate 37.1 *B*); and they range in size from a neutrophil up to a small parabasal cell (neutrophils in *upper part of left picture*). When a florid vaginitis is not present, they are best found in endocervical material Fast smear (single slide, vaginopancervical). Papanicolaou stain, ($\times 1,100$).

however, most of the latter latent infections go unnoticed by both patient and examining physician. A cervical smear or the routine Fast smear, as indicated in Figures 37.18, 19, will contain the organism where it can usually be identified diagnostically. In this latent phase, it can also be cultured from either endocervical or urethral material, depending upon the site of continuing infection. The hanging drop examination of vaginal material is usually negative in the latent phase, unless adequate endocervical or urethral material contaminates it or is specifically examined.

Identification of the organism should not be made lightly. It must be definite, or it should not be reported, because of therapeutic reasons and possible venereal implications. For positive identification one must be careful to rule out a bare epithelial cell nucleus, neutrophile histiocyte, or parabasal cell with a small pyknotic nucleus. Each of these can mimic a trichomonad in certain circumstances. Flagella, undulating membrane, axostyle, and specific cytoplasmic structures are rarely identified in the routine cytological smear. There are three principal morphological characteristics, however, which are present and are most important for a diagnostic identification (Fig. 37.5): a nucleus must be present, but it must be small, pale, and nonpyknotic; the rest of the organism must be definitely cytoplasmic, neither vague mucus nor a bare epithelial nucleus (Plate 37.1*B*); and the size of the organism falls between that of a neutrophile and a parabasal cell.

There is an association of *Trichomonas vaginalis* with cervical cancer and epithelial atypias, but how much of its role is saprophitic and how much pathogenic has not been completely ascertained. A few investigators have well demonstrated that *Trichomonas vaginalis* is identified significantly more frequently with the more serious epithelial lesions of the cervix. Furthermore, the trichomonal strains isolated from patients with severe dysplasias and in situ carcinomas of the cervix are more pathogenic in laboratory animals, as adjudged by the Honigberg mouse assay, than those strains isolated from women with minor atypias, simple inflammation and repair, or lack of apparent disease. Their role may be merely opportunistic, living off of serous exudate but there is increasing evidence that they may prepare and maintain epithelium in a state which is more receptive and susceptible to carcinogens.

Although there is an extremely high association of the presence of the more virulent strains of this organism with those bizarre epithelial cell changes within the endocervix which are nondegenerative in nature (*i.e.*, severe atypia, dysplasia, carcinoma), the *most* frequent cellular changes associated with trichomonas infection are merely those of degeneration, simple inflammation, and repair. A severe trichomonas infection with cellular degeneration, on the one hand, can cause diagnostic changes in *cancer* cells to be modified and rendered nondiagnostic; on the other hand, it can produce serious cytological degenerative alterations in *benign* cells, which can be sufficiently bizarre as to be confused with cancer (Fig. 37.6). In such an obscuring and necrotizing infection, cancer cells can be hidden and remain unrecognized.

The presence of alarming cells bears the same indications for intensive cytological and histological studies when trichomonads are present, as it does in the absence of the organism. If no cancer is found on apparently *adequate tissue* examination in the presence of a severe dysplasia and trichomonas infection, one must not be lulled into a false security of benignancy. By directing intensive therapy (*i.e.*, flagyl, *not* cautery), a clearer interpretation of the most severe lesion becomes possible, with identification of its malignant or benign character.

Helminthic Infestation

Pinworm and other ova can be found in the vaginal vault or picked up on a specimen from the labia. They must not be confused with some pollens or plant

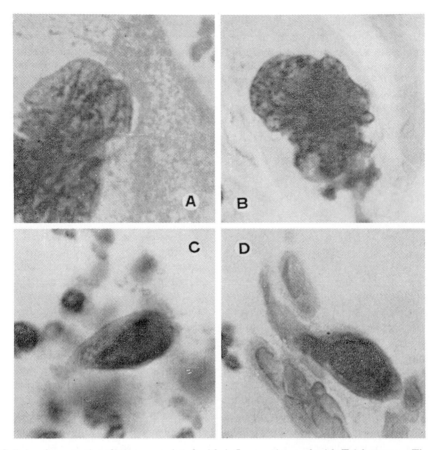

37.6. Cellular degenerative changes associated with inflammation and with Trichomonas. These changes can cause benign cells (A and C) to take on some neoplastic morphology, while causing malignant cells (B and D) to lose many diagnostic criteria. A, nuclear size increase and hyperchromasia in a benign cell with degenerative early chromatin smudging, perinuclear "halo," and abundant cytoplasm. The bizarre changes approach those of the malignant cell (in B). B, a malignant cell with degenerative chromatin smudging in its nucleus. The diagnostic value of the nuclear irregularities, abnormally cleared areas, gigantism, and hyperchromasia is greatly diminished by the loss of sharp detail from degenerative chromatin smudging. C, intense nuclear hyperchromasia from chromatin degeneration in a benign cell with scant cytoplasm. The extreme peripheral smudging and central laking of chromatin bespeak degenerative changes (compare with D). D, degenerative smudging in the nucleus of a malignant tadpole cell from squamous cell carcinoma. The malignant chromatin clumps are so smudged by degeneration that their criteria are inconclusive and are mimicked by the degenerative processes of the benign cell (in C).

cells which might contaminate and which appear morphologically similar. They are usually contaminants from the perineum, but pinworm endomyometritis does occur rarely. Schistosomes are found in the vaginal pool and cervical scrapings in cases of Bilharziasis involving the bladder, colon, uterus, or placenta. Even filaria have been reported.

Mixed and Nonspecific Infections

Most of the gynecologic infections are mixed. One agent might initiate the process of develop into the major cause of the inflammation, but many are involved in any given case. In spite of some apparently efficacious "shotgun" therapy now available, which may needlessly destroy useful symbiotic microorganisms (*i.e.,* Doederlein's bacillus), it is advantageous to identify the key etiological agents or states in order to direct specific therapy which otherwise might not be included in a general broad spectrum approach. Such is the case for Trichomonas and Candida, where effective and more specific therapy is available. Furthermore, recognition of teleatrophy of the aged or the child, so prone to mixed or nonspecific infections, allows for the production of a lush and resistent vaginal epithelium by estrogens with subsequent disappearance of infection and associated disturbing epithelial reactions. It is important also to recognize the predilection to infection in the pregnant and diabetic states so that appropriate vaginal and cervical therapy may be instituted.

RADIATION CHANGES

General Changes

Many general changes are produced by ionizing irradiation. It may cause tissue and cellular *damage* of general nature, more specific *radiation response, teleatrophy* with decreased resistance to infections, *repair,* and *atypias* or *dysplasias.*

The former, tissue *radiation damage,* ranges from mild and reversible to severe and irreversible leading to death of tissues. It evokes a general inflammatory reaction with leukocytic and fluid outpouring, reflected in the vaginal pool cellular spread as a nonspecific acute inflammation. On the other hand, tissue *radiation response* reflects the host's response peculiar to such energy and, more specifically, may herald its pattern of reaction to, and cure of, the neoplasm it harbors.

Repair and *atypias,* coupled with damage and response, may give morphological changes most difficult to differentiate from recurring neoplasm. Multiple cellular studies may be necessary with tissue biopsies of any suspicious lesions. Local estrogen therapy with broad spectrum antibiotics (*i.e.,* triple sulfa cream, tetracycline) and specific therapy (*i.e.,* Flagyl for Trichomonas) will markedly decrease the inflammation and promote healing. In this way, serial cellular studies every week or biweekly will note either healing and decrease of atypia, or unequivocal malignancy.

Cytology at times provides the only *early* evidence of recurring or newly developing cancer. Continuing *severe* postirradiation dysplasia should be viewed with alarm due to high recurrence rates, and is to be followed carefully with frequent cytologic examinations and adequate tissue studies of any suspicious lesion.

Cellular Response Patterns

Radiation Response

Striking changes occur in cells of benign and malignant tissue *following* irradiation. In therapy for carcinoma of the cervix, changes occur in the *nonmalignant* squamous cells (Fig. 37.7) which have considerable prognostic correlation. Of greatest significance are these findings when evaluated in vaginal pool material 10 to 14 days after radium application, and on the five days around the last day of external therapy. When good radiation response (RR) (over 70%) is found in patients treated for Stage II carcinoma of the cervix, approximately 80% are alive and well after 5 years. When poor RR is found in the same Stage II group of patients, about 80% are dead within 5 years. The highest degree of RR correlation with salvage is found in Stage II. First worked out well by the Grahams, many workers have corroborated these findings. It has no clinical application at the present time, however.

Sensitization Response

Prior to irradiation for cervical carcinoma, morphological changes may be discerned in normal parabasal cells which Graham named "sensitivity to radiation" (SR). She found a high correlation of this and the host response to subsequent irradiation (RR), as well as with the prognosis of host ability to overcome its tumor (survival).

Since the initial work, many investigators have repeated various studies of radiation response. Very careful and meticulous cytological observation and correlation with follow-up has clearly established certain relationships—others remain obscure. The significance of the SR in Graham's hands is high; others' results are disappointing and probably represent subjective differences in

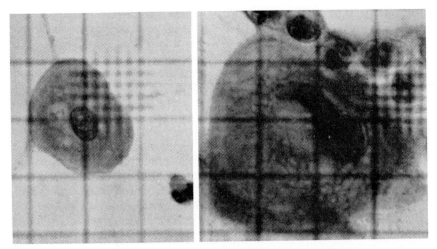

37.7. Cellular response to irradiation in carcinoma of the cervix. Many of the important features of radiation response (RR) are present in these two nonmalignant parabasal cells from a vaginal pool smear, Papanicolaou stained. *Left,* an untreated parabasal cell and neutrophil taken on first day of therapy. *Right,* parabasal cell and neutrophils following external irradiation therapy. The cytoplasm has swollen and is vacuolated. The nucleus has also swollen, is folded and distorted. The cell is *not* pale. Neutrophils have swollen (×1100).

cellular evaluation. On the other hand, results of RR when carefully done appear to be consistently corroborative.

Buccal Irradiation

Cellular changes on a buccal smear, following single dose irradiation of the buccal mucosa at the start of cervical irradiation, closely correlate with survival in carcinoma of the cervix. By using this method, some disadvantages of vaginal smears are overcome. Of perhaps greater importance, however, this clearly indicates a basic host factor complex taking place in the patients overcoming cancer with the help of irradiation. Normal epithelial cells of the buccal mucosa react in manners which herald the ability of this host to handle its carcinoma in the pelvis—a "body" away.

Endocrine-Radiation Host Response Relationships

The cytohormonal patterns, both *before* radiation therapy and during the months *following* therapy, have some correlation with patient survival. Patients with an M.I. shift to the left, with increased parabasal cell exfoliation *before* radiation therapy, have a somewhat better cellular

RR during therapy and a higher survival rate.

After radiation therapy to the cervix, the M.I. usually shifts to the left toward teleatrophy $(\overline{100/0/0})$. If this were due merely to ovarian irradiation with functional oophorectomy, the M.I. shift would be to the midzone producing estratrophy $(\overline{0/100/0})$ (see Chap. 36). That it progresses toward teleatrophy is, at least in part, due to direct radiation injury to the vaginal epithelium. It is significant to note that this pattern of teleatrophy is usually present in those patients whose tumor is conquered, whereas a persistent M.I. shift to the right is found in patients harboring residual cancer. Wachtel and others find a high correlation between this persistence of the M.I. to the right following full therapy, and tumor recurrence.

NEOPLASIAS AND RELATED LESIONS

In the detection, diagnosis, and study of the biological behavior of neoplastic lesions of the genital tract, exfoliative cytology offers many unique advantages and opportunities.

First, a properly taken cellular sample

provides surface biopsy material from a *wide* area of epithelium, rather than the restricted limits of a small excised bit of tissue. This makes possible the detection of early, small, or hidden lesions.

Second, when proper cellular material is available which is adequate, well preserved, and evaluated by qualified individuals, definitive *diagnoses* may be rendered which can be made to be as reliable as those based upon proper tissue biopsy, and frequently more comprehensive in biological information. Therapy is to be based upon tissue biopsy study of the disease whenever possible; however, to determine its exact anatomical *location* and to assure as complete evaluation as is possible concerning the *nature* and *extent* of the most serious lesion present is important.

Third, as a lesion is not altered from a cytologic specimen as it is from biopsy interference, it can be left intact to continue its normal growth during the study of exfoliated elements. In this way, biological behavior can be closely observed and followed without fear of biopsy disturbance or even removal of essential parts of the lesion. As knowledge and experience with the exfoliated elements from lesions grow, our correlation of cellular pattern with existing tissue pattern becomes definite and closer to absolute.

The Cellular Specimen

A completely *satisfactory* and *adequate* specimen is essential for highest quality clinical cytology. For study of tissue, either cytological or surgical, one must carefully choose the material as to *site,* adequacy of *amount,* and quality of *preservation.* Many techniques are available, some designed for routine cancer detection and others for specific tasks.

A cellular specimen for *routine* use should be adequate, containing material from both the vaginal pool (for endometrial lesions, ovarian lesions, and endocrine evaluation) and pancervical areas (*endo*cervical, *external os, ecto*cervical) for cervical lesions.

For routine gynecological work the Fast smear (single slide, combined vagino-pancervical) has been very satisfactory (Figs. 37.1B, 19). It provides more material for examination from the most important areas than most techniques, with less time expended by the clinician, laboratory, and pathologist. Other techniques are available for special circumstances (pp. 806–9).

Immediate fixation is necessary for the fine nuclear detail of adequate, satisfactory specimens. *Ethyl* alcohol, 95%, has been found to be most satisfactory. Certain spray and dropper fixatives are very satisfactory if applied *immediately,* so that not even slight drying begins to occur. It can be disastrous to dry *before* fixation, even for fractions of a second, as there is no satisfactory method for reconstitution without sacrificing quality. One needs all the assistance possible to extract every bit of evidence from the cells, and should not be handicapped with material degenerated by drying or improper fixation. On the other hand, *after* immediate and proper fixation, the specimens can then be air-dried for transportation without sacrifice in quality (Fig. 37–21).

Cervix Uteri

The *location* and character of the *early* neoplasms of the cervix are of extreme importance to the clinician in obtaining *both* cellular and tissue specimens for adequate examination leading to diagnosis, therapy, and cure. The junctional zone of the stratified squamous epithelium with the columnar epithelium is present *near* the external os. At times columnar epithelium presents itself on the pars vaginalis (ectropion, etc.) bringing portions of the squamocolumnar junction into view. In the presence of persistent and chronic cervicitis, areas of columnar epithelium in the endocervical canal may become tongues and islands of stratified squamous epithelium through the process of *metaplasia.* Also the squamous epithelium of the ectocervix may extend up the canal, through the process of *epidermidization.* Thus by both processes, squamocolumnar junctions may exist high up in the canal, even centimeters above the external os. Most are confined to the distal 2 cm. of the endocervical canal, but still remain hidden from even the experienced and careful examiner's view. These areas may even be hidden from careful colposcopic examination.

Early carcinomas and *severe dysplasias* are found in these important areas near the squamocolumnar junction, hidden from the clinician's view but easily accessible to proper cellular examination (Fig. 37.8).

A satisfactory cellular sample for cervical disease, therefore, must contain adequate material from this *endo*cervical area. It should contain adequate sampling from as *high* up the canal as a properly designed cervical scraper will allow (Figs. 37.16, 17). Lesions on the ectocervix, or portio vaginalis, are visible and easily available for biopsy. It is the first 1 or 2 cm. of the *endo*cervical canal *proximal* to the external os, however, which may be incompletely evaluated unless carefully examined cytologically.

Atypia, Dysplasia, Carcinoma in Situ, and Invasive Squamous Cell Carcinoma

Atypia and dysplasia include such processes as atypical, regenerative, defensive, and neoplastic epithelial reactions. Morphologically, they include such "shades-of-gray" lesions as epidermidization and squamous metaplasia with varying degrees of atypia, transitional metaplasia, atypical hyperplasia, proso-

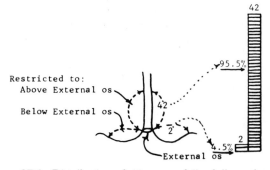

37.8. Distribution of 44 cases of "early" carcinoma of the cervix restricted to *either* above *or* below the external os, but not involving both (data from Marsh).

plasia, pseudoepitheliomatous hyperplasia, squamous cell hyperactivity, basal cell hyperactivity, reserve cell hyperplasia, subcolumnar cell hyperplasia, and subcylindrical cell anaplasia. Dysplasia is usually considered the more severe lesion, bordering on in situ carcinoma.

Although this "shades-of-gray" spectrum morphologically runs imperceptibly into carcinoma in situ, their separation must be attempted morphologically and correlated on the biological basis of reversibility *versus* irreversibility. As this is true with the histopathological study of surgically removed tissues, so it is true with the cytopathological study of cellular specimens.

One of the most valuable features which is well correlated with biological behavior in the critical zone between severe dysplasia and carcinoma in situ, is the ability for cells to *mature* in *orderly* fashion throughout *all* layers of the epithelium. Thus carcinoma in situ tissue sections have extremely scanty cytoplasm with extreme cellular crowding in all layers, loss of stratification as the cells reach the surface, and loss of polarity in the germinal layer.

In exfoliated material, this phenomenon of loss of orderly maturation is reflected in the lack of cytoplasmic maturation with extremely scant cytoplasm, high nucleocytoplasmic (N/C) ratio, and loss of squamification or columnarization in individual cells (Figs. 37.9, 10).

Cells of this *"shades-of-gray"* spectrum and of carcinoma in situ have a peculiar type of nucleus, to which Papanicolaou gave the name of dyskaryotic. Although some cells shed from an invasive squamous cell carcinoma are also of this dyskaryotic type, others have a characteristically different nucleus (Figs. 37.11, 12 and Plate 37.1 C, D) which provides some of the cellular evidence used in cytologically separating the lesions to diagnose the presence of invasive cancer.

Epithelial changes in a cervix are usually not of only one type but consist of collections of different "shades-of-gray"

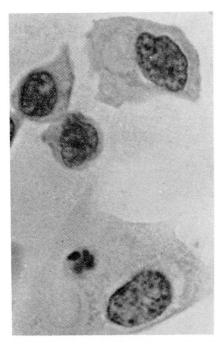

37.9. Dyskaryotic cells shed from a "shades-of-gray" lesion (severe dysplasia) of the cervix. Many malignant criteria are present in these dyskaryotic nuclei, such as coarse granularity of the chromatin, increase in nuclear size, nuclear membrane irregularities and hyperchromasia; but each whole cell does not admit to a diagnosis of malignancy. The *bottom* cell with mature squamous cytoplasm, is a mature squamous dyskaryotic cell; the cell in the *upper right* has moderately mature cytoplasm, a moderately mature dyskaryotic cell; the two cells in the *upper left* have scanty immature cytoplasm and are immature dyskaryotic cells (×1200).

a small area of in situ carcinoma can be missed while the surrounding dysplasia is diagnosed.

Likewise, if cells from dysplasia and from carcinoma in situ are present in a cellular sample, they indicate the presence of carcinoma in situ but do *not* rule out invasive cancer, which could be present yet inadequately sampled.

Experience has shown, however, that with *adequate* cellular samples there is 95% correlation of the highest lesion represented on the cell spread with the highest lesion histologically demonstrable.

Accuracy of this correlation is directly proportional to *adequacy* of cellular sample *and* interpretation, as well as ade-

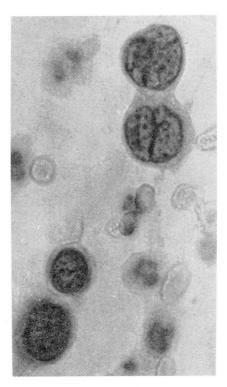

37.10. Diagnostic cells shed from a carcinoma in situ of the cervix. Essentially the same malignant criteria are present in these nuclei as are present in the "shades-of-gray" lesions (see Fig. 37.9) but they are more severe. Furthermore, the cytoplasm is completely immature with a nucleocytoplasmic ratio high enough for the whole cell to admit to a diagnosis of malignancy. Note the extremely scanty cytoplasm and nuclear hyperchromasia of the cell in the *upper right* (×1200).

lesions, at times including carcinoma in situ and, less often, invasive carcinoma. This has been well established by many workers, who have serially sectioned cervices and plotted the anatomical distribution of these lesion variants. The mixture of epithelial lesions which is present in a given cervix is directly reflected in the *adequate* cellular spread.

The presence of *only* diagnostic cells of severe dysplasia in a patient's smear does *not* rule out carcinoma, especially if the specimen is less than adequate, as exfoliated material from carcinoma in situ also contains such cells in addition to those diagnostic of in situ carcinoma. Thus, with an *in*adequate cellular sample,

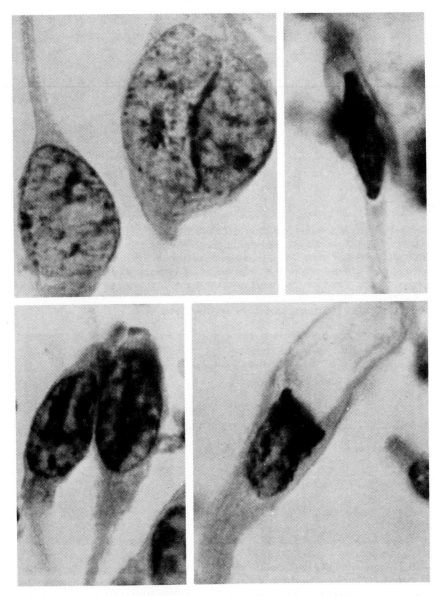

37.11. Cells shed from invasive squamous cell carcinoma. The nuclei are of bizarre shapes, have angular and distorted membranes and varying thickness of the chromatinic rim, contain huge and irregular chromatin aggregates and nucleoli, and have abnormally cleared areas of parachromatin. Nuclei in cells shown in *upper right* and *lower right* photomicrographs are becoming pyknotic. The cytoplasm is asymmetrical, with bizarre and uncontrolled squamous cell maturation of thinning and keratinization with, in the *lower right,* ectoendoplasm and beginning formation of a fibrillar apparatus of the tail extending downward (×1200).

quacy and interpretation of histologic sample. The clinical preparation of an adequate and satisfactory specimen is thus of fundamental importance (see "Clinical Preparation of Specimens", p. 806).

Adenocarcinoma of the cervix usually has a fairly characteristic cell type (Fig. 37.13), which can frequently be separated not only from cervical epidermoid carcinoma but also, at times, from adenocarcinoma of the endometrium and of the ovary. When this is possible, it can greatly aid the clinician in guiding his biopsies for tissue studies, for the lesion can lie high

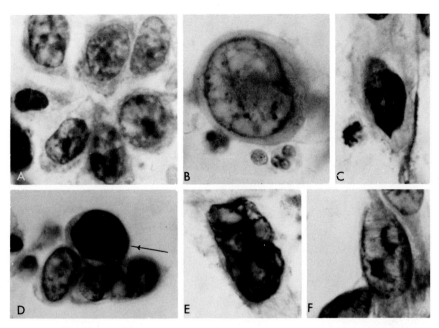

37.12. General criteria of malignancy. *A,* undifferentiated cells with scant cytoplasm and indistinct borders. There is a moderate nuclear size variation. Note irregular chromatin patterns with large cleared areas and chromatin clumps with sharp points and angles. Nuclear rims vary abruptly in thickness. *B,* nucleocytoplasmic ratio high in a large cell. Although the nuclear pattern is bland, the total chromatin is increased and there are large, abnormally cleared areas and chromatin spindles. *C,* the nuclear outline is irregular with a sharp, pointed angle protruding. *D,* prominent chromatin clumping with abnormally cleared areas; sharp, angled nucleolus to the right of the largest nucleus; very scant cytoplasm with poor borders and resultant crowding. *E,* marked hyperchromasia with chromatin clumping and sharply delineated parachromatin. Two nucleoli are large and prominent, indicating protein production. They are perfectly round, however, and offer no diagnostic assistance. *F,* well preserved sharp, pointed nucleoli and chromatin clumps with abnormal clearing. Marked cytoplasmic attenuation over nuclear sides (×700).

up in the canal rather than nearer the external os as does the more usual squamous cervial carcinoma.

Cytological pick-up of the early, curable endocervical adenocarcinomas is good, especially with adequately *high* endocervical specimens. Mixed or mucoepidermoid carcinomas enjoy the same high degree of cellular detection.

Pregnancy is an extremely critical time for the detection and diagnosis of the early, curable neoplasms of the cervix. A pregnancy visit is the only time many women see a physician, until later when lesions become advanced and symptomatic.

The optimum time to obtain a cytological specimen is the *earliest* in the pregnancy. Cervical infections increase as pregnancy progresses, with resulting ob-

scuring and degeneration of cellular samples. An early cellular examination obviates much of this cellular distortion. It also gives more opportunity to clear inflammation, if necessary to arrive at a diagnosis, or to carry out any therapeutic or diagnostic procedures indicated.

Even though pregnant patients as a group are of a young age, they have an appreciable incidence of cervical carcinoma which is higher, age for age, than nonpregnant women. Spjut *et al.* found 7 carcinomas in situ among 3,000 pregnant women, 2.3 per 1,000. Schmitz, Isaacs, and Fetherston found 12 invasive and 13 in situ carcinomas among 10,369 obstetrical patients, 2.4 per 1,000.

Among 2,828 consecutive private and clinic patients at The Johns Hopkins Hospital, 10 were found by a routine Fast

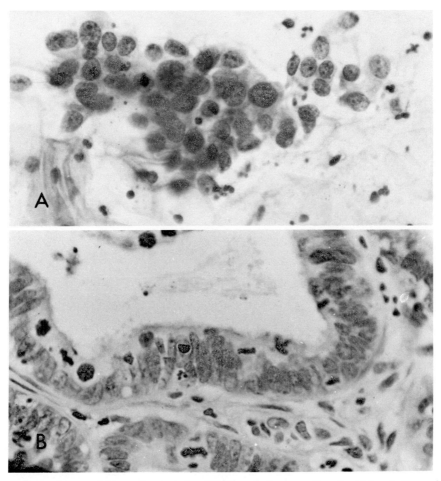

37.13. Adenocarcinoma of the cervix uteri. Age 35. These lesions usually arise higher in the endocervical canal than do the squamous cell carcinomas of the cervix and, many times, lie near the internal os. This makes both cellular and tissue sampling of the endocervical canal mandatory.

A. Fast smear. There is a large pointed nucleolus near mid-field, marked variation in the numbers of nucleoli throughout this tissue fragment, and other malignant criteria. Note the great similarity between these cancer cells and the normal endocervical cells in Plate 37.1*A, i.e.,* vesicular nuclei, abundant columnar-shaped cytoplasm, a distinct epithelial luminal border of the cells near mid-field. (Papanicolaou stain, ×480.)

B. Tissue biopsy of the same lesion. Note numerous mitoses and loss of orientation. Many cellular features (*i.e.,* prominent epithelial luminal border, vesicular nuclei) resemble those in the illustration above. (H & E, ×480.)

smear to have carcinoma of the cervix, 3.5 per 1,000. On tissue examination, 6 of these were in situ, 2 were in situ with questionable invasion, and 2 were frankly invasive. In another patient outside of this consecutive series, invasive squamous carcinoma of the cervix was cytologically detected in a 16-year-old pregnant girl with one previous child who, in spite of prompt and full therapy, died 2 years later of recurrent disease.

Dysplasias in pregnancy are basically no different from those in the non-pregnant patient. They do tend, however, to progress in *degree* of atypicality during pregnancy and then regress in the post-partum months. This regression usually is not complete and with each subsequent pregnancy the cervical dysplasia may begin at a more atypical level.

There appears to be *no* innocuous atypical cellular change which is specific for, characteristic of, or caused by pregnancy. In the presence of an atypia, a careful cytological and histological evaluation to determine the exact nature of the most severe epithelial lesions present is as indicated in pregnant patients as it is in the nonpregnant. Present knowledge of these sinister lesions is far too meager for dogmatism.

Other cellular atypias resembling those shed from dysplasia are encountered. At times they are associated with severe *folic acid* deficiency in pregnancy. They are reversible with proper therapy. Similar epithelial atypias of varying degrees of severity occur with the use of some anticancer *chemotherapeutic* agents (*i.e.,* busulfan, methotrexate) and *immunosuppressive* drugs (*i.e.,* immuran).

Recurrence of Carcinoma after Therapy

Following therapy for carcinoma of the cervix, recurrences *within* the lumen of the genital tract are cytologically detected to a high degree, provided sufficient and proper cellular specimens are examined. This is frequently accomplished before gross evidence of recurrence is present. Extraluminal recurrences are, of course, not detected vaginally.

Usually the recurrences are of the original histological variety. Frequently, however, they can recur as an extremely small and undifferentiated type (small celled non-keratinized) which may be difficult to distinguish from reactive histiocytes and are easily missed in rapid or careless screening.

Occasionally an invasive carcinoma recurs as an in situ lesion. The question of a recurrence *versus* a second primary thus arises. Because of persisting radiation cellular changes and atypias (see p. 789), interpretation of postradiation specimens may be most difficult and the unwary may overcall reaction or healing. On the other hand, however, undercalling may

occur when the small undifferentiated carcinoma cells are missed or are mistaken for histiocytes. This small celled non-keratinizing carcinoma is a very frequent cell type, unfortunatedly, in recurring or residual carcinoma.

Carefully done cytopathology can, and frequently does, provide the first real evidence of recurrence and serves to guide localization biopsies and therapy.

Vulva and Vagina

Vaginal and labial dermatoses, dysplasias, carcinoma in situ, and invasive carcinoma are usually easily detected clinically, and diagnosed by biopsy of suspicious areas. At times, the lesion is diffuse, obscured, or, for some other reasons, not clinically obvious. Depending upon the site of the lesion, either a vaginal pool smear or a direct scraping yields valuable cytological diagnosis.

Squamous cell carcinoma and its preceding lesions are the most frequently encountered (see p. 792). A direct scraping of a leukoplakic or condylomatous lesion may be necessary to insure cellular representation of the entire lesion. Such a specimen, taken in conjunction with tissue examination of the lesion, augments and tends to compensate for the patchy nature of biopsies. In lesions of the labia and in dry or keratotic lesions of the vagina, physiological saline should be used to moisten growing margins of the lesion before scraping, and to remove keratotic and necrotic debris. A cotton swab dipped in egg albumen or serum, or a wooden or plastic spatula, are good instruments for preparing these specimens. The use of frosted slides increases cell adherence, especially following saline moistening of the lesion.

Adenosis vaginae and *adenocarcinoma* of the vagina have increased in frequency, particularly among those in their early twenties. This latter incidence is due mainly to diethylstilbesterol therapy while in utero. The lesion is frequently "hobnailed" in morphology, resembling mesonephroma (Fig. 37.14). These

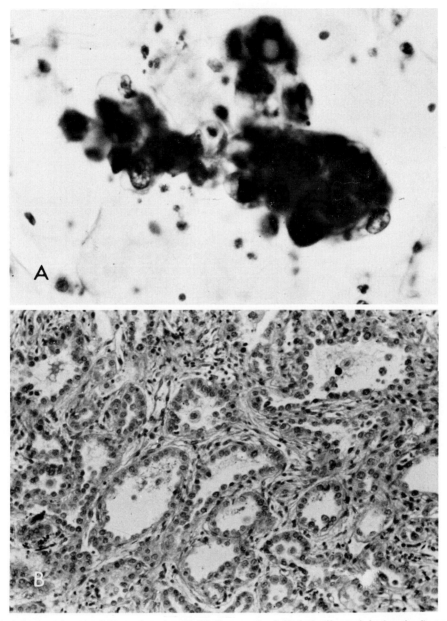

37.14. Adenocarcinoma of the vagina. Age 20. Mother received diethylstilbestrol during the first trimester of the pregnancy.

A. Fast smear with vaginal cell scraping. Note the youthful cytohormonal pattern. There is a hob-nail pattern of the cells as they pouch out from the edges of the tissue fragment. (Papanicolaou stain, ×480.)

B. Tissue biopsy of the same lesion. There is a mesonephric pattern to this adenocarcinoma with pouching-out into the lumen in hob-nail fashion, resembling that of the cell spread in the illustration above. (H & E, ×120.)

cellular features in the presence of a youthful cytohormonal pattern are distinctive. Cellular samples will be negative if the lesion does not involve the vaginal surface or if the clinician does not scrape adequately.

Endometrium

Cancer cells (Fig. 37.15) are recognized in vaginal pool material in about 75% of endometrial adenocarcinomas. An additional 15 to 20% of the patients shed abnormal cells resembling *atypical* histiocytes, endometrial cells, endocervical cells, or even dyskaryotic cells from cervical dysplasia. Furthermore, if postmenopausal, the abnormal presence of even *typical* endometrial cells, or an abnormal cytohormonal pattern with an unexplained estrogenic effect (M.I. to the

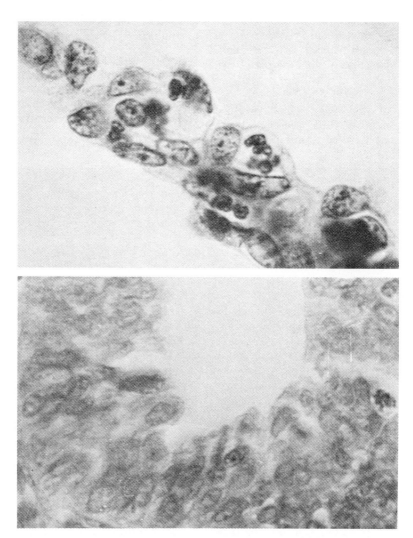

37.15. Adenocarcinoma of the endometrium, in an 80-year-old patient. The cytohormonal pattern was distinctly abnormal with a maturation index of $\overrightarrow{0/77}/\overleftarrow{23}$ shifted toward the right. *Upper,* cells present on a Fast smear. Nuclear malignant criteria marked. Hyperdistended secretory vacuoles contain neutrophils which are phagocytosing the mucus in the otherwise intact secretory cells. *Lower,* tissue obtained at dilatation and curettage of the same patient. This malignant gland is lined by cells having many malignant criteria. The whole cells are not available, as in the cellular spread, so that malignant criteria are less pronounced. Note mitosis on *right* and hyperdistended secretory cell at lumen on *left* (×1200).

right) may be the only finding present to lead to an early diagnosis of endometrial adenocarcinoma.

Atypical hyperplasia and adenocarcinoma are not usually associated with teleatrophy, even in the very aged. At times the associated *cytohormonal pattern* is bizarre enough for the M.I. to fall to the right of normal limits. Women over 60 or 65 usually shed under 10% superficial cells. When over 10% are present in the *absence* of significant *inflammation* and after carefully ruling out exogenous *estrogens* (*i.e.,* therapy, face creams, geriatric vitamin preparations) one must carefully consider endometrial hyperplasia, endometrial adenocarcinoma, and ovarian neoplasms, both primary and metastatic to the ovary.

The finding of *endometrial cells* at a time in the cycle *other* than during menses is abnormal. Degenerated endometrial cells may be found 3 or 4 days after bleeding stops. In the luteal phase, however, their presence is distinctly abnormal. It is not possible to set a definite day after which it is abnormal to find endometrial type cells, but after the 10th day of the cycle one becomes concerned over their presence, especially with a patient in her forties.

The cytological distinction between these degenerating endometrial cells shed at the end of menses, poorly preserved cells from endometrial hyperplasia, and degenerating adenocarcinoma can be very difficult at times. This may reflect a poor state of preservation resulting from long travel down the canal, a difficult histological differentiation in the given case, or both.

The term *"endometrial-type cell"* is used to connote this group of cells (including: atypical endocervical, atypical endometrial, bizarre histiocytes, and some types of dyskaryotic cells) whose exact identity is not obvious, but one cannot definitely rule out endometrial disease. When found in the cell spread, further identification and studies are necessary to rule out endometrial adenocarcinoma.

Bleeding is a frequent occurrence with endometrial lesions, benign as well as malignant. It is important, thus, that cellular specimens be taken at any time the patient is seen, menstruating or not; however, as a bloody smear may be less than satisfactory and may have to be repeated later, the patient should be alerted for the possible necessity of repeating the specimen to allay anxiety if that should become necessary. To take a smear when bleeding is present is well worth the possibility of an occasional unsatisfactory specimen. Many times the bloody smear is the only one to contain diagnostic cells.

Cervical scrapings yield a *poor* detection of endometrial carcinoma, as opposed to cervical carcinoma. Vaginal pool specimens and endocervical aspirations are better for endometrial carcinoma, whereas endometrial cavity specimens (*i.e.,* aspiration, lavage, brush jet) are optimal but not usually employed routinely.

As a routine procedure in the study of *endometrial* disease, *vaginal pool* material is best suited either as a separate smear or in the combined Fast smear, due to its cellular contents, cytohormonal evaluation, and clinical simplicity.

Endometrial specimens obtained *directly* from the endometrial cavity (*i.e.,* aspiration, brush, irrigation jet) yield superb cellular samples. They are sufficiently more difficult and time-consuming that they do not lend themselves well as a *routine* screening procedure of all asymptomatic women. Furthermore, they should *never* replace a dilatation and curettage, when that procedure is indicated. They are very valuable in detecting over 97% of endometrial carcinomas and in adding information and understanding of other diseases. They should be in everyone's armamentarium. Before their use, of course, intrauterine pregnancy must be excluded.

For a *routine* examination specimen, a well prepared Fast combined vagino-cervical smear is thus well suited (Figs. 37.18, 19). It contains not only a cellular scraping of the endocervical canal and external os for *cervical* disease, but also a vaginal pool sample for *cytohormonal* evalulation and for *endometrial* and *ovarian* disease. Both components, the *vaginal pool* and the *pancervical scraping,* must be adequate.

Placenta

Trophoblast cells can be present in vaginal pool specimens, especially during the first trimester. Their presence may indicate a low lying placenta or a threatened abortion, but they are also present in some pregnancies which continue as apparently perfectly normal.

They have been found with hydatidiform moles. Cytology, however, has been of very little assistance in predicting the grade of mole or the presence of a choriocarcinoma because of the paucity or unpredictability of the cells in the lumen. When present, however, they can be diagnostic of the cancer, yielding both malignant syncytiotrophoblast and cytotrophoblast.

Multinucleated cells from herpes simplex (Fig. 37.2) are easily mistaken by the unwary for syncytiotrophoblast. Decidual cells are at times shed, and are to be distinguished from dyskaryotic cells shed from cervical atypias.

Miscellaneous Uterine Lesions

At times, myomas and endometriosis are associated with a peculiar cytohormonal pattern, with the M.I. shifted to the right for the age and clinical history. Most of the cases, however, fall within normal limits.

Leiomyosarcomas, mixed mesodermal sarcomas, and carcinosarcomas may shed diagnostic cells into the vaginal pool. Usually there is quite a bit of necrosis with cellular breakdown, so that cytological pick-up of sarcomas is discouraging unless the cervix or vault is involved to allow a surface scraping to yield intact cells.

Sarcomas usually shed pleomorphic cells which are undifferentiated and have prominent nucleoli. On occasion the exfoliated cells do manifest differentiating characteristics such as fat, myofibrils, cross striations, etc., sufficient to suspect, or even diagnose, tumor-type.

The finding of a *biphasic* cellular pattern with both sarcomal cells and adenocarcinoma cells, should make one consider a mixed mesodermal tumor or a carcinosarcoma.

Fallopian Tubes

At times, adenocarcinoma of the oviducts will shed diagnostic cells into the endometrial cavity and into the vaginal pool. It is usually associated with a watery or bloody discharge cytologically or even clinically. The vaginal cytohormonal pattern may show an abnormal M.I. shift to the right.

Unexplained adenocarcinoma cells or an abnormal cytohormonal pattern in a *vaginal* specimen should provoke consideration of a lesion of the Fallopian tube, even though its occurrence is rare. Cells from it may present in endometrial cavity samples.

Ovaries

Tumors of the ovary may be considered in three categories, the primary neoplasms which produce their own hormones (*i.e.,* granulosa cell tumors), those which do not (*i.e.,* adenocarcinoma), and secondary cancers metastatic to the ovary (*i.e.,* Krukenberg tumors).

The *hormone producing* tumors express their presence by a cytohormonal pattern characteristic for the endocrine substances being secreted. Granulosa cell tumors shift the M.I. to the right (toward $\overrightarrow{0/0/100}$), the degree of shift depending upon the amount of circulating estrogens, biologic activity of these estrogens, and the age of the patient. Luteinized mesenchymal tumors shift the M.I. toward the midzone (toward $\overline{0/100/0}$) if progesterone alone is being produced, or give a mixed pattern resembling pregnancy, if estrogens are also secreted. Hilar cell tumors and arrhenoblastomas may show the effect of androgen, such as its M.I. "spread" pattern (toward $\overleftrightarrow{33/34/33}$) or its shift to the left (toward $\overleftarrow{100/0/0}$).

These hormone-producing tumors of

the ovary do *not* shed diagnostic cells into the vaginal pool, the abnormal cytohormonal pattern being all that is present. Abnormal columnar cells, however, frequently do appear in the vaginal specimen, shed from the endometrial hyperplasia which is often associated with the abnormal endocrine milieu, and may be noted as atypical or "endometrial-type cells."

Tumors *without known hormone* production involving the ovary, paradoxically, are also frequently found in an abnormal cytohormonal M.I. shift to the right, but to a lesser degree. These not only include the solid and cystic adenomas and adenocarcinomas, but benign lesions (*i.e.,* Brenner) and tumors metastatic to the ovary. There is evidence that the ovarian stroma is stimulated into increased steroid production by the presence of such lesions (Chapt. 24).

Furthermore, individuals differ in their sensitivity to estrogens. When the tissues of Müllerian origin have increased sensitivity to estrogens, an otherwise normal endocrine milieu can produce an abnormal response of these structures. This can result in a shift to the right of the M.I. and hyperplastic lesions of the endometrium, tubes, and ovaries.

In about one-half of the patients with ovarian tumors, the M.I. is sufficiently shifted to the right to fall outside of normal.

Cells exfoliate from these tumors into the peritoneal cavity. Here they can be detected "early" by culdocentesis, or travel down the tubes to appear in the vaginal pool. The serous cystadenocarcinomas may shed psammoma bodies with their cellular tissue fragments (Fig. 37.16). They frequently have "pouched-out" secretory vacuoles and at times have single, prominent, cherry-red nucleoli with perinucleolar clearing, or "Howdon" halos.

Characteristically, ovarian tumors are found with a "clean" background to the vaginal spread. These patterns may serve to indicate an ovarian origin in the presence of a negative D. & C.

About one-third of the patients with ovarian cancer shed recognizably ab-

normal cells into the vaginal pool specimen, while an additional third of the postmenopausal patients have an abnormal M.I. only. By observing *both* abnormal cells and abnormal cytohormonal pattern, over 60% of the ovarian lesions are detectable in this age group by using specimens with vaginal pool component.

ABNORMAL PATTERNS ASSOCIATED WITH MALIGNANCIES

Cytohormonal Patterns

An abnormal *cytohormonal pattern* should arouse suspicion of neoplasm, even in the absence of cells exfoliated from a tumor surface. One must be alerted for adrenal, hypophysial, and mammary tumors (see Chap. 36), in addition to the ovarian, tubal, and endometrial lesions just noted above.

Serous, Bloody, Degenerating, and Obscuring Patterns

These nonspecific patterns frequently accompany neoplasms without diagnostic cells being present. Paradoxically, some of the largest and most invasive tumors present themselves in this fashion, with necrotic cellular debris and serosanguineous fluid the only material from the lesion.

These patterns are *serious warnings* which mandate repeat cellular examinations, attempts to clear the condition sufficiently to identify cellular elements, and/or adequate biopsy or dilatation and curettage, depending upon the nature of the case.

Microscopic Aspects

Because of limited space and the clinical nature of this text, more detailed diagnostic microscopic aspects will not be dealt with here but can be found elsewhere (see references: Frost, Graham, Koss, Patton, Reagan).

CLINICAL PREPARATION OF SPECIMENS

When to Take Specimens for Routine Detection and Diagnosis

A gynecological specimen may be obtained at virtually *any* time, as long as it

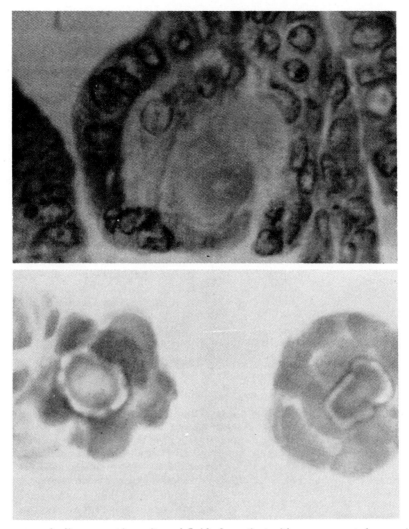

37.16. Psammoma bodies present in peritoneal fluid of a patient with a serous cystadenocarcinoma of the ovary. *Upper,* a papillary frond in tissue section with one psammoma body. *Lower,* two psammoma bodies and associated cellular groups which exfoliated into the peritoneal cavity. The peritoneal fluid was extremely bloody and, as this was the first paracentesis, the cells had sat in this degenerating fluid for a period of time sufficient to lose their fine nuclear detail. Their general nuclear outline is evident enough, however, to demonstrate severe molding and size variation (×1200).

is properly taken. It should be obtained when the opportunity arises and repeated if indicated, rather than being postponed for minor reasons (ie: bleeding, douching).

If there is any doubt whether a satisfactory specimen will result, the smear should be taken and a repeat, with proper preparation, arranged for.

Thus, sampling during active menstrual flow does yield a higher percentage of unsatisfactory specimens; however, menses or apparent menses may be the *only* time

that cancer cells are shed. In such situations, therefore, one should take a specimen with full understanding that it may have to be repeated, inform the patient of that possibility, and arrange with her for a repeat cellular examination later, at the proper time in the month.

Bleeding is thus *not* a contraindication, although sometimes a repeat cellular sample may be necessary for a satisfactory examination. Harsh scraping to produce excessive hemorrhage or trauma to the tissues is to be avoided. Bleeding, however, rather than being a contraindication to cell examination, is itself a strong indication for the consultation.

Douching also is *not* a contraindication. Whereas for certain things it is preferable that the patient refrain from douching for about 24 hours, cell spreads should be prepared even if it is determined that she had just douched. Remarks should be made on the consultation request to that effect, and the patient should be advised that another specimen should be obtained after an interval of 24 hours without a douche. Very little change is usually made in the endocervical scraping specimen, but the vaginal pool is frequently useless for cytohormonal evaluation, endometrial lesions, and ovarian disease in a postdouche specimen.

Pregnancy

The best time for a cell examination of a pregnant patient is the *first visit* of her pregnancy. It should include a *high* endocervical scraping component, unless specifically contraindicated by an obstetrical difficulty, as many early lesions of pregnancy lie within the canal.

The cervix everts and cervical infections tend to increase in severity as the pregnancy progresses, causing increased difficulty of interpretation and obscuring of diagnostic material. Furthermore, examination *early* in pregnancy will allow adequate time to clear any confusing conditions, determine underlying lesions, and institute proper therapy.

After delivery, cervical lacerations and infections take many weeks or even months to heal sufficiently to provide a satisfactory cellular examination of cervical lesions. At the 6-week visit a repeat cellular examination should be performed, especially if any atypia was noted during the pregnancy. Biopsies or conization should be contemplated at that visit, depending upon the degree of severity of the atypia.

Frequency of Repeat Examination

After completely negative cellular examinations, the frequency with which routine cytopathology consultation should be requested must be individualized. The interval to be considered for any one *asymptomatic* patient following *negative* (repeated twice) cellular examination and with a history devoid of abnormalities, usually falls between six months and two years. The chosen interval mainly depends upon age, but also upon various other factors such as parity, previous or present disease, dependability of revisit, etc. The availability of cytopathological consultation should *not* have to be a factor for the clinician to consider at this time.

Biopsy, Conization, Dilatation, and Curettage

Cytopathology and histopathology are complementary, not competitive. Thus, tissue confirmation of cytological findings should be sought at *all* times for determination of extent, degree of invasiveness, and localization of the lesion.

As the early endocervical lesions (dysplasias and in situ) are extremely friable and easily rub off on even gentle manipulation, endocervical biopsies or conization should be obtained *before* any instrumentation or dilatation of the canal. The vaginal epithelium and the pars vaginalis of the cervix should be well cleansed, but the external os and the endocervical canal should *not* be touched by anything for cleansing (Fig. 37.17), for dilatation, or for curettage before obtaining the cervical biopsy.

Obtain cellular specimens *before* D. & C. Minimal clean-up and trauma of any kind to the cervix must be the rule in obtaining cytological and pathological specimens.

Technique for Proper Cellular Specimen

So many methods have been devised and advocated for preparation of specimens for cellular examination that it may at first seem unnecessarily complicated to the clinician. A few simple guidelines only, however, need to be understood.

Before deciding upon the form of gynecological cell specimen to prepare, one must first have clearly in mind what type of information he wishes to obtain. Then

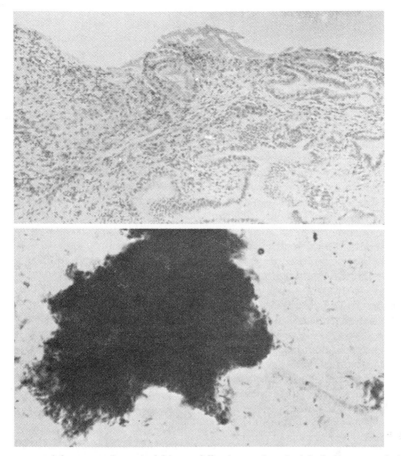

37.17. *Upper, unsatisfactory* endocervical biopsy following antiseptic (alcohol) cotton pledget "gently" placed in canal to reduce bacterial contamination before procedure. Lumen, *above*; stroma, *below.* The lumenal epithelium, for which the biopsy was obtained, is entirely missing; the endocervical glands and stroma, only, are intact. *Lower,* same patient; the cotton pledget was rinsed in saline, which was then passed through a Millipore-SM cellulose membrane filter. A large sheet of markedly atypical epithelium (marked dysplasia), and numerous endocervical cells are present, which should have been intact on the biopsy (*upper*), for a satisfactory histopathologic epithelial diagnosis (×30).

the best technique for that information should be performed to obtain the best specimen.

Routine and Specific Information

The *ideal* procedure should encompass all realms of desired information adequately, and yet be sufficiently simple and straitforward to be used in a general gynecological examination for *routine* all-inclusive gynecological cellular examination. A few combined techniques best perform this.

The *Fast smear* (Figs. 37.18, 19) obtains two specimens: one the vaginal pool material and the other *pan*cervical (endo-cervical, ectocervical, and external os) scraping material. These are then mixed *on* the slide and one cellular spread is made therefrom.

It helps to keep the *upper* portion of the cell spread along the edge of the slide away from the endocervical mixture for mainly *vaginal pool* material to provide an accurate hormonal evaluation, adjudgment of radiation response, determination of sex, detection of endometrial hyperplasia and cancer (90%), and detection of salpingeal and ovarian lesions (60%). In this way, the lower portion of the cell spread contains a rich endocervical component. This is better preserved from drying on spreading by the vaginal pool mucus than it is in separate cervical smear spreads, and yields a high detection of carcinoma of the cervix (97%) and associated lesions.

Special Indications

A few techniques have proved themselves to be of outstanding value in well chosen instances: cervical neoplasia (endocervical scraping, swab, aspiration), endometrial neoplasia (vaginal pool; endometrial aspiration, irrigation, brush jet wash), salpingeal and ovarian neoplasia (vaginal pool, culdocentesis), localization of inflammatory site and determination of etiological agents (V-C-E, differential direct swabs), endocrine evaluation (vaginal pool, lateral vaginal wall), daily cytohormonal evaluation and determination of ovulation (serial vaginal pool aspirations by patient), evaluation of tissue capacity for response to irradiation (vaginal pool, buccal scraping), determination of chromosomal sex (vaginal pool, buccal scraping), population surveys (irrigation smear). They are described here more in detail.

Clinical Techniques

Fixation

Immediate wet-fixation gives highest diagnostic accuracy. The best and simplest fixative is 95% ethyl alcohol in a wide-mouth jar. The specimen is *rapidly* and *uniformly* spread onto a slide and *immediately* immersed into the fixative. Alcohols other than ethyl (*e.g.,* methyl, iso-

propyl) are to be avoided due to their tinctorial artifacts and morphological distortions, at times obliterating valuable diagnostic nuclear detail.

Air drying *before* fixation is far inferior, and *not* to be used. There is *no* technique available to rehydrate back to the original form, regardless of numerous methods reported to do so. Air drying *after* adequate immediate fixation, however, is entirely satisfactory (Fig. 37.21).

Some commercial spray and dropper fixatives are satisfactory, if *immediately* applied by a waiting assistant. A fraction of a second of drying may ruin the diagnostic material.

Fast Smear (Routine Single Slide Combined Vaginal Pool-Pancervical)

The simple procedure to obtain this specimen, shown in Figures 37.18, 19, is as follows:

(*A*) Obtain mucus from posterior vaginal pool with spatula.

(*B*) Place upon slide as a thick drop. Do *not* smear.

(*C*) Scrape *high* up endocervical canal, 360° around, with cervical end of spatula.

(*D*) Mix on the slide all of endocervical scraping with *lower* portion of vaginal pool mucus drop. Do *not* smear with cervical end of spatula (uneven, inferior cell spreads result).

(*E*) Holding *over open* bottle of fixative (or with spray can or dropper bottle of fixative *poised*), smear drop with (Fig. 37.18) two lengthwise *light* strokes of gloved fifth finger or (Fig. 37.19) one

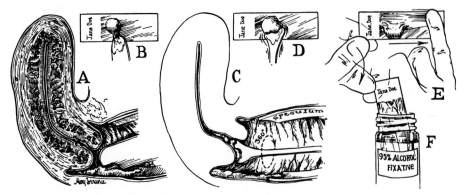

37.18. Fast smear routine, using *wooden* spatula

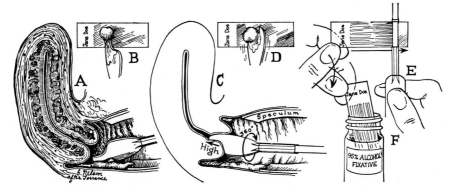

37.19. Fast smear routine, using *plastic* spatula with *cell spreader* (see text)

stroke of cell spreader, holding spatula handle parallel to the glass slide.

(*F*) *Immediately* drop slide into fixative (or spray or drop fixatives onto slide). Fix slides from only *one* patient per bottle to keep from having cross contamination of cells between patients.

Vaginal Pool Smear

Follow steps *A, B, E,* and *F* in Figures 37.18 or 19. A glass pipette and aspirating bulb is excellent to obtain posterior pool mucus (*A*) with or with*out* a speculum for the simple vaginal pool specimen.

Lateral Vaginal Wall Specimen (Cytohormonal Evaluation Only)

With the use of a spatula or saline-moistened cotton swab, the midportion of the lateral vaginal wall (slightly distal to the tip of the cervix) is gently scraped. The material so removed is spread rapidly onto a glass slide which is held *over* an *open* bottle of 95% ethyl alcohol and *immediately* dropped into the fixative.

Spray or dropper commercial fixatives can be used if they are held (by an assistant) *poised* over the slide and *immediately* applied for preservation of nuclear detail. Immediate fixation is critical to accurate cytohormonal evaluation to assess karyopyknosis.

Serial Vaginal Pool Smears (Complete Cytohormonal Evaluation)

Daily or frequent smears made by the *patient* herself provide the most complete cytohormonal evaluation. The glass or plastic pipette method of vaginal pool aspiration is preferred, simplest for the patient to use on herself, and least expensive.

The bulb is slightly expressed, the pipette is introduced to the posterior fornix, the bulb is released and rotated about 30° back and forth to obtain secretions. The bulb is again gently pressed to equalize pressure (so vacuum will not blow material against pipette wall upon withdrawal), pipette is withdrawn, material blown onto slide, smeared with pipette, and fixed in ethyl alcohol. The previous day's smear is removed, air dried, and placed in a slide box until all are returned at the patient's next office visit.

The number and date of the slide are recorded by the patient (*e.g.,* on her basal body temperature chart) with menstrual data. In the same fashion, serial vaginal irrigation smears can be obtained by the patient. A separate pipette is provided for each day and all are returned by the patient at her next office visit with their accompanying record.

Pediatric Gynecologic Smear

In the *child,* a small, thin nonabsorbent cotton swab is used. It is first soaked in saline and expressed against the bottle neck. It must *not* touch the examiner's *or* patient's skin lest a *false* cytohormonal evaluation result.

The swab is introduced through either a speculum (*i.e.,* nasal, otic, pediatric gynecologic) or a drinking straw. This important protection is to keep from labial contamination of the specimen. The swab is advanced into the vaginal vault and posterior pool area, where it is rotated against the vaginal epithelium. It is then carefully withdrawn *through* the speculum or within the drinking straw, rapidly rolled onto a slide, and fixed *immediately.*

Direct Lesion Scraping

If a lesion is visible in the vaginal vault or on the labia, it is best to obtain a direct smear in addition to a routine Fast smear. A direct scraping with a wooden blade is usually sufficient, unless the lesion is dry or necrotic. Hold a slide *over* an open bottle of fixative, quickly smear the material from the blade onto the slide, and *immediately* drop slide into fixative.

If the lesion is dry, keratotic, or has a necrotic and purulent surface, a different technique is needed. A nonabsorbent cotton swab, liberally soaked in physiological saline, is used to moisten and gently remove the necrotic debris which is then discarded. A second nonabsorbent cotton swab or a tongue blade is then moistened in saline (preferably containing some protein, *e.g.,* serum, egg albumin) and used to gently scrape the growing margins of the lesion. Hold a slide *over* an open bottle of fixative, quickly smear the material onto the slide, and *immediately* drop slide into fixative.

Pancervical Scraping Smears

Gently remove excess material lying at the os (without touching the epithelium) and *discard.* Follow Figs. 37.18, 19, *C, E,* and *F.* The spatula can be used to make the smear (*E*) if material is very scanty, but it does not make a satisfactorily uniform smear quickly enough to keep drying from occurring so that it should *not* be used in place of the finger or the cell spreader when sufficient material is present. This contains ectocervical, external os, and endocervical material.

Endocervical Swab Smear

Gently remove and *discard* excess material lying at the os. With the use of a moistened nonabsorbent cotton swab in place of the cervical spatula (Fig. 37.19 *C*) obtain material from the endocervical canal, roll it onto the slide, and fix *immediately* (Fig. 37.19 *F*).

Cervical material tends to dry and to be unsatisfactory, if there is the least delay in immediate fixation. This is most marked when there is inflammation (cervicitis), serum, or bleeding—all present in both the neoplasias and severe epithelial atypias, where cytology can help the most clinically if it is well preserved. The mucus of the vaginal pool serves to protect the cervical material when mixed together, as in a Fast smear, yielding more consistently satisfactory and clinically valuable results than pure endocervical swab smears.

Endocervical Aspiration Smear

Gently remove and discard excess material lying at the os. By the use of a plastic or glass pipette, material in the endocervical canal is aspirated, blown upon a glass slide, a second slide is placed upon it and then drawn apart, and both slides are *immediately* immersed in 95% ethyl alcohol.

Endometrial Aspiration Smear

The ectocervix is gently cleansed. A sterile endometrial aspirating cannula (or antral sinus cannula) with syringe attached is *gently* introduced, through the external os and internal os, into the endometrial cavity. The endometrial cavity is aspirated and the cannula is withdrawn. The material is blown upon a slide, spread with a second slide, and both are immediately immersed in 95% alcohol. The syringe and canula can then be flushed out with physiologic saline for filter preparations.

Endometrial Brush Smear

The brush is retracted into its cannula for protection from cervical contamination, and then extruded when in the endometrial cavity. All areas of the cavity are brushed (*i.e.,* both cornus, fundus, walls), the brush retracted into its cannula, and withdrawn. The brush and its material are extruded onto a slide, spreads made of the material, and *im-*

mediately fixed. The brush is then rinsed in physiologic solution which is then filtered (i.e., millipore-SM) for cell capture.

Jet Washings

The jet wash yields a valuable endometrial sample. Follow directions with the instrument.

V-C-E Smear

The lateral vaginal wall is first scraped by a cotton swab or spatula, the ectocervix is then scraped with a second spatula, and, finally a cotton swab is gently inserted into the endocervical canal. They are then *rapidly* smeared in inverse succession upon a single glass slide, the endocervical portions nearest the far end of the slide, the exocervical portion next, and the vaginal portion nearest the label. The slide is then immersed *immediately* into fixative.

Because of momentary drying which is unavoidable before smearing, and between smearings and fixation, cell preservation frequently is not optimum. This technique, however, gives valuable information as to the sites of disease processes, and the vaginal wall scraping affords excellent cytohormonal evaluation.

Vaginal Irrigation Smear

Irrigation of the vaginal vault with a physiological solution provides a satisfactory sample of the vaginal pool material. This can then be prepared or it can be placed with a preservative for preparation at a later time.

A large quantity of uniform slides can be prepared from one patient in this manner, each of which is high in diagnostic and teaching value. As it is a blind procedure, it can be performed either by medical personnel or by the patient in her own home. Either of these has satisfactory cytological characteristics, as both are processed uniformly in the laboratory.

Its microscopic examination and interpretation vary slightly from the usual cytopathological specimen due to preservation (partial fixation) before smearing. This makes the spread cells thicker with both nuclear detail preservation and

staining qualities less optimal. With experience, however, its interpretation can be made to approach that of the classical specimens, above, in quality.

For population screening a higher sensitivity is placed in the reporting, recalling far more patients with minor disease for a physician's workup than the more diagnostic cytopathology specimens (Figs. 37.18, 19) taken by the clinician.

This technique allows for a uniformity and quality in teaching material. For *mass* population screening it is unequaled by other methods, but is *inferior* to the classical specimens obtained as above.

Buccal Scraping Smears

Following Figure 37.20, hold slide with thumb and forefinger of left hand. Have open bottle of 95% ethyl alcohol fixative near.

(*A*) Hold angle of mouth laterally with left little finger. Firmly draw tongue blade forward a few times along the mucosa covering the buccal pouch *above* the dentate line (linea alba), collecting milky cellular fluid. Be careful not to contaminate sample with material from the linea alba.

(*B*) *Quickly* smear onto the glass slide in one motion, and

(*C*) *Immediately* immerse in 95% *ethyl* alcohol fixative. Make multiple smears.

Fixative and Transporting Specimen

After immediate fixation, cellular specimens can be dried in the air (Fig. 37.21). If they are protected from mechanical harm, they can be kept dry (with*out* glycerin, etc.) with virtually no harm to cytological detail. Drying *before* fixation, however, gives *inferior* specimens and can be disastrous.

The best possible cellular preservation must be obtained for properly identifying many early lesions, especially those present in inflammation, infection, bleeding, and serous oozing. In these conditions even momentary drying ruins the nuclear detail.

For this, *immediate* fixation in 95% *ethyl* alcohol has been found most satisfactory. The original Papanicolaou fixative, ethyl alcohol and ether, is equally

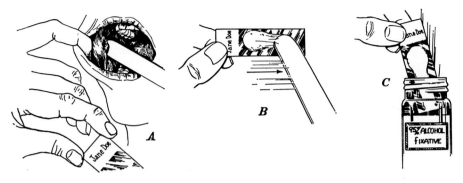

37.20. Buccal smear (see text)

excellent, but the ethyl ether is too flammable and volatile to be as practical. Because of the tax on ethyl alcohol, numerous types of other alcohols, various methods for reconstituting after drying without fixation, etc., have been tried and advocated; but quality is compromised. Price is of little concern if the alcohol is reused over and over *after* simple filtration in the office (Fig. 37.21 *B*).

After the material has been *immediately* placed in 95% ethyl alcohol and fixed at least one-half hour, it can then be air-dried (Fig. 37.21) and properly stored for years without deteriorating, if the cellular surface is physically protected (*i.e.,* facial tissue, slide box).

Various forms of administering proper fixatives have been developed such as the open bottle, dropper bottle, aerosol spray, and one-use miniature plastic ampulla. These all give satisfactory results if the two basic principles are adhered to: the *proper type* of fixative, and *immediate* immersion of the specimen in or under fixative.

SUMMARY

As a cellular sample is a *microbiopsy,* it must be representative, adequate, and properly prepared. The consultation requested upon this specimen should be as highly skilled with as experienced an interpretation as it is possible to obtain. Today, through wide postgraduate education, this is available in all areas of the country and, virtually, of the world. There should exist *no* logical excuse of

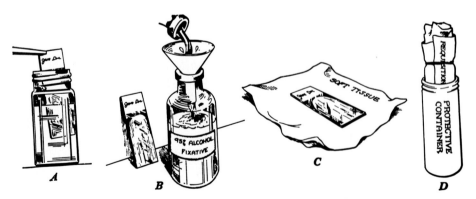

37.21. Air-dry technique for transporting specimens. *A,* after adequate fixation, preferably overnight, the smear is removed and allowed to dry in the air. *B,* the fixative is filtered and ready for reuse. *C,* when thoroughly dry, the slide is wrapped in soft tissue. *D,* the requisition is attached and the specimen protected for transit.

inadequate facilities for lack of obtaining clinical specimens for cellular interpretation.

Complete *understanding* of the patient and *liaison* between the two physicians are mandatory for a wise and thorough interpretation. This is basic to *all* consultations; but is especially essential to the proper handling of the borderline or questionable lesions, where free and complete exchange of ideas are mandatory for *proper* diagnosis, therapy, follow-up, and prognosis of the patient.

Clinical cytology can be of great assistance if properly understood and utilized. As with any potent tool, it is dangerous if misused or abused. When expertly utilized by clinician and pathologist working together as a team with complete inter-liaison, it makes otherwise impossible diagnoses commonplace and life-saving.

REFERENCES

Bechtold, E., and Reicher, N. B.: The relationship of *Trichomonas* infestations to false diagnoses of squamous carcinoma of the cervix. Cancer, 5: 442, 1952.

Berg, J. W., Durfee, G. R., and Bader, G. M.: The cellular detection of uterine adenocarcinoma. Trans. I.C.C.C., 1: 285, 1956.

Berry, A.: A cytopathological and histopathological study of bilharziasis of the female genital tract. J. Path. Bact., 91: 325, 1966.

Bibbo, M., Keebler, C. M., and Wied, G. L.: The cytologic diagnosis of tissue repair in the female genital tract. Acta Cytol., 15: 133, 1971.

Brewer, J. K., and Guderian, A. M.: Diagnosis of uterine-tube carcinoma by vaginal cytology. Obstet. Gynec., 8: 664, 1956.

Carson, R. P., and Gall, E. A.: Preinvasive carcinoma and precancerous metaplasia of the cervix. Amer. J. Path., 30: 15, 1954.

Coman, D. R.: Decreased mutual adhesiveness, a property of cells from squamous cell carcinomas. Cancer Res., 4: 625, 1944.

Davis, H. J.: The irrigation smear: accuracy in detection of cervical cancer. Acta Cytol., 6: 459, 1962.

Fennell, R. H., Jr., Carcinoma *in situ* of the cervix with early invasive changes. Cancer, 8: 302, 1955.

Fluhmann, C. F.: Carcinoma *in situ* and the transitional zone of the cervix uteri. Obstet. Gynec., 16: 424, 1960.

Frost, J. K.: *Concepts Basic to General Cytopathology.* The Johns Hopkins Press, Baltimore, 4th ed., 1972.

Frost, J. K.: *Trichomonas vaginalis* and cervical epithelial changes. Ann. N. Y. Acad. Sci., 97: 792, 1962.

Frost, J. K.: Gynecologic and obstetric cytopathology, Chapter 35 in *Novak's Gynecologic and Obstetric Pathology,* Novak, E. R., and Woodruff, J. D. (Eds.). W. B. Saunders Company, Philadelphia, 7th ed., 1974.

Frost, J. K.: *The Cell in Health and Disease.* S. Karger, Basel, and Williams and Wilkins Company, Baltimore, 1969.

Frost, J. K.: Diagnostic accuracy of "cervical smears." Obstet. Gynec. Survey, 24: 893, 1969.

Frost, J. K., Honigberg, B. M., and McLure, M. T.: Intracellular *Trichomonas vaginalis* and *Trichomonas gallinae* in natural and experimental infections. J. Parasit., 47: 302, 1961.

Galvin, G. A., Jones, H. W., and TeLinde, R. W.: The significance of basal-cell-hyperactivity in cervical biopsies. Amer. J. Obstet. Gynec., 70: 808, 1955.

Galvin, G. A., Jones, H. W., Jr., and TeLinde, R. W.: Clinical relationship of carcinoma *in situ* and invasive carcinoma of the cervix. J.A.M.A., 149: 744, 1952.

Graham, J. B., and Graham, R. M.: The sensitization response in patients with cancer of the uterine cervix. Cancer, 13: 5, 1960.

Graham, R. M.: Cytologic prognosis in cancer of the cervix. Amer. J. Obstet. Gynec., 79: 700, 1960.

Graham, R. M.: *The Cytologic Diagnosis of Cancer.* W. B. Saunders Company, Philadelphia, 3rd. ed., 1972.

Graham, R. M.: Accuracy of cytologic diagnosis in the treated cancer. Acta Cytol., 8: 3, 1964.

Hertig, A. T., and Gore, H.: Tumors of the female sex organs. II. Tumors of the vulva, vagina, and uterus. Chapter 33 in *Atlas of Tumor Pathology.* Armed Forces Institute of Pathology, Washington, D.C., 1960.

Hertig, A. T., and Mansell, H.: What is carcinoma *in situ* of the cervix?, p. 520 in *Progress in Gynecology,* Vol. III, Meigs, J. V., and Sturgis, S. H. (Eds.). Grune and Stratton, New York, 1957.

Hesseltine, H. C.: Factors relating to mycotic and trichomonal infections. Ann. N. Y. Acad. Sci., 83: 245, 1959.

Honigberg, B. M., Livingston, M. C., and Frost, J. K.: Pathogenicity of fresh isolates of *Trichomonas vaginalis*: "the mouse assay" versus clinical and pathologic findings. Acta Cytol., 10: 353, 1966.

Howdon, W. M., Howdon, A., Frost, J. K., and Woodruff, J. D.: Cyto- and histopathologic correlation in mixed mesenchymal tumors of the uterus. Amer. J. Obstet. Gynec., 89: 670, 1964.

Johnson, L. D.: The histopathological approach to early cervical neoplasia. Obstet. Gynec. Survey, 24: 735, 1969.

Johnson, L. D., Easterday, C. L., Gore, H., and Hertig, A. T.: The histogenesis of carcinoma *in situ* of the uterine cervix; a preliminary report of the origin of carcinoma *in situ* in subcylindrical cell anaplasia. Cancer, 17: 213, 1964.

Jones, H. W., Jr., Davis, H. J., Frost, J. K., Park, I., Salimi, R., Tseng, P., and Woodruff, J. D.: The value of the assay of chromosomes in the diagnosis of cervical neoplasia. Amer. J. Obstet. Gynec., 102: 624, 1968.

Jones, H. W., Jr., Goldberg, B., Davis, H. J., and Burns, B. C., Jr.: Cellular changes in vaginal and buccal smears after radiation: an index of the radiocurability of carcinoma of the cervix. Amer. J. Obstet. Gynec., 78: 1083, 1959.

Jordan, M. J., Bader, G. M., and Nemazie, A. S.: Comparative accuracy of preoperative cytologic and histologic diagnosis in endometrial lesions. Obstet. Gynec., 7: 646, 1956.

Kean, B. H., and Day, E.: *Trichomonas vaginalis* infection; an evaluation of three diagnostic techniques with data on incidence. Amer. J. Obstet. Gynec., 68: 1510, 1954.

Kjellgren, O.: The radiation reaction in the vaginal smear and its prognostic significance; studies on radiologically treated cases of cancer of the uterine cervix. Acta Radiol. (Stockholm) Suppl., 168: 1, 1958.

Koss, L. G.: *Diagnostic Cytology.* J. B. Lippincott Company, Philadelphia, 2nd ed., 1968.

Koss, L. G., and Durfee, G. R.: Cytological changes preceding the appearance of *in situ* carcinoma of the uterine cervix. Cancer, *8:* 295, 1955.

Koss, L. G., and Wolinska, W. H.: *Trichomonas vaginalis* cervicitis and its relationship to cervical cancer. A histological study. Cancer, *12:* 1171, 1959.

Krantz, K. E.: The gross and microscopic anatomy of the human vagina. Ann. N. Y. Acad. Sci., *83:* 89, 1959.

Kulda, J., Honigberg, B. M., Frost, J. K., and Hollander, D. H.: Pathogenicity of *Trichomonas vaginalis:* a clinical and biological study. Amer. J. Obstet. Gynec. *108:* 908, 1970.

Mardh, P.-A., Stormby, N., and Weström, L.: Mycoplasma and vaginal cytology. Acta Cytol., *15:* 310, 1971.

Marsh, M.: Original site of cervical carcinoma; topographical relationship of carcinoma of the cervix to the external os and to the squamocolumnar junction. Obstet. Gynec., *7:* 444, 1956.

McKay, D. G., Terjanian, B., Poschyachinda, D., Younge, P. A., and Hertig, A. T.: Clinical and pathologic significance of anaplasia (atypical hyperplasia) of the cervix uteri. Obstet. Gynec., *14:* 2, 1959.

Meisels, A.: Dysplasia and carcinoma of the uterine cervix. IV. A correlated cytologic and histologic study with special emphasis on vaginal microbiology. Acta Cytol., *13:* 224, 1969.

Merrill, J. A., and Wood, D. A.: Comparative studies on histologic and cytologic technics of radiosensitivity testing in carcinoma of the cervix. Trans. I.S.C.C., *7:* 85, 1959.

Naib, Z. M., and Masukawa, N. K.: The identification of condyloma acuminata cells in routine vaginal smears. Obstet. Gynec., *18:* 735, 1961.

Nesbitt, R. E., Jr., and Brack, C. B.: Role of cytology in detection of carcinoma of cervix. J.A.M.A., *161:* 183, 1956.

Ng, A. B. P., Reagan, J. W., and Lindner, E. A.: The cellular manifestations of microinvasive squamous cell carcinoma of the uterine cervix. Acta Cytol., *16:* 5, 1972.

Ng, A. B. P., Teeple, D., Lindner, E. A., and Reagan, J. W.: The cellular manifestations of extrauterine cancer. Acta Cytol., *18:* 108, 1974.

Nieburgs, H. E.: *Diagnostic Cell Pathology in Tissue and Smears,* Grune and Stratton, New York and London, 1967.

Nieburgs, H. E.: Tissue and cell pathology of uterine cervix dysplasias and carcinoma in situ. Acta Cytol., *15:* 513, 1971.

Nieburgs, H. E., Stergus, I., Stephenson, E. M., and Harbin, B. L.: Mass screening of the total female population of a county for cervical carcinoma. J.A.M.A., *164:* 1546, 1957.

Nielsen, A. M.: The value of the cyto-prognostic test in the treatment of carcinoma of the cervix, p. 293 in *First International Cancer Cytology Congress Transactions.* Chicago, 1956.

Papanicolaou, G. N.: *Atlas of Exfoliative Cytology.* Published for The Commonwealth Fund by Harvard University Press, Cambridge, 1954, with supplements.

Papanicolaou, G. N., and Traut, H. F.: *Diagnosis of Uterine Cancer by the Vaginal Smear.* The Commonwealth Fund, New York, 1943.

Papanicolaou, G. N., Traut, H. F., and Marchetti, A. A.: *The Epithelia of Woman's Reproductive Organs. A Cor-*

relative Study of Cyclic Changes. The Commonwealth Fund, New York, 1948.

Patten, S. F., Jr.: *Diagnostic Cytology of the Uterine Cervix.* S. Karger. Basel, and Williams and Wilkins Company, Baltimore, 1969.

Patten, S. F., Jr., Hughes, C. P., and Reagan, J. W.: An experimental study of the relationship between *Trichomonas vaginalis* and dysplasia in the uterine cervix. Acta Cytol., *7:* 187, 1963.

Potter, J. F., Longenbaugh, G., Chu, E., Dillon, J., Romsdahl, M., and Malmgren, R. A.: The relationship of tumor type and resectability to the incidence of cancer cells in blood. Surg. Gynec. Obstet., *110:* 734, 1960.

Przybora, L. A., and Plutowa, A.: Histological topography of carcinoma *in situ* of the cervix uteri. Cancer, *12:* 263, 1959.

Reagan, J. W.: A cytologic study of incipient carcinoma. Amer. J. Clin. Path., *22:* 231, 1952.

Reagan, J. W., and Hamonic, M. J.: Dysplasia of the uterine cervix. Ann. N. Y. Acad. Sci., *63:* 1236, 1956.

Reagan, J. W., Hamonic, M. J., and Wentz, W. B.: Analytical study of the cells in cervical squamous-cell cancer. Lab. Invest., *6:* 241, 1957.

Reagan, J. W., and Ng, A. P. B.: *The Cells of Uterine Adenocarcinoma.* S. Karger, Basel, and Williams and Wilkins Company, Baltimore, 1965.

Reagan, J. W., and Patton, S. F., Jr.: Dysplasia: a basic reaction to injury in the uterine cervix. Ann. N. Y. Acad. Sci., *97:* 662, 1962.

Rubin, D. K., and Frost, J. K.: The cytologic detection of ovarian cancer. Acta Cytol., *7:* 191, 1963.

Sedlis, A., Walters, A. T., Balin, H., Hontz, A., and LoSciuto, L.: Evaluation of two simultaneously obtained cervical cytological smears. Acta Cytol. *18:* 291, 1974.

Simon, T. R., Durfee, G. R., and Ricci, A.: The value of the vaginal aspiration smear as compared with the cervical swab smear in the detection of *in situ* carcinoma of the cervix and adenocarcinoma of the fundus. Trans. I.S.C.C., *3:* 77, 1955.

Sonek, M.: Vaginal cytology during puberty. Acta Cytol., *11:* 41, 1967.

Stern, E., and Longo, L. D.: Identification of herpes simplex virus in a case showing cytological features of viral vaginitis. Acta Cytol., *7:* 295, 1963.

Sutherland, J. C., Berry, A., Hynd, N. M., and Proctor, N. S. F.: Placental Bilharziasis—report of a case. Afr. J. Obstet. Gynaec., *3:* 76, 1965.

Takeuchi, A., and McKay, D. G.: A study of the area of the cervix involved by carcinoma-*in-situ* and anaplasia (atypical hyperplasia). Trans. I.S.C.C., *7:* 61, 1959.

Taft, P. D., Robboy, S. J., Herbst, A. L., and Scully, R. E.: Cytology of clear-cell adenocarcinoma of genital tract in young females; review of 95 cases from the Registry. Acta Cytol., *18:* 279, 1974.

Trichomoniasis, p. 246 in *Control of Communicable Diseases in Man.* American Public Health Association, Inc., New York, 10th ed., 1965.

Varga, A., and Browell, B.: Viral inclusion bodies in vaginal smears. Obstet. Gynec., *16:* 441, 1960.

Wachtel, E.: A simple cytological test for cancer cure. Brit. Med. J., *5061:* 20, 1958.

Wentz, W. B., and Reagan, J. W.: Survival in cervical cancer with respect to cell type. Cancer, *12:* 384, 1959.

Index

RAILWAYS

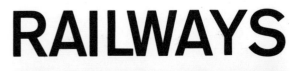

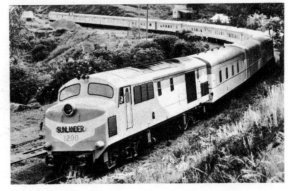

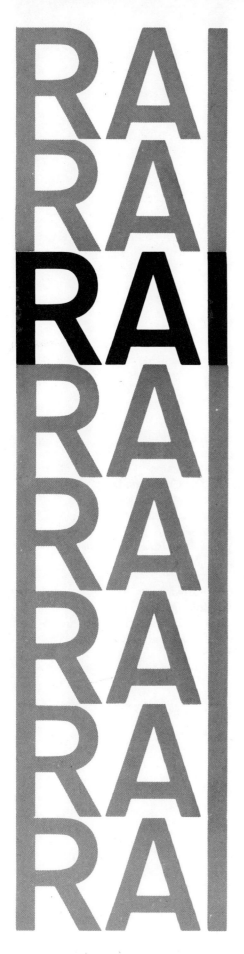
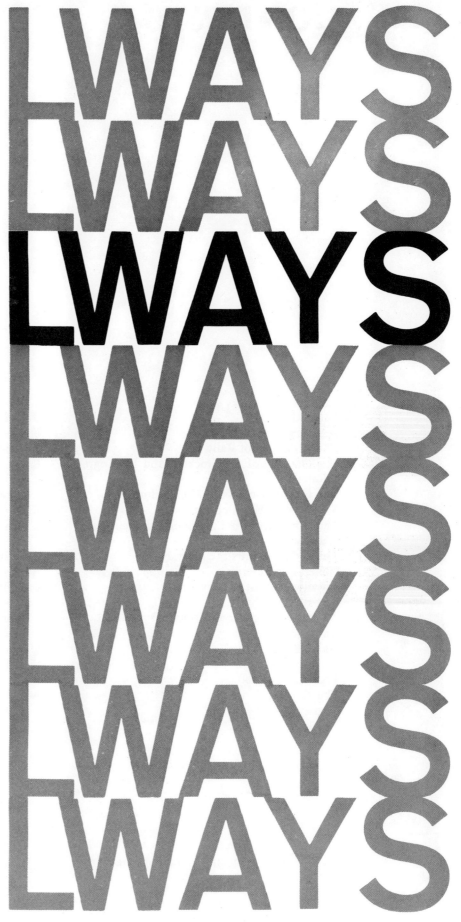

RAILWAYS

HOWARD LOXTON

PAUL HAMLYN
LONDON · NEW YORK · SYDNEY · TORONTO

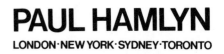

CONTENTS

Published by
THE HAMLYN PUBLISHING GROUP LIMITED
LONDON ● NEW YORK ● SYDNEY ● TORONTO
Hamlyn House, Feltham, Middlesex, England
© The Hamlyn Publishing Group Ltd 1963
Revised edition 1970

Imprimé en France par Brodard et Taupin. 3289/2.

38513

ABOUT THIS BOOK

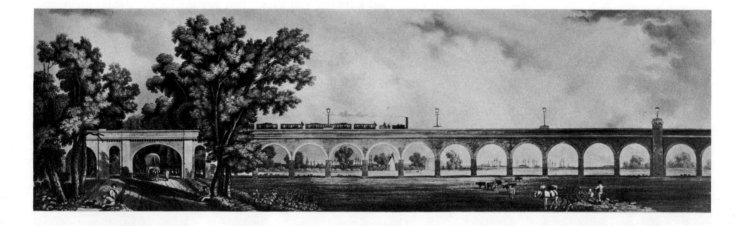

THE CHANGES which railways brought to the economic and social life of the world were so far-reaching that the first railways seem to have belonged to a time remote from our own, yet, only 150 years ago, no public railway existed. Those early railways were a symbol of modernity to contemporary people and epitomised the aggressively advancing spirit of their age. Today, although earthworks, tunnels, viaducts and stations built by the pioneers are still in use, the railways themselves are going through a great period of change: new forms of power and automation are transforming their appearance and operation.

Railways combine past and present, and with every train that passes they link our thoughts with places far away. The locomotive itself is a personification of speed and power. As a small boy I remember being taken, for the first time, to meet the driver at the end of a railway journey, and I was so frightened of the monster of steel and steam that I would not go on to the footplate.

The railways have romance, but they have too a fascination for the technically and mechanically minded, with their complex organisation and operation and the excitement of new developments in locomotives, permanent way and signalling.

This book reflects all these facets of the railway's character. It adds to the historic record of the first railways and the stimulating picture of the railways' future, the comments in words and pictures of writers and artists both of those early days and our own times. However, it is not the writers, artists and historians who have made the railways what they are, but the engineers and architects, the railwaymen — drivers, firemen, signalmen, cleaners, station masters, ticket clerks — everyone who helps in running them. It is their achievement that this book records.

THE SONG OF THE IRON ROAD

Engine driving's got to be in your blood for a start. If it's not in your blood to stand the erratic hours you'll never stand the pace. The railway life, to my mind—to the proper railwayman—it always comes first, it's in his blood. (ALEC WATTS — Chargeman Cleaner)

The old railwayman, it was a tradition, it was part of your life—railways went through the back of your spine like Blackpool went through rock. (JIM HOWARTH—Driver)

What a feeling you have when you get off the shed; you've got the engine, you've got the control of it, and what a feeling—'I'm cock of the bank, there's nobody can take a rise out of me now, she's mine.' Come on, me old beauty, and off we go. The moon's out and the countryside—it's lovely. On we go, what a feeling—she answers to every touch. 'Some more rock on, lad.' Yes—it's grand. (JACK PICKFORD—Driver)

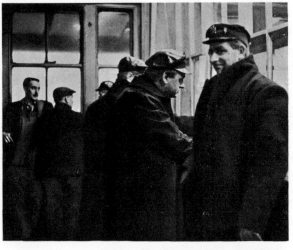
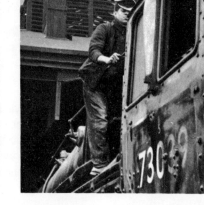
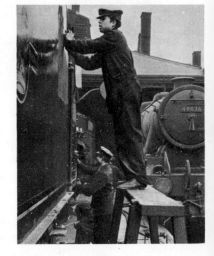

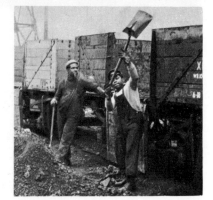

The iron road is a hard road and the work is never-ending,
Working night and day on the iron way
We're the boys who keep the engines rolling.

You sign on at the loco-shed, they put you on the cleaning . . .
In your dungarees cleaning super Dees . . . . you're a
Sweeper-upper, brewer-upper, shovel-slinger, spanner-bringer,
Steam-raiser, fire-dropper, general cook and bottle-washer,
Learning how to keep 'em rolling.

'Here, lad, fetch me a bucket of red oil for a red tail lamp!'
Charlie!
'Charlie!'
On your toes!
Clean that muck out of number five.
'Look alive there.'
Get weaving!
'Where you going for that oil? Arabia?'
See the job on number three,
They're gonna strip her.
'Hey, Ginger!'
Leave the job you're working on,
Help the Fitter.
Hold the light,
The one inch spanner off the bench,
The one inch reamer!

'Hey, cleaner!'

Do this! Do that!
Get me this! Get me that!
A rush job on number eight
Working late, got a date,
I'll never make it.

You'll have to break it!
'JUST A BLOODY SKIVVY THAT'S ME!'
Two years,
Five years,
Ten years,
Fifteen years a cleaner.

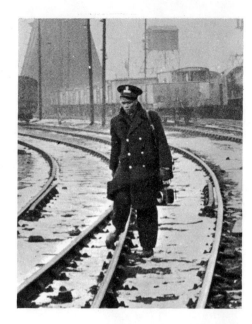

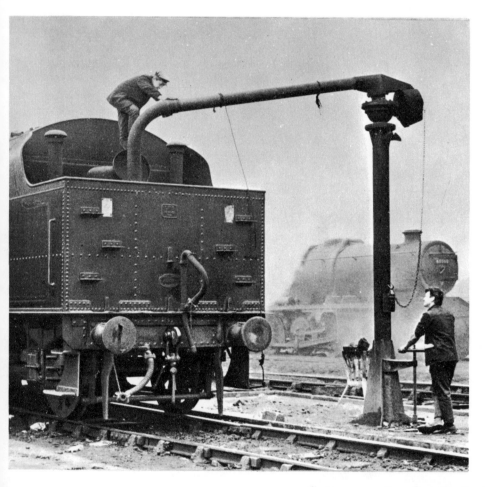

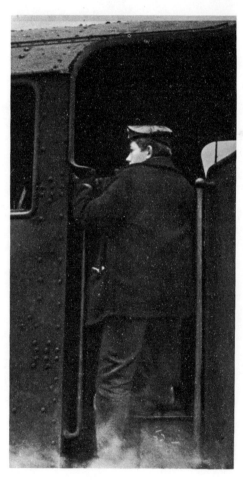

When you've done your time at the loco shed
And had your share of trouble,
On the old footplate you're the driver's mate,
And you're married to a lousy shovel.

It's check the water, check the tools,
And chuck the blooming coal in;
Give the gauge a wipe, check injector-pipe,
Now it's:

Swing your shovel at the double,
Give her rock, watch the clock,
Steam raising, sweat running,
Back aching, bone shaking,
Fireman, fireman, keep her rolling.

When you've shovelled a million tons of coal
Some ten or twelve years later;
And your only dream is of raising steam,
Then they hand to you your driver's papers.

You're on your own mate,
King of the footplate.
You've got a load mate,
Watch the road mate.
Get her through mate,
It's up to you mate.

She's a class eight engine
She's as tough as they come.
Weighs well over a hundred tons.

She's a puller,
An iron horse.
You've got nine tons of coal
You've got four thousand gallons of water.

You've got her measure,
Her boiler pressure is
Two hundred and twenty-five pounds an inch.

You've got a snorter.

You've got to watch the line
And get her there on time
And keep her rolling.

Keep your hand on the brake
She's a monster mate,
That you're controlling.

The iron road is a hard road and the work is never-ending
Working night and day on the iron way we're the

Loco-drivers, early risers, lodging turners, mile burners,
Eleven-quid-a-week earners,
We're the boys who keep'em rolling.

(FROM THE BALLAD OF JOHN AXON
by Ewan MacColl, Peggy Seeger and Charles Parker)

THE BEGINNING OF RAILWAYS

NO ONE KNOWS who first invented railways, but we do know that the ancient civilisations realised that wheels moved more easily over a smooth surface, and that the Greeks, Romans and Assyrians used grooves cut in stone slabs as guide tracks for their vehicles, for the grooves have outlasted their makers by two thousand years.

Heavy carts with wooden wheels soon wore ruts into the soft roads of Elizabethan times. Someone discovered that if boards were put into the ruts before they became too deep horses could haul their carts much more easily. Lines of wooden rails came into use in Britain's mines some time after 1600. Roger Worth described tramroads at Newcastle in 1680: 'The manner of the carriage is by laying rails

wheels to give greater strength they soon wore out the wooden rails, which then had to have iron plates fixed to them. As early as 1738 there is a report of cast iron rails being substituted for wooden ones, but the wagons were too heavy for them. The use of smaller wagons linked together dispersed the weight and solved this problem. In 1765, however, wooden rails were still being laid: 'When the road has been traced at six feet in breadth, and where the declivities are fixed, an excavation is made of the breadth of the said road, more or less deep according as the levelling of the road requires. There are afterwards arranged along the whole breadth of this excavation, pieces of oak wood of the thickness of four, five, six, and even eight inches square: these are placed

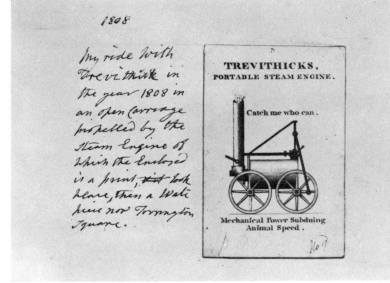

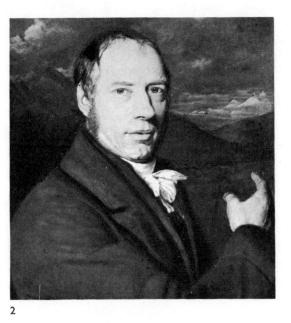

of timber from the colliery down to the river, exactly straight and parallel, and bulky carts are made with four rowlets fitting these rails, whereby the carriage is so easy, that one horse will draw down four or five chaldron of coals, and is an immense benefit to the coal merchants.'

When iron tyres were added to the wooden

1 Richard Trevithick's *Catch Me Who Can,* a print kept as a souvenir by one of the passengers on the experimental railway.
2 A portrait of the inventor painted by Linnell in 1816 when Trevithick was forty-five.

across and at the distance of two or three feet from each other: these pieces need only be squared at their extremities, and upon these are fixed other pieces of wood, well squared and sawed, of about six or seven inches breadth by five in depth, with pegs of wood; these pieces are placed on each side of the road along its whole length; they are commonly placed at four feet distance from each other, which forms the interior breadth of the road.'

With the harnessing of steam power in the mines, iron became cheaper and cast iron rails became more usual. These railways operated by man-power, horse-power, or sometimes by a rope attached to a stationary engine. In 1759

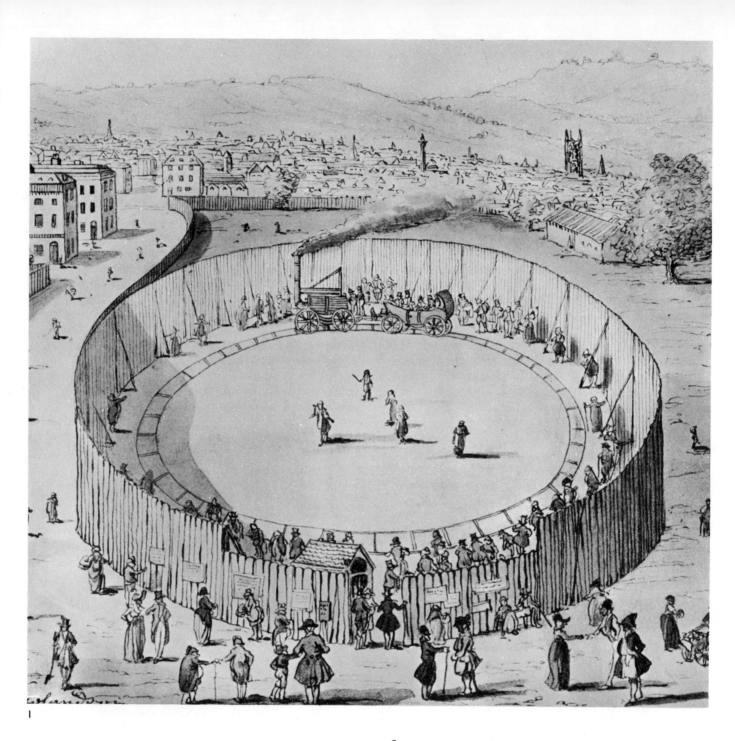

1

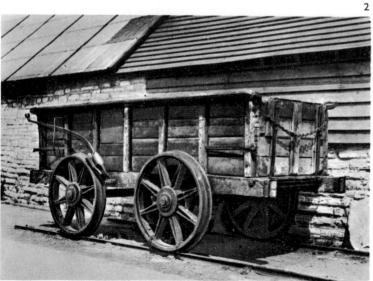

2

1 A drawing by Thomas Rowlandson showing the circular railway at Euston Square in 1809.
2 A tram wagon from the horse-drawn railway from Stratford to Moreton-in-the Marsh dating from 1826, the year the line was opened. It stands on a section of the original line which was fastened to square blocks, not wooden sleepers.
3 A poster giving charges on the Surrey Iron Railway.
4 William Hedley's locomotive *Puffing Billy* of 1813.

James Watt, who had developed the steam engine, is believed to have experimented with steam power in a locomotive, and his assistant William Murdock made a working model which is still preserved in the Birmingham Museum of Science and Industry. In France, Joseph Cugnot built a steam engine for operation on the highway in 1769, but the first locomotive to run on rails was built by an Englishman, Richard Trevithick. Trevithick developed his own road vehicle (which when first tried out in 1801 broke down after 300 yards and later set fire to the coach-house of the hotel where Trevithick was recovering) and then built a locomotive which he demonstrated in 1804 on Pen-y-Darran Ironworks Railway in Wales. It carried ten tons of iron ore and seventy passengers in five wagons, at five miles per hour along a ten mile line. Four years later Trevithick tried to rouse public interest by building a circular track on some waste land near where Euston Station stands today. For a shilling Londoners could travel in open carriages pulled by a locomotive called *Catch Me Who Can*.

All the early railways were operated for private use, but three years before Richard Trevithick's success at Pen-y-Darran the World's first public railway was chartered by an Act of Parliament — on 26th July 1803 it was opened between Wandsworth Wharf and Croydon. Although flanged wheels had been known in Germany since the mid-sixteenth century and were used in Great Britain at Bath as early as 1731, these cars had smooth wheels and ran on angled rails.

Others followed Trevithick's lead; one man, called Brunton, tried to make a locomotive which walked like a horse! William Hedley, at one time Trevithick's agent and a director of Wylam Colliery, Durham, designed a locomotive very like the *Catch Me Who Can* and took out a patent in 1813 with Mr. Blackett, owner of the colliery. They called the locomotive *Puffing Billy*.

George Stephenson, an engineer from Wylam, at this time working at a Killingworth colliery, saw Trevithick and Hedley's machines and with the encouragement of Lord Ravensworth built a locomotive which, on 25th July 1814, drew eight carriages weighing twenty tons up a slight ascent. In 1815, he took out a patent for his locomotive, which he named the *Blücher*.

Stephenson became technical manager of the Stockton and Darlington Railway in 1823. The company was formed in 1821 and the line was opened publicly on 27th September, 1825, with a train drawn by 'Locomotive No. 1.'

3
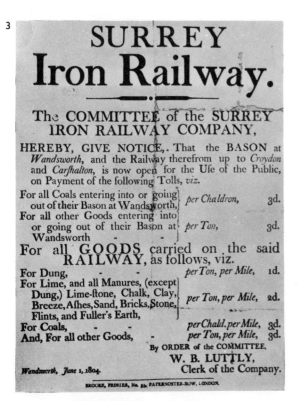

SURREY
Iron Railway.

The COMMITTEE of the SURREY IRON RAILWAY COMPANY,

HEREBY, GIVE NOTICE, . That the BASON at *Wandsworth*, and the Railway therefrom up to *Croydon* and *Carshalton*, is now open for the Use of the Public, on Payment of the following Tolls, *viz.*

For all Coals entering into or going out of their Bason at Wandsworth,	*per Chaldron*,	3d.
For all other Goods entering into or going out of their Bason at Wandsworth - -	*per Ton*,	3d.

For all GOODS carried on the said RAILWAY, as follows, viz.

For Dung,	*per Ton, per Mile*,	1d.
For Lime, and all Manures, (except Dung,) Lime-stone, Chalk, Clay, Breeze, Ashes, Sand, Bricks, Stone, Flints, and Fuller's Earth,	*per Ton, per Mile*,	2d.
For Coals,	*per Chald. per Mile*,	3d.
And, For all other Goods, -	*per Ton, per Mile*,	3d.

By ORDER of the COMMITTEE.
W. B. LUTTLY,
Wandsworth, June 1, 1804. Clerk of the Company.

BROOKE, PRINTER, No. 35, PATERNOSTER-ROW, LONDON.

4
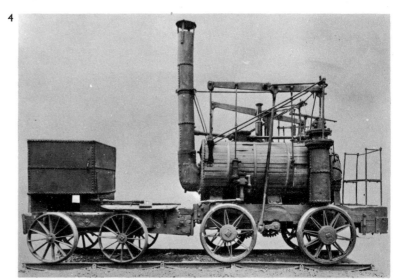

THE OPENING OF THE STOCKTON AND DARLINGTON RAILWAY

THE 'NEWCASTLE COURANT,' 1st OCTOBER 1825

ON TUESDAY LAST, September 27th, 1825, that great work, the Stockton and Darlington Rail-Way, was formally opened by the proprietors, for the use of the public. It is a single Rail-Way of 25 miles in length, and will open the London market to collieries in the western part of the county of Durham, as well as facilitate the obtaining of fuel to the country along its line and the northern parts of Yorkshire.

The line of Rail-Way extends from the collieries in a direction nearly from west to east, from Witton Park and Etherly, near West Auckland, to Stockton upon Tees, with branches to Darlington, Yarm, etc., and is chiefly composed of Malleable Iron Rails. At the western extremity of the line, a deep ravine

occurs at the river Gaunless; on the summit of the hills on each side of which permanent steam-engines are fixed for the purpose of conveying the goods across the two ridges. The engine on the western side of the vale is called the Etherly Engine, and that on the eastern side the Brusselton Engine; the latter of which, in addition to conveying the goods up from West Auckland, also continues the transit down the eastern side of the ridge: below this, to the east, the country, though undulating, is pretty flat, and the conveyance is performed by locomotive engines. To give eclat to the public opening of the road, a programme was issued, stating that the proprietors would assemble at the permanent

1

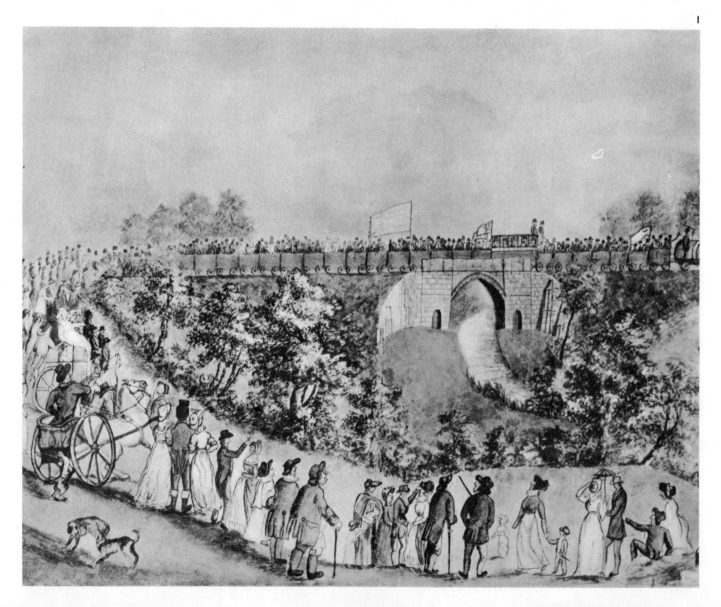

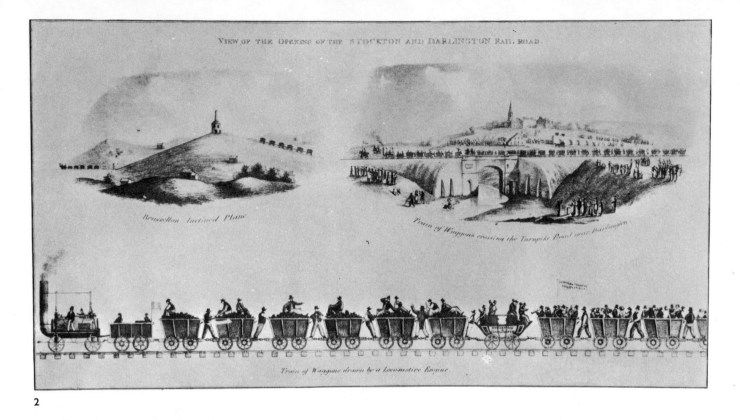

VIEW OF THE OPENING OF THE STOCKTON AND DARLINGTON RAIL ROAD.

Brusselton Inclined Plane.

Train of Waggons crossing the Turnpike Road near Darlington.

Train of Waggons drawn by a Locomotive Engine.

2

1 Dobbin's contemporary sketch of the opening of the Stockton and Darlington Railway in 1825.
2 Scenes on the railway: the Brusselton tower and inclined plane; a train of wagons crossing the turnpike road near Darlington (note the mounted rider leading the procession); a train of wagons drawn by a locomotive.
3 The world's first railway ticket office: this cottage was used as a booking office for the Stockton and Darlington Railway.
4 Locomotive No. I: *Locomotion.*

steam-engine below Brusselton Tower, about nine miles west of Darlington, at eight o'clock. Accordingly, the committee, after inspecting the Etherly Engine Plane, assembled at the bottom of Brusselton Engine Plane, near West Auckland, and here the carriages, loaded with coal and merchandise, were drawn up the eastern ridge by the Brusselton Engine, a distance of 1960 yards, in seven and a half minutes, and then lowered down the plane on the east side of the hill 880 yards in five minutes. At the foot of the plane the locomotive engine was ready to receive the carriages; and here the novelty of the scene and the fineness of the day had attracted an immense concourse of spectators—the fields on each side of the Rail-Way being literally covered with ladies and gentlemen on horseback, and pedestrians of all kinds. The train of carriages was then attached to a locomotive engine, of the most improved construction, and built by Mr. George Stephenson, in the following order:

1. Locomotive engine, with the Engineer, (Mr. Stephenson,) and assistants. 2. Tender, with coals and water; next, six waggons loaded

3

4

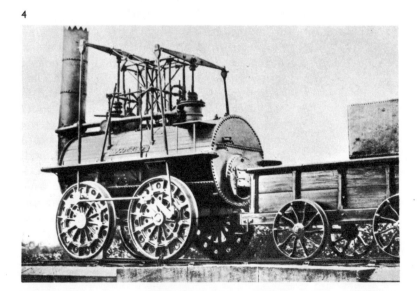

with coals and flour; then an elegant covered coach, with the committee and other proprietors of the Rail-Way; then 21 waggons, fitted up on the occasion for passengers; and last of all, six waggons loaded with coals, making altogether a train of 38 carriages, exclusive of the engine and tender.

Tickets were distributed to the number of near 300, for those whom it was intended should occupy the coach and waggons; but such was the pressure and crowd, that both loaded and empty carriages were instantly filled with passengers. The signal being given, the engine started off with this immense train of carriages, and here the scene became most interesting—the horsemen galloping across the fields to accompany the engine, and the people on foot running on each side of the road, endeavouring in vain to keep up with the cavalcade. The Rail-Way descending with a gentle inclination towards Darlington, though not uniform, the rate of speed was consequently variable. On this part of the Rail-Way it was wished to ascertain at what rate of speed the engine could travel with safety. In some parts the speed was frequently twelve miles per hour, and in one place, for a short distance, near Darlington, fifteen miles per hour; and at that time the number of passengers was counted to four hundred and fifty, which, together with the coals, merchandise, and carriages, would amount to near ninety tons.

After some little delay in arranging the procession, the engine with her load arrived at Darlington, a distance of eight miles and three quarters, in sixty-five minutes, exclusive of stops, averaging about eight miles an hour. Six carriages, loaded with coals, intended for Darlington, were then left behind; and after obtaining a fresh supply of water, and arranging the procession to accommodate a band of music and passengers from Darlington, the engine set off again. Part of the Rail-Way from Darlington to Stockton has little declivity, and in one place is quite level; and as in the upper part, it was intended to try the speed of the engine; in this part it was proposed to prove her capability of dragging a heavy load, and, certainly, the performance excited the astonishment of all present, and exceeded the most sanguine expectations of every one conversant with the subject. The engine arrived at Stockton in three hours and seven minutes after

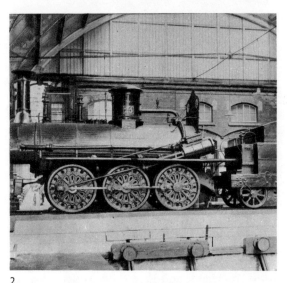

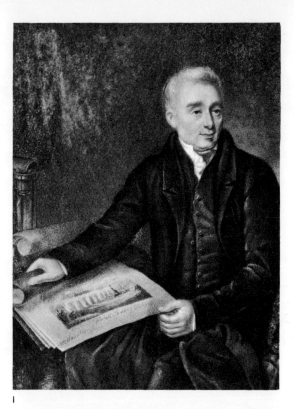

leaving Darlington, including stops, the distance being nearly twelve miles, which is at the rate of four miles an hour; and upon the level part of the Rail-Way, the number of passengers in the waggons was counted about five hundred and fifty, and several more clung to the carriages on each side, so that the whole number could not be less than six hundred, which, with the other load, would amount to about eighty

1 A watercolour portrait of George Stephenson, painted in 1836.
2 Locomotive No. 25, the *Derwent,* which went into service in 1845.

tons. Nothing could exceed the beauty and grandeur of the scene. Throughout the whole distance, the fields and lanes were covered with elegantly dressed females, and all descriptions of spectators.

Numerous horses, carriages, gigs, carts, and other vehicles travelled along with the engine, and her immense train of carriages, and in some places within a few yards, without the horses seeming the least frightened; and at one time the passengers by the engine had the pleasure of accompanying and cheering their brother passengers by the stage coach, which passed alongside, and of observing the striking contrast exhibited by the power of the engine and of horses; the engine with her six hundred passengers and load, and the coach with four horses, and only sixteen passengers.

In contemplating the events of the day, either in a national point of view, or as the efforts of a company of individuals furnishing a speedy, efficacious, and certain means of traffic to a wide and extended district, it alike excites the deepest interest and admiration; and the immense train of carriages covered with people, forming a load of from eighty to ninety tons, gliding, as it were, smoothly and majestically along the Rail-Way through files of spectators, at such an astonishing rate of speed, left an impression on those who witnessed it, that will never be forgotten.

Part of the workmen were entertained at Stockton, and part at Yarm, and there was a grand dinner for the proprietors and their more distinguished guests at the Town Hall, in Stockton. Mr. Meynell, of Yarm, was in the chair, and the Mayor of the town acted as vice-president.

LOCOMOTION NO. 1 was the first steam locomotive to run on a public railway but most of the Stockton and Darlington's regular traffic at this time was horse-drawn. The first line built for, and operated solely by, steam haulage was the Liverpool and Manchester Railway.

This project was first discussed in 1822, but opposition to railways was so great that the necessary Act of Parliament was not passed until 1826. George Stephenson, who was appointed Chief Engineer, had considerable difficulties to face in constructing the 31 miles of double line. Apart from tunnels, bridges and viaducts he had to make a way across the

marshland of Chat Moss, four miles of bog more than thirty feet in depth.

In 1829, before the line was finished, the directors of the railway held a competition at Rainhill, near Liverpool, to find 'the most improved locomotive engine', laying down strict conditions to which the entrants must conform:

1829 GRAND COMPETITION OF LOCOMOTIVES ON THE LIVERPOOL & MANCHESTER RAILWAY

Stipulations & Conditions on which the Directors of the Liverpool and Manchester Railway offer a Premium of £500 for the most improved locomotive engine.

I. The said Engine must 'effectually consume its own smoke' according to the provisions of the Railway Act, 7th Geo. IV.

II. The Engine, if it weighs six Tons, must be capable of drawing after it, day by day, on a well-constructed Railway, on a level plane, a Train of Carriages of the gross weight of Twenty Tons, including the Tender and Water Tank, at the rate of Ten Miles per Hour, with a pressure of steam in the boiler not exceeding Fifty Pounds on the square inch.

III. There must be Two Safety Valves, one of which must be completely out of the reach or control of the Engine-man, and neither of which must be fastened down while the Engine is working.

IV. The Engine and Boiler must be supported on Springs, and rest on Six Wheels; and the height from the ground to the top of the Chimney must not exceed Fifteen Feet.

V. The weight of the Machine, WITH ITS COMPLEMENT OF WATER in the Boiler, must at most, not exceed Six Tons, and a Machine of less weight will be preferred if it draw AFTER it a PROPORTIONATE weight; and if the weight of the Engine, & c., do not exceed FIVE TONS, then the gross weight to be drawn need not exceed Fifteen Tons; and in that proportion for Machines of still smaller weight — provided that the Engine, & c., shall still be on six wheels, unless the weight (as above) be reduced to Four Tons and a Half, or under, in which case the Boiler, & c., may be placed on four wheels. And the Company shall be at liberty to put the Boiler, Tube, Cylinders, & c., to the test of a pressure of water not exceeding 150 Pounds per square inch, without being answerable for any damage the machine may receive in consequence.

VI. There must be a Mercurial Gauge affixed to the Machine, with Index Rod, showing the Steam Pressure above 45 Pounds per square inch; and constructed to blow out a Pressure of 60 Pounds per inch.

VII. The Engine to be delivered complete for trial, at the Liverpool end of the Railway, not later than the 1st of October next.

VIII. The price of the Engine which may be accepted not to exceed £550, delivered on the Railway; and any Engine not approved to be taken back by the Owner. N. B. — The Railway Company will provide the Engine Tender with a supply of Water and Fuel for the experiment. The distance within the Rails is four feet eight inches and a half.

THE GRAND LOCOMOTIVE COMPETITION

THE 'LIVERPOOL TIMES,' 13th OCTOBER 1829
ON TUESDAY, the first day of trial, the race-ground presented a scene of extraordinary gaiety and bustle. The day being remarkably fine, thousands of persons of all ranks were assembled from the surrounding towns and districts. Upwards of 10,000 persons were computed to have been present, among whom were a greater number of scientific men, and practical engineers, than have been assembled on any previous occasion.

During the whole of the day the different carriages were exhibiting on the Rail-Way, and it is scarcely possible for any one who has not seen them in motion to form any conception of their astonishing speed. In the early part of the day, the carriage of Mr. Robert Stephenson, of Newcastle, attracted great attention. It ran without any weight attached to it, at the rate of 24 miles in the hour, rushing past the spectators with amazing velocity. It has been stated by several of the papers that it emitted very little smoke; but the fact is, that during the trial it emitted none. Previous to the trial, a little coal was put into it, and then it sent forth a smoke; but after the trial had commenced, it used coke, which as it does not produce any smoke, of course could not emit any. We know that there were some persons on the ground who mistook steam for smoke. After this carriage had moved about for some time, without any weight, cars, containing stones, were attached to it, weighing, together with its own weight, upwards of 17 tons, preparatory to the trial of its speed being made. The precise distance between the point of starting, at or near the weighing shed, to the point of returning, was $1\frac{3}{4}$ mile; but in the adjudication of distances, we are given to understand the judges allowed a furlong at each end for the acquirement and abatement of speed. Our observations apply, however, to the whole distance. With a load of $12\frac{1}{2}$ tons gross, the *Rocket* travelled the above space of $1\frac{3}{4}$ mile, four times forward and backward, equal to 14 miles, in the space of 75 minutes, exclusive of stoppages; but, including the stoppages, the average rate was $10\frac{1}{2}$ miles per hour. In the fifth course, the rate of speed, with a load, augmented by passengers, until equal to 13 tons was full 15 miles an hour.

Mr. Hackworth, of Darlington, ran his carriage along the course during the day; but no trial of its speed with weights took place.

Mr. Winan's machine, worked by two men, and carrying six passengers, was also on the ground. It moved with no great velocity compared to the Locomotive Steam-Carriages, but with considerable speed considering that it was put in motion by human power. One of the

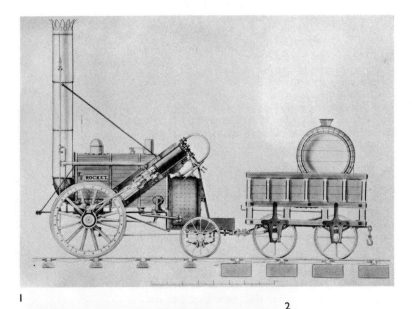

1

2

1 Robert Stephenson's *Rocket* as it appeared at the Rainhill Trials.
2 Timothy Hackworth, an assistant to the Stephensons, subsequently Engine Superintendent of the Stockton and Darlington Railway, who built many fine locomotives.
3 Hackworth's entry for the Rainhill Trials, the *Sans Pareil*.
4 A reproduction of the *Novelty* locomotive incorporating the wheels and one cylinder of the original engine.

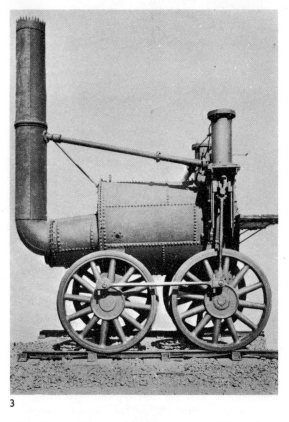

3

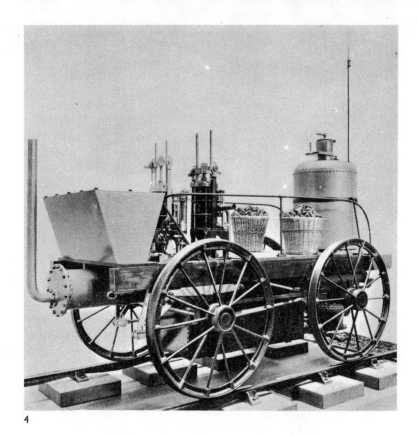

4

wheels was damaged in the course of the afternoon, by Mr. Hackworth's Locomotive Steam-Carriage.

Mr. Brandreth's horse-power Locomotive Engine exhibited, not in the way of competition, but as exercise. About fifty persons clung round the waggons, giving a gross weight, with the machine, of about 5 tons, and with this weight, the horses (themselves moving scarcely one mile and a quarter an hour) propelled the waggons and load exactly at the rate of five miles an hour.

The engine of Messrs. Braithwaite and Erickson, of London, was universally allowed to exhibit, in appearance and compactness, the beau-ideal of a Locomotive Carriage. Its performance, whilst exercising without a load was most astonishing, passing over a space of $2\frac{3}{4}$ miles in seven minutes and a quarter, including a stop-space of one minute and thirty-three seconds! Had the Rail-Way been completed, the engine would, at this rate, have gone nearly the whole way from Liverpool to Manchester within the hour. Mr. Braithwaite, has, indeed, publicly offered to stake £1000, that as soon as the road is opened, he will perform the entire distance in that time. The velocity with which the *Novelty* moved, surprised and amazed every beholder. It seemed indeed to fly, presenting one of the most sublime spectacles of mechanical ingenuity and human daring the world ever beheld. It actually made one giddy to look at it, and filled the breasts of thousands with lively fears for the safety of the

individuals who were on it, and who seemed not to run along the earth, but to fly, as it were, 'on the wings of the wind.'

On Wednesday Braithwaite and Erickson's carriage drew the weight assigned by the judges, namely, 6 tons 2 cwt., at the rate of $20\frac{3}{4}$ miles per hour. Unfortunately, however, the bellows burst after the first trip, so that the experiment had to be postponed.

The first systematic trial of the power of the engines, under the inspection of the judges, took place on Thursday, when Mr. Stephenson's carriage, the *Rocket*, was brought out to perform the task assigned. This engine has a boiler of a new construction, adapted for coke, the invention of Mr. Henry Booth, the treasurer to the Railway Company. The distance appointed to be run was 70 miles; and it was a condition that, when fairly started, the engine was to travel on the road at a speed of not less than 10 miles per hour, drawing after it a gross weight of 3 tons, for every ton weight of itself. Before starting, the machine was weighed, and the weight ascertained to be 4 tons 5 cwt. the gross weight to be drawn, therefore, was 12 tons 15 cwt., which was accordingly placed behind the engine, part of the said weight consisting of the engine tender, with the needful supply of water and fuel. The prescribed distance of 70 miles, it must be remembered, was to be accomplished by moving backwards and forwards, on a level plane of one mile and three-quarters in length; of course the engine had to pass along this plane 40 times, having

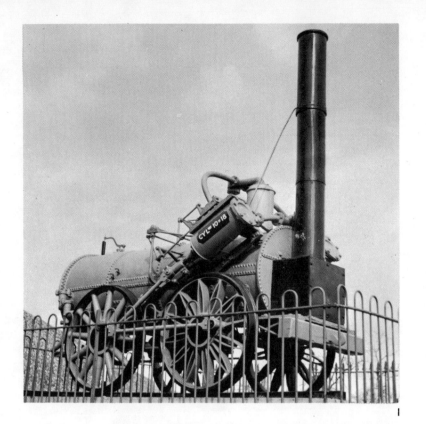

to make as many stops, and each time to regain the lost speed and momentum. She started on her journey about half-past ten in the morning, and performed the first 35 miles in 3 hours and 10 minutes, being upwards of 11 miles an hour. About a quarter of an hour was then consumed in filling the water tank, and obtaining a fresh supply of coke. The second 35 miles were accomplished in less time than the first, being performed in 2 hours and 52 minutes, which is at the rate of upwards of 12 miles an hour, including stoppages, the whole time from the first starting to the final arrival being under six hours and a half. The speed of the carriage over the ground was frequently 18 miles per hour, and sometimes more, and the motion is represented by the gentlemen who accompanied it, as particularly easy and agreable. The engine having to return and stop at the same point so frequently, opportunity was thereby afforded for a considerable number of gentlemen to have the pleasure of a ride; amongst others mounted behind the engine, we noticed Dr. Traill, Mr. Robert Gladstone, Mr. Henry Moss, etc. etc. On the whole, the performance gave great satisfaction, and the work done was far more than the quantum prescribed by the Directors of the Rail-Way.

On saturday morning ... the *Novelty* with her appointed load, started, and performed the first trip of three miles and a half in good style. On the second journey, however, owing to an accident to one of the pipes, all

locomotion was suspended; and before the injury, though unimportant, could be repaired, the day was too far advanced to recommence her allotted task. It was evident, from the frequent, though slight, derangements which had occurred to this engine, that a little further time was desirable before her performance should be again brought under the special notice of the judges. Accordingly, it was arranged by mutual consent that the London engine should run the 70 miles with her load on Wednesday (tomorrow). On the Saturday afternoon, however, the injury sustained being repaired, she appeared again on the course, with the Directors' carriage attached to her, in which were about forty ladies and gentlemen, and with which she moved along in beautiful style at the almost incredible speed of upwards of 30 miles per hour! In the course of the day, Mr. Stephenson's engine also performed an equally brilliant feat. Between the occurrence and the repair of the accident to Messrs. Braithwaite's carriage, that of Mr. Stephenson's the *Rocket,* ran, without load or tender, 7 miles in 14 minutes, which is at the rate of 30 miles an hour; and one of the trips of $3\frac{1}{2}$ miles was performed in 6 minutes and 37 seconds, which is at the rate of 32 miles an hour!

The trials lasted eight days altogether and at the end there was no doubt about it, Stephenson's *Rocket* was the winner, although some people felt that had there been a railway near London where the *Novelty* could have been tried out, and perhaps improved before the Trials, the result might have been different.

On 14th June 1830 a locomotive called the *Arrow* drew the first train from Liverpool to Manchester.

A month earlier, on 3rd May 1830, the Canterbury and Whitstable Railway was opened, to become the first railway on which passenger trains were hauled by steam locomotives. However, while technically the Kent line can claim historic precedence it was only worked by locomotive for the last two miles into Whitstable, the four miles at the Canterbury end being operated by fixed engines. Even then the incline out of Whitstable proved too much for the locomotive and a stationary engine was installed, leaving only a single mile worked by the locomotive.

A TRIP WITH MR. STEPHENSON

described by Fanny Kemble

IN AUGUST 1830 Fanny Kemble was playing at a Liverpool theatre. This famous niece of Sarah Siddons, who married a Philadelphian and fought for the emancipation of the slaves in Georgia, visited the railroad. She wrote to a friend:

My dear Harriet,

A common sheet of paper is enough for love, but a foolscap extra can alone contain a railroad and my ecstasies. There was once a man, who was born at Newcastle-upon-Tyne, who was a common coal-digger! this man had an immense constructiveness, which displayed itself in pulling his watch to pieces and putting it together again; in making a pair of white shoes when he happened to be some days without occupation; finally—here there is a great gap in my story it brought him in the capacity of an engineer before a committee of the House of Commons, with his head full of plans for constructing a railroad from Liverpool to Manchester. It so happened that to the quickest and most powerful perceptions, to the most indefatigable industry and perseverance, and the most accurate knowledge of the phenomena of nature as they affect his peculiar labours, this man joined an utter want of the 'gift of the gab.' He could no more explain to others what he meant to do and how he meant to do it, than he could fly; and therefore the members of the House of Commons, after saying 'There is rock to be excavated to a depth of more than sixty feet, there are embankments to be made nearly to the same height, there is a swamp of five miles in length to be traversed, in which if you drop an iron rod it sinks and disappears: how will you do all this?' and receiving no answer but a broad Northumbrian 'I can't tell you how I'll do it, but I can tell you I will do it,' dismissed Stephenson as a visionary. Having prevailed upon a company of Liverpool gentlemen to be less incredulous, and having raised funds for his great undertaking, in December of 1826 the first spade was struck into the ground.

And now I will give you an account of my yesterday's excursion. A party of sixteen persons was ushered into a large courtyard, where, under cover, stood several carriages of a peculiar construction, one of which was prepared for our reception. It was a long-bodied vehicle with seats placed across it, back to back; the one we were in had six of these benches and was a sort of uncovered char-a-banc. The wheels were placed upon two iron bands, which formed the road, and to which they are fitted, being so constructed as to slide along without any danger of hitching or becoming displaced, on the same principle as a thing sliding on a concave groove. The carriage was set in motion by a mere push, and, having received this impetus, rolled with us down an inclined plane into a tunnel which forms the entrance to the railroad. This tunnel is four hundred yards long (I believe) and will be lighted by gas. At the end of it we emerged from darkness, and, the ground becoming level, we stopped. There is another tunnel parallel with this, only much wider and longer, for it extends from the place which we had now reached, and where the steam-carriages start, and which is quite out of Liverpool, the whole way under the town, to the docks. This tunnel is for waggons and other heavy carriages; and as the engines which are to draw the trains along the railroad do not enter these tunnels, there is a large building at this entrance which is to be inhabited by steam-engines of a stationary turn of mind, and different construction from the travelling ones, which are to propel the trains through the tunnels to the terminus in the town, without going out of their houses themselves. The length of the tunnel parallel

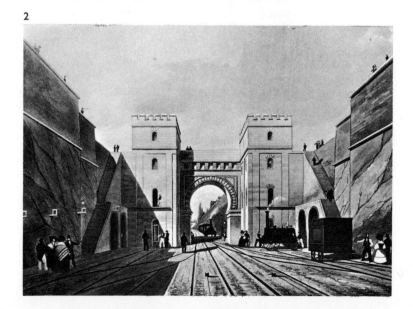

2

1 The *Invicta* locomotive driven by Edward Fletcher at the opening of the Canterbury and Whitstable Railway in 1830. (*Opposite*)
2 The Moorish arch at Edgehill, the exotic Liverpool entrance to the Liverpool and Manchester Railway, from a print by Ackermann and Co.

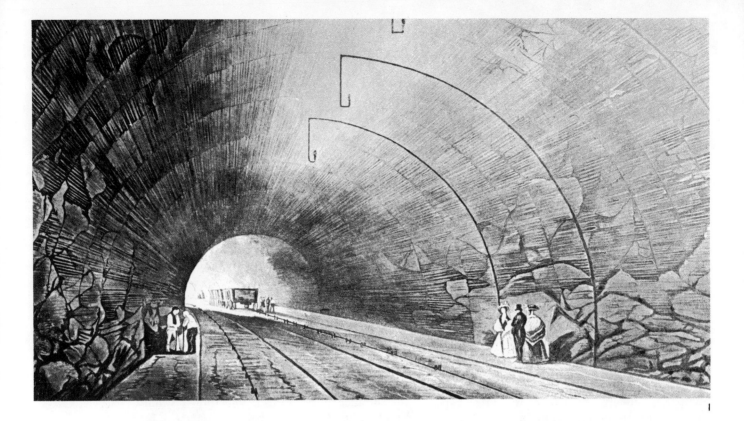

to the one we passed through is (I believe) two thousand two hundred yards.

I wonder if you are understanding one word of what I am saying all this while!

We were introduced to the little engine which was to drag us along the rails. She (for they make these curious little firehorses all mares) consisted of a boiler, a stove, a small platform, a bench, and behind the bench a barrel containing enough water to prevent her being thirsty for fifteen miles—the whole machine not bigger than a common fire-engine. She goes upon two pairs of wheels, which are her feet, and are moved by bright steel legs called pistons. These are propelled by steam, and in proportion as more steam is applied to the upper extremities (the hip-joints, I suppose) of these pistons, the faster they move the wheels; and when it is desirable to diminish the speed, the steam, which unless suffered to escape would burst the boiler, evaporates through a safety-valve into the air. The reins, bit, and bridle of this wonderful beast — a small handle which applies or withdraws the steam from its legs or pistons, so that a child could manage it. The coals, which are its oats, were under the bench, and there was a small glass tube affixed to the boiler, with water in it, which indicates by its fullness or emptiness when the creature wants water, which is immediately conveyed to it from its reservoirs. There is a chimney to the stove, but as they burn coke there is none of the dreadful black smoke which accompanies the progress of

a steam-vessel. This snorting little animal, which I felt rather inclined to pat, was then harnessed to our carriage, and, Mr. Stephenson having taken me on the bench of the engine with him, we started at about ten miles an hour.

The steam-horse being ill-adapted for going up and down hill, the road was kept at a certain level, and appeared sometimes to sink below the surface of the earth and sometimes to rise above it. Almost at starting it was cut through the solid rock, which formed a wall on either side of it, about sixty feet high. You can't imagine how strange it seemed to be journeying on thus, without any visible cause of progress other than the magical machine, with its flying white breath and rhythmical, unvarying pace, between these rocky walls, which are already clothed with moss and ferns and grasses. When I reflected that these great masses of stone had been cut asunder to allow our passage thus far below the surface of the earth, I felt as if no fairy tale was ever half so wonderful as what I saw. Bridges were thrown from side to side across the top of these cliffs, and the people looking down upon us from them seemed like pygmies standing in the sky.

I must be more concise, though, or I shall want room. We were to go only fifteen miles, that distance being sufficient to show the speed of the engine and take us to the most beautiful and wonderful object on the road. After proceeding through this rocky defile, we presently found ourselves raised upon embankments ten or twelve feet high. We then came to a moss

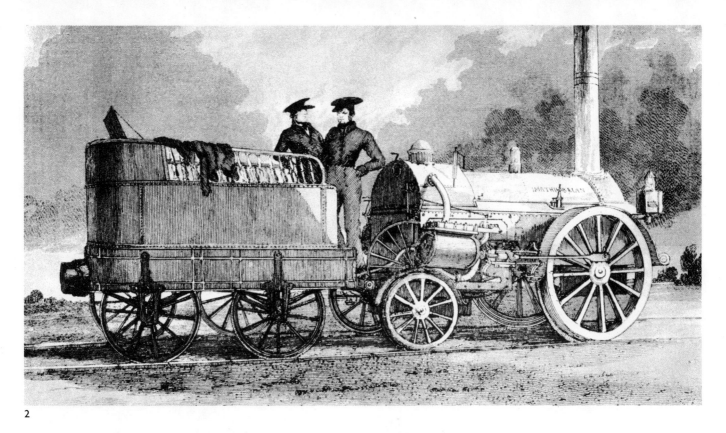

2

or swamp of considerable extent, on which no human feet could tread without sinking, and yet it bore the road which bore us. This had been the great stumbling-block in the minds of the committee of the House of Commons, but Mr. Stephenson had succeeded in overcoming it. A foundation of hurdles, or, as he called it, basket-work, was thrown over the morass, and the interstices were filled with moss and other elastic matter. Upon this the clay and soil were laid down and the road does float, for we passed over it at the rate of five and twenty miles an hour, and saw the stagnant swamp trembling on the surface of the soil on either side of us. I hope you understand me. The embankment had gradually been rising higher and higher, and in one place, where the soil was not settled enough to form banks, Stephenson had constructed artificial ones of wood-work, over which the mounds of earth would lie, for he said that though the wood-work would rot, before it did so the banks of earth which covered it would be sufficiently consolidated to support the road.

We had now come fifteen miles and stopped where the road traversed a wide and deep valley. Stephenson made me alight and led me down to the bottom of this ravine, over which, in order to keep his road level, he had thrown a magnificent viaduct of nine arches, the middle one of which is seventy feet high, through which we saw the whole of this beautiful little valley. It was lovely and wonderful beyond all words. Here he told me many curious things respecting this ravine; how he believed the Mersey had once rolled through it; how the soil had proved so unfavourable for the foundations of his bridge that it was built upon piles which had been driven into the earth to an enormous depth; how, while digging for a foundation, he had come to a tree bedded in the earth fourteen feet below the surface of the ground; how tides are caused, and how another flood might be caused; all of which I have remembered and noted down at much greater length than I can here enter upon it. He explained to me the whole construction of the steam-engine, and said he could soon make a famous engineer of me, which, considering the wonderful things he has achieved, I dare not say is impossible. His way of explaining himself is peculiar, but very striking, and I understood, without difficulty, all that he said to me. We then rejoined the rest of the party, and the engine having received its supply of water, the carriage was placed behind it, for it cannot turn, and was set off at its utmost speed, thirty-five miles an hour, swifter than a bird flies (for they tried the experiment with a snipe).

1 *The Tunnel,* from an Ackermann print. Locomotives were not used through the gas-lit tunnel, trains were rope-hauled by a stationary engine.
2 The *Northumbrian* locomotive built by the Stephensons for service on the Liverpool and Manchester Railway in 1831.

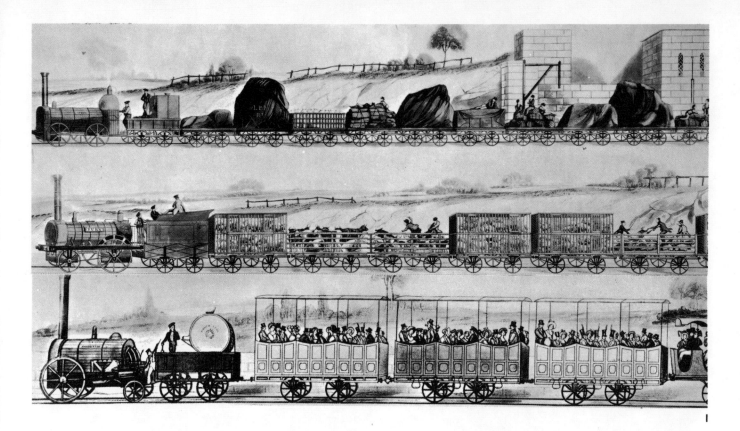

You cannot conceive what that sensation of cutting the air was; the motion is as smooth as possible too. I could either have read or written; and as it was, I stood up, and with my bonnet off 'drank the air before me.' The wind, which was strong, or perhaps the force of our own thrusting against it, absolutely weighed my eyelids down. When I closed my eyes this sensation of flying was quite delightful, and strange beyond description, yet, strange as it was, I had a perfect sense of security and not the slightest fear. At one time, to exhibit the power of the engine, Mr. Stephenson caused it to be fastened in front of ours; moreover, a waggon laden with timber was also chained to us, and thus propelling the idle steam engine, and dragging the loaded waggon which was beside it, and our own carriage full of people behind, this brave little she-dragon of ours flew on. Farther on she met three carts, which [were] fastened in front of her without the slightest delay or difficulty. When I add that this pretty little creature can run with equal facility either backwards or forwards, I believe I have given you an account of all her capacities.

Now for a word or two about the master of all these marvels, with whom I am most horribly in love. He is a man from fifty to fifty-five years of age. [Stephenson was then forty-nine.] His face is fine, though careworn, and bears an expression of deep thoughtfulness. His mode of explaining his ideas is peculiar and very original, striking, and forcible. Al-

though his accent indicates strongly his north country birth, his language has not the slightest touch of vulgarity or coarseness. He has certainly turned my head.

Four years have sufficed to bring this great undertaking to an end. The railroad will be opened upon the 15th of next month. The Duke of Wellington is coming down to be present on the occasion, and, I suppose, what with the thousands of spectators and the novelty of the spectacle, there will never have been a scene of more striking interest. The whole cost of the work (including the engine and carriages) will have been eight hundred and thirty thousand pounds. It is already worth double that sum. The directors have kindly offered us three places for the opening, which is a great favour, for people are bidding almost anything for a place, I understand!

Fanny managed to break her tour to return for the opening by the Duke of Wellington and described the occasion in another letter.

1 Goods trains and a second-class passenger train on the Liverpool and Manchester Railway, from prints published by the Ackermann Company in 1831-3.
2 The scene at Edgehill at the opening of the railway on 15th September 1830.

THE OPENING OF LIVERPOOL AND MANCHESTER RAILWAY

described by Fanny Kemble

WE STARTED [from Liverpool] on Wednesday last, to the number of about eight hundred people. The most intense curiosity and excitement prevailed. Though the weather was uncertain, enormous crowds of densely packed people lined the road, shouting and waving hats and handkerchiefs as we flew by them. What with the sight and sound of these cheering multitudes and the tremendous velocity with which we were borne past them, my spirits rose to the true champagne height, and I never enjoyed anything so much as the first hour of our progress.

I had been unluckily separated from my mother in the first distribution of places, but by an exchange of seats which she was enabled to make she rejoined me when I was at the height of my ecstasy, which was considerably dampened by finding that she was frightened to death, and intent upon nothing but devising means of escaping from a situation which appeared to her to threaten with instant annihilation herself and all her travelling companions.

While I was chewing the cud of this disappointment, which was rather bitter, as I had expected her to be as delighted as myself with our excursion, a man flew by us, calling out through a speaking trumpet to stop the engine, for that somebody in the directors' carriage had sustained an injury. We were all stopped accordingly, and presently a hundred voices were heard exclaiming that Mr. Huskisson was killed. The confusion that ensued is indescribable: the calling out from carriage to carriage to ascertain the truth, the

contrary reports which were sent back to us, the hundred questions eagerly uttered at once, and the repeated and urgent demands for surgical assistance, created a sudden turmoil that was quite sickening. At last we distinctly ascertained that the unfortunate man's thigh was broken.

From Lady Wilton, who was in the Duke's carriage, and within three yards of the spot where the accident happened, I had the following details, the horror of witnessing which we were spared through our situation behind the great carriage. The engine had stopped to take in a supply of water, and several of the gentlemen in the directors' carriage had jumped out to look about them. Lord Wilton, Count Batthyany, Count Matuscewitz, and Mr. Huskisson among the rest were standing talking on the middle of the road, when an engine on the other line, which was parading up and down merely to show its speed, was seen coming down upon them like lightning. The most active of those in peril sprang back into their seats. Lord Wilton saved his life only by rushing behind the Duke's [Wellington's] carriage, and Count Matuscewitz had but just leaped into it, with the engine all but touching his heels as he did so. Poor Mr. Huskisson, less active from the effects of age and ill health, bewildered too, by the frantic cries of 'Stop the engine! Clear the track!' that resounded on all sides, completely lost his head, looked helplessly to the right and left, and was instantaneously prostrated by the fatal machine, which dashed down like a thunderbolt upon him, and passed over his

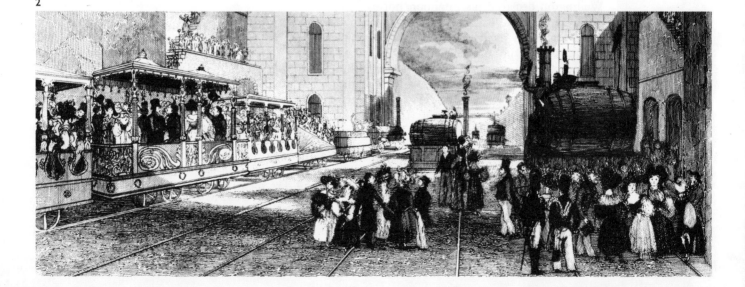

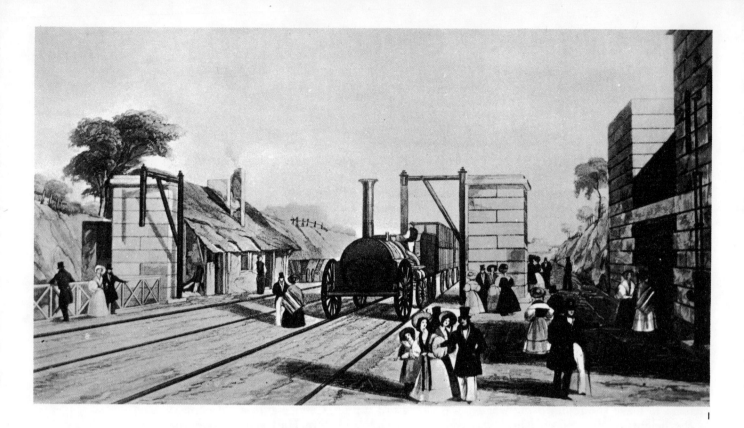

leg, smashing and mangling it in the most horrible way. (Lady Wilton said she distinctly heard the crushing of the bone.) So terrible was the effect of the appalling incident that, except for that ghastly 'crushing' and poor Mr. Huskisson's piercing shriek, not a sound was heard or a word uttered among the immediate spectators of the catastrophe.

Lord Wilton was the first to raise the poor sufferer, and calling to aid his surgical skill, which is considerable, he tied up the severed artery, and for a time, at least, prevented death by loss of blood. Mr. Huskisson was then placed in a carriage with his wife and Lord Wilton, and the engine, having been detached from the directors' carriage, conveyed them to Manchester.

So great was the shock produced upon the whole party by this event that the Duke of Wellington declared his intention not to proceed, but return immediately to Liverpool. However, upon its being represented to him that the whole population of Manchester had turned out to witness the procession, and that a disappointment might give rise to riots and disturbances, he consented to go on, and gloomily enough the rest of the journey was accomplished.

One Manchester man saw in the opening of the railway to Liverpool the beginning not only of economic but of political change. He wrote:

'Parliamentary Reform must follow soon after the opening of this road. A million of persons will pass over it in the course of this year, and see that hitherto unseen village of Newton; and they must be convinced of the absurdity of its sending two members to Parliament whilst Manchester sends none.'

During the years that followed, Britain became covered with a network of railways. Between 1825 and 1835 fifty-four Railway Acts were passed through Parliament — one of them for Robert Stephenson's London and Birmingham line. In the next two years thirty-nine received the royal assent, and then again in 1844—47 there was another boom in railway building. Through these arteries the development of industry was hastened and much of Britain changed from a rural to an urban society.

1 Parkside Station, where Mr. Huskisson's fatal accident took place.
2 Viaduct across the Sankey Valley, Lancashire.
3 The entrance to the railway at Edgehill, Liverpool. (2) and (3) drawn by T. T. Bury and published by Ackermann and Co. in 1831.

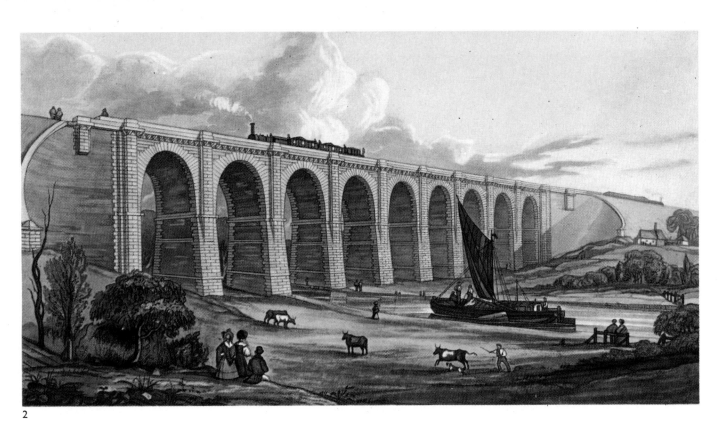

2

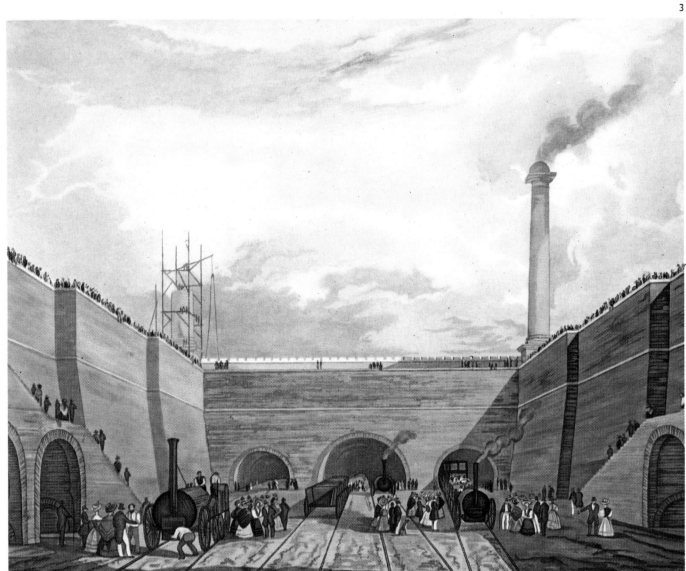

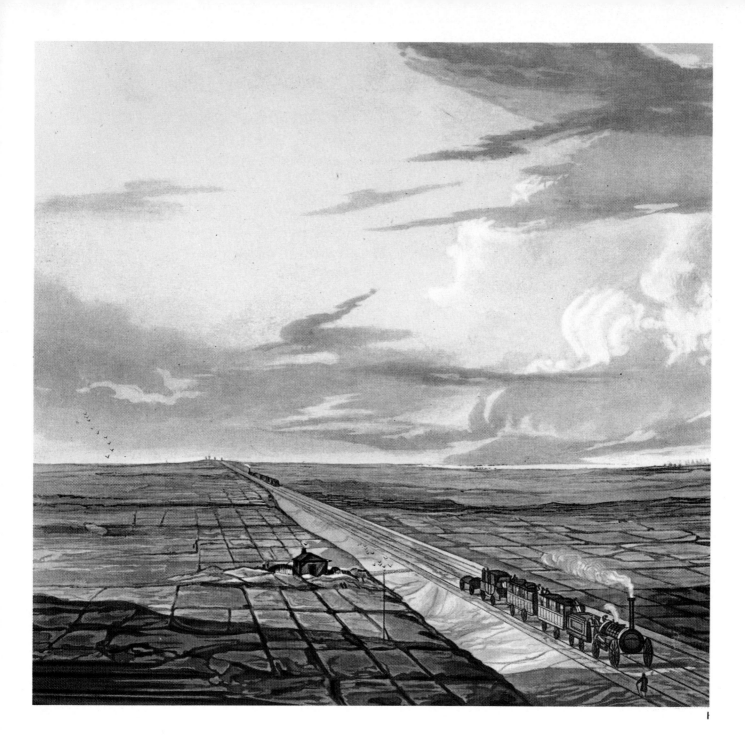

1 A view of the railway across Chat Moss.
2 The excavation of Olive Mount, four miles from
Liverpool. Both from Ackermann prints drawn by
T. T. Bury and engraved by H. Pyall.
3 A view of the Manchester and Liverpool Railway
taken at Newton in 1885, drawn by Calvert, aquatint
by Havell.

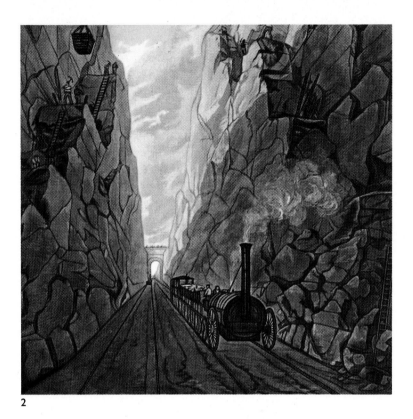

2

3

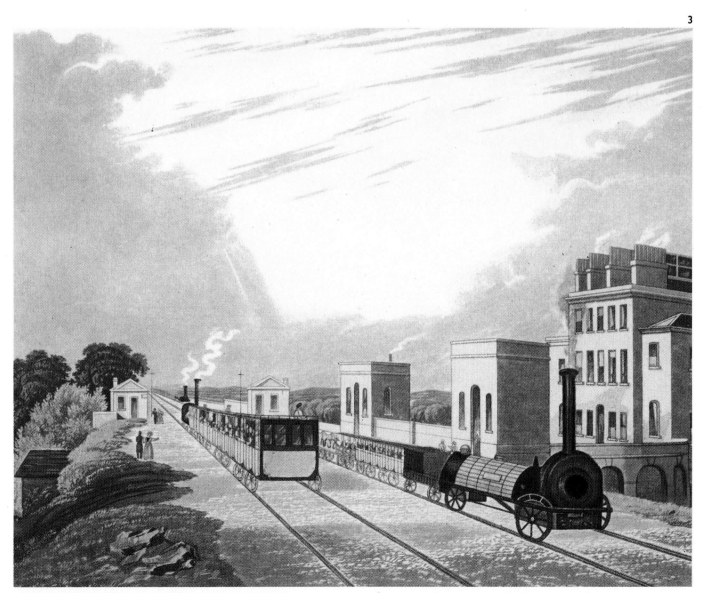

1

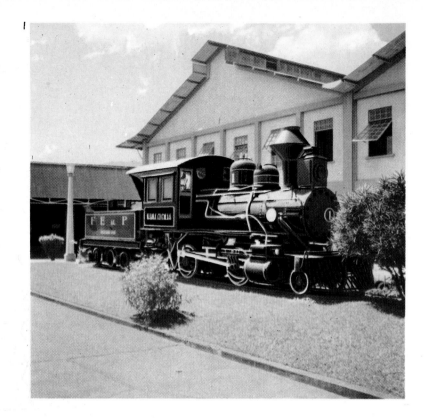

2

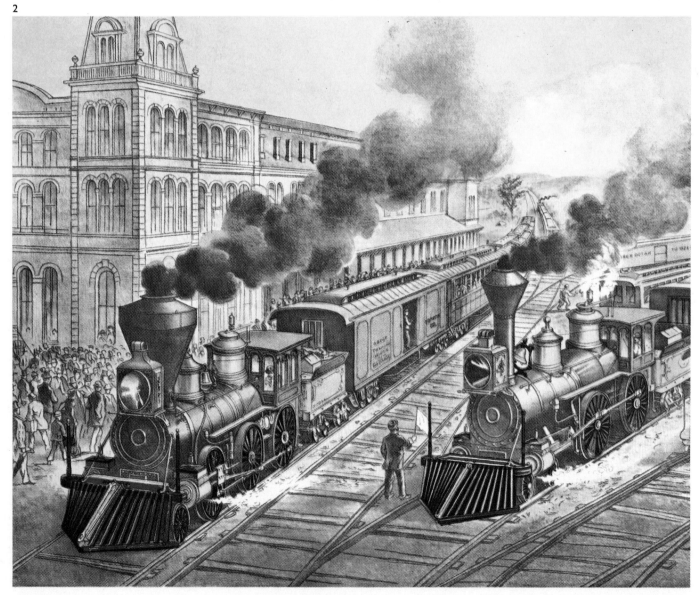

THE WORLD ADOPTS THE RAILWAY

THE SUCCESS of the Liverpool and Manchester Railway gave encouragement to railway enthusiasts elsewhere. More and more railways were built in Britain: the Leicester and Swannington, the Grand Junction Railway, the London and Birmingham, and in Scotland lines from Monkland to Kirkintilloch and from Glasgow to Garnkirk; and overseas the lines began to appear.

Steam locomotion was first introduced to France in 1832 on a mine railway which had been opened in 1823. The Dublin and Kingstown Railway in Ireland was opened in 1834. The same year the Belgian Government began construction of a line from Brussels to Malines which was opened in 1835 with two locomotives built by Stephenson. In December 1835 *Der Adler*, another Stephenson locomotive, opened the Ludwigsbahn from Nuremberg to Fürth.

A line from St. Petersburg to Pavlovsk was opened in 1837, although later development in Russia was slow. That year, too, the first steam locomotive, sent out from England, began work on the Kaiser Ferdinands Nordbahn near Vienna, though Austria had had horse railways since 1832.

In Holland a line from Amsterdam to Haarlem was opened on 24th September 1839 and ten days later five miles of line from Naples to Portici were opened in Italy. The first railway in Scandinavia, a privately owned line from Copenhagen to Roskilde, did not come until 1847 and railways in Norway and

3

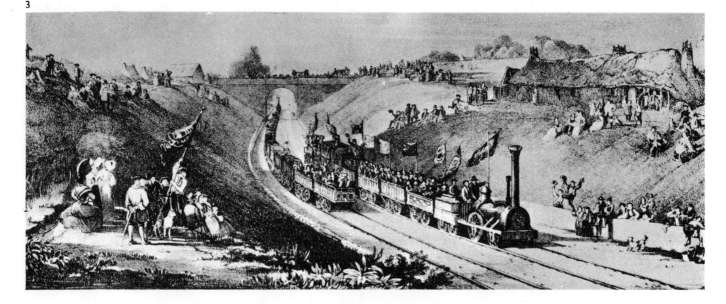

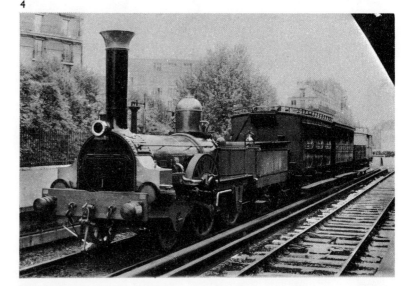

1 The first locomotive in Costa Rica.
2 American express trains, from a lithograph by Currie and Ives.
3 The opening of the Glasgow and Garnkirk Railway.
4 The *Buddicombe* locomotive which was in use on French railways in 1854.

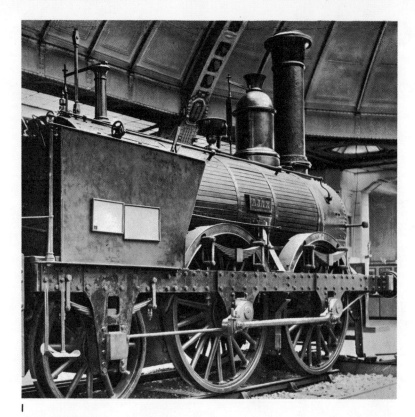

1

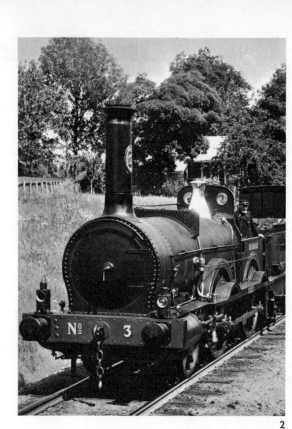

2

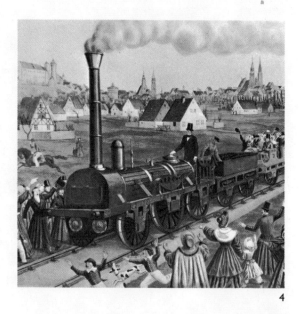

3

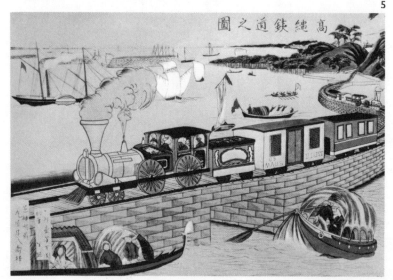

4

5

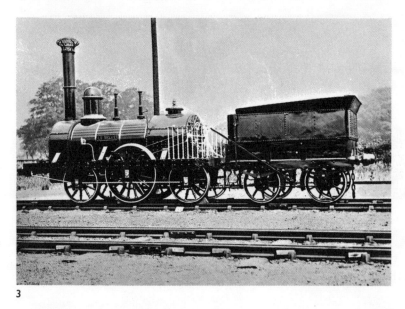

1—8 (1) Austria's oldest locomotive, the *Ajax*, was built by James Turner Evans at Newton. It first ran between Floridsdorf and Stokerau in July 1841. (2) An early Swedish train. (3) *La Belge,* built for the Belgian State Railway in 1835. (4) The opening of the Ludwigsbahn (from a painting). (5) Japanese print showing the railway at Takanawa in 1880. (6) Built by Stephenson, this locomotive was among the first imported into New South Wales in 1855. (7) A Fairlie type locomotive in use on the Port Chalmers Railway, New Zealand, in 1872. (8) Students inspecting a modern Chinese train. The Chinese Government of 1876 did not like railways but the People's Republic is today engaged on an enormous railway building programme.

Sweden did not appear until the next decade — and in Finland not until 1862.

Switzerland, which since 1844 had had a mile-long extension of the Alsace Railway linking Basle with the French frontier, built a line between Zürich and Baden in 1847. In 1849 Robert Stephenson was called in to advise on the country's railway development.

In 1848 the first Spanish line, from Barcelona to Mataró, was inaugurated with a ceremony, attended by the full court, at which the Cardinal Archbishop of Toledo blessed the locomotive.

As the rails spread across the Continent the European powers built railways in their overseas possessions. Indeed there was a railway in Cuba eleven years before the first line in Spain. In India there was strong pressure in favour of using waterways for communications, but railways were developed from 1853.

For Australia the British Government recommended a standard gauge of 4 ft. 8½ in. but in 1852 and 1853 New South Wales and Victoria went ahead with lines on a 5 ft. 3 in. gauge. The next year New South Wales converted to 4 ft. 8½ in. Later Queensland and Western Australia built lines at 3 ft. 6 in. — and South Australia had all three gauges! The result, still with us, is that travellers across Australia must change trains as they pass from state to state.

In New Zealand the Lyttelton and Christchurch Railway was commenced in 1860 to a gauge of 5 ft. 3 in. but an Act of Parliament in 1870 set down a gauge of 3 ft. 6 in. for all future railways, thereby preventing the confusion which grew up in Australia.

In Africa, Egypt's first railway dated from 1852, and at the other end of the Continent the first line, two miles long from Durban to the Point, opened in 1860. In 1862 the first steam trains began to run in South Africa between Cape Town and Eerste, and after the discovery of diamonds in 1867 the railway system grew rapidly.

Japan's first railway, between Yokohama, Tokyo and Shimbashi, was not opened until 1872; and the first railway in China, a nine-mile line from Shanghai to Woosung, begun in 1876, was torn up by the authorities — although four years later another line was opened.

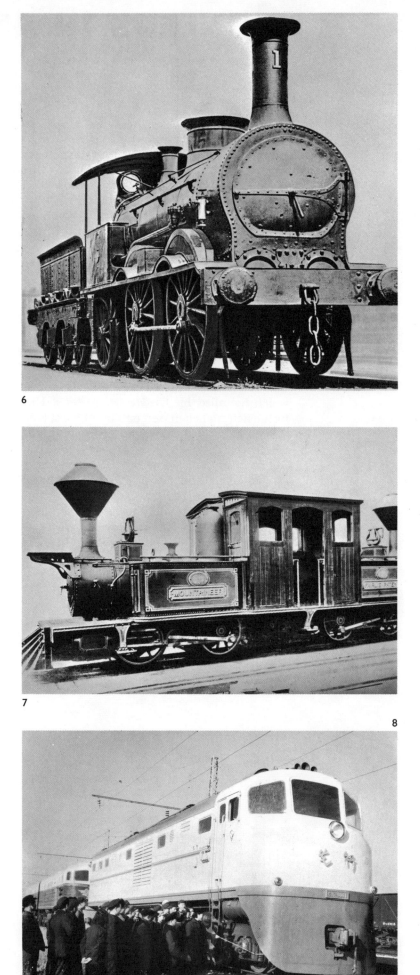

6

7

8

PIONEERS IN AMERICA

AS EARLY as 1764 there was a cable-operated tramway of grooved logs in operation in the United States at Lewiston, New York, where it hauled supplies for a military camp. Other similar tramways followed, including, in 1826, the horse-hauled Granite Railway in Quincey, Massachusetts. The wooden track of this railway was iron faced. Some people claim that this should be considered the 'first railroad in the United States'.

While Richard Trevithick was demonstrating his first locomotive in Europe, inventors were also at work in America. Oliver Evans, a Philadelphia blacksmith, was commissioned to build a dredge, but it ended up as a steam-operated dredge plus wheels and a propeller—the first steam-powered amphibious craft—which he called his *Orukter Amphibolos*. Unfortunately, when it set out on the cobbled streets of Philadelphia the axles and the wheels collapsed.

The first steam locomotive to run on tracks in the United States was built by Colonel John Stevens, a farsighted advocate of railways who, in 1812, published a paper entitled *Documents relating to the superior advantage of Railways over Canal Navigation*. In 1825 he built a circular track with a racked rail on his estate at Hoboken, New Jersey. On this track his locomotive reached a speed of twelve miles per hour carrying six passengers.

Although Stevens, by this time seventy-six, made no further active contribution to American railroad history, his demonstrations stimulated the interest of others. Among them was John Jervis, chief engineer of the Delaware and Hudson Canal Company. In 1828 his company built a nine-mile stretch of horse-operated track between their mines and the end of their canal at Honesdale, Pennsylvania. The same year Jervis sent his assistant, Horatio B. Allen, to England, where he was a witness of the Rainhill Trials. Allen was commissioned to purchase locomotives for the company.

One of them, the *Stourbridge Lion*, arrived in New York in May 1829 and was tried out at Honesdale on 8th August 1829 with Allen at the controls. A festive crowd turned up for the occasion and a cannon was fired for the official start (overcharged, it tore the arm off the man who discharged it). The locomotive, with a red and gold lion's head on the front of the boiler, weighed nearly eight tons—five tons more than had been thought at the time of its purchase.

Three hundred yards from the start the track crossed a rickety trestle bridge thirty feet above Lackawaxen Creek. Allen took it at full speed, twenty miles an hour, and reached the other side. Three miles farther on he reversed and came back to the start. The *Lion* had proved itself, but it was immediately decided that it was too heavy for the track and its active life was brought to a rapid close.

The following year a one-horse-power engine, called *Tom Thumb*, was tried out on the Baltimore and Ohio Railroad and hauled a car-load of thirty-six people at a maximum speed of eighteen miles per hour.

British engineers had advised that the curves

1

2

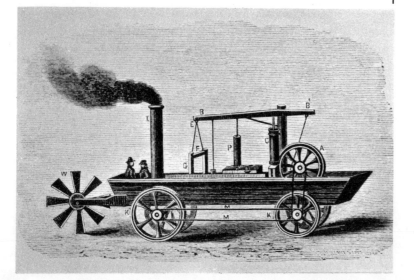

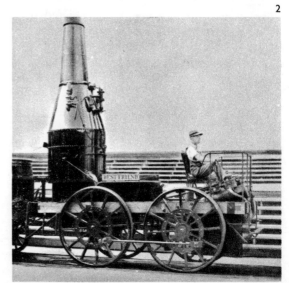

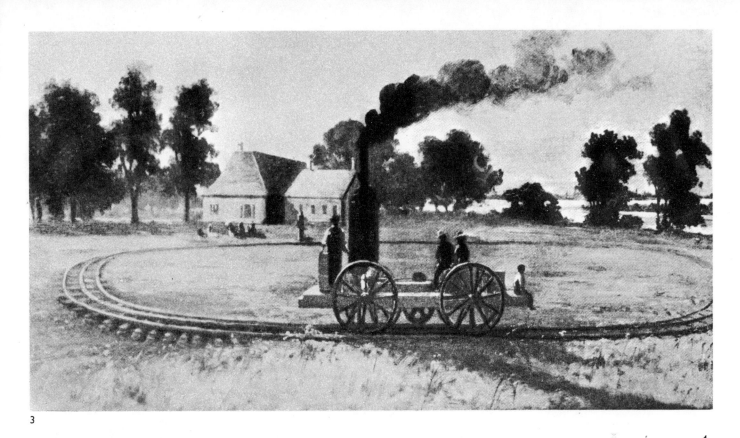

3

4

1 Evans's *Orukter Amphibolos*.
2 The *Best Friend of Charleston*.
3 John Stevens's Experimental Railway.
4 The *Stourbridge Lion*, built by Poster and Rastrick.
5 Peter Cooper's *Tom Thumb* (1829-30).
6 The *Atlantic* locomotive.

of the Baltimore and Ohio's track, which included one on a 150-foot radius, made it impossible to use steam power on the railroad. Shareholders began to withdraw. Peter Cooper, a man who had bought land along the track, was worried about his own investment. As he told it later in the *Boston Herald*, the directors of the railroad 'had a fit of the blues. I had naturally a knack of contriving, and I told the

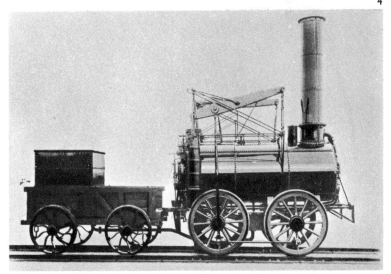

5

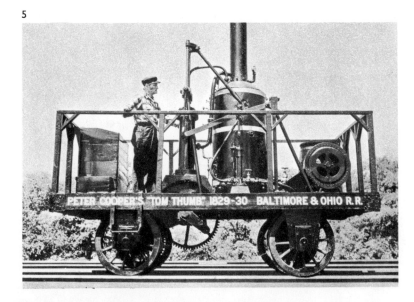

6

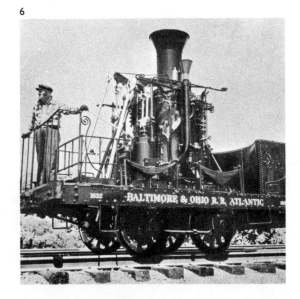

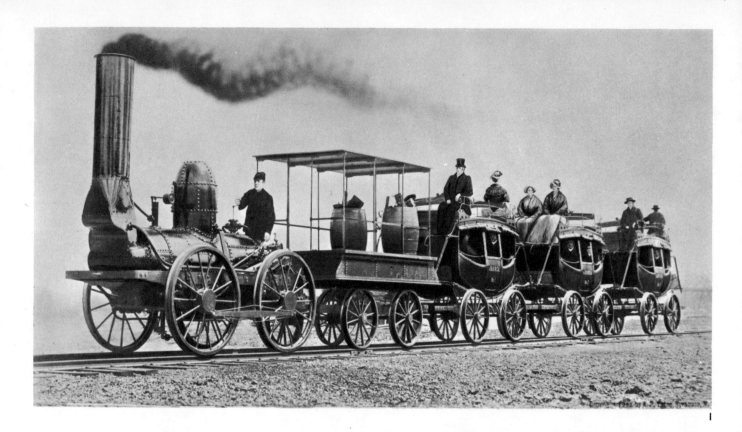

directors I believed I could knock together a locomotive that would get around that curve . . .

'So I came to New York and got a bit of an engine, about one horse-power (three and one-half cylinder and fourteen-inch stroke), and carried it back to Baltimore.'

Cooper added a boiler and set his engine up on wheels—and it worked. The trial on 28th August 1830 attracted little attention in the press, but it perturbed the local stage-coach operators. The largest firm challenged Cooper to a race. On a double track their finest grey was set against the *Tom Thumb*.

The horse soon had the lead, but the locomotive built up power and speed and overtook the horse. It was well ahead when the belt

which operated the fan for the fire slipped from its pulley. As the steam pressure fell the speed of the locomotive dropped, and the horse came galloping past to win, to the delight of the supporters of the horse-drawn train. But their jubilation did not prevent the Baltimore and Ohio directors from deciding to adopt steam power. As far as they were concerned the little *Tom Thumb* had amply proved itself.

Like the Liverpool and Manchester Railway in Britain the company announced a competition for a steam engine, which was won in 1831 by the *Atlantic*, the first 'grasshopper'-type locomotive, built at York, Pennsylvania, by Phineas Davis.

Late in 1829, Horatio Allen, driver of the *Lion*, took charge of the building of a railroad

2

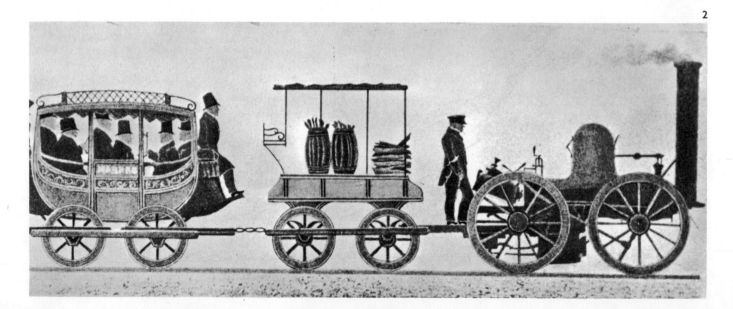

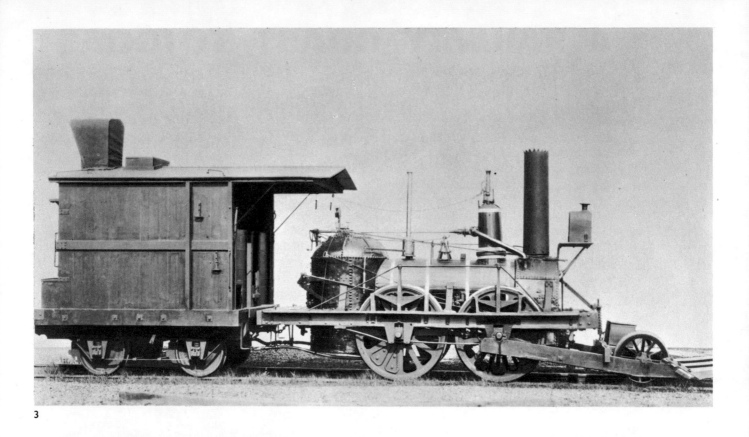

3

1 *De Witt Clinton, the third successful locomotive to be built in America.*
2 This print shows it pulling its first train from Albany to Schenectady. It covered the 14 miles in 46 minutes. Horse-drawn cars took about 1½ hours.
3 The *John Bull*, built by Robert Stephenson for the Camden and Amboy Railroad (1831), was the first locomotive to have a cowcatcher, added after its arrival in the United States.

for the South Carolina Canal and Railroad Company. The seaport of Charleston saw how the Baltimore and Ohio line would increase Baltimore's trade at their expense, and so planned a railway of its own.

Allen ordered two locomotives to be built by the West Point Foundry in New York City, and this railroad can claim to be the first in the United States built expressly for steam locomotion. The first locomotive, named *The Best Friend of Charleston*, arrived by sea in October and, after undergoing trials, drew the first train out of Charleston on Christmas Day 1830. Behind the locomotive was a flat wagon with a detachment of artillerymen and the cannon used to signal the opening, then came two covered coaches full of celebrities and dignitaries. Great crowds came to watch, and there were bands and fireworks.

The locomotive gave excellent service for six months, then one day her fireman shut off the safety valve and the boiler exploded, making an end of him and of his *Best Friend*. To dispel the fears this incident put in passengers' heads the line thereafter placed a flat car piled with bales of cotton immediately behind the locomotive. The cotton was to shield the passengers should a similar accident occur.

The makers of *The Best Friend* supplied the first locomotive, the *De Witt Clinton*, for the Mohawk and Hudson Railroad. A charter for the railroad had been given in 1826, but various delays prevented the completion of the seventeen-mile track until 1831.

On the inauguratory trip the passengers came under a rain of smoke, sparks and cinders from the chimney stack. Those in the open carriages protected themselves with their umbrellas — only to find that the umbrella covers disappeared in flames. Soon the passengers found their clothes were on fire and most of them spent the journey trying to put each other out! However, not one person who set out failed to complete both the outward and the return journeys.

Within ten years of the opening of these first American railroads there were nearly three thousand miles of track in operation in the United States, and by the outbreak of the Civil War the total had increased tenfold. Unfortunately, these lines were not to a standard gauge, which made through traffic impossible.

A RAILWAY COAST TO COAST

IN 1835 Senator Chase of Ohio introduced a Bill to the United States Congress to provide a survey of four routes for a railroad to link the nation from coast to coast; Jefferson Davis, Secretary of War, initiated reconnaissance for five other routes; and two years later Stephen A. Douglas promoted another Bill to provide three further routes—but, though interest and speculation was considerable and much research was done, no positive action was taken to build a railroad to link the eastern and western states of the United States.

In 1861 the beginning of the Civil War made clear the vulnerability of the nearly isolated west coast. It was national defence, rather than anything else, that led to the passing of the Enabling Act, signed by Abraham Lincoln

help finance the railway. The railway received a strip of land, 130 yards wide, along its whole length, and in addition a further grant of 3,000 acres of land, to be freely selected by the railway authorities within ten miles of the tracks, was made for every mile of line. There was still difficulty in raising money and by Act of 2nd July 1864 Lincoln doubled the land grants.

There was disagreement from the start. The engineers thought that the line should connect with a 4 ft. $8\frac{1}{2}$ in. gauge line east of Missouri, but California already had a five-foot gauge railway. Lincoln supported their demand for a five-foot gauge on the new line, but Congress prescribed the standard gauge. (In the circumstances Congress was right, but if the choice

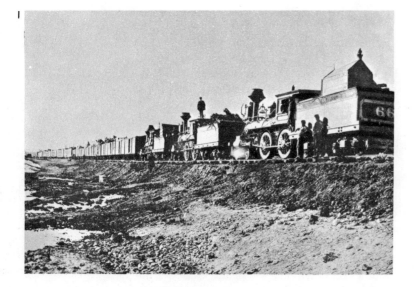

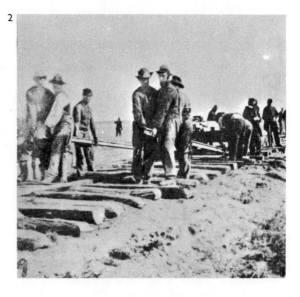

on 1st July 1862, which created the 'Union Pacific Railroad Company, authorising it to 'lay out, construct, furnish and maintain and enjoy a continuous railroad and telegraph line, with the appurtenances, from a point on the 100th meridian of longitude west from Greenwich between the south margin of the valley of the Republican river and the north margin of the valley of the Platte in the Territory of Nebraska to the western boundary of Nevada Territory.'

The Act also provided for a connection between a point on the western boundary of the state of Iowa and the 100th meridian, and provided for land grants and bond issues to

1 A construction train for the trans-American railway. The workers lived in, and on top of, the long cars which were also used as store rooms for food and dining cars. The train moved forward as building progressed.
2 Track-laying in Wyoming.
THE TRANSCONTINENTAL LINE TODAY
3 A diesel freight train of the Union Pacific Railroad in the Columbia River Gorge, Oregon.
4 Southern Pacific streamliner *Golden State* near Picacho Peak, Arizona.

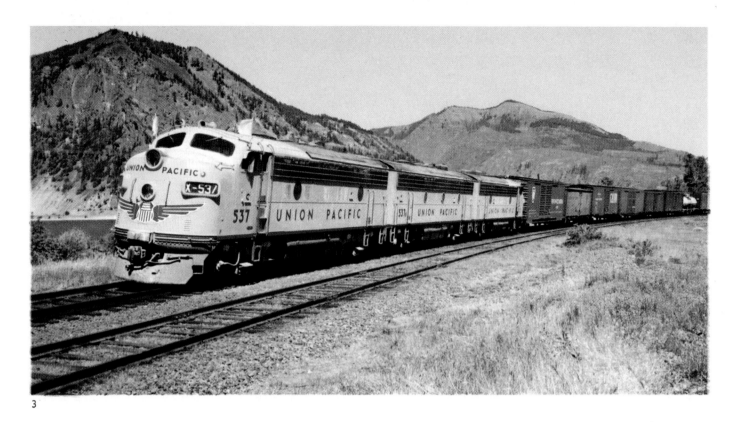

3

4

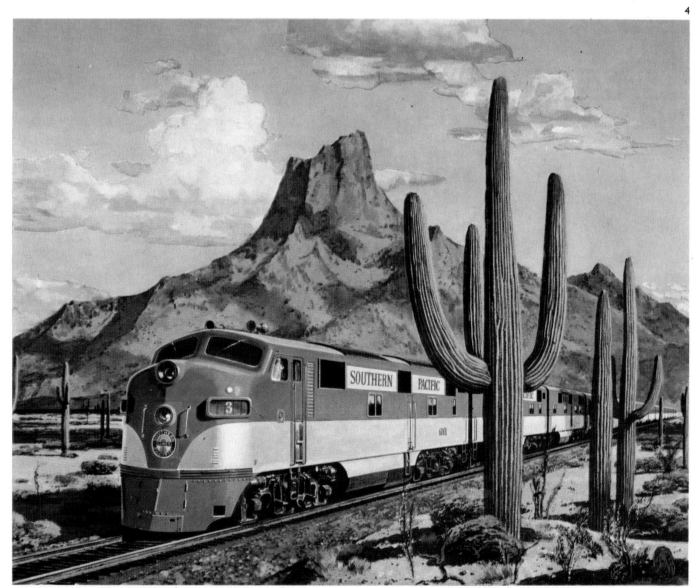

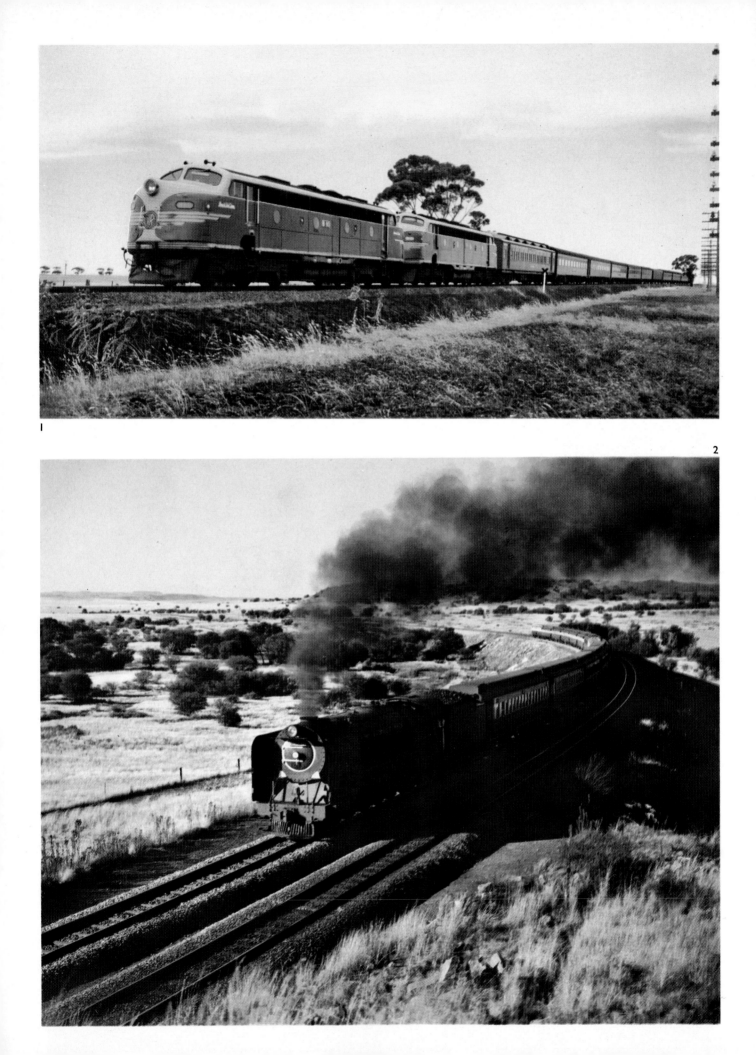

1

2

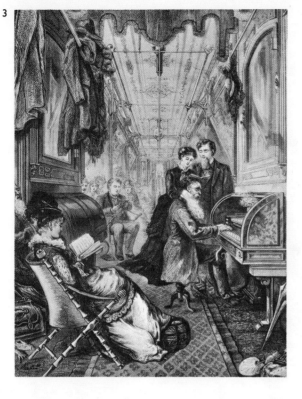

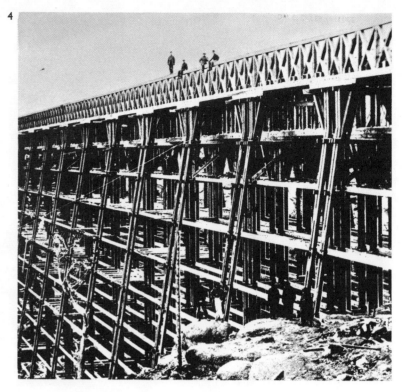

could be made today a wide gauge would probably be chosen.)

The first sod was cut at Sacramento, California on 22nd February 1863. But in the east there were more complications. Lincoln had specified a place called Council Bluffs, across river from Omaha, as the Missouri railhead. The engineers preferred Bellevue, a few miles farther south, and started construction there. $100,000 had been spent before the President forced them to stop. Construction from Council Bluffs began on 2nd December 1863, but the first rail was not laid until July 1865. The task was formidable. Raw materials, including 6,250 sleepers and 50,000 tons of rails, had to be carried over hundreds of miles from the east by ox cart, or by boat up the Missouri River.

As the railway grew the rails were brought up to the end of the line on an open truck drawn by two horses, which were then unhitched and a single small horse used. A crew of five men stood on each side of the track. At a command from the foreman each crew seized a rail from the back of the truck, pulled it out to its full

length and, at the foreman's shout of 'Down,' placed it on the sleepers. A man at the far end checked and adjusted the width between the rails and the horse moved forward pulling the truck over the newly laid rail, the process being repeated until the load of thirty rails had all been laid. Following close behind the layers came the teams who spiked the rails to the sleepers. An average of two miles was laid each day.

When they reached the plains the construction teams came under Indian attack. The Indians were right in seeing the railroad as an enemy. It opened up new territory and made possible the extinction of the bison herds, destroying the Indians' hunting grounds and rapidly leading to their confinement in reservations. But the Indians made pioneering a railroad a dangerous occupation.

The construction gangs had to take everything they needed with them, and every few miles a new 'end of track' town sprang up, complete with saloons and gambling houses operated by hangers-on who saw an easy way of making money out of the isolated railroad men. This travelling community was given the name of 'Hell on Wheels', and at one stage got so rough that the army at Fort D. A. Russell in Wyoming was called in to restore order. The entire 'population' was run out of town and only permitted to return when arrangements had been made to ensure that in future the community would be orderly.

In 1867 the line reached an altitude of 8,247 feet at Sherman Hill as it crossed the Rocky

1 Australia today: a double-headed diesel passenger train of the Victorian State Railways.
2 The *Orange Express* near Brandfort, Orange Free State, South Africa.
3 Sunday on the Union Pacific Railway about 1875.
4 Dale Creek Bridge in Wyoming was built of timber and later replaced by a 'spider web' bridge of steel, only to be abandoned for a more direct route.

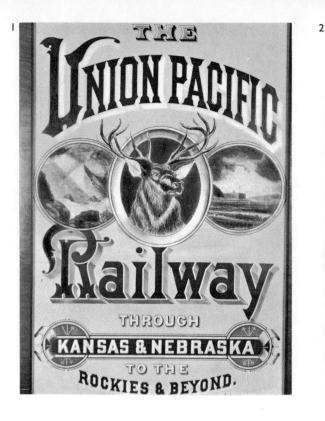

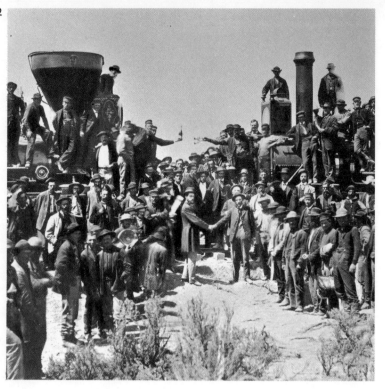

Mountains. Meanwhile the Central Pacific Company was following the watercourses up the western slopes of the Sierra Nevada. Originally it had been planned that they should only build the line as far as the boundary of California, but permission was obtained to continue eastward to meet the other company and they pressed on across Nevada to the Great Salt Lake.

Both companies pushed forward, eager for the grants of land that more line built would give. They met early in 1869 in Western Utah, but neither company would acknowledge the fact. Both went on building line at speed. Congress debated ways of stopping this pointless competition. After 225 miles of double track had been laid agreement was reached and the link was made on 10th May 1869.

The ceremony opened with a prayer, then the spikes of silver and gold and a special sleeper, which were to be used for the formal completion of the line, were presented and all except the final golden spike were driven home.

Governor Sandford, the President of Central Pacific, raised his maul, which had been wired so that by telegraph its blows would ring the fire alarm of the Tower in San Francisco and the bell of the Capitol in Washington, signalling to all America that the railway was complete. Governor Sandford struck; and missed, as did Dr. Durant who struck the next blow. Other guests were invited to tap the spike and it fell into place in the hole bored for it.

Two locomotives, *Jupiter* and 119, were unhooked from their trains and moved forward until their cowcatchers touched and bottles of champagne were broken. Then, hooked up again, the trains took it in turns to cross the rails. The ceremonial spikes and sleeper were then quickly removed and replaced by conventional materials; but the new sleeper was soon torn to pieces by souvenir hunters, and half a dozen more—and two rails—had to be replaced in the next six months.

1 An early poster advertising the transcontinental route.
2 The scene at Promontory, Utah, on 10th May 1869. The railroad is complete — shaking hands in the centre are Mr. Montague (left), Chief Engineer of the Central Pacific and Mr. Dodge (right), Chief Engineer of the Union Pacific Railroad.
3 *Across the Continent,* a Currier and Ives lithograph (1868).

ACROSS THE PLAINS

I MADE MY OBSERVATORY on the top of a fruit-waggon, and sat by the hour upon that perch to spy about me, and to spy in vain for something new. It was a world almost without a feature; an empty sky, an empty earth; front and back, the line of railway stretched from horizon to horizon, like a cue across a billiard-board; on either hand, the green plain ran till it touched the skirts of heaven.

Along the track innumerable wild sunflowers, no bigger than a crown-piece, bloomed in a continuous flowerbed; grazing beasts were seen upon the prairie at all degrees of distance and diminution; and now and again we might perceive a few dots beside the railroad which grew more and more distinct as we drew nearer till they turned into wooden cabins, and then dwindled and dwindled in our wake until they melted into their surroundings, and we were once more alone upon the billiard-board. The train toiled over this infinity like a snail; and being the one thing moving, it was wonderful what huge proportions it began to assume in our regard. It seemed miles in length, and either end of it within but a step of the horizon. Even my own body or my own head seemed a great thing in that emptiness. I note the feeling the more readily as it is the contrary of what I have read of in the experience of others. Day and night, above the roar of the train, our ears were kept busy with the incessant chirp of grasshoppers—a noise like the winding up of countless clocks and watches,

3

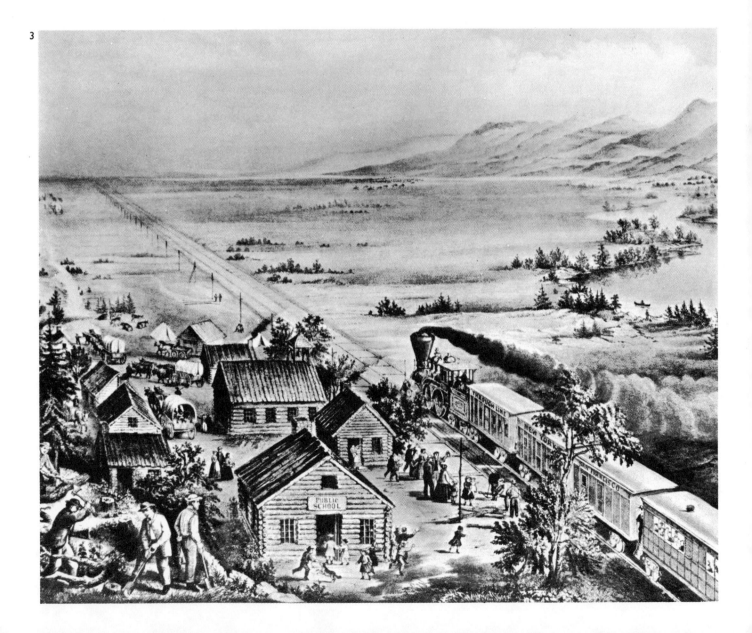

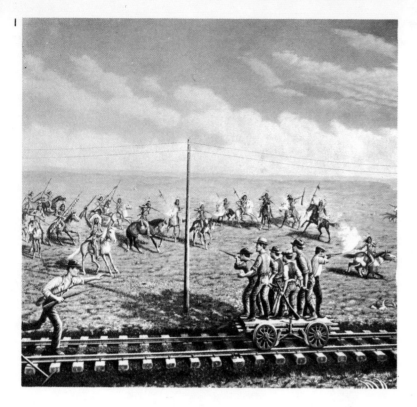

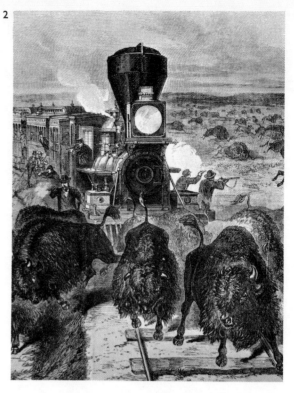

which began after a while to seem proper to that land.

To one hurrying through by steam there was a certain exhilaration in this spacious vacancy, this greatness of the air, this discovery of the whole arch of heaven, this straight, unbroken, prison-line of the horizon.

Although it was chill, I was obliged to open my window, for the degradation of the air soon became intolerable to one who was awake and using the full supply of life. Outside, in a glimmering night, I saw the black, amorphous hills shoot by unweariedly into our wake. They that long for morning have never longed for it more earnestly than I.

And yet when day came, it was to shine upon the same broken and unsightly quarter of the world. Mile upon mile, and not a tree, a bird, or a river. Only down the long, sterile canyons, the train shot hooting and awoke the resting echo. That train was the one piece of life in all the deadly land; it was the one actor, the one spectacle fit to be observed in this paralysis of man and nature. And when I think how the railroad has been pushed through this unwatered wilderness and haunt of savage tribes and now will bear an emigrant for some £12 from the Atlantic to the Golden Gates, how at each stage of the construction, roaring, impromptu cities, full of gold and lust and death, sprang up and then died away

again, and are now but wayside stations in the desert; how in these uncouth places pigtailed Chinese pirates worked side by side with border ruffians and broken men from Europe, talking together in a mixed dialect, mostly oaths, gambling, drinking, quarrelling and murdering like wolves; how the plumed hereditary lord of all America heard, in this last fastness, the scream of the 'bad medicine waggon' charioting his foes; and then when I go on to remember that all this epical turmoil was conducted by gentlemen in frock coats, and with a view to nothing more extraordinary than a fortune and a subsequent visit to the one typical achievement of the age in which we live, as if it brought together into one plot all the ends of the world and all the degrees of social rank, and offered to some great writer the busiest, the most extended, and the most varied subject for an enduring literary work. If it be romance, if it be contrast, if it be heroism that we require, what was Troy town to this? But, alas! it is not these things that are necessary —it is only Homer.

Here also we are grateful to the train, as to some god who conducts us swiftly through these shades and by so many hidden perils. Thirst, hunger, the sleight and ferocity of Indians are all no more feared, so lightly do we skim these horrible lands; as the gull, who wings safely through the hurricane and past the shark.

FROM 'ACROSS THE PLAINS'
BY ROBERT LOUIS STEVENSON.

RAILWAYS ACROSS THE CONTINENTS

IN 1870 a start was made on a railway from Callao, in Peru, across the highlands of Oraya to the navigable part of the Amazon, which would link the Pacific and Atlantic coasts of South America. The railway itself was only a small part of the route, most of which would have been by water, but the difficulties in building it were considerable, for the line had to cross the Andean Cordillera.

The mountains rose sheer above deep valleys to sharp ridges and pointed peaks, and it took all the skill of the engineer, the heroic pioneer Henry Meiggs, to find a route. He blasted his way along the mountainside, and when he could go no farther doubled back and zigzagged higher. He used two hundred and fifty tons of dynamite every month and in one ten-mile stretch alone had to drill out fifty tunnels.

When the line reached 6,000 feet a fever epidemic broke out among the crews. When, in 1877, it had reached an altitude of 12,000 feet Meiggs himself died, worn out. The cost of the line over those seven years was 7,000 dead from a labour force of 8,000—a high price to pay.

Fourteen years later the line was completed. At an altitude of 15,694 feet the Galera Tunnel, the highest in the world, was driven through the mountains. Because of the rarefied air it was only possible to work for about three hours a day.

Farther south in Chile and Bolivia the line between Antofagasta and La Paz reaches a height of 13,000 feet. The 729-mile journey takes about forty-eight hours. The line between La Paz and Arica, part of which is racked, has the highest station in the world—General Lagos, at an altitude of 13,900 feet.

On all these routes trains have to be stopped for a time around 7,000 feet to enable passen-

1 Cheyenne Indians, led by Tall Bull, attack a hand-car crew near Fossil Creek, Kansas, on 28th May 1869.
2 Shooting buffaloes in the far west in 1871.
3 The Marquis Viaduct on the Valparaiso and Santiago Railway, 120 ft. high and 600 ft. in length.
4 The line of the Canadian Pacific Railway penetrates the prairies south of Moose Jaw Amulet, Saskatchewan.
5 Driving in the golden spike on the Canadian Pacific Railway, 7th November 1885.

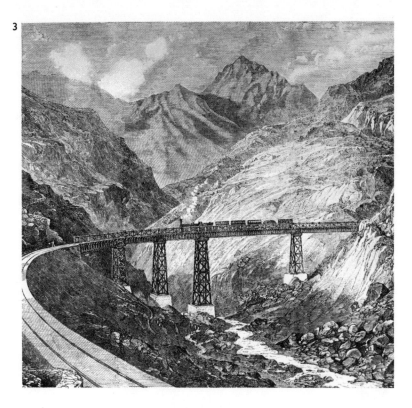

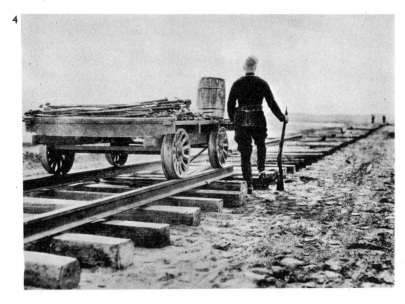

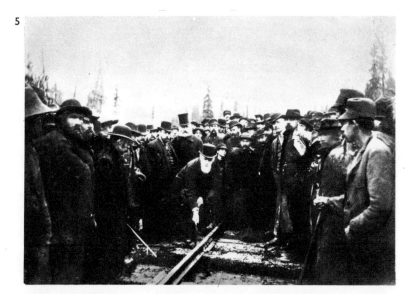

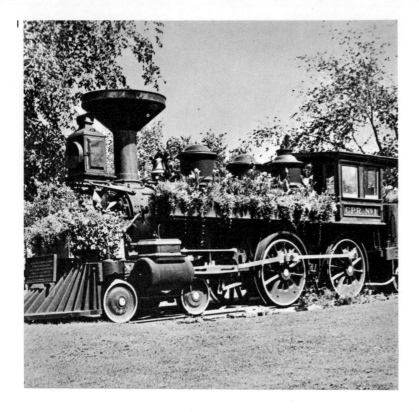

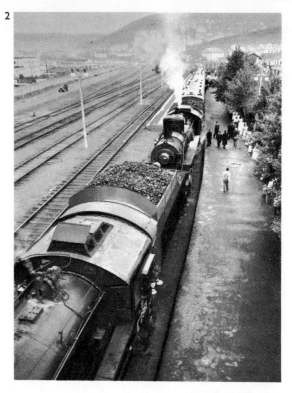

gers not used to the rarefied air to get accustomed to it.

In 1871 a promise of a transcontinental line played a major part in the creation of the modern Dominion of Canada, for the building of such a line was one of the conditions on which British Columbia and the Maritime Provinces insisted before agreeing to enter the confederation. The Intercolonial Railway to the East was completed by 1876. The Pacific Line, although started in 1874, was so delayed that British Columbia talked of secession. In 1880 the building of the line was taken over by the Canadian Pacific Company, and it was completed in 1885. The engineering achievement not only involved the conquest of the Rockies but meant taking the line across the swamps north of Lake Superior, which sucked up an immeasurable quantity of trees and rock. Even when the line was finally laid across them, sleepers forty feet long had to be used to spread the load. Two other trans-Canadian railways grew out of the Grand Trunk Railway and the Northern Railway. Both are now part of the Canadian National system.

The longest railway journey in the world is from Moscow to Vladivostock on the Trans-Siberian Railway, a distance equivalent to that between London and the tip of Africa.

As early as 1851 the Governor of Eastern Siberia had suggested that a road (on which a railway could later be laid) should be built to link his territories with European Russia,

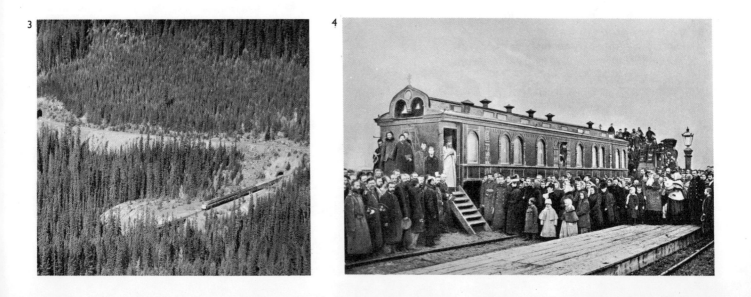

but it was not until March 1891 that the construction of the line was authorised by Tsar Alexander III. His son, Tsarevich Nicholas, was made chairman of the construction committee. 'The fulfilment of this essential peaceful work,' he said, '. . . is my sacred duty and my sincere desire. I hope to complete the construction of the Siberian line and to have it done cheaply and—most important of all—quickly and solidly.'

Construction began from Vladivostock, in the east, in May 1891 and from Chelyabinsk, in the Urals 4,627 miles away, in July 1892. Materials for the Pacific end of the line had to be shipped right round Asia via the Suez Canal or right round Africa as well. In the west the great Siberian rivers could be used for transportation—during those months of the year when they were not frozen over. Cold, rain, disease and shortage of labour all slowed down what was already a superhuman task of engineering. West of Lake Baikal alone eight massive bridges over 1,000 feet wide had to be built, including ones of 2,800 feet, 2,670 feet and 2,100 feet. They had solid masonry piers and metal spans. When the line reached Lake Baikal the construction of the railway around the lake was postponed, and a combined ferry-boat and ice-breaker was ordered from Britain to carry trains across. The dismantled vessel was delivered in six months, but it was two years later before it was assembled on the lake. The section of line which circled the Manchurian border was not built as planned, because under the Russo-Chinese treaty of 1896 China allowed a more direct route to be constructed through Manchurian territory. However, after the Russo-Japanese war work on the original section was begun, but it was not completed until 1916.

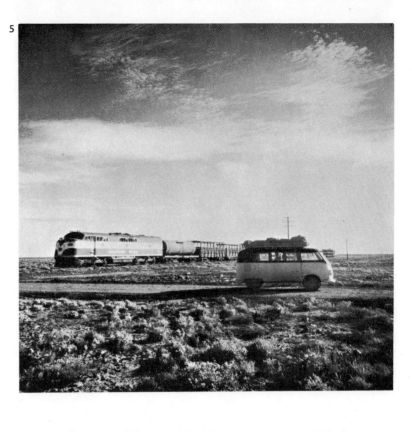

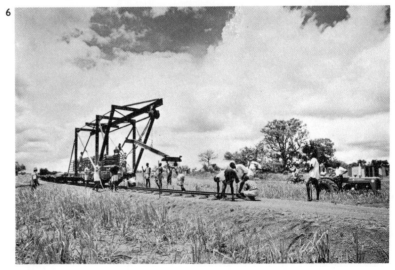

---

1 *The Countess of Dufferin,* the Canadian Pacific Railway's first locomotive.
2 A modern Trans-Siberian train in the station at Tomsk.
3 This length of track in the Canadian Rockies enters a spiral tunnel at the opening far left and emerges where the train is seen on the right.
4 A church service in Siberia in 1906. Church carriages were part of Trans-Siberian trains.
5 An Australian transcontinental train crossing the Nullarbor Plain near Woomera.
6 Platelaying on the new Soroti to Lira line, Uganda.

Supplies to Russian forces during that war were held up at the Lake Baikal bottle-neck because the ferry could only carry three trains each way daily. As a remedy rails were laid across the ice of the lake itself and wagons hauled across by horses. When the line around the lake was finally completed a ledge had to be cut into the side of the lake, and in one forty-two-mile stretch thirty-eight tunnels had to be bored through the rock.

The Trans-Siberian Railway was a great stimulus to the opening-up of Siberia. Between 1887 and 1892 about 40,000 colonists moved east each year. In 1896 this figure had risen to 200,000.

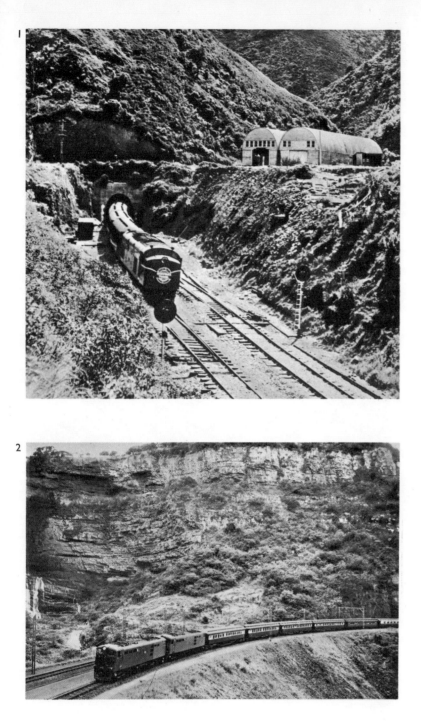

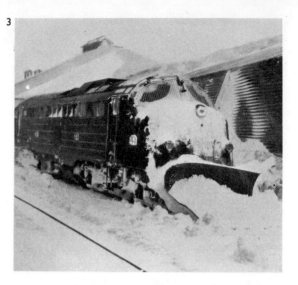

A transcontinental railway was one of the inducements held out to Western Australia to encourage the state to join the Australian Federation, but it was not until 1911 that the work was authorised by the Commonwealth Parliament. The first sod was turned on 14th September 1912, and track-laying commenced in 1913. Most of the construction work was done during the First World War, but, despite shortages of materials, the Commonwealth Railways of Australia had completed the whole line from Kalgoorlie to Port Augusta within four years, and the first passenger train was run on 22nd October 1917.

The building of the Trans-Australian line did not involve great engineering difficulties, there were no mountains or rivers, and most of the way is a level plain—a flat, waterless desert. In the whole 1,051 miles of the route there is not a single running stream. Wells, bores and reservoirs had to be built at enormous cost for all water requirements. Until the change in recent years to diesel-electric operation this meant that water and coal for locomotives had to be stored along the line, and the railway administration still has to supply the needs of all its staff. A supply train known as the 'Tea and Sugar' operates along the whole line, providing continual fresh supplies of meat, fruit, vegetables, bread, groceries, clothing and household goods. Drinking and domestic water and firewood are carried to areas where they are not obtainable locally—water is carried up to 537 miles.

The Trans-Australian Railway includes the longest stretch of straight railway track in the world. For three hundred miles the line continues, without a single curve, across the dry, treeless Nullarbor Plain.

The building of each great transcontinental line has been a tremendous achievement but short routes can pose equal difficulties. Railway engineers have continually achieved

1 Headed by a diesel-electric locomotive, the inauguratory train leaves the Rimutaka Tunnel, New Zealand. Five and a half miles long, it eliminated the 1 in 15 Rimutaka Incline which was worked on the Fell system.
2 The *Orange Express* passes through Shonweni Gorge, Natal.
3 A diesel locomotive clears its own way on the Bergen Railway, Norway, and helps to stop drifts from forming on the line.
4 A snow-plough at work in northern Scotland.
5 A treble-rotor snow-plough at work on the Orenburg Railway, U.S.S.R. These machines can clear snow up to 6 feet deep.

4

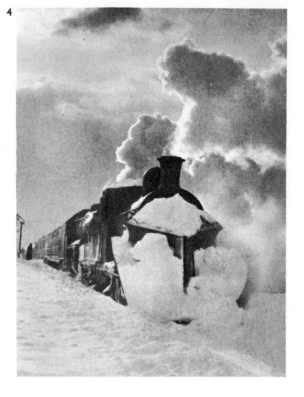

5

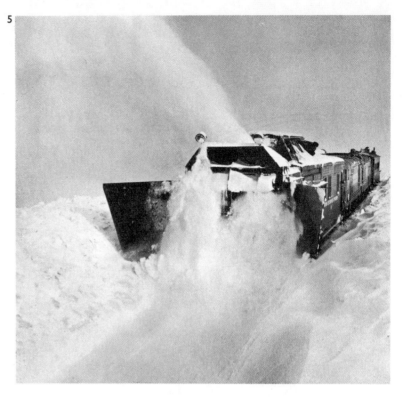

the impossible. Tunnels have been built with fantastic accuracy. As long ago as 1857 the Mont Cenis Tunnel between Italy and France, $7\frac{1}{2}$ miles long, was built without the aid of dynamite or gelignite, with no horizontal error and with a vertical divergence of only 11.8 inches. Sometimes a way has been made where none existed—as in the Feather River Canyon in the Californian Sierra Nevada, originally thought of as a route for the Central Pacific Railway. For 150 miles this perpendicular cleft cuts its way through the mountains. The torrent at its bottom rises forty-six feet above its normal level when the snow melts in the spring. Experts said it was madness to try to build a railway there, but surveyors worked out routes which gradually reduced the planned gradient from 1 in 43 to 1 in 81. Eventually the Western Pacific's line was built, at fantastic cost, with a gradient of only 1 in 100. To achieve this a ledge 75 miles long was blasted from the solid rock.

Ravines, swamps, deserts, rivers—all are crossed. The Copper River and North West Railroad in Alaska is even laid across a glacier, though one which has not been known to move in living memory. In building this line a bridge was built near to the end of Child Glacier. With the aid of steam jets piles were sunk through the ice of the frozen Copper River. With the bridge already partly built, an unexpected thaw set the glacier moving and its three-mile-wide, 500-feet-high face began to calve iceblocks which threatened to destroy the

bridge. The builders fought to keep the piles in place and repair the damage as fast as it was done, and the bridge was saved.

It is not only the physical features of a terrain which set problems for the engineer, whether in building or maintaining his railway. Snow can block the line and avalanches carry with them track and trains. Snow-sheds are built to carry the danger over them, snow-fences sometimes used to deflect the snow and prevent drifts building up on the line. Rain and floods can wash away embankments and bridges; in mountainous country rock falls can be a danger; in deserts sandstorms can bury the track. Animals can prove dangerous too. Teams building the railway from Mombasa to Kisumu on Lake Victoria were continually attacked by man-eating lions. Herds of buffalo often held up trains crossing the American prairies in pioneer days, but small animals can sometimes do worse damage. In Norway the burrowing teledu undermines the permanent way to such an extent that repair teams have to go out and repair the tracks each spring. A swarm of locusts can stop a train; killed or knocked senseless by their impact with the locomotive they are crushed upon the rails to form a mushy pulp which stops the wheels from getting a grip upon the track.

Heat, cold and disease have all taken their heavy toll of the construction gangs who have built our railways. Engineers and maintenance gangs still fight a constant battle against Nature to keep the permanent way open.

NIGHT MAIL

This is the night mail crossing the border,
Bringing the cheque and the postal order,
Letters for the rich, letters for the poor,
The shop at the corner and the girl next door,
Pulling up Beattock, a steady climb —
The gradient's against her but she's on time.

Past cotton grass and moorland boulder,
Shovelling white steam over her shoulder,
Snorting noisily as she passes
Silent miles of wind-bent grasses;
Birds turn their heads as she approaches,
Stare from the bushes at her blank-faced coaches;
Sheepdogs cannot turn her course
They slumber on with paws across,
In the farm she passes no one wakes,
But a jug in a bedroom gently shakes.

Dawn freshens, the climb is done.
Down towards Glasgow she descends,
Towards the steam tugs, yelping down the glade of cranes
Towards the fields of apparatus, the furnaces
Set on the dark plain like gigantic chessmen.
All Scotland waits for her;
In the dark glens, beside the pale-green sea lochs,
Men long for news.

Letters of thanks, letters from banks,
Letters of joy from the girl and boy,
Receipted bills and invitations
To inspect new stock or visit relations,
And applications for situations,
And timid lovers' declarations,
And gossip, gossip from all the nations,
News circumstantial, news financial,
Letters with holiday snaps to enlarge in,
Letters with faces scrawled on the margin.
Letters from uncles, cousins and aunts,
Letters to Scotland from the South of France,
Letters of condolence to Highlands and Lowlands,
Notes from overseas to the Hebrides;
Written on paper of every hue
The pink, the violet, the white and the blue
The chatty, the catty, the boring, adoring,
The cold and official and the heart's outpouring,
Clever, stupid, short and long,
The typed and the printed and the spelt all wrong.

Thousands are still asleep
Dreaming of terrifying monsters
Or a friendly tea beside the band at Cranston's or Crawford's;
Asleep in working Glasgow, asleep in well-set Edinburgh,
Asleep in granite Aberdeen.
They continue their dreams
But shall wake soon and long for letters.
And none will hear the postman's knock
Without a quickening of the heart,
For who can bear to feel himself forgotten?

W. H. AUDEN

Originally written for the G. P. O.
film NIGHT MAIL

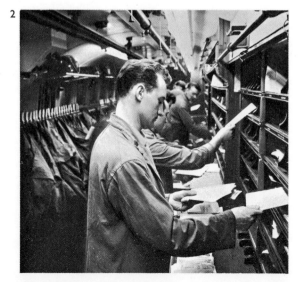

1 Picking up mail: the light string ties break and the bags are carried off their hooks into the van's net.
2 A modern sorting-coach of British Rail.
3 A replica of a Post Office van on the London and Birmingham Railway (1838).
Postal authorities were quick to make use of the railways. In England the Liverpool and Manchester Line began to carry mail in November 1830. In 1838 letter-sorting carriages, automatic pick-up systems and set-down systems all made their appearance. The demands of the Postal authorities were one reason for increased speeds.

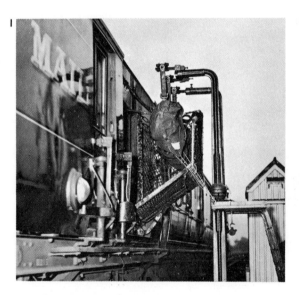

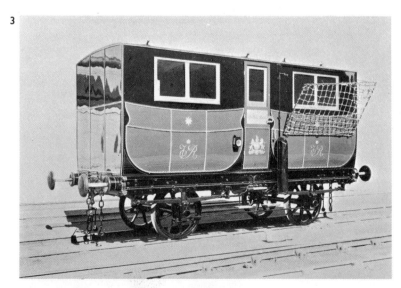

SPEED KINGS

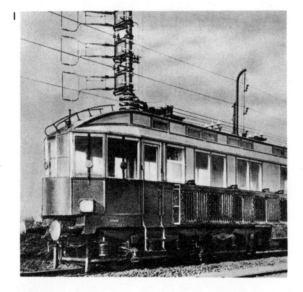

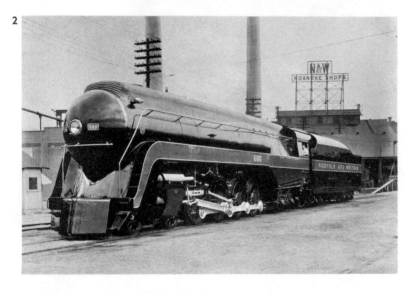

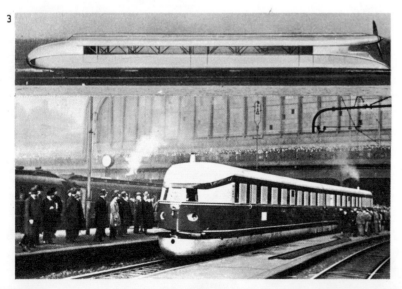

IT IS EXCITING to travel very fast, but breaking records is of less practical importance than are regular sustained fast services. Although the track itself makes the railway the safest means of transport, bends, gradients and other features of the permanent way may regulate the safe speed on a certain stretch. In some places the nature of the terrain will make very high speeds impossible, but where it is possible to level and to straighten out the track the record-breaking locomotives give some indication of what may one day become possible in regular service.

An electrically powered locomotive set the first great record of this century when in 1903 a German locomotive reached the then fantastic speed of 130 m.p.h.

In six decades, this speed has not been equalled by a steam locomotive. It was beaten in 1931 when Germany set up a new record of 143 m.p.h. with the Kruckenburg rail-car. This was an experimental vehicle, driven by a rear-mounted aeroplane propeller. From it were developed the streamlined diesel-electric trains, the *Flying Hamburger* and the *Flying Frankfurter,* which often exceeded 100 m.p.h. and sustained average speeds approaching 80 m.p.h. in regular passenger service: but to reach these speeds the German State Railways had to rebuild most of the track over which the expresses ran.

Streamlining was applied with great success to steam locomotives. In Britain Sir Nigel Gresley built his famous Pacific locomotives. Gresley designed a wedge-shaped front which kept smoke and steam well clear of the driver's cab so that it should not obscure his view. Internal streamlining of the flow of steam, developed by André Chapelon in France, also helped to increase speed.

It was a Gresley locomotive, *the Mallard* A.4 Class Pacific, then No. 4468, which set up an unbeaten record for a steam locomotive

1 The Siemens and Halska electric locomotive which set up a record of 130 m.p.h. in 1903.
2 United States streamliner placed in service in 1942.
3 *The Kruckenburg* rail-car (above) and the *Flying Hamburger* which developed from it.
4 S.N.C.F. locomotive BB. 9004 at the speed trials.
5 United States streamliner *Silver Streak.*
6 205.6 m.p.h.! Electric locomotive CC. 7107.

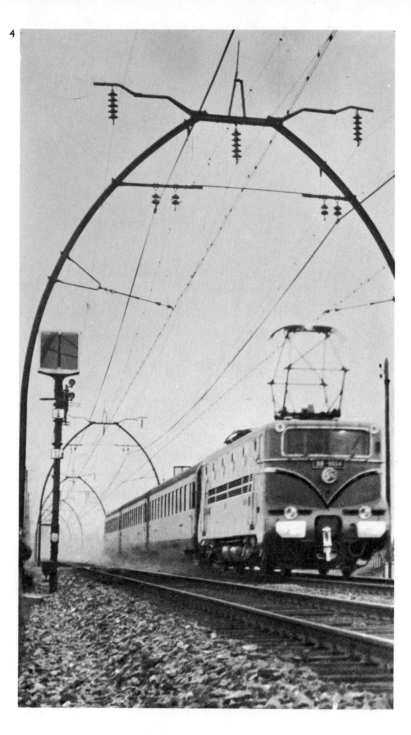

when on 3rd July 1938, it reached a top speed of 126 m.p.h. It still bears a plaque to commemorate the achievement. The maximum permissible speed on most British main lines is about 90 m.p.h. and the advantages of streamlining at this speed are offset by the difficulties of maintenance when streamlining covers the working parts. For this reason, some British Pacifics have had their streamlining removed until such time as it is possible to operate at increased speeds.

Steam, however, can never hope to catch up with electric traction. On 21st February 1954, CC. 7121, an electric locomotive of French Railways, set up a record of 151 m.p.h. without any special modification. The following year, the S.N.C.F. made preparations for another speed trial, to test the potential of locomotive CC. 7107 of the same class (the type used to haul the *Mistral* express daily between Paris and Lyons at an average speed of 80 m.p.h. and BB. 9004 of a lighter and less powerful class. The transmission system of both locomotives was modified so as to raise the gear ratio to achieve speeds in the neighbourhood of 185 m.p.h.

Preparations for these trials, which included the close inspection of all equipment involved and the making of many special arrangements, lasted nearly a year. To give some idea of what was involved, it was calculated that if 4,000 h.p. was sufficient for a speed of 151 m.p.h., over 10,000 h.p. would be required for 185 m.p.h. To pick up a current of 4,000 amperes at that speed, a special pantograph

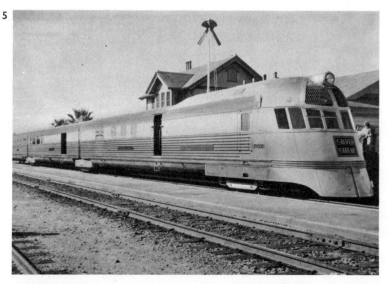

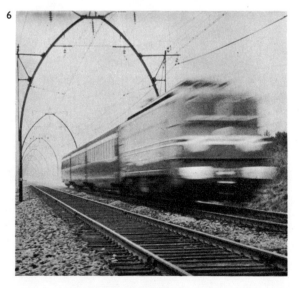

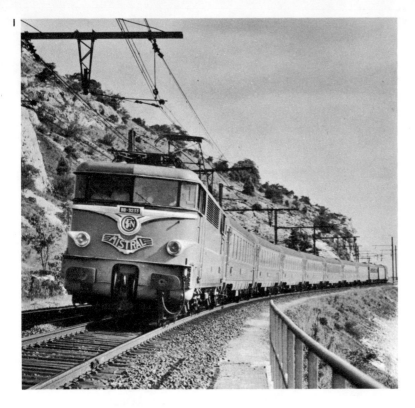

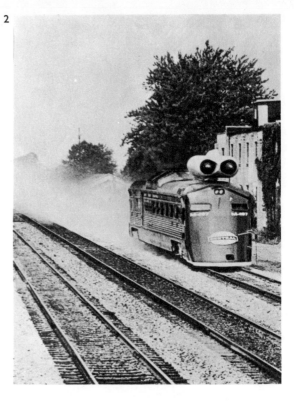

had to be designed. Tests were made in a wind tunnel to study the effects of an air current of 185 m.p.h. on the pressure of the pantograph against the traction wire. Locomotives and coaches were fitted with solid monobloc wheels so as to avoid the effects of centrifugal force and of braking on the normal steel-tyred wheel.

All parts which had to rotate at high speeds were tested in workshop pits where they were subjected to rotary speeds equivalent to 280 m.p.h. A two-way radio link was provided between the control post and the driver's cab of each of the locomotives.

The trials took place on the morning of 28th March for the CC. 7107 and on the morning of the 29th the BB. 9004. A speed of 185 m.p.h. was reached after travelling 13 miles. The two locomotives travelled at over 185 m.p.h. for $7\frac{1}{2}$ miles and at over 199 m.p.h. for nearly 4 miles. The speed of 205.6 m.p.h. was maintained over nearly $1\frac{1}{4}$ miles—a new world record!

The power reached exceeded the estimated figure, and at top speed the locomotives were using 12,000 h.p., which shows the considerable effect of wind resistance at high speeds. Special instruments showed their stability to be very satisfactory.

The United States rail speed record was set by a New York Central Railroad test vehicle, a single passenger coach with two turbo-jet engines mounted on the roof, which reached a speed of 183.85 m.p.h. on 23rd July, 1966.

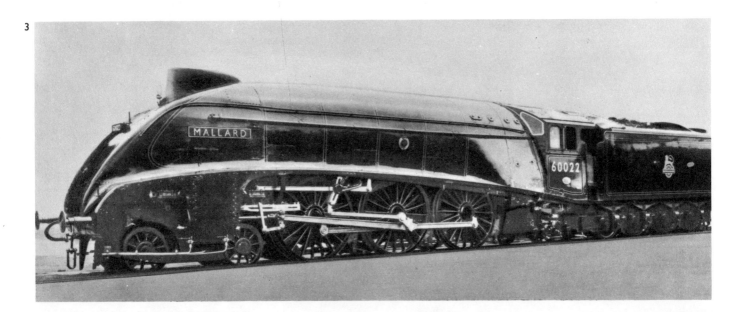

RACK RAILWAYS

IN THE EARLY DAYS of railways many people doubted whether a locomotive with smooth wheels was capable of propelling itself along a smooth track. They thought some more positive grip was required. In 1811 John Blenkinsop patented a system using a pinion on the locomotive which fitted into teeth at the side of the rails, a system which greatly increased the hauling power of the locomotive. In 1812—13 this system was installed on the Middleton, Kenton and Coxlodge Colliery lines. The laying of the Blenkinsop rails and the adoption of steam traction on 12th August 1812 probably made the Leeds-Middleton Colliery line the first steam railway in Britain.

The first American railway locomotive, built by Colonel John Stevens of Hoboken, New Jersey, in 1825, combined a rack-and-pinion system between the rails with guide wheels. The circular demonstration track was America's first steam railway.

In 1831—2 the Neath Abbey Ironworks designed a locomotive combining adhesion and rack operation for Dowlais Ironworks which operated with a rack running parallel to the tramplates.

Thirty years later in America Sylvester Marsh was planning rack railways up the slopes of Mount Washington and Mount Lafayette in New Hampshire. In 1858 he had built a model locomotive and been granted a charter to proceed, and in 1866 he gave a demonstration on a section of track built at his own expense. It was not until a year later, however, that

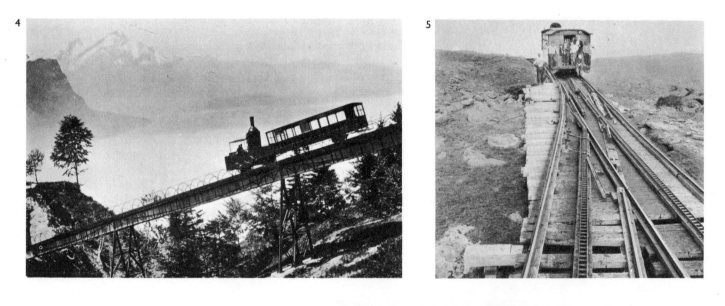

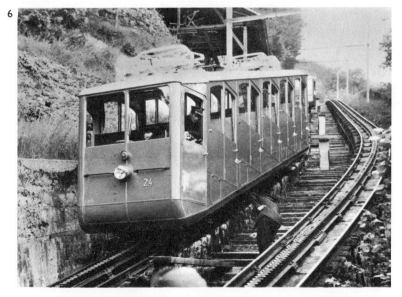

1 BB. 9233, of the same class as one of the record-holding locomotives, hauling the *Mistral* express in the Valley of the Rhône.
2 New York Central Railroad's jet-powered test car during a run between Butler, Indiana, and Stryker, Ohio.
3 The *Mallard*, which set up an unbeaten record of 126 m.p.h., for a steam locomotive, in 1938.
RACK RAILWAYS
4 The Rigi Railway in 1873.
5 Mount Washington Cog Railway.
6 The Locher system on Mount Pilatus, Switzerland.

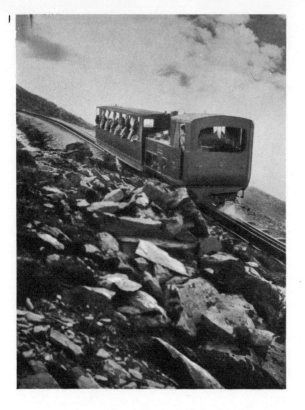

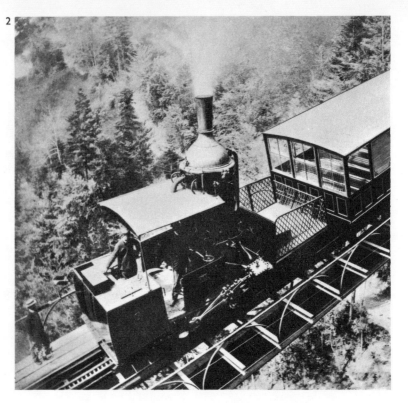

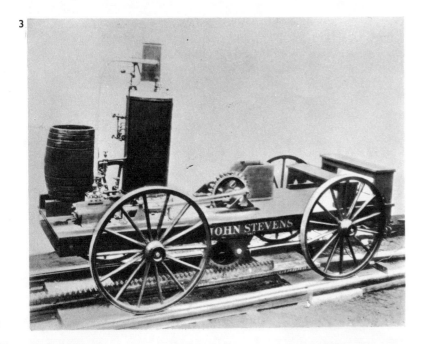

sufficient money was raised, and in July 1869 the Mount Washington Cog Railway was carrying passengers to the summit. Today it is very much as when it was built.

In 1863 Nicholas Riggenbach of the Central Swiss Railway patented a system for a rack railway. When he heard of Marsh's system he went to see it in America and found it very like his own.

Back in Europe he and two other engineers (Naeff and Zschokke) obtained a concession to build a rack railway up the 5,905-foot Rigi Mountain. Finally two railways were built, both using his principle, one from the Canton of Lucerne and one from the Canton of Schwyz.

Other railways using the Riggenbach rack were built elsewhere in Switzerland, by Lake Constance from Rorschach to Heiden, up the Kahlenberg near Vienna, up the Corcovado Mountain, Rio de Janiero, and in Angola.

Other systems using racks were devised by a Swiss engineer called Wetli in 1868 and an Italian called Agudio whose rope-worked system was first used on a steep slope on the Turin and Alessandria Railway in 1862.

In 1882 another rack system was patented, by Dr. Roman Abt, consisting of a double pinion running in two stepped tracks arranged so that the teeth of one are opposite the gaps of the other. This system was designed for a line built at Blankenburg in 1884, and has since been used in America, Australia, Japan and India. A line in Colorado, U.S.A., climbs to the summit of Pike's Peak, 14,147 feet above sea level.

The Snowdon Mountain Railway, the only rack railway now operating in Great Britain, works on the Abt principle.

Another system consisting of pairs of pinion wheels mounted horizontally which engage with a flat rack rail with teeth cut in both sides was devised by E. Locher specially for the railway from Alpanachstad up Mount Pilatus in Switzerland, where the gradient is 1 in 3 and sometimes 1 in 2.

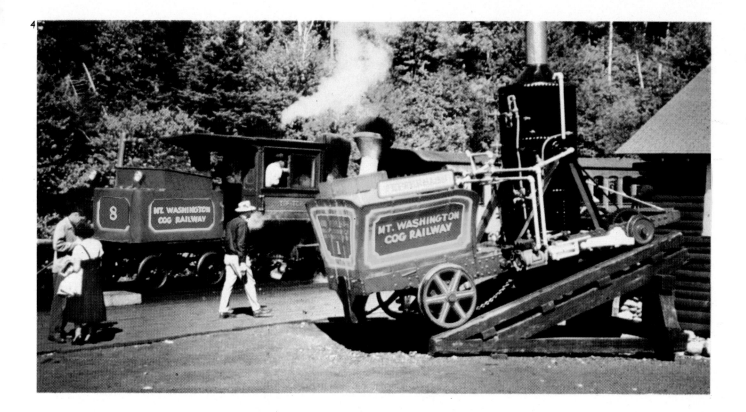

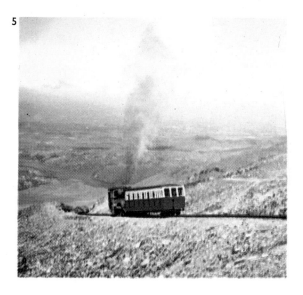

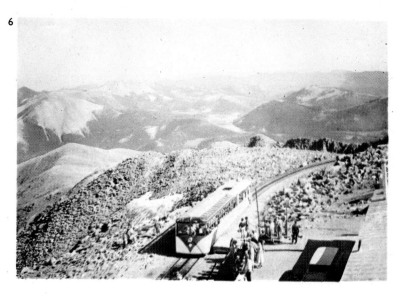

1 & 5 Snowdon Mountain Railway, opened in 1896.
2 The Rigi Railway.
3 A model of John Stevens' locomotive and rail.
4 The new and the old *Old Peppersass* on the Mount Washington Cog Railway, New Hampshire.
6 A narrow-gauge train on Pike's Peak Railway.

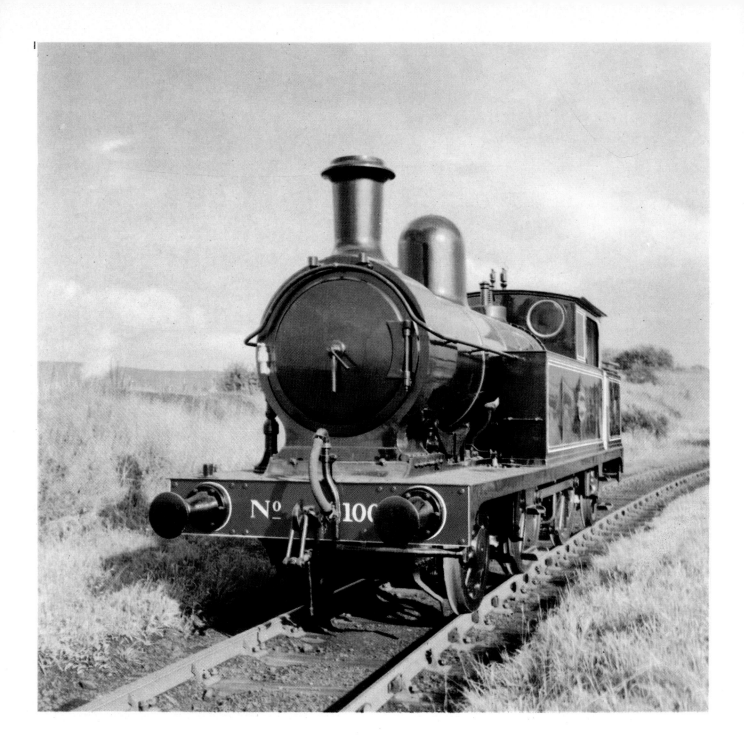

1 Locomotive No. 1008 of the Lancashire and Yorkshire Railway. This 2-4-2 was built in 1889.
2 Great Eastern Railway 0-6-0 locomotive No. 87, built in 1904 and run on the line to Alexandra Palace.
3 Furness Railway 0-4-0 locomotive No. 3, *Coppernob,* built in 1846.
4 Great Central Railway 4-4-0 locomotive No. 506, *Butler Henderson,* built in 1920.
All these locomotives are now in the Museum of British Transport, London.

2

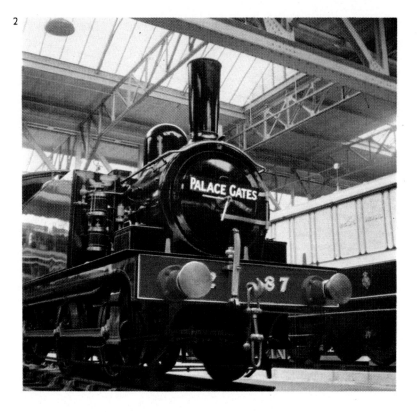

3

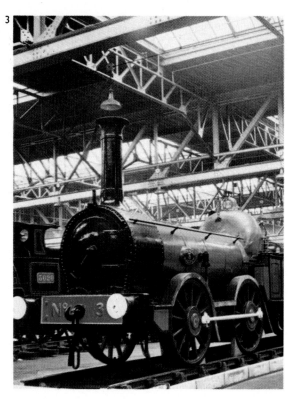

4

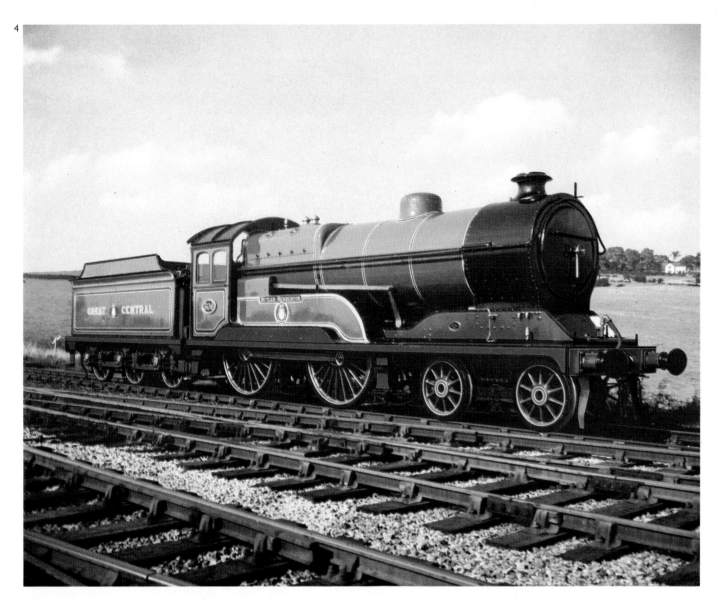

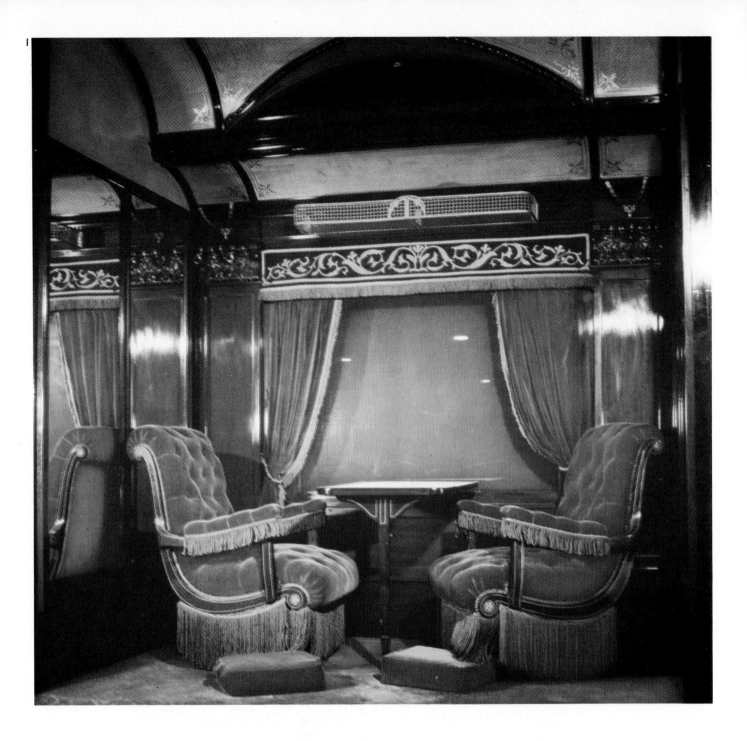

1 A Pullman car of about 1890. A facsimile in the
Museum of British Transport.

TRAVEL IN COMFORT

'DIED FROM EXPOSURE in a second-class carriage of the Great Western Railway' — that was the verdict of an early Victorian inquest on the death of a railway traveller. What happened to the poor devils travelling third or fourth? On this particular line third-class travellers were carried by the night goods trains in ordinary, open wagons with planks laid across to serve as seats and holes bored in the floor to let out the rain. Sometimes passengers simply stood in open boxes.

In 1844 Gladstone, then President of the Board of Trade, pushed the Regulation of Railways Bill through Parliament. It became known as the Cheap Trains Act because, among its provisions, it required that all railway companies should, once a day on each of their lines, provide accommodation for third-class passengers which afforded light, air and protection from the weather at a charge of one penny per mile. These 'cheap trains' were also required to provide a service at an average speed of at least twelve miles per hour.

Some second-class carriages were open with wooden seats; others, 'second-class closed,' were covered boxes with drop windows in the doors—but for anything like comfort it was necessary to travel first-class.

If you owned your own coach you could have it mounted on a truck and travel in that, the horses travelling in a special horse-box. If you travelled in the company's first-class carriages, it was very similar to travelling in a coach. The well-padded seats had head-and-elbow-rests and your luggage was out of the way on top. At first, solid padded buffers and linking-chains made every stop and start a very jerky business but, as spring buffers and screw couplings were introduced, the journey became more smooth. For a supplement you could travel in the mail-coach, which seated only two passengers each side, instead of three (or on the broad-gauge Great Western, four).

There were no food facilities on these early trains or toilets (except for some special carriages available for hire by incontinent invalids of ample means), no corridors, no heating (foot-warmers filled with hotwater were provided later) and only oil lamps dropped in through the roof for light. There was, however, a primitive form of sleeper formed by placing two sticks and a cushion across the space between the seats as a sort of stretcher. The sticks could be hired from the guard. Where this was still too short to lie down, a boot was built out beyond the compartment to accommodate the feet. A 'bed-carriage' of this kind was built for Queen Adelaide in 1842.

North American emigrant trains used a similar arrangement, with a board and cushions laid across the seats which could be purchased from the railway staff; but other amenities were available. They had to be, for American trains were unable to go very fast, their track was not designed for speed; distances were considerable and journeys long, so some provision was necessary for passengers to move up and down the train. American carriages soon developed from a simple stage-coach on rails to a long saloon. They were not cut up into separate small compartments but arranged with seats on either side of a central gangway. Stoves for heating, toilets, and mounting on bogies soon became general. Clerestory roofs were used more frequently than in Europe and gave better lighting and ventilation.

Despite these improvements American trains could hardly have been called comfortable. One man, making a night journey in 1853, found conditions so intolerable that he set about devising a comfortable type of sleeping-car. In 1857 George M. Pullman built his first sleeper, a remodelled car called No. 9. It was a primitive affair but, in 1864, after experimenting with sleeping-cars of various designs on the Chicago and Alton Railroad for some years, he produced an elaborate car which he called *The Pioneer*. It cost twenty-thousand dollars and was lavishly fitted—but no one used it. *The Pioneer* was higher and wider than any car then in service on American railroads. It posed clearance problems where station platforms, tunnels and bridges were concerned. But in 1865 it was made part of Abraham Lincoln's funeral train and platforms and bridges from Chicago to Springfield were hurriedly changed to allow for its extra size. From then on *The Pioneer* was a success. In 1867 Pullman joined forces with his competitors, Andrew Carnegie's Central Transportation Company, to form Pullman's Palace Car Company. The same year they produced an 'hotel' car for eating and sleeping and one of these, on the Great Western Railroad of Canada, was the first dining-car.

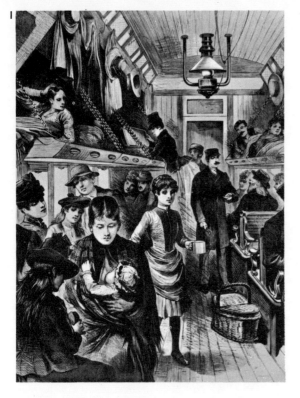

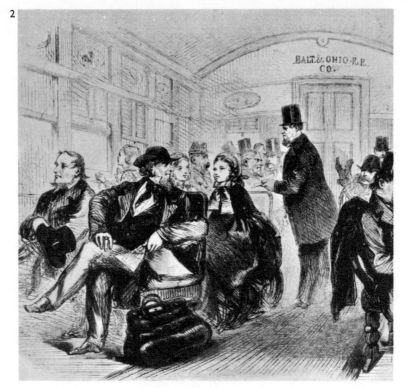

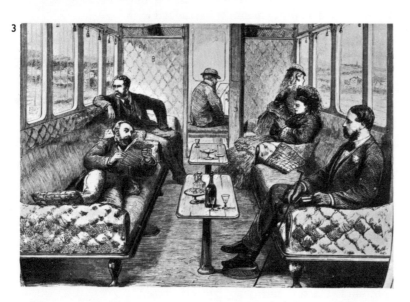

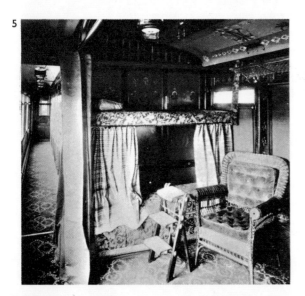

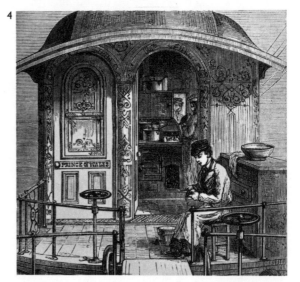

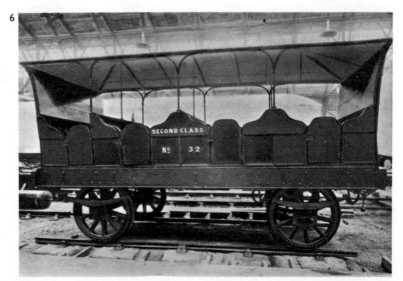

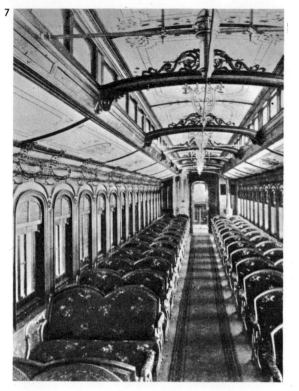

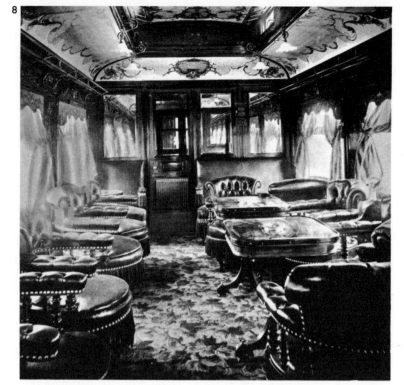

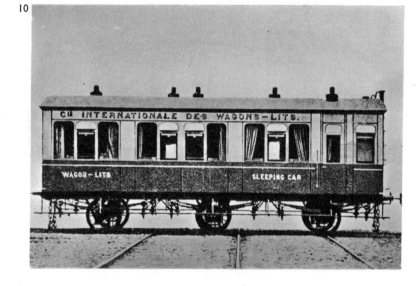

1—11 (1) Colonial sleeping-car of the Canadian Pacific Railway, 1888. (2) Travel on the Baltimore and Ohio Railroad in 1861. (3) A saloon carriage of the London, Brighton and South Coast Railway, 1873. (4) The kitchen of the Pullman dining-car introduced on the British Great Northern Railway in 1879. (5) European wagon-lit in 1888. (6) Second-class carriage on the Dublin and Kingstown Railway, Ireland, 1837. (7) Early passenger car on the Union Pacific Railway. (8) Wagon-salon in 1889. (9) A train with 'Hotel Sleeping Cars,' 1875. (10) Wagon-lit in 1877. (11) Great Western Railway third-class carriage, *circa* 1855.

In 1874 the Midland Railway in England imported Pullman cars from America. Mounted on four-wheeled bogies, these long-bodied carriages had central passageways, lavatories, hot-water radiators running from a stove and kerosene lamps for illumination. Day travel was in drawing-room cars with a row of pivoted armchairs on each side of the gangway. Sleeping accommodation was in two-tier curtained berths. The upper berths folded up to the roof and the lower ones turned into two comfortable seats for day-time use.

In 1879 a Pullman car running between London and Leeds on the Great Northern Railway provided the first regular dining service on a British train, with the meals cooked on board.

On 4th December 1876, two years after the first Pullman in Great Britain, a Belgian engineer, Georges Nagelmackers, founded the Compagnie Internationale des Wagons-Lits. Reassured by the success of Pullman in America, Nagelmackers sought to provide 'vehicles which would carry travellers making long journeys with the maximum of comfort, notably by making it possible to have complete rest in real beds put at their disposal for the night.' The complexity of European rail systems and the difficulties encountered with Customs and Police at every frontier made innumerable changes of train necessary. The company was planned on an international basis, outside the various railway administrations, and aimed to provide comfortable through-coaches in which passengers could travel throughout their journey without having to change trains.

By the beginning of 1877 contracts had been signed with twenty-one different railway companies for wagons-lits. To the wagons-lits were added wagons-restaurants and, despite the obstacles presented by the lack of standardisation, either of equipment or regulations, the first great international express ran in 1883: the *Orient Express*.

In May 1883 the C.I.W.L. signed agreements with the different companies over whose lines the *Orient Express* would have to pass.

The first train ran on 5th June. The journey from Paris to Constantinople (Istanbul) took eighty-one hours and thirty minutes. Following a route north of the Alps (the Simplon Tunnel was not opened until 1906), passengers tra-velled direct to Vienna, Budapest and Bucharest but at Giurgeva, a little port on the Danube, they crossed from the Rumanian to the Bulgarian bank in a ferry-steamer and then boarded another train for a seven-hour journey to Varna, on the Black Sea. There they took a packet of the Lloyd-Austria Line and after another fifteen hours docked in Constantinople.

Meanwhile, in Britain, native-built coaches were becoming more comfortable. In January 1875 the Midland Railway, followed later by the other companies, abolished the second class and began to build its third class with upholstered seats. Coaches were mounted on four- or six-wheel bogies; clerestory roofs were built and, to improve illumination, coal gas, oil gas and, in 1881, electricity were used. The year 1881 also saw, on the Great Northern Railway, the first ordinary British train to have a corridor. It led only to the toilet, there was no connection with the adjoining coach. Eight years later the Midland Railway had gone so far as to install lavatories in its third class, and by 1891 the Great Western Railway had built a through-corridor train.

One interesting feature of British railways in the latter half of the nineteenth century was the family saloon—consisting of a main saloon furnished with armchairs, a table and sofa seats, smaller compartments, including perhaps a smoking-room, a second-class compartment for servants, baggage room, toilet, and sometimes a kitchen. These carriages were made available to parties who made a block booking above a certain number of tickets. The railway companies would undertake to take one to any destination without disturbance to the occupants, providing the sort of direct service which Nagelmackers sought to give to travellers on the Continent.

1 and 2 A three-tier compartment in a modern sleeping-car which converts from (1) to (2) for day use.
3 Restaurant car in 1908, interior.
4 Restaurant car in 1906, exterior.
5 A single compartment in a modern sleeping-car.
6 A modern wagon-lit.

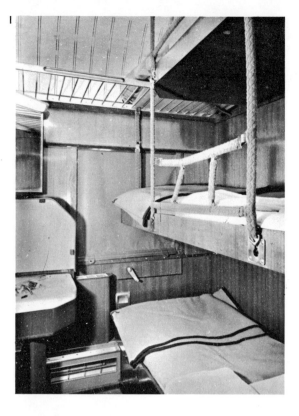

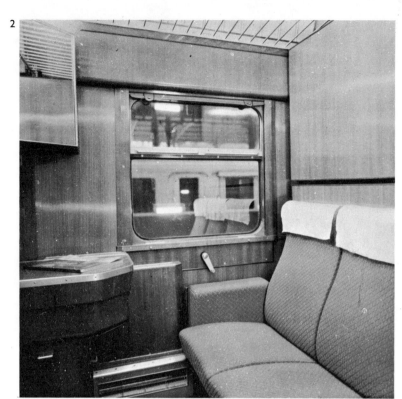

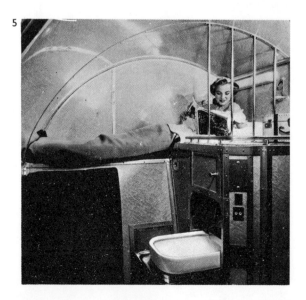

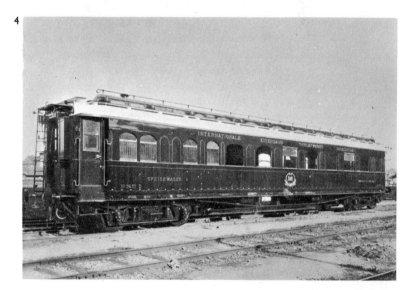

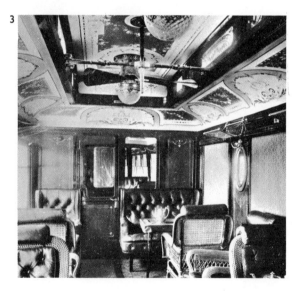

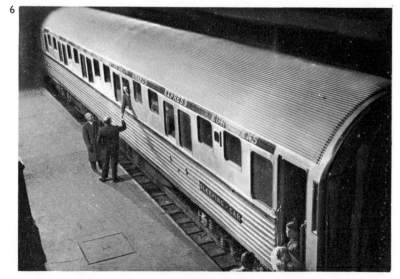

EMIGRANT'S BED

I SUPPOSE the reader has some notion of an American railroad-car, that long narrow wooden box, like a flat-roofed Noah's ark, with a stove and a convenience, one at either end, a passage down the middle, and transverse benches upon either hand. Those destined for emigrants on the Union Pacific are only remarkable for their extreme plainness, nothing but wood entering in any part into their constitution, and for the usual inefficacy of the lamps, which often went out and shed but a dying glimmer even while they burned. The benches are too short for anything but a young child. Where there is scarce elbow-room for two to sit, there will not be space enough for one to lie. Hence the Company, or rather, as it appears from certain bills about the Transfer Station, the Company's servants, have conceived a plan for the better accommodation of travellers. They prevail on every two to chum together. To each of the chums they sell a board and three square cushions stuffed with straw, and covered with thin cotton. The benches can be made to face each other in pairs, for the backs are reversible. On the approach of night the boards are laid from bench to bench, making a couch wide enough for two, and long enough for a man of the middle height; and the chums lie down side by side upon the cushions with the head to the conductor's van and the feet to the engine. When the train is full, of course this plan is impossible, for there must not be more than one to every bench, neither can it be carried out unless the chums agree. It was to bring about this last condition that our white-haired official now bestirred himself. He made a most active master of ceremonies, introducing likely couples, and even guaranteeing the amiability and honesty of each. The greater the number of happy couples the better for his pocket, for it was he who sold the raw material of the beds. His price for one board and three straw cushions began with two dollars and a half; but before the train left, and, I am sorry to say, long after I had purchased mine, it had fallen to one dollar and a half.

FROM 'ACROSS THE PLAINS'
BY ROBERT LOUIS STEVENSON

1 A carriage used for emigrants, 1883.
2 Interior of an emigrant carriage, 1884.
3—6 Fast and comfortable diesel Pullman trains are bringing back passengers to British Rail services. Operating on several different routes, they offer air-conditioning, adjustable seats and fine food.

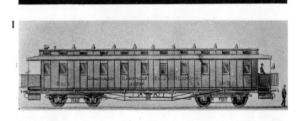

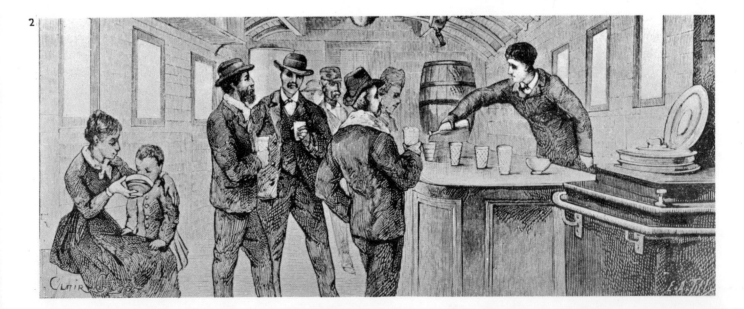

LUXURY TODAY

AS THE YEARS have passed passenger accommodation has improved for all classes, but recent years have seen particular efforts by the railways to compete with other forms of transport by providing extra comforts and services.

Long-distance routes, such as American transcontinental expresses which take two days to complete the journey, have upheld the tradition of Pullman's Palace Cars and counter the attraction of airliner speeds with a level of comfort and luxury impossible in the air. Restaurants, lounges, bars, domed compartments for better sightseeing, and a much greater variety of sleeper accommodation than the European first and second class and couchette make the trip a pleasant holiday for the traveller who does not demand the speed of jet aeroplanes.

One of these luxury trains, the Great Northern Railway's *Empire Builder*, which takes 43 hours 50 minutes to complete the 2,210 miles from Chicago to Seattle, cost £1¼ million to equip and has a staff of 25, not counting the locomotive crew, to look after only 323 passengers.

Services directed at the businessman have been another field, particularly in Europe, where the railways have been at pains to attract and increase custom. In 1954 the railway authorities of Belgium, France, West Germany, Italy, Luxembourg, the Netherlands and Switzerland planned a new service of comfortable, high-speed trains linking 90 of the major cities and industrial centres of Western Europe. These *Trans-Europ-Expresses* are scheduled to suit the businessman's convenience, with

3

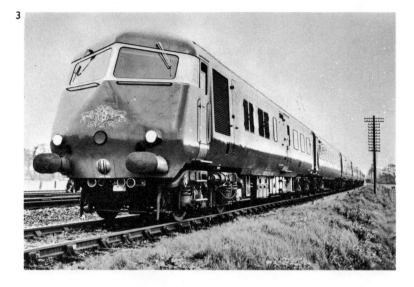

4

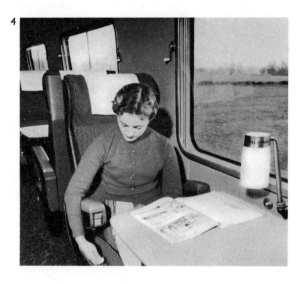

5

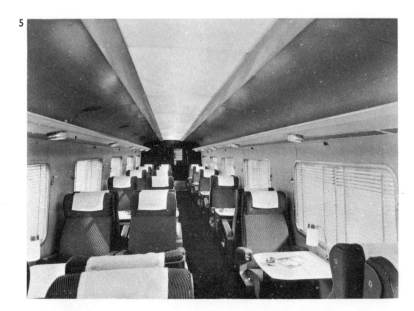

6

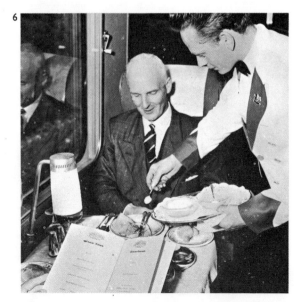

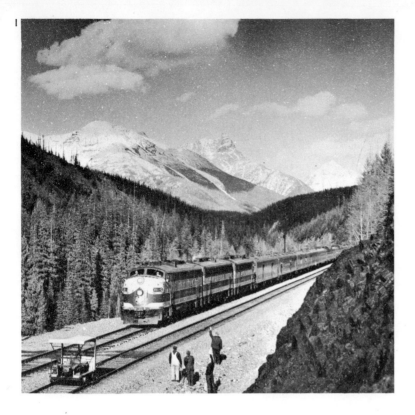

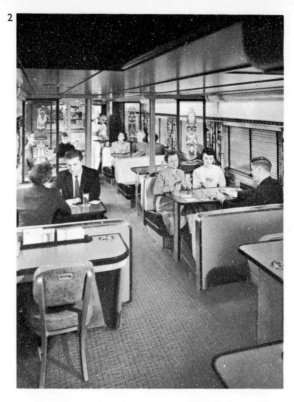

timings that compare favourably with those for road transport or for air travel plus in and out of city times. They have proved a great success. The same principle is now being applied to freight with *Trans-Europ-Express Marchandises* which operates fast scheduled freight services between eighteen countries, aided by simplified Customs procedures.

Facilities for the traveller today do not stop at providing excellent restaurant and sleeping accommodation. Secretarial services, radio, relayed music, radio telephones, film shows—all these can be found on wheels, and so long as the present competition for the traveller's custom continues no doubt more services will become available.

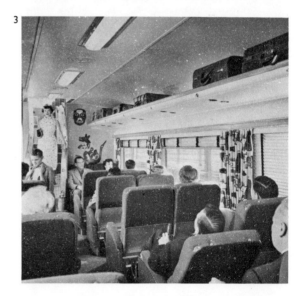

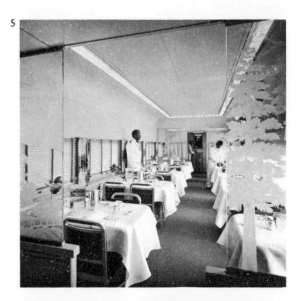

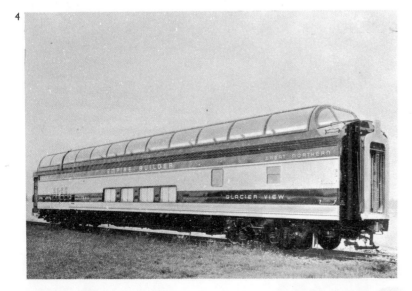

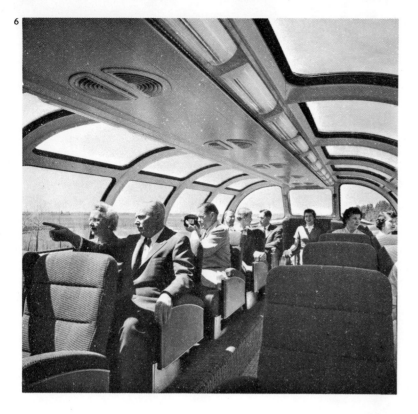

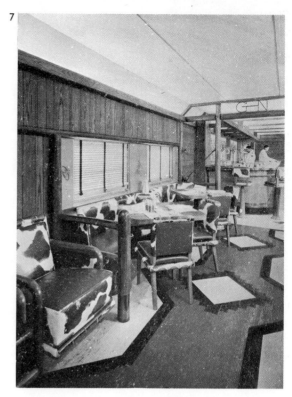

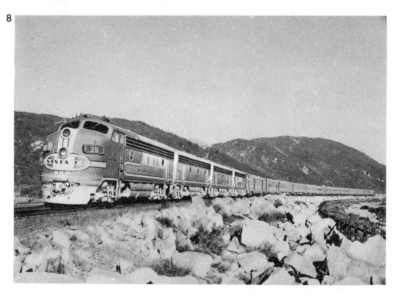

1—7 The Great Northern Railway of America's transcontinental streamliner which departs daily from Chicago for Seattle and Portland, provides three domed sections, and a full-length domed lounge for sight-seeing (which provide spectacular views of the Montana Rockies. Dining-cars and lounges are decorated with Indian and ranch motifs.

8—10 The Santa Fé Railroad's express running between Chicago and Los Angeles has comfortable reclining seats set four feet above the rails giving a smoother ride with less noise and vibration. There is a sight-seeing 'pleasure dome' and a special feature is the Turquoise Room (9), one of the first private dining-rooms on any railroad.

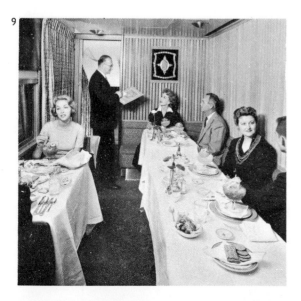

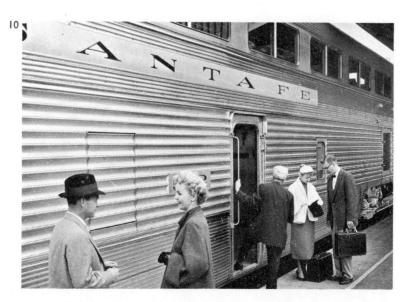

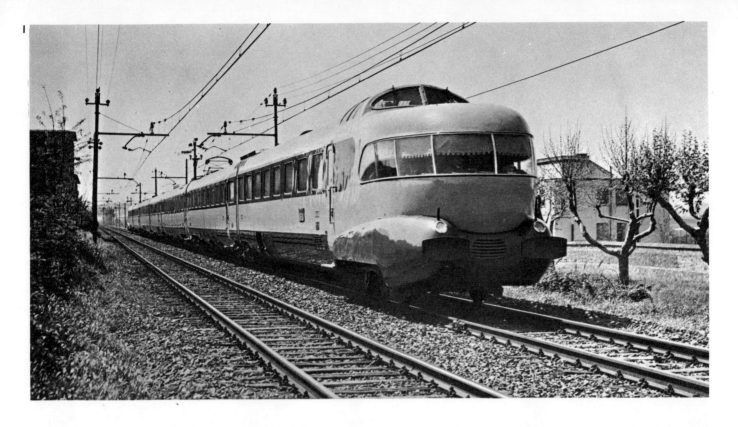

1

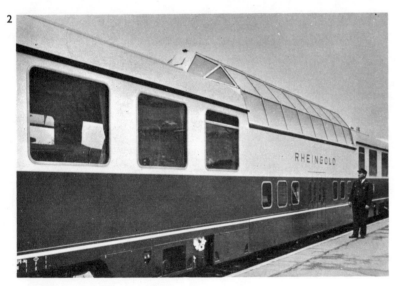

2

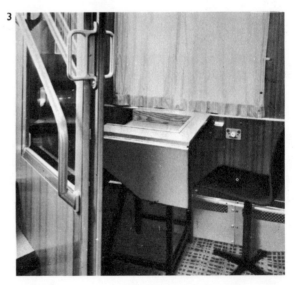

3

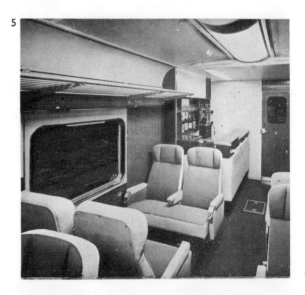

4

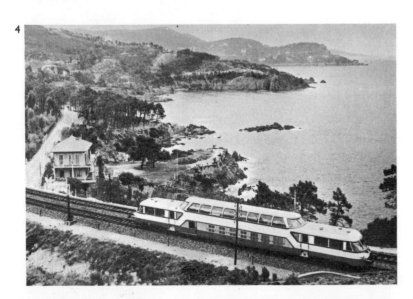

5

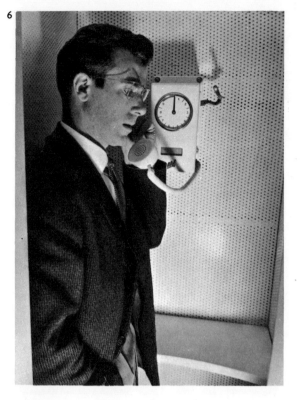

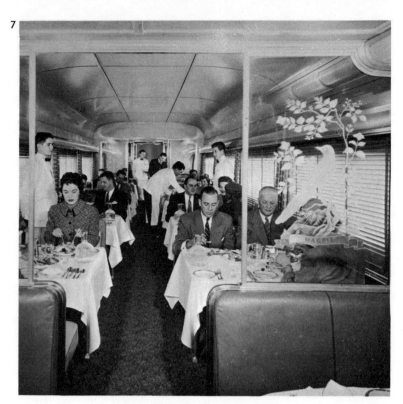

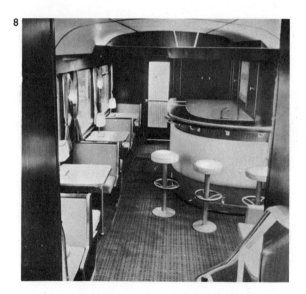

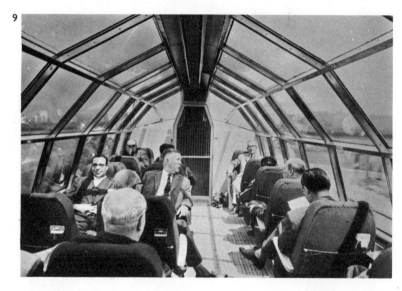

1 The Italian State Railways' *Settebello* has a forward observation car; the driver's cab is mounted above the observation department.

2, 3, 8, 9. The West German *Rheingold* express features provision for secretaries (3), a comfortable bar and an observation car.

4 A panoramic car of the French Railways.

5 The bar in a diesel train-set on Cuba's rail system.

6 Radio-telephones are now available on some French routes.

7 A dining-car on the *Canadian Pacific Express*.

10 A buffet-car on British Rail's diesel 'Trans-Pennine' service.

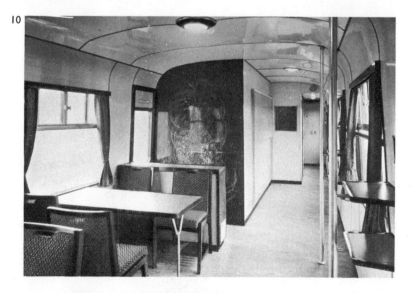

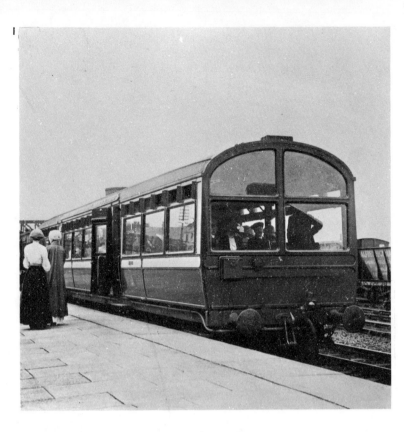

1, 2 Observation cars are not a new idea, this one was photographed in service on the Llandudno—Llanberis line in Wales in 1912, but modern observation domes like that of the *Canadian* (2) give an even better view.

3—7 *Trans-Europ-Express* service of (3) Swiss Railways, (4) Italian State Railways, (5) German State Railways, (6) French Railways. The Swiss electric train seen here on the shores of Lake Geneva is able to run on any of four different line currents. All the other train-sets are diesel powered. Trans-Europe inter-city routes are shown in (7). The building of a Channel Tunnel will make it possible to extend the TEE and TEEM services to major British cities. Although some difficulties will be encountered because British routes were built for smaller rolling stock and often do not give sufficient clearance for continental vehicles, and the slight difference in gauge is critical at high speeds, ways will be found of overcoming these difficulties.

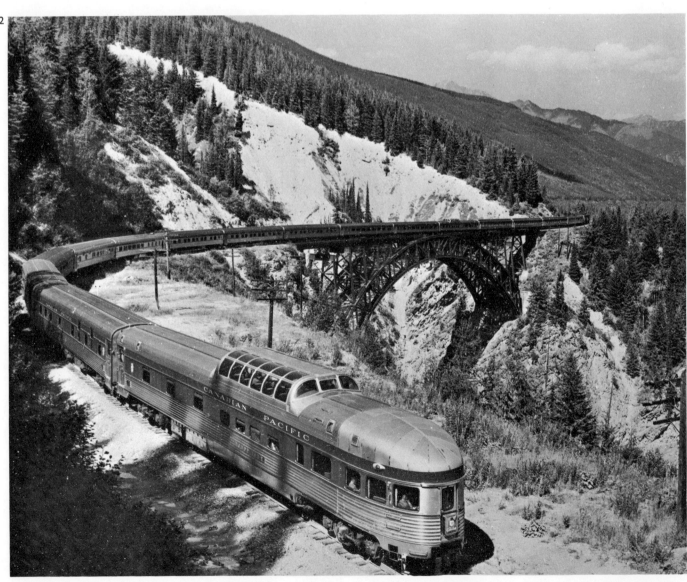

3

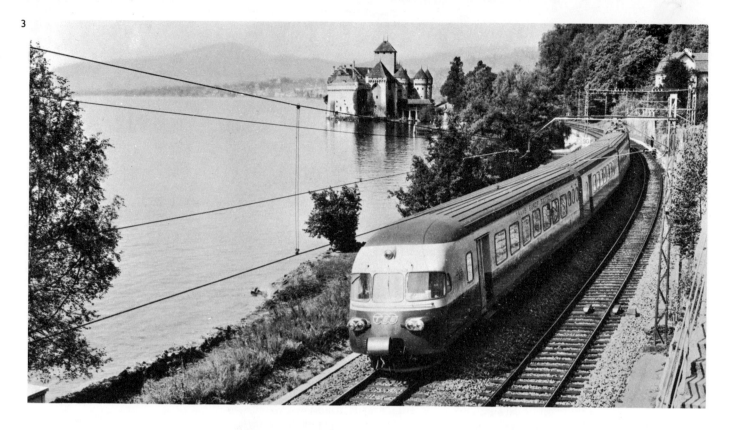

4

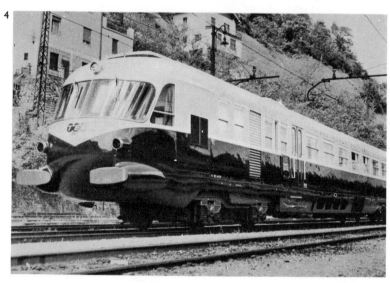

5

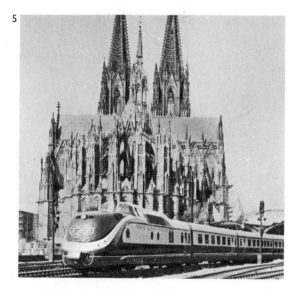

6

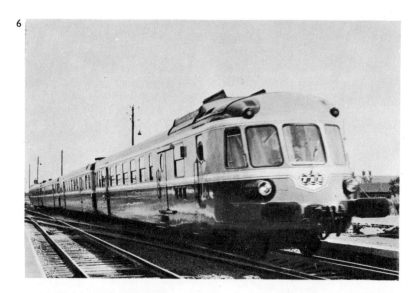

7

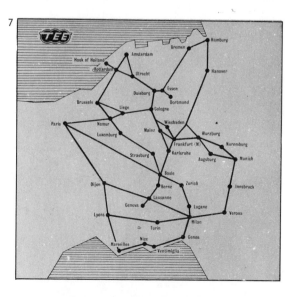

TO A LOCOMOTIVE IN WINTER

THEE for my recitative,
Thee in the driving storm even as now, the snow, the winter-day
    declining,
Thee in thy panoply, thy measur'd dual throbbing and thy beat
    convulsive,
Thy black cylindric body, golden brass and silvery steel,
Thy ponderous side-bars, parallel and connecting rods, gyrating,
    shuttling at thy sides,
Thy matrical, now swelling pant and roar, now tapering in the
    distance,
Thy great protruding head-light fix'd in front,
Thy long, pale, floating vapor-pennants, tinged with delicate
    purple,
The dense and murky clouds out-belching from thy smoke-
    stack,
Thy knitted frame, thy springs and valves, the tremulous twinkle
    of thy wheels,
Thy train of cars behind, obedient, merrily following,
Through gale or calm, now swift, now slack, yet steadily
    careering;
Type of the modern—emblem of motion and power—pulse of
    the continent,
For once come serve the Muse and merge in verse, even as here
    I see thee,
With storm and buffeting gusts of wind and falling snow,
By day thy warning ringing bell to sound its notes,
By night thy silent signal lamps to swing.

Fierce-throated beauty!
Roll through my chant with all thy lawless music, thy swinging
    lamps at night,
Thy madly-whistled laughter, echoing, rumbling like an earth-
    quake, rousing all,
Law of thyself complete, thine own track firmly holding,
(No sweetness debonair of tearful harp or glib piano thine,)
Thy trills of shrieks by rocks and hills return'd,
Launch'd o'er the prairies wide, across the lakes,
To the free skies unpent and glad and strong.

WALT WHITMAN

NARROW-GAUGE RAILWAYS

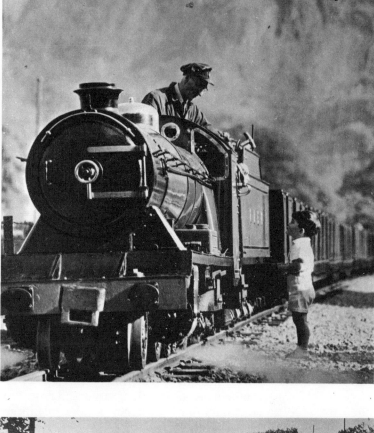

TO MOST PEOPLE in Europe and America the 'standard' gauge for railways today is 4 ft. $8\frac{1}{2}$ in. and they consider anything less as 'narrow gauge,' but in some countries (the U.S.S.R., India, Brazil, Spain, Ireland and Australia, for instance, who have a wider gauge) 4 ft. $8\frac{1}{2}$ in. would be considered narrow. Indeed, many early American and British railways were built to wider gauges than today. Isambard Kingdom Brunel, the great engineer, built his Great Western line to a 7-foot gauge. When a standardised gauge became imperative in Britain, pressure from the 4 ft. $8\frac{1}{2}$ in. lines caused Parliament to declare for the present standard and Brunel's line first had a narrow track laid between its metals, and then was taken up altogether. The last Great Western wide-gauge locomotive ran in 1892.

Wide gauge gives greater stability because a lower centre of gravity is possible in the rolling-stock, but it requires more solid support, wider bridges and smoother bends—all of which can add enormously to the cost of line construction. Some people think that the demands of modern heavy, high-speed traffic will lead to the adoption of a broader gauge.

A narrow gauge can also have great advantages, provided that very high speeds are not required. A narrow gauge can take sharp bends and follow natural gradients much more easily, so that the engineering difficulties and expenses of construction are reduced, and the rolling-stock is lighter, and therefore cheaper. These advantages led to the adoption of narrow-gauge track for mine and quarry railways and other industrial closed systems, for railways in very difficult terrain, and for small local lines even in countries where a larger gauge was standard. In other countries a narrow gauge was adopted as the usual size.

Those railways which are narrower than their country's standard gauge are usually either used for industrial purposes or have become pleasure lines. Many of the local pas-

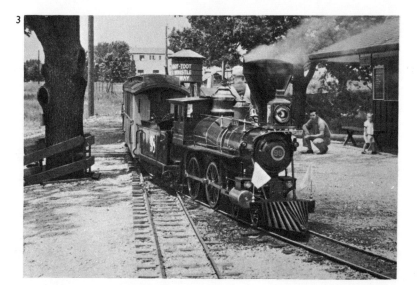

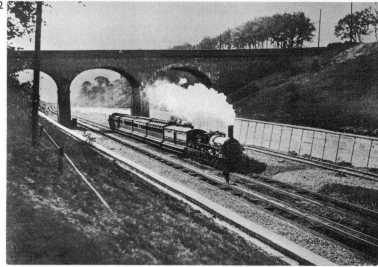

1 A would-be engine driver on the Ravenglass and Eskdale Railway, Cumberland.
2 The last broad-gauge train in Britain, seen in Sonning Cutting.
3 The Hoot, Toot and Whistle Railway, near Chicago.

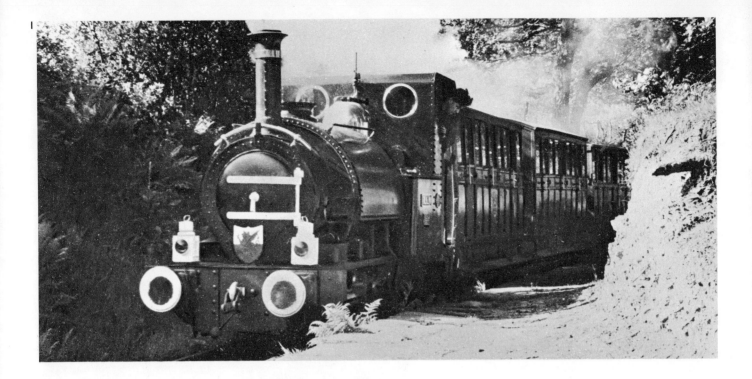

senger lines have been forced to close by the competition of road transport. Those that remain do so because they are the only means of reaching a particular beauty spot or because they have sufficient interest in themselves to attract passengers 'just for the ride'.

The miniature and the oddity are always fascinating and many narrow-gauge lines have both, for their locomotives and rolling-stock are far from standard patterns. In many places miniature lines have been specially built as an attraction in themselves and these are frequently operated by locomotives and stock which are scaled-down replicas of standard equipment. Some lines have rolling-stock which reproduces historic locomotives and carriages—the Hoot, Toot and Whistle Railway, for instance, has everything in the style of 1860 and a miniature version of the famous locomotive *The General*.

In the U.S.S.R., Czechoslovakia and Hun-gary there are a number of narrow-gauge railways which are run by boys and girls. Here there is an opportunity for every boy to satisfy his ambition to be an engine driver and they play a valuable part in training young people for railway work.

1 *Talyllyn* Locomotive No. 1, pulls a train into Dolgoch station on the Talyllyn line, originally a quarry railway.
2 The 2 ft. gauge Darjeeling Railway in the Himalayas. The men on the front of the locomotive drop sand on the rails to stop slipping.
3 A young engine driver on the Young Pioneers' Railway at Kharkov in the Ukraine.
4 French Railways' 1300 h.p. Z. 7100 rail-car, in use on the electrified line between Lyons and Saint-Etienne. Its maximum speed is 74 m.p.h. It can seat 70 passengers and haul three trailers.
5 An electric train entering Castellamare di Stabia Station on the narrow-gauge Circum-Vesuviana Railway between Naples and Sorrento.

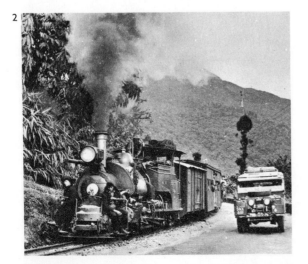

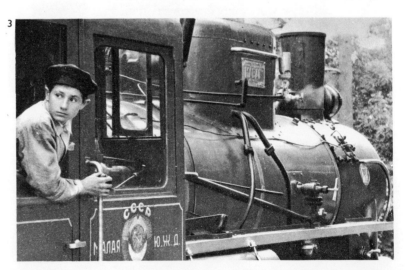

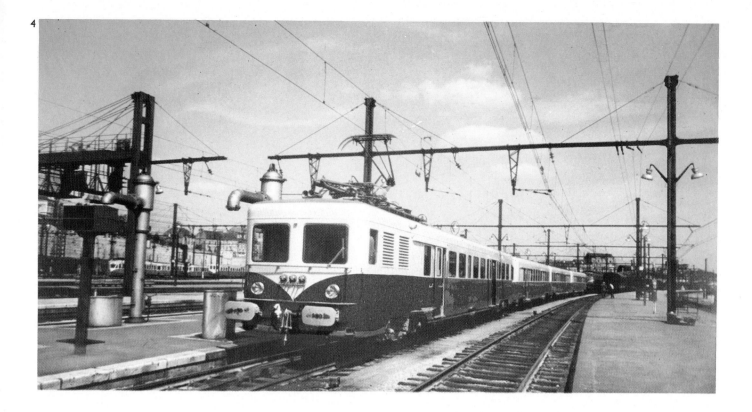

4

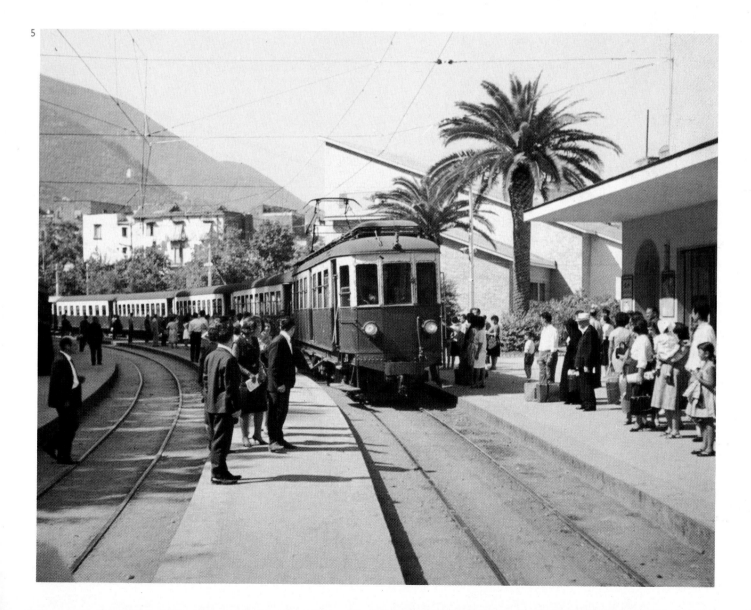

5

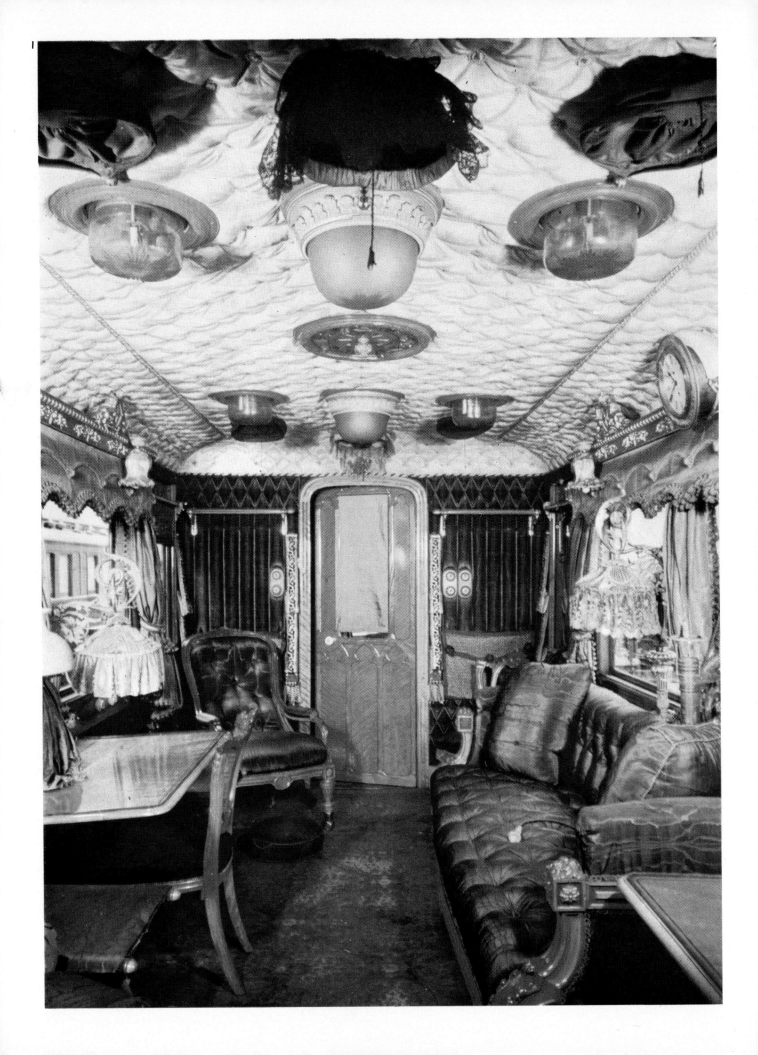

ROYAL AND STATE TRAINS

AT TWENTY-FIVE PAST TWELVE on 11th June 1842 a young woman of twenty-three stepped down from a carriage at Paddington Station to join her husband on the platform. Railway travel had become respectable. Queen Victoria had made her first train journey.

Two years before, the Great Western Railway 'anticipating the Patronage of the Queen and her illustrious Consort, Prince Albert, and of the members of the Royal Family,' had ordered a 'splendid railway carriage' from the famous London coach-builder David Davies.

'It is a very handsome vehicle 21 feet in length and divided into three compartments, the two end ones being four feet six inches long and nine feet wide, while the centre forms a noble saloon, twelve feet long, nine feet wide and six feet six inches high. The exterior is painted of the same brown colour as the others of the Company's carriages, and at each end is a large window affording a view of the whole of the line. The interior has been most magnificently fitted up by Mr. Webb, upholsterer, Old Bond Street. The saloon is handsomely decorated with hanging sofas in the rich style of Louis XIV, and the walls are panelled out in the same elegant manner, and fitted up with rich crimson and white silk and exquisitely executed paintings representing the four elements by Parris. The end compartments are also fitted up in the same style, each apartment having in the centre a useful and ornamental rose-wood table; and the floors of the whole are covered with chequered India matting.'

Originally designed to run on four wheels, it was modified to run on eight—perhaps at the suggestion of Prince Albert or Queen Adelaide, who were already railway travellers.

When the railway company received unexpected instructions that the Queen wished to be conveyed by rail from Slough to London, they assembled a train for the royal party

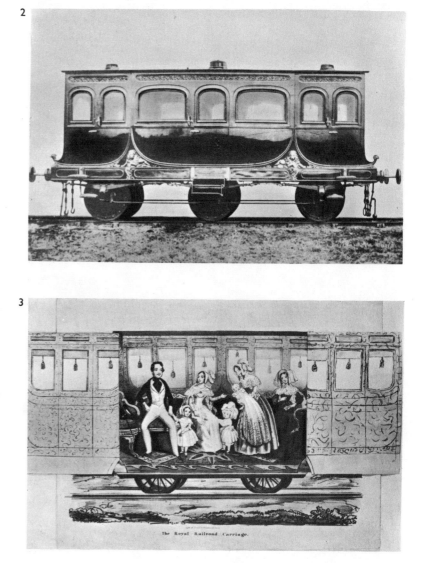

The Royal Railroad Carriage.

1 Queen Victoria's saloon, built by the London and North Western Railway in 1869, now in the Museum of British Transport.
2 The Queen's saloon carriage designed by Richard Mansell for the South Eastern Railway and built in 1851.
3 A coloured print of the Queen's carriage which opened to show the Royal Family inside.

drawn by *Phlegethon,* an almost new locomotive with seven-foot driving wheels.

The Queen drove by coach from Windsor Castle and while the royal coaches were being loaded on to flat cars she inspected the line. The locomotive was driven by Daniel Gooch, its designer, who was Locomotive Superintendent of the line, accompanied by Brunel, the company's Engineer.

The Queen enjoyed her first rail journey and wrote to her uncle, the King of the Belgians: 'We arrived here yesterday morning having come by railroad, from Windsor, in half an hour, free from dust and crowd and heat, and I am quite charmed by it.'

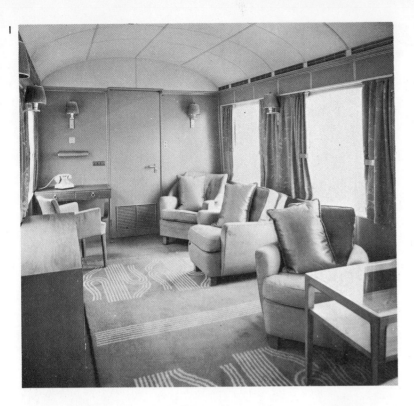

1 The Royal Saloon built at Wolverton Works in 1941 and still used by Elizabeth II.
2 Queen Adelaide's coach, built by the London and Birmingham Railway in 1842.
3 The sleeping arrangements in Queen Adelaide's coach. Note the padded stretcher between the seats and the 'boot' to accommodate the royal feet.
4 Twin saloons built for Queen Victoria in 1869 were joined on a single frame to form this carriage in 1895.
5 The carriage used by Oscar II of Sweden for official trips.
6 The bedroom in Queen Alexandra's 1903 saloon.
7 A locomotive decorated for a royal tour of Cardiff Docks in 1907.
8 The papal train of Pope Pius IX.

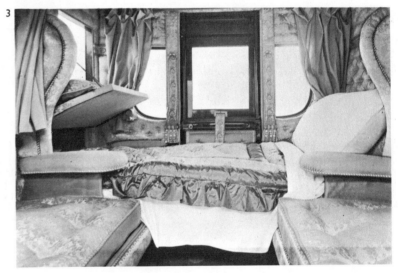

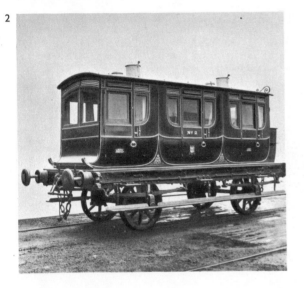

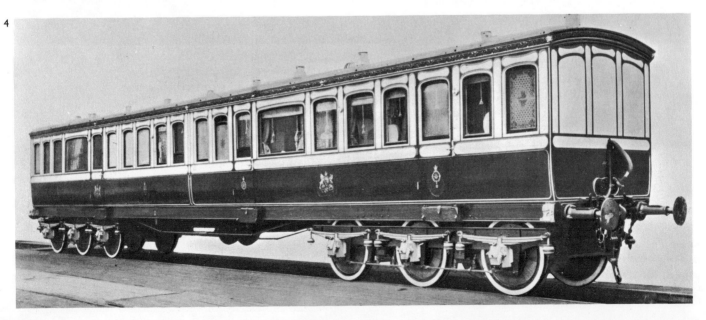

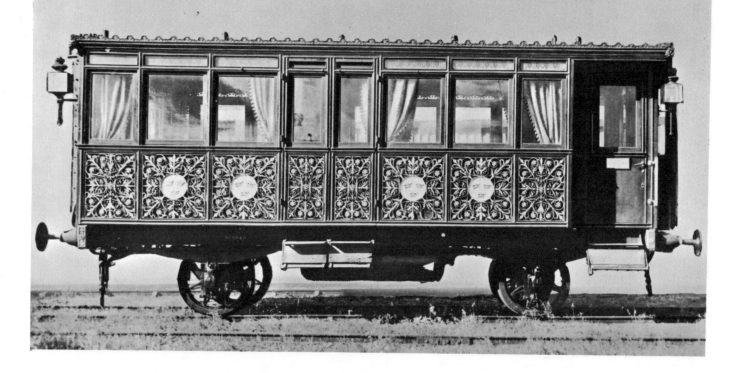

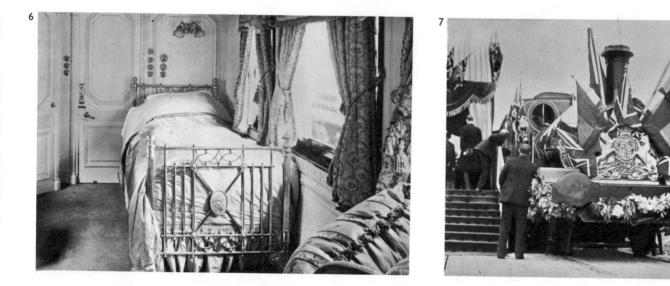

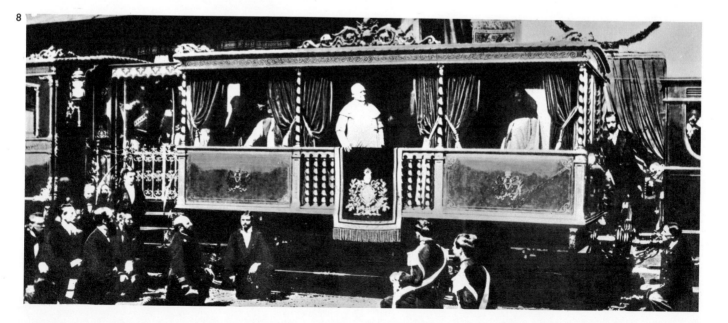

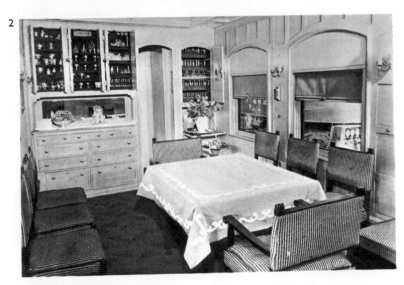

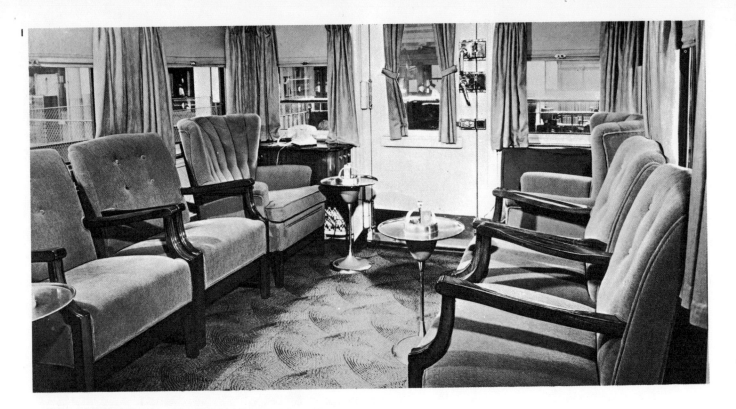

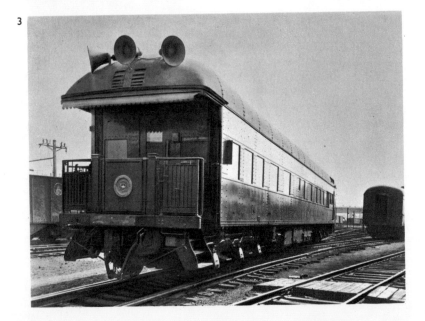

United States Car No. 1: the Official Carriage of the President.
1 The Lounge.
2 The Dining Room.
3 Exterior.

RAILWAYS AND THE COUNTRYSIDE

TOO OFTEN the railways have been associated with grimy buildings and dirty back-to-back houses huddled beneath embankments. These things exist, it is true; however, they are not caused by the railway but by the sudden development of industry which railways made possible, and the urbanisation which followed. Indeed, in the early days, when locomotives burned coke, not coal, there was no dirty smoke, nor will there be in the future when our railways are diesel- or electric-powered. Another charge which has been brought is that they have defaced the countryside. Wordsworth was among the people who decried the railways; an angry Ruskin said, 'I detest railways. Your railway has cut through some of the loveliest bits of scenery in the country,' and many landowners opposed them, though more, perhaps, for fear of damage to their hunting than fear of damage to the natural scene.

However, after a century which had seen the drastic change following the increasing enclosure of the land, the building of turnpike roads and of canals cutting across the countryside, many people thought of the new cuttings and embankments not as scars but as arteries carrying life to the countryside.

The author of *Osborne's London and Birmingham Railway Guide* describes that railway as '...a piece of human workmanship of the most stupendous kind; which, when considered with respect to its scientific character, magnitude, utility, its harmony of arrangement, and mechanical contrivance, eclipses all former works of art. Compared to it, how shabby a structure would be the celebrated Roman Wall, or even the more extensive one of the Chinese; as for the Egyptian pyramids, they so far from being fit to be mentioned in comparison with the railway, are merely uncouth monuments...' A guide book to Surrey, describing the view from the North Downs in 1865, says: 'The railway lines from Redhill to Dorking, from East Grinstead to Three Bridges and from Redhill far on the way to Brighton, are visible from this point; the wreaths of white smoke that float above the deep foliage of the Weald marking the progress of the trains across the old country of the Iguanodon and the Plesiosaurus.'

George Eliot, too, seems to have found pleasure in the sight of the railways:

'Our Midland plains have never lost their familiar impression and conservative spirit for me; yet at every other mile, since I first looked on them some sign of world-wide change some new direction of human labour, has wrought itself into what one may call the speech of the landscape... While hardly a wrinkle is made in the fading mother's face, or a new curve of health in the blooming girl's, the hills are cut through, or the breaches between them spanned, we choose our level, and the white steam-pennon flies along it.'

1 The Avon Viaduct, Wolston, Warwickshire. From a drawing by John Bourne.
2 A cutting near Roade, Northamptonshire.

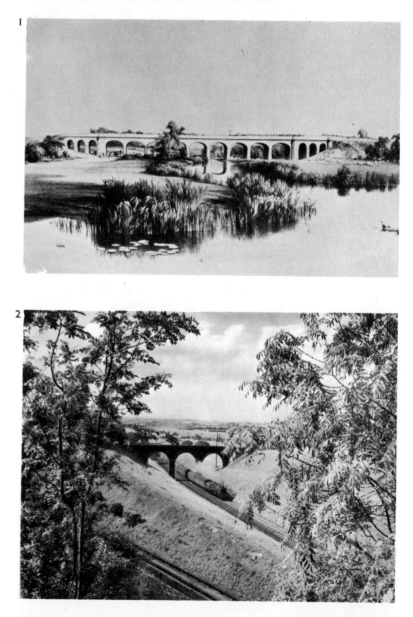

THE ARCHITECTURE OF THE RAILWAYS

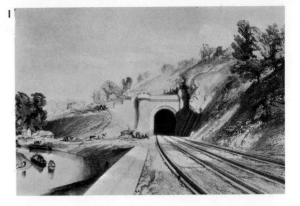

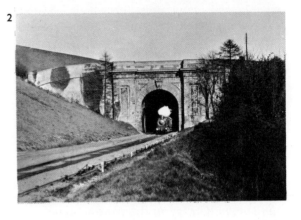

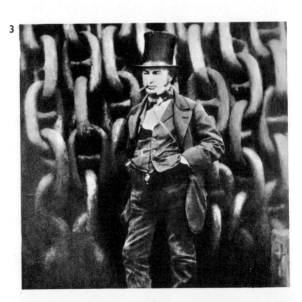

THE RAILWAYS cut across the countryside, but the taste and skill of the great railway architects and engineers ensured that they contributed to the shape of the countryside. Change was unavoidable, but as much was gained as lost. Pioneers like George and Robert Stephenson and Isambard Kingdom Brunel, building without the use of steel, designed so well that their bridges and viaducts can still be used today, and for much heavier traffic than they were ever intended to carry. Their earthworks, cuttings and embankments were among their greatest achievements, although perhaps least noticed by the traveller today.

Aware of the magnitude of their task they decorated their tunnel entrances with fine arches, some grandly classical, others more fanciful with gothick crenellations or exotic shapes. Set at the end of stark cuttings (since softened by a century's vegetation), they must have been even more imposing than they are today.

At first Robert Stephenson thought that locomotives should not be expected to haul on gradients steeper than 1 in 330, so viaducts were built to carry the line at an even level. These viaducts, and the many bridges to carry the line over waterways and roads, were often a graceful addition to the scene and bear comparison with the fine aqueducts of Imperial Rome.

But such features had been seen before. One thing the railway demanded for which no other form of transport had shown a need— a proper station building. The stage-coach had used a convenient inn as a departure point or relay station where its passengers could shelter, but the railway had to have a building on its tracks. The requirements were a place where passengers could buy their tickets and await the departure of the train and have easy access to the carriages themselves.

Mount Clare, the first station in the United States, provided little more than a booking office with no other shelter for the passenger; but the first British station, at Crown Street, Liverpool, embodied many features of the modern station. There was a vehicle court, separated from street traffic by a wall, a combined ticket-selling and waiting room and both covered access to the carriages and a train-shed right across the tracks.

Many variations in station buildings were

1 The entrance to Bristol Long Tunnel at Foxes' Wood.
2 The entrance to Box Tunnel.
3 Isambard Kingdom Brunel, the great rival of the Stephensons; among his achievements were the Royal Albert Bridge at Saltash, the steam ship *Great Eastern*— and the Great Western broad-gauge line.
4 The Conway Bridge was dressed up to match the castle by order of Act of Parliament.
5 The Britannia Tubular Bridge across the Menai Straits, built by Robert Stephenson.
6 Wharncliffe Viaduct, a drawing by J. C. Bourne.
7 The viaduct across the Rhine at Eglisau.

tried. The first, of which Crown Street was an example, had a single platform on one side of the tracks only. Next came two facing platforms for arriving and departing passengers, as at the first Euston Station (1835—9) with waiting, baggage and booking facilities on the departure side. The great drawback of this type was that when the volume of traffic became too great to be handled by one platform at each side, intermediate platforms had to be added. To reach them, cross-platforms or footbridges were necessary. At Paddington, where there was no space for a cross-platform, Brunel installed a sort of drawbridge which could be withdrawn and stored under the platforms when not in use. Naturally, while in position these got in the way of the trains, but passengers preferred them to using footbridges.

Another plan was that of the head-type station with the offices in a building at the head of the tracks and platforms perpendicular to it—a scheme particularly suited to terminal stations but equally suited for use where the tracks can be made to pass below the station building.

The European railway companies and their architects sought to make their stations, and particularly the terminals, a symbol of the importance of their enterprise. The grand scale of Euston, with its imposing Doric 'propylaeum' forming, as it were, a gateway to the railways of England, made a great impression on the departing traveller, and many stations boasted a classically styled portico.

In some towns the architect tried to harmonise his building with the aspect and the spirit of the town itself. It is interesting to note that Brunel took the medieval abbey at Bath as the model for his station there, not the 'classical' architecture of the Georgian town.

Not every station was built on imposing lines. Small stations, sometimes built of local stone, fitted comfortably into the countryside. Frequently seeking to emulate a domestic style, they suggested a chalet or *cottage orné*. An Italianate style became very popular; in smaller stations looking like villas and in larger ones, to which a campanile was often added, suggesting an Italian palace. The *Illustrated London News* in 1844 stated that the South East Railway Company had selected the 'Italian Palazzo style' for its buildings: 'the choice having been determined by the convenience

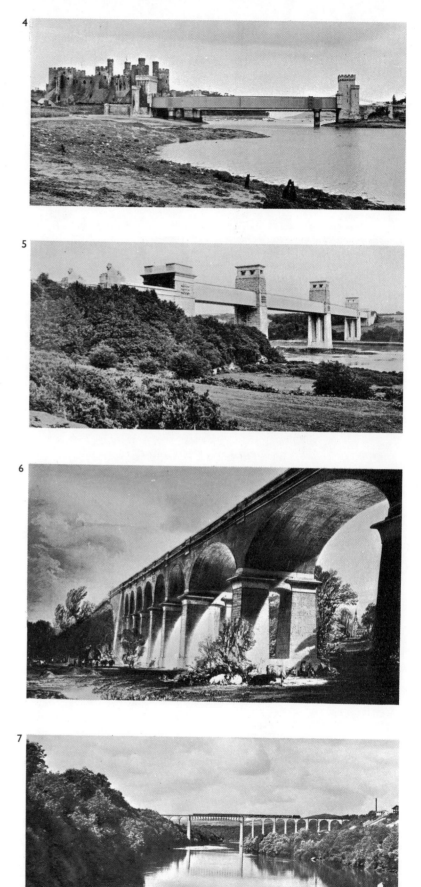

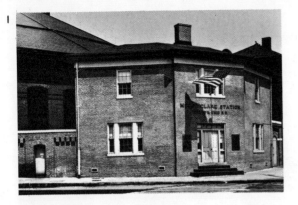

1

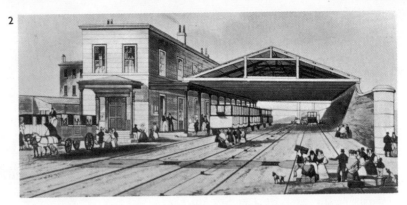

2

3

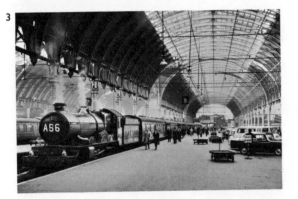

4

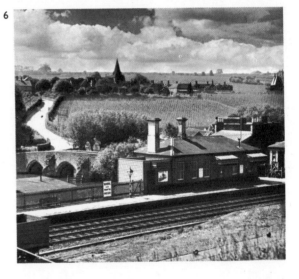

COMPLETION OF THE SOUTH-EASTERN RAILWAY.

5

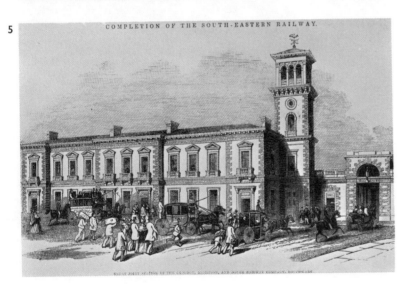

6

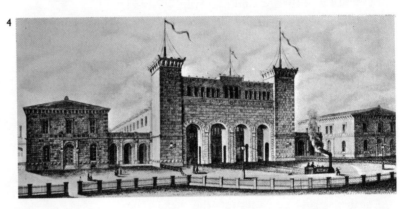

of its general arrangement, its cheapness and the suitability of its picturesque decorations to the bustling character of a railway site . . . the campanile made here to serve the useful purpose of a clock tower—is certainly a striking and appropriate feature.'

In the New World the station buildings took second place. The capital was all needed for the building of the line itself. Many stations consisted of only a single room, and until the building of the Old Grand Central Station in New York in 1869, there was nothing in America to compare with the great European stations.

Not everyone agreed that railway stations

should be either monumental or highly decorated. While people flocked to see Hardwick's Euston arch, Pugin thought: 'The architects have evidently considered it an opportunity for *showing off what they could do* instead of *carrying out what required*. Hence the colossal Grecian portico or gateway, 100 feet high [an exaggeration—the overall height was only 72 feet] for the cabs to drive through, and set down a few feet further at the 14-inch brick wall and sash window booking office. This piece of Brobdignaggian absurdity must have cost the company a sum which would have built a first-rate station replete with convenience and which would have been really grand from its simplicity.'

William Cubitt said: 'A good station could be built at King's Cross for less than the cost of the ornamental archway at Euston Square.'

Considering some of Pugin's own highly gothic designs, it is a little difficult to understand his wish for simplicity. King's Cross, however, was built in 1851–2 by Cubitt's brother in an effectively simple style at a cost of £123,000 (the Euston arch cost £35,000).

The first station at Liverpool embodied the idea of a roof covering all the tracks, a concept more often rejected now in favour of separate platform covers. This idea of the 'train-shed' gave the architects an opportunity to join a competition which has been going on since the first arch was built—to construct the widest possible unsupported span.

Crown Street had a modest wooden shed 30 feet wide, but within a few years sheds were being supported on iron columns and then, when it was seen how quickly wood deteriorated from the smoke and steam of the locomotives, were made entirely of iron.

In 1854 a single span of 211 feet at New Street Station, Birmingham, exceeded the span of the dome of St. Peter's Basilica in Rome and every other earlier vault.

The great arched roof was by no means the only form of train-shed, but it was the most spectacular. At St. Pancras, London, a span of 243 feet was built in 1863–76, not to be exceeded until 1888 when the Pennsylvania

1 Mount Clare Station of the Baltimore and Ohio Railroad, America's first railway station.
2 Crown Street, Liverpool, a print by Bury, dated 1831. Note the turntables for reversing locomotives and rolling-stock, and the cable working of the centre track.
3 Paddington Station, which replaced the Bishop's Road terminus of Brunel's Great Western Railway. The original roof arches still stand.
4 The First Thüringer Banhof, Leipzig (1840-4), architect Eduard Pötsch. The tracks meet at a turntable in front of the forecourt.
5 London Bridge Station, terminus of the Brighton, Dover and Croydon Railway (1844).
6 The village station at East Farleigh, Kent.
7 The 'new station house' at Washington, D.C., built in 1852.
8 The Euston 'propylaeum' designed by Philip Hardwick was built of Yorkshire stone and cost £35,000. It has been demolished to make way for a new Euston.
9 Cubitt's station at King's Cross.
10 New Street Station, Birmingham, about 1905.

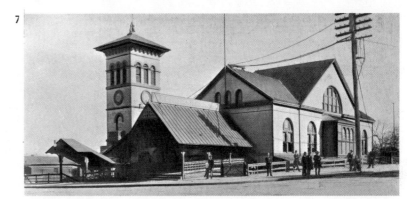

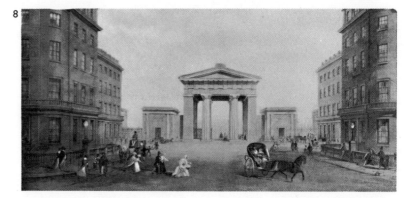

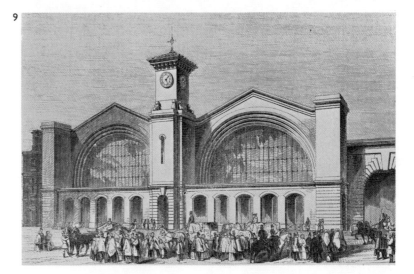

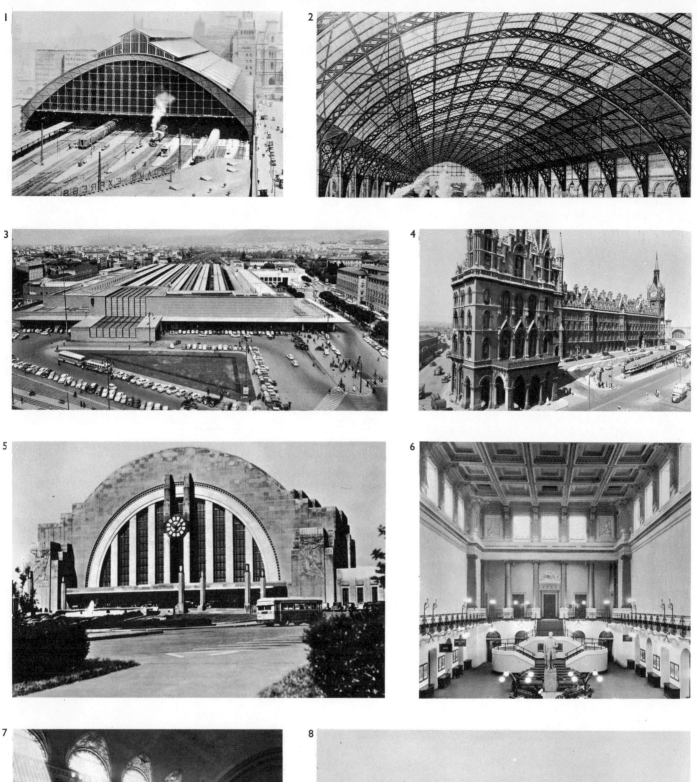

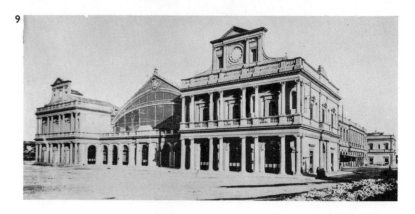

Railroad's station at Jersey City was built with a span of 252 feet. The climax was reached with 300 feet at the second Broad Street Station, Philadelphia, in 1892—30.

Not only did the train-shed grow larger as the traffic and the number of platforms increased, the head-block also became larger and more complex. Sometimes fronted by an imposing façade, sometimes sheltering behind a great hotel, as at Paddington or St. Pancras, there had to be provision for additional passenger services, offices for company staff and often the opportunity was taken to add grandeur for its own sake.

Euston was once more in the lead when Philip Charles Hardwick, son of the original architect, added the richly decorated 'Great Hall' which was soon copied by other designers.

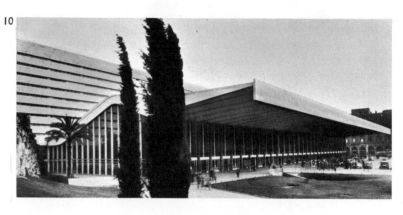

The head-buildings began to incorporate shops, restaurants, barbers' shops, bathrooms, in later years even cinemas, as well as the necessary booking, waiting, baggage and toilet facilities for the passenger. Instead of proceeding directly via the ticket office to the platform, with a waiting-room near by if he was early for his train, the passenger had to find his way through an assemblage of halls, corridors, concourses, arcades and staircases. The simpler utilitarian functions of the station were hidden under vast masonry designed chiefly to impress. In North America particularly many opulent buildings were erected, some of them railway cities where all the requirements of life could be found without ever leaving the station building.

One American station which uses a colossal scale without loss of functional efficiency is the Grand Central Station in New York, built 1903—13. However, highly satisfactory though the planning of this station is, the cost of operating it is proving uneconomic today.

The great glass-arch train-shed was going out of favour in the United States by 1914. Ten years before, Lincoln Bush had patented his form of shedding of low-reinforced concrete spans with slots to allow fumes and smoke to escape. This style in turn was supplanted by the simple platform canopy making no attempt to cover the lines or provide protection from stormy weather.

Train-sheds continued to be built in Europe. In 1930 the new Stazione Centrale at Milan

1 The second Broad Street Station, Philadelphia.
2 The train-shed of St. Pancras.
3 Stazione Santa Maria Novella, Florence.
4 The front of St. Pancras, originally designed as a great hotel.
5 Ohio Union Terminal, Cincinnati.
6 The Great Hall at Euston (now demolished).
7 The main concourse, Grand Central Terminal, New York City.
8 Roma Termini in 1869.
9 Roma Termini in 1874.
10 and 11. The magnificent modern Roma Termini has platforms running directly from a wide internal piazza which stretches the full width of the building, forming a thoroughfare with shops and restaurants. The dramatic curve of the roof echoes the line of the remains of the wall of Septimius Serverus, seen at the end of the booking hall (11).

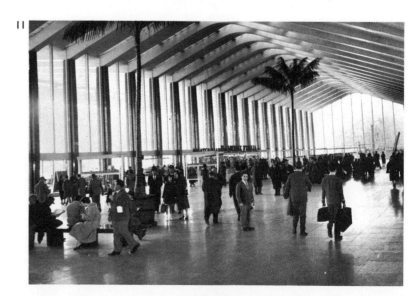

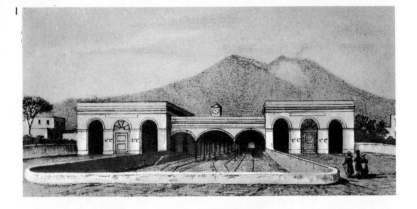

1

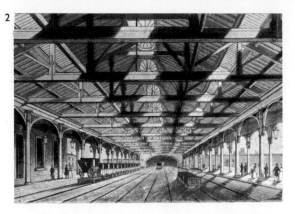

2

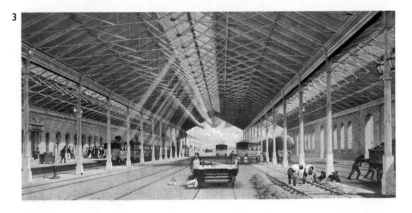

3

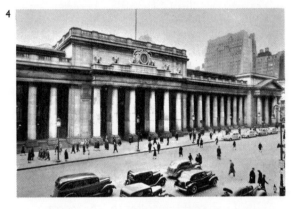

4

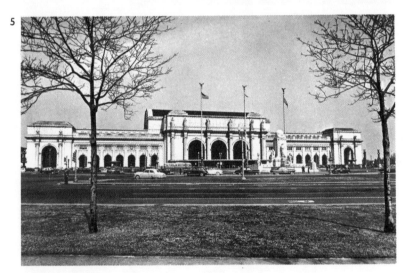

5

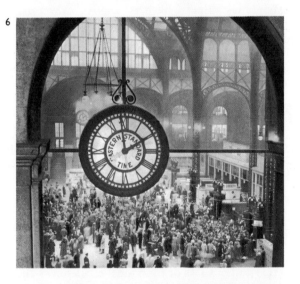

6

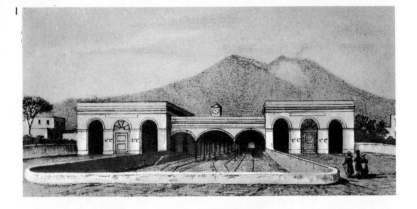

7

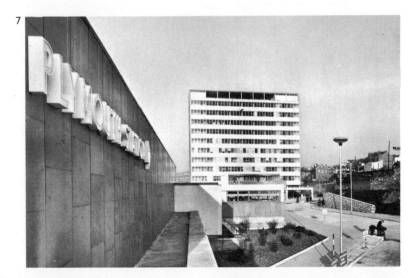

8

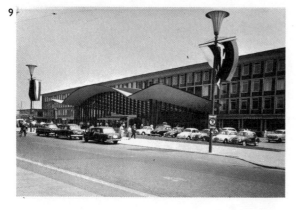

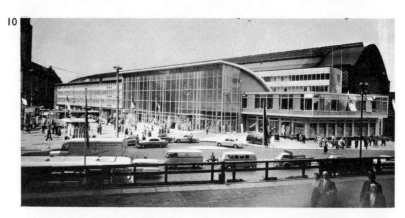

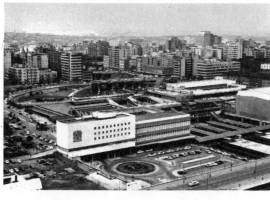

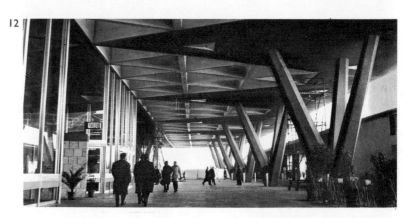

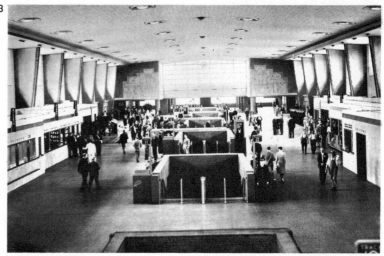

1 Naples (1839).
2 Lime Street, Liverpool (1836).
3 Derby (1839), architect Francis Thompson. Note the graceful fluted columns with their ribbon motif.
4 & 6 Pennsylvania Station, New York City: façade and main concourse.
5 Union Terminal, Washington, D.C.
7 New station at Plymouth, Devon.
8 Stairs and bridges at Coventry, Warwickshire (1962).
9 Bochum, West Germany (1956).
10 Cologne, main station.
11 Johannesburg, South Africa.
12 Napoli Centrale.
13 Concourse of Montreal Central.
14 Kuala Lumpur, Malaya.
15 S. Lucia, Venice. The steps of this new station lead straight down to the Grand Canal.

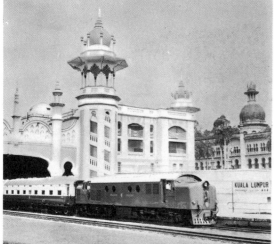

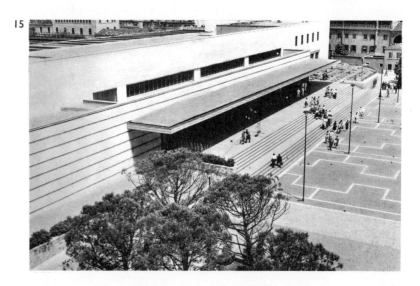

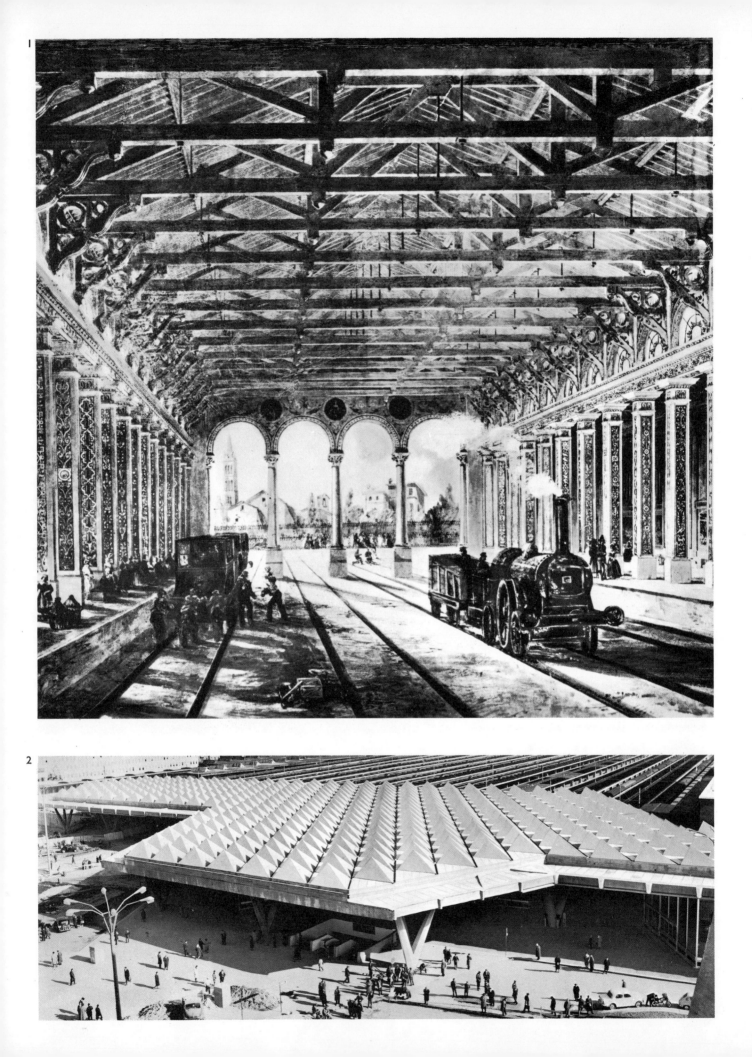

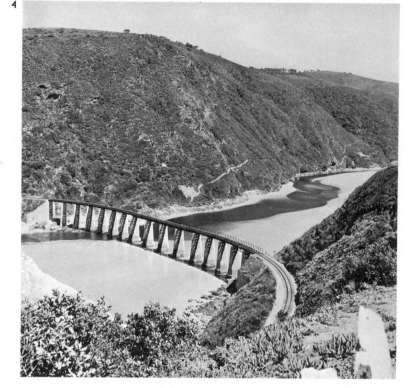

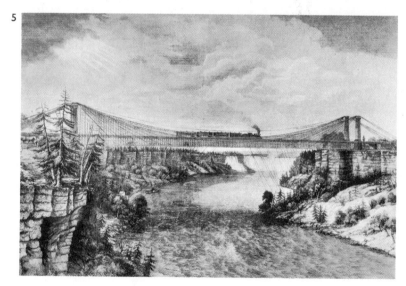

1 S. Maria Novella, Florence, arrival platform (1848).
2 The new Napoli Centrale station features this vigorous roof treatment.

MORE BRIDGES

3 Forth Bridge, Scotland. Each of the centre spans is 1,710 feet long.
4 Kaaimans River Bridge, Cape Province, South Africa.
5 & 7. Niagara Falls, 1861 and 1897.
6 Joise River Bridge, South Africa.

was completed. Built from designs by Ulisse Stacchini which won a competition in 1913 it has a beautiful series of five simple arched spans, the largest of which is 236 feet wide. Unfortunately, this simplicity is not carried through to the head-building, which is probably

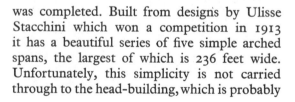

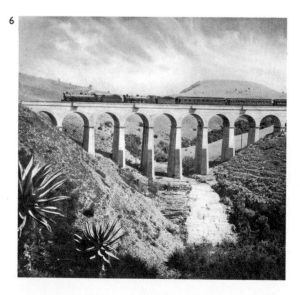

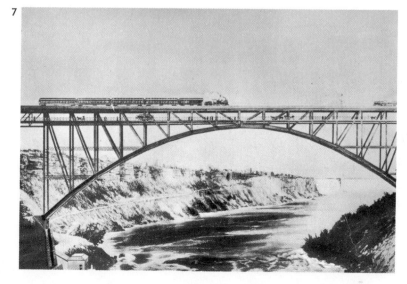

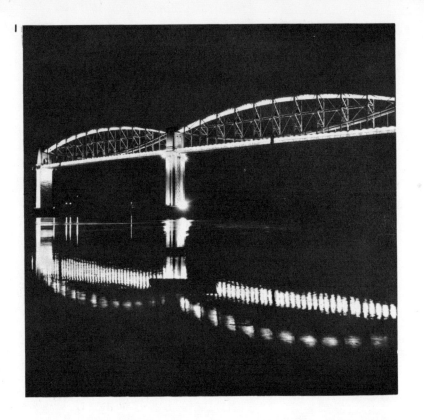

the most pompous and grandiose of its kind. Compare it with the stark simplicity of the Stazione Santa Maria Novella designed by G. Michelucci and finished only six years later. Here the function and direction of the platforms and tracks are expressed in the lines of the head-building and the glassed panel of the porte-cochère.

Scandinavia, Holland, Germany, Austria and Great Britain have all produced good station designs in recent years but, to my mind, the most satisfying station in the world today is again in Italy—the fine Stazione Termini in Rome.

This, perhaps, is the type of station we shall see in the future.

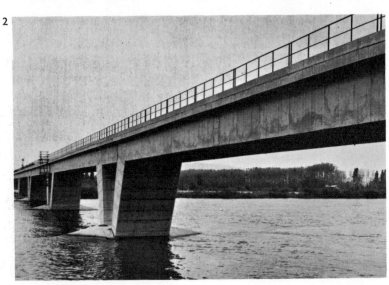

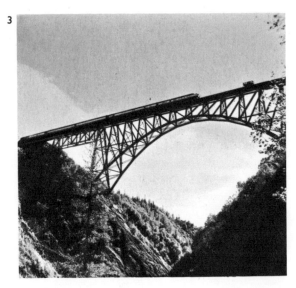

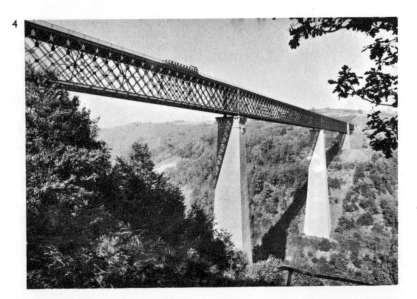

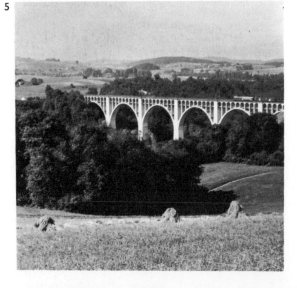

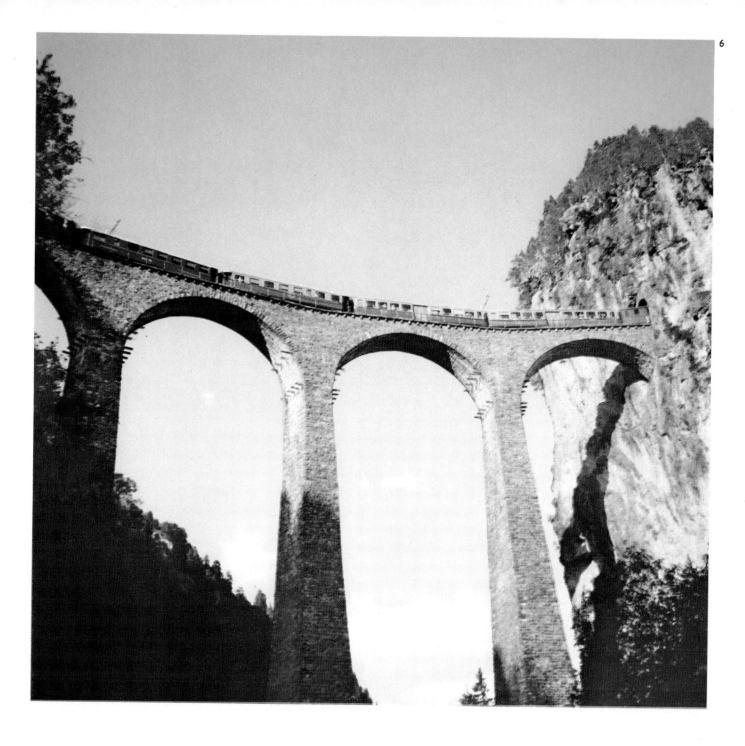

1 Royal Albert Bridge across the River Tamar at Saltash, Cornwall, built by Brunel and opened in 1859.
2 La Voulte Viaduct across the Rhône in France, is the longest railway structure in pre-stressed concrete.
3 Hurricane Gulch Bridge, Alaska.
4 Fades Viaduct, France, the highest in the world.
5 Grandfey Viaduct, Switzerland.
6 The Landwasser Viaduct on the Rhaetian Railway's main line from Chur to St. Moritz, Switzerland.

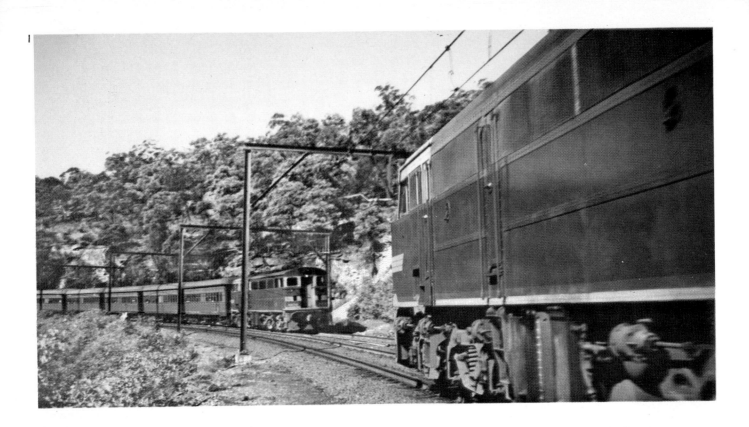

1

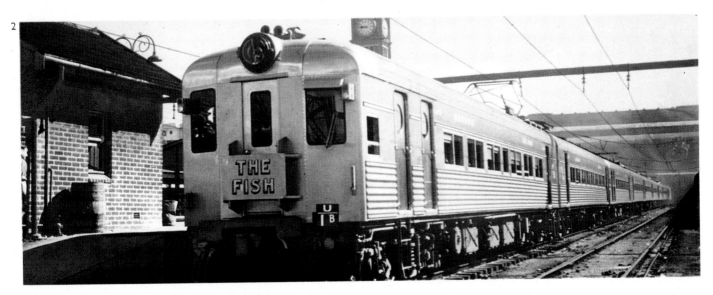

2

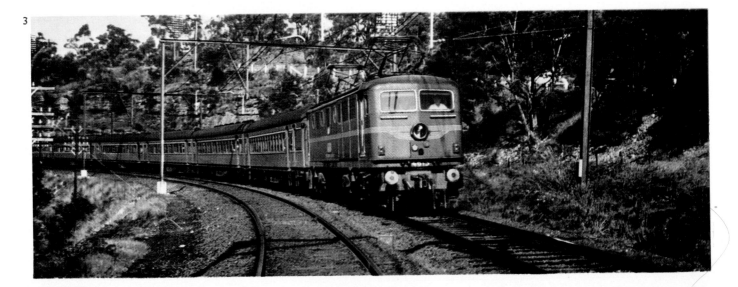

3

LONDON TO BIRMINGHAM IN 1838

TICKET IN HAND we pass through to the departure platform and find our numbered seats. We have a five and a half hour journey ahead of us in an open second-class carriage, single fare twenty shillings. If we paid more we could travel in one of the six-seater, closed-in first-class carriages or even in one of the four-seater mail carriages, but second-class *closed* carriages only run at night.

The officials are already shouting for us to take our places and as soon as we are settled some of the railway staff push the train of carriages to the end of the departure platform where they are attached to a continuous cable by which we are hauled up to Chalk Farm by a powerful winding engine. There the locomotive, one of Edward Bury's little engines with a tall chimney and shining brass dome, is attached.

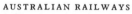

AUSTRALIAN RAILWAYS
1 Two '44' class diesel-electric locomotives.
2 An inter-urban electric train leaving Sydney Station.
3 A '46' class electric locomotive in the Blue Mountain region of New South Wales.

LONDON AND BIRMINGHAM RAILWAY
4 Philip Hardwick's great Doric arch was the gateway to the London and Birmingham Railway. Passengers entering through it were set down under a colonnaded covered way. First-class passengers entered through the north door, bought their tickets at the booking office and then went down a corridor to their waiting-room. Second-class passengers used another door to a combined waiting-room and booking office. Hand baggage was carried to the waiting-room and heavy trunks and cases loaded on to the train from a baggage dock at the end of the lines.
To the right of the 'propylaeum' a gate led to the carriage dock. The nobility and gentry could arrive in their own carriages, which were then placed on flat wagons, the horses travelling in a special horse-box. The passenger could either travel in his own carriage or in the company's. When he reached the end of his journey the carriage was taken down, the horses harnessed, and milord could drive off straight away.
5 The departure platform, Euston.
6 The fixed engine station at Camden Town. To cross the Regent's Canal, near Chalk Farm, the line had to be given a gradient of 1 in 70. This section, known as the Camden Inclined Plane, was thought too steep for locomotive operation and until 1844 was worked by cable. The trains were attached to an endless rope, 4,080 yards long and $2\frac{1}{4}$ inches thick, which was operated by two 60 h.p. engines at the top of the incline. Men known as 'bankriders' travelled on incoming trains to manipulate the brakes and prevent the speed exceeding 10 m.p.h.

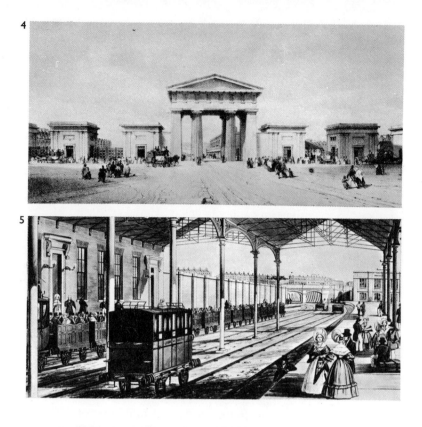

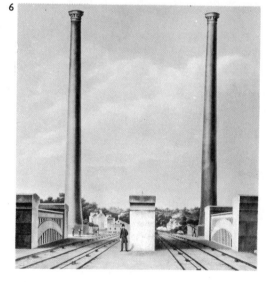

With a jerk we are really on our way. 'The noise made by the engine is at first somewhat between a pant and a cough; but this becomes less distinct as our rapidity increases, for the motion of the piston which occasions the coughing sound, when it becomes rapid, connects the sound into a continuous burring noise . . . by no means so unpleasant as the noise of the stage coach.'

We are approaching the Primrose Hill Tunnel, 1,154 yards long, so we put on our gauze spectacles to protect our eyes against the soot and smoke—anyone without spectacles should keep their eyes closed when passing through tunnels. A railway constable at the lineside shows a white flag to indicate that the line is clear and into the darkness we go. A rain of sparks bounces back off the roof but we are soon out in the air again, passing the villages of Hampstead and Highgate away on the right, and on through Kilburn.

By now we must be rushing at a speed of at least twenty miles an hour and we roar through Kensal Green Tunnel in no time at all, past the place where Willesden Junction, one of the largest railway centres in the country, will appear in later years; but now the open fields and farmsteads give no sign that they are so soon to be swallowed up by the spread of London's houses and factories.

The train rushes on, up the long gradient to Hatch End with the buildings of Harrow School away on the crest of Harrow Hill to the left, and then down through Bushey and over a magnificent viaduct into Watford. Here, whilst the train makes its first stop and takes water to refill the thirsty boiler, we may admire the neat 'Gothic building, the residence of the inspector of the station.'

Soon we are jolting into motion again and entering Watford Tunnel, 1,817 yards long, with five ventilation shafts. We can feel quite safe for 'great attention is paid by the policemen to detect any obstruction on the rails in the tunnel.' From the tunnel we reach the lower slopes of the Chilterns and pound through Boxmoor (the original terminus when the first section of the line was opened last year). The calm waters of the Grand Junction Canal run alongside us until we top the rise at Tring and roll downhill into the great Tring Cutting, its white chalk walls agleam in the September sunshine.

The Stephensons, father and son, can be proud of this achievement. Two and a half miles long, in places sixty feet deep, it took 400 men three and a half years to make, excavating one and three-quarter million tons of soil. Another few miles, then through the tunnel at Leighton and on to Denbigh Hall where, since April until only the other day, passengers had to transfer to a horse-coach for the trip to Rugby; but now the Kilsby Tunnel is all complete and we go straight through.

Our next stop is at Wolverton and here, fifty-two and a half miles from London, the engines are changed. 'The trains stop at this station 10 minutes, and a female attendant has been placed here for the convenience of ladies.' Here too are workshops, artisans, etc., and every convenience, to repair accidents, or to obtain any requisite which the trains may require.'

Seven miles further on we reach Roade, from which horse-coaches connect with Northampton (fare 1s 6d), then on to Blisworth through a great cutting which, though not the largest on the line, was the most difficult and expensive. The ground consists largely of hard blue limestone and this had to be drained by pumping. A mile and a quarter long and an average of fifty feet deep, the excavation required 300,000 pounds of gunpowder which at £2 10s. per cwt. cost £8,000. It is estimated that the whole operation cost about £200,000.

Ten miles beyond Roade we reach Weedon, then up Buckby Bank, across the Grand Junction Canal to Welton Station. With a warning shriek on the whistle we plunge into Kilsby Tunnel. It is 2,398 yards long, 28 feet high and 25 feet wide, with two huge ventilating shafts, each sixty feet in diameter, one of them 120 feet deep the other 90 feet.

The original contractor undertook to build the tunnel for £99,000 but the workmen struck a hidden spring which flooded the tunnel so rapidly that they only escaped by improvising a raft out of timbers which, it is said, one of the engineers towed to safety by means of a rope held in his teeth. The contractor gave up and died of a broken heart. Robert Stephenson carried on with the company's money. It took eight months of continuous pumping, night and day, at the rate of 2,000 gallons a minute and from a depth of 120 feet, before the quicksand spring was conquered and the tunnel finished. The total cost was £300,000, 36 million bricks were used to line the tunnel and 1,250 men, 200 horses and 13 steam engines were employed.

Out of Kilsby Tunnel we roll down a gentle slope into the town of Rugby, to stop at a station built in the style of a Swiss chalet. Then on across the Warwickshire countryside, where the leaves have not yet begun to fall, to Coventry. The spires of Grey Friars, Holy Trinity and St. Michael's (not yet a cathedral) dominate the skyline and soon we are in the station. Only eighteen more miles to go. We speed on through Hampton-in-Arden but before we

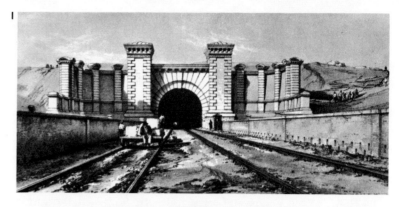

reach the Birmingham terminal we halt for
a moment and a clerk of the railway company
comes along the train to collect our tickets.
A short while more and we have stopped under
the roof of the station in Curzon Street.
The $112\frac{1}{2}$ mile journey is over.

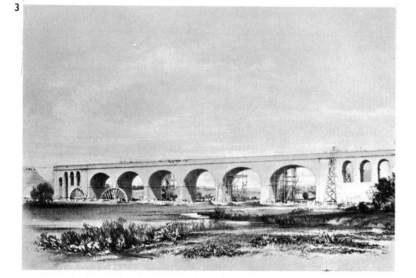

1 Entrance to the tunnel at Primrose Hill.
2 Entrance to the tunnel at Watford (the train here
seems to be going backwards).
3 Wolverton Viaduct under construction.
4 The 'Great Ventilating Shaft' in Kilsby Tunnel.
5 Blisworth Cutting (there is a railway policeman, with
signal flag, left).
6 The Birmingham terminus at Curzon Street.

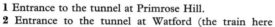

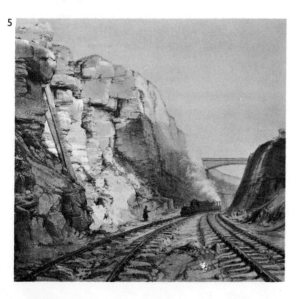

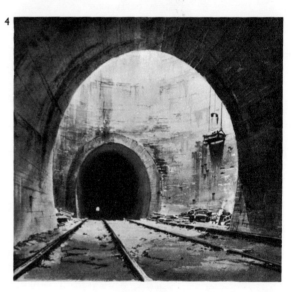

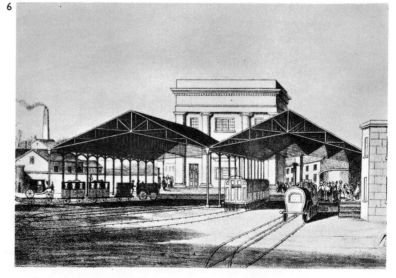

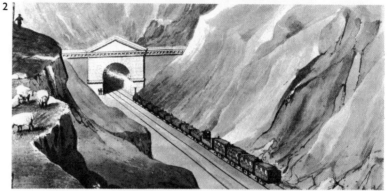

RAILWAYS IN THE ARTS

FROM THEIR BEGINNING railways have exerted a strange fascination over people of all kinds. The fascination of something new, a machine which could draw men, animals and goods at twelve miles an hour, a contraption which enthusiasts saw as a means to all kinds of ends: economic, social and political. It was a challenge to the engineer, a speculation for the financier and to the general public a sometimes frightening symbol of a changing world.

The very scale of railway engineering caught the imagination and there was a popular demand for prints and drawings such as those in which J. C. Bourne recorded the construction of the London and Birmingham Railway and the Great Western Railway. Outstanding as pictures, Bourne's work also shows amazing technical accuracy and is a reliable record of those early years.

But there was more than engineering to attract the artist. The railway combined the elemental powers of fire and water—steam, speed, power—here was a stimulus few could resist.

To a painter like the English artist J. M. W. Turner who was working in terms of coloured light—what Constable called 'tinted steam'—here was a perfect subject. To anyone who thinks of railway travel on a stormy day as a depressing rain-washed window, Turner's *Rain, Steam, Speed* may seem a romantic overstatement; but another traveller, a certain Mrs. Simon, was able to confirm its truth. While travelling one rainy day, she was surprised to see the kindly looking old gentleman opposite put his head out of the window during a torrential downpour—and keep it there for nearly nine minutes! Then he drew back into the compartment, well and truly soaked, and sat with his eyes shut for another quarter of an hour. Mrs. Simon was so curious to know what had prompted this strange action that she put *her* head out of the window and was so fascinated that she too received a thorough drenching.

Next year she went to see the exhibition at the Royal Academy and overheard a visitor near by saying, 'Just like Turner, ain't it? Whoever saw such a ridiculous conglomeration?' Mrs. Simon looked at the picture he was talking about. It was *Rain, Steam, Speed*. 'I did,' she said.

During 1877 Claude Monet painted a series of pictures of the Gare St. Lazare in Paris. They show how the effects of steam and smoke must have interested this artist, who was so eager to record the changing effects of light.

The people and situations of railways have been the inspiration for many artists. Honoré Daumier produced a splendid series of railway drawings, full of character and incident. W. P. Frith, painter of the famous *Derby Day*, painted an equally animated scene set on the departure platform at Paddington Station.

Other artists were more interested in showing the excitement of the railway and suggesting the power of the locomotive. The American print-makers Nathaniel Currier and James Ives must have produced hundreds of coloured lithographs which combined dramatic effect with accurate representation of the railway. For more than fifty years their company produced about three prints a week on every aspect of American life. The lithographs were hand coloured on a mass-production system—one girl per colour—and they were in great demand all over the States and abroad. The same excitement has been caught, though perhaps with more sophisticated technique, by the modern English painter Terence Cuneo who has been particularly successful at evoking the fiery heat of the footplate and the pent-up energy of the steam locomotive. He has also been able to suggest the power behind the much less dramatic exterior of the diesel or electric locomotive. Much of Cuneo's work has appeared in posters commissioned by the railway companies.

Railway posters, whether depicting railway operations or places served by the railway—or in special designs to promote a particular service—have often led the way in poster design. London Transport in particular has produced designs of such high quality that many people wanted to hang them in their

1 Detail from W. P. Frith's *The Railway Station* (1862). The locomotive is the *Great Britain*, built in 1847.
2 Part of a poster by Terence Cuneo advertising a night freight service.
3 Third-class passenger travel, drawn by Honoré Daumier (1808-79).
4 The great train accident scene in *The Whip* (1909).
5 Illustration from the sheet music for *The Excursion Train Galop*, showing a South Eastern Railway excursion.

1

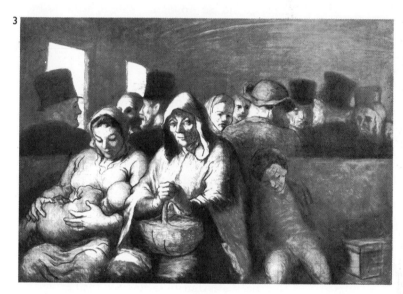

2

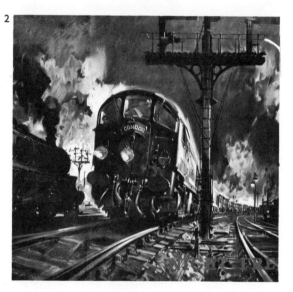

3

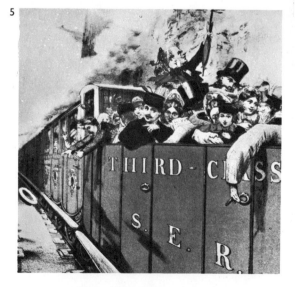

4

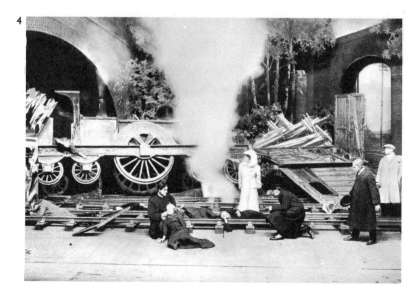

5

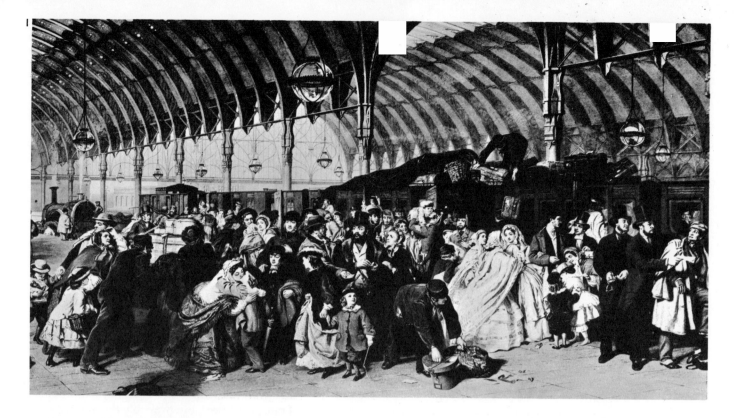

homes and copies had to be made available to the public. London Transport also led the way in commissioning work from sculptors Epstein, Gill and Henry Moore to decorate their headquarters building near St. James's Park.

Essayists have taken railways as their subject and poets have found railways an inspiration, and the railway has been the background to many plays from Ivanov's *The Armoured Train* and Afinogenov's *Distant Point* to *The Ghost Train*. Spectacular settings have ranged from the crash in *The Whip* in Victorian times to the Underground in Lionel Bart's *Blitz*.

Writers, dramatists and poets have all used the railway station setting. Apart from the steam, noise, crowds and atmospheric lighting which provide an excellent dramatic foil, a railway journey is a time between places, a time apart, and so to some extent is a railway station a place apart from the world around. It was for this reason that Jean Anouilh chose a provincial railway station for his setting of the Orpheus legend *Eurydice*. In Noel Coward's *Brief Encounter*, the refreshment room becomes a place outside society.

Massine based a ballet on the building of the Union Pacific Railroad, but *Terminal* merely used a station as a means of stringing a series of divertissements together and the Cocteau-Milhaud-Nijinska *Le Train Bleu*, named after the famous French train to the Riviera, was set on a bathing beach!

A railway journey gives the traveller an opportunity to reconsider, the writer a chance to ruminate or recapitulate. It can also throw people together without escape. A railway train has been a favourite setting for thriller-writers or film-makers.

The image of a great express rushing towards them was one of the first thrills for the kinematograph audience and America's earliest attempt at a narrative film was *The Great Train Robbery*, and anxious spectators in the nickelodeon would see Pearl White, or another favourite cliff-hanger heroine, tied to the rails with an express thundering round the bend. (But there is real tragedy in the death of Tolstoy's Anna Karenina beneath the wheels of a goods wagon.) From Hitchcock's *Strangers on a Train* to James Bond grappling with an enemy in *From Russia with Love*, the French resistance movie *The Train* or the zany humour of *The Great St. Trinian's Train Robbery*,

railways have been a gift to the film maker.

The cinema has also taken the story of the railroad itself and made such movies as Cecil B. de Mille's *Union Pacific*, the story of the building of the railroad, or John Ford's *The Iron Horse*, and of course the railroad played a major part in *The Way the West was Won*. The famous Civil War story of the locomotive called *The General* was used for Buster Keaton's classic film and retold by Walt Disney in *The Great Locomotive Chase*.

There have been several very fine films about railways. In 1944 Sidney Newman made *Trans-Canada Express* for the National Film Board of Canada, in 1960 John Schlesinger made *Terminus*, a film about a day on Waterloo Station, London, for British Transport Films, but probably the most famous of all railway films was made for the G.P.O. by Basil Wright and Harry Watt in 1935: *Night Mail*. This classic film has music by Benjamin Britten and specially written verse by W. H. Auden which reflects and continues the rhythm of the wheels on the natural sound track—the whole film is an exciting and romantic presentation of a mail train from London to Perth in Scotland.

Night Mail had a romantic treatment. Another exercise in combined documentary actuality, music and verse, this time in radio, did not. Ewan MacColl and Charles Parker's radio programme *The Ballad of John Axon* had an epic quality. Among the finest works ever devised for radio, this production from the B.B.C.'s Midland Region was inspired by the heroism of an engine driver.

Ewan MacColl's folk-song style music for this programme was in a long tradition of railway songs. In the United States in particular the railroad builders had sung their way

---

1 Buster Keaton in *The General*, the story of the *Great Locomotive Chase*.
2 A scene from *The Iron Horse*, directed by John Ford.
3 The *Coronation Scot* at speed.
4 Vittorio de Sica's *Stazione Termini* was set entirely within the confines of a railway station.
5 A lost child at Waterloo Station—in John Schlesinger's film *Terminus*, about a day at the station.
6 The British comedy *The Titfield Thunderbolt* (directed by Charles Crichton) told the story of an attempt to save a local line.

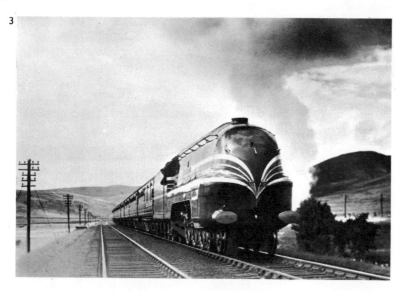

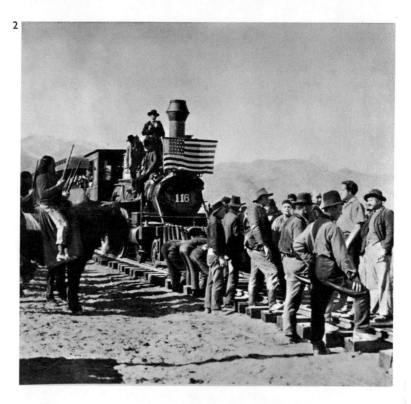

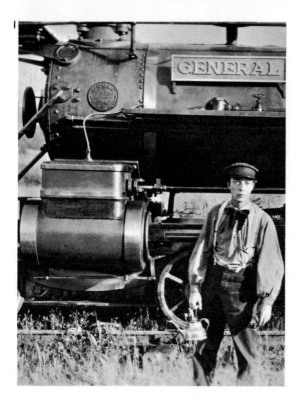

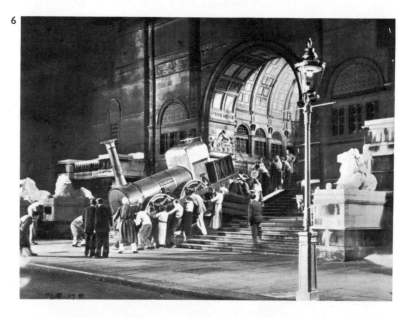

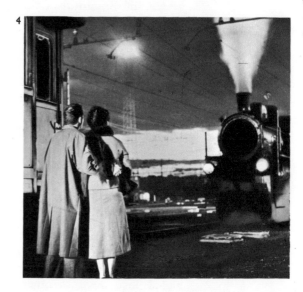

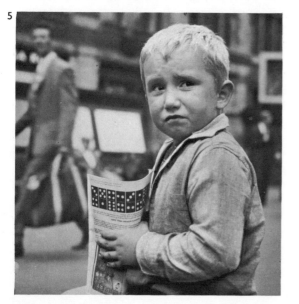

across the continent with ballads like *John Henry* and *Locomotive Bill* and railwaymen were celebrated in songs like *Casey Jones*. MacColl and Parker had been excited by Millard Campbell and Earl Robinson's radio ballad for *The Lonesome Train* but to this form they added actual recordings of people close to John Axon talking about the man and about life on the railway.

Work songs were not the only popular music to feature the railway. During the 1840's a piece called the *Excursion Train Galop* was extremely popular. There was an *Express Train Galop* too.

Many railways have found their place in popular songs. Crewe Junction has achieved fame less for its importance in the railway system of Britain than for its place in the music-hall song:

Oh Mr. Porter, what shall I do?
I wanted to go to Birmingham
And they've taken me on to Crewe.

Eric Coates' more recent *Coronation Scot* has a real feel of the railway about it.

It is not only lightweight composers who have found the railway interesting. Arthur Honegger, one of Les Six, in his *Pacific 231* written in 1923, has composed what must be the best-known musical work inspired by the railway. A quotation from an interview with Honegger which was published in the Geneva journal *Dissonance* forms a preface to the full score:

'I have always had a passionate liking for locomotives; for me they are living things, and I love them as others love women or horses. What I have endeavoured to describe in *Pacific 231* is not an imitation of the sounds of the locomotive, but the translation into musical terms of the visual impression and the physical sensation of it. It shows the objective contemplation; the tranquil breathing of the machine in repose, the effort to start, the progressive gathering of speed, leading from the lyric state to the pathetic, of a train of 300 tons hurling itself through the night at 120 miles an hour.

'For my subject I have chosen the locomotive type 'Pacific 231' for heavy trains of great speed.'

Honegger certainly succeeded in his intention. We feel the thrust of the powerful pistons, the driving rods beginning to move round with great force and then the free movement as the great locomotive speeds across the plains.

The Brazilian composer Heitor Villa-Lobos found inspiration in a very different train. A journey on a tiny Brazilian railway gave him the idea for his musical sketch *The Little Train of the Caipara,* a delightful, cheerful piece which he later incorporated in the second of his *Bachianas Brasileiras.*

Even Gioacchino Rossini, who refused to travel by train, wrote an amusing piano piece which he called *The Little Excursion 'Train.* One of the sections is headed 'The Derailment', which probably explains his dislike of railway travel.

The trains which inspired these composers —the big Pacific or the little Brazilian locomotive—were steam trains and the sounds which they evoke will soon be missing from many of our railways as the snort and hiss of the steam locomotive give way to the sound of the diesel and the rhythm of wheels over the joins in the track is lost as welded rail is laid. A railway journey will not sound the same; but these noises will not be lost, for enthusiasts in Britain and America have been carefully recording the sounds of the steam era and they are now available on gramophone records.

These recordings do not merely offer the exitement of an express train rushing stereophonically through your home (though you can have that too if you wish), the best of them really catch the railway atmosphere. Folkways in America and Transacord in Britain have issued some first-rate discs. As long ago as 1954 Peter Handford of Transacord set himself the task of recording as many steam locomotive types as possible before they were withdrawn. His aim is to record the railway's natural sound and he never asks a driver to produce spectacular effects; his sleeve notes too, help to create the exact atmosphere. One of his most exciting records, *Trains at Night,* must have involved many cold sessions waiting patiently by lonely stretches of track, but the results, recorded in stereo, are well worth while: we hear the locomotives slip on icy rails on a December night, we can feel the damp and smell the fog and hear not only the locomotives pounding past, or echoing off the hills, but the midnight owls, the signal levers, the fireman's conversation and the dawn chorus of moor and forest birds in the high fells.

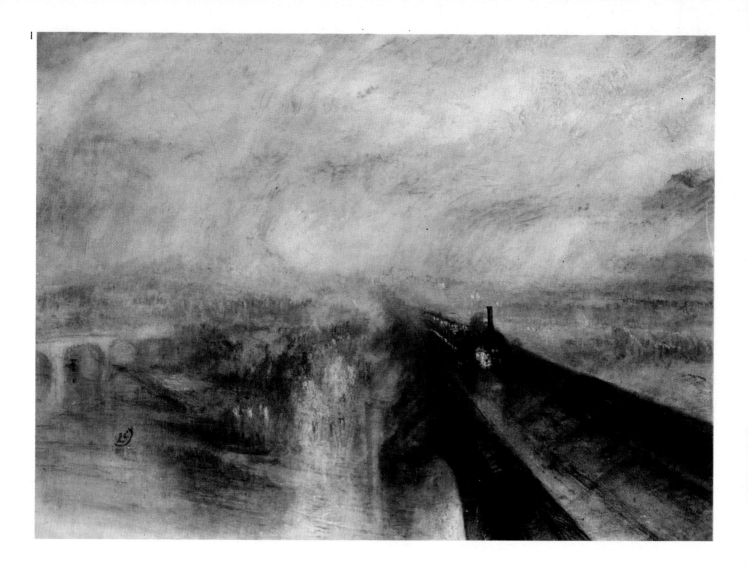

1 *Rain, Steam, Speed,* by J. M. W. Turner (National Gallery, London).
Overleaf:
2 *Le pont de l'Europe, Gare St. Lazare,* by Claude Monet (Musée Marmottan).
3 *Le train dans la neige,* by Claude Monet (Musée Marmottan).
4 *The 'Lightning Express' Trains,* a Currier and Ives lithograph.
5 *The Return,* showing a first-class compartment, painted by Abram Solomon in 1855.

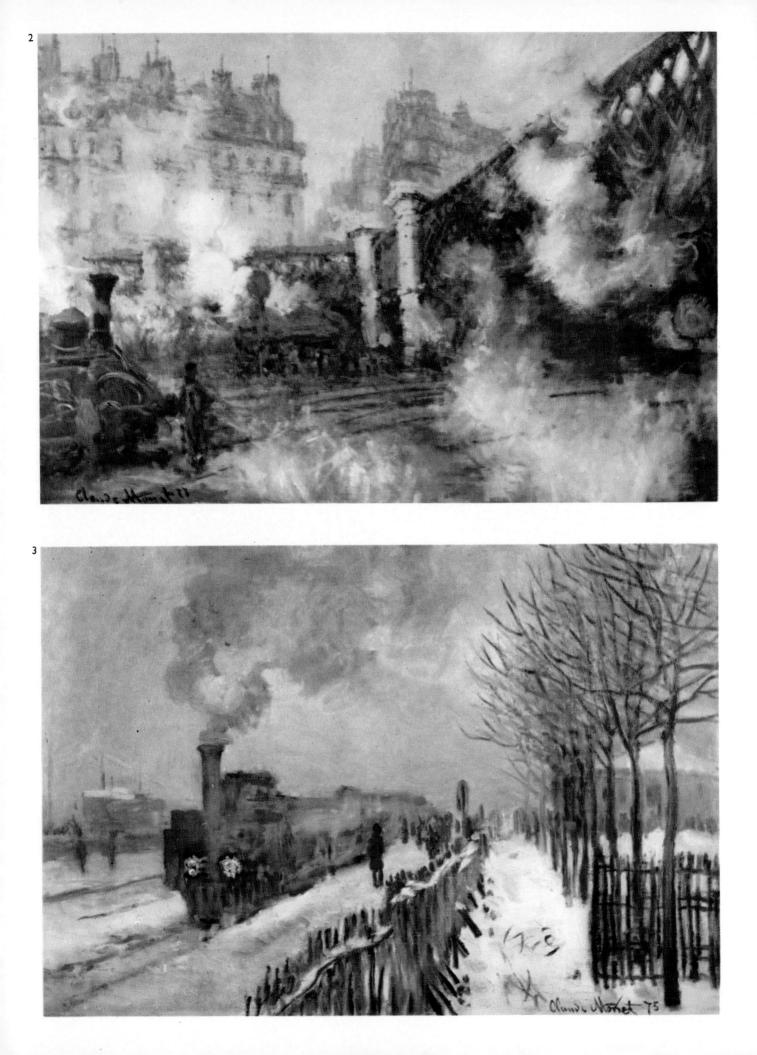

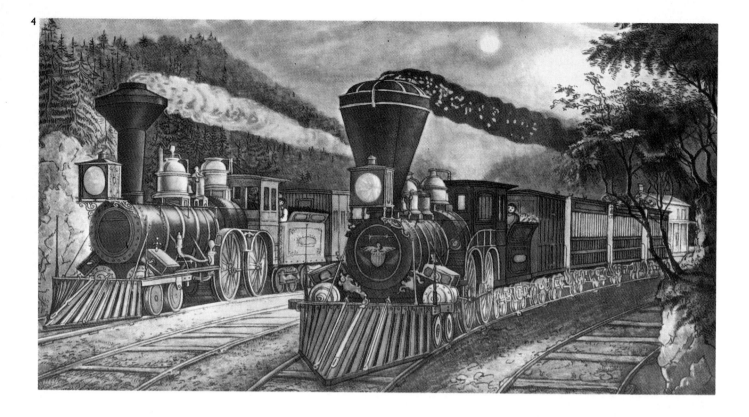

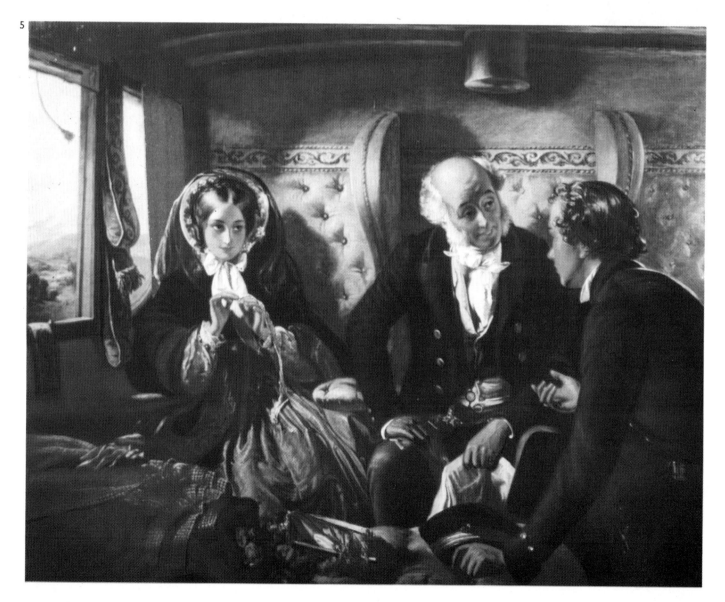

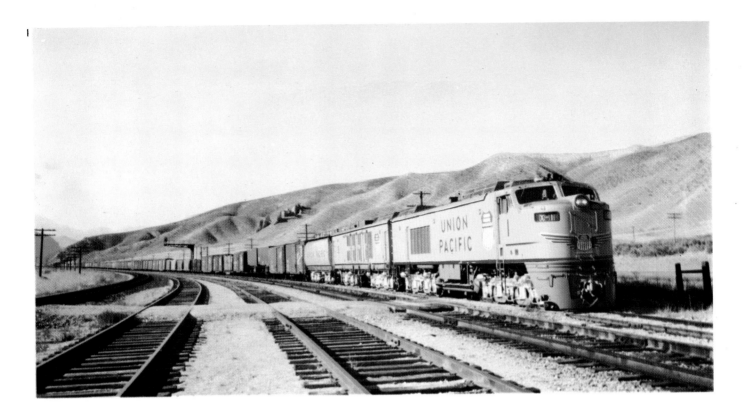

2

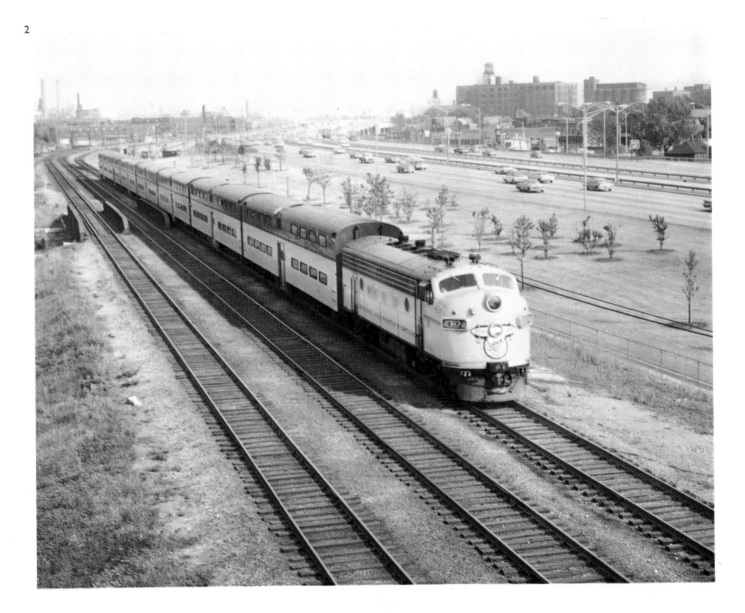

THE STORY OF CASEY JONES

Come all you rounders, I want you to hear
The story of a brave engineer,
Casey Jones was the rounder's name,
On a big eight-wheeler of a mighty fame.

Casey Jones, he pushed on the throttler,
Casey Jones was a brave engineer,
Come on, Casey, and blow the whistler,
Blow the whistle so they all can hear.

JOHN LUTHER JONES, from Cayce, Kentucky, was the original of the Casey Jones in the popular ballad. A fine railwayman, he was killed on 30th April 1900 when the train he was driving was wrecked at Vaughan, Mississippi.

On the evening of Sunday, April 29th, Casey and his fireman Sim Webb brought the No. 4 train from Canton into Poplar Street Station, Memphis, and were ready to go off duty; but the driver who was to take the No. 1 train south at 11.15 had reported sick and, since no other crew was available, Casey and Sim were asked to take over the trip.

No. 1 was an hour late getting into Memphis and another thirty-five minutes had been lost loading and switching before Casey was able to steam out of Poplar Street on his way south to New Orleans.

Jones was determined to make up the time. The locomotive ran beautifully and they were in Sardis in sixty-two minutes—thirty-five minutes already made up—by Grenada they had gained an hour. They sped on at speeds of over seventy miles an hour. They drew out of Winona only fifteen minutes late and at Durant were only five minutes behind: with only thirty-five miles ahead they would be in Canton on the scheduled time.

Ahead at Vaughan two goods trains had pulled off the single main track onto a double section to let Casey past, but together they were too long. A flagman was sent up-line and warning detonators set on the track to signal Casey that he was to 'saw by', that is cut speed and pull slowly down past the north points so that once he was clear the trains on the passing track could move north and clear the south end of the section.

At 3.50 a.m., only two minutes behind time, No. 1 swung into the long double 's' curve approaching Vaughan with the north set of points about the middle of the first 's'. As the train came rushing around the bend Sim Webb heard a detonator go off on the rail, and felt the air-brakes go on beneath his feet. Leaping to the right side of the cab he saw the flagman's lantern waving behind him, but ahead—where the first set of points should have been completely clear—were the red tail lights of a train on the main line. Casey could not see them because of the curve. Webb called out a warning and Casey told him to jump, pulled on the whistle and slammed on the emergency brakes. But it was too late.

They found Casey under the tender, still clutching the broken end of his whistle cord.

At the south end of the siding a local passenger train had drawn in with orders to get on the house-track at Vaughan station, out of the way of No. 1. But the points on to this track were blocked by the overhanging wagons of one of the goods trains. They had to pull north to let it through and as they moved back to clear the northern points for No. 1 an air-coupling broke bringing both trains to a stop. It was quickly replaced and pumping up the air pressure was begun but no one realised how fast No. 1 was running. Before they could get the remaining wagons off the main line Casey had ploughed into them.

Another wreck, another engineer dead—it had happened before on the railroad. But that was not the end of Casey Jones. Wallace Saunders and Ike Wentworth, railwaymen who had looked after Casey's engine at Canton, put their grief into a song which was soon being sung and whistled up and down all Mississippi with new verses being added day by day. By the time it was published in 1902 it was very different from the original version.

Nevertheless, however distorted the song may be it is still a great song of the railroad and gives lasting fame to Casey's name.

U. S. RAILWAYS TODAY

1 A gas-turbine-hauled goods train near Echo, Utah, on the Union Pacific Railroad.
2 A diesel-hauled train on the Chicago and North Western Railway which has double-decker carriages for commuter traffic. The locomotive operates on a push-pull basis; when pushing it is controlled from a cab in the forward coach.

THE BALLAD OF JOHN AXON

John Axon was a railwayman
To steam trains born and bred,
He was an engine driver
At Edgeley loco shed.
For forty years he followed
And served the iron way;
He lost his life upon the track
One February day.

At four a.m. that Saturday
John Axon left his bed;
At five he drew his time-card
At Edgeley loco-shed.
Just after six Ron Scanlon
His fireman, cried 'Away';
It was a day no different
From any other day.

The rain was gently falling
When they started down the line,
And on the way to Buxton
The sun began to shine.
From out the steam-brake pipe valve
A wisp of steam did rise,
And Axon he reported this
When in Buxton he arrived.

Under the large injector steam-valve
There's a length of one and one-eighth piping
Which connects with the driver's brake-valve.
The connecting point is a joint of brass.

A one and one-eighth steam-pipe
Fixed in a theaded joint,
Rests on asbestos packing,
And is sealed . . .
. . . sealed with brazing metal.

The repair was done and the train made up
When they left the Buxton sidings,
And the time was just eleven five
And the sun it was a-shining.

Four eight one double eight was her number
Scanlon was the fireman,
And the guard in the van was Alfred Ball,
And the driver was John Axon.

Her wagons numbered thirty-three,
And a twenty-ton rear brake van,
She was carrying coke, woodpulp and coal,
And firebricks and pig-iron.

The down line out of Buxton climbs,
She was pulling nice and steady,
And the bank engine was pushing behind,
And the guard's brake-stick was ready.

John Axon looked at the rolling hills
And he found them to his liking,
And he thought of his early courting days.
The days when he went hiking.

John Axon smiled at the thought that later
He'd be celebrating;
And he smiled when he thought of the Stockport pub,
Where a pint of mild was waiting.

John Axon was a dancing man,
On his pins he was light and nimble,
And often he'd stand on the old footplate
Whistling an olde-time jingle.

The joint of the driver's steam-brake pipe
Began to sweat a little,
By the time they were half way up the hill
It was coming in a steady trickle.

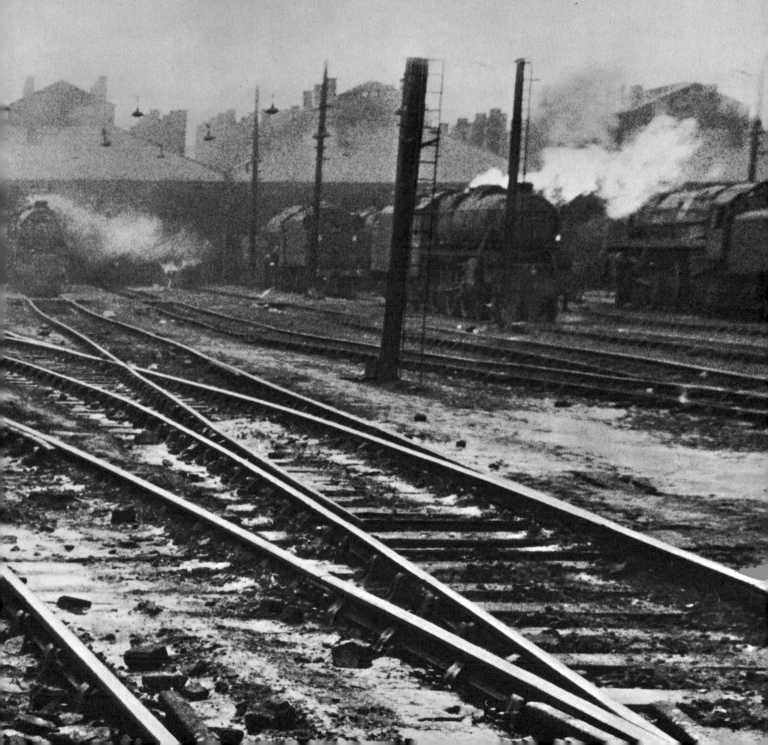

A hundred and twenty-five tons of engine,
Six hundred and fifty tons behind!
And the boiler pressure . . .
Two twenty-five pounds an inch!

And the men —
Two fragile bodies,
Flesh and blood,
And brittle bone.
Carbon and water,
Nerves and dreams.
Nerves and dreams.

Power from coal,
Power from water,
Power imprisoned
In a one and one-eighth pipe.

The restless steam
Watches the tired metal,
Explores the worn thread,
Watching,
Watching,

Every turn of the four-foot wheels
Every lunge of the smooth-armed piston,
Every thrust in the two great cylinders
Weakens the joint's resistance.

And the brazed flange crumbles,
The pipe is parted.
It **BLOWS!**

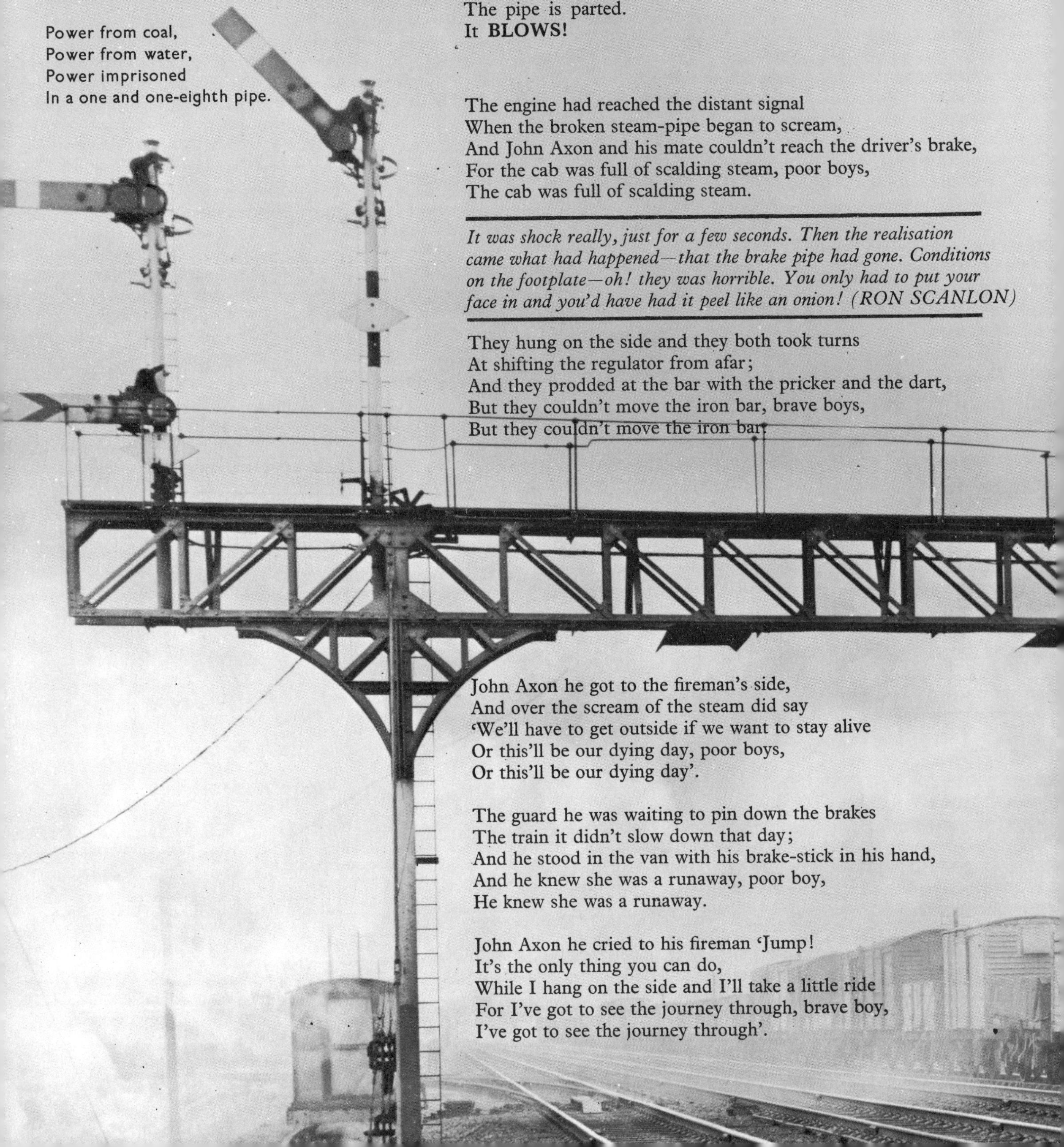

The engine had reached the distant signal
When the broken steam-pipe began to scream,
And John Axon and his mate couldn't reach the driver's brake,
For the cab was full of scalding steam, poor boys,
The cab was full of scalding steam.

*It was shock really, just for a few seconds. Then the realisation
came what had happened—that the brake pipe had gone. Conditions
on the footplate—oh! they was horrible. You only had to put your
face in and you'd have had it peel like an onion! (RON SCANLON)*

They hung on the side and they both took turns
At shifting the regulator from afar;
And they prodded at the bar with the pricker and the dart,
But they couldn't move the iron bar, brave boys,
But they couldn't move the iron bar.

John Axon he got to the fireman's side,
And over the scream of the steam did say
'We'll have to get outside if we want to stay alive
Or this'll be our dying day, poor boys,
Or this'll be our dying day'.

The guard he was waiting to pin down the brakes
The train it didn't slow down that day;
And he stood in the van with his brake-stick in his hand,
And he knew she was a runaway, poor boy,
He knew she was a runaway.

John Axon he cried to his fireman 'Jump!
It's the only thing you can do,
While I hang on the side and I'll take a little ride
For I've got to see the journey through, brave boy,
I've got to see the journey through'.

John Axon he was all alone, there on the engine side,
The train it reached the hilltop and began the downhill ride,
The sun it was still shining, the sky was still of blue,
He gambled with his life that day and this John Axon knew.

It's a seven-mile drop from Bibbington top,
O Johnny!
It's one in fifty-eight and you've no steam brake,
O Johnny!

She's picking up speed,
And the power is freed,
It's prayer you need,
But you'll never make it, Johnny!

Every yard of the track says you won't come back,
O Johnny!
She's a fist of steel, every turn of the wheels
Cries 'Johnny'!

There isn't a chance
You'll get to your dance,
You can see at a glance
That you'll never make it, Johnny!

There's a tunnel ahead, you can't cover your head,
O Johnny!
Doing sixty an hour and she's gaining power,
O Johnny!
Watch out for the wall,
Bunch yourself up small
In the smoky pall . . .
O, you'll never make it, Johnny!

It's hell on the plate, it's a funeral freight,
O Johnny!
It's the end of a dream in steel and steam,
O Johnny!
There's a world in your head,
And you're due at the shed,
And there's life ahead,
But you'll never see it, Johnny!

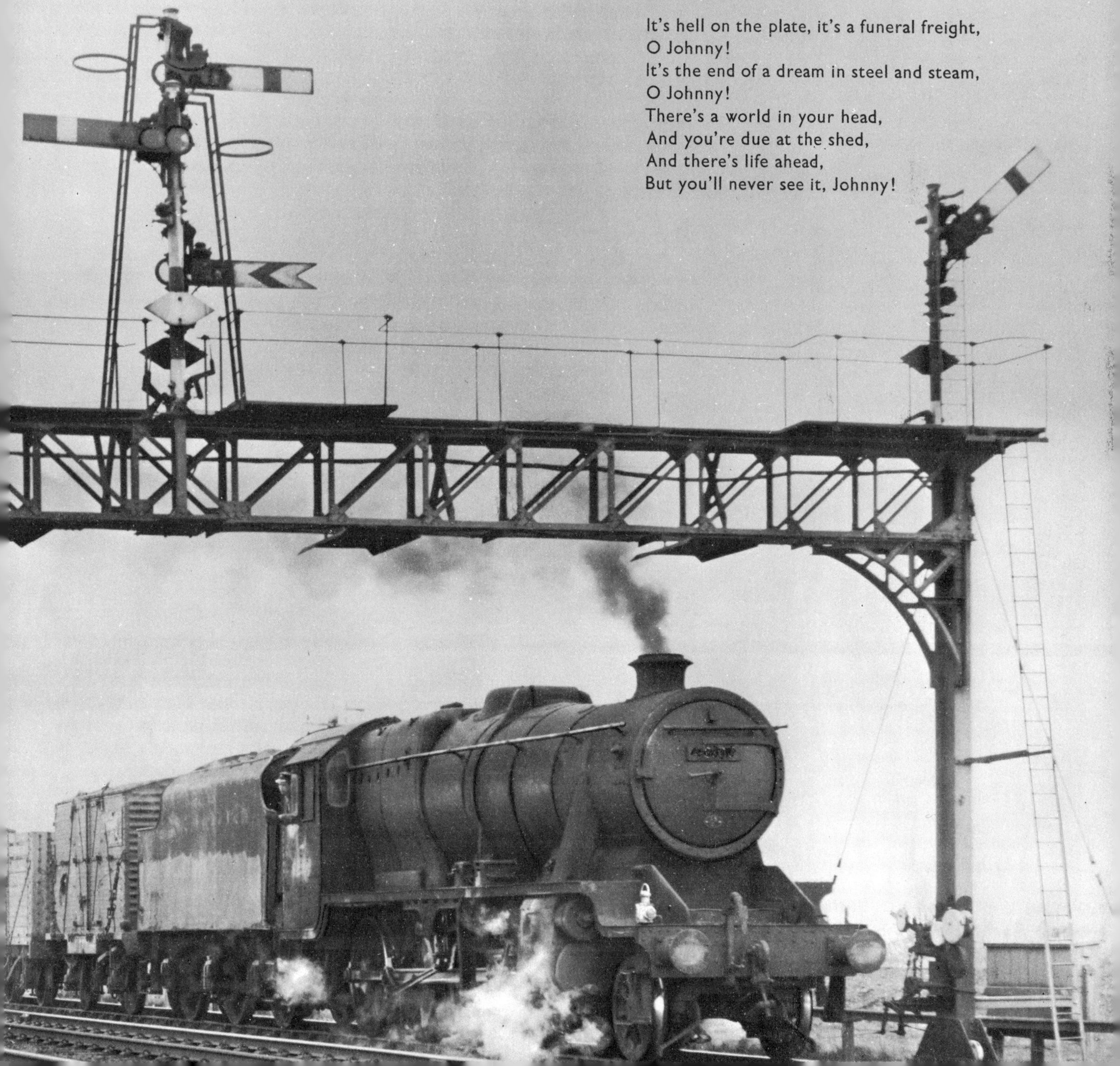

Every turn of the four foot wheels,
Every lunge of the smooth-armed piston,
Every thrust of the two great cylinders . . . .
Sings of a man's destruction.

What was it Jim said?
One day in the shed . . . .
Jim said . . . .
Or was it in the pub?
What was it that Jim said . . . .
About steam?
About power?

With a steam locomotive you make the
power, you direct the power and you control
the power.
You make the power, you direct the POWER
and you control the POWER.
CURSE the power!

The run it is finished,
The shift's nearly ended.
So long, mates!
So long . . . .
Remember
A man is a man
He must do what he can
For his brothers.

By his deeds you shall know him,
By the work of his hands,
By his friends who will mourn him,
By the love that he bore,
By the gift of his courage,
And the life that he gave.

On the 3rd May 1957 Mrs. Gladys Axon
received the following letter:

10 Downing Street,
Whitehall
2nd May 1957

Madam,

*I have the honour to inform you that the Queen
has been graciously pleased to approve the Prime Minister's
recommendation that the George Cross be awarded posthumously
to your husband John Axon . . .*

John Axon was a railwayman
To steam trains born and bred,
He was an engine driver
At Edgeley loco shed.
He was a man of courage
And served the iron way,
He gave his life upon the track
One February day.

*From THE BALLAD OF JOHN AXON, a radio
ballad by Ewan MacColl, Peggy Seeger, and
Charles Parker, first broadcast by the B.B.C.
Midland Region 2nd July 1958.*

THE END OF STEAM

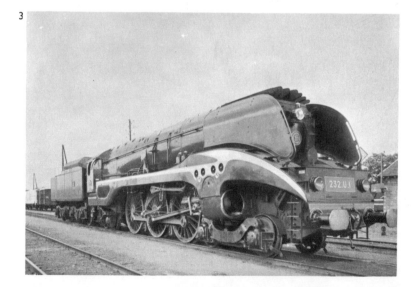

THE DAYS of the steam locomotive are numbered. Steam power, to which the whole development of the railways was due, which has given them their shape and their emotional appeal, is inefficient when set against its successors.

Although initially diesel and electric locomotives cost much more than steam locomotives to build, they are much cheaper to operate. Not only are their fuel costs lower, they also require much less maintenance and therefore have a fuller working life.

From the time its boiler is lit, a steam locomotive needs three to five hours to build up sufficient steam power to be put to work. At the end of its trip, if it has been of any length, it must go into a depot to have its fire raked clear of ash and clinker and the smoke-box cleaned of soot. It will probably have to stop to be refuelled. At the end of the day the fire will be dropped, the engine allowed to cool and more maintenance work done. Then, at regular intervals, the engine's boiler has to be washed out. No matter how smoothly and efficiently these things are done, they all take time and staff. Time which, with a diesel or an electric locomotive, can be added to their working day, and staff who may prefer the cleaner working conditions of modern industry to the soot and grime that goes with coal-fired locomotives.

No, the electric- or diesel-hauled trains may seem coldly clinical to those of us who miss the dramatic atmosphere of smoke and steam, but they are cleaner and more efficient, and both they and their crews can complete far more traffic work. Steam has to go.

Coal, particularly the lower grades available today, is more effectively used at the power

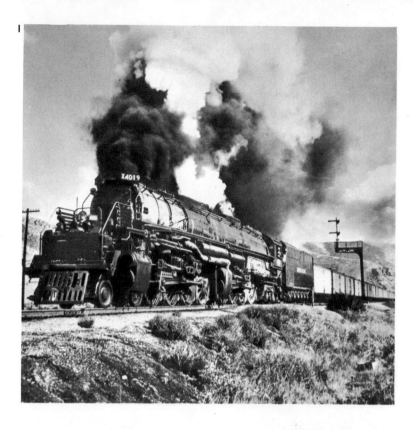

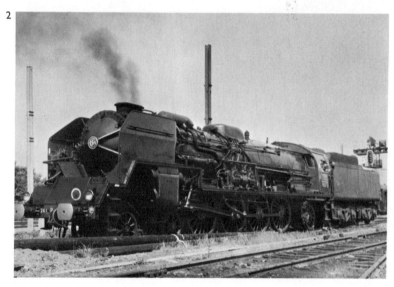

1 One of the Union Pacific Railroad's 'Big Boys' hauling a long freight. These 132³/₄-feet-long 4-8-8-4s were built to handle fast freight traffic on heavy gradients at speeds up to 80 m.p.h. They rank among the greatest steam locomotives ever built.
2 A Class 241P four-cylinder comound of French Railways, equipped with mechanical stoker. Locomotives of this class were built between 1947 and 1949 for express passenger work.
3 The final development in French steamers was this Class U 4-6-4 four-cylinder compound passenger locomotive built in 1949.

1
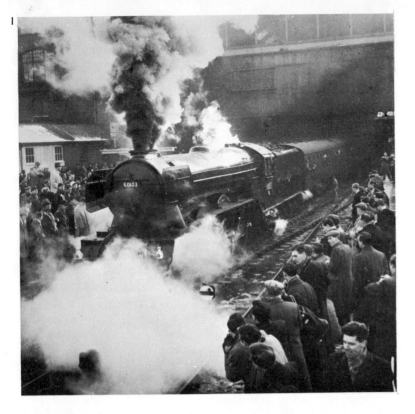

2
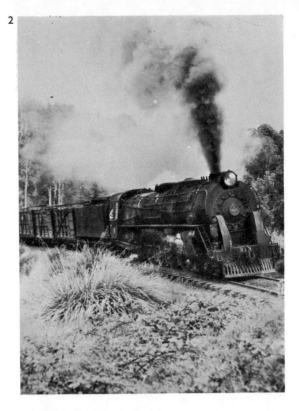

3
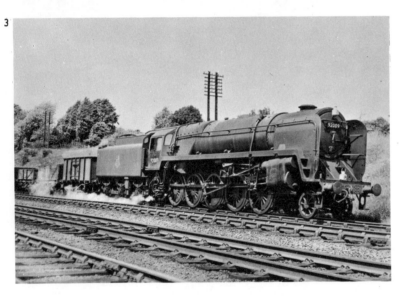

4
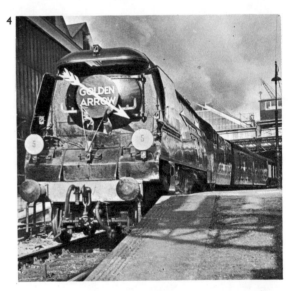

5
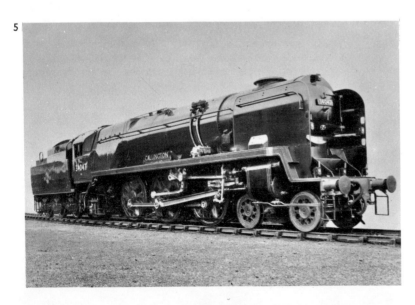

6
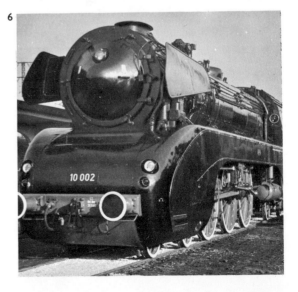

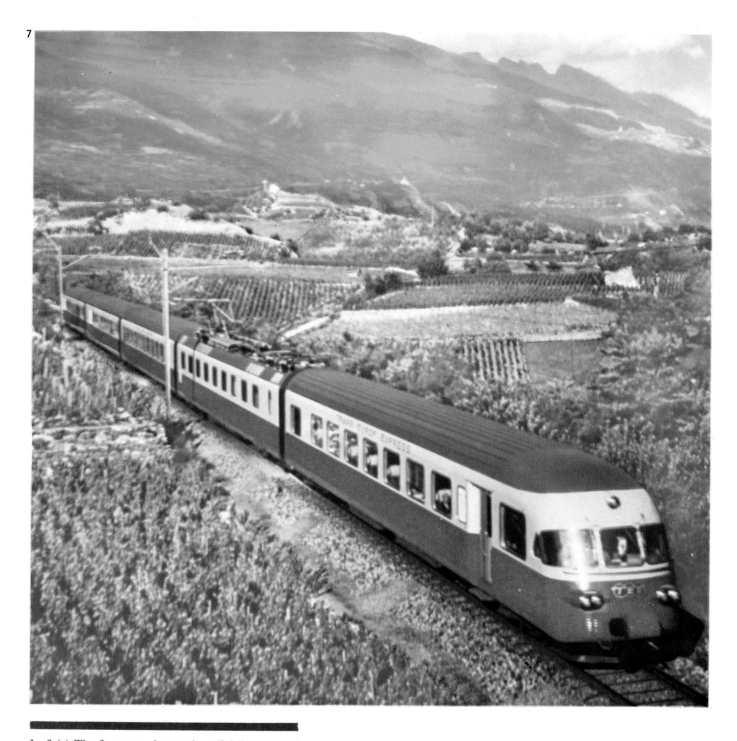

1—6 (1) The first steam locomotive officially to record a speed of 100 m.p.h., *The Flying Scotsman,* built at Doncaster in 1923, here hauling its last train out of King's Cross before retirement on 14th January 1963. (2) A New Zealand-built 3 ft. 6 in. gauge 'K' type locomotive hauling a goods train near the top of the Spiral, Raumiru. (3) British Rail Class 9F 2-10-O, a versatile locomotive used mainly for heavy freight but also used for express passenger work. (4) A Merchant Navy class Bulleid heavy Pacific leaving Victoria with the *Golden Arrow.* This famous train is now electric hauled. (5) A West Country class light Bulleid Pacific. Locomotives of this class have the streamlining removed as in this picture. (6) The ultimate in German express passenger steam locomotives was this 4-6-2 No. 10,002; only two locomotives of the type were built (1956).

TRANS-EUROP-EXPRESS TRAIN-SETS

7 Swiss electric train-set. **8** German diesel train-set. This pattern has now been replaced by a standard German electric locomotive.

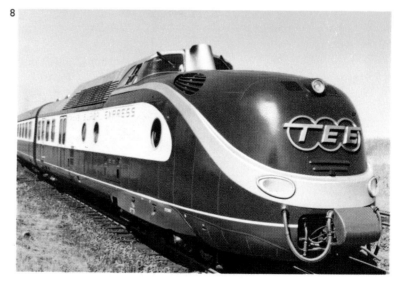

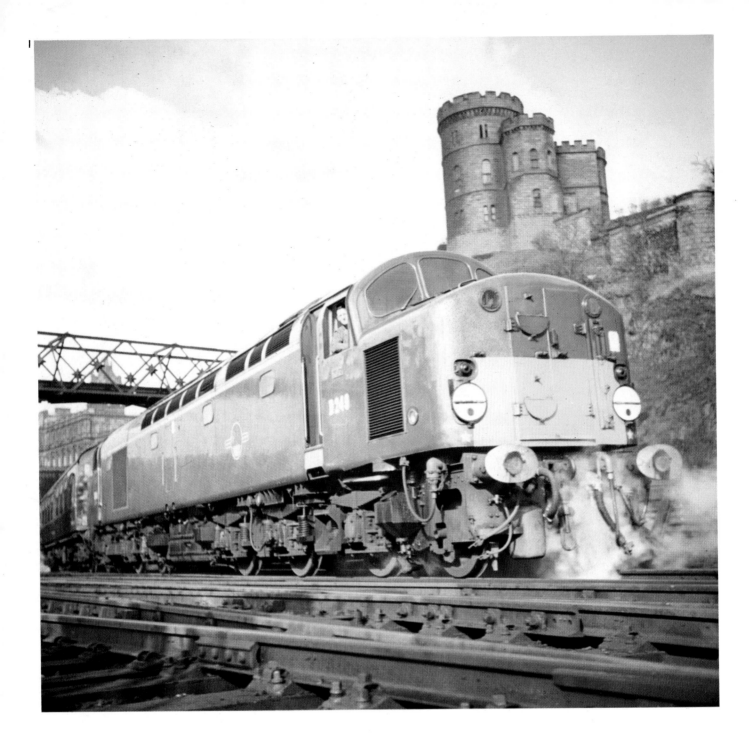

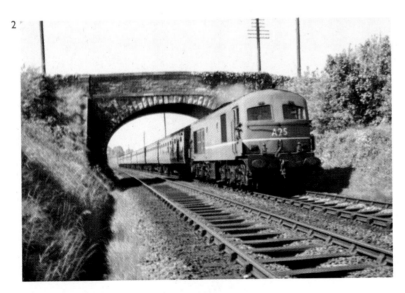

1 British Rail's diesel-electric type 4 number D 249.
2 Irish Railways' diesel-powered *Failte* express at Hazelhatch.
3, 4 British Rail's 3,300 h.p. electric locomotive for operation on 25,000 volts A.C. overhead supply.

3

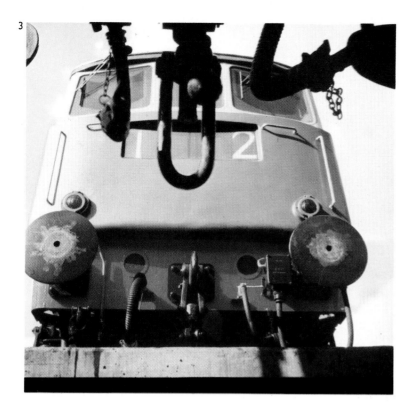

4

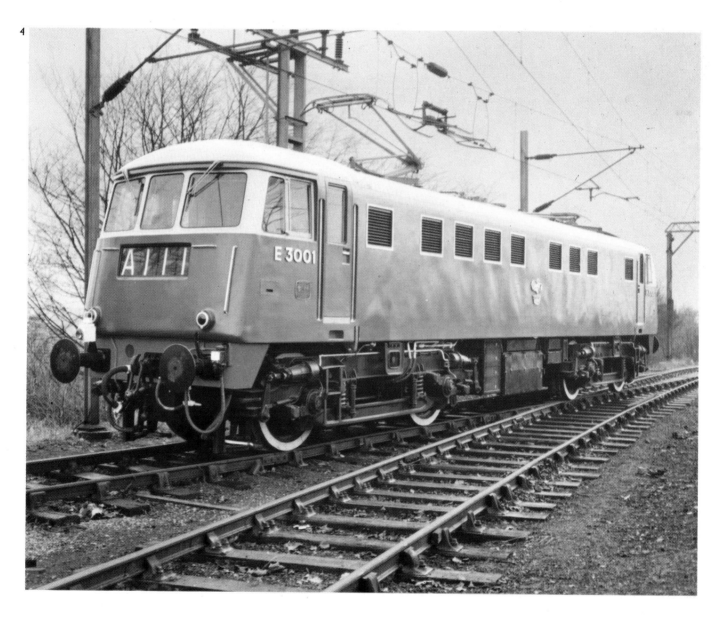

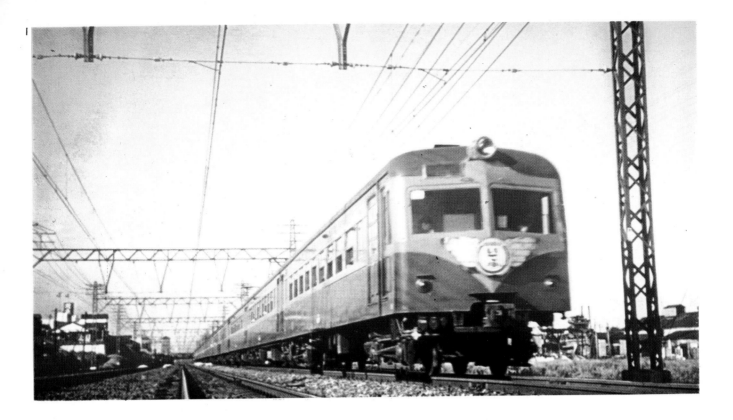

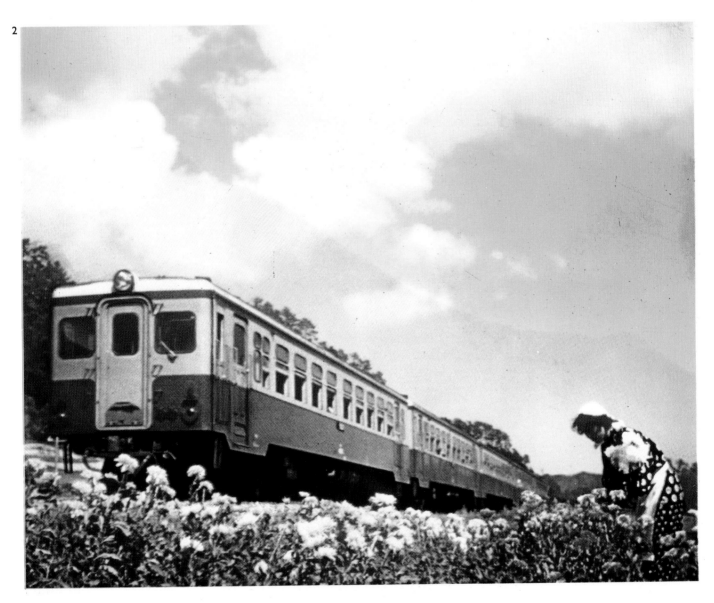

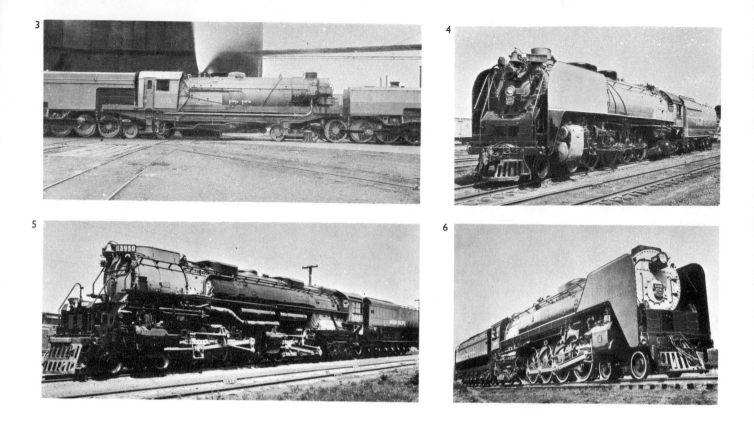

3

4

5

6

station, generating electricity. And diesel power is the obvious choice where the capital cost, or other reasons, prevent electrification. The diesel power may be used either to drive an electric traction engine (diesel-electric) or the power may be passed on by hydraulic transmission, developed in Germany. Although electric transmission is more easily installed and maintained, hydraulic transmission is much less bulky—the weight saved can be added to the load hauled or the saving can be effected in lower fuel consumption.

Another choice for traction power is the gas-turbine, but gas-turbines work best when worked hardest, and if not required to work 'full-out' only give about the same ratio

7

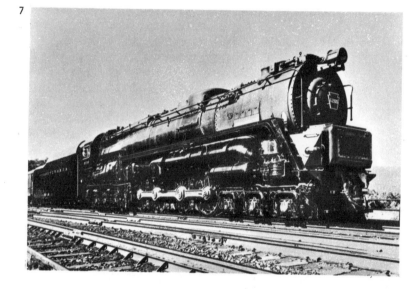

JAPANESE NATIONAL RAILWAYS

1 Electric train-set for inter-city services.

2 Diesel car KI-HA 45000 for local services.

STEAM LOCOMOTIVES

3 An articulated Garratt locomotive by Beyer Peacock. The central boiler is free of all driving wheels and can therefore be bigger than is otherwise possible.

4 Union Pacific 4-8-4 Northern class.

5 Union Pacific 4-6-6-4 Challenger class.

6 New York Central Railroad Niagara S-10.

7 A Pennsylvania Railroad coal-burning locomotive powered by a steam-turbine instead of cylinders, pistons and driving rods. The engine and tender weigh nearly one million pounds and cover 123 feet of track.

8 A Franco-Crosti boilered locomotive of Italian State Railways. There is no chimney in the usual place; exhaust steam passes through the cylinders at either side of the boiler (which are in fact preheaters) and out through the stove pipes towards the rear.

8

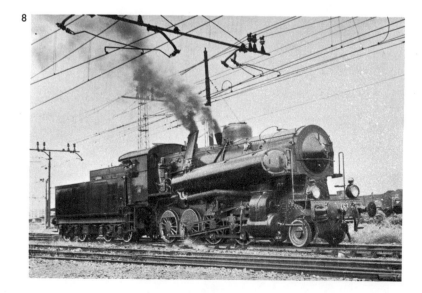

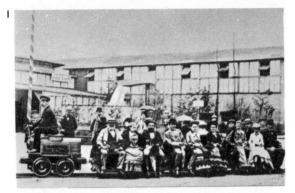

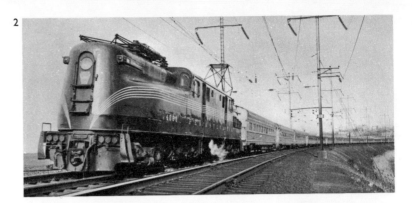

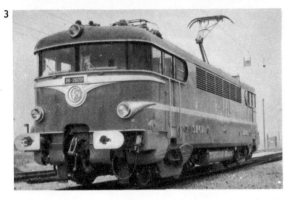

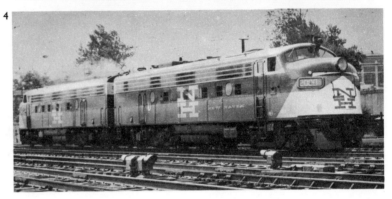

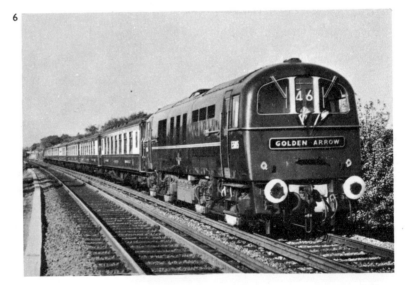

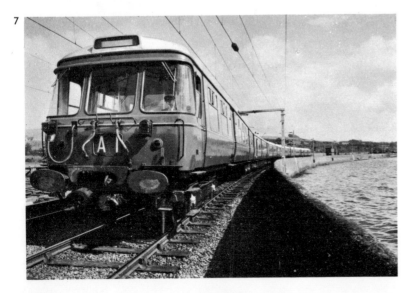

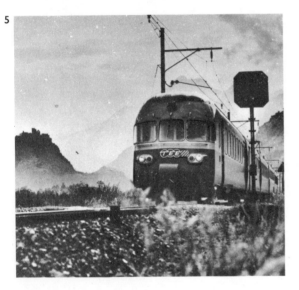

ELECTRIC LOCOMOTIVES

1 The first electric train made by Werner Siemens in operation at the Berlin Trade Fair (1879).

2 Pennsylvania Railroad locomotive hauling the *Congressional*, operated daily in both directions between New York and Washington.

3 French Railways' locomotive, which operates on three different currents: 1,500 and 3,000 volts D.C. and 25,000 volts A.C.

4 New Haven Railroad two-unit 3,500 h.p. FL-9 locomotive which combines diesel and third-rail operation. Designed for routes which are only partially electrified, it can switch from one system to the other without loss of speed.

5 Swiss Federal Railways TEE train-set takes the 'Cisalpin' through the Rhône valley. This express links Milan, Lausanne and Paris in 8 hours.

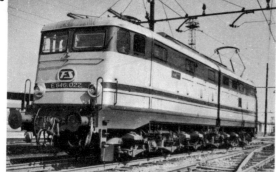

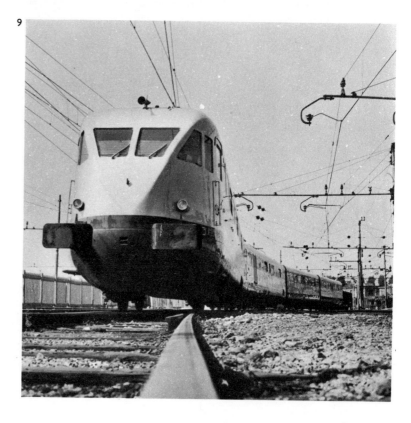

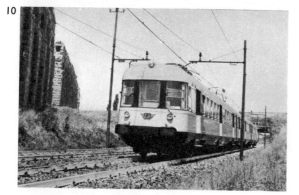

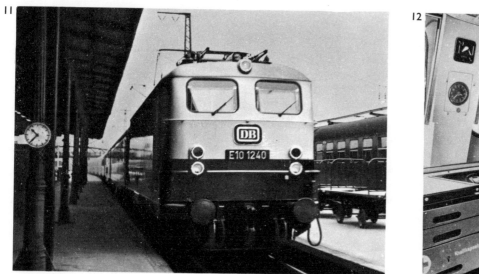

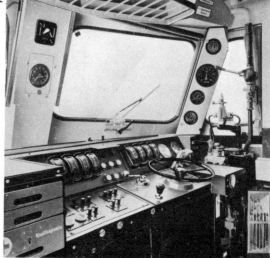

6 The *Golden Arrow* is now electric hauled on the third-rail system, but this locomotive has a pantograph which can take current from overhead supply in sheds and sidings.

7 A train-set operating on overhead supply on a Glasgow suburban service.

8 An E 646 locomotive of Italian State Railways.

9 An ALE 803 train-set in suburban service near Rome.

10 Italian State Railways' beautiful ETR 220 locomotive.

11 German State Railways' E 10 locomotive hauling the *Rheingold* express.

12 Inside the cab of the restyled E 10 locomotive.

13 A 3,600 h.p. D.C. locomotive in service with Spanish National Railways.

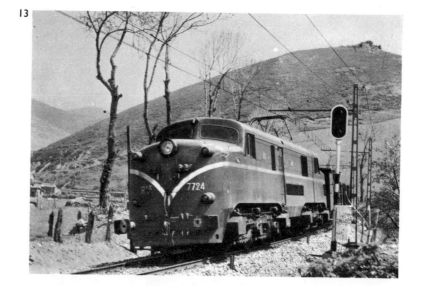

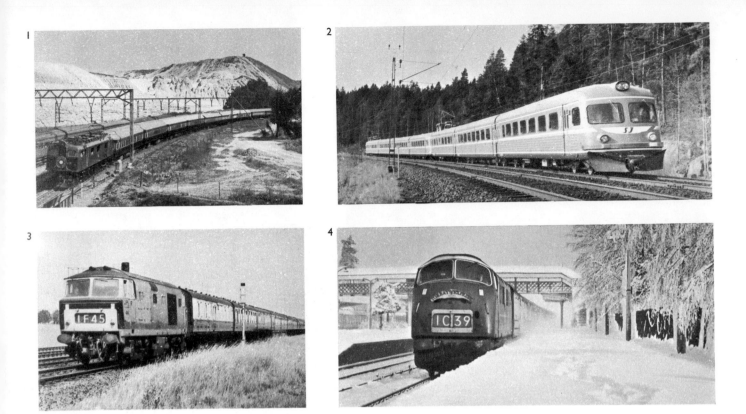

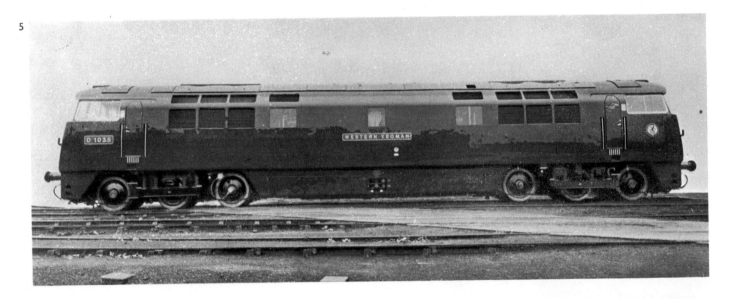

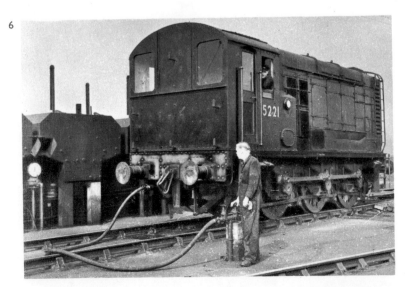

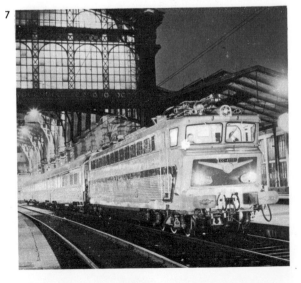

of work for fuel as a steam engine. They were tried out by British Rail but until recently only one railway system made much use of them — the Union Pacific Railroad, whose line between San Francisco and Chicago is particularly suited to their characteristics. Hauling heavy freight trains of up to 5,000 tons, locomotives climb to a height of 8,013 feet over a line which for 65 miles has a continuous gradient of more than 1 in 100. Under these conditions the locomotive is working full-out (and for technical reasons the cold air of these high altitudes makes for even greater efficiency). When the locomotive passes the high point of the route the gas-turbine is cut off and the train rolls down the long slope of the other side.

Now the ST6 gas-turbine, developed from an aircraft turbine, which overcomes many of the difficulties of operating at low speeds by using a free-power turbine, is being used in conjunction with lightweight rolling stock on the New Haven Railroad. The same turbine provides the motive power for Canadian National Railroad's 'Turbotrains', introduced in 1967 between Toronto and Montreal. Weighing only 250 pounds, and burning conventional diesel fuel, they are capable of developing 400 h.p. each. They can be started in temperatures as low as 60 degrees below zero and the Turbotrains are able to reach a speed of 100 m.p.h. within five minutes of starting. Designing on aerodynamic lines with many new features they look forward to the train of the future (see pages 150—1).

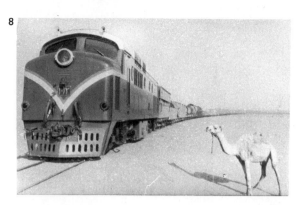

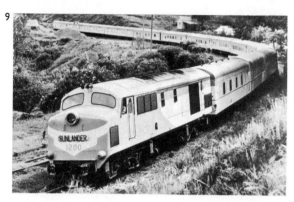

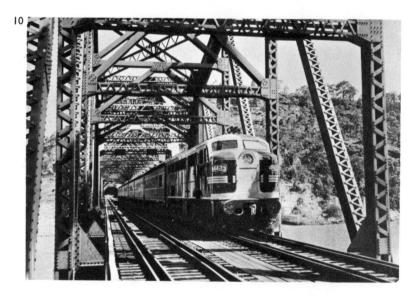

ELECTRIC LOCOMOTIVES
1 South African Railways' *Blue Train.*
2 A locomotive of Swedish Railways
7 French Railways' CC 40 100 class electric locomotive used for TEE Paris-Brussels-Amsterdam service.
DIESEL TRAIN-SETS AND
LOCOMOTIVES
3 A British Rail D 7000 class locomotive.
4 The *Torbay Express,* from London to the West Country.
5 British Rail Type 4 2,700 h.p. locomotive.
6 350 h.p. shunting locomotive being refuelled.
8 1,850 h.p. locomotive of Sudan Railways.
9 Queensland Government Railways' *Sunlander* express on the narrow-gauge route from Brisbane to Cairns, hauled by a 1,500 h.p. locomotive.
10 New South Wales train crossing Hawkesbury River Bridge.
11 2,000 h.p. train-set of Rhodesian Railways.

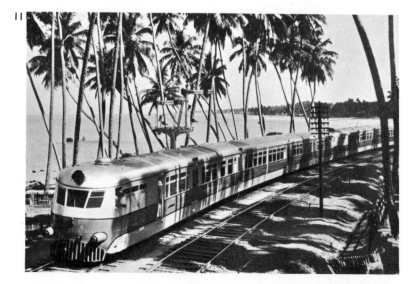

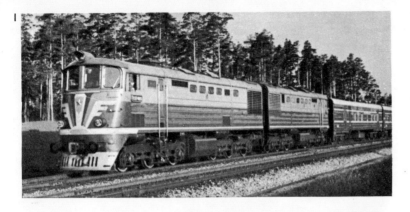

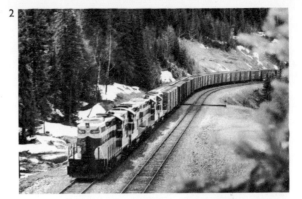

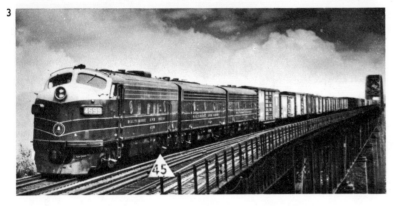

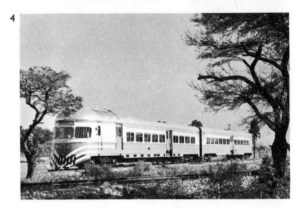

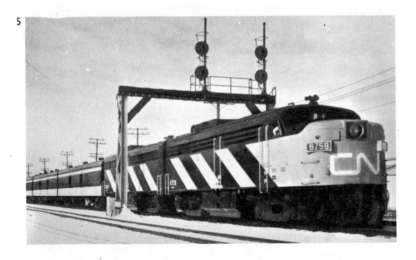

MORE DIESELS

1 A two-unit locomotive on the Moscow-Leningrad line, U.S.S.R.

2 Four GP-20 units provide 8,000 h.p. to speed this fast freight over the Montana Rockies.

3 A Baltimore and Ohio freight crossing the Susquehanna River.

4 A Fiat Type 131 rail car for Argentine State Railways.

5 A diesel-hauled passenger express of Canadian National Railways.

6 A locomotive of Italian State Railways.

7 A diesel-hauled train at Haifa, Israel.

GAS-TURBINE

8 One of Union Pacific's 8,500 h.p. gas-turbine locomotives hauling a heavy freight.

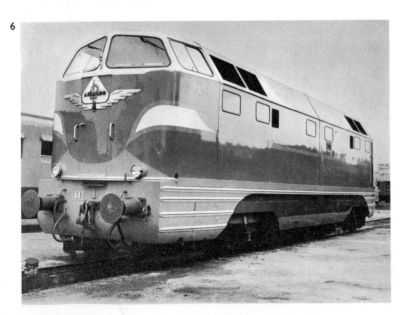

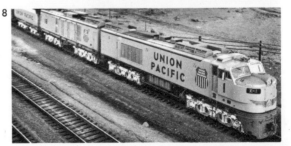

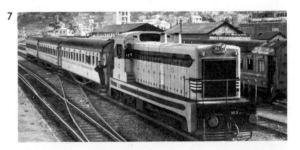

ATMOSPHERIC RAILWAYS

THE IDEA of propelling carriages by means of air pressure in an air-tight tunnel was proposed by George Medhurst in a pamphlet published in 1827 and an experimental system was tried out by a Mr. Vallance at Brighton but it had little popular appeal. The idea of being sucked through a dark tunnel was not attractive, particularly as Mr. Vallance proposed that his system should be used between London and Brighton.

Henry Pinkus, an American living in London, took out a patent in 1835 for a pneumatic system by which a piston pushed by air through a cylinder should propel a vehicle by means of a rod passing through a valve-sealed slit. He exhibited a model in Cavendish Square and the following year set up a full-scale trial. Others took up the idea and Samuel Clegg and Jacob and Joseph Samuda patented a version, with one edge of the valve fastened down, which they tried out at Wormwood Scrubs.

Various atmospheric railways, worked either by air pressure or vacuum, were proposed and lines were built for an extension of the Dublin and Kingstown Railway to Dalkey, for a line from New Cross (in London) to West Croydon, for a section of the Paris—Saint-Germain Railway, for a line between Geneva and Plainpalais

and for the extension of the Bristol and Exeter Railway to Plymouth.

The effect of wear and weather on the valves and other difficulties caused the system to be eventually given up, but not before it had been used for an underground Post Office railway in London. The first underground line in the United States, running 312 feet under Broadway from Warren Street, was also pneumatically operated.

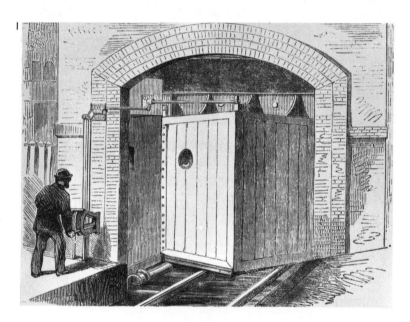

1 & 2 An experimental pneumatic railway opened at the Crystal Palace, London, in 1846. These contemporary engravings show the starting of the train and its arrival at the other end of the tube.

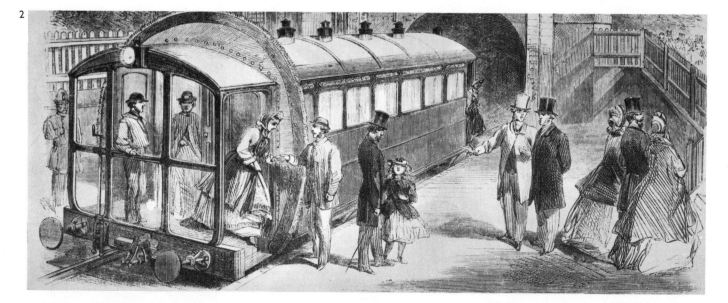

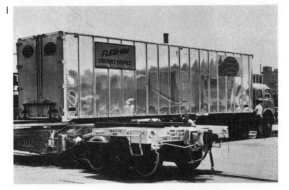

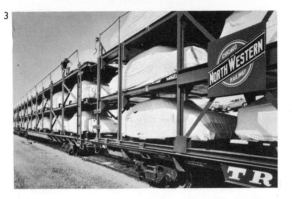

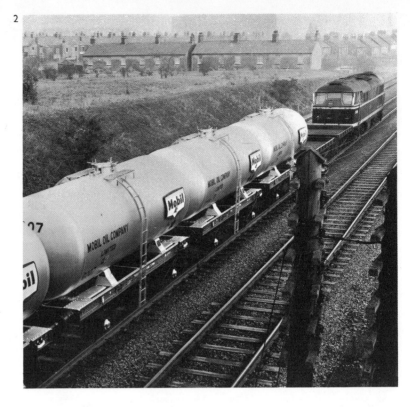

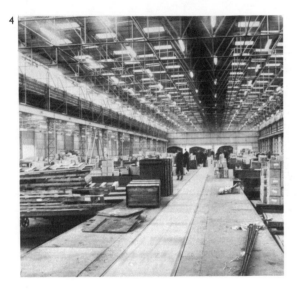

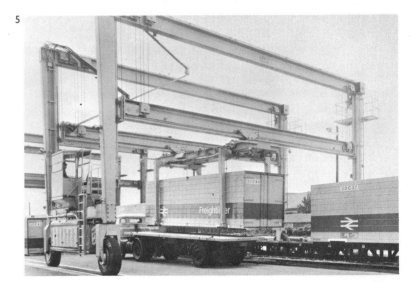

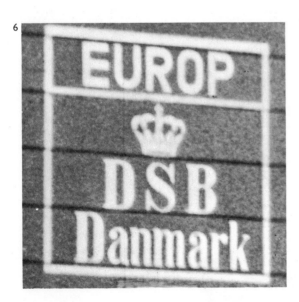

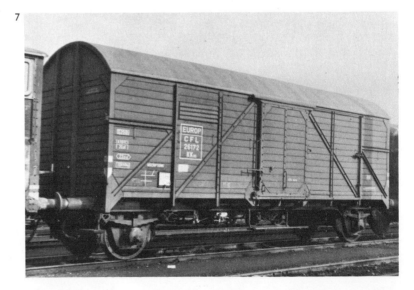

FREIGHT AND ROLLING STOCK

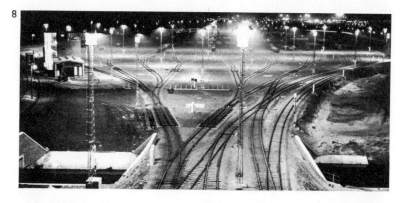

Measures to speed freight and attract more custom to the railways include specialist bulk containers, like the 37,000 gallon tank car (10) the largest ever built to carry oil, 'piggy-back' arrangements carrying highway trailers on flat cars (9), 'flexi-vans' (1) and other types of road-rail containers, such as those used in British Rail's high-speed Freightliner service (5), and specialist services like the car-sleeper service for private motorists operated in Britain and on the continent (11). Increased efficiency is aided by modern automated marshalling yards (8), palettisation of loading (12), conveyor belts (4) and, in Europe, by the creation of a pool of wagons for international use through T.E.E.M. (6 and 7).

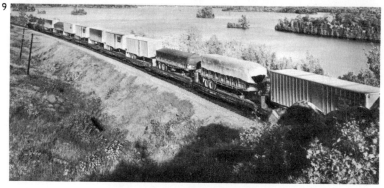

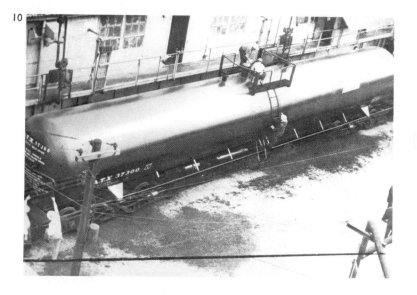

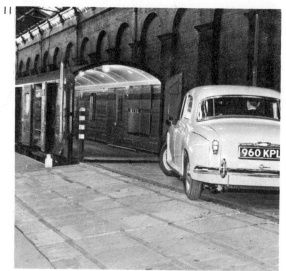

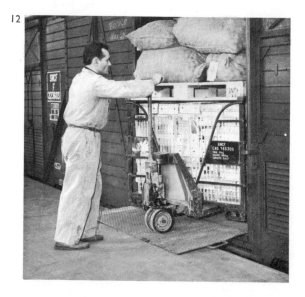

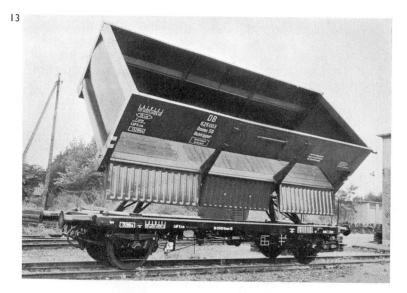

CABLE-WORKED RAILWAYS AND FUNICULARS

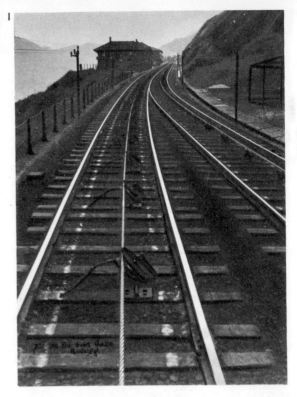

FIXED ENGINES and rope haulage were proposed for the Liverpool and Manchester railway until the success of the *Rocket* at the Rainhill Trials won favour for the locomotive. However, it was still thought impracticable for locomotives to manage steep gradients on their own and the system of endless rope haulage which had been used for many years in mines was adopted on some of the new railways and on the steeper parts of others, including the approach from Edge Hill to Liverpool and the rise from Euston to Camden Town on the London and Midland Line.

One of London's earliest railways, the London and Blackwall, was cable-worked for the whole of its $3\frac{1}{2}$ mile length; it was authorised in 1836 and Robert Stephenson and George Bidder were the engineers.

In 1841 the Düsseldorf-Elberfeld line was opened with a continuous incline of $1\frac{3}{4}$ miles cable-worked. Part of the Brussels-Liège main line was rope-worked for a section where the gradient is 1 in 32.

In the Peak District of England two of the nine cable-worked inclines which formed part of a line from Cromford to Whaley Bridge are still in operation.

London's first tube railway beneath the river from Tower Hill to Southwark was cable-operated, as was the Glasgow subway until electrified in 1935.

Until the 1930's there was a cable-worked railway at Jim Thorpe, Pennsylvania, the Mauch Chunk Switch-Back, which had originally been a coal-mine railway.

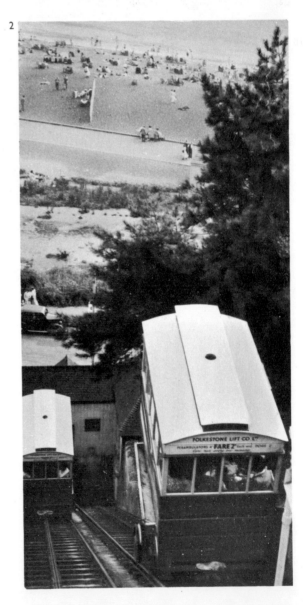

The most spectacular railway in the world with cable working must be one in South America: the Santos-Jundiai Railway of Brazil. The concession to build it was granted in 1856 and the line opened in 1867. Four cable-worked inclines each have a gradient of 1 in 9.75. To save expense one end of the hauling rope was attached to the ascending and one to the descending car, thereby reducing the power required from the stationary engines— a system used in funicular.

Funiculars, which are really ordinary rope railways worked on this principle over short steep gradients, are used all over the world whether to climb mountains, as in Switzerland, Norway or Japan, seaside cliffs as at Scarborough, Hastings, Folkestone and the Isle of Man, or just to climb steep hills as at

3

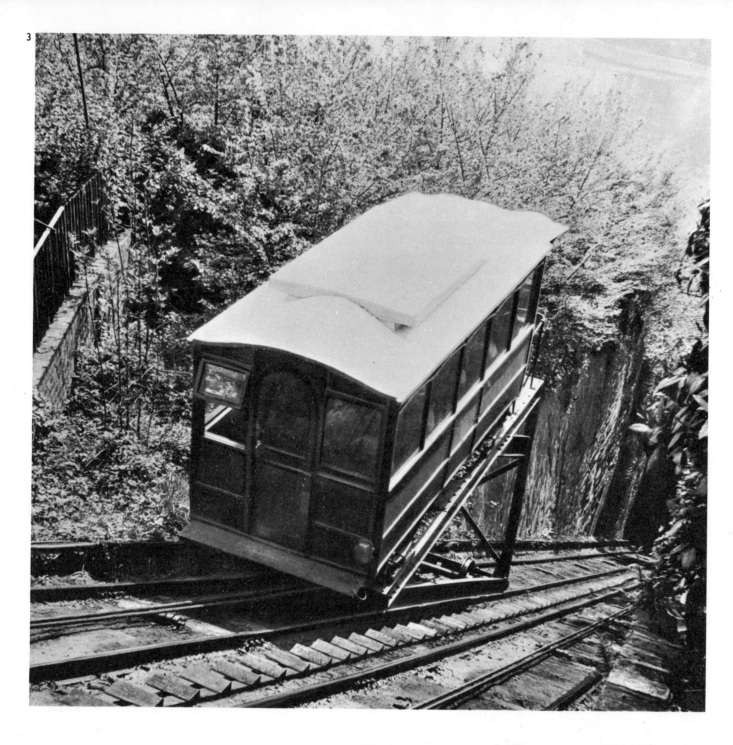

Montmartre in Paris or the Castle Hill at Bridgnorth.

Cable railways are by no means out of date: because of its steep gradient the underground railway recently built at Haifa in Israel is cable hauled.

4

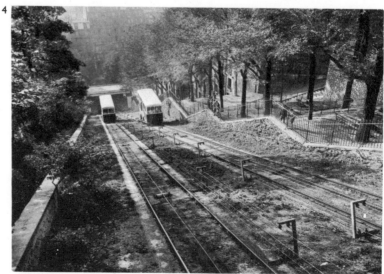

1 A section of cable-operated track between Santos and Sao Paulo, Brazil.
2 The 'lifts' at Folkestone, Kent.
3 The cable car which connects the High Town and the Low Town at Bridgnorth, Shropshire.
4 The funicular at Montmartre, Paris.

MONORAILS AND SUSPENDED RAILWAYS

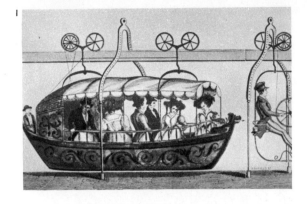

THE IDEA of self-supporting trains riding completely above the track was developed in the systems invented by Louis Brennan, August Scherl and Peter Schilovsky, which depend on gyroscopes to maintain equilibrium. If power failed the gyroscopes had sufficient momentum to keep their cars upright long enough for supports to be put in place or emergency rods with rollers to be lowered. Brakes could be applied for normal stops.

Brennan, an Irishman, was experimenting with monorails in 1896 and took out a patent in 1903, exhibiting a model in 1907. Scherl, a German pioneer, took out a patent in 1907 and gave a public demonstration of his car in the Berlin Zoological Gardens on 10th November 1909. Prior news of this reached Brennan, who quickly arranged a demonstration of his car for the same day followed by a more elaborate performance three months later. The invention excited great interest and won Brennan a Grand Prize when it was shown at the Japan-British Exhibition in 1910. The same year an agreement was drawn up which granted Scherl the right to use Brennan patents in Germany and to exhibit his car in the U.S.A.

Various systems of operation on a single rail had been developed, either with vehicles balanced by the man or animal pushing them along, by subsidiary supporting rails at the sides, or by carefully balanced panniers.

An alternative form of single-rail operation consists of suspending the train from the rail, and a horse-drawn form was in operation in London Docks as early as 1825.

A system of this kind invented by C. F. M. T. Lartigue was used for many years in North Africa. In 1894 an electrically operated Lartigue line was opened in Central France and others followed in Russia, Guatemala and Peru. An elaborate steam version was shown in London in 1886. In 1888 a $9\frac{1}{2}$ mile line was opened from Listowel to Ballybunion in Co. Kerry, Ireland, which ran successfully until 1924. The Managing Director of the Lartigue Railway Construction Company, Fritz Behr, developed the idea of a high-speed monorail and had a great success with a demonstration of his streamlined car at the Brussels Exhibition of 1897, and at the St. Louis World's Fair in 1904. There were plans for Behr railways between Liverpool and Manchester and between London and Brighton which eventually had to be dropped due to

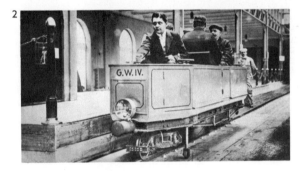

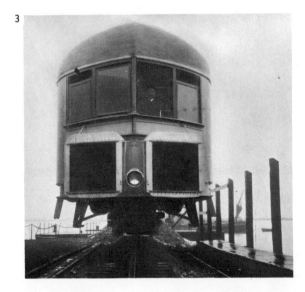

1 The suspension railway at the Royal Panarmonion Gardens, St. Pancras, invented by a Mr. H. Torrington. 'The admittance to the Gardens is one shilling each person, entitling the parties to ride round the gardens in the car or on the Hobby Horse. Refreshments may be obtained on the premises.'
2 The demonstration of Scherl's monorail car in 1909.
3 A demonstration of the Brennan system in 1910.
4 Meigg's system proposed for an overhead railway in New York in 1886.
5 The Wuppertal Schwebebahn between Barmen and Elberfeld in Germany.
6 The *Skyway* monorail at Dallas.
7 The Safege system developed in France.

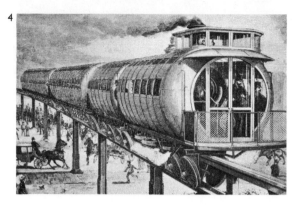

lack of capital and the opposition of the conventional railways.

A system particularly suited to underground railways was publicly presented by E. W. Chalmers Kearney in 1908, after six years of experiments. Trains ran on one rail with a second rail above the train to keep its balance. Kearney proposed that platforms could be sited immediately below the street, with a steep gradient to working depth which would assist acceleration on leaving a station and increase deceleration on coming into one. A railway was very nearly built beneath the Tyne between North and South Shields and there were proposals to use the system between Venice and the Lido and between Nice and Monte Carlo. The system was also suggested for an elevated railway in New York.

Of the many projects proposed for a suspended monorail the most important is that built and still in operation between Barmen and Elberfeld in Germany, the Wuppertal Schwebebahn, opened in 1901.

A British system invented by George Bennie, which combined the Wuppertal system with airscrew propulsion, was tried out in 1930. Economic and safe operation at speeds of 200 m.p.h. was claimed but despite various proposals for its development no regular service has been built on this system.

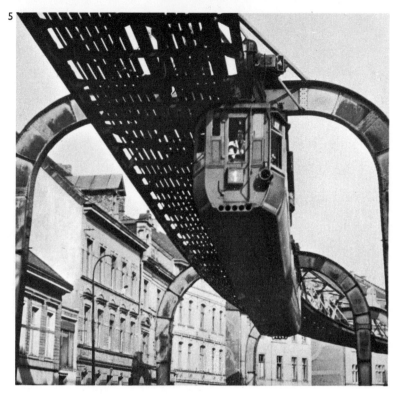

In the United States, Monorail Incorporated opened a test line for their Skyway system in Texas in 1956. An experimental saddle design was abandoned in favour of a suspended version which was built at the State Fair grounds in Dallas.

Two other systems seem the most likely to be developed in the near future: the Alweg system developed in Germany by the Swedish-born industrialist Dr. Axel Gren and the French Safege system.

A scaled-down experimental track and train of the Alweg saddle design were built near Cologne and demonstrated in 1952 and the first regularly operated track was opened at Disneyland, California in 1959. Another track was built with the co-operation of Fiat for

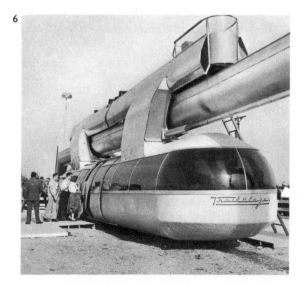

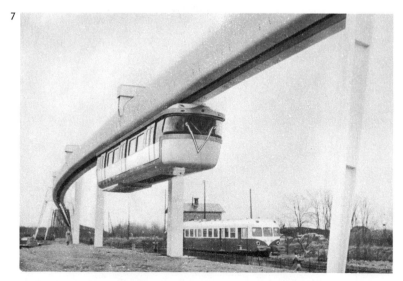

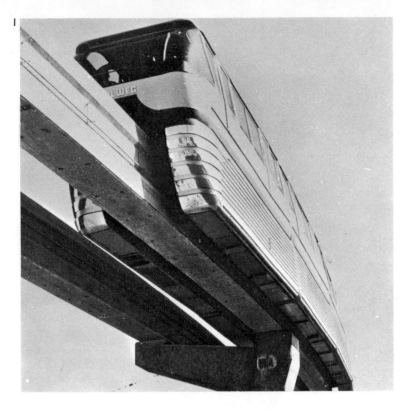

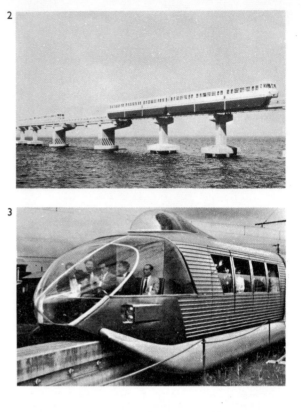

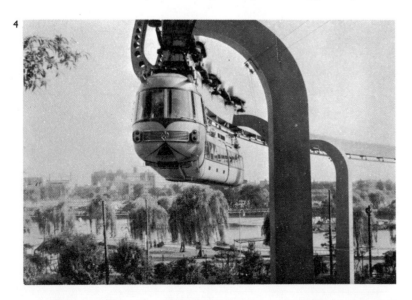

the Italia 61 Exhibition at Turin, and this system was also used for the mile-long link between Seattle and the Century 21 Exposition in 1962.

In the Safege system the car is suspended from pneumatic-tyred bogies, with carrying wheels and horizontal guide wheels (rather like those used on the Paris Mètro) which run within a hollow box girder. The designers claim to have developed a servo-mechanism which overcomes the tendency of suspended systems to sway. An experimental section of Safege track began operation near Orleans in 1960, and in 1966 work began on a line between Charenton and Creteil in the suburbs of Paris.

Monorails are being taken very seriously in Japan where a suspended system using bogies running *on top* of a supporting beam

has been developed. A line of this kind was built at Tokyo Zoological Gardens in 1957. A straddle system has been built in an amusement park at Nara and another straddle design, developed by the Lockheed Corporation of America, links the city of Nikko with the mountain resort of Kirifuri $2\frac{1}{2}$ miles away.

In 1964, in time for the Tokyo Olympic Games, an Alweg monorail, similar to that in Seattle, was opened between Haneda International Airport and central Tokyo. The train is carried on prestressed concrete beams 1.8 metres deep and 0.8 metres wide, cast in 10-20 metre sections. Two guiding wheels follow the track on top of the beam, two driving wheels operate horizontally on the sides of the beam and two other horizontal wheels act as stabilisers. All are pneumatic tyred and air sprung. Electric power is picked up from a track laid in the concave section on each side of the beam. The beam is supported by concrete pylons. The minimum radius of curves is 120 metres. Alweg claim that their trains can be used on slopes with an incline of 1 in 1 but the maximum on the Tokyo line is 6 in 10.

A monorail has often been proposed to link London airport with the city centre but the decision has continually been deferred and the building of a motorway link with west London puts it even further into the future.

1 The monorail built for the World Fair in Seattle.
2 The Tokyo-Haneda Airport line, the journey of over 13 kilometres takes 15 minutes.
3 The monorail at Nara.
4 The suspended monorail at Tokyo Zoo.

RAILWAY RELICS

In museums and collections all over the world all kinds of relics still survive to remind us of the colourful history of the railways.

1 An advertisement of 1833.

2 A warning to horse-cab drivers.

3 A china mug commemorating the opening of the Liverpool and Manchester Railway in 1830.

4 A section of Blenkinsop patent rack rail and wheel (1812).

5 Fish-bellied rail from the Stourton Tramway (1837), built from the original rails of the Liverpool and Manchester Railway.

6 Fish-bellied rails. This type of rail, used 1816—48, was made in four-foot lengths which clipped into connecting clogs.

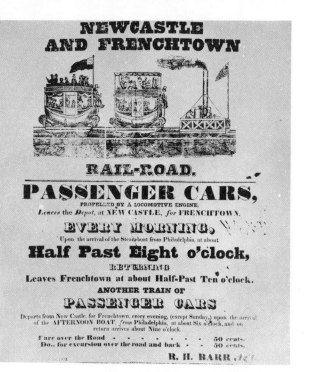

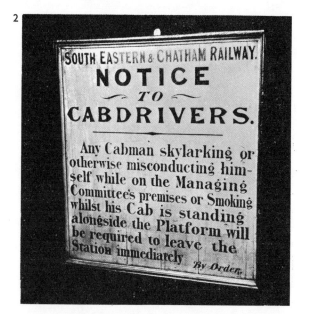

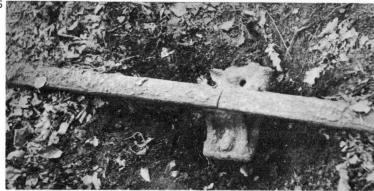

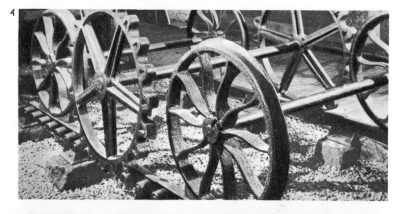

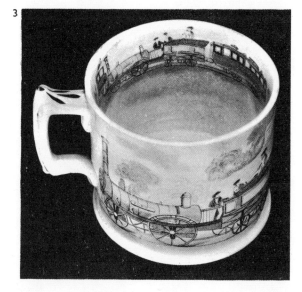

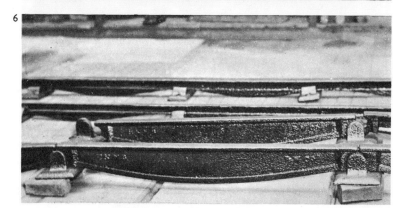

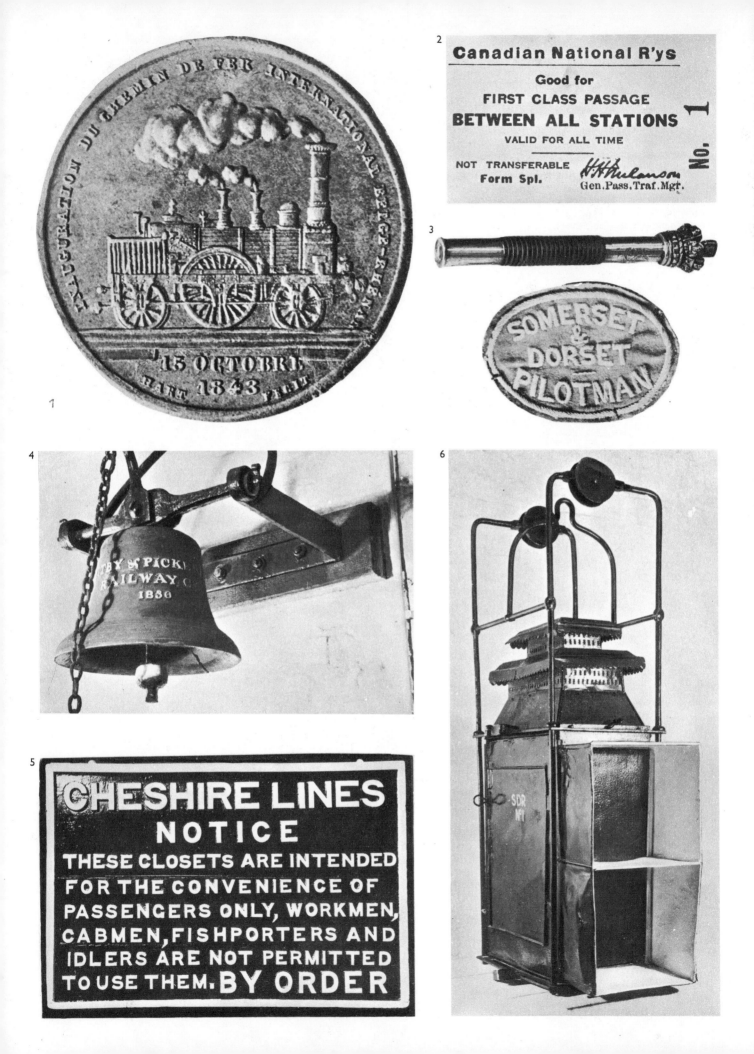

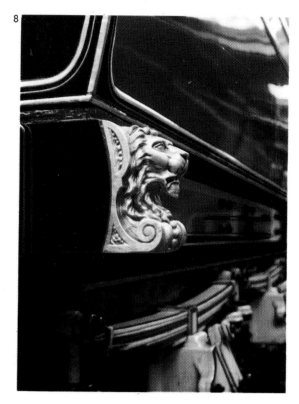

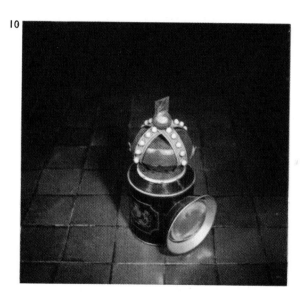

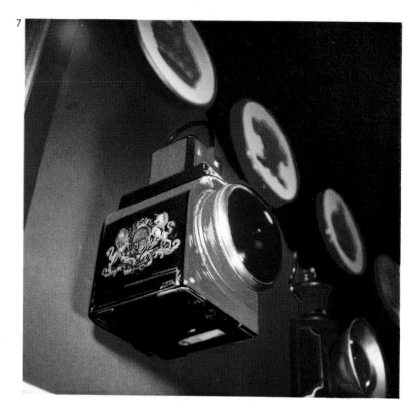

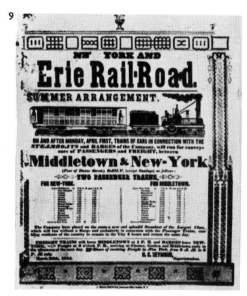

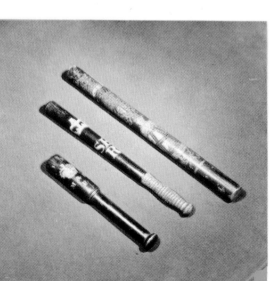

1—11 (1) Medal cast for the opening of the International Railway, Belgium and the Rhine (1843). (2) Ticket No. 1 on Canadian National Railways. (3) A pilotman's badge (the pilotman travelled on the footplate of all trains on a single track section) and an inspector's baton of office (the crown unscrews and his warrant was kept inside). (4) Station bell of 1836. (5) Station notice. (6) First signal lamp used on the Stockton and Darlington Railway (1840). (7) and (10) Rear and front lamps used on royal trains. (8) Headstock of Queen Victoria's 1869 saloon. (9) Poster of 1844. (11) Police truncheons of the Manchester and Liverpool and South Eastern Railways and a signal baton of the London and Birmingham Railway.

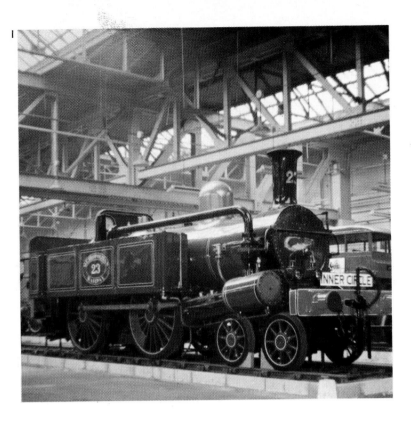

1 The Metropolitan Railway's steam locomotive No. 23, used on the Inner Circle Line. The pipes at the side of the boiler carried exhaust steam back to the water tanks where it was condensed.
2 A London Underground train at the platform at Bethnal Green Station.

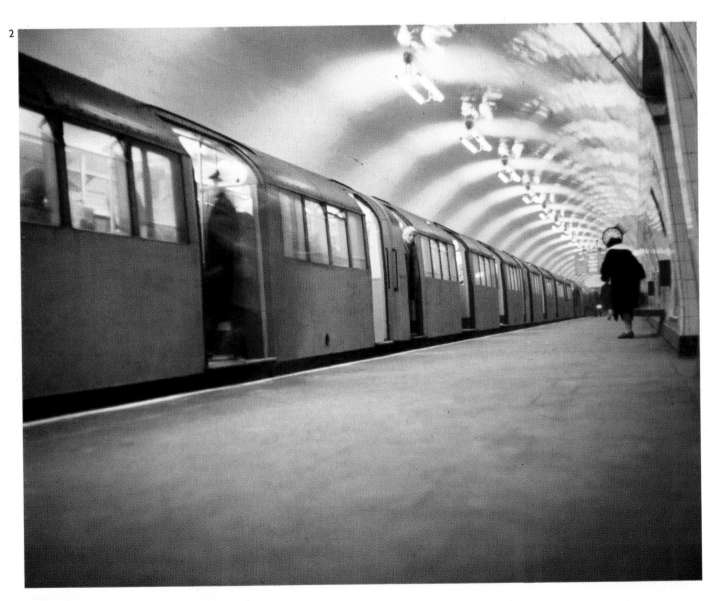

UNDERGROUND RAILWAYS

WHEN AN URBAN TRANSPORT SYSTEM becomes inadequate and the streets are too congested to increase services, what is to be done? As London and New York grew in size and their populations mushroomed in the middle of the last century, people saw railways as a solution—but as there was no room to lay tracks in the streets the railway had to be overhead or underground.

In New York the Elevated Railway was first to be tried out (in 1867) but by then an underground railway had been in operation in London for more than four years. People had begun to make proposals for underground lines in London after the successful opening of a pedestrian subway beneath the Thames in 1843. By 1850 there was a crying need for a transport link between the main-line railway termini which were already handling a quarter of a million passengers a day. The answer was an underground railway from Bishop's Road, Paddington, to Farringdon Street via Euston and King's Cross.

In 1853 Parliament gave approval for the construction of the $3\frac{3}{4}$-mile-long line but work on its construction did not start until 1860. Most of the line was built by the 'cut-and-cover' method, following wherever possible the line of the existing street pattern. A great trench was dug down the centre of the street, the railway laid at its bottom and roofed with a brick arch and then the roadway relaid again on top.

On 9th January 1863, after a banquet at Farringdon Street, the Prime Minister, Mr. Gladstone, and members of the Cabinet travelled along the line in an open truck. The next day the Metropolitan Railway was opened to the public and carried 30,000 passengers.

Siemens's electric railway was still sixteen years away and this first underground was hauled by coal-burning steam locomotives. To keep the air as clean as possible these were designed to consume their own steam, which was passed into a condenser. The carriages, which earned the nick-name 'padded cells,' were lit by flickering oil lamps, passengers wanting to read on the journey would stick candles on the side of the compartments, but despite all the disadvantages 9,050,000 passengers travelled on the Metropolitan Railway during its first year. The Underground was successful and the lines were soon extended

north to Finchley Road, south to Kensington, east to Aldgate, west to Hammersmith. Another company was formed to build the District Line, and together the two companies created the Circle Line.

In New York in 1867 the editor of the *Scientific American*, Alfred Beach, was secretly tunnelling an Underground from a basement at the corner of Murray Street. Without bothering to obtain official permission he built New York's first subway, on which a single train was propelled by air pressure the 312 feet between Murray Street and Warren Street, under Lower Broadway. In 1869 the public were invited to try it out.

In 1870 a tunnel was cut beneath the Thames near the Tower for a rope-hauled railway of two foot six inches gauge. The seven-foot diameter tunnel was cut with a 'shield' developed by James Greathead from one Peter Barlow had patented in 1863. This could tunnel through the London clay and its invention made the cutting of deep 'Tube' lines a possibility.

In 1886 excavations began for the first deep-level 'Tube,' using the Greathead shield operated by hydraulic pressure. The three and a half mile line, known as the City and South London, linked the Monument north of the Thames with London Bridge Station and Stockwell to the south. The original plan was that the trains should be cable-hauled but before the tunnel was completed it was decided that they should be electrically driven. The City and South London was opened in 1890. It now forms part of the Northern Line. Other tube lines followed, including the famous 'Tuppeny Tube,' the Central London Railway from Shepherd's Bush to the Bank which was opened in 1900. The smoke-free 'Tubes' proved stiff competition for the underground lines and these were gradually converted to electric traction. The whole of London's underground and tube railways are now part of the London Transport underground system except for the line linking the Bank and Waterloo Station (opened in 1898), which is operated by the Southern Region of British Railways, and the completely independent Post Office Tube Railway used exclusively for the transfer of mails between the London District Offices, which is automatically operated.

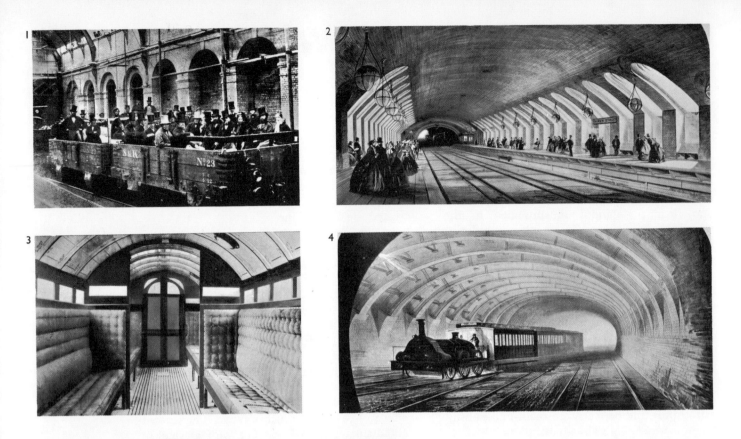

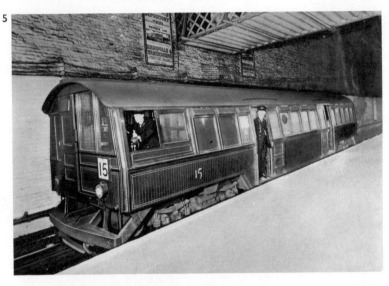

1—11 (1) The opening of the Metropolitan Railway, 9th January 1863. Mr. and Mrs. Gladstone are seated in the first truck. (2) Baker Street Station in 1863. (3) Inside a 'padded-cell' carriage. (4) In the tunnel at Praed Street, 1863. (5) A coach built for the Waterloo and City Line in 1899. (6) A Glasgow Corporation rail-car. The whole Glasgow line is below ground but cars are hauled to the surface for repairs and maintenance. (7) An electric locomotive used on the City and South London Railway in 1890. (8) A pre-war Paris Métro carriage. (9) A pneumatic-tyred train on the Paris Métro. (10) Rome Metropolitana underground, which uses overhead current collection. (11) New York's fully automated service between Grand Central and Times Square. The devices on posts (right) help control the train's speed as it approaches passenger platforms.

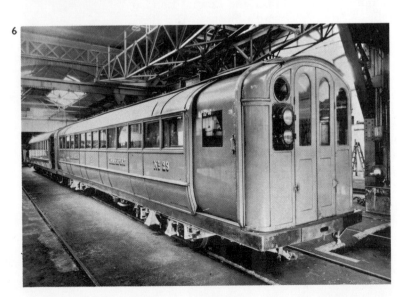

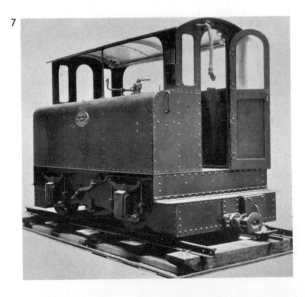

The first underground railway on the European continent was the Franz Josef Electric Underground in Budapest, opened in May 1896. Two miles long, it was the first Underground to be given a flat roof. Built by the 'cut-and-cover' method, the double-track tunnel is rectangular with central supports.

The next city to have an Underground was Glasgow, where a circular line in two concentric tunnels was begun in 1891 and opened in January 1897. Until 1935 the motive power consisted of endless wire ropes which were gripped by the carriages. They were driven by static steam engines which gave the ropes a speed of 15 miles per hour. Electric working was substituted in 1935.

In 1898 a one and a half mile long cut-and-cover line was built under Tremont Street, Boston. Although it was originally used by street-cars only, it was America's first public subway line. In Europe that same year the Stadtwerk system was opened in Vienna with steam traction and work was begun in Paris on the Métro. In July 1900 the first section, from Porte Vincennes to Porte Maillot, was opened to the public. This ten-kilometre line linked the Place de la Bastille, the Louvre, the Place de la Concorde, and the Arc de Triomphe. The engineer, M. Bienvenue, and the contractor, M. Chagnaud, used their own version of the cut-and-cover system to build the line. They excavated from the street down to the planned roof level, built the roof, replaced the street and then constructed the underground underneath the roof.

In 1902 the U-Bahn was opened in Berlin, the first section from Potsdamer Platz to the Zoo having only 2.3 kilometres in tunnel, the rest being on viaducts.

In March 1900 work had started on New York's first public subway line from City Hall to Grand Central, Times Square and West 145th Street. Long before the line was finished approval was given to extend it out to Brooklyn and contracts were being invited for other lines. The official opening was on 27th October 1904 when the first train pulled out of City Hall full of city notables.

Philadelphia followed with 4¼ miles of Underground in 1908. Hamburg opened a circular line, of which about a quarter was underground in 1912. In 1913 a completely underground line was opened in Buenos Aires.

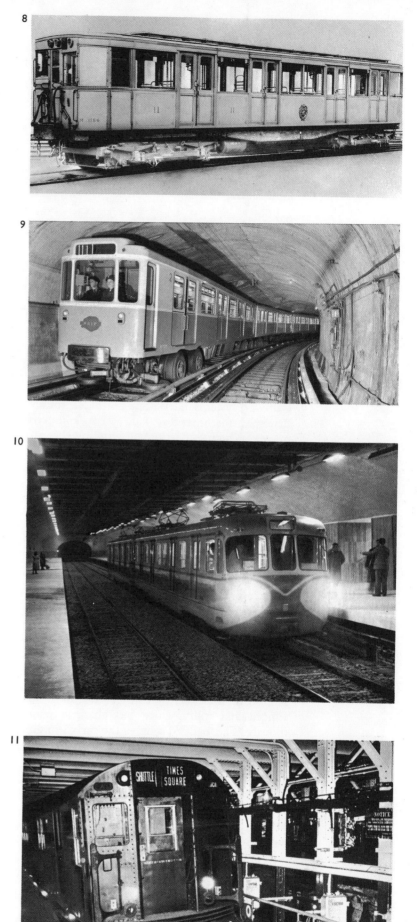

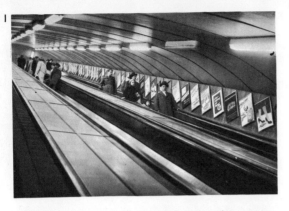

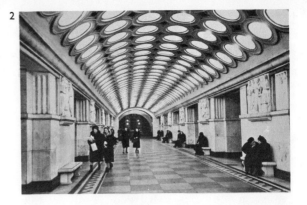

Since then more and more cities have seen underground systems as a necessary addition to their transport services: Madrid (opened 1919), Barcelona (1924), Sydney (1926), Tokyo (1927), Moscow (1933), Osaka (1933), Chicago (1943), Stockholm (1950, the first tunnel converted from a tramway system), Toronto (1954), Rome (1954), Leningrad (1955), Cleveland, Ohio (1956), Nagoya (1957), Lisbon (1959), Haifa (1959, cable hauled), Kiev (1960), Milan (1964), Montreal (1966). There are several other cities where conventional railway or tramway systems have sections underground: Brussels, for instance, has a two-kilometre tunnel section six tracks wide linking the two mainrail termini. Copenhagen, Liverpool, Oslo, Warsaw and San Francisco all have sections underground.

Undergrounds are being built in Baku, Tbilisi, Washington and Rotterdam and lines are projected in many other cities; meanwhile the older lines are being continually extended. The Paris Métro, for instance, is building a new express line between St. Germain-en-Laye and Boissy-St. Leger, and London Transport will add $10\frac{1}{2}$ miles to the 258-mile route length of its system when the new Victoria line is completed.

Underground development has by no means been limited to extensions of track. Efficiency of operation and comfort have been continually increased. Methods of construction have advanced and rolling-stock has changed enormously. The 'padded cells' of the early London Underground have given way to lightweight aluminium carriages with comfortable seats and automatic doors. Automation has been introduced everywhere from the ticket-vending machines the escalators and automatic lifts to the destination indicators, the automatic signalling and the 'programming machines' which control the automatic signalling of several sections of the London Transport system. These carry information of the train service as a series of punched holes on a roll like that of an old fashioned pianola. The coded information is 'read' by a row of feelers and signals and points are set automatically according to the existence, or lack, of a hole. As each train leaves the section controlled by the machine it moves the roll on a line. Should a delay cause a train to get out of schedule a 'time-machine,' similar to the programming machine, but with an information sheet moving according to the official timings, works in operation with the programming machine to put through another train if necessary and then signal the first train through out of schedule. If trains get very much out of order the central control room is automatically informed and human operators can take over on push-button controls

In New York one public line is already completely automatic. A shuttle service between Grand Central Station and Times Square is operated with driverless trains operated by electronic signals passed along the rails.

The Paris Métro has introduced pneumatic-tyred trains on its No. I and No. II lines. Pneumatic tyres are claimed to give much smoother running and, by improving the adhesion of the motor bogies, increase acceleration and braking, thus cutting journey times and increasing route capacity. The tyred wheels are mounted outside the normal flanged wheels and are a little larger. Horizontal wheels also press sideways against a side rail. At points and cross-overs the running surface of the pneumatic wheel drops, lowering the flanged wheel onto the normal rails.

Surface congestion has led to the construc-

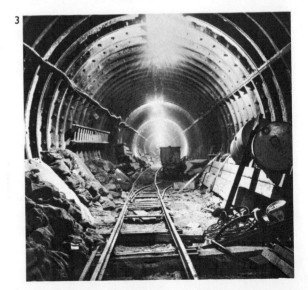

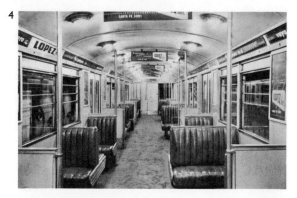

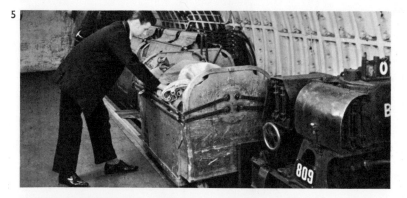

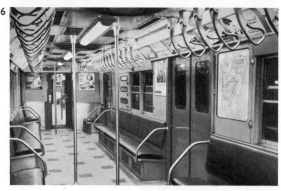

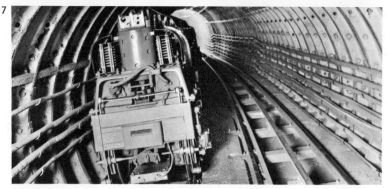

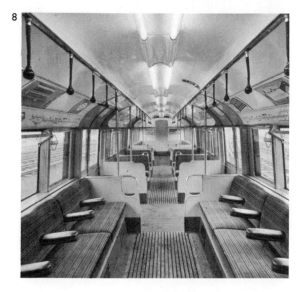

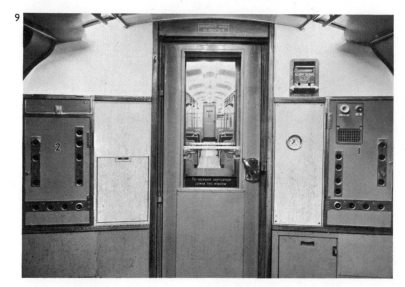

1—10 (1) Lifts and escalators are an essential part of all underground systems. This one is in Stockholm. (2) The vestibule of Electrozavodskaya Station, Moscow. Many of the Moscow Metro stations are lavishly decorated. (3) Tunnelling work on London's Victoria Line. (4), (6) and (8) Carriages from Buenos Aires, New York and London. New York caters for more standing passengers, Buenos Aires has no straphangers. (5) and (7) The London Post Office Railway driverless trains are controlled by switching on and off the current. The mail bag containers roll on and off the cars. (9) The guard's controls on a London Underground train. He is in microphone contact with the driver (panel, right) and controls the doors by push-buttons. (10) Programme machines on London Underground.

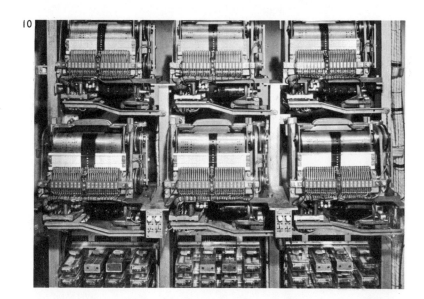

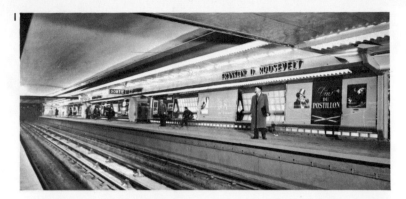

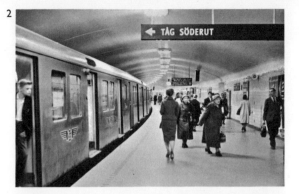

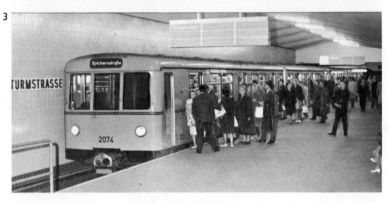

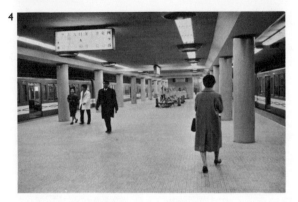

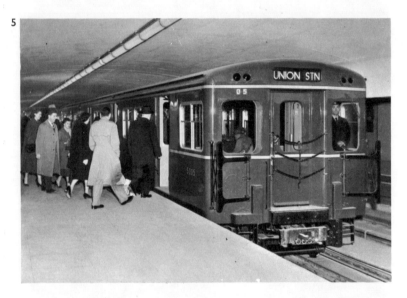

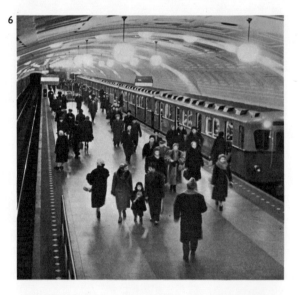

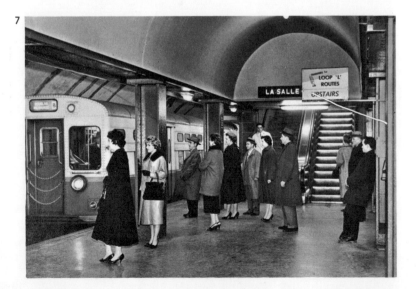

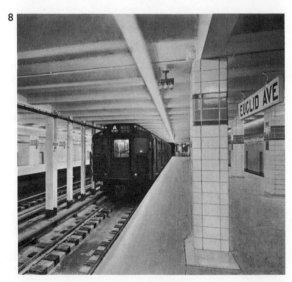

SIGNALS

tion of more and more passenger lines, but as long as urban conditions include rush-hour transport peaks that require the provision of rolling-stock and staff that are used for only a small part of the day, these and high construction costs mean that the Underground must be viewed as a public service rather than a commercial undertaking. Many routes lose money, but far less than the transport snarl-ups they prevent would cost. Perhaps the day will come when transport, like streets, will be considered a necessary provision to be paid for from the public purse. A survey of the Paris Métro showed that the cost of selling tickets and checking passengers was greater than the income from fares—it would be cheaper to operate the Métro free.

On some systems, in Paris, New York, Moscow and Rome for instance, there is a standard fare payable whatever the distance travelled; on others, such as the London Underground, the fare is proportionate to the distance travelled. Each system seems to have its own peculiarities and it is as well to discover them — many American visitors to London, for instance, will have been surprised to find they should have kept their ticket to give up at the end of their journey (this applies to surface railway travel too). In London you buy a ticket from the ticket office or an automatic vending machine and may be asked to show it for the whole length of the journey. In Paris you buy a ticket or, to save money and time, a block (*carnet*) of tickets from the ticket office and may be asked to show it to an inspector on the journey but do not have to show it at the exit. The Métro has both first- and second-class carriages. In New York you buy a token from the subway office and put it in a turnstile to get into the subway. On the Roman Metropolitana you buy a token from a stand which also sells newspapers and magazines and put it in a turnstile which issues a paper ticket.

One system for which you can never buy a ticket is the Post Office underground railway in London, for it carries no passengers, only mail bags. It has no drivers, and is controlled by the switching on and off of the power supply.

Without their signs underground platforms would be difficult to tell apart: **1** Paris. **2** Stockholm. **3** Berlin. **4** Tokyo. **5** Toronto. **6** Moscow. **7** Chicago. **8** New York.

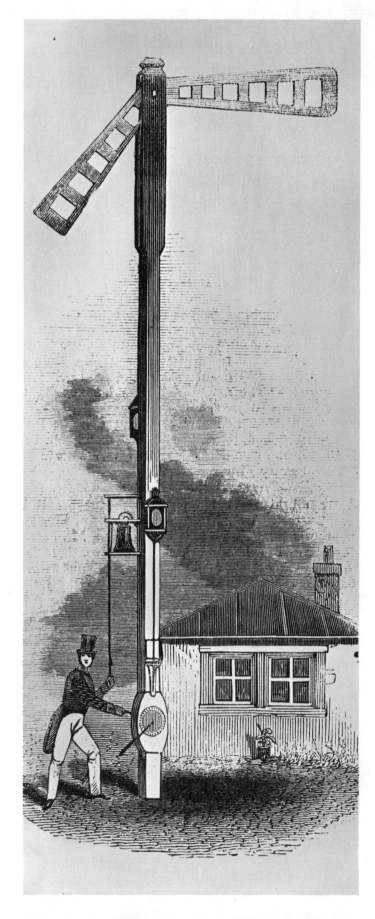

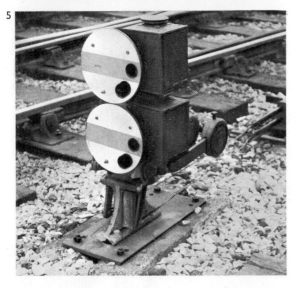

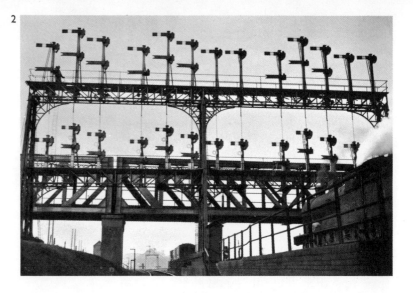

The safety of a railway depends upon careful maintenance and efficient signalling. Signal forms have changed a great deal from the policeman with a flag to the automatic systems of today.

Preceding page Station post signal (1844) set at caution and danger.

1 Railway policemen (1844). The flag position left indicates slacken speed because of a defect in the rails, that right slow down — another train ahead.

2 Forty signals at stop. The biggest gantry in Britain (1934).

3 Modern colour-light signals.

4 Upper quadrant distant signal at clear.

5 Ground disc signals.

6 Models of revolving disc signal (London and South Western Railway, 1840), ball signal (Great Western, 1837) and disc and crossbar signal (Great Western, 1841).

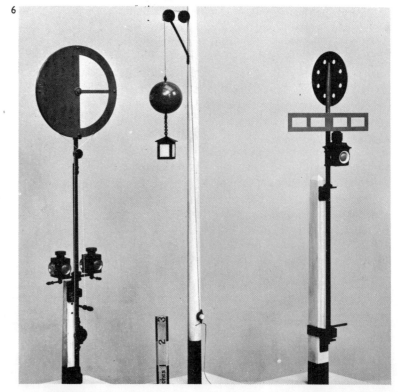

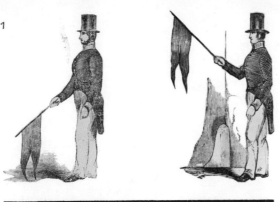

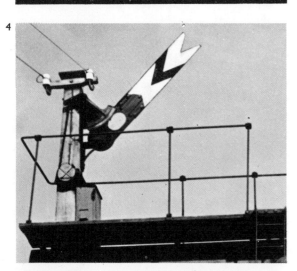

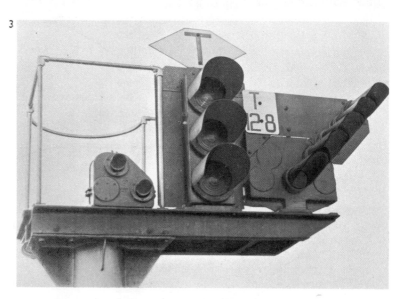

ELEVATED RAILWAYS

ELEVATED RAILWAYS were the obvious alternative to Undergrounds for city transportation. They found favour because they were much cheaper to construct and because it was thought that Undergrounds would damage the foundations of buildings which they passed beneath.

By the mid-1850's people were proposing overhead railways for New York, horse-drawn, rope-hauled, atmospheric, suspended—but it was not until July 1867 that the money was found for the first experimental track, from Greenwich Street, Manhattan, up Ninth Avenue to 30th Street. In December that year the inventor, Charles Harvey, made the first trip on the world's first elevated track. In 1868 the State Commissioners and the Governor approved the venture and the system was rapidly extended.

In 1893 the overhead railway along the Mersey shore in Liverpool became the first elevated railway to use electric traction.

The drawbacks of the Elevated running through city streets and the increasing development of Undergrounds led to the system losing favour and the Liverpool Overhead and most of the New York system have now been dismantled. In recent years there has been a renewal of interest in overhead monorails, such as the one built for the Century 21 Exposition at Seattle, particularly as links between airports and city terminals.

1 The 'El' near the waterfront in 1884.
2 A trial trip on the first elevated railway (1867).
3 On Third Avenue near 10th Street.
4 The Liverpool Overhead Railway, opened in 1893, was the first to use electric traction.

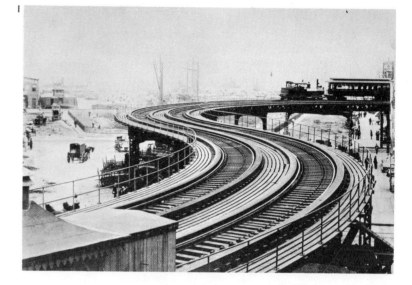

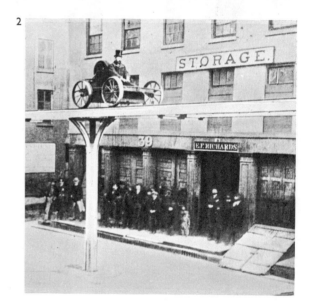

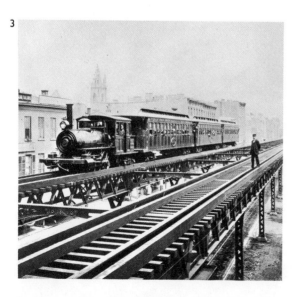

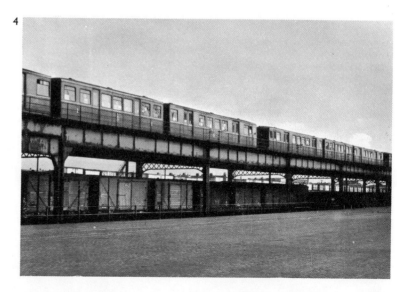

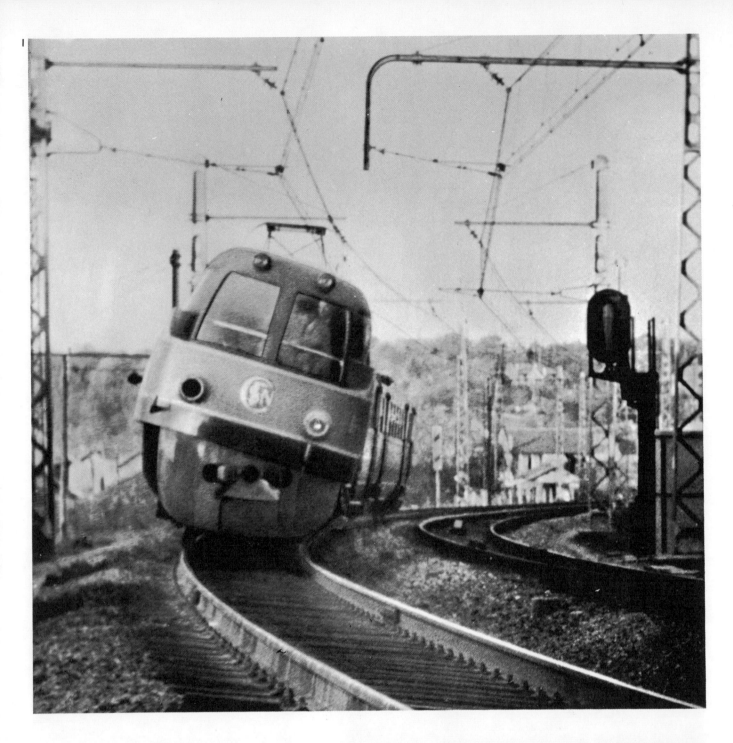

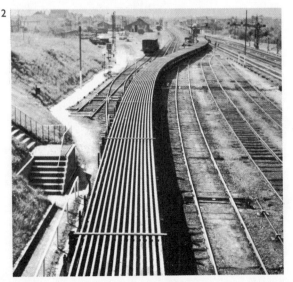

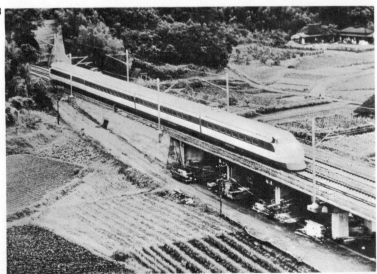

A GLIMPSE OF THE FUTURE

'RAILWAYS ARE FINISHED as a means of transport.' What utter nonsense! The railways were developed before the invention of the internal combustion engine and the aeroplane but that does not make them obsolete now. The railways cannot compete with the supersonic speeds of jet aircraft or with the door-to-door manoeuvrability of the family motor-car, but they can offer much greater safety and comfortable direct travel from city centre to city centre. Even with the development of vertical take-off it seems unlikely that airports will ever be sited in a central, easily accessible position, and the strain of driving cannot be removed from the private motorist.

Many railways have lost ground in the economic field. Saddled with heavy upkeep costs for permanent way and depot facilities, often with accumulated debts and committed by law in many cases to run uneconomic services, they must compete with road services having minimal overheads. But think what a railway train can do—haul hundreds of sleeping passengers and thousands of tons of freight, in safety and at speed, almost regardless of weather and with a single driver, instead of the innumerable lorries or motor-coaches which would otherwise be required.

As the world's industrial conurbations grow ever larger and traffic congestion increases, transport planning will become imperative, and in many areas efficient and frequent public services may replace the one-man-one-vehicle attitude prevalent today. If placed on an equal footing with other transport methods the railways will be able to offer an incomparable service wherever regular, large-scale transport is required, and a service which modern technical developments are daily improving.

What changes are these technical develop-ments bringing about on the railways themselves?

Steam will be replaced, first by diesel or electric power, then perhaps, much farther in the future, by atomic power.

Speeds will increase, and this will mean that track will be laid or relaid straighter (though a slight curve makes the wheel flange press against the side of the rail and increases safety).

Bends there still will be, and when rounding bends at high speeds vehicles tend to be pushed outwards by the centrifugal force. This could be countered by sloping the track inwards, as on a motor-racing circuit, but to do so would cause considerable difficulties where slow traffic used the same line, or if a train had to stop on the curve. The strain placed upon the inner rail makes a super-elevation of six inches the maximum possible.

American engineers were working on this problem in the early 'forties and devised a carriage called the 'Precopendulum' which inclined as it rounded corners in the same way as a cyclist leans when going round a corner on a bicycle. In this carriage the inclination was obtained by using flexible springs, but in 1957 French Railways built an experimental prototype of a pendulum carriage with two bogies on which the body could oscillate. The body was built on to a steel girder, each end of which was shaped like a swan's neck and the ends of the girder rested on raised supports on the bogies.

1 French Railways' 'pendulum' train.
2 Enormous lengths of rail for welded track are themselves a tricky transport problem.
3 One of the super-expresses on the new Tokaido line, Japan. Capable of 130 m.p.h. they complete the 320 mile journey at an average speed of 101 m.p.h.
4 The suspension system on Canadian National Railway's Turbotrains which banks cars inwards on curves instead of outwards. The solid line shows the position on a curve, the dotted line the train on level track.

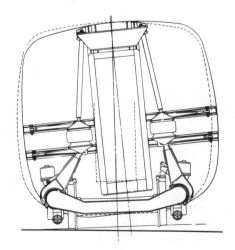

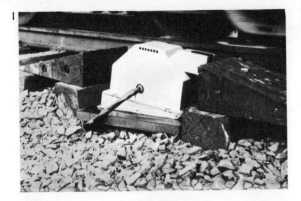

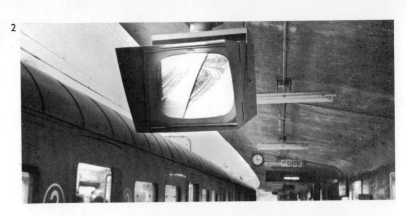

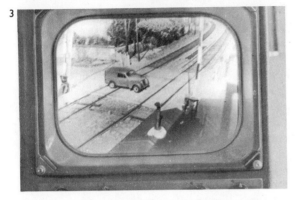

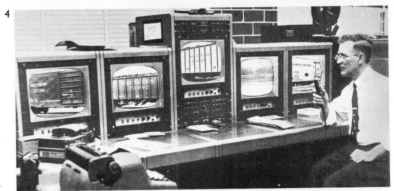

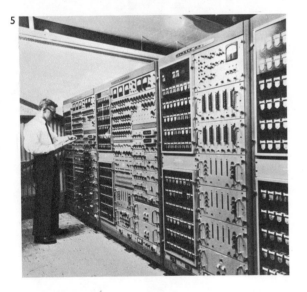

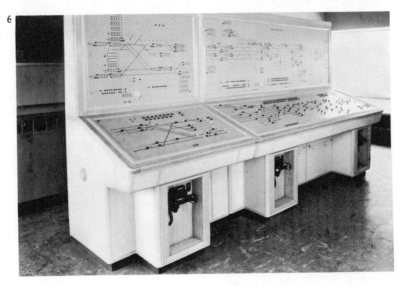

1 Pennsylvania Railroad's 'hot box' detector is so sensitive that it can detect the warmth of a human hand 200 yards away. An overheated bearing on a passing train causes a sudden leap to be marked on a linked graph roll at the signal box.

2—4 Television used on the Paris Ligne de Sceaux to enable station staff to see the whole length of a long curving platform (2), in the remote control of a level crossing on French Railways (3) and to identify numbers of freight trucks in the U.S.A. (4).

5 An electronic brain at Elkart, Indiana, which 're-members' and supplies information on each freight car, or group of cars, during marshalling.

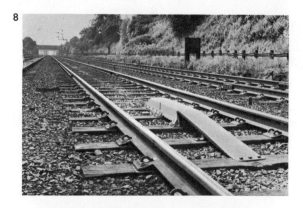

Canadian National Railroad's new Turbo-trains use a pendulum system which, combined with a guided axle system and a low centre of gravity (floors are 10 inches lower than in their usual rolling-stock) give smoother riding. Carriage building of this kind will make sure that fast travel is still comfortable travel for the passenger.

Locomotives are becoming more powerful and, as more powerful locomotives haul heavier loads, it may become necessary to resort to a wider gauge. The Soviet scientist, Professor Vassili Vassilievich Zvonkov, considers the Russian 1.524 metre gauge already inadequate and 9—15 feet gauges necessary to allow for roomier trucks, 40—50,000 h.p. locomotives and speeds from 150—200 m.p.h. He thinks even wider gauge tracks across the Continent may prove necessary in later years.

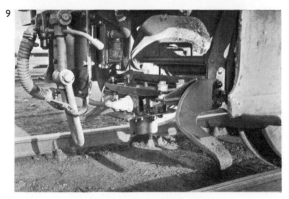

Electrical traction and steel rails make the railway an ideal subject for automation and remote control. Instructions can be transmitted along the metals themselves. France, Germany, the U.S.A. and the U.S.S.R. have all made successful experiments in radio control. New York Subway already has one automatic shuttle service and London Underground a section of automatic signalling controlled by a programming machine.

Modern colour light signalling has already made the semaphore old-fashioned and the installation of various types of Automatic Warning Systems has increased the effectiveness of signalling by reproducing signal information in the driver's cab and automatically applying the brakes if it is ignored.

Low currents passed through the running

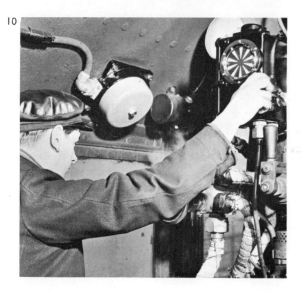

6 The control panel at Old Oak Common signal box.
7 Mills propane gas heaters at York station stop points from freezing.
8, 9, 10 The induction equipment of British Rail's Automatic Warning System (8) foreground, is connected with the signal seen ahead. Through the magnet carried beneath the locomotive (9) it activates the striped dial and the bell within the cab (10) and automatically applies the brakes if they are ignored.
11 A British Rail automatic carriage-cleaning plant.

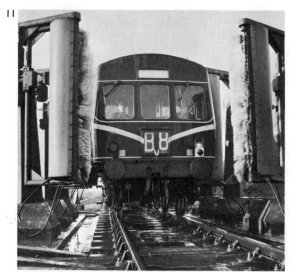

rails of a section of track (each section being insulated from the next) are short-circuited by the wheels and axles of passing trains. This can be used to stop signals being cleared behind the train, or points being changed in front of it. To go a stage farther, it can actually operate the signal behind it, clearing the signal as the train passes out of the section, and it can operate level crossings in the same way. Track circuiting also operates a series of lights along the track diagram at signal boxes to show the signalmen the position of the train. By a code system of letters and numbers, which can be set at the train's point of origin and automatically transferred to signal-box diagrams along the route, the train can be identified by the signalman in charge. These train description codes can also be used to automatically set the correct route ahead of the train by incorporating a symbol indicating the required route.

In Germany half the mileage of the Federal Republic's rail system is controlled by Automatic Train Control. This not only applies the brakes if the driver passes a distant signal at caution without pressing a button to disengage the mechanism, but will also apply them if he does not reduce speed to 56 m.p.h. within 22 seconds of passing the signal, if the train is travelling at more than 41 m.p.h. 160 yards ahead of the home signal, or if the train overruns the home signal. With this system trains cannot overrun a stop signal by more than one-eighth of a mile, even if travelling at 100 m.p.h. when the A.T.C. comes into operation.

Different frequency impulses passed through the running rails can be used to transmit varied information. On the Pennsylvania Railroad where the breaking of the circuit when a locomotive passes sends electric messages back along the track to set the previous signal, the frequency is raised and sets the signal before that to the right position, increasing the frequency at each signal until it reaches a level at which it sets a signal clear. This information is also picked up by the locomotive and shows the setting of other signals ahead.

In 1955 French Railways began experiments with radio-controlled, driverless trains with locomotive BB. 9003, of the same type as the rail-speed record-holder. From a diesel rail-car on a parallel track orders to release brakes,

control the supply of current to the traction motors of the locomotive and apply the brakes at the end of the run were given verbally by radio-telephone to a radio-control post. From there signals were sent out to the receiving set on the locomotive, which in turn set the necessary mechanisms in motion.

The aerial on the train was quite short, the receiving set very light in weight and the relay could be placed in the waistcoat pocket. Starting and acceleration up to maximum speed are automatic on this type of locomotive and the only things which had to be operated by remote control were the brakes and the supply of current. This system did not even use the rails to transmit signals.

British Rail have been experimenting with a system where two conductor wires are laid between the rails and connected to an alternating current source. One is parallel to the rails, the other follows a zig zag which varies in length of wave according to the speed required on that section of track. Induction from one wire to the other creates a magnetic field and the effect of the zig zag is to vary its intensity along the line of movement. As the locomotive runs along the track this fluctuation is picked up as pulses increasing or decreasing according to the length of wave—and apparatus on the train causes it to brake or accelerate. A refinement uses a square-wave in binary code.

Many countries are experimenting with the use of computors, both in the locomotive and at central control. (They are, of course, already an essential part of the administrative apparatus of many railway systems.)

Illogically, many people seem to prefer a fallible human driver to an almost infallible machine which, if it fails, automatically fails safe—it stops—but the problem of the future is likely to be a different human one. The driver travelling on an automatic train will have nothing to do unless there is a breakdown. Will it be possible to find a person capable of coping with an emergency situation who will be able to tolerate the boredom of normal running? However they develop, railways in the future are going to be very different from those we have known for the last hundred years. Dr. Sydney Jones of British Rail looked forward in these words:

We can envisage a transport system which

would be capable of speeds of 200 and 300 m.p.h. on track that was largely if not entirely separate from existing railway track, running on silent steel wheels and signalled by a continuous system of communication between the train and control. The track construction would probably be different from the conventional railway, the construction techniques embodied in vehicles would be similar to those found in aircraft practice, and the shape would be dictated by aerodynamic considerations to reduce the drag at full speed. 'The tractive power would probably be electric, and at these speeds the linear could well come into its own . . . Such a transport system would no longer have to be compatible with conventional railways, and the railway designers would for the first time be free from the straightjacket which has inhibited innovation in the railway.'

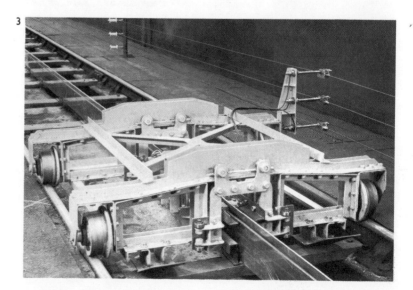

1 Canadian National Railroad's *Turbotrains* combine aluminium structure, pendulum suspension and a low centre of gravity with guided axles and gas-turbine engines to create a very fast and very comfortable train.
2 The *Talgo* train, a Spanish development, is an articulated whole with the front end of each trailer resting on the rear end of the preceding coach. The wheels supporting the rear maintain an imaginary axle at right-angles to the longitudinal axis and the carriage surrounds them, giving a low centre of gravity. This form of suspension enables a higher speed at curves than is possible with an ordinary train.

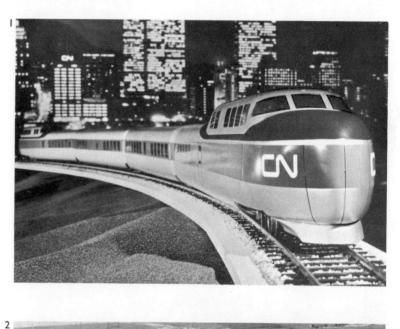

3 The train of the future? Research prototype for a *Limpet* (linear induction motor propelled train), developed by Professor E. R. Laithwaite of Manchester University and British Rail's Research Department. A vertical metal plate along the centre of the track is sandwiched by the windings of the motor. Current from overhead is supplied to the motor windings in three-phase form, corresponding currents are induced in the plate and the reaction between the two propels the train along the track. Tractive effort is not limited by adhesion and there are no moving parts, so both acceleration and braking (by reversing the current) are much greater than in other land vehicles. Running speeds up to 200 m.p.h. are possible.

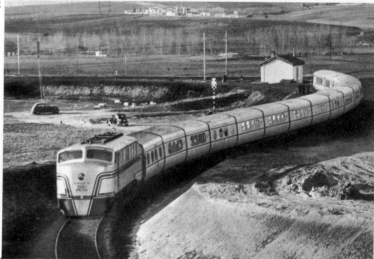

ACKNOWLEDGMENTS

The author and publishers are indebted to the Central Office of Information for permission to reproduce W. H. Auden's verses from the film *Night Mail* and to the writers and the British Broadcasting Corporation for the extracts from *The Ballad of John Axon*, which was the first of a series of radio ballads written by Ewan MacColl and Peggy Seeger, and edited and produced by Charles Parker, Senior Features Producer in the B.B.C.'s Midland Region. Our thanks are also due to Mrs. Gladys Axon, Mr. Alec Watts, Mr. Jack Pickford, Mr. Roy Howarth and Mr. Ron Scanlon. This radio programme has now been issued on a gramophone record by Argo Records. *London to Birmingham 1836* is based on material supplied by British Rail. (London Midland Region). *The Story of Casey Jones* includes material supplied by Mr. Jim Sullivan of the New York Central System.

We should also like to thank the staff of the Museum of British Transport and the many railway companies throughout the world who have given assistance in the preparation of this book, and the following for permission to reproduce illustrations. (Figure in roman type is page on which caption appears, figure in **bold** is number of illustration).

Ab Stockholm Sparvägar 140 **1**, 142 **2**
Alaska Railroad 91 **3**
Association of American Railroads 33 **3**, 35 **1**, 55 **9**, 80 **1—3**, 87 **5**, 89, 5 127 **11**, 133 **1**, 135 **9**
Atchison, Topeka & Santa Fé Railway 67 **8—10**
Australian News and Information Bureau 39 **1**, 45 **5**
Baltimore & Ohio Railroad 61 **2**, 84 **1, 7**, 124 **3**
B. T. Batsford Ltd. 77 **3** (from *British Trains* by O. S. Nock)
Berliner Verkehrs-Betriebe 142 **3**
Black Star 130 **7**, 132 **1**, 45 **2** *(John Launois)*
British Rail 13 **4**, 14 **2**, 19 **2**, 21 **1**, 22 **2**, 24 **2**, 49 **1, 3**, 53 **3**, 56 **1, 4**, 64 **3—6**, 73 **2**, 77 **1—2**, 78 **2—4**, 81 **1**, 82 **1, 2, 4—6**, 84 **3, 8, 10**, 87 **4**, 89 **2, 7—8**, 91 **3**, 92 **1**, 95 **4—6**, 97 **1—6**, 98 **2, 5**, 101 **3**, 110—111, 114 **3—5**, 116 **3—4**, 120 **6—7**, 123 **3—6**, 127 **4—5, 9**, 133 **3—4**, 135 **4, 6**, 148 **1, 7, 9, 11, 13—15**, 150 **3—7**
British Transport Films 101 **5**
Maurice Broomfield 116 **3**
Camera Press 30 **8**, 74 **2**
Canadian National Railways 89 **13**, 91 **7**, 124 **5**
Canadian Pacific Railway 45 **3**, 69 **6**, 70 **2**, 127 **10**
Central Press 53 **2**
Chicago Transit Authority 142 **6**
Cie. Internationale des Wagons-Lits 61 **5, 8, 10**, 62 **1—6**
Delaware & Hudson Railroad 33 **4**
Deutsche Bundesbahn 50 **1, 3**, 69 **2—3, 8—9**, 70 **5**, 89 **9—10**, 114 **6, 8**, 120 **4**, 121 **11**, 127 **12**, 148 **8, 12**
East African Railways & Harbours 45 **6**
English Electric 46 **1**, 89 **14**, 121 **5**, 123 **1, 7—8, 10**
F.I.A.T. 69 **5**, 124 **4**
Ferrovie dello Stato Italia 69 **1**, 70 **4**, 78 **7**, 87 **3, 8—11**, 89 **1, 12, 15**, 91 **1—2**
H. G. Forsythe 144 **3, 4**
French Embassy 28 **4**
C. L. Fry 116 **2**
Giraudon 103 **2—3**
Glasgow Corporation Transport 138 **6**
Great Northern Railway 67 **1—7**, 124 **2**
Gulf Oil Co. 33 **2**
H. M. Postmaster-General 49 **2**, 140 **5, 7**
High Commissioner for New Zealand 114 **2**
Israel Tourist Office 124 **7**

Japanese Embassy 130 **8**, 132 **2**
Japanese National Railways 119 **1—2**
Järvägsmuseum, Stockholm 78 **5**
Chas. E. Keevil 73 **3**
Keystone 116 **1**
E. R. Laithwaite 150 **1**
London Transport Executive 138 **3**, 140 **8—11**
Raymond Mander & Joe Mitcheson Collection 98 **4**
Mansell Collection 10 **1**, 26 **3**, 28 **2**, 30 **5**, 35 **2**, 39 **3**, 40 **3**, 43 **2**, 61 **1**, 64 **1—2**, 84 **2**, 87 **2**, 91 **5**, 98 **3**, 103 **4**, 125 **1—2**
John Masey-Stewart 74 **3**
J. Meredith 53 **6**, 74 **4**, 130 **4**
Mobil Oil Co. 127 **3**
Mount Washington Cog Railway 53 **5**, 55 **4**
Musée Marmottan (Giraudon) 103 **2—3**
Museum of British Transport 78 **1**
Museum of the City of New York 142 **10** (J. Clarence Davis Collection)
Mustograph 10 **4**, 13 **3**, 19 **1**, 55 **5**, 81 **2**, 84 **6**, 128 **2—3**, 133 **5**, 145 **4**
Nairn's Photo Services 46 **3**
National Gallery, London 103 **1** (Photo: M. Holford)
New York, New Haven & Hartford Railroad 120 **4**
New South Wales Government 30 **6**
New York Central System 87 **7**, 119 **6**, 127 **1**, 148 **5**
New York City Transit Authority 138 **11**, 140 **6**, 142 **7**
Norfolk & Delaware Railroad 50 **2**
Norges Statsbane 46 **5**
Novosti Press Agency 140 **3**
Österreichische Bundesbahnen 30 **4**
Pennsylvania Railroad 35 **3**, 55 **3**, 87 **1**, 89 **4, 6**, 119 **7**, 120 **2**, 150 **2**
Paul Popper 28 **1**, 30 **1**, 45 **1**, 55 **5**, 73 **1**, 130 **6**, 132 **2**, 138 **10**
Radio Times Hulton Picture Library 10 **3**, 13 **1**, 21 **2**, 24 **1—3**, 26 **1—2**, 30 **3, 7**, 33 **1**, 39 **4**, 43 **3—5**, 45 **4**, 53 **4**, 55 **2**, 61 **3**, 70 **1**, 78 **6**, 84 **4**, 101 **1**, 120 **1**, 128 **1**, 130 **1—3, 5**, 133 **6**, 138 **1**, 142 **8—9**, 144 **2**
Red Nacional de los Ferrocarriles Espanole 148 **6**
Regie Autonome des Transports Parisiens 128 **4**, 138 **8—9**, 142 **1**, 148 **2**
Lewis Robertson 74 **1**
Schweizerische Bundesbahnen 70 **3**, 92 **5**, 114 **3**
Science Museum, London 5, 9 **1—2**, 10 **2**, 13 **2**, 14 **1**, 16 **1—4**, 22 **1**, 55 **3, 6**, 82 **3**, 89 **3**, 138 **2, 4, 7**, 144 **6**
Société Nationale des Chemins de Fer Français 50 **4, 6**, 53 **1**, 69 **4, 7**, 70 **6**, 91 **2, 4**, 113 **2, 3**, 120 **3**, 123 **7**, 127 **6—7**, 146 **1—2**, 148 **3**
S.C.R. 46 **4**, 124 **1**
South African Railways 39 **2**, 46 **2**, 89 **11**, 91 **4, 6**
Southern Pacific Co., 36 **4**
Southern Railway 148 **4**
Standard Oil Co 36 **4**
Statens Järnvägar 12 **32**
Swedish Travel Bureau 30 **2**
Swiss Railways 120, **5**
Swiss Tourist Office 82 **7**, 92 **6**
Teito Rapid Transit Authority 142 **4**
Toronto Transit Commission 142 **5**
Transportes de Buenos Aires 140 **4**
Union Pacific Railroad 36 **1—3**, 40 **1—2**, 43 **1**, 107 **1**, 113 **1**, 119 **4—5**, 124 **8**
United Press 114 **1**
Viewpoint Project (Norman Tozer) 6, 7, 8, 65 **5**, 56 **2—3**, 58 **1**, 74 **5**, 84 **5**, 84 **9**, 103 **5**, 108—**9**, 133 **2**, 135 **3, 5**, 7—**8, 10—11**, 136 **1—2**
Alex Wilson *jacket*

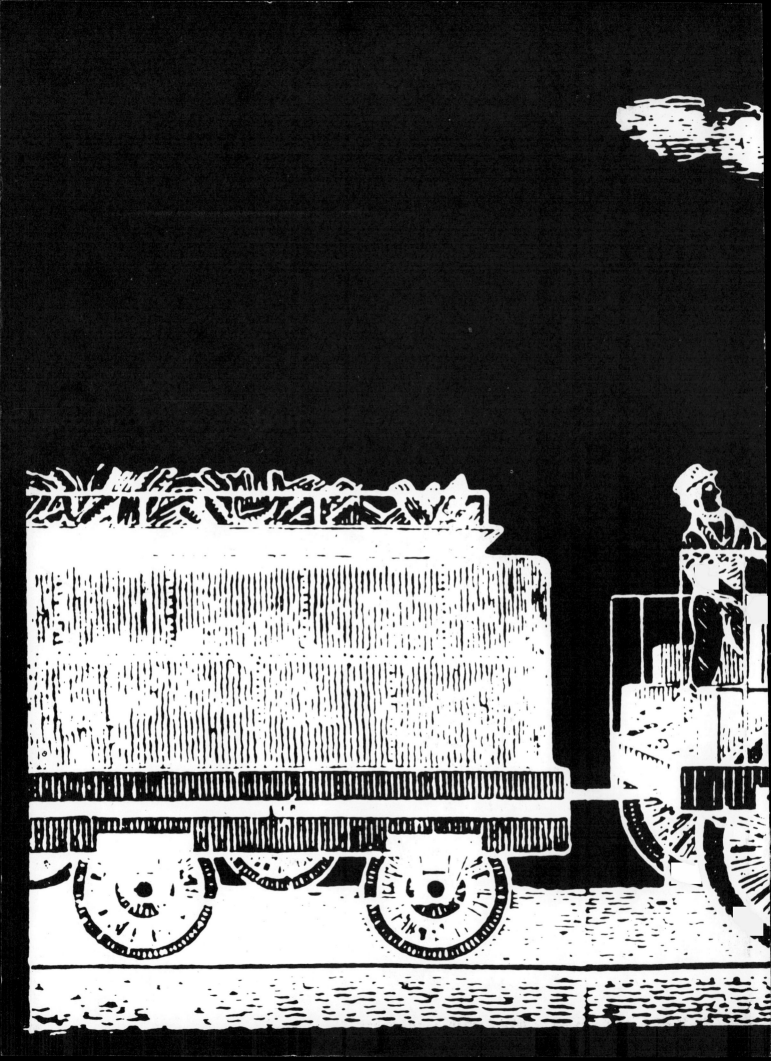